# Rosen's
# Breast Pathology

*Second Edition*

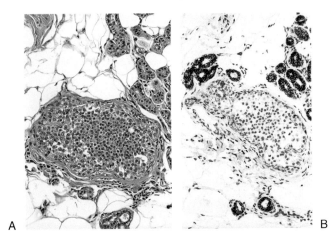

**FIG. 1.** *Lobular carcinoma* in situ. **A:** *In situ* carcinoma in duct (*left*) next to lobule. **B:** E-cadherin immunoreactivity is seen in lobule, but not in *in situ* carcinoma (avidin-biotin).

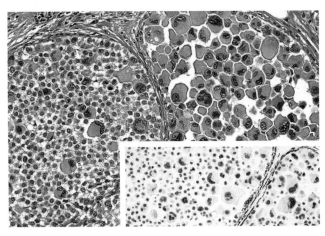

**FIG. 2.** *Florid lobular carcinoma* in situ, *classical and pleomorphic cytology.* Classical (*left*) and pleomorphic (*right*) cell types. *Inset:* E-cadherin immunoreactivity is not present in either carcinoma cell type (avidin-biotin).

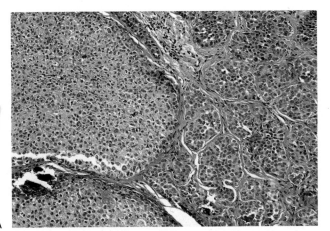

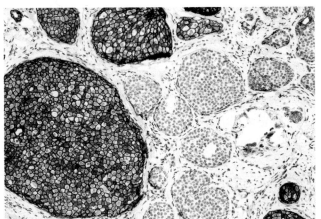

**FIG. 3.** *Intraductal carcinoma and lobular carcinoma* in situ. **A:** Two enlarged ducts filled with cohesive carcinoma cells and one calcification (*left*) next to lobular carcinoma *in situ* composed of dyscohesive cells (*right*). **B:** E-cadherin reactivity is present in intraductal carcinoma and absent in lobular carcinoma *in situ* in a parallel section from the tissue shown in **A.**

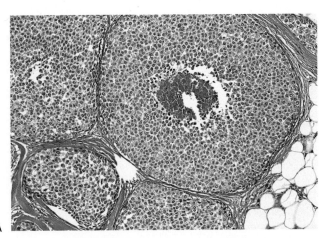

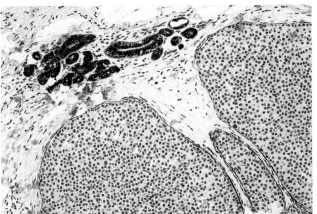

**FIG. 4.** *Florid lobular carcinoma* in situ. **A:** Marked duct enlargement with focal necrosis. **B:** E-cadherin immunoreactivity is present in normal lobule and in myoepithelial cells around florid lobular carcinoma *in situ*, but not in carcinoma cells (avidin-biotin).

# ROSEN'S BREAST PATHOLOGY

## Second Edition

**PAUL PETER ROSEN, M.D.**
*Professor*
*Department of Pathology*
*New York Weill Cornell Medical College*
*Chief of Breast Pathology*
*Breast Pathology Consultation Service*
*Department of Pathology*
*New York Presbyterian Hospital–Cornell Medical Center*
*New York, New York*

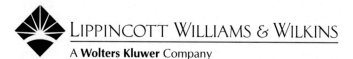

LIPPINCOTT WILLIAMS & WILKINS
A **Wolters Kluwer** Company
Philadelphia · Baltimore · New York · London
Buenos Aires · Hong Kong · Sydney · Tokyo

*Acquisitions Editor: Ruth W. Weinberg*
*Developmental Editor: Keith Donnellan*
*Production Editor: Rosemary Palumbo*
*Manufacturing Manager: Tim Reynolds*
*Cover Designer: Mark Lerner*
*Compositor: Maryland Composition Company, Inc.*

**© 2001 by LIPPINCOTT WILLIAMS & WILKINS**
**530 Walnut Street**
**Philadelphia, PA 19106 USA**
**LWW.com**

Printed and bound in China

---

**Library of Congress Cataloging-in-Publication Data**

Rosen, Paul Peter.
    Rosen's breast pathology / Paul Peter Rosen.—2nd ed.
        p. cm.
    Includes bibliographical references and index.
    ISBN 0-7817-2379-5
        1. Breast—Cancer—Pathophysiology. 2. Breast—Pathophysiology. I. Title: Breast pathology. II. Title.

RC280.B8 R67 2001
616.99'44907—dc21                                    00-052058

---

10 9 8 7 6 5 4 3 2 1

*To my parents, Beate Caspari-Rosen, M.D., and George Rosen, M.D.,*
*and to the ineffable Mary Sue Rosen.*

# Contents

Preface . . . . . . . . . . . . . . . . . . . . . . . . . . . . . . . . . . . . . . . . . . . . . . . . . . . . . . . . . . ix

Preface to the First Edition . . . . . . . . . . . . . . . . . . . . . . . . . . . . . . . . . . . . . . . . . xi

Acknowledgments . . . . . . . . . . . . . . . . . . . . . . . . . . . . . . . . . . . . . . . . . . . . . . . . . xiii

Introduction . . . . . . . . . . . . . . . . . . . . . . . . . . . . . . . . . . . . . . . . . . . . . . . . . . . . . xv

1  Anatomy and Physiologic Morphology . . . . . . . . . . . . . . . . . . . . . . . . . . 1

2  Abnormalities of Mammary Growth and Development . . . . . . . . . . . . . . 23

3  Inflammatory and Reactive Tumors . . . . . . . . . . . . . . . . . . . . . . . . . . . . 29

4  Specific Infections . . . . . . . . . . . . . . . . . . . . . . . . . . . . . . . . . . . . . . . . . 65

5  Papilloma and Related Benign Tumors . . . . . . . . . . . . . . . . . . . . . . . . . 77

6  Myoepithelial Neoplasms . . . . . . . . . . . . . . . . . . . . . . . . . . . . . . . . . . . 121

7  Adenosis and Microglandular Adenosis . . . . . . . . . . . . . . . . . . . . . . . . 139

8  Fibroepithelial Neoplasms . . . . . . . . . . . . . . . . . . . . . . . . . . . . . . . . . . 163

9  Ductal Hyperplasia: Ordinary and Atypical . . . . . . . . . . . . . . . . . . . . . 201

10  Precancerous Breast Disease: Epidemiologic, Pathologic,
    and Clinical Considerations . . . . . . . . . . . . . . . . . . . . . . . . . . . . . . . . 229

11  *In Situ* (Intraepithelial) Carcinoma: An Overview . . . . . . . . . . . . . . . . 249

12  Staging of Breast Carcinoma . . . . . . . . . . . . . . . . . . . . . . . . . . . . . . . . 253

13  Intraductal Carcinoma . . . . . . . . . . . . . . . . . . . . . . . . . . . . . . . . . . . . . 257

14  Invasive Duct Carcinoma: Assessment of Prognosis, Morphologic
    Prognostic Markers, and Tumor Growth Rate . . . . . . . . . . . . . . . . . . . 325

15  Tubular Carcinoma . . . . . . . . . . . . . . . . . . . . . . . . . . . . . . . . . . . . . . . . 365

16  Papillary Carcinoma . . . . . . . . . . . . . . . . . . . . . . . . . . . . . . . . . . . . . . 381

17  Medullary Carcinoma . . . . . . . . . . . . . . . . . . . . . . . . . . . . . . . . . . . . . 405

18  Carcinoma with Metaplasia . . . . . . . . . . . . . . . . . . . . . . . . . . . . . . . . . 425

19  Squamous Carcinoma . . . . . . . . . . . . . . . . . . . . . . . . . . . . . . . . . . . . . . 455

20  Mucinous Carcinoma . . . . . . . . . . . . . . . . . . . . . . . . . . . . . . . . . . . . . . 463

21  Apocrine Carcinoma . . . . . . . . . . . . . . . . . . . . . . . . . . . . . . . . . . . . . . . 483

22  Mammary Carcinoma with Endocrine Features . . . . . . . . . . . . . . . . . . 497

23  Small Cell (Oat Cell) Carcinoma . . . . . . . . . . . . . . . . . . . . . . . . . . . . . 503

**24**  Secretory Carcinoma . . . . . . . . . . . . . . . . . . . . . . . . . . . . . . . . . . . . . . . . . . . 509

**25**  Mammary Carcinoma with Osteoclast-like Giant Cells . . . . . . . . . . . . . . . . . . 517

**26**  Cystic Hypersecretory Carcinoma and Cystic Hypersecretory Hyperplasia . . . . . . . 527

**27**  Adenoid Cystic Carcinoma . . . . . . . . . . . . . . . . . . . . . . . . . . . . . . . . . . . . . 535

**28**  Cribriform Carcinoma . . . . . . . . . . . . . . . . . . . . . . . . . . . . . . . . . . . . . . . . 551

**29**  Lipid-rich Carcinoma . . . . . . . . . . . . . . . . . . . . . . . . . . . . . . . . . . . . . . . . 555

**30**  Glycogen-rich Carcinoma . . . . . . . . . . . . . . . . . . . . . . . . . . . . . . . . . . . . . 557

**31**  Invasive Micropapillary Carcinoma . . . . . . . . . . . . . . . . . . . . . . . . . . . . . . 561

**32**  Paget's Disease of the Nipple . . . . . . . . . . . . . . . . . . . . . . . . . . . . . . . . . . 565

**33**  Lobular Carcinoma *In Situ* and Atypical Lobular Hyperplasia . . . . . . . . . . . . . 581

**34**  Invasive Lobular Carcinoma . . . . . . . . . . . . . . . . . . . . . . . . . . . . . . . . . . . 627

**35**  Unusual Clinical Presentations of Carcinoma . . . . . . . . . . . . . . . . . . . . . . . 653

**36**  Metastases in the Breast from Nonmammary Malignant Neoplasms . . . . . . . . . . 689

**37**  Benign Proliferative Lesions of the Male Breast . . . . . . . . . . . . . . . . . . . . . . 703

**38**  Carcinoma of the Male Breast . . . . . . . . . . . . . . . . . . . . . . . . . . . . . . . . . . 713

**39**  Breast Tumors in Children . . . . . . . . . . . . . . . . . . . . . . . . . . . . . . . . . . . . 729

**40**  Benign Mesenchymal Neoplasms . . . . . . . . . . . . . . . . . . . . . . . . . . . . . . . . 749

**41**  Sarcoma . . . . . . . . . . . . . . . . . . . . . . . . . . . . . . . . . . . . . . . . . . . . . . . . 813

**42**  Lymphoid and Hematopoietic Tumors . . . . . . . . . . . . . . . . . . . . . . . . . . . . 863

**43**  Pathologic Effects of Therapy . . . . . . . . . . . . . . . . . . . . . . . . . . . . . . . . . . 887

**44**  Cutaneous Neoplasms . . . . . . . . . . . . . . . . . . . . . . . . . . . . . . . . . . . . . . . 899

**45**  The Pathology of Axillary and Intramammary Lymph Nodes . . . . . . . . . . . . . . 913

**46**  Pathologic Examination of Breast and Lymph Node Specimens . . . . . . . . . . . . 931

Subject Index . . . . . . . . . . . . . . . . . . . . . . . . . . . . . . . . . . . . . . . . . . . . . . . . 991

# Preface

This volume updates the comprehensive, extensively illustrated description of breast pathology in a clinical context that was offered in the First Edition. The reader of the Second Edition will find more color illustrations, as well as substantially expanded discussions of most topics, with emphasis on precancerous lesions, atypical hyperplasia, intraductal carcinoma, needle core biopsies, and sentinel lymph node pathology. In order to create space for the new material, especially additional illustrations, chapters on important but somewhat peripheral subjects which appeared in the First Edition have been omitted. These include chapters covering an historical overview of *in situ* carcinoma, biomarkers of prognosis, cytology and pathology consultation issues. Each of the 46 chapters which comprise the Second Edition has been thoroughly revised to incorporate new information and references available until completion of the manuscript in the year 2000.

I am grateful to readers of the First Edition who drew my attention to deficiencies in the labelling of illustrations and in reference citations. It was encouraging that very few corrections were needed. The Second Edition has been subjected to careful scrutiny by the author and at various stages of production by the outstanding diligent staff of Lippincott Williams & Wilkins. Any residual or new errors remain the responsibility of the author. The selection of references and illustrations, the citation of data from published sources and the conclusions expressed herein, reflect the author's experience and opinions.

# Preface to the First Edition

*He will manage to cure best who has foreseen what is to happen from the present state of matters.*

Hippocrates (1)

The management of diseases of the breast is a multidisciplinary endeavor dependent on the skill and expertise of an array of clinical specialists. In this complex effort, the importance of one or another member of the team for a given patient will vary depending upon the clinical circumstances. At the outset and often at later critical points, an accurate pathological diagnosis is the crucial element for determining the course of treatment and for estimating prognosis. A thorough knowledge of the pathology of the breast is essential for physicians and other medical personnel who take care of patients with breast diseases. Conversely, the pathologist cloistered in a laboratory, out of touch with patient care, will not be able to provide the clinically meaningful information currently expected of practitioners of this specialty.

The breast appears structurally and functionally to be relatively uncomplicated, but it is the site of a surprisingly broad array of pathological alterations, many of which are organ-specific. New entities continue to be identified. Our understanding of breast pathology has been substantially amplified by the application of new technology to this effort. Particularly rapid progress has occurred in the past decade as a result of the availability of immunohistochemistry and *in situ* hybridization that have made it possible to observe the tissue-specific and cell-specific localization of molecular and genetic processes associated with physiological and pathological conditions. Yet, it is important not to be blinded by the blizzard of information and to avoid being swept away in the annual flood of "hot topics." All too often, today's hot topic becomes tomorrow's footnote. Ultimately, our understanding of breast pathology is remodeled and enriched by the ongoing process of discovery and thoughtful analysis that contributes to a growing body of knowledge composed of many bits of information from innumerable contributors. This vision embodies the precept of Hippocrates who wrote:

> But all these requisites belong of old to Medicine, and an origin and way have been found out, by which many and elegant discoveries have been made, during a length of time, and others will yet be found out, if a person possessed of the proper ability, and knowing those discoveries which have been made, should proceed from them to prosecute his investigations (2).

This book provides a comprehensive, extensively illustrated description of breast pathology in a clinical context. Most of the chapters are devoted to specific diseases or disease groupings. The discussion of each topic consists, where relevant, of sections detailing clinical presentation and mammography, epidemiology, gross pathology, microscopic pathology including electron microscopy and immunohistochemistry, differential diagnosis, treatment, and prognosis. Several chapters deal with broad subjects, such as precancerous breast pathology, staging of carcinoma, biological markers of prognosis, the pathological effects of therapy, cytologic and needle core diagnosis, and the pathological examination of breast specimens.

Illustrations have been selected to demonstrate not only the standard appearance of lesions but also to emphasize the heterogeneity represented by variant forms. Following the manner in which the pathologist encounters them in daily practice, many entities are shown as they appear grossly, in whole mount histological sections and, finally, at progressively higher magnification, amplified with immunohistochemistry and other diagnostic procedures.

It is my hope that there is no "pathomythology" in this book. A myth is defined as "an idea that forms part of the beliefs of a group or class but is not founded on fact" (3). Pathomythology is a term I use to describe the persistent repetition of hypotheses relating to pathology that are completely contradicted by existing data. Perpetrators of this activity frequently reinforce their myth by quoting themselves or other followers of their belief, eschewing facts that can easily be confirmed by direct observation. One example of pathomythology is the seemingly indestructible idea that the carcinomatous cells of mammary Paget's disease arise by transformation of squamous cells in the squamous epithelium that harbors Paget's disease. Intraductal carcinoma, which is the source of these carcinoma cells, is detected in virtually every patient with Paget's disease but the pathomythologists rest their case on the very few instances in which duct carcinoma is not discovered. A reasonable explanation for these exceptional cases is offered in this book. Another example of pathomythology is the inaccurate statement that an intraductal component is not found in true medullary carcinoma. Intraductal carcinoma can be found at the periphery of most medullary carcinomas, but the presence or absence of intraductal carcinoma has been shown not to be a criterion for the diagnosis of medullary carcinoma.

Despite diligent attention to detail, it is likely that some errors of omission or commission have occurred in the preparation of this book. The author is responsible for the selection of references and illustrations, the citation of data from published sources, and for conclusions expressed herein, based on his personal experience and his interpretation of the literature.

## REFERENCES

1. Adams F. The book of prognostics. *The genuine works of Hippocrates.* Baltimore: The Williams & Wilkins Co.; 1939:42.
2. Adams F. On ancient medicine. *The genuine works of Hippocrates.* Baltimore: The Williams & Wilkins Co.; 1939:1–2.
3. Stein J, ed. *The Random House dictionary of the English language.* New York: Random House; 1973:946.

# Acknowledgments

The Second Edition of *Rosen's Breast Pathology* is based on the foundation laid in the previous edition. With few exceptions, the contributions made by individuals acknowledged in the First Edition remain and I hereby salute them once more. I am particularly grateful for the outstanding assistance of Tammy Son in preparing the groundwork for the Second Edition.

Many of the illustrations in the book were taken from cases received in consultation. An extraordinary phenomenon of the consultation practice is the tendency of types or categories of pathology to arrive in temporal clusters, although they originate from totally independent and geographically diverse sources. The theme may be papillary lesions one day, and the next day may be dominated by fibroepithelial tumors. I am deeply indebted to the pathologists who have sent and continue to submit diagnostic consultations, since this is an invaluable source of material for research and teaching. In return for the nearly 100% cooperation of pathology colleagues when further material or information has been requested for academic purposes, I hope that the results of these studies over nearly three decades have been useful to them and have benefited their patients. Thousands of adult women, as well as many hundreds of men and children afflicted with breast diseases who cannot be recognized individually, are the fundamental contributors to this work and they are acknowledged for their anonymous contributions.

In addition to individuals acknowledged in the First Edition, the following physicians provided data, case material or illustrations which have been added to the Second Edition: R. Adelsberg, B. Ben-Dor, F. Braza, G. Bussolati, H.A. Evans, A. Fortin, R. Heimann, S. Hellman, K. Kapila, H. Kim, J. Kracht, L. Liberman, P.J. Pickhardt, A. Sapino, and K. Verma.

The assembly of much of the new illustrative material, and the initial stages of revising the manuscript for the Second Edition were accomplished during my tenure as Senior Consulting Pathologist at the White Plains Hospital Center and the Dickstein Cancer Center. Drs. Christine Honig, Astrid Quish, and Diane Schechter, members of the Pathology Department under the Directorship of Dr. Deena Shah, and Dr. Arthur Lerner, Director of the Cancer Program, remain esteemed colleagues. Joan Kansas deserves a special accolade for creating and managing the Breast Pathologist Consultation Service from which some of this material was drawn.

Final preparation of the Second Edition was accomplished at the Weill-Cornell Medical College and New York-Presbyterian Hospital where the Breast Pathology Consultation Service is now located. Under the Chairmanship of Dr. Daniel M. Knowles, it has been possible to establish an academic program providing specialized breast pathology diagnostic service combined with teaching and research. The strong support of Dr. Knowles and of Dr. Ronald A. DeLellis, Vice Chair for Anatomic Pathology were instrumental in enabling the completion of this work. I have also been very pleased to have Drs. Sandra Shin, Sunati Sahoo, and Erica Resetkova as Fellowship trainees on the Breast Pathology Service. Their high level of enthusiasm, dedication to clinical and academic excellence and meticulous work reflect the highest medical standards and auger well for the future of pathology. The results of studies accomplished by Drs. Shin and Sahoo have been included in this volume.

The Breast Pathology Consultation Service at the Weill-Cornell Center of the New York-Presbyterian Hospital continues to be a source of challenging diagnostic material that serves as a basis for ongoing investigation and teaching. I have been extremely fortunate to have Lori Billingsley as the Office Assistant, to manage the service. Special thanks are due to Ms. Billingsley for her exemplary dedication to this program.

The experience of turning the manuscript into a finished book has been a cooperative enterprise with the superb staff of Lippincott Williams & Wilkins. Starting with the agreement to prepare the Second Edition, I have had the very strong support of Ruth W. Weinberg, Senior Editor, in making this a comprehensive, up-to-date book. Andrea Post, assistant to Ms. Weinberg, made many constructive contributions to the manuscript. Keith Donnellan, Senior Developmental Editor, performed the vital service of sifting through the nooks and crannies of the final manuscript for misplaced or missing parts of which there were thankfully but few. Timothy Reynolds, Manufacturing Manager, succeeded in the tricky task of improving color balance in some of the images. The final editing and production phase was masterfully managed with meticulous care by Rosemary Palumbo. Credit for the excellent cover design goes to Diana Andrews.

# Introduction

## CONSULTATIONS AND SECOND OPINIONS IN BREAST PATHOLOGY

Surgical pathologists in general practice provide accurate diagnoses on the great majority of the breast specimens they encounter without the assistance of intramural or extramural consultation. Nonetheless, pathology departments should have a built-in mechanism for obtaining second opinions internally, through conferencing or other quality assurance programs. In this setting, the individual pathologist, or the pathology group in a department, may seek an extramural opinion from an expert consultant. This typically occurs when there is a difference of interpretation among pathologists in an institution or the diagnosis is uncertain after internal review. Consultation may be obtained when the probable diagnosis is one with which there is little or no experience. Another category of consultation results from uncertainty about the diagnosis engendered by a limited or unrepresentative sample, poor histologic preparation, or a pathologic change that appears to be on the borderline between two or more diagnoses. As noted by Leslie et al., "second opinions in anatomic pathology are an integral part of quality practice. . .frequent consultation between pathologists should be fostered in all practice settings and documented as part of the quality assurance process" (1).

Several studies have demonstrated the important contribution of second opinion pathology consultations to patient care, generally in the context of referrals seen at academic centers. A very positive aspect of this practice is the high degree to which the primary diagnosis has been confirmed by the consultant. Epstein et al. reported concordant diagnoses (cancer vs. noncancer) in 98.7% of 535 prostatic needle biopsies diagnosed as cancer (2). Nonetheless, the six diagnoses not sustained as cancer were critically important for the 1.3% of patients. A cost analysis of these results suggested that the saving in medical expenses for the 6 patients who did not undergo surgery substantially exceeded the cost of reviewing all 535 biopsies. A higher rate of discrepancies was found by Abt et al., who compared the original and second opinion diagnoses in a broad range of pathology among 777 patients referred to an academic center (3). Forty-five diagnostic disagreements (6%) were regarded as clinically significant, and overall the level of agreement was 92.1%.

The need to ship glass slides for consultation will be with us for some time to come. It is unlikely that complete microscopic pathology samples will be routinely converted to electronic images in the foreseeable future given the time and cost of this undertaking and the fact that much of the information will be a record of "normal" or nonlesional tissue. Within the United States, several factors have contributed to the growing number of pathology consultations. Much of the increase is generated by patients who seek multiple clinical opinions from different physicians and institutions. Some patients are primarily concerned with confirmation of their diagnosis, and one or more consultations may be obtained directly from pathologists for this reason alone. Most of the remainder of consultations are initiated by pathologists seeking opinions from their colleagues. Surgeons, medical oncologists, and other physicians generate some second opinion reviews.

Slides sent for consultation, regardless of the reason, must be accompanied by documents that: (a) confirm the identity of the specimen with the patient; (b) explain why the material has been sent; (c) provide complete information about who should receive the report; (d) designate who will pay for the consultation and how billing should be submitted; and (e) indicate the disposition of materials.

There is no evident advantage to sending slides separately from the documents. This procedure, which seems to be routinely followed in some laboratories, can cause considerable problems, especially if the correspondence and slides do not arrive coincidentally. The correspondence may take many forms, but it is essential that the information cited above be provided. This must include a copy of the pathology/cytology report for each specimen represented, clearly displaying the anatomic source, the name of the patient, and the accession number corresponding to the slides enclosed.

It is unacceptable and substandard practice to withhold the pathology report from a consultant or second opinion institution so as not to "bias" the second review. In addition to confirming the anatomic source and patient identity of the slides, the pathology report provides essential information such as an index of the specific location(s) of the specimen(s) in individual slides, a description of the gross appearance of the specimen(s), clinical information provided with the specimen, frozen section interpretations, and details of the pathologist's diagnosis that should be evaluated. The pathology report must be included even if the final diagnosis will depend upon the consultation. When the slides are sent directly from one laboratory to another in relation to a clinical consultation at the recipient institution, the correspondence should include the pathology report, the name of the clinical physician who is being consulted (if it is known), and the patient's address, with available insurance information. When more than one consultant is involved it is vital that all consultants examine the same or equivalent material.

## THE PATHOLOGIST AS A SPECIALIST IN BREAST CANCER CARE

The development and application of a concept of localized pathology laid the groundwork for modern specialism by providing a number of foci of interest in the field of medicine. Each such focus of interest, that is, a disease or the diseases of an organ or region of the body, provided a nucleus around which could gather the results of clinical and pathological investigation.

On the technological side the influences represented in specialization manifest themselves in the multiplicity of technical skills, devices, and theories applied to the achievement of human aims in the field of medicine.

*The Specialization of Medicine* by George Rosen, M.D., 1944

Impressive advances have been made in the past 50 years in the effort to prevent, treat, and cure breast cancer. Major milestones include the development of mammography for early detection, the shift from mastectomy to breast conservation therapy for many patients, advances in chemotherapy as an adjuvant modality, the demonstration that antiestrogenic compounds can inhibit the development and progression of breast cancer, and the introduction of sentinel lymph node mapping for axillary staging. The growth of medical specialization in the second half of the twentieth century has had a profound influence on these accomplishments by fostering multidisciplinary clinical practice and research.

Specialism in all aspects of medical care has revolutionized the role of the Surgical Pathologist. Rather than fostering professional independence, specialization in medicine has created circumstances in which the specialist delivering a limited segment of medical care is increasingly dependent on the assistance of colleagues who have acquired complimentary expertise. This situation is epitomized by the multidisciplinary approach now standard for treating breast diseases. Inherent in this circumstance is the expectation that each member of the team is capable of delivering optimal specialty care. A corollary effect is growing pressure for subspecialization in diagnostic pathology, especially in academic centers. Breast pathology has largely remained in the domain of generalists except for a few referral centers. The recent formation of the International Society of Breast Pathology heralds recognition of subspecialization in Breast Pathology. A year-2000 position paper of the European Society of Mastology setting forth guidelines for a clinical program devoted to providing a "high quality specialist Breast Service" included among the physicians "a lead pathologist plus usually not more than one other nominated pathologist, specializing in Breast Disease . . . [to be] responsible for all breast pathology and cytology" (5). This process will be furthered by growing awareness on the part of patients and patient advocacy organizations that accurate and comprehensive pathology diagnosis is fundamental to effective treatment and research in breast diseases.

Major advances that have contributed to the role of the pathologist as a key member of the breast cancer team include:

- Widespread use of mammography which detects nonpalpable lesions;
- Image-guided needle core biopsy that acquires samples from nonpalpable lesions;
- Breast conservation therapy which requires more detailed pathologic assessment of breast specimens;
- The availability of histologically-based methods for detecting markers used to assess prognosis and to plan therapy; and
- Sentinel lymph node mapping and bone marrow sampling for micrometastases.

Pathologists generate an important part of the information used for therapeutic decisions. The complex, multifactorial description of breast pathology now considered to be standard practice has expanded the diagnostic report from a brief one- or two-line statement to a catalogue of data sometimes several pages in length. Immunohistochemistry makes it possible to determine the presence of prognostic and therapeutic markers by microscopic examination, and these observations are part of the pathologist's report.

Coincidental with these medical developments has been the growing involvement of patients in making decisions about their treatment. This has led to greater public awareness of the importance of information contained in pathology reports. For the untrained lay person to read and interpret a pathology report, it is necessary to learn and understand a new vocabulary. This is a daunting task, even more difficult for the patient whose name appears on the document. Books and literature provided by medical and lay societies or associations are helpful, as is the bottomless well of information that appears on the Internet. The radiologist, surgeon, oncologist, and radiotherapist are expert at interpreting pathology reports for their patients, and in explaining the significance of the data. Nonetheless, a substantial number of patients with breast diseases want an explanation from the pathologist who issued the report or they seek out another pathologist, often with specialized expertise, for a second opinion review. Many more patients are aware that a pathology consultant is involved in their case. In this way pathologists participate increasingly in direct patient care and also in education, a vital public service.

## PROGRESS AND UNCERTAINTY IN BREAST PATHOLOGY

Extraordinary progress has been made in linking anatomic pathology, the study of normal and diseased tissues, to patient care throughout the spectrum of human ailments. The twentieth century has been marked by great advances in defining the pathology of breast diseases and in relating these observations to the development of more effective therapy tailored to the specific type and extent of disease in the individual patient.

The stage was set in the latter half of the nineteenth and first decades of the twentieth centuries, with the flowering of classical pathology based largely on the postmortem examination of the gross and microscopic changes found in diseased tissues. The principle objectives of these investigations were to describe and catalogue diseases in an effort to detect clues to their pathogenesis and to better understand their clinical manifestations. Surgical pathology, the study of tissues from the living, emerged from classical anatomic pathology as advances in surgery, made possible by effective anesthesia and antisepsis, focused greater attention on pathologic diagnosis as a critical element in the treatment of many diseases. The study of breast pathology has been a model of interdisciplinary investigation involving clinical and laboratory science. Pathologists are in a unique position to meet the challenge of developing and adapting innovative laboratory methods to better understand and to improve the treatment of breast diseases.

Despite the perceptions of the public and some medical colleagues that diagnostic pathology lacks ambiguity and subtlety, pathologists are repeatedly faced with the need to deal with uncertainty. The usually blunt, seemingly "black and white" recitation of a final pathology report actually represents a synthesis of possibilities which constitute the "differential diagnosis." We strive to reduce uncertainty by constant study leading to the development and application of new insights or improved techniques. Yet, each advance brings with it a new horizon of uncertainty, a new confidence interval. One manifestation of uncertainty in the study of breast cancer and precancerous breast disease is our limited ability to separate "the drivers from the hitchhikers," that is "to distinguish between silent alterations acquired by the malignant cell and those that truly contribute to the malignant phenotype" (4).

In the clinical arena, the phenomenon of advances creating new uncertainty is illustrated by the procedure for axillary lymph node staging by sentinel lymph node mapping. The coincidence of improved surgical techniques to localize the lymph node or nodes most likely to harbor metastatic carcinoma and the application of immunohistochemistry to the lymph nodes by the pathologist makes it possible to detect metastases in selected lymph nodes without the need for more extensive axillary dissection. Sentinel lymph node staging therefore documents axillary nodal status with less morbidity than conventional axillary dissection. Nonetheless, the procedure has raised new questions about the prognostic significance of the micrometastases so elegantly uncovered, leaving uncertainty about therapy based on this finding.

Pathologists have unique opportunities in breast cancer research. Technical advances now make it possible to apply the extraordinarily powerful techniques of molecular and genetic analysis directly to tissues visualized with the microscope. This is truly the intersection of the classical microscopic pathology of the nineteenth and twentieth centuries with the molecular science of the twenty-first century. By microdissection the pathologist can select small groups of cells and even individual cells from normal and abnormal tissues that are identified and diagnosed with the microscope. DNA extracted from these minute samples can be amplified and studied for molecular alterations by a variety of techniques. This approach holds great promise for furthering our understanding of precancerous and cancerous breast diseases and for finding clues to improved prevention and therapeutic strategies. Microdissection is presently too costly and laborious for widespread clinical application. Nonetheless, I expect that only a decade or two hence, pathologists will routinely employ microdissection and molecular analysis in the diagnosis of breast tissues and that robotic instrumentation will contribute substantially to making this a clinically feasible enterprise. The ability of pathologists to distinguish between structurally normal and abnormal tissues will remain a fundamental step in diagnosis in the foreseeable future, but technological advances will require greater sophistication on the part of pathologists and continue to foster subspecialization in Breast Pathology.

## REFERENCES

1. Leslie KO, Fechner RE, Kempson RL. Second opinions in surgical pathology. *Am J Clin Pathol* 1996;106:S58–S64.
2. Epstein JI, Walsh PC, Sanfilippo F. Clinical and cost impact of second-opinion pathology. Review of prostate biopsies prior to radical prostatectomy. *Am J Surg Pathol* 1996;20:851–857.
3. Abt AB, Abt LG, Olt GJ. The effect of interinstitution anatomic pathology consultation on patient care. *Arch Pathol Lab Med* 1995;119:514–517.
4. Cordon-Cardo C. At the crossroad of tumorigenesis: drivers and hitchhikers. *Hum Pathol* 1999;20:1001–1003.
5. EUSOMA (European Society of Mastology). Position paper. The requirements of a specialist breast unit. *Europ J Cancer* 2000;36:2288–2293.

# ROSEN'S BREAST PATHOLOGY

*Second Edition*

# CHAPTER 1

# Anatomy and Physiologic Morphology

## EMBRYOLOGY AND INFANTILE BREAST DEVELOPMENT

The mammary glands develop from the mammary ridges or milk lines, which are thickenings of the epidermis that first appear on the ventral surface of the 5-week fetus, extending from the axilla to the upper medial region of the thigh. In the human, most of the ridge does not develop further and disappears during fetal development. Persistence of segments of the milk line is the embryologic anlage for ectopic mammary glandular tissue, which occurs most often at the extreme ends of the mammary ridge in the axilla or vulva.

On the chest wall, mesenchymal condensation occurs around an epithelial stalk, the breast bud, at the site of mammary development in the fifteenth week of gestation. Growth of cords of epithelium into the mesenchyme produces a group of solid epithelial columns, each of which gives rise to a lobe in the mammary gland. The papillary layer of the fetal dermis continues to encase these growing epithelial cords, and it ultimately gives rise to the vascularized fibrous tissue surrounding individual ducts and their branches into lobules. In the fetal breast, epithelial cells that form the breast bud express transforming growth factor $\alpha$, a mitogen and differentiation factor that may mediate the growth-promoting effect of estrogen on the developing breast (1). Stromal tissue surrounding the breast bud is rich in transforming growth factor $\beta_1$, a protein involved in modulating cell–matrix interaction. The basement membrane protein, collagen type IV, is distributed around the basal layer of cells in the breast bud. Early in fetal development, proliferative activity measured by Ki67 immunoreactivity is maximal in the region of the neck of the breast bud, involving epithelial and stromal cells.

Less cellular, more collagenized stroma that originates in the reticular dermis extends into the breast to encompass lobes and subdivisions of lobes, forming the suspensory ligaments of Cooper, which attach the breast parenchyma to the skin (2). Coincidentally, differentiation of the mesenchyme into fat within the collagenous stroma occurs between weeks 20 and 32. In the last 2 months of gestation, canalization of the epithelial cords occurs, followed by development of

branching lobuloalveolar glandular structures. The mammary pit is a depression in the epidermis where the lactiferous ducts converge. Near birth, the nipple is formed by evagination of the mammary pit. A congenitally inverted nipple is the result of failure of this normal process to occur.

The earliest stages of fetal mammary gland formation appear not to be dependent on steroid hormones, whereas the actual development of the breast structure after the fifteenth week is largely influenced by testosterone. Estrogen receptor alpha has been detected by immunohistochemistry in epithelial cell nuclei in the fetal breast during and after the thirtieth week of gestation (2a). Estrogen receptor alpha is up-regulated shortly after birth, accompanied by progesterone receptor, a finding indicating that the estrogen receptor is functional. In the last weeks of gestation, the fetal breast is responsive to maternal and placental steroid hormones and to prolactin, which induce secretory activity. This is manifested after birth by the secretion of colostrum and palpable enlargement of the breast bud. The secretory activity typically subsides and ceases during the first or second month after birth due to disappearance of maternal hormones from the infant's bloodstream. The gland shrinks and returns to an inactive state in which it is composed of lactiferous ducts that branch somewhat without progressive alveolar differentiation, although lobular structures may persist (Fig. 1.1).

The protein product of the *bcl*-2 gene, which acts to inhibit apoptosis, is maximally expressed in the fetal breast (3). Immunohistochemical localization of *bcl*-2 has been detected in the basal epithelium of the developing breast bud and in the surrounding stroma. Similar patterns of staining have been reported in male and female breast tissue. *Bcl*-2 reactivity is lost soon after birth, and it is not present in the epithelium of the normal adult breast. These observations suggest that up-regulation of *bcl*-2 contributes to morphogenesis of the fetal breast by its inhibitory effect on apoptosis.

Further normal breast development does not begin until puberty. *Premature thelarche* is the unilateral or bilateral appearance of a discoid subareolar thickening prior to puberty. The incidence of premature thelarche in white female infants

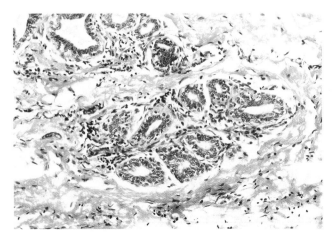

**FIG. 1.1.** *Infantile breast with lobule.* Persistent lobule in the breast of a 6-month-old girl who had an intraductal papilloma excised.

and children up to 7 years old in the United States in 1980 was 20.8 per 100,000 (4). This condition probably is a response to aberrant levels of endogenous hormones. The mean basal follicle-stimulating hormone level in girls with premature thelarche is higher than in normal controls, and these girls have a greater response to gonadotrophin-releasing hormone (5). Patients with precocious puberty tend to have normal follicle-stimulating hormone levels and a normal response to luteinizing hormone-releasing hormone (6). Klein et al. (7) reported that girls with premature thelarche have significantly higher levels of estradiol than normal prepubertal girls.

The nodular breast tissue measuring 1.0 to 6.5 cm tends to regress slowly over the subsequent 6 months to 6 years, but in some instances, the hyperplastic breast bud persists until puberty (4). Volta et al. (8) reported that 60% of girls with premature thelarche that began before age 2 years had complete regression before the onset of puberty. Excision of this tissue results in amastia. van Winter et al. (4) reported that

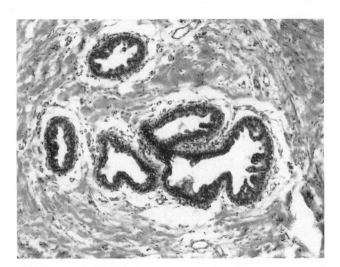

**FIG. 1.2.** *Premature thelarche.* Mild papillary epithelial hyperplasia in a biopsy from a 1-year-old girl with unilateral breast enlargement.

follow-up of women who had premature thelarche revealed no predisposition to breast carcinoma and a normal age of menarche. In another series, 14% of girls with premature thelarche developed precocious puberty (9), a circumstance more likely to occur if the onset of premature thelarche is after age 2 years (5).

Histologically, the breast tissue in premature thelarche resembles gynecomastia, because it is characterized by epithelial hyperplasia in the duct system with a solid and micropapillary configuration (Fig. 1.2). Growth and branching of the proliferating ducts result in an increased number of duct cross sections surrounded by moderately cellular stroma. Fine needle aspiration cytology reveals a background of myxoid stroma, bipolar stromal cells, and sparse sheets of benign ductal cells (10). Premature thelarche should be distinguished from prepubertal breast enlargement, which typically occurs as a result of the accumulation of excess mammary fat and connective tissue.

## ADOLESCENT BREAST DEVELOPMENT

With the onset of cyclical estrogen and progesterone secretion at puberty, adolescent female breast development commences. Growth of ducts that elongate and acquire a thickened epithelium is dependent on estrogens (11). Differentiation of hormonally responsive periductal stroma, which is estrogen dependent, also occurs at this time. Growth hormone and glucocorticoids contribute to ductal growth. Lobuloalveolar differentiation and growth during this period are enhanced primarily by insulin, progesterone, and growth hormone. The lobules are derived from solid masses of cells that form at the ends of terminal ducts. The greatest amount of breast glandular differentiation occurs during puberty, but the process continues for at least a decade and is enhanced by pregnancy (Fig. 1.3). The adolescent male breast consists of fibrofatty tissue and ducts lined by a thin layer of small cuboidal cells (Fig. 1.4).

## GROSS ANATOMY OF THE ADULT BREAST

The mature breast has an eccentric configuration, with the long axis diagonally placed on the chest wall largely over the pectoralis major muscle and extending into the axilla as the tail of Spence. The peripheral anatomic boundaries of the breast are not precisely defined, except at the deep surface where the gland overlies the pectoralis fascia. Superficially, the breast extends over portions of the serratus anterior muscle laterally, inferiorly over the external oblique muscle and superior rectus sheath, and medially to the sternum.

Anatomically, the breast lies in a space within the superficial fascia, although microscopic extensions of glandular parenchyma sometimes traverse these boundaries. Superiorly this layer is continuous with the cervical fascia and inferiorly with the superficial abdominal fascia of Cooper. Fibrous strands extend from the dermis into the breast, forming the suspensory ligaments of Cooper, which attach the skin and nipple to the breast. Cooper's ligaments are more

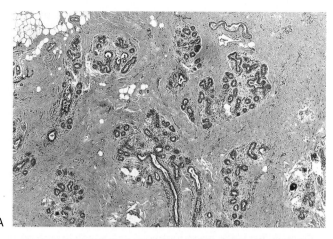

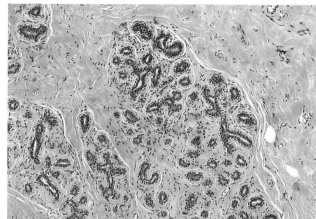

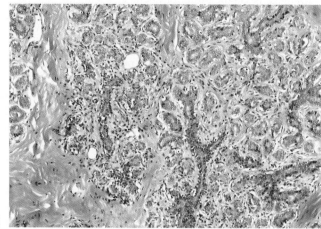

**FIG. 1.3.** *Pubertal and adolescent female breast.* **A:** Biopsy from a 12-year-old girl who had a juvenile fibroadenoma. Menarche was less than 1 year earlier. Lobular architecture is present. **B:** Lobules in a 15-year-old girl consistent with the follicular phase of the menstrual cycle. **C:** Lobules consistent with the luteal phase of the menstrual cycle in a 16-year-old girl.

extensive in the upper part of the breast. Distortion or contraction of the suspensory ligaments by parenchymal lesions may be manifested by skin dimpling or nipple retraction.

The deep membranous layer of the superficial fascia is separated from the fascia of the pectoralis major and serratus anterior muscles by the retromammary or submammary

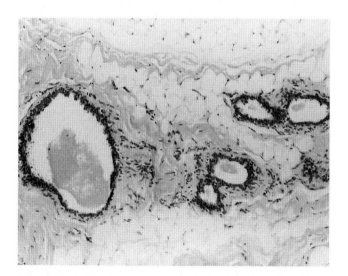

**FIG. 1.4.** *Adolescent male breast.* The thin layer of epithelium shows characteristic cellular crowding, and there is slight dilatation of ducts.

space, which contains loose areolar tissue. Extensions of the membranous superficial fascia that traverse the retromammary space act as posterior suspensory ligaments. Microscopic extensions of glandular breast tissue may be found in conjunction with the posterior suspensory ligaments in the retromammary space and rarely in the underlying pectoral fascia. Neoplastic or inflammatory infiltration of the retromammary space is associated clinically with fixation of the breast to the chest wall.

The axillary fascia at the dome of the pyramidal axillary space is formed by an extension of the pectoralis major muscle. A fascial layer arising from the lower border of the pectoralis minor joins an extension of the pectoralis major fascia to form the suspensory ligament of the axilla in continuity with the fascia of the latissimus dorsi muscle. An inconstant muscle band in this fascial plane is referred to as the suspensory muscle of the axilla. The fascial boundaries of the axilla provide important landmarks for the *en bloc* dissection of the axillary contents.

## ARTERIAL AND VENOUS CIRCULATION

The arterial circulation of the breast is derived from the internal thoracic, axillary, and intercostal arteries (12). There are many individual variations in the relative contributions of these vessels, and patterns of circulation are not necessarily symmetric in the left and right breast of an individual (13). Branches of the internal thoracic artery provide the major source of arterial circulation in most cases. These perforating branches traverse the thoracic wall at the sternal border in the first four intercostal spaces. The largest vessel usually lies in the second intercostal space. In about 30% of individuals, the axillary artery is of minor consequence, and in 50% there is little or no dependence on the intercostal arteries (14). Branches of the arterial circulation within the breast parenchyma do not specifically follow the major duct system (13).

Venous drainage is more variable than the arterial supply, but it tends to follow the distribution of the arterial circulation (13). The superficial venous complex consists largely of transverse veins corresponding to branches of the internal thoracic artery. These vessels drain medially into the internal thoracic veins. A minor superficial venous system flows longitudinally toward the suprasternal notch to drain into superficial veins of the neck. Deep venous drainage is largely via perforating branches of the internal thoracic vein. Branches of the axillary vein also contribute to deep venous drainage and are especially prone to variable distribution. Tributaries of the intercostal veins provide a third route for venous drainage, with direct access to the vertebral veins and vertebral plexus.

## LYMPHATIC DRAINAGE

Seventeenth-century studies of the mammary lymphatic system took note of the similarity between milk and chyle in the lymphatic drainage of the intestine. This led to studies intended to demonstrate the anatomic basis for the transport of chyle to the breast as the mechanism for lactation. A thorough description of the mammary lymphatics was first provided in 1786 by Cruikshank (15), who referred to lymphatic vessels as "absorbents." He was able to identify the major routes of lymphatic flow from the breast as being along the course of the branches of the external thoracic and internal thoracic veins toward the axilla and internal mammary regions, respectively. Nearly a century later, Sappey (16) used mercury injection to demonstrate the lymphatic system of the lactating breast and observed drainage that appeared to flow from the parenchyma to the plexus of vessels in the subareolar region, now referred to as the subareolar plexus of Sappey. It has subsequently been appreciated that this plexus serves as a pathway for cutaneous lymphatic drainage to the interlobular connective tissue of the breast and thence to the parenchymal lymphatic flow.

Various techniques have been used to study the pathways for lymphatic flow leaving the breast. These include dissection of static injected specimens, x-ray studies of thorotrast-injected specimens (17), *in vivo* injection of colloidal gold (18), and *in vivo* injection of a vital dye (19). These investigations have resulted in conflicting observations with respect to the pattern and amount of flow from different regions of the breast. In all likelihood, these differences observed by investigators reflect limitations of the techniques used and the intrinsic variability in lymphatic drainage between individuals.

Nonetheless, three routes for mammary lymphatic drainage have been identified. The most important of these is to the axilla, which receives 75% or more of lymphatic flow into the axillary lymph nodes. Lymph nodes located in the interpectoral fascia constitute Rotter's nodes. The most medial group lymph nodes occur at the apex of the axilla or level 3. Drainage via internal lymphatics is 25% or less of lymph flow. These vessels penetrate the pectoralis major and intercostal muscles to the internal thoracic mammary lymph nodes located along the sternal borders of the internal thoracic trunks. The third and least important route for lymph drainage is via the posterior intercostal lymphatics to posterior intercostal lymph nodes in the chest where the ribs and vertebrae articulate.

There is evidence that lymph drainage from any given region in the breast is not limited to one of the foregoing pathways (18,19). Nonetheless, correlation of patterns of lymph node metastases with the location of primary tumors in the breast suggests that preferential flow exists. For example, in the absence of axillary nodal metastases, the internal mammary lymph nodes are rarely affected, except when the primary tumor arises in the medial or central part of the breast. Conversely, tumors located in the upper outer quadrant are very unlikely to metastasize only to internal mammary lymph nodes. Carcinomas that give rise to metastases in Rotter's interpectoral lymph nodes typically are located in the upper outer and upper central regions.

Very little lymphatic drainage traverses the deep fascia of the breast and the retromammary space. Although minute lymphatic channels have been identified in this fascia, minimal lymph from the mammary gland flows in this system under normal circumstances. There also is no significant lymphatic flow to the contralateral internal mammary or axillary lymph nodes, but flow via these pathways may be augmented if ipsilateral drainage is obstructed as a result of therapy or by carcinoma.

Studies of sentinel lymph node mapping have provided additional information about mammary lymphatic drainage in a physiologic setting. The existence of one or more sentinel lymph nodes that appear to the initial site of nodal metastases implies that a hierarchy exists in the anatomic and functional distribution of the lymph nodes in the axilla as they relate to the breast. It is remarkable that this phenomenon can be demonstrated with seemingly equal specificity by injection of a tracer substance in the skin of the breast or in the parenchyma in the vicinity of a carcinoma. For a more complete discussion of sentinel lymph node mapping, see Chapters 45 and 46.

## FUNCTIONAL GROSS ANATOMY

The mature adult female breast is composed of 15 to 25 grossly defined lobes corresponding to parenchyma associated with each of the major lactiferous ducts that terminate in the nipple. These anatomic subdivisions may be appreciated after injection of visible or radiopaque dye into the duct system. No obvious landmarks defining the extent of individual lobes are found on gross inspection at operation or on dissection of the resected breast, and they are not evident in histologic sections. Three-dimensional reconstruction of the duct system in the breast of a 19-year-old woman revealed that each duct drained an independent territory or "catchment" (20). The total volume drained by a duct and the length of the duct were highly variable. The existence of this functional lobar architecture provides an anatomic framework for treating some benign conditions by major duct excision and certain types of carcinoma by quadrantectomy.

The nipple is covered by stratified squamous epithelium that is unpigmented in the prepubertal breast. Melanin pigmentation develops after menarche, increases during pregnancy, and persists to a variable degree thereafter. Sebaceous glands are present in the skin of the nipple. The areola surrounding the nipple is a ring of skin that undergoes pigmentary changes similar to the nipple. This specialized zone of mammary skin contains the glands of Montgomery, which are modified sebaceous glands that open on the surface of the areola via the tubercles of Morgagni. The latter structures are visible, especially during pregnancy, around the base of the nipple, which appears to be "studded over and rendered unequal by the prominence of glandular follicles, which, varying in number from twelve to twenty, project from the surface a sixteenth to an eighth of an inch" (21). The glands of Montgomery enlarge and contribute to a milk-like secretion that moistens the nipple and areola skin. These glands atrophy after menopause.

The functional glandular and ductal elements are embedded in fibrofatty tissue in most of the mammary gland. The relative proportions of fat and collagenous stroma vary greatly among individuals and with age. The combination of stromal and epithelial components is responsible for the radiographic appearance of breast structure in normal and pathologic states. Analysis of mammographic images was used to develop a classification scheme based on parenchymal density to predict cancer risk (22,23). The lowest risk was associated with the N1 or radiolucent pattern attributed to a predominantly fatty breast. The highest risk was attributed to the most dense images classified as D4, presumed to reflect less fat and greater glandular components. Intermediate risk was associated with P1 and P2 patterns with intermediate density. The concept that mammographic pattern provides a guide to breast cancer risk has not been widely validated and does not appear to be sufficiently reliable to be used in current clinical practice as a basis for recommending preventative therapy.

Magnetic resonance imaging (MRI) provides a more precise method for discriminating between fatty and fibroglandular tissue in the breast. By comparing images obtained with mammography and MRI, Lee et al. (24) found a mean fat content of 42.5% (SD ±30.3%) in mammograms and 66.5% (SD ±18%) in magnetic resonance images. The ranges of fat content obtained by mammography and MRI

were 7.5% to 90% and 17% to 89%, respectively. The correlation coefficient for estimates of fat content obtained by both methods was 0.63, with the strongest correlation ($r = 0.81$) in postmenopausal women. Breast density determined by mammography is increased by exogenous hormone administration (25), with the greatest effect in postmenopausal women who receive continuous combined estrogen-progesterone hormone replacement therapy (26). Estrogen alone causes appreciably less increase in fibroglandular tissue when assessed by mammography (27) or MRI (28) than does combined estrogen-progesterone treatment. Decreased breast parenchyma has been demonstrated by mammography after tamoxifen treatment (29).

## MICROSCOPIC ANATOMY OF THE ADULT BREAST

Each of the major lactiferous ducts terminates in and exits from the breast at the nipple via a secretory pore forming the lactiferous duct orifice. The superficial portion of the duct orifice is lined by squamous cells where the duct traverses the epidermis, and squamous epithelium may extend for a short distance into the most terminal portion of the lactiferous duct. The squamocolumnar junction, where the squamous epithelium joins the glandular duct epithelium, normally is distal to a dilated segment of the lactiferous duct, referred to as the lactiferous sinus. Extension of squamous epithelium into or beyond the lactiferous sinus is a pathologic condition termed *squamous metaplasia* (Fig. 1.5). This may result in obstruction of the affected duct system. The

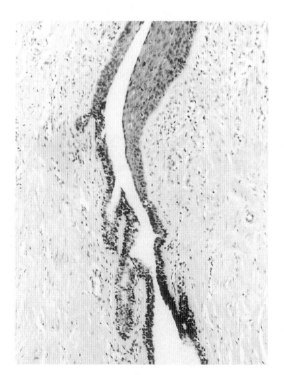

**FIG. 1.5.** *Major lactiferous duct in nipple with squamous metaplasia.*

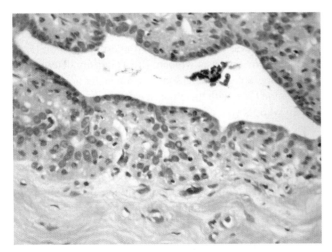

**FIG. 1.6.** *Major lactiferous duct with ductular bay-like branches.*

squamocolumnar junction also is an important landmark in the pathogenesis of Paget's disease.

Lactiferous ducts in the nipple are surrounded by circular and longitudinal arrays of smooth muscle fibers embedded in fibrocollagenous stroma. Some of these muscle fibers attach to the skin of the nipple and areola. Sebaceous glands associated with the overlying skin protrude downward into the superficial stroma of the nipple. The lactiferous ducts extend into the breast through a series of branches that diminish in caliber from the nipple to the terminal ductal-lobular units, which are embedded in specialized, hormonally responsive stroma. Extralobular ducts are lined by columnar epithelium that is supported by myoepithelial cells, a basement membrane, and surrounding elastic fibers. In the nonlactating breast, the major ducts cut in cross section have contours marked by folds or indentations that create a foliate or serrate appearance (Fig. 1.6). The epithelium in the bay-like branches of the duct lumen can give rise to ductules (Fig. 1.7). Fully

formed lobules can originate directly from this anatomic arrangement in the nipple and at deeper levels of the mammary duct system (Fig. 1.8) (30).

Cells that form the duct epithelium are of two types that are best distinguished by electron microscopy. The majority are columnar cells lining the lumen. They have cytoplasm endowed with abundant organelles involved in secretion. Basal cells thought to be capable of differentiating into columnar or myoepithelial cells are distributed in a discontinuous manner in the epithelium. Conversion of luminal epithelial cells to myoepithelial cells was documented by Péchoux et al. (31). Myoepithelial cells lie between the epithelial layer and the basal lamina, where they form a network of slender processes investing the overlying epithelial cells. The branching network of myoepithelial cell cytoplasmic processes can be seen especially well in scanning micrographs of lobules taken after the basal lamina and surrounding collagen have been removed by enzyme digestion (Fig. 1.9) (32). The histologic appearance and immunoreactivity of myoepithelial cells is variable, especially in pathologic conditions, and depends on the degree to which the myoid or epithelial phenotype is accentuated in a particular situation (Figs. 1.10 and 1.11). The myoepithelial layer is continuous in larger ducts, but it normally becomes attenuated and discontinuous in smaller branches of the ductal system.

The epithelial–stromal junction consists of the epithelial–myoepithelial layer within the duct, the basal lamina, and a surrounding zone of delimiting fibroblasts and capillaries (Fig. 1.12). Elastic tissue fibers are variably present around normal ducts, and these fibers tend to be less pronounced in the premenopausal breast. Farahmand and Cowan (33) were able to detect periductal elastic fibers in 71% of patients younger than 50 years and in 89% of patients older than 50 years. Marked periductal elastic fiber deposi-

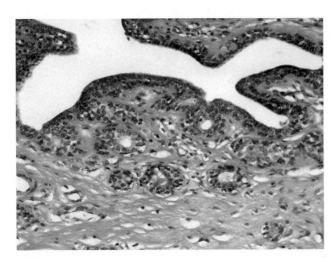

**FIG. 1.7.** *Major lactiferous duct with ductular branches and early acinar formation.*

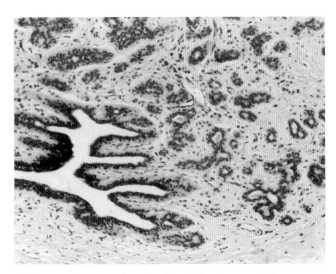

**FIG. 1.8.** *Lobules in nipple.* Major lactiferous duct in nipple with adjacent lobules. Note the specialized intralobular stroma.

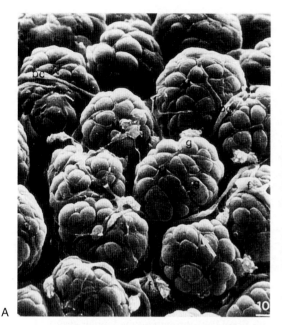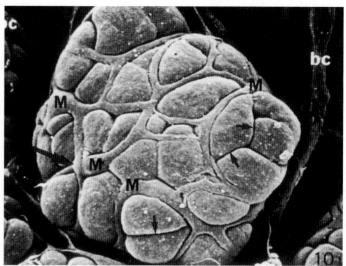

**FIG. 1.9.** *Scanning electron microscopy of lobules in the rat breast.* **A:** Connective tissue has been removed by enzyme-HCl digestion to expose rounded glandular cells *(g)* and stellate myoepithelial cells *(large arrow).* Blood capillaries *(bc)* and fibroblasts *(f)* can be seen. **B:** Magnified view of a lobule with a network of myoepithelial cells *(M). Small arrows* indicate boundaries between glandular cells. (From Nagato T, Yoshida H, Yoshida A, et al. A scanning electron microscope study of myoepithelial cells in exocrine glands. *Cell Tissue Res* 1980;209:1–10, with permission.)

tion was found in only 3% of normal specimens from women younger than 50 years and in 17% older than 50 years. Elastic fibers are largely absent at the lobular level; when present, they surround but do not extend into the lobular unit.

In addition to elastic fibers, the normal periductal stroma contains a sparse scattering of lymphocytes, plasma cells, mast cells, and histiocytes. Ochrocytes are periductal histiocytes with cytoplasmic accumulation of lipofuscin pigment. These pigmented cells become more numerous in the postmenopausal breast and in association with inflammatory or proliferative conditions (Fig. 1.13) (34).

The histologic appearance of the ducts and glands of Montgomery in the subareolar tissues resembles the major lactiferous ducts of the nipple (35,36), except that the contour tends to be smoother (Fig. 1.14). Serial sections have demonstrated direct connections between lactiferous ducts draining lobular parenchyma and the ducts of Montgomery glands in the tubercle of Morgagni (37). The epithelium of the ducts connecting breast lobules to the glands of Montgomery is subject to proliferative changes that occur in the lactiferous ducts, including hyperplasia and *in situ* carcinoma (37).

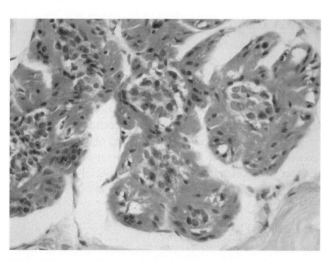

**FIG. 1.10.** *Myoid metaplasia in lobule.* Myoepithelial cells with a myoid phenotype around lobular glands.

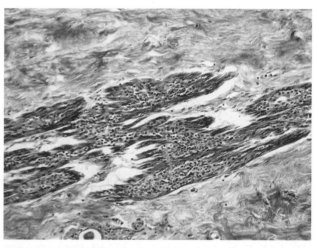

**FIG. 1.11.** *Myoid metaplasia in terminal duct lobular unit.* Myoid myoepithelial cells are red in this section stained with Masson's trichrome.

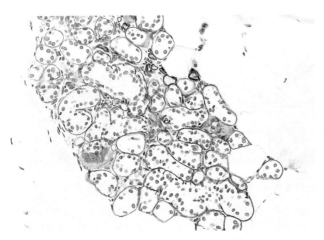

**FIG. 1.12.** *Basement membrane in lobule.* This immuno-stained section of a normal lobule shows the basement membrane surrounding all glands (antilaminin, avidin-biotin).

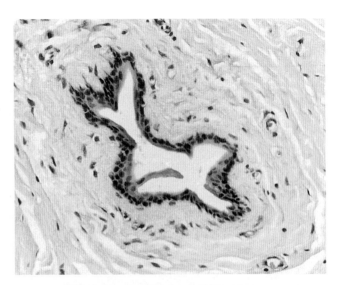

**FIG. 1.14.** *Duct of gland of Montgomery.*

Mammary secretion occurs in the lobules, which consist of groups of alveolar glands encompassed by specialized stroma. Alveoli are connected by intralobular ductules combined to form a single terminal lobular duct that drains into the extralobular duct system. In lobules, alveolar glands are formed along and at the end of intralobular ductules. In whole-mount preparations and in histologic sections, these glandular structures appear as blunt or round saccules protruding from the duct lumen.

The resting lobular gland is lined by a single layer of cuboidal epithelial cells supported by underlying, loosely connected myoepithelial cells. The intralobular stroma contains more capillaries and is less densely collagenized than the interlobular stroma. Ultrastructural studies suggest that, in addition to providing support, the cells in the intralobular stroma have a paracrine effect on the epithelium. Intralobular stromal fibroblasts are characterized by attenuated cytoplasmic processes that create a network of cell-to-cell connections (38). These link the delimiting fibroblasts that cover the basement mem-

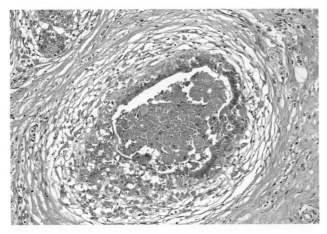

**FIG. 1.13.** *Ochrocytes in periductal stroma.* Histiocytes with granular, lipofuscin-containing cytoplasm are present in the periductal stroma and in the ductal epithelium in an example of periductal mastitis.

brane with fibroblasts throughout the lobular stroma. Delimiting and other fibroblasts in the lobule are ultrastructurally similar. Both cell types have a well-developed rough endoplasmic reticulum, numerous mitochondria, and a prominent Golgi apparatus, features that suggest synthetic activity. Lymphocytes, plasma cells, macrophages, and mast cells, which normally reside in the lobular stroma, are distributed within the interstices of this fibroblastic network in a manner that results in close apposition of cell surfaces to facilitate cell–cell interaction (38). Intralobular fibroblasts are immunoreactive for CD34, an endothelial-associated ligand involved in cellular attachment of leukocytes in inflammation and immune responses (39).

The normal microscopic anatomy of the lobules is not constant, because the structure and histologic appearance of the lobule in the mature breast are subject to changes associated with the menstrual cycle, pregnancy, lactation, exogenous hormone administration, and menopause. Furthermore, there is variation in the functional state of individual lobules regardless of physiologic circumstances, an observation that suggests that individual lobules or lobules in regions of the breast have intrinsic differences in response to hormonal stimuli. This is reflected in the substantial variability in labeling indices indicating different proliferative rates among lobules in a given individual (40).

Genetic alterations manifested by loss of heterozygosity have been detected in histologically normal-appearing lobular epithelium (41). Genetic changes have been found in epithelial and myoepithelial cells. The frequency of these alterations has not been established, but existing data suggest that they are detected more often in histologically normal lobules from patients with carcinoma than in breasts without carcinoma.

## THE MENSTRUAL CYCLE

The structural effects of cyclic hormonal changes are manifested clinically by fluctuations in breast size and texture. In general, the breast tends to be the least nodular at mid-cycle in the latter part of the follicular phase, making this the optimal time for clinical breast examination. A study of mammograms obtained from women 40 to 49 years of age revealed significantly lower parenchymal density during the follicular phase than during the luteal phase of the menstrual cycle (42). Studies based on water displacement demonstrated an increase in breast volume during the second half of the normal menstrual cycle of about 100 mL and in the contraceptive-controlled cycle of about 60 mL (43). Examination by MRI revealed that breast volume was least in the interval from days 6 to 15 of the menstrual cycle, a time characterized by low parenchymal and low water volumes (44,45). An increase in breast volume between days 16 and 28 was marked by a rise in parenchymal volume and water content that peaked on day 25. A sharp decline in parenchymal and water volume occurred just prior to menses in one study (44), but other studies reported elevated water content and fibroglandular content "during menses" (45). These observations indicate that cyclical changes in breast volume involve parenchymal growth as well as fluctuations in water content (40).

Nodular and diffuse contrast medium (gadolinium) enhancement has been observed in clinically normal breasts during the course of the menstrual cycle (46). These foci of enhancement were more frequent in weeks 1 and 4. The rate of enhancement may meet the criteria for a malignant lesion resulting in a false-positive interpretation in a premenopausal woman. This finding is consistent with data obtained by Müller-Schimpfle et al. (47), who reported that overall parenchymal contrast medium enhancement was greatest during days 21 to 6 of the cycle, corresponding to the first and fourth weeks, and that enhancement was significantly less during days 7 to 20. This effect was maximal in women 35 to 50 years of age.

The cellular and structural alterations observed histologically in the normal breast during the menstrual cycle were described in detail by Vogel et al. (48). These investigators divided the changes into five phases. However, they noted "that different lobules within the same breast may vary in morphologic appearance. Placing a specimen within a phase required that the most consistent morphology among a population of lobules within several sections be determined. Lobules that varied from the dominant pattern often expressed the morphologic features of the adjacent phase" (48).

An *in vitro* study of purified populations of epithelial and myoepithelial cells obtained from reduction mammoplasty specimens revealed notable differences in growth requirements between the cell types (49). Epidermal growth factor and basic fibroblast growth factor had a mitogenic effect on epithelial cells but not on myoepithelial cells. Insulin was necessary for myoepithelial growth, whereas epithelial cells required fetal calf serum. Reconstitution of lobuloalveolar structures was observed when the two cell types were mixed in a basement membrane matrix. These differences in growth factor requirements probably reflect different physiologic functions that also are expressed morphologically during the menstrual cycle.

The proliferative phase (days 3 to 7) features the highest

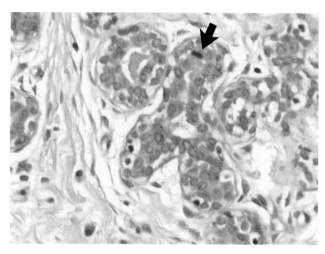

**FIG. 1.15.** *Normal lobule: proliferative phase of menstrual cycle.* A metaphase mitotic figure *(arrow)* and several pyknotic nuclei are evident.

rates of epithelial mitoses and of apoptosis (50,51). This corresponds to a marked decrease in *bcl*-2 expression detected immunohistochemically in lobular gland epithelium at the end of the menstrual cycle in comparison to maximal expression at mid-cycle (52). The peak time of apoptosis is about 3 days after the peak for mitotic activity (53). Lobular glands at this time are lined by crowded, poorly oriented epithelial cells with little or no lumen formation and secretion (Fig. 1.15). Myoepithelial cells are inconspicuous. Epithelial cells have eosinophilic cytoplasm and round nuclei with prominent nucleoli. The lobular stroma is relatively dense and hypovascular, with plump fibroblasts ringing lobular glands.

Mitotic activity is decreased in the follicular phase (days 8 to 14). The myoepithelial cells have a polygonal shape and clear cytoplasm. Epithelial cells become columnar, with increasingly basophilic cytoplasm and basally oriented, darkly stained nuclei (Fig. 1.16). Intermediate basal cells with pale

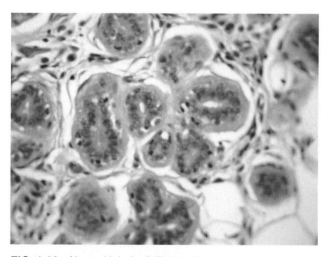

**FIG. 1.16.** *Normal lobule: follicular phase of menstrual cycle.* Lumens are beginning to appear in lobular glands, and the basal lamina is prominent.

cytoplasm are present in small numbers. These cells are thought to serve as progenitor cells for myoepithelial and epithelial cells (54). An acinar lumen without secretion is evident. The basal lamina is prominent, and there is slight loosening of intralobular stroma.

During the luteal phase (days 15 to 20), myoepithelial cells become more prominent due to increased glycogen accumulation that results in cytoplasmic clearing. Intermediate basal cells are more evident. The glandular lumen is clearly defined by columnar epithelial cells with basophilic cytoplasm. A small amount of secretion is present in a few glands. The basement membrane is attenuated and less prominent, and there is coincidental further loosening of the stroma (Fig. 1.17).

Immunohistochemical study of normal breast tissue during the menstrual cycle revealed peak expression of epidermal growth factor receptor and HER2/*neu* during the luteal phase (55). When quantitated by image analysis, the differences in expression between the luteal and follicular phases were statistically significant. Epidermal growth factor receptor was mainly expressed in the stroma and myoepithelial cells, whereas HER2/*neu* was localized to epithelial cells. These observations may reflect a promoting effect of hormones, especially progestins, and suggest that these tyrosine kinase receptors play a role in the normal growth and differentiation of mammary glandular epithelium in response to cyclical hormonal stimulation. Short-term administration of tamoxifen during the luteal phase significantly reduces mitotic activity in normal breast tissue (56).

The secretory phase (days 21 to 27) features heightened apocrine secretion with distention of glandular lumens by accumulated secretory material (Fig. 1.18). The epithelium consists of columnar epithelial cells and myoepithelial cells with clear cytoplasm. The basal lamina is thin, and the lobular stroma exhibits maximal edema. Ultrastructural examination of lobular epithelial cells reveals an increase in endo-

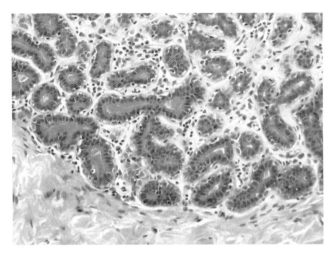

**FIG. 1.18.** *Normal lobule: secretory phase of menstrual cycle.* Stromal edema is evident with a modest mononuclear cell infiltrate.

plasmic reticulum, an enlarged Golgi, and other changes in organelles, indicative of active secretion (57).

In the menstrual phase (days 28 to 2), the stroma once again becomes compact with loss of intralobular edema. Lymphocytes, macrophages, and plasma cells are most conspicuous in the lobular stroma (50). Some glandular lumens remain and others appear collapsed. Mitotic activity is absent (Fig. 1.19).

Cyclical variation in immunoglobulin localization in lobules has been described (58). Intraluminal immunoglobulin A (IgA) and immunoglobulin M are present in significantly more lobules in the preovulatory proliferative and follicular phases (days 4 to 14) than in the postovulatory luteal, secretory, and menstrual phases (days 15 to 3). No strong intraluminal localization of immunoglobulin G was found, and weak intraluminal immunoglobulin G staining was present throughout the menstrual cycle, with no significant differ-

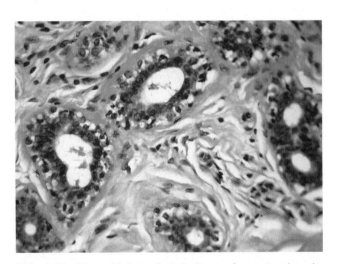

**FIG. 1.17.** *Normal lobule: luteal phase of menstrual cycle.* Myoepithelial cells are conspicuous, and glandular lumens contain scant secretion.

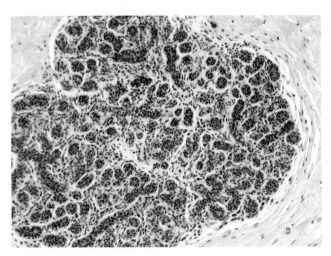

**FIG. 1.19.** *Normal lobule: menstrual phase of cycle.* Collapse of lobular glands, decreased stromal edema, and intralobular round cell infiltration are present.

ence between preovulatory and postovulatory phases. There was not a strong correlation between luminal IgA concentration and the number of stromal plasma cells.

Thymidine labeling index (TLI) studies of lobules isolated from normal human breast tissue revealed that the proliferative rate in epithelial cells is higher in the luteal than in the follicular phase of the menstrual cycle (59,60). This effect is seen largely in parous women, and other investigators reported little difference in TLI during the menstrual cycle in nulliparous women (61). The difference in TLI between the luteal and follicular phases decreases with age (62), and there is an overall inverse relationship between TLI and age (63,64). Analysis of the synthesis phase fraction (SPF) in epithelial cells from normal breast tissue samples by flow cytometry revealed a decreasing SPF with advancing age, such that SPF in atrophic tissue was approximately 50% less than in samples from premenopausal women (65). Similar results were obtained with 5-bromodeoxyuridine (BrdU) labeling (40) and by using the immunohistochemical proliferation marker Ki67 (MIB1) on cytologic preparations obtained by fine needle aspiration from normal volunteers (66). Mean TLI throughout the menstrual cycle varies from 0% to 11.5% (59,63). Measurements of paired samples obtained simultaneously from the left and right breast revealed a highly significant correlation between SPF determinations in the two breasts (65). Proliferation detected by TLI is limited to epithelial cells and intermediate basal cells with pale cytoplasm in explants of normal breast tissue studied in culture (67). Under normal circumstances, mature myoepithelial cells are not mitotically active.

Meyer (60) reported that cyclical changes in the TLI of the epithelium in fibroadenomas and ductal hyperplasias paralleled the status of the normal breast. Mean turnover time for a normal ductal epithelial cell was calculated to be 22 days at age 20 years and 147 days at age 40 years. A study of normal parenchyma from breast specimens that contained carcinoma found no difference in proliferative activity reflected in the TLI of samples near and at a distance from the neoplasm (40) or in samples of benign tissue from breasts harboring carcinoma studied for SPF by flow cytometry (65). The proliferative rate in normal tissue determined by BrdU labeling was not correlated with the TLI of the coexisting carcinoma. Labeling indices decreased in lobules and ducts with age.

Estrogen and progesterone receptors are localized to the nuclei of epithelial cells. Nuclei of approximately 7% of epithelial cells are immunoreactive for estrogen receptor in normal resting breast tissue, with a higher proportion in lobular than in ductal cells (68). Considerable heterogeneity exists in nuclear hormone receptor activity among lobules. Estrogen receptor-positive cells typically are distributed singly, surrounded by receptor-negative nuclei in lobules (69). A significant correlation with increasing age was observed by Shoker et al. (69), who reported a tendency for positive cells to be "contiguous in patches of variable size." The increase in estrogen receptor-positive cells remained relatively stable after menopause.

Several groups of investigators studied the expression of estrogen and progesterone receptors in noncancerous breast tissue during different phases of the menstrual cycle in premenopausal women. Using biochemical analyses of grossly normal-appearing tissue, Silva et al. (70) reported that the greatest frequency of estrogen receptor positivity and the highest mean concentrations were found during the proliferative phase of the cycle (days 3 to 7), whereas progesterone receptor was highly expressed in the follicular phase (days 8 to 14). A study of benign epithelial cells obtained by fine needle aspiration revealed immunocytochemically detectable evidence of nuclear estrogen receptor in 31% of samples taken during the first half of the menstrual cycle and no estrogen receptor-positive cells in 33 samples taken during the second half of the cycle (71). Other investigators reported that nuclear estrogen and progesterone receptor activity demonstrated by immunohistochemistry in lobular epithelial cells was maximal in the follicular phase (72). Decreased expression of estrogen receptor in the luteal phase may be due to down-regulation of this protein by the rise in progesterone produced by the corpus luteum (63). Pujol et al. (73) studied 575 women with breast carcinoma in whom menstrual cycle phases were determined by serum measurements of estradiol, progesterone, follicle-stimulating hormone, and luteinizing hormone. Expression of estrogen receptors in the carcinoma was significantly more frequent in the follicular phase (62%) than in the ovulatory (52%) and luteal (53%) phases. In contrast, progesterone receptor expression was positive more often in the ovulatory phase (85%) than in the follicular (78%) and luteal (72%) phases, but these differences were not statistically significant. Other investigators did not find a consistent menstrual cycle-related pattern in the expression of estrogen and progesterone receptors in breast carcinomas from premenopausal women (71,74,75).

## PREGNANCY

Secretory changes associated with pregnancy occur unevenly throughout the breast. Localized adenomatous lactational hyperplasia, usually encountered it the third trimester, is an extreme manifestation of this phenomenon that may result in one or more palpable and radiologically detectable masses called lactational adenomas (76).

Progressive recruitment of lobules occurs with successive pregnancies. Early in pregnancy, terminal ducts and lobules grow rapidly, resulting in lobular enlargement with variable coincidental depletion of the fibrofatty stroma (77–81). Stromal vascularity increases, accompanied by infiltration by mononuclear inflammatory cells. More pronounced areolar pigmentation and dilation of superficial cutaneous veins are apparent by the end of the first trimester. At this time, a small amount of colostrum may be found in lobular glands (Fig. 1.20).

During the second and third trimesters, lobular growth progresses through enlargement of cells as well as by cellular proliferation (Fig. 1.21). Myoepithelial cells remain evident in ducts, but they are largely obscured by the greatly

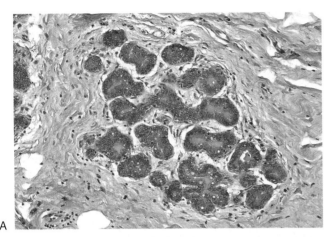
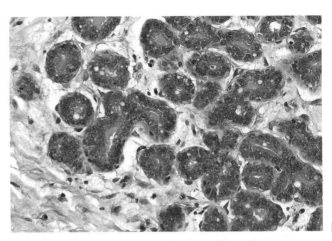

A

B

**FIG. 1.20.** *Lobular hyperplasia in pregnancy: first trimester.* **A,B:** Increased metabolic activity is manifested by cytoplasmic hyperchromasia and nuclear enlargement with nucleoli in this specimen from a 34-year-old woman who was 3 months pregnant.

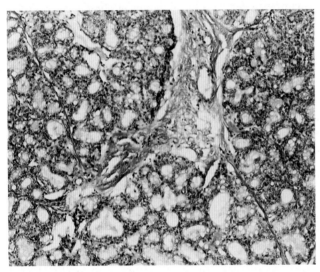

**FIG. 1.21.** *Lobular hyperplasia in pregnancy: early third trimester.* Greatly enlarged lobules efface the intervening stroma.

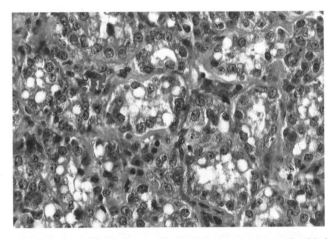

**FIG. 1.22.** *Lobular hyperplasia in pregnancy: early third trimester.* Cells forming the lobular glands have abundant vacuolated cytoplasm. There is little secretion, and the nuclei have punctate nucleoli.

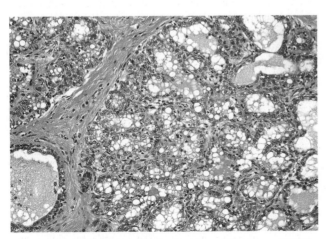

**FIG. 1.23.** *Lobular hyperplasia in pregnancy: late third trimester.* Enlarged nuclei with nucleoli are present. Lactation is evident.

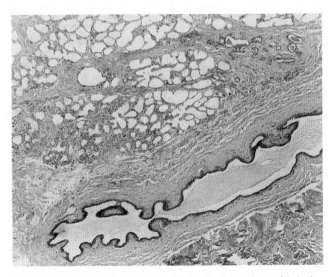

**FIG. 1.24.** *Lactating breast.* Marked distention of lobular glands and accumulation of secretion in a duct.

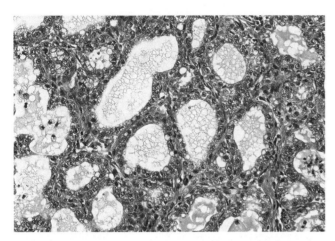

**FIG. 1.25.** *Lactating breast.* Ectatic lobular glands contain vacuolated secretion.

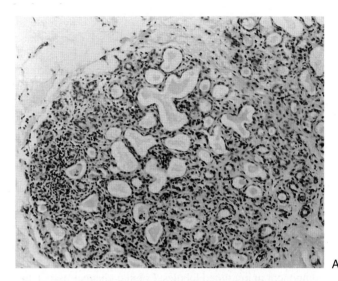

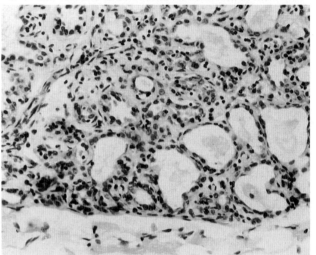

**FIG. 1.27.** *Postlactational lobular involution.* **A:** Some dilated lobular glands with secretion persist. The patient was 6 months postpartum and stopped nursing 3 weeks before surgery. **B:** Glandular epithelium is quiescent, and myoepithelial cells are apparent.

expanded epithelial cells (Fig. 1.22). The cytoplasm of lobular epithelial cells becomes vacuolated, and secretion is progressively accumulated in distended lobular glands (Figs. 1.23–1.25). Glandular expansion through pregnancy and lactation is accompanied by a relative decrease in fibrofatty stroma. Fine needle aspiration of the lactating breast yields a highly cellular specimen that can contain cohesive glandular clusters as well as dispersed cells (Fig. 1.26). Nuclei are hyperchromatic and often have small nucleoli.

Electron microscopic examination of lactating epithelium reveals organelle-rich cytoplasm with a prominent endoplasmic reticulum, hypertrophied Golgi apparatus, swollen mitochondria, and abundant secretory material (80). Myoepithelial cells are flattened and attenuated.

Involution of the breast, after lactation ceases, occurs over a period of about 3 months. Initially, lobular glands are further distended by additional accumulation of milk, which results in attenuation of the epithelial lining (Fig. 1.27). As prolactin levels decrease, secretion of milk ceases, and desquamated, degenerated, lobular epithelial cells are

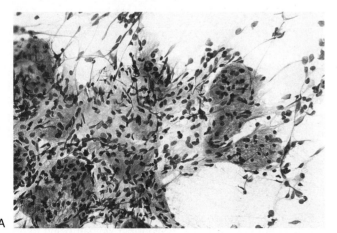

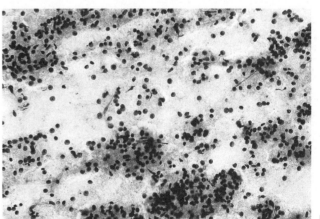

**FIG. 1.26.** *Lactating breast: fine needle aspiration cytology.* **A,B:** The specimen consists of cohesive glandular elements and abundant dispersed cells. Note that many nuclei appear isolated from cytoplasm and the presence of background secretion.

phagocytized. Involution is accompanied by a decrease in the number and size of lobular glands and the reappearance of myoepithelial cells in the lobular epithelium. Fat and collagen are redeposited in the stroma, accompanied by diminished vascularity. Increased numbers of macrophages appear in the stroma during postlactational involution.

Battersby and Anderson (82) described histologic changes that they determined to be characteristic of the postpartum involuted lobule. Compared with the "normal" lobules of women who were not recently pregnant, the postpartum lobule appeared to be irregularly shaped, with a partially angular rather than rounded contour. Intralobular stroma tended to be less distinct in the involuted lobule than in the normal lobule, resulting in a poorly defined border. Intralobular ductules were prominent and, because of concomitant atrophy of lobular epithelium, were the most conspicuous epithelial component in involuted lobules. Lobular changes associated with recent pregnancy were most noticeable within 18 months postpartum. The authors observed that postpartum lobules that appeared to be relatively atrophic could exhibit a histologic response to a subsequent pregnancy in as little as 6 weeks.

## MENOPAUSE

Parenchymal changes during and after menopause reflect hormonal alterations that occur at this time. Plasma levels of estrogen and progesterone decline, whereas androgen levels, largely testosterone, are not diminished. The major structural alteration is a decrease in the cellularity and number of lobules, mainly as a result of epithelial atrophy (83). Coincidental with loss of glandular epithelium, there is a tendency for thickening of lobular basement membranes and collagenization of intralobular stroma (Fig. 1.28). The process of menopausal atrophy occurs in a heterogeneous fashion, which often leaves some lobules relatively unaffected com-

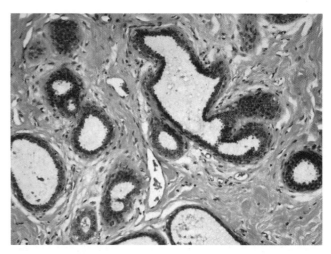

**FIG. 1.29.** *Menopausal atrophy of lobule.* This stage features microcystic dilation of lobular glands and collagenized intralobular stroma.

pared with neighboring glands. Atrophy tends to spare myoepithelial cells, which frequently persist even in a late stage of the process. Most lobular glands appear to collapse and shrink, but cystic distention also may occur (Fig. 1.29). Small calcifications sometimes are deposited in atrophic lobular glands. In many women over 65 years of age, lobular integrity is progressively lost, leaving small ducts and glands embedded in fibrocollagenous stroma. The relative proportions of fat and stroma vary greatly in the atrophic breast.

Menopausal mammary atrophy can be attenuated and substantially diminished by administration of exogenous estrogen or estrogen-progesterone preparations after menopause. The morphologic effects of these increasingly widely administered medications have not been thoroughly documented (Fig. 1.30).

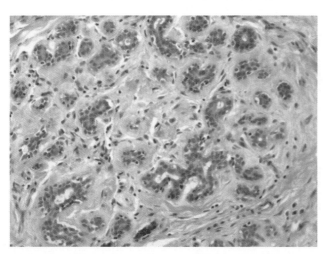

**FIG. 1.28.** *Menopausal atrophy of lobule.* Collagenized intralobular stroma and thickened basement membranes around lobular glands.

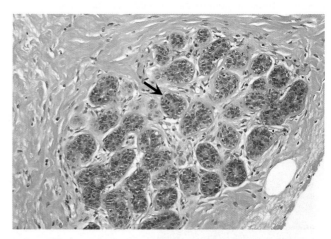

**FIG. 1.30.** *Postmenopausal breast: estrogen replacement.* Lobule in the breast of a 72-year-old woman being treated with hormone replacement therapy that included estrogen. Differentiation of intralobular stroma is evident, and the glandular epithelium is hyperplastic with a mitosis *(arrow).*

Mammographic changes suggestive of physiologic proliferative alterations have been observed in women receiving postmenopausal hormone replacement therapy (84,85). The effect of hormone replacement therapy on the mammographic appearance of the breast is substantially less in women who have undergone prior breast irradiation (86). The effect of hormone replacement on the nonradiated breast, manifested mainly by increased parenchymal density, has been observed after treatment with estrogen alone and with estrogen-progesterone combination therapy. Histologic examination does not reveal a consistent pattern. Some patients have lobular differentiation comparable to the premenopausal state, whereas other patients have prominent cystic or proliferative alterations of ducts and lobules. The findings suggest that the existing epithelial status of the breast is accentuated by exogenous hormone administration. Hargreaves et al. (87) studied the effect of hormone replacement therapy, which consisted of estrogens alone or estrogen-progesterone combination, on proliferation and progesterone receptor expression in the postmenopausal breast. Proliferation was assessed by Ki67 expression. In untreated women, the median Ki67 and progesterone receptor labeling indices of 0.19 and 4.75, respectively, were unrelated to patient age, duration of menopause, or presence of either benign or carcinomatous breast disease. Hormone treatment caused a significant increase in progesterone receptor expression but did not significantly alter the Ki67 index.

Arteries in the breast undergo sclerotic changes comparable to those seen throughout the body with increasing age (88). Arterial calcification is most likely to be encountered in the postmenopausal breast (89,90). Some patients with mammographically detected calcifications have diabetes mellitus, coronary artery disease, and hypertension (91,92). Arterial calcifications were found in the breasts of 9.1% of 12,239 women aged 50 to 69 years studied in one screening mammography program (93). This finding was associated with a significantly increased risk of associated arteriosclerotic disease, hypertension, and diabetes mellitus. In another screening program, arterial calcification occurred more often in hypertensive than in normotensive women, but the difference was not statistically significant (89). Calcific arterial sclerosis usually is readily distinguishable from epithelial-associated calcifications in mammograms.

## PREGNANCY-LIKE CHANGE

This structural alteration affecting lobules resembles lactational hyperplasia. It occurs in breast tissue from patients who are neither pregnant nor lactating when the specimen is obtained. Most of the patients are premenopausal or postmenopausal women who had been pregnant, but similar changes have been observed in women who are nulliparous (94,95) and in breast tissue from men treated with estrogens (96). The reported frequency of finding pregnancy-like change is 1.7% to about 3% in surgical pathology and autopsy series (94,95,97,98).

The etiology of pregnancy-like change is unknown. Consequently, it is uncertain whether this is a normal physiologic alteration. Recent studies documented hyperplasia associated with this lesion (99). Speculation as to the cause of pregnancy-like change centers on the possibility that the affected lobules remain in a persistent lactating state after pregnancy, or that they are lobules that exhibit an idiosyncratic reaction to endogenous hormones, exogenous hormones, medication, or other unidentified substances. Pregnancy-like change can be induced in the rat mammary gland by administering phenothiazine (100), and similar changes have been found in breast tissue from women receiving this and other medications (101,102).

Glands and terminal ducts with pregnancy-like change usually contain little secretion, although they are dilated (Fig. 1.31). The glandular cells are swollen, with abundant pale-to-clear, finely granular, or vacuolated cytoplasm. The nuclei usually are round and darkly stained, and intranuclear vacuoles may be present. The luminal cytoplasmic borders of glandular cells are frayed, and small cytoplasmic blebs are formed. The nucleus may be contained in blebs of cytoplasm extruded into the glandular lumen. Periodic acid-Schiff (PAS)–positive diastase-resistant granules are present in the cytoplasm, which also is immunoreactive for α-lactalbumin and S-100 (98). The cells express secretory component and IgA in their cytoplasm, as well as lysozyme and lactoferrin (103). These features resemble the findings in normal breast lobules in late pregnancy and lactation.

In most instances, the epithelium in lobules altered by pregnancy-like change remains one or two cell layers thick, thus simulating the architecture of the truly lactating breast. *Pregnancy-like hyperplasia* is the occurrence of pregnancy-like change in hyperplastic epithelium (Fig. 1.32). The epithelium is arranged in irregular fronds composed entirely of glandular cells. The glandular lumens in pregnancy-like hyperplasia often contain secretion that may accumulate in a laminated fashion and undergo calcification (Figs. 1.33 and 1.34). This lesion may be detected by mammography, leading to sampling by needle core biopsy (99).

Some examples of pregnancy-like hyperplasia feature more florid atypical epithelial proliferation with substantial nuclear pleomorphism (Fig. 1.35). These instances of *atypical pregnancy-like hyperplasia* have been seen most commonly in association with cystic hypersecretory lesions (Figs. 1.36 and 1.37) (99) (see Chapter 26).

Ultrastructural study of pregnancy-like hyperplasia revealed some features similar to the findings in active lactation (98). However, cells in pregnancy-like hyperplasia lack well-organized parallel arrays of rough endoplasmic reticulum and abundant swollen mitochondria characteristic of the lactating cell. The mitochondria appear to be shrunken, which is a feature of postlactational involution (104). Decapitation secretion, which is responsible for the formation of cytoplasmic blebs in pregnancy-like change, is also an involutional feature that differs from the formation of membrane-bound vacuoles.

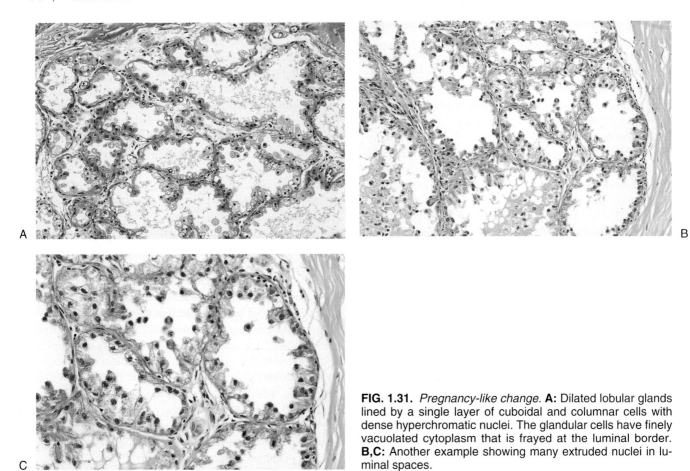

**FIG. 1.31.** *Pregnancy-like change.* **A:** Dilated lobular glands lined by a single layer of cuboidal and columnar cells with dense hyperchromatic nuclei. The glandular cells have finely vacuolated cytoplasm that is frayed at the luminal border. **B,C:** Another example showing many extruded nuclei in luminal spaces.

**FIG. 1.32.** *Pregnancy-like hyperplasia.* **A:** Hyperplastic cells fill most of the lobular glands, and some secretion is present. **B:** Secretion is present in an intralobular duct. Note the partially involved hyperplastic lobule on the *upper right* in this specimen from a 60-year-old woman.

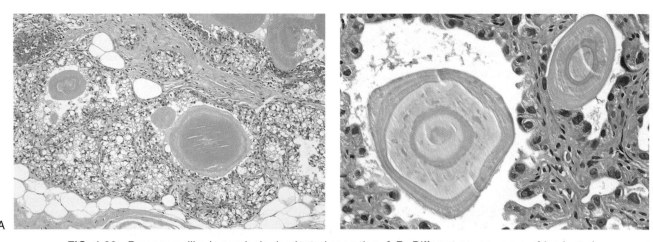

**FIG. 1.33.** *Pregnancy-like hyperplasia, laminated secretion.* **A,B:** Different appearances of laminated deposits of secretion. Cytologic atypia is shown in **B**.

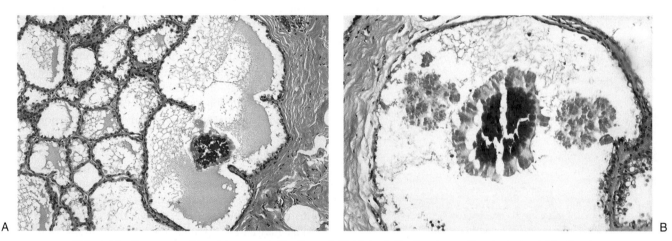

**FIG. 1.34.** *Pregnancy-like change, calcifications.* **A,B:** This distinctive type of laminated calcification is very characteristic for pregnancy-like lesions.

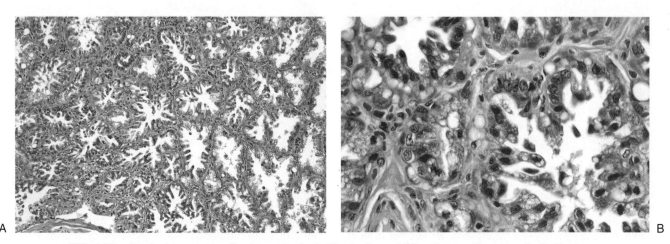

**FIG. 1.35.** *Atypical pregnancy-like hyperplasia.* **A:** The lesion exhibits micropapillary growth. **B:** Nuclear atypia is evident. The patient was 57 years old.

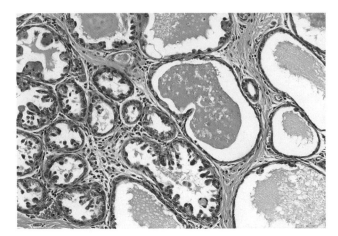

**FIG. 1.36.** *Atypical pregnancy-like hyperplasia and cystic hypersecretory hyperplasia.*

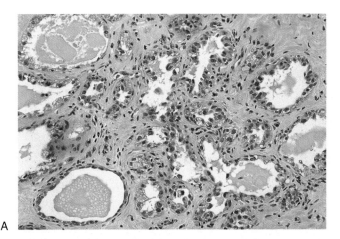

A

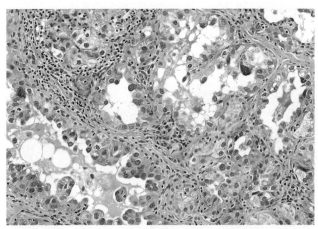

B

**FIG. 1.37.** *Atypical pregnancy-like hyperplasia and cystic hypersecretory hyperplasia.* This biopsy from a 41-year-old woman was performed for mammographically detected calcifications. **A:** Some of the glands contain retracted secretion typical for cystic hypersecretory hyperplasia. Note nuclear atypia in the pregnancy-like hyperplasia. **B:** Another area in the same biopsy with very severe cytologic abnormalities bordering on intraductal carcinoma.

## CLEAR CELL CHANGE

This cytologic alteration in lobular and terminal duct epithelium differs microscopically from pregnancy-like change. It also has been referred to as "lamprocytosis," and the term "hellenzellen," meaning clear cells, has been used in the German literature (105). The affected lobules tend to be larger than adjacent uninvolved lobules. The lobular gland epithelium is composed of swollen cells with abundant clear or pale, finely granular cytoplasm (Fig. 1.38). The cells have well-defined borders. Some glands have dilated lumens with PAS-positive, diastase-resistant secretion, but more often the lobular gland lumens are obliterated by the swollen cells (106). The small, round, and darkly stained nuclei often are displaced toward the center of the gland. The clear cells are immunoreactive for cytokeratin (Fig. 1.39) but not for actin (Fig. 1.40). The cytoplasm of the clear cells contains diastase-sensitive, PAS-positive glycogen and usually is S-100 positive. The mucicarmine stain is negative, and there is no immunoreactivity for α-lactalbumin.

The etiology and histogenesis of clear cell change are uncertain. The results of special stains and immunohistochemistry suggest that the clear cells are altered epithelial cells. However, clear cell alterations of a less extreme degree affecting myoepithelial cells are not uncommon, leaving open the possibility that fully developed clear cell change is an extreme form of this abnormality (Fig. 1.41). Clear cell change is encountered in premenopausal and postmenopausal women. There is no association with pregnancy or exogenous hormone use (102,106). Foci of clear cell change have been identified retrospectively in breast tissue obtained in the 1940s before exogenous hormones were available. Viña and Wells (98) reported finding clear cell change in 15 (1.6%) of 934 biopsies. Specimens that contain clear cell change may harbor carcinoma or benign changes, as there is no association with any other particular breast lesions (98).

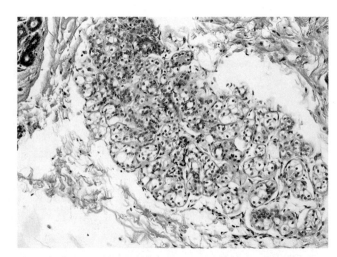

**FIG. 1.38.** *Clear cell change in a lobule.* Almost all glands in the lobule are composed of cells with clear cytoplasm. Part of an unaffected lobule is present at the left edge of the photograph.

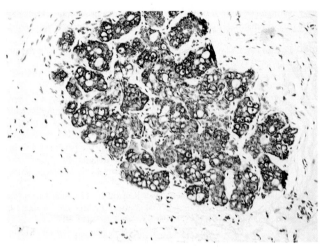

**FIG. 1.39.** *Clear cell change in a lobule.* The clear cells are immunoreactive for cytokeratin (CAM 5.2, avidin-biotin).

Clear cell change and pregnancy-like change may coexist in the same breast; rarely, the two abnormalities seem to overlap in their histologic appearance.

Electron microscopy revealed that the cytoplasm of clear cells contained lipid and protein granules (106). Dissolution of the former in tissue processing could explain the cytoplasmic clearing, whereas luminal accumulation of protein-associated secretion is the probable source of the PAS-positive material.

The differential diagnosis of clear cell change includes pregnancy-like change, cytoplasmic clearing in apocrine metaplasia, cytoplasmic clearing in myoepithelial cells, and lobular involvement by clear cell carcinoma. These lesions usually can be distinguished in surgical biopsy specimens, but difficulty can be encountered in a needle core biopsy sample. Pregnancy-like change is most readily distinguished from clear cell change because it features "decapitation" secretion at the luminal borders of the cells. Cytoplasmic clear-

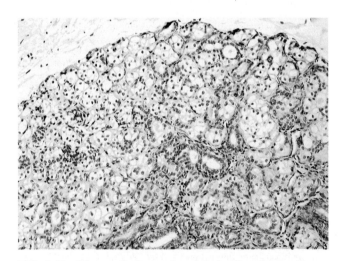

**FIG. 1.40.** *Clear cell change in a lobule.* The clear cells are not immunoreactive for actin (anti-smooth muscle actin, avidin-biotin). Faint staining of myoepithelial cells is apparent.

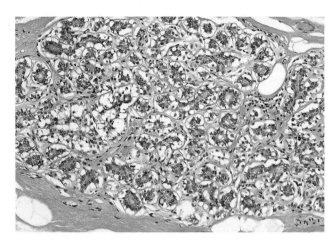

**FIG. 1.41.** *Clear cell change in myoepithelial cells.*

ing in apocrine metaplasia is usually a focal change in epithelium that otherwise has the typical features of apocrine metaplasia. Myoepithelial cells with clear cell change retain their position as a layer between the epithelium and basement membrane. Most instances of clear cell carcinoma have a pronounced ductal component.

## REFERENCES

1. Osin PP, Anbazhagan R, Bartkova J, et al. Breast development gives insights into breast disease. *Histopathology* 1998;33:275–283.
2. Ham AW, Cormack DH. *The breast. Histology,* 8th ed. Philadelphia: JB Lippincott, 1979:866–874.
2a. Keeling JW, Ozer E, King G, et al. Oestrogen receptor alpha in female fetal, infant and child mammary tissue. *J Pathol* 2000;191:449–451.
3. Nathan B, Anbazhagan R, Clarkson P, et al. Expression of BCL-2 in the developing human fetal and infant breast. *Histopathology* 1994;24:73–76.
4. van Winter JT, Noller KL, Zimmerman D, et al. Natural history of premature thelarche in Olmsted County, Minnesota, 1940 to 1984. *J Pediatr* 1990;116:278–280.
5. Verrotti A, Ferrari M, Morgese G, et al. Premature thelarche: a long-term follow-up. *Gynecol Endocrinol* 1996;10:241–247.
6. Aritaki S, Takagi T, Someya H, et al. A comparison of patients with premature thelarche and idiopathic true precocious puberty in the initial stage of illness. *Acta Paediatr Jpn* 1997;39:21–27.
7. Klein KO, Mericq V, Brown-Dawson JM, et al. Estrogen levels in girls with premature thelarche compared with normal prepubertal girls as determined by an ultrasensitive recombinant cell bioassay. *J Pediatr* 1999;134:190–192.
8. Volta C, Bernasconi S, Cisternino M, et al. Isolated premature thelarche and thelarche variant: clinical and auxological follow-up of 119 girls. *J Endocrinol Invest* 1998;21:180–183.
9. Pasquino AM, Pucarelli I, Passeri F, et al. Progression of premature thelarche to central precocious puberty. *J Pediatr* 1995;126:11–14.
10. Pangarkar MA, Poflee SV, Lele VR. Fine needle aspiration cytology of juvenile hypertrophy of the breast. *Acta Cytol* 1997;41:940–941.
11. Topper YJ, Freeman CS. Multiple hormone interactions in the developmental biology of the mammary gland. *Physiol Rev* 1980;60:1049–1106.
12. Salmon M. Les artères de la glande mammaire. *Ann Anat Pathol* 1939;16:477–500.
13. Cunningham L. The anatomy of the arteries and veins of the breast. *J Surg Oncol* 1977;9:71–85.
14. Skandalakis JE, Grey SW, Rowe JS Jr. *Anatomical complications in general surgery.* New York: McGraw-Hill, 1983;43.
15. Cruikshank WC. *Anatomy of the absorbing vessels,* 2nd ed. London: G. Nicol, 1790.

16. Sappey MPC. *Description et ichonographie des vaisseaux lymphatiques.* Paris: A. Delahaye, 1885.
17. Gray JH. Relation of lymphatic vessels to spread of cancer. *Br J Surg* 1939;26:462–495.
18. Hultborn KA, Larsson LG, Ragnhult I. Lymph drainage from breast to axillary and parasternal lymph nodes, studied with aid of colloidal. *Acta Radiol* 1955;43:52–64.
19. Turner-Warwick RT. The lymphatics of the breast. *Br J Surg* 1959;46:574–582.
20. Moffat DF, Going JJ. Three dimensional anatomy of complete duct systems in human breast: pathological and developmental implications. *J Clin Pathol* 1996;49:48–52.
21. Montgomery WF. *An exposition of the signs and symptoms of pregnancy, the period of human gestation, and the signs of delivery.* London: Sherwood, Gilbert and Piper, 1837.
22. Wolfe JN. Breast patterns as an index of risk for developing breast cancer. *AJR Am J Roentgenol* 1976;126:1130–1139.
23. Saftlas AF, Wolfe JN, Hoover RN, et al. Mammographic parenchymal patterns as indicators of breast cancer risk. *Am J Epidemiol* 1989;129:518–526.
24. Lee NA, Rusinek H, Weinreb J, et al. Fatty and fibroglandular tissue volumes in the breasts of women 20–83 years old: comparison of x-ray mammography and computer-assisted MR imaging. *AJR Am J Roentgenol* 1997;168:501–506.
25. Rand T, Heytmanek G, Seifert M, et al. Mammography in women undergoing hormone replacement therapy. Possible effects revealed at routine examination. *Acta Radiol* 1997;38:228–231.
26. Persson I, Thurfjell E, Holmberg L. Effect of estrogen and estrogen-progestin replacement regimens on mammographic breast parenchymal density. *J Clin Oncol* 1997;15:3201–3207.
27. Marugg RC, van der Mooren MJ, Hendriks JHCL, et al. Mammographic changes in postmenopausal women on hormonal replacement therapy. *Eur Radiol* 1997;7:749–755.
28. Reichenbach JR, Przetak C, Klinger G, et al. Assessment of breast tissue changes on hormonal replacement therapy using MRI: a pilot study. *J Comput Assist Tomogr* 1999;23:407–413.
29. Son HJ, Oh KK. Significance of follow-up mammography in estimating the effect of tamoxifen in breast cancer patients who have undergone surgery. *AJR Am J Roentgenol* 1999;173:905–909.
30. Rosen PP, Tench W. Lobules in the nipple. *Pathol Annu* 1985;20[Pt 1]:317–322.
31. Péchoux C, Gudjonsson T, Rønnov-Jessen L, et al. Human mammary luminal epithelial cells contain progenitors to myoepithelial cells. *Dev Biol* 1999;206:88–99.
32. Nagato T, Yoshida H, Yoshida A, et al. A scanning electron microscope study of myoepithelial cells in exocrine glands. *Cell Tissue Res* 1980;209:1–10.
33. Farahmand S, Cowan DF. Elastosis in the normal aging breast. *Arch Pathol Lab Med* 1991;115:1241–1246.
34. Davies JD. Pigmented periductal cells (ochrocytes) in mammary dysplasias: their nature and significance. *J Pathol* 1974;114:205–216.
35. Montagna W, Macpherson EE. Some neglected aspects of the anatomy of human breasts. *J Invest Dermatol* 1974;63:10–16.
36. Schnitt SJ, Goldwyn RM, Slavin SA. Mammary ducts in the areola: implications for patients undergoing reconstructive surgery of the breast. *Plast Reconstr Surg* 1993;92:1290–1293.
37. Smith DM Jr, Peters TG, Donegan WL. Montgomery's areolar tubercle. *Arch Pathol Lab Med* 1982;106:60–63.
38. Eyden BP, Watson RJ, Harris M, et al. Intralobular stromal fibroblasts in the resting human mammary gland: ultrastructural properties and intercellular relationships. *J Submicrosc Cytol* 1986;18:397–408.
39. Yamazaki K, Eyden BP. Ultrastructural and immunohistochemical observations on intralobular fibroblasts on human breast, with observations on the CD34 antigen. *J Submicrosc Cytol Pathol* 1995;27:309–323.
40. Christov K, Chew KL, Ljung B-M, et al. Proliferation of normal breast epithelial cells as shown by *in vivo* labeling with bromodeoxyuridine. *Am J Pathol* 1991;138:1371–1377.
41. Lakhani SR, Chaggar R, Davies S, et al. Genetic alterations in "normal" luminal and myoepithelial cells of the breast. *J Pathol* 1999;189:496–503.
42. White E, Velentgas P, Mandelson MT, et al. Variation in mammographic breast density by time in menstrual cycle among women aged 40–49 years. *J Natl Cancer Inst* 1998;90:906–910.
43. Milligan D, Drife JO, Short RV. Changes in breast volume during normal menstrual cycle and after oral contraceptives. *Br Med J* 1975;4:494–496.
44. Fowler PA, Casey CE, Cameron GG, et al. Cyclic changes in composition and volume of the breast during the menstrual cycle, measured by magnetic resonance imaging. *Br J Obstet Gynecol* 1990;97:595–602.
45. Graham SJ, Stanchev PL, Lloyd-Smith JOA, et al. Changes in fibroglandular volume and water content of breast tissue during the menstrual cycle observed by MR imaging at 1.5T. *J Magn Reson Imaging* 1995;5:695–701.
46. Kuhl CK, Bieling HB, Gieseke J, et al. Healthy premenopausal breast parenchyma in dynamic contrast-enhanced MR imaging of the breast: normal contrast medium enhancement and cyclical-phase dependency. *Radiology* 1997;203:137–144.
47. Müller-Schimpfle M, Ohmenhäuser K, Stoll P, et al. Menstrual cycle and age: influence on parenchymal contrast medium enhancement in MR imaging of the breast. *Radiology* 1997;203:145–149.
48. Vogel PM, Georgiade NG, Fetter BF, et al. The correlation of histologic changes in the human breast with the menstrual cycle. *Am J Pathol* 1981;104:23–34.
49. Gomm JJ, Coope RC, Browne PJ, et al. Separated human breast epithelial and myoepithelial cells have different growth factor requirements in vitro but can reconstitute normal breast lobuloalveolar structure. *J Cell Physiol* 1997;171:11–19.
50. Longacre TA, Bartow SA. A correlative morphologic study of human breast and endometrium in the menstrual cycle. *Am J Surg Pathol* 1986;10:382–393.
51. Ferguson DJP, Anderson TJ. Morphological evaluation of cell turnover in relation to the menstrual cycle in the "resting" human breast. *Br J Cancer* 1981;4:177–181.
52. Sabourin JC, Martin A, Baruch J, et al. bcl-2 expression in normal breast tissue during the menstrual cycle. *Int J Cancer* 1994;59:1–6.
53. Anderson TJ, Ferguson JP, Raab GM. Cell turnover in the "resting" human breast: influence of parity, contraceptive pill, age and laterality. *Br J Cancer* 1982;46:376–382.
54. Bassler R. The morphology of hormone induced structural changes in the female breast. *Curr Top Pathol* 1970;53:1–89.
55. Gompel A, Martin A, Simon P, et al. Epidermal growth factor receptor and c-erbB-2 expression in normal breast tissue during the menstrual cycle. *Breast Cancer Res Treat* 1996;38:227–235.
56. Uehara J, Nazário AC, Rodrigues de Lima G, et al. Effects of tamoxifen on the breast in the luteal phase of the menstrual cycle. *Int J Gynaecol Obstet* 1998;62:77–82.
57. Fanger H, Ree HJ. Cyclic changes of human mammary gland epithelium in relation to the menstrual cycle—an ultrastructural study. *Cancer* 1974;34:574–585.
58. McCarty KS Jr, Sasso R, Budwit D, et al. Immunoglobulin localization in the normal human mammary gland: variation with the menstrual cycle. *Am J Pathol* 1982;107:322–326.
59. Potten CS, Watson RJ, Williams GT, et al. The effect of age and menstrual cycle upon proliferative activity of the normal human breast. *Br J Cancer* 1988;58:163–170.
60. Meyer JS. Cell proliferation in normal human breast ducts, fibroadenomas, and other ductal hyperplasias measured by nuclear labeling with tritiated thymidine. Effects of menstrual phase, age, and oral contraceptive hormones. *Hum Pathol* 1977;8:67–81.
61. Masters JRW, Drife JO, Scarisbrick JJ. Cyclic variation of DNA synthesis in human breast epithelium. *J Natl Cancer Inst* 1977;58:1283–1285.
62. Anderson TJ, Battersby S, King RJB, et al. Oral contraceptive use influences resting breast proliferation. *Hum Pathol* 1989;20:1139–1144.
63. Going JJ, Anderson TJ, Battersby S, et al. Proliferative and secretory activity in human breast during natural and artificial menstrual cycles. *Am J Pathol* 1988;130:193–204.
64. Russo J, Calaf G, Roi L, et al. Influence of age and gland topography on cell kinetics of normal human breast tissue. *J Natl Cancer Inst* 1987;72:413–418.
65. Visscher DW, Gingrich DS, Buckley J, et al. Cell cycle analysis of normal, atrophic, and hyperplastic breast epithelium using two-color multiparametric flow cytometry. *Anal Cell Pathol* 1996;12:115–124.
66. Söderqvist G, Isaksson E, von Schoultz B, et al. Proliferation of breast epithelial cells in healthy women during the menstrual cycle. *Am J Obstet Gynecol* 1997;176:123–128.

67. Joshi K, Smith JA, Perusinghe N, et al. Cell proliferation in the human mammary epithelium. Differential contribution by epithelial and myoepithelial cells. *Am J Pathol* 1986;124:199–206.

68. Petersen OW, Hoyer PE, van Deurs B. Frequency and distribution of estrogen receptor-positive cells in normal, nonlactating human breast tissue. *Cancer Res* 1987;47:5748–5751.

69. Shoker BS, Jarvis C, Sibson DR, et al. Oestrogen receptor expression in the normal and pre-cancerous breast. *J Pathol* 1999;188:237–244.

70. Silva JS, Georgiade GS, Dilley WG, et al. Menstrual cycle-dependent variations of breast cyst fluid proteins and sex steroid receptors in the normal human breast. *Cancer* 1983;51:1297–1302.

71. Markopoulos C, Berger U, Wilson P, et al. Oestrogen receptor content of normal breast cells and breast carcinoma throughout the menstrual cycle. *Br Med J* 1988;296:1349–1351.

72. Fabris G, Marchetti E, Marzola A, et al. Pathophysiology of estrogen receptors in mammary tissue by monoclonal antibodies. *J Steroid Biochem* 1987;27:171–176.

73. Pujol P, Daures JP, Thezenas S, et al. Changing estrogen and progesterone receptor patterns in breast carcinoma during the menstrual cycle and menopause. *Cancer* 1998;83:698–705.

74. Weimer DA, Donegan WL. Changes in estrogen and progesterone receptor content of primary breast carcinoma during the menstrual cycle. *Breast Cancer Res Treat* 1987;10:271–278.

75. Smyth CM, Benn DE, Reeve TS. Influence of the menstrual cycle on the concentrations of estrogen and progesterone receptors in primary brest cancer biopsies. *Breast Cancer Res Treat* 1988;11:45–50.

76. Tobin CE, Hendrix TM, Geyer SJ, et al. Breast imaging case of the day. Lobular hyperplasia of pregnancy. *Radiographics* 1996;16:1225–1226.

77. Dawson EK. A histological study of the normal mamma in relation to tumour growth. II. The mature gland in pregnancy and lactation. *Edinburgh Med J* 1935;42:569–598.

78. McCarty KS Jr, Tucker JA. Breast. In: Sternberg SS, ed. *Histology for pathologists.* New York: Raven Press, 1992:893–902.

79. Pitelka DR. The mammary gland. In: Weiss L, ed. *Cell and tissue biology. A textbook of histology,* 6th ed. Baltimore: Urban & Schwarzenberg, 1988:881–898.

80. Salazar H, Tobon H, Josimovich JB. Developmental gestational and postgestational modifications of the human breast. *Clin Obstet Gynecol* 1975;18:113–137.

81. Vorherr H. Human lactation and breast feeding. In: Larson BI, ed. *Lactation,* vol. IV. New York: Academic Press, 1978:182.

82. Battersby S, Anderson TJ. Histological changes in breast tissue that characterize recent pregnancy. *Histopathology* 1989;15:415–433.

83. Huseby RA, Thomas LB. Histological and histochemical alterations in the normal breast tissues of patients with advanced breast cancer being treated with estrogenic hormones. *Cancer* 1954;7:54–74.

84. Rand T, Heytmanek G, Seifert M, et al. Mammography in women undergoing hormone replacement therapy. Possible effects revealed at routine examination. *Acta Radiol* 1997;38:228–231.

85. Laya MB, Gallagher JC, Schreiman JS, et al. Effect of postmenopausal hormonal replacement therapy on mammographic density and parenchymal pattern. *Radiology* 1995;196:433–437.

86. Margolin FR, Denny SR, Gelfand CA, et al. Mammographic changes after hormone replacement therapy in patients who have undergone breast irradiation. *AJR Am J Roentgenol* 1999;172:147–150.

87. Hargreaves DF, Knox F, Swindell R, et al. Epithelial proliferation and hormone receptor status in the normal post-menopausal breast and the effects of hormone replacement therapy. *Br J Cancer* 1998;78:945–949.

88. Sickles EA, Galvin HB. Breast arterial calcification in association with diabetes mellitus: too weak a correlation to have clinical utility. *Radiology* 1985;155:577–579.

89. Leinster SJ, Whitehouse GH. Factors which influence the occurrence of vascular calcification in the breast. *Br J Radiol* 1987;60:457–458.

90. Kragel PJ, Aquino MO, Fiorella R, et al. Clinical, radiographic, and pathologic features of medial calcific sclerosis in the breast. *South Med J* 1997;90:518–521.

91. Baum JK, Comstock CH, Joseph L. Intramammary arterial calcifications associated with diabetes. *Radiology* 1980;136:61–62.

92. Moshyedi AC, Puthawala AH, Kurland RJ, et al. Breast arterial calcification: association with coronary artery disease. *Radiology* 1995;194:181–183.

93. van Noord PAH, Beijerinck D, Kemmeren JM, et al. Mammograms may convey more than breast cancer risk: breast arterial calcification and arterio-sclerotic related diseases in women of the DOM cohort. *Eur J Cancer Prev* 1996;5:483–487.

94. Kiaer HW, Andersen JA. Focal pregnancy-like changes in the breast. *Acta Pathol Microbiol Scand [A]* 1977;85:931–941.

95. Frantz VK, Pickren JW, Melcher GW, et al. Incidence of chronic cystic disease in so-called normal breasts: a study based on 225 postmortem examinations. *Cancer* 1951;4:762–783.

96. Schwartz IS, Wilens SL. The formation of acinar tissue in gynecomastia. *Am J Pathol* 1963;43:797–807.

97. Sandison AT. An autopsy study of the adult human breast. *Natl Cancer Inst Monogr* 1962;8:58–59.

98. Viña M, Wells CA. Clear cell metaplasia of the breast: a lesion showing eccrine differentiation. *Histopathology* 1989;15:85–92.

99. Shin SJ, Rosen PP. Pregnancy-like (pseudolactational) hyperplasia: a primary diagnosis in mammographically detected lesions of the breast and its relationship to cystic hypersecretory hyperplasia. *Am J Surg Pathol* 2000;24:1670–1674.

100. Pier WJ Jr, Garancis JC, Kuzma JF. Fine structure of tranquilizer-induced changes in rat mammary gland. *Am J Pathol* 1970;60:119–130.

101. Hooper JH, Welch VC, Shackelford RT. Abnormal lactation associated with tranquilizing drug therapy. *JAMA* 1961;178:506–507.

102. Tavassoli FA, Yeh IT. Lactational and clear cell changes of the breast in nonlactating, nonpregnant women. *Am J Clin Pathol* 1987;87:23–29.

103. Al-Sam SZ, Davies JD. Phenotypic expression of immunosecretory function in focal pregnancy-like change in the human breast. *Virchows Arch [A]* 1987;410:515–521.

104. Mills SE, Fraire AE. Pregnancy-like change of the breast. An ultrastructural study. *Diagn Gynecol Obstet* 1981;3:187–191.

105. Skorpil F. Uber das Vorkommen von sog. Hellen Zellen (Lamprocyten) in der Milchdruse. *Beitr Pathol Anat* 1943;108:378–393.

106. Barwick KW, Kashigarian M, Rosen PP. "Clear-cell" change within duct and lobular epithelium of the human breast. *Pathol Annu* 1982;17[Pt 1]:319–328.

# CHAPTER 2

# Abnormalities of Mammary Growth and Development

## HYPOPLASIA AND AMASTIA

The most extreme form of mammary hypoplasia is amastia, the complete absence of one or both breasts, including the nipple (1,2). As one of the least common developmental abnormalities, amastia is encountered more often in females than in males. Familial amastia has been documented in instances in which a brother and sister (3) and mother and daughter (4) have been affected. It may be accompanied by developmental defects of the ipsilateral shoulder, chest, and/or arm (5). Amastia has been reported in the complex genetic defect of acrorenal ectodermal dysplasia with lipotrophic diabetes (AREDYLD syndrome) (6). In addition to amastia, developmental abnormalities in these young women include skeletal and renal defects and hypodontia.

Mammary hypoplasia can occur as a congenital or acquired defect and may be unilateral or bilateral. A diagnosis of unilateral hypoplasia may be made if there is a substantial difference in breast size that far exceeds the mild asymmetry commonly present, and the larger breast is not macromastic. The breast tissue consists of fibrous stroma and ductal structures without acinar differentiation (Fig. 2.1).

Ipsilateral mammary hypoplasia has been reported in conjunction with Becker's nevus, a unilateral hairy hyperpigmented lesion (7,8), although breast abnormalities were not described in Becker's original report (9). Concurrent hypoplasia of the ipsilateral pectoralis major muscle also has been reported (10). The pigmented lesions and accompanying mammary hypoplasia occur in males and females (11). High androgen receptor levels have been detected in Becker's nevi (7,12) but not in the skin from the unaffected contralateral chest (7).

Hypoplasia or aplasia of the mammary glands and hypoplasia of the nipples occur in the ulnar-mammary syndrome, a familial genetic abnormality with autosomal dominant inheritance (13–15). Commonly associated defects include skeletal abnormalities affecting the ulnar rays of the hands, hypoplasia of apocrine glands, and genital anomalies in males. Poland's syndrome includes severe congenital defects of the chest and arm combined with mammary hypoplasia, amastia, or athelia (16). Carcinoma can arise in the hypoplastic breast of women with Poland's syndrome (17). Mammary hypoplasia also occurs in Turner's syndrome and in congenital adrenal hyperplasia. Familial hypoplasia of the nipples and athelia associated with mammary hypoplasia have been described in a father and his daughters (18). Hosokawa et al. (19) described the occurrence of a subcutaneous squamous cyst at the site of unilateral athelia, which suggested that the cystic lesion arose from a maldeveloped nipple.

Acquired mammary hypoplasia has been observed in women who received irradiation of the mammary region during infancy or childhood (20,21). The most frequent clinical reason for radiation in this age group was the treatment of cutaneous hemangiomas. The severity of hypoplasia was directly related to the dose of radiation. Surgical excision of the prepubertal breast bud, which enlarges in precocious and early breast development, will result in mammary hypoplasia or amastia by removing part or all of the infantile breast anlage. Unilateral atrophy of a previously normal breast has been described in a 17-year-old girl associated with infectious mononucleosis (22). Biopsy revealed "normal" breast tissue. The rare occurrence of carcinoma arising in an irradiated hypomastic breast has been reported (23).

## MACROMASTIA

Several types of excessive breast growth have been described as forms of macromastia. *Adolescent macromastia* occurs as a result of progressive growth over 1 to 2 years during adolescence, resulting in breast size that far exceeds normal limits. The breasts do not decrease in size in subsequent years, and breast reduction surgery invariably is required. Although the condition usually is relatively symmetric, there are instances in which there is substantial disparity in breast size.

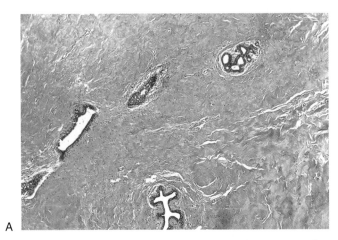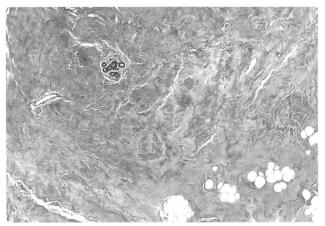

A                                                                                                              B

**FIG. 2.1.** *Mammary hypoplasia.* Breast tissue from a 23-year-old woman with unilateral hypoplasia. **A:** Ducts that resemble prepubertal breast in collagenous stroma. **B:** Minimal lobular differentiation.

Histologic examination reveals greatly increased stromal collagen and fat (Fig. 2.2). Epithelial hyperplasia of ducts is present in a minority of cases (24). Pseudoangiomatous stromal hyperplasia is evident in a minority of these individuals. The stromal cells in one instance of adolescent macromastia, which appears to be pseudoangiomatous stromal hyperplasia in the published illustrations, lacked nuclear estrogen receptor but were positive for nuclear progesterone receptor (25). Biochemical estrogen receptor assays on tissues from a series of 25 patients (aged 17 to 77 years) with macromastia not associated with pregnancy were negative (26).

*Gravid macromastia* develops rapidly, shortly after the onset of pregnancy in the affected individual (27–29). It occurs in less than 0.01% of pregnancies (27). The etiology is unknown. Onset very early in pregnancy in some cases has implicated chorionic gonadotrophin, possibly through a hypersensitivity mechanism. Fetal sex does not appear to be a factor.

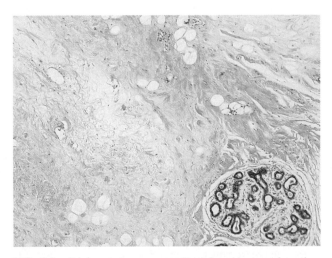

**FIG. 2.2.** *Adolescent macromastia.* A broad area of moderately edematous interlobular stroma surrounding a normal lobule.

The majority of women are primiparous, but in some individuals macromastia does not occur until the second or third pregnancy (27,29,30). Once established, the condition is likely to recur in successive pregnancies, even if the pregnancy terminates in a miscarriage. The chance of recurrence is decreased by reduction mammoplasty, but some patients have required additional surgery for regrowth of breast tissue after mastectomy (29,31). In one case, gravid macromastia involved bilateral axillary breasts and one ectopic thoracic breast, as well as both normally situated glands (32).

A variety of pathologic changes has been reported in gravid macromastia. Leis et al. (30) described a case in which the stroma exhibited "marked fibrosis, with bands of dense collagenous tissue and thickening of the intralobular fibrous tissue." Thickening of basement membranes was noted, whereas "ducts and acini demonstrated a two-layered epithelium with apparently inactive cuboidal cells." Fibrosis and collagenization also were noted by Beischer et al. (27) and Kullander (33). Others have reported fibroadenomas (31,34) and lactational hyperplasia (35). Several authors have commented on the presence of dilated lymphatics in the breast tissue. Pseudoangiomatous stromal hyperplasia often is a prominent feature that is evident in retrospect in published illustrations (36), although the condition was not described in the reports by this recently introduced term (see Chapter 40). In most instances, the diagnosis can be made clinically. Rarely, the clinical presentation of neoplastic conditions, such as angiosarcoma or lymphoma in the breast, may mimic gravid macromastia. Pseudohyperparathyroidism has been associated with gravid macromastia (36). Mastectomy results in prompt remission of the hypercalcemia.

Mastectomy or breast reduction usually is undertaken after delivery to ameliorate the incapacitating effects of gravid macromastia, which include pain, depression, and, in some cases, altered pulmonary function. Necrosis of the skin or parenchyma complicated by infection or bleeding may necessitate mastectomy during pregnancy. The concept that hormonal disturbances contribute to the development of gravid macromastia has led to attempts at endocrine treatment, although none have been uniformly effective. There have not been consistent hormonal abnormalities in the patients who were studied, and it presently appears likely that the fundamental problem lies in abnormal responsiveness of the breast tissues (37). Bromocriptine has been administered and has resulted in reduced prolactin levels in some cases but inconsistent clinical responses (33,37,38). Treatment with tamoxifen was not effective in one case (39).

*Penicillamine-induced macromastia* has been reported in patients receiving this drug for treatment of rheumatoid arthritis (40), and marked breast enlargement or "hypertrophy" has been observed in women with human immunodeficiency virus infection after treatment with indinavir (41).

## ECTOPIC BREAST TISSUE

There are two general patterns of ectopic mammary tissue: supernumerary breasts and aberrant breast tissue. In most instances these types are distinguishable, but there are situations in which the distinction is arbitrary.

*Supernumerary breast tissue* occurs along the milk lines extending bilaterally from the mid-axilla through the normal breasts and then inferiorly to the medial groins (42). In women, the inferior extensions of the milk lines traverse the vulva bilaterally. The embryologic anlage of the milk line is the milk ridge, which later undergoes complete atrophy except for short segments that remain in the pectoral region to give rise to normal breasts. Supernumerary breasts develop from portions of the milk ridges that fail to atrophy.

A study of neonates revealed supernumerary nipples in 49 (2.4%) of 2,035 infants (43). The abnormality was more frequent in black than in white neonates. Male and female infants were equally affected. Clinically, supernumerary breasts are encountered in 1% to 6% of adult women and considerably less frequently in men (42,44–46). Rare instances of familial supernumerary breasts and nipples have been described (47–49). In one report, the condition consisted of bilateral axillary breasts limited to females in two generations (49). Another report described a male child who had accessory breasts on the thorax and abdomen along the milk lines and whose mother also had accessory breast tissue (47). A study of 156 white patients with aberrant mammary tissue diagnosed in a dermatology clinic revealed that 18 (11.5%) patients had a relative with the same condition (50). Aberrant breast tissue was more frequent on the left side than on the right side.

Supernumerary nipples often are located on the anterior chest above or below the normal breast. Alterations in the size of accessory breasts was noted with the menstrual cycle and pregnancy. The majority of patients with clinically apparent supernumerary breast tissue have unilateral axillary involvement. Bilateral axillary breasts are the second most frequent presentation. Thoracic, abdominal, inguinal, and vulvar supernumerary breasts, whether isolated, multiple, or

in conjunction with axillary breast tissue, are much less frequent. An association between supernumerary nipples and renal anomalies has been described (51). However, this relationship has not been confirmed by other investigators (50). Kenny et al. (43) found ultrasound evidence of a renal abnormality in only one of 49 neonates with supernumerary nipples. The latter study included a high proportion of African-American children, whereas the former study described Hungarian children (51). The differing results of these investigators may reflect inherent genetic differences in the populations studied.

The clinical presentation of supernumerary breasts is highly variable. Intraareolar polythelia is a form of accessory breast in which two or more nipples, usually appearing deformed or "dysplastic," occur within the areola (52). The reported occurrence of intraareolar polythelia in patients with neurofibromatosis (53) may be the result of mistaking cutaneous neurofibromas of the skin of the areola for accessory nipples (54).

In some of these cases, the glandular tissue of supernumerary breast is partly or entirely replaced by fat and may be diagnosed clinically as a lipoma, especially if the nipple and areola are absent (44,55). A complete supernumerary mammary gland with nipple-areola complex is uncommon (56). Physiologic changes may occur during the menstrual cycle, causing swelling of the gland that occasionally can be painful. Lactation from supernumerary breast tissue has been reported during pregnancy and postpartum (42,57). Spontaneous galactorrhea from an ectopic axillary mammary gland with fully developed nipple was attributed to a pituitary microadenoma in a 28-year-old woman (58). Her serum prolactin level decreased to normal after treatment with bromocriptine.

The presence of ectopic breast tissue can be confirmed and lesions arising in these sites can be diagnosed by fine needle aspiration (59). The findings in an aspiration smear are variable, depending on the state of development of the tissue. Typically, there are clumps and sheets of uniform, cytologically benign duct cells distributed in a monolayered fashion (60). Proteinaceous material, secretion, and small groups of acinar cells are found in the aspirate of axillary tissue from a lactating patient. Monolayered sheets of benign ductal cells and bipolar stromal cells characterize the specimen obtained from an axillary fibroadenoma. Histologic sections reveal duct and lobular mammary structures (Fig. 2.3).

Most examples of supernumerary nipples (polythelia) occur along the milk line without the development of a supernumerary breast. Supernumerary breasts are more common on the left side (45,56). Examination of 1,691 consecutive neonates in one study revealed supernumerary nipples in 24 of 1,000 live births (61). Other studies report frequencies ranging from 1.7% (56) to 3.75% (45). There are a number of reports of polythelia, with and without familial occurrence involving men and women, associated with congenital abnormalities (62,63). An unusual syndrome is the familial occurrence of intraareolar polythelia (dysplastic divided nipples) in hypoplastic breasts (53).

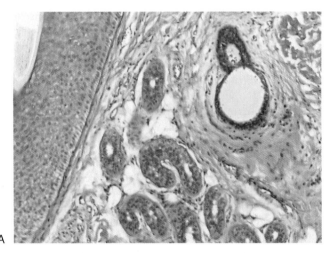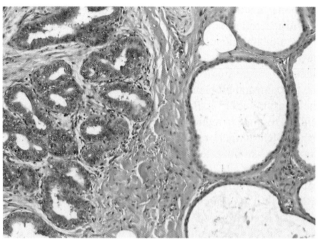

**FIG. 2.3.** *Ectopic breast in axilla.* **A:** Deep dermis of axillary skin showing, from left to right, a hair follicle, a sweat gland, and an ectopic mammary duct. **B:** Mammary lobule with mild epithelial hyperplasia next to a dilated axillary apocrine gland.

Mehregan (64) described the microscopic pathology of 51 examples of supernumerary nipple among 360,000 consecutive skin biopsy specimens. The microscopic components of a normal nipple, including lactiferous ducts and smooth muscle and epidermal thickening with pilosebaceous structures, were present. Almost all specimens included mammary glandular tissue in the deep dermis.

## ABERRANT BREAST TISSUE

Aberrant breast tissue is defined as mammary glandular parenchyma found in the region of, but beyond, the usual anatomic extent of the breast. Ducts and lobules that make up aberrant breast are structurally normal, but they are not as well organized as in normal or supernumerary breasts. By definition, aberrant breast is anatomically separate from the duct system of the breast and differs in this respect from peripheral extensions of the breast (4,65). Microscopically, aberrant and peripheral breast tissue are histologically indistinguishable. Aberrant breast tissue does not form a nipple and/or areola and rarely is clinically apparent unless it becomes the site of a pathologic process (see Chapter 35).

## THE TRANSSEXUAL BREAST

Female-to-male transsexual conversion involves prolonged androgen administration that usually begins prior to mastectomy. When compared with normal female breast tissue obtained from reduction mammoplasty operations, the androgen-treated breast had more frequent calcifications (66). No significant difference in the prevalence of ducts and lobules, cysts, or apocrine metaplasia was observed. The expression of estrogen and progesterone receptors and gross cystic disease fluid protein 15 was not significantly different in transsexual specimens when compared with normals.

Male-to-female transsexuals undergo surgical or chemical castration and estrogen therapy. Chemical castration using cyproterone, a progestational medication, is accomplished by blocking androgen receptors. Breast tissue obtained from six patients after 18 months of combined therapy revealed well-developed lobular structures in all cases and pregnancy-like hyperplasia in two patients (67). Breast carcinoma has been reported in male-to-female transsexuals (68).

## REFERENCES

1. Pierre M, Bureau H. A propos de deux case d'absence congenitale d'une glande mammaire. *Ann Chir Plast* 1960;5:137.
2. Trier WC. Complete breast absence. Case report and review of the literature. *Plast Reconstr Surg* 1965;36:430–439.
3. Kowlessar M, Orti E. Complete breast absence in siblings. *Am J Dis Child* 1968;115:91–92.
4. Goldenring H, Crelin ES. Mother and daughter with bilateral congenital amastia. *Yale J Biol Med* 1961;33:466.
5. Zilli L, Stephani G. Unilateral agenesis of the pectoralis muscles associated with mammary hypoplasia. *Friuli Med* 1960;15:1522.
6. Breslau-Siderius EJ, Toonstra J, Baart JA, et al. Ectodermal dysplasia, lipoatrophy, diabetes mellitus, and amastia: a second case of the AREDYLD syndrome. *Am J Med Genet* 1992;44:374–377.
7. Formigón M, Alsina MM, Mascaró JM, et al. Becker's nevus and ipsilateral breast hypoplasia androgen-receptor study in two patients. *Arch Dermatol* 1992;128:992–993.
8. Glinick SE, Alper JC, Bogaars H, et al. Becker's melanosis: associated abnormalities. *J Am Acad Dermatol* 1988;9:509–514.
9. Becker SW. Concurrent melanosis and hypertrichosis in distribution of nevus unis lateris. *Arch Dermatol Syphil* 1949;60:155–160.
10. Moore JA, Schosser RH. Becker's melanosis and hypoplasia of the breast and pectoralis major muscle. *Pediatr Dermatol* 1985;3:34–37.
11. Sharma R, Mishra A. Becker's naevus with ipsilateral areolar hypoplasia in three males. *Br J Dermatol* 1997;136:471–472.
12. Person JR, Longcope C. Becker's nevus: an androgen-mediated hyperplasia with increased androgen receptors. *J Am Acad Dermatol* 1984;10:235–238.
13. Franceschini P, Vardeu MP, Dalforno L, et al. Possible relationship between ulnar-mammary syndrome and split hand with aplasia of the ulna syndrome. *Am J Med Genet* 1992;44:807–812.
14. Gilly E. Absence complête des mammeles chez une femme mere. Atrophie du membre superieur droit. *Courier Med* 1882;32:27–28.
15. Schinzel A. Ulnar-mammary syndrome. *J Med Genet* 1987;24: 778–781.
16. Shamberger RC, Welch KJ, Upton J III. Surgical treatment of thoracic deformity in Poland's syndrome. *J Pediatr Surg* 1989;24:760–765.

17. Fukushima T, Otake T, Yashima R, et al. Breast cancer in two patients with Poland's syndrome. *Breast Cancer* 1998;6:127–130.

18. Nelson MM, Cooper CK. Congenital defects of the breast—an autosomal dominant trait. *S Afr Med J* 1982;61:434–436.

19. Hosokawa K, Hata Y, Yano K, et al. Unilateral athelia with a subcutaneous dermoid cyst. *Plast Reconstr Surg* 1987;80:732–733.

20. Fürst CJ, Lundell M, Ahlbäck SO, et al. Breast hypoplasia following irradiation of the female breast in infancy and early childhood. *Acta Oncol* 1989;28:519–523.

21. Kolar J, Bek V, Vrabec R. Hypoplasia of the growing breast after contact x-ray therapy for cutaneous angiomas. *Arch Dermatol* 1967;96:427–430.

22. Haramis HT, Collins RE. Unilateral breast atrophy. *Plast Reconstr Surg* 1995;95:916–919.

23. Funicello A, De Sandre R, Salloum L, et al. Infiltrating ductal carcinoma of the hypomastic breast: a case report. *Am Surg* 1998;64:1037–1039.

24. Sagot P, Mainguené C, Barrière P, et al. Virginal breast hypertrophy at puberty: a case report. *Eur J Obstet Gynecol Reprod Biol* 1990;34:289–292.

25. Hugh JC, Friedman MH, Danyluk JM, et al. Absence of estrogen receptors in a case of virginal hypertrophy of the breasts related to oral contraceptives. *Breast Dis* 1993;6:143–148.

26. Jabs AD, Frantz AG, Smith-Vaniz A, et al. Mammary hypertrophy is not associated with increased estrogen receptors. *Plast Reconstr Surg* 1990;86:64–66.

27. Beischer NA, Hueston JH, Pepperell RJ. Massive hypertrophy of the breasts in pregnancy: report of 3 cases and review of the literature, "never think you have seen everything." *Obstet Gynecol* 1989;44:234–243.

28. Ship AG, Shulman J. Virginal and gravid mammary gigantism—recurrence after reduction mammaplasty. *Br J Plast Surg* 1971;24:396–401.

29. Williams PC. Massive hypertrophy of the breasts and axillary breasts in successive pregnancies. *Am J Obstet Gynecol* 1957;74:1326–1341.

30. Leis SN, Palmer B, Östberg G. Gravid macromastia: case report. *Scand J Plast Reconstr Surg* 1974;8:247.

31. Nolan JJ. Gigantomastia. Report of a case. *Obstet Gynecol* 1962;19:526.

32. Barreto AU. Juvenile mammary hypertrophy. *Plast Reconstr Surg* 1991;87:583–584.

33. Kullander S. Effect of 2 Br-alpha-ergocryptin (CB 154) on serum prolactin and the clinical picture in a case of progressive gigantomastia in pregnancy. *Ann Chir Gynaecol* 1976;65:227.

34. Lewison EF, Jones GS, Trimble FH, et al. Gigantomastia complicating pregnancy. *Surg Gynecol Obstet* 1960;110:215.

35. Wølner-Hanssen P, Palmer B, Sjöberg NO, et al. Case report. Gigantomastia. *Acta Obstet Gynecol Scand* 1981;60:525.

36. Van Heerden JA, Gharib H, Jackson IT. Pseudohyperparathyroidism secondary to gigantic mammary hypertrophy. *Arch Surg* 1988;123:80–82.

37. Taylor PJ, Cumming DC, Corenblum B. Successful treatment of D-penicillamine–induced breast giantism with danazol. *Br Med J* 1981;282:362.

38. Szczurowicz A, Szymula A. Gravidic macromastia. A problem for the patient and for the doctor. *Clin Exp Obstet Gynecol* 1996;23:177–180.

39. Hedberg K, Karlsson K, Lindstedt G. Gigantomastia during pregnancy: effect of a dopamine agonist. *Am J Obstet Gynecol* 1979;133:928–931.

40. Wolf Y, Pauzner D, Groutz A, et al. Gigantomastia complicating pregnancy. Case report and review of the literature. *Acta Obstet Gynecol Scand* 1995;74:159–163.

41. Lui A, Karter D, Turett G. Another case of breast hypertrophy in a patient treated with indinavir. *Clin Infect Dis* 1998;26:1482.

42. DeCholnoky T. Supernumerary breast. *Arch Surg* 1939;39:926–941.

43. Kenny RD, Filippo JK, Black EB. Supernumerary nipples and anomalies in neonates. *Am J Dis Child* 1987;141:987–988.

44. DeCholnoky T. Accessory breast tissue in the axilla. *N Y State J Med* 1951;5:2245–2248.

45. Iwai T. A statistical study of the polymastia of the Japanese. *Lancet* 1907;2:753–759.

46. Petrek J, Rosen PP, Robbins GF. Carcinoma of aberrant breast tissue. *Clin Bull* 1980;10:13–15.

47. Cellini A, Offidavi A. Familial supernumerary nipples and breasts. *Dermatology* 1992;185:56–58.

48. Leung AKC. Familial supernumerary nipples. *Am J Med Genet* 1988;31:631–635.

49. Weinberg SK, Motulsky AG. Aberrant axillary breast tissue: a report of a family with six affected women in two generations. *Clin Genet* 1976;10:325–328.

50. Urbani CE, Betti R. Familial aberrant mammary tissue: a clinicoepidermiological survey of 18 cases. *Dermatology* 1995;190:207–209.

51. Meggyessy V, Mehes K. Association of supernumerary nipples with renal anomalies. *J Pediatr* 1987;111:412–413.

52. Brightmore T. Bilateral paired nipples. *Br J Surg* 1972;59:55–57.

53. Rintala A, Norio R. Familial intra-areolar polythelia with mammary hypoplasia. *Scand J Plast Reconstr Surg* 1982;16:287–291.

54. Haagensen CD. Anatomy of the mammary gland. In: Haagensen CD. *Diseases of the breast*, 3rd ed. Philadelphia: WB Saunders, 1986:1–46.

55. Shrotria S, Ghilchik MW. Axillary accessory breasts: a clinicopathological study of 35 patients with axillary masses. *Breast Dis* 1994;7:43–52.

56. Kajava Y. The proportions of supernumerary nipples in the Finnish population. *Duodecim* 1915;31:143–170.

57. O'Hara MF, Page DL. Adenomas of the breast and ectopic breast under lactational influences. *Hum Pathol* 1985;16:707–712.

58. Ünlühizaraci K, Bayram F, Öztürk M, et al. Unusual presentation of prolactinoma with spontaneous galactorrhoea from ectopic breast tissue. *Clin Endocrinol* 1998;49:136.

59. Das DK, Gupta SK, Mathew SV, et al. Fine needle aspiration cytologic diagnosis of axillary accessory breast tissue, including its physiologic changes and pathologic lesions. *Acta Cytol* 1994;38:130–135.

60. Dey P, Karmakar T. Fine needle aspiration cytology of accessory axillary breasts and their lesions. *Acta Cytol* 1994;38:915–916.

61. Mimouni F, Merlob P, Reisner SH. Occurrence of supernumerary nipples in newborns. *Am J Dis Child* 1983;137:952–953.

62. Hersh JH, Bloom AS, Cromer AO, et al. Does a supernumerary nipple/renal field defect exist? *Am J Dis Child* 1987;141:989–991.

63. Toumbis-Ioannou E, Cohen PR. Familial polythelia. *J Am Acad Dermatol* 1994;30:667–668.

64. Mehregan AH. Supernumerary nipple. A histologic study. *J Cutan Pathol* 1981;8:96–104.

65. Hicken NF. Mastectomy: clinical and pathological study demonstrating why most mastectomies result in incomplete removal of the mammary gland. *Arch Surg* 1940;40:6–14.

66. Burgess HE, Shousha S. An immunohistochemical study of the long-term effects of androgen administration on female-to-male transsexual breast: a comparison with normal female breast and male breast showing gynaecomastia. *J Pathol* 1993;170:37–43.

67. Kanhai RCJ, Hage JJ, van Diest PJ, et al. Short-term and long-term histologic effects of castration and estrogen treatment on breast tissue of 14 male-to-female transsexuals in comparison with two chemically castrated men. *Am J Surg Pathol* 2000;24:74–80.

68. Ganly I, Taylor EW. Breast cancer in a trans-sexual man receiving hormone replacement therapy. *Br J Surg* 1995;82:341.

# CHAPTER 3

# Inflammatory and Reactive Tumors

## FAT NECROSIS

Fat necrosis in the breast may result from trauma, but presently the majority of instances follow surgery or radiation therapy. In the era prior to breast-conserving therapy, no specific, antecedent, exogenous cause was reported in many instances. Trauma was described in 32% of patients reported by Haagensen (1) and in 44% of women reported by Adair and Munger (2). The observation that clinical features mimic carcinoma, first emphasized by Lee and Adair (3) in 1920, was confirmed in numerous later reports. Mammographic findings initially were characterized by Leborgne (4).

### Clinical Presentation

Traumatic fat necrosis occurs most frequently in overweight women and in women with pendulous breasts. Haagensen (1) reported a mean patient age of 52 years, with a range from 27 to 80 years. The youngest patient in the series reported by Adair and Munger (2) was 14 years old, with a median age in the 50s.

Patients typically present with a painless mass located superficially in the breast, often accompanied by retraction or dimpling of the overlying skin. The skin may be thickened clinically and radiologically. The lesion most frequently occurs in the subareolar and periareolar regions, but any part of the breast may be affected. Tumors formed by fat necrosis tend to be small, averaging 2 cm. They are firm and relatively circumscribed on palpation. The clinical problem of distinguishing between fat necrosis and recurrent carcinoma is especially difficult in patients who have undergone breast-conserving surgery and radiation therapy (5). Fat necrosis has been reported after external beam therapy (6) and at the site of iridium implantation (7). Massive fat necrosis of the breast has been described as a complication of secondary hyperparathyroidism with mural arterial calcification (8).

Mammography usually reveals a spiculated, often poorly defined mass that may contain punctate or large irregular calcifications (9). Less frequently, the lesion consists of a circumscribed, oil-filled, partly calcified cyst (4,10,11).

Both patterns may coexist in a single lesion. Attachment to the skin with dimpling and thickening of the skin often are evident on the mammogram. Fat necrosis with calcifications has been detected by mammography in axillary lymph nodes (12). Sonography demonstrates a discrete mass in almost all cases (13). The sonographic appearance is variable and usually is accompanied by distortion of the parenchymal architecture. Follow-up examination reveals evolution of the lesion, which decreases in size and becomes solid.

### Gross Findings

Early in its development, fat necrosis has the appearance of hemorrhage in indurated fat. After several weeks, the affected area becomes demarcated, forming a distinct yellow-gray and focally reddish tumor. Cystic degeneration may develop in the center, resulting in a cavity that contains oily fluid or necrotic fat. Calcification frequently develops in the cyst wall.

### Microscopic Findings

The initial change in fat necrosis is disruption of fat cells accompanied by hemorrhage and an influx of histiocytes. Progression of the lesion is marked by the formation of multinucleated histiocytes, hemosiderin deposition, and calcification (Fig. 3.1). A variable infiltrate of lymphocytes and plasma cells, sometimes with eosinophils, is present at this stage. Fibrosis develops peripherally as the lesion demarcates, enclosing an area of necrotic fat and cellular debris that may become cystic (Fig. 3.2). In late lesions, reactive inflammatory components replaced by fibrosis contract into a scar. Loculated degenerated fat or oil may persist for months or years within a cyst surrounded by such a scar. Squamous metaplasia can develop in the epithelium of ducts and lobules in the area of fat necrosis. Among patients who develop fat necrosis after radiation therapy, cytologic changes attributable to this treatment may be found in contiguous ducts, lobules, and blood vessels.

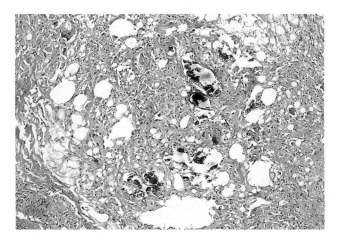

**FIG. 3.1.** *"Spontaneous" fat necrosis.* Histocytes, multinucleated cells, and calcification in necrotic fat.

## Treatment

Excisional biopsy is required when the clinical and radiologic features resemble carcinoma. If there is a distinct history of trauma or prior surgery and characteristic radiologic findings of a demarcated cystic lesion with typical calcifications, excision may not be performed after the diagnosis has been established by fine needle aspiration (FNA) or needle core biopsy. In such cases, the patient should be monitored by clinical examination and mammography to detect occult carcinoma masked by coexisting fat necrosis.

## HEMORRHAGIC NECROSIS AND ANTICOAGULANT THERAPY

Localized hemorrhagic necrosis of the skin and subcutaneous tissue occurs as a complication of anticoagulant therapy (14). The first description of this condition in the breast

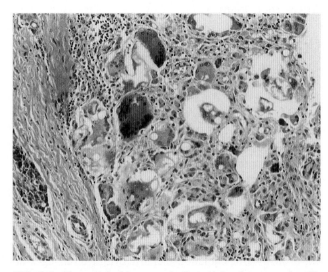

**FIG. 3.2.** *Traumatic fat necrosis.* Organizing fat necrosis with numerous multinucleated histiocytes. The lesion is demarcated by fibrosis on the left.

was reported by Flood et al. (15) in 1943. Hemorrhagic necrosis of the breast most often occurs in middle-aged or elderly women treated for thrombophlebitis with warfarin (Coumadin). Within a week after anticoagulation therapy begins, the patient complains of pain and swelling accompanied by blue-black discoloration of the breast. The condition usually progresses despite discontinuation of anticoagulant medication or administration of vitamin K, eventuating in gangrene of part or all of the breast (16). After the area of necrosis has become demarcated, surgical treatment consists of local resection or mastectomy.

Hemorrhagic necrosis in the skin and subcutaneous tissue or in the breast has been associated specifically with warfarin anticoagulant therapy. The prothrombin time usually is within the therapeutic range. Heparin does not appear to be a predisposing agent. The clinical features and pathologic findings suggest a hypersensitivity reaction to the medication, affecting small vessels in the skin and subcutaneous tissue. Recent studies determined that this syndrome occurs in patients with heterozygous protein C deficiency. In this setting, warfarin diminishes the formation of vitamin-K–dependent coagulation factors. It also interferes with the synthesis of proteins C and S and of vitamin-K–dependent inhibitors of clotting (17). In some patients, the net effect of these alterations is to promote thrombosis, a situation that leads to hemorrhagic necrosis. Histologic examination of the acutely affected tissue reveals hemorrhagic necrosis and infarction diffusely involving the skin, subcutaneous tissue, and breast parenchyma. Fibrin thrombi are present in small blood vessels, and neutrophils infiltrate the walls of arteries and veins (18,19). At a later stage, fibrosis and granulomatous inflammation appear as part of the healing process.

## BREAST INFARCT

### Clinical Presentation

The most frequent form of breast infarct occurs during pregnancy or postpartum. Infarction may develop in lactating glandular parenchyma or in a lactational adenoma. The lesion presents clinically as a discrete mass that usually is asymptomatic, although pain and tenderness sometimes are reported. Because of the association with pregnancy, breast infarcts usually occur in women less than 35 years of age. The firm mass produced by infarcted mammary parenchyma can suggest carcinoma clinically. Axillary lymph node enlargement may coexist with infarcts presumably resulting from the inflammatory reaction to necrosis. Infarction of accessory breast tissue during pregnancy has been described (20).

Robitaille et al. (21) found that mammary infarcts could be grouped into broad categories that included lesions that simulated carcinoma and those that did not suggest carcinoma. The former group included infarcts in sclerosing adenosis, papillomas, fibroadenomas, and pregnancy. Infarcts that did not mimic carcinoma were associated with anticoagulant therapy, infections with abscess formation, and superficial thrombophlebitis.

### Gross Pathology

The gross appearance of the excised infarcted tissue is variable. Hemorrhage is seen in lesions of recent onset, whereas older infarcts typically are characterized by one or more areas of relative pallor or yellow discoloration, sometimes bounded by a hyperemic border.

### Microscopic Pathology

Microscopic findings are influenced by the duration of the infarct. Hemorrhage and ischemic degeneration with little or no inflammation characterize early lesions. Later stages feature coagulative necrosis with loss of nuclear detail, pallor, and retention of architectural integrity. Liquefactive necrosis is very rarely encountered. Infarction is demarcated by a zone of granulation tissue with variable inflammatory reaction, hemosiderin deposition, and fibrosis. Some authors described organized or organizing thrombi in areas of infarction or in adjacent tissue (22,23), but this has not been a constant finding (24).

The specimen obtained by FNA from a mammary infarct during pregnancy may present a very challenging diagnostic problem. The nuclear atypia that reflects the physiologic hyperplasia of lactation may be accentuated in cells that are in early states of ischemic necrosis. Nuclear enlargement and hyperchromasia may be encountered in such cells. At a later stage, these cells will appear poorly preserved and fragmented.

Infarction can occur in proliferative lesions other than fibroadenomas. Foci of necrosis may be found in florid sclerosing adenosis (Fig. 3.3). This is most likely to occur during pregnancy, when the epithelium in sclerosing adenosis may exhibit pronounced hyperplasia, cytologic atypia, and mitotic activity.

Papillomas are susceptible to partial or complete infarction, especially lesions in major lactiferous ducts. Infarction occurs in papillomas at any age, but it tends to be more frequent in postmenopausal women and there is no association with pregnancy (25). Bloody nipple discharge is the most frequent symptom of an infarcted papilloma with or without a mass. Pain is rarely reported. Although infarction of papillomas has been ascribed to ischemia, clinical factors predisposing to this alteration have rarely been documented. One 19-year-old woman with serous nipple discharge and hyperprolactinemia developed bloody nipple discharge after treatment with bromocriptine. Duct excision revealed a partially infarcted papilloma (26).

Acutely infarcted regions in a papilloma exhibit ischemic coagulative necrosis. Structural integrity usually is maintained in such foci despite progressive loss of cytologic detail. At a late stage, fragmentation of superficial portions of the infarcted tissue occurs. Occasionally, portions of an infarcted papilloma are reduced to intraductal inflammatory polyps consisting of granulation tissue with little or no epithelium. Chronic ischemia and healing of infarcts are marked by fibrosis, which may cause considerable distortion of residual entrapped epithelium, producing a pattern that may be mistaken histologically for carcinoma (25). Squamous metaplasia sometimes develops in the reparative epithelium that proliferates after infarction, and calcification may form in the infarcted tissue (25).

Infarcted carcinoma can be distinguished from infarction of a benign lesion if there is a residual intact component of *in situ* or invasive carcinoma (Fig. 3.4) (27). The occurrence of rare instances of seemingly totally infarcted carcinoma is more problematic, but most of these lesions have a ghost architecture that is recognizable with a reticulin stain or cytokeratin immunostain. A sclerotic or thrombosed blood vessel

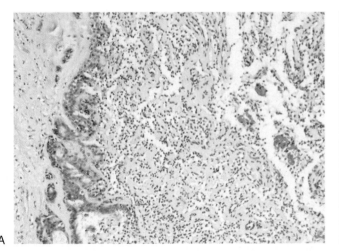
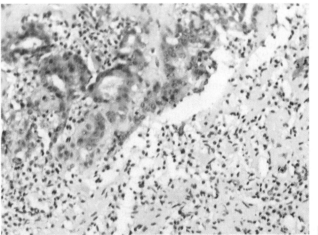

A                                                                                                                    B

**FIG. 3.3.** *Postpartum infarct in sclerosing adenosis.* **A:** A zone of residual epithelium on the left borders on the infarct. **B:** Only the nuclei of myoepithelial cells remain in the infarct on the right to outline the spaces formerly occupied by adenosis glands. A few partially preserved glands persist on the left.

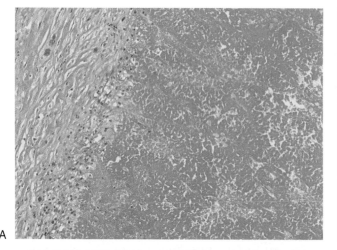

A

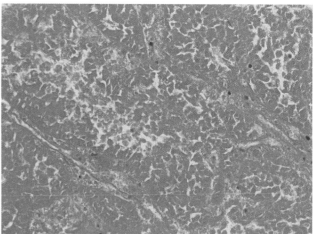

B

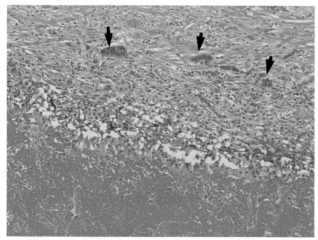

C

**FIG. 3.4.** *Infarcted papillary carcinoma.* **A:** The entire lesion is necrotic and surrounded by a granulomatous reaction. **B:** The ghost architecture of the tumor is evident. The abundant epithelial component suggests papillary carcinoma. **C:** Invasive carcinoma persisting in the wall of the tumor *(arrows).*

sometimes is identified in the surrounding tissue (27). Whereas focal necrosis is considered to be an unfavorable prognostic feature of ordinary invasive carcinoma, the prognosis of nearly or totally infarcted carcinoma is not well characterized. Two patients described by Jones et al. (27) had negative lymph nodes and were free of disease 12 months after diagnosis.

**Treatment and Prognosis**

Biopsy, usually excision of the lesion, is required for the diagnosis of a mammary infarct, although the findings in a needle core biopsy may be suggestive. Infarction occurs more often in benign papillary tumors than in papillary carcinoma. Instances of totally infarcted solid papillary carcinoma have been encountered. In these cases, the nature of the tumor was determined from the characteristic distribution of fibrovascular stroma. Follow-up data for patients with totally infarcted carcinomas are anecdotal. A favorable prognosis would be expected for a patient with noninvasive, infarcted, solid papillary carcinoma.

Epithelial hyperplasia that is reparative may be found in or near infarcts. Squamous metaplasia also occurs in association with these lesions. There is no documented evidence that proliferative changes related to infarcts are associated with an increased risk for carcinoma.

**INFLAMMATORY LESIONS IN PREGNANCY AND LACTATION**

*Puerperal mastitis* typically occurs within 2 to 3 weeks of the start of lactation and usually is the result of infection via the mammary duct system. The most common organism is *Staphylococcus aureus* transmitted from the infant (28). Accumulation of milk in ducts and lobules creates a microenvironment that fosters bacterial growth. Without prompt antibiotic treatment, the condition may progress to form an abscess. At a chronic stage, fistulas can develop that require drainage. The histologic appearance of specimens from these lesions depends on the chronicity of the process, varying from acute inflammation that may be accompanied by focal necrosis, to organized chronic abscesses. Excisional biopsy may be required to control chronic lesions with fistula formation.

*Mammary infarcts* formed during pregnancy present as discrete, firm tumors that may or may not be tender. The lesion usually is detected in the third trimester or shortly after delivery. The affected area forms a well-demarcated tumor

1 cm or more in diameter that appears distinct from the surrounding hyperplastic parenchyma. Multiple infarcts are uncommon (29). On the cut surface, part or all of the tissue has the yellow color of coagulative necrosis. Grossly and microscopically, the distinction between infarction in a lactational fibroadenoma and breast parenchyma with lactational hyperplasia is not always clear. Infarcts that presumably have been present for several weeks before detection are likely to be surrounded by a granulation tissue reaction in which calcification may occur (29).

The pathogenesis of pregnancy-related infarcts is uncertain. Although the finding of thrombi in some cases suggests that this may be a factor, no consistent explanation for vascular occlusion has been established, and it is possible that the vascular changes are secondary to infarction initiated by some other mechanism.

Most *galactoceles* occur in adult women during pregnancy, but the lesion has been described in male and female infants (30). Galactocele associated with chronic galactorrhea caused by a pituitary adenoma has been reported (31). The tumors present as solitary or multiple circumscribed masses that may be unilateral or bilateral. The lesions average about 2 cm in diameter, but galactoceles 5 cm or larger have been described (31). Mammography reveals a circumscribed density that, in many instances, has a characteristic appearance consisting of a hypodense upper area and a lower area with density close to that of the surrounding tissue (32,33). The interface tends to remain horizontal as the patient changes position. The two zones consist of lighter lipid-containing components above the water-based constituents of the fluid. Comparable differences in echogenicity are observed on ultrasound examination (32).

Necrotic cells and nuclear debris, possibly accompanied by inflammatory cells, are seen in an FNA specimen (34). Cells with hyperchromatic, atypical-appearing nuclei may suggest carcinoma, but in this inflammatory background such changes should not be considered definitive. Birefringent crystals were found in the aspirate from one galactocele (35). Needle core biopsy cannot be relied on in all cases. Excisional biopsy is diagnostic and provides adequate therapy.

On gross inspection, a galactocele is composed of cysts that contain fluid contents resembling milk and are lined by smooth epithelium. Inspissated secretion may be present in the form of soft caseous material. The cysts appear to be formed as a result of duct dilation. Microscopically, the cysts are lined by cuboidal or flat epithelial cells with cytoplasmic vacuolization due to lipid accumulation (Fig. 3.5). Apocrine metaplasia may be seen (30). When intact, the cysts are encompassed by a fibrous wall of varying thickness with little or no inflammatory reaction. Leakage from a cyst elicits a chronic inflammatory reaction that may be accompanied by fat necrosis.

Most patients are treated by aspiration of the cyst contents. A milk fistula is a rare complication of incomplete surgical excision (31).

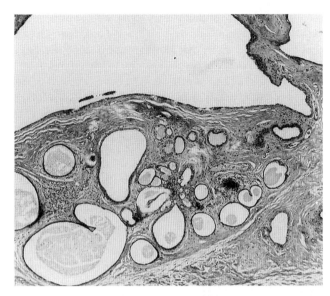

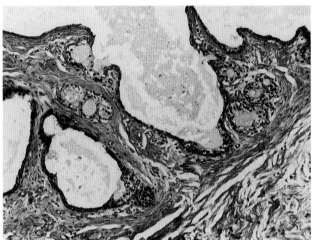

**FIG. 3.5.** *Galactocele.* **A:** Intact cysts. **B:** Cuboidal epithelium and secretion in the cysts.

*Raynaud's phenomenon* has been described in the nipple, especially in breast-feeding women (36). The resultant pain leads to cessation of breast-feeding. Clinical manifestations precipitated by cold and breast-feeding includes pain, blanching of the nipple, as well as cracked nipples, and ulcers or blisters of the nipple surface.

## PLASMA CELL MASTITIS

### Clinical Presentation

This condition is an extreme form of periductal mastitis that features an intense plasmacytic reaction to retained secretion in ducts. Ten patients described by Adair (37) were 29 to 44 years old, average 36 years, and all had been pregnant. The average interval between cessation of lactation and the onset of symptoms was 4 years. In the early phase, patients experienced the acute onset of mild pain, tenderness, redness, and nipple discharge consisting usually of thick secretion. After the inflammatory symptoms subsided, the skin appeared edematous over a firm-to-hard mass several centimeters in diameter that remained at the same site. Nipple discharge usually persisted, and nipple retraction was observed in the majority of patients. The mass occurred in the periphery of the breast or in a subareolar location. Axillary lymph nodes often were enlarged.

### Gross Pathology

The affected ill-defined area consists of indurated, mammary parenchyma in which there are dilated ducts containing thick, creamy secretion. Some of the affected ducts appear to be cysts. Punctate yellow or golden areas of xanthomatous granuloma may be observed.

### Microscopic Pathology

On histologic examination, two features that distinguish plasma cell mastitis are hyperplasia of ductal epithelium and a marked, diffuse, plasma cell infiltrate surrounding these ducts as well as the lobules. A histiocytic reaction, sometimes with granulomatous features, to the desquamated epithelium and lipid material in the ducts is responsible for areas that grossly appear to be xanthomatous and for the comedo-like character of the duct contents (Fig. 3.6) (38). Lymphocytes and neutrophils are variably present, but not in sufficient numbers to obscure the plasmacytic reaction. Periductal fibrosis and obliterative proliferation of granulation tissue are not prominent features of plasma cell mastitis.

### Prognosis and Treatment

Plasma cell mastitis in its acute and mature phases is difficult to distinguish clinically from mammary carcinoma (35,39). Redness and edema in the early stage are suggestive of inflammatory carcinoma. The residual nontender mass is easily mistaken for carcinoma on palpation, and the radio-

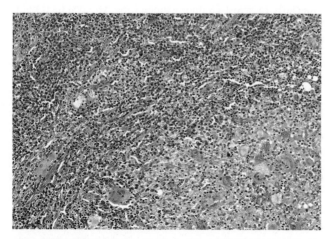

**FIG. 3.6.** *Plasma cell mastitis.* An intense infiltrate of lymphocytes and plasma cells surrounding a zone of histiocytic infiltration with xanthomatous features (*lower right*).

logic findings may be interpreted as indicative of carcinoma, especially when calcifications are present. FNA biopsy yields a specimen consisting of inflammatory cells in which plasma cells and histiocytes are especially conspicuous. Hyperplastic epithelial cells, which may appear very atypical, can be mistaken for carcinoma in this setting. Similar difficulty is likely to be encountered if the tissue is examined by frozen section. Ultimately, the histologic distinction between plasma cell mastitis and comedocarcinoma depends on careful analysis of paraffin sections.

Excisional biopsy is the recommended treatment for plasma cell mastitis because cutaneous ulceration and fistulas may develop after the lesion has been incised or only partially removed. Generally, surgery to remove the mass is performed after the acute phase has subsided. On occasion, the acute stage may resolve without a persistent tumor.

## MAMMARY DUCT ECTASIA

The term *mammary duct ectasia* (MDE) was introduced by Haagensen (40) in 1951, but the disease had been recognized at least 30 years earlier. In 1921, Bloodgood (41) included this condition, characterized as "diffuse dilatation of the ducts," under the heading of "chronic cystic mastitis," and he described assisting Halsted in operating on such a patient in 1897. At surgery, a clinically "indefinite palpable tumor beneath the nipple . . . proved to be a dilated duct with a thick wall about the size of a slate pencil (5 mm), tortuous and filled with a brown, granular mass." They did not regard this to be a malignant condition but ". . . concluded that it was safer to perform the complete operation for cancer." Bloodgood (42) later used the term *varicocele of the breast* for cases with prominent subareolar duct dilation. Other names such as mastitis obliterans and comedomastitis (43) have not been as widely used as MDE, which is the preferred diagnostic term. The clinical and pathologic features of MDE, granulomatous lobular mastitis, and plasma cell mastitis are sufficiently different in most cases that these lesions should be distinguishable. In instances where the findings lack specificity, the condition may be diagnosed as mastitis, modified by appropriate descriptive terms.

The etiology of MDE is not known. Some authors believe that duct dilation caused by glandular atrophy and involution in older women is the primary pathologic process leading to stasis of secretion, which is followed by leakage of lipid material through the walls of the ducts to elicit periductal inflammation (40,44). Other authors have concluded that periductal inflammation is the underlying abnormality responsible for duct sclerosis, obliteration, and ectasia (43,45,46). The latter authors considered stasis caused by duct obstruction to be the process responsible for inciting the inflammatory reaction that contributed to further obstructive changes as well as to duct dilation. Parity and breast-feeding are not factors predisposing to the development of MDE (47). In some cases, squamous metaplasia of the terminal lactiferous duct epithelium results in obstruction that contributes to the development of duct ectasia and eventually to the formation of lactiferous duct fistulas (Fig. 3.7) (48,49).

Cigarette smoking has been associated with the development of periductal mastitis and MDE and with an increased risk for fistula formation (50,51). The mechanism is thought to be mediated through the effects of smoking on the bacterial flora of the mammary ducts.

MDE, galactorrhea, and lipogranulomatous mastitis have been associated with prolonged phenothiazine treatment (52). MDE was found in three patients who had hyperprolactinemia caused by pituitary adenomas (53). Slightly elevated serum prolactin was detected in a 3-year-old boy with bilateral MDE (54). These isolated cases suggest that hyperprolactinemia may play a role in the development of MDE in some patients. Galactorrhea and lactational hyperplasia do not ordinarily precede the development of MDE. The relationship has not been studied sufficiently to determine if this is more than a sporadic association.

## Clinical Presentation

The earliest symptom is spontaneous, intermittent nipple discharge that usually is clear, yellow, green, or brown. There may be no palpable abnormality. The discharge gives a positive test for blood in about 50% of patients. In more advanced cases, subareolar induration progresses to the formation of a mass. Occasionally, dilated ducts may be palpable as "one or more doughy, worm-like masses beneath the nipple" (42). Pain usually is reported among the early symptoms and tends to be more frequent in young women, whereas nipple inversion or retraction is described more often at a later age (55). The mean age of patients with pain (39.9 years) or a lump (42.7 years) was younger than that of patients who had painless (47.1 years) and nonpalpable (42.7 years) MDE. On the other hand, women with nipple retraction (53.4 years) were older than those without this abnor-

mality (43.4 years). The presence of nipple inversion generally is associated with periductal fibrosis and contracture. Well-established mass lesions may be painful and tender, with the symptoms accentuated in the premenstrual phase of the cycle. When the onset is acute, the clinical findings suggest an abscess. If allowed to persist, the subareolar inflammatory lesion may develop into a mamillary or lactiferous duct fistula (56).

MDE has been found in women younger than 30 (47,57) and in patients over 80 years of age (47), but rarely in men (58). Approximately two-thirds of the female patients are between 40 and 70 years old. The median age in one series of 34 patients was 44 years (57).

Mammography reveals a variety of changes associated with MDE. Sweeney and Wylie (59) reported that 12 of 1,437 women who underwent biopsy in a series of screened women had MDE. The mammographic abnormalities included microcalcifications, spiculated masses, and lobulated partially smooth masses. In some instances, the mammographic findings suggested carcinoma.

## Gross Pathology

At surgery, obviously dilated ducts are identified through a circumareolar incision and removed in a segmental excision with the apex in the nipple. The specimen usually consists of firm breast tissue in which there are prominent ducts that contain pasty or granular secretion. The duct contents vary greatly in color, but most often the secretion is white, cream colored, or brown. Many ducts appear dilated and thick walled as a consequence of periductal fibrosis. Calcification sometimes is apparent grossly in the dilated ducts. Abscess-like yellow necrotic areas can be found in the most severe cases, and these areas may be the site of cholesterol granulomas and calcification (38). In addition, the stroma between ducts may be fibrotic and contain cysts.

## Microscopic Pathology

The microscopic composition of the duct contents often is varied in a given case. In its most bland form, it consists of eosinophilic, granular or amorphous, proteinaceous material. Usually, there is an admixture of lipid-containing foam cells (so-called colostrum cells) and desquamated duct epithelial cells (Fig. 3.8). The origin of foam cells remains controversial. Davies (60,61) concluded that they were macrophages derived from the periductal mononuclear inflammatory infiltrate. Other authors have suggested that the foam cells are altered epithelial or myoepithelial cells (62). Derivation of foam cells from altered epithelial or myoepithelial cells may be suggested by the way in which foam cells sometimes are found distributed in the epithelial layer (Fig. 3.9). Myoepithelial and apocrine cells with cytoplasmic clearing bear a superficial resemblance to foam cells. Immunohistochemical study has demonstrated the histiocytic character of some foam cells with reactivity for CD68,

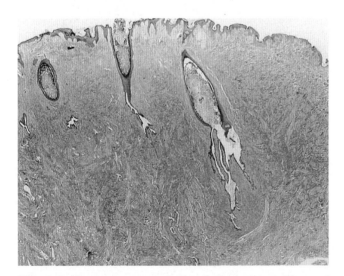

**FIG. 3.7.** *Squamous metaplasia of nipple ducts.* Plugs of desquamated keratin fill the terminal portions of the lactiferous ducts in the nipple at sites of squamous metaplasia.

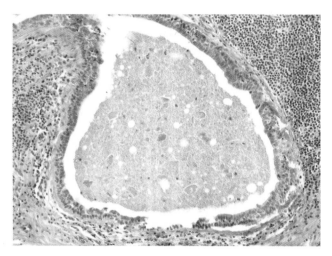

**FIG. 3.8.** *Duct stasis.* The lumen of this dilated duct contains granular secretion and degenerated epithelial cells. A lymphocytic reaction surrounds the duct.

HAM56, MAC387, lysozyme, and $\alpha_1$-antitrypsin, and absence of staining for cytokeratins (63).

A detailed study of mammary foam cells in the epithelium, stroma, and gland lumens was reported by Damiani et al. (64). Immunohistochemistry revealed that three types of cells were described by the term foam cell. Some were epithelial cells, immunoreactive for epithelial membrane antigen and cytokeratin, with apocrine differentiation manifested by the presence of gross cystic disease fluid protein 15 (GCDFP-15) demonstrated by immunohistochemistry and *in situ* hybridization. Another group of cells consisted of macrophages with immunoreactivity for MAC387 and CD68. A third cell type with intermediate features was immunoreactive for CD68 and GCDFP-15. These cells also had a peripheral rim of cytokeratin positivity. This latter group of cells lacked GCDFP-15 mRNA when examined by *in situ* hybridization. Epithelial foam cells were within glandular lumens and apparently originated in the surrounding

epithelium. Macrophage foam cells were stromal, intraluminal, or pagetoid in their distribution, whereas intermediate foam cells were pagetoid and intraluminal. The authors were unable to determine whether intermediate cells were histogenetically macrophagic or epithelial.

Histiocytes that contain ceroid pigment were termed ochrocytes by Davies (65) (Fig. 3.10). These cells are immunoreactive with markers of macrophage differentiation (66). Hamperl (62) described these foam cells as "fluorocytes" because the pigment is autofluorescent in ultraviolet light. Ochrocytes and foam cells occur within the epithelial–myoepithelial layer of ducts, in periductal tissue, and in duct lumens.

Inflammatory changes in the walls of ducts and periductal tissues are a prominent part of the pathologic findings in MDE (Fig. 3.11). Inflammation featuring lymphocytes with smaller numbers of plasma cells, neutrophils, and histiocytes is present circumferentially throughout the thickness of the duct and in the periductal stroma. Disruption of ducts is accompanied by discharge of stasis material into the breast, causing more intense periductal reaction and resulting in abscess formation (Fig. 3.12). There usually is an abundant lipid component, which elicits a prominent lipophagic histiocytic reaction bordered by an infiltrate of lymphocytes, plasma cells, neutrophils, and variable numbers of multinucleated histiocytes. Plasma cells and granulomas are not conspicuous features of the lesion in most cases.

Cholesterol granuloma is an uncommon complication of periductal mastitis (38,67). Findings on clinical examination and mammography may suggest carcinoma because of the localized nature of the lesion. Histologic examination reveals groups of cholesterol crystals encased by histocytes

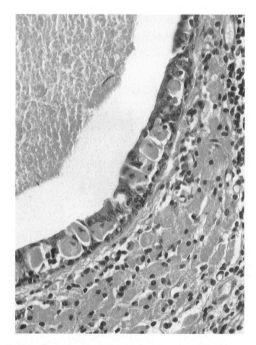

**FIG. 3.10.** *Ochrocytes in duct stasis.* Histiocytes with eosinophilic cytoplasm (ochrocytes) in the stroma around an ectatic duct and in the epithelium of the duct.

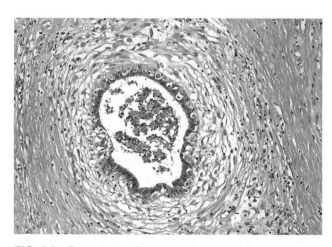

**FIG. 3.9.** *Duct stasis.* Histiocytes (ochrocytes) with granular cytoplasm are present within the duct epithelium and in the surrounding stroma.

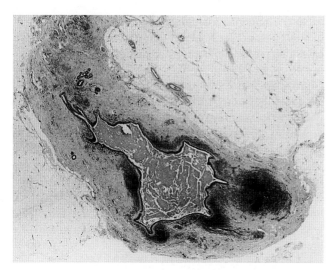

**FIG. 3.11.** *Duct ectasia and stasis.* A dilated duct containing stasis material with nodular periductal lymphocytic infiltrates. (From Rosen PP, Oberman HA. Tumors of the mammary gland. In: *Atlas of tumor pathology.* Washington, DC: Armed Forces Institute of Pathology, 1993, with permission.)

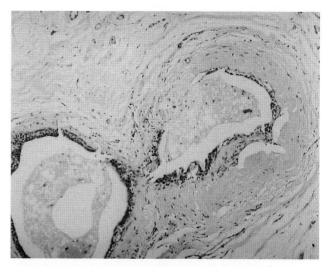

**FIG. 3.13.** *Duct ectasia.* Focal disruption of an ectatic duct with discharge of duct contents into the periductal stroma. (From Rosen PP, Oberman HA. Tumors of the mammary gland. In: *Atlas of tumor pathology.* Washington, DC: Armed Forces Institute of Pathology, 1993, with permission.)

and giant cells with surrounding granulomatous zones of histiocytes, lymphocytes, plasma cells, and fibroblastic reaction. The remnants of ectatic ducts sometimes can be identified within cholesterol granulomas as well as in the surrounding tissue.

Periductal fibrosis and hyperelastosis, often with a lamellar distribution, lead to mural thickening. The inflammatory reaction typically spreads throughout the fibrous periductal collar into the surrounding breast stroma (Fig. 3.13). The duct epithelium is atrophic, flat, and inconspicuous. Epithelial hyperplasia is not a feature of MDE, but it may be found as a component of proliferative breast changes that are coincidentally present.

In a late phase, the inflammatory reaction is less conspicuous but the ducts become encased in a thick laminated layer of hyaline fibrous and elastic tissue (Fig. 3.14) (45). The duct lumen may be patulous, but in some instances the sclerotic process includes actively proliferating granulation tissue and hyperelastosis, which narrows and may totally occlude ducts (68). The latter configuration has been termed *mastitis obliterans* (Fig. 3.15) (46). Remnants of persisting epithelium may proliferate to form secondary glands within the sclerotic duct, creating a pattern that resembles a recanalized, healed thrombus in a blood vessel. When the epithelium is totally absent, the duct is reduced to a linear fibrous scar. Residual hyperelastotic tissue and histiocytes sometimes are evident,

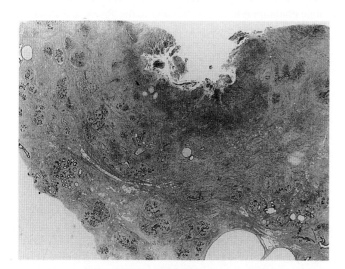

**FIG. 3.12.** *Duct ectasia with abscess.* An abscess associated with duct ectasia is evident in the lower central part of this photograph from the same case as shown Fig. 3.5B.

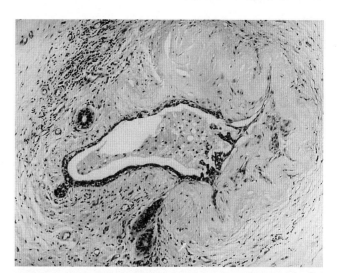

**FIG. 3.14.** *Duct ectasia with fibrosis.* Reactive fibrosis formed in the region of prior duct disruption. Histiocytes are present in the duct lumen.

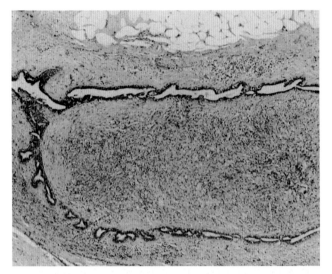

**FIG. 3.15.** *Duct ectasia with mastitis obliterans.* A polyp composed of granulation tissue has obliterated most of the duct lumen.

but on occasion the only evidence is a band or ring of eosinophilic collagenous tissue.

The inflammatory reaction is concentrated in and around major lactiferous ducts, but it also extends into peripheral ducts and lobules. This lobulitis typically features a lymphocytic reaction without granulomas. Plasma cells, acinar dilation, and stasis of intralobular secretion are not conspicuous. There is no evidence of lobular hyperplasia or increased secretory activity in such lobules. Stasis of secretion with mild ectasia may occur in the terminal duct.

An unusual variant of duct stasis and periductal mastitis features multinucleated histiocytic reaction within the duct lumen, apparently elicited by secretion (Fig. 3.16).

### Treatment and Prognosis

The diagnosis of MDE may be suggested by symptoms and clinical findings, but these are not sufficiently specific to

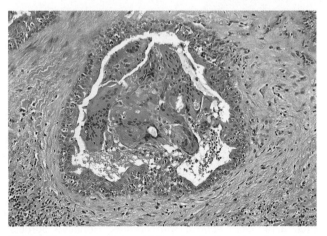

**FIG. 3.16.** *Duct ectasia with intraluminal multinucleated histiocytes.*

exclude carcinoma. Mammography can be helpful, but a radiologic distinction between comedocarcinoma and MDE cannot be made with confidence in all cases. The diagnosis usually is established by excising the affected area. A circumareolar incision is used to expose the dilated ducts. These are transected at the base of the nipple and excised with a conical segment of the surrounding tissue. In more severe cases, the mass formed by reaction to ruptured ducts also is excised with the affected segmental ducts. Incision and drainage of MDE that has been mistaken clinically for an infection with abscess formation may lead to fistula formation (57). Asynchronous involvement of the contralateral breast sometimes is encountered. MDE is not associated with an increased risk for subsequent carcinoma of the breast.

## GRANULOMATOUS LOBULAR MASTITIS

Numerous pathogenic processes responsible for granulomatous inflammation of the breast can be included under the generic heading of granulomatous mastitis (69). In the absence of a specific etiologic agent, the term granulomatous lobular mastitis has been adopted for these lesions (70–73). Kessler and Wolloch (74) drew attention to the distinction between granulomatous and plasma cell mastitis. Going et al. (72) recommended the term *granulomatous lobular mastitis* (GLM) to separate the lesion from granulomatous forms of periductal mastitis. The diagnosis of postlactational granulomatous mastitis (75) is less satisfactory, because the lesion may develop as long as 15 years postpartum (72).

The etiology of GLM is unknown. No microorganism has been consistently isolated from the tissue, and histochemical stains for pathogens are routinely negative. The perilobular distribution and granulomatous character of the inflammation suggest a cell-mediated reaction to one or more substances concentrated in the mammary secretion or lobular cells, but no specific antigen has been identified. An autoimmune phenomenon seems unlikely in the absence of vasculitis or a prominent plasma cell component in the reactive infiltrate (75).

### Clinical Presentation

The lesion usually appears after, rather than during, pregnancy. Because the mean interval between the last pregnancy and the diagnosis of GLM is 2 years, there does not appear to be an association with breast-feeding. A relationship to oral contraceptive use was suggested in one study in which eight of nine patients had used these medications (72), and other authors reported an increased incidence of GLM in women taking oral contraceptives (76). It is thought that oral contraceptives induce hyperplasia in lobular ductules leading to obstructive desquamation of ductular epithelial cells, distention of ductules, and ultimately a perilobular inflammatory reaction. One patient had hyperprolactinemia associated with phenothiazine treatment, and prolactin levels reportedly were normal in two other patients (72). Coexistent erythema nodosum was present in one patient (77).

The age at diagnosis ranged from 17 to 42 years, with a mean of about 33 years (72). Virtually all patients were parous. Women with GLM typically presented with a distinct, firm-to-hard mass that involved any part of the breast but tended to spare the subareolar region. Bilateral involvement was uncommon (75). Nipple discharge usually was not present. The tumor sometimes was tender. Axillary nodal enlargement or tenderness were rarely encountered. The breast tumors reportedly measured from 1 cm to as much as 8 cm, averaging nearly 6 cm. The clinical findings often suggested carcinoma, and mammography also was described as "suspicious" (75). Variable mammographic findings in one study included multiple small masses or asymmetric density without calcification or spiculation (78). The lesions were hypoechoic on sonography, and more of them were detected by the latter method than by mammography. The sonograms were characterized by "multiple clustered, often contiguous tubular hypoechoic lesions" (78).

## Gross Pathology

The specimen typically consists of firm-to-hard mammary parenchyma that contains a palpably distinct mass. The margins are less apparent on visual inspection of the cut surface where the gray-to-tan tissue appears to have a faintly nodular architecture. In some cases, the nodules appear to be small foci of abscess formation, but confluent abscesses are not a characteristic feature of GLM.

## Microscopic Pathology

The primary pathologic change in GLM is a granulomatous inflammatory reaction centered on lobules, a granulomatous lobulitis (Fig. 3.17). Granulomas composed of epithelioid histiocytes, Langhans giant cells accompanied by

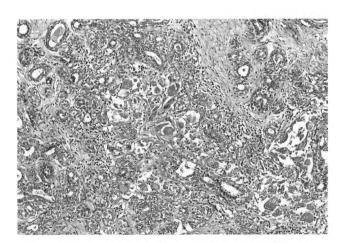

**FIG. 3.17.** *Granulomatous lobular mastitis.* Lobular inflammation with a lymphocytic component involving a lobule. Multinucleated histiocytes are present in the center of the lesion.

lymphocytes, plasma cells, and occasional eosinophils are found within and around lobules. The same cellular components are present in FNA smears from these lesions (79,80). Asteroid bodies are unusual, and Schaumann bodies have not been reported in the giant cells formed in GLM.

With progression of the inflammatory process, confluent granulomas may obscure or obliterate the lobulocentric distribution of the process, particularly toward the central portion of the tumor. Fat necrosis, abscess formation, and fibrosis contribute to effacement of the lobular distribution in confluent lesions (Fig. 3.18) (75). A space that develops in the center of the abscesses contains no foreign material or demonstrable secretion. It is likely that lipid from degenerating cells contained in these spaces is dissolved during histologic processing of the tissue. A narrow zone of neutrophils usually outlines this space. No microorganisms are demonstrable with special stains. Focal lactational changes can be encountered in lobules in recently parous women. Ducts incorporated in the lesion may become dilated and exhibit periductal or intraductal inflammation, but usually this is relatively inconspicuous. Affected ducts and lobules do not ordinarily contain refractile or birefringent crystalline material or calcifications in GLM. Squamous metaplasia of duct and lobular epithelium is unusual. Vasculitis is not seen in GLM. Stains and cultures for bacteria, acid-fast organisms, and fungi are negative. *S. aureus* was isolated from one patient (72).

The differential diagnosis includes a variety of lesions. The distinction between GLM and various other granulomatous inflammatory conditions, such as tuberculosis, sarcoidosis, and cat scratch disease, usually can be made by correlating the clinical and pathologic findings. It is critically important that granulomatous reaction in carcinoma also be considered. Whereas most examples of this unusual complex have areas composed of easily identified intraductal or invasive carcinoma, the associated carcinoma sometimes is obscured by this reaction (81). In rare cases, immunohistochemical stains for cytokeratin or other epithelial markers may be necessary to identify carcinoma in this background.

## Prognosis and Treatment

When the diagnosis of GLM has not been suspected clinically, primary treatment often has been excisional biopsy. Persistence or recurrence of the inflammatory process that may lead to skin ulceration have been described after biopsy (71,72), but in many patients, the disease is self-limiting and controlled by a single operation. Antibiotics may be helpful, especially if secondary infection occurs. Corticosteroids have been effective in resolving the lesions after a specific infectious etiology has been ruled out (82,83). In some cases, prolonged treatment with steroids is necessary to prevent or control recurrences (83). Sarcoidosis also should be considered in the differential diagnosis clinically. Patients presenting with the characteristic clinical and pathologic features of

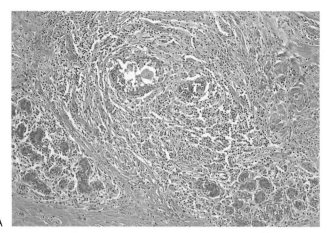

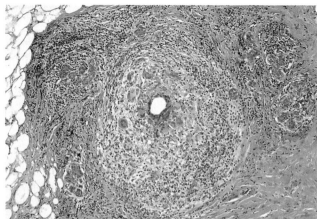

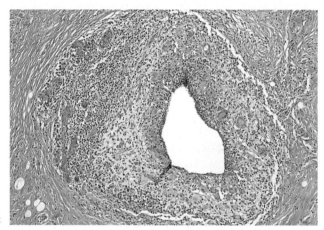

**FIG. 3.18.** *Abscesses in granulomatous lobular mastitis.* These images from a single specimen illustrate progressive destruction of lobules leading to abscess formation. **A:** An early stage where the inflammatory reaction consists mainly of lymphocytes. **B:** The lobule shown here is entirely engulfed by inflammation with a characteristic lamellar distribution. The lymphoplasmacytic reaction at the periphery surrounds a histiocytic zone with giant cells. A thin layer of neutrophils outlines a central, empty lumen. **C:** Part of the lobule remains on the left in this lesion with a large central vacuole.

GLM have not had evidence of systemic granulomatous inflammation, and Kveim tests in a minority of patients were negative (72).

## SARCOIDOSIS

### Clinical Presentation

Systemic sarcoidosis may affect the breast. The women tend to be in their 20s and 30s, reflecting the age distribution of sarcoidosis. One patient was 65 years old (84). Mammary lesions usually are detected after the diagnosis has been established on the basis of the typical clinical manifestations of the disease. Only very rarely does sarcoidosis present as a primary breast tumor, usually accompanied by lymph node enlargement (84,85). Early reports published before the distinction between sarcoidosis and tuberculosis was well recognized may have misclassified some cases of tuberculosis as sarcoidosis. The breast lesion caused by mammary sarcoidosis is a firm-to-hard mass that may be mistaken clinically for carcinoma (86). The mammographic, ultrasound, and magnetic resonance imaging (MRI) characteristics of mammary sarcoidosis are not specific and can be interpreted as suggestive of carcinoma (87), especially if a spiculated lesion is seen on mammography (88).

### Gross Pathology

The excised specimen consists of firm-to-hard, tan tissue that may have well-defined or indistinct borders. Calcification and necrosis are not features of sarcoidosis involving the breast. Tumors up to 5 cm in diameter have been reported.

### Microscopic Pathology

Microscopic examination reveals epithelioid granulomas forming nodules in the mammary parenchyma among lobules and ducts (Fig. 3.19). Multinucleated Langhans giant cells that accompany the granulomas may form asteroid or Schaumann bodies. The lesions do not have caseous necrosis or calcification, and fat necrosis is not found in the surrounding breast. Traces of fibrinoid necrosis may be found in cellular lesions. A lymphoplasmacytic reaction and fibrosis are present in varying amounts. Small, isolated granulomas with a sparse lymphocytic reaction can be found in breast tissue that appears grossly to be unaffected. These inconspicuous granulomatous foci tend to be associated with ducts or lobules.

The differential diagnosis includes many specific agents, such as tuberculosis, leprosy, brucellosis, and other bacterial infections, various fungi, parasitic infestations (70), and

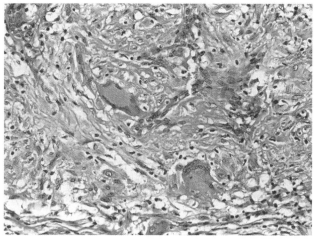

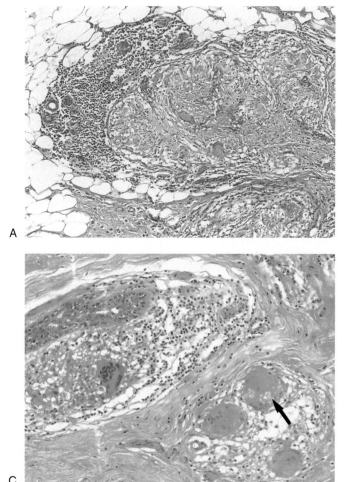

**FIG. 3.19.** *Sarcoidosis.* **A:** Confluent nonnecrotizing granulomas with giant cells involving a lobule. **B:** Remnants of an intralobular ductule surrounded by granulomatous inflammation. **C:** Granulomas next to a duct and in the stroma. An asteroid body is present in a histiocyte on the *right (arrow).*

rheumatoid nodules (89). Lesions caused by miliary tuberculosis may lack caseous necrosis. It is necessary to exclude the presence of acid-fast or other bacteria and fungi with cultures, histochemical stains, and appropriate clinical tests. These studies are indicated even in patients with previously diagnosed sarcoidosis, because they can develop secondary infections, especially when receiving corticosteroid treatment. The diagnosis of mammary sarcoidosis is established by excluding other potential etiologic agents.

Nonnecrotizing sarcoid-like granulomatous inflammation can develop in lymph nodes draining organs that harbor carcinoma (90). This phenomenon has been documented in the lymph nodes of patients with mammary carcinoma who have no clinical evidence of sarcoidosis (90–92). Bässler and Birke (91) reported sarcoid-like granulomas in axillary lymph nodes from 0.7% of patients with breast carcinoma. Similar granulomatous foci were found in the stroma of 0.3% of mammary carcinomas (Fig. 3.20) (91). Some patients who have sarcoid-like granulomas associated with a carcinoma develop similar lesions in their axillary lymph nodes (91); other patients do not manifest granulomatous lymphadenitis (93). Systemic manifestations of sarcoidosis may be mistaken clinically or radiologically for metastatic

carcinoma in a patient with known mammary carcinoma (94).

Histologically, it can be difficult to distinguish carcinoma-associated sarcoid-like reactions from coexistent carcinoma in a patient with sarcoidosis (95,96). The lymph node lesions of Boeck's sarcoid and sarcoid-like reactions are identical, especially when the granulomas are composed entirely of epithelioid histiocytes. Both have Langhans giant cells, asteroid and Schaumann bodies, and focal fibrinoid necrosis (90). However, little or no fibrosis is encountered in carcinoma-associated axillary lymph node granulomas, whereas long-standing sarcoidosis is likely to be accompanied by fibrosis.

Within the breast, the carcinoma-associated granulomatous reaction is restricted to the tumor and immediately surrounding mammary parenchyma. Necrosis has been noted in a minority of the carcinomas that had sarcoid-like granulomas. In one case, amyloid deposition accompanied the granulomatous reaction associated with a poorly differentiated carcinoma (97). Electron microscopy confirmed the presence of tubular amyloid. Collagenization has been described in mammary sarcoid granulomas (95). Sarcoid-like granulomas were found associated with both tumors in two patients who developed bilateral asynchronous carcinomas within

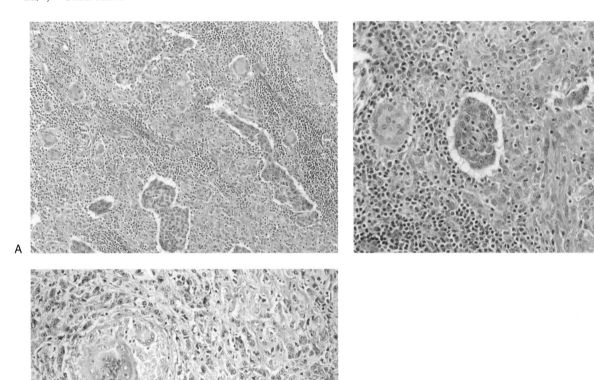

**FIG. 3.20.** *Sarcoid-like granulomas in carcinoma.* **A:** Infiltrating duct carcinoma with granulomatous inflammation. **B:** Histiocytes, lymphocytes, and a giant cell around infiltrating carcinoma. **C:** Granulomatous reaction in metastatic carcinoma in an axillary lymph node.

intervals of 1 and 4 years, respectively (91). A granulomatous reaction accompanied the chest wall recurrence in one of these patients.

### Prognosis and Treatment

The clinical course of women who have generalized sarcoidosis involving the breast depends on the extent of the underlying disease. The presence of granulomatous inflammation may be suggested in a needle aspirate of the breast, but the cytologic features are not sufficiently specific to distinguish sarcoidosis from other granulomatous lesions (98). Mammary lesions are adequately managed by excisional biopsy, which is necessary to rule out carcinoma. Patients with advanced sarcoidosis may develop multiple, bilateral lesions. Despite significant impairment of cellular immunity associated with sarcoidosis and an increased incidence of malignant lymphoma and pulmonary carcinoma, there is no evidence that sarcoidosis influences the risk of developing

mammary carcinoma or the prognosis of carcinoma that develops in these women (99).

### INFLAMMATORY PSEUDOTUMOR

There is no well-characterized lesion of the breast that qualifies for this diagnosis. The diagnosis has been mistakenly applied to metaplastic carcinoma, granulomatous mastitis, fibromatosis and infarcts. Localized nodular lesions in the breast consisting of fibrovascular stroma with a prominent infiltrate composed mainly of plasma cells and lymphocytes have been diagnosed as inflammatory pseudotumors (Fig. 3.21) (100–102). Chetty and Govender (102) described three histologic patterns: nodular fasciitis, interlacing fascicles of spindle cells in variably collagenized stroma, and a hypocellular variant composed mainly of hyalinized collagen resembling a scar. The three cases described in their report had varied appearances with differing proportions of these elements.

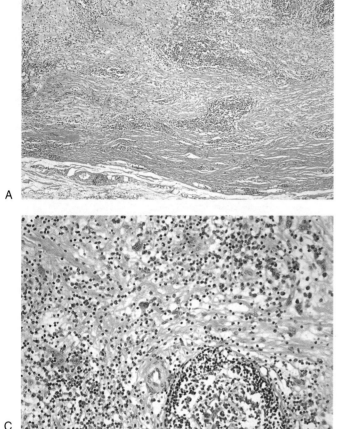

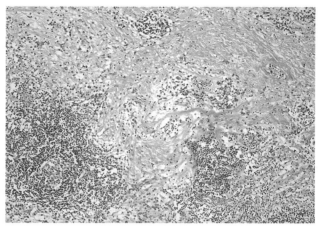

**FIG. 3.21.** *Inflammatory pseudotumor.* **A:** Peripheral fibrosis outlines the lesion. **B:** Lymphocytic infiltrates with germinal center formation in the midst of variably collagenized stroma. **C:** A few multinucleated histiocytes and scattered plasma cells are shown.

Four reported patients had a unilateral lesion that did not recur after excision, but follow-up rarely exceeded 1 year (101,102). Another patient with bilateral tumors developed recurrences in both breasts (100).

## VASCULITIS

Inflammatory lesions of blood vessels, particularly arteries, are encountered in a variety of systemic disorders which are broadly grouped under the heading of collagen-vascular disease. The breasts may be affected as an isolated manifestation or as part of multiorgan involvement. The mammary lesions caused by vasculitis often clinically resemble carcinoma. Although there are differences in the histopathologic features of the vasculitides associated with various collagen-vascular diseases, the diagnosis of a specific condition is made on the basis of both the clinical and pathologic findings.

### Giant Cell Arteritis

This condition typically involves the cranial arteries of elderly women who present with temporal headaches, visual impairment, fever, and other symptoms. Anemia and an ele-

vated erythrocyte sedimentation rate usually are present. In patients with appropriate symptoms, the diagnosis is confirmed by finding granulomatous arteritis with giant cells and destruction of elastica in a temporal artery biopsy specimen.

Giant cell arteritis limited clinically to the breast was first described by Waugh (103) in 1950, and there have been a number of subsequent case reports (104–109). The patients have been women 52 to 72 years of age. Almost all presented with one or more palpable breast tumors. An exceptional patient complained of pain and erythema in the upper outer quadrant of one breast (105). No mass was palpable or evident on a mammogram, and inflammatory carcinoma was suspected clinically. She also had palpable nontender temporal arteries. Biopsy of the breast revealed arteritis. The temporal arteries were not biopsied.

The lesions were bilateral in nearly 50% of cases. The firm-to-hard tender or painful tumors have measured from less than 1 to 4 cm, and carcinoma was suspected in most cases. Fixation to the skin was described in several cases; one patient had nipple retraction, and axillary nodal enlargement was noted in some cases (108,110). These features may suggest carcinoma clinically (108,111). Temporal artery biopsy revealed giant cell arteritis in one patient who had concomitant invasive mammary duct carcinoma and mammary arteritis (106). A 72-year-old woman with giant cell arteritis of the breast and polymyalgia was found to have necrotizing polyarteritis in a muscle biopsy (112).

Most patients with giant cell arteritis of the breast had few systemic symptoms, which may include headache, muscle and joint pain, fever, and night sweats. Mild anemia (hemoglobin 10 to 12 g/dL) and elevated erythrocyte sedimentation rate are found in most cases.

The excised specimen consists of ill-defined, rubbery, firm tissue. In one patient with bilateral lesions, each focus of arteritis contained a grossly enlarged, thickened, and thrombosed artery (103), but in most reports the vascular changes were not grossly evident. Microscopically, granulomatous inflammation involves small- and medium-sized arteries throughout the affected tissue (Fig. 3.22) (107,109). Veins and arterioles are spared. The reactive process consists of a transmural and perivascular infiltrate composed mainly of lymphocytes, histiocytes, and giant cells. Plasma cells, eosinophils, and scattered neutrophils also are seen. Fibrinoid necrosis is not a consistent feature, but fragmentation of the mural elastic fibers is demonstrable with an elastic tissue stain (Fig. 3.23). Multinucleated giant cells tend to be oriented around these disrupted elastic fibers. In some cases, giant cells are sparse and difficult to detect. The lumen may be narrowed or occluded by a recent blood clot, organizing thrombus, or laminated subintimal fibrosis. Calcification commonly develops in vessels that are the site of healed arteritis. The surrounding fibrofatty tissue exhibits changes as a consequence of the vascular lesions, which include fibrosis, edema, fat necrosis, and atrophy of glandular elements.

The diagnosis of giant cell arteritis of the breast is made by excisional biopsy. The differential diagnosis includes other types of arteritis, phlebitis, infarction related to preg-

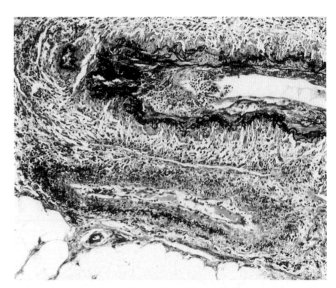

**FIG. 3.23.** *Giant cell arteritis.* Fragmentation of the internal elastica is evident in the artery. The inflammatory reaction involves a small adjacent vein (elastic van Gieson stain). (From Rosen PP, Oberman HA. Tumors of the mammary gland. In: *Atlas of tumor pathology.* Washington, DC: Armed Forces Institute of Pathology, 1993, with permission.)

nancy or lactation, and traumatic fat necrosis. Most patients were treated with adrenal corticosteroids and remained free of systemic symptoms with follow-up of 2 years or less. One patient had arteritis in a thyroid lobectomy performed for an adenoma shortly after a breast biopsy demonstrated arteritis (113). Complete resolution of systemic symptoms was reported without steroid therapy in one woman who had bilateral breast involvement (108).

### Wegener's Granulomatosis

This disease is characterized by necrotizing vasculitis affecting the upper and lower respiratory tract accompanied by glomerulonephritis (114). Rarely, the skin, joints, and visceral organs also are involved (115). The first case of Wegener's granulomatosis of the breast was reported by Elsner and Harper (116) in 1969. Additional patients described have been women 40 to 69 years of age (117–122) and a 40-year-old man with bilateral, ulcerated painless breast lesions (123). The tumor was unilateral in all but one female patient. In two women, the breast tumor was the initial indication of Wegener's granulomatosis (119,121). In four other patients, systemic manifestations were evident coincidental with (119) or shortly before (116,117,121) detection of a breast mass. Late onset of breast involvement 1 and 6 years after other symptoms has been described (120).

The clinical manifestations of Wegener's granulomatosis in the breast can mimic mammary carcinoma (124). The breast tumor usually is tender. In one case, nipple retraction and *peau d'orange* suggested inflammatory carcinoma (117). The presence of a breast mass and lung nodules may be regarded as evidence of advanced breast carcinoma.

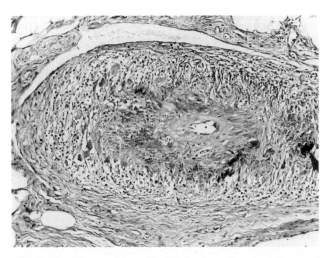

**FIG. 3.22.** *Giant cell arteritis.* Histiocytes, lymphocytes, and giant cells in the wall of an artery. The lumen is almost entirely occluded. Irregular calcifications are present *(arrow).* (From Rosen PP, Oberman HA. Tumors of the mammary gland. In: *Atlas of tumor pathology.* Washington, DC: Armed Forces Institute of Pathology, 1993, with permission.)

Mammography reveals a distinct dense lesion with irregular or stellate borders (117). Calcifications are absent. Regression following steroid and immunosuppressive treatment of unresected lesions diagnosed by FNA has been documented with mammography (117). However, the cytologic findings, consisting of inflammatory cells and evidence of necrosis, are nonspecific. Surgical biopsy is necessary to demonstrate necrotizing vasculitis affecting arteries and veins that characterizes this condition. The presence of the underlying vas-

culitis may not be appreciated when the specimen exhibits prominent fat necrosis (118). Infarcted portions of the lesion may resemble a carcinoma grossly (124).

Microscopic examination of the biopsy reveals acute and chronic inflammation of the mammary parenchyma and fat. Vessels in necrotic areas and in the surrounding breast exhibit inflammatory changes. Granulomatous foci are present in the surrounding breast and at the periphery of areas of infarcted breast tissue (Fig. 3.24).

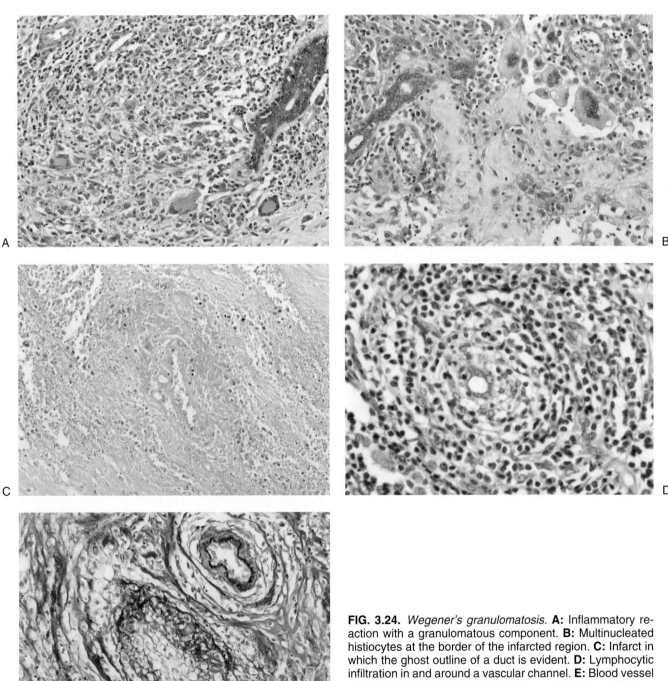

**FIG. 3.24.** *Wegener's granulomatosis.* **A:** Inflammatory reaction with a granulomatous component. **B:** Multinucleated histiocytes at the border of the infarcted region. **C:** Infarct in which the ghost outline of a duct is evident. **D:** Lymphocytic infiltration in and around a vascular channel. **E:** Blood vessel obstructed by the inflammatory process (elastic van Gieson stain). (Courtesy of Dr. Wolfgang Schneider). (From Göbel U, Kettritz R, Kettritz U, et al. Wegener's granulomatosis masquerading as breast cancer. *Arch Intern Med* 1995;155: 205–207, with permission.)

Treatment directed at systemic manifestations of the disease involves steroids, immunosuppressive drugs, and supportive management. Prognosis depends on the severity and extent of systemic involvement. Two of 10 patients described in the literature died of rapidly progressive systemic vasculitis within 6 months (116,120). The other patients were reportedly alive with or without evidence of Wegener's granulomatosis 2 to 6 years after diagnosis (117–121).

### Polyarteritis

There are several case reports of mammary involvement in polyarteritis (124–128). In most patients, a unilateral breast lesion was the initial manifestation. One woman with chronic polyarteritis developed a unilateral breast mass 18 years after the onset of her illness (127). In another case, bilateral involvement caused multiple painful breast nodules and became apparent after several months (126). Mammography revealed arterial calcification in a 37-year-old woman who had localized mammary arteritis (128). Postpartum development of a breast mass and cutaneous lesions have been reported in a 34-year-old woman (128a).

Microscopic examination of the breast biopsy reveals transmural necrotizing vasculitis without a giant cell reaction in the breast parenchyma. Eosinophils may be a prominent component of the mixed inflammatory cell infiltrate. The process involves arterial vessels of varying size, including arterioles, but spares venous channels (Fig. 3.25). Obliteration of vascular lumens during the acute phase is mainly due to the inflammatory process with secondary thrombosis. Fibrinoid necrosis may be evident as well. Secondary effects in the surrounding breast resulting from ischemic degeneration include acute and chronic inflammation and fat necrosis.

After a relatively brief follow-up period, all of the patients remained alive, with improvement in systemic symptoms after treatment with corticosteroids. A woman who did not have systemic manifestations of arteritis remained asymptomatic after no treatment other than excision of the breast tumor (128).

### Scleroderma

Scleroderma or systemic sclerosis usually presents with cutaneous and/or visceral symptoms secondary to the effect of the underlying disorder on blood vessels and collagen. Cutaneous involvement of the breast may occur as part of progressive systemic disease. One case report appears to describe an instance of scleroderma diffusely involving the skin and parenchyma of one breast (129). The patient had no systemic manifestations of scleroderma and no follow-up was given. There are several case reports of patients with breast carcinoma who developed scleroderma (130–132). The skin of the breast was involved in at least one of these cases as part of the diffuse cutaneous manifestations of scleroderma (130). The association between breast carcinoma and scleroderma may be coincidental. However, there is evidence for an established relationship between scleroderma and pulmonary carcinoma (132,133). Scleroderma also has been observed in women following breast augmentation with silicone implants after intervals of 2 to 19 years (134–136). In one case, symptoms of scleroderma regressed after silicone implants were replaced with saline-filled implants (135). Smooth muscle differentiation has been described in the fibroblastic cells present in cutaneous and visceral sclerodermal lesions (137).

### Dermatomyositis

Calcification of blood vessels and soft tissues, especially in the extremities, is an important manifestation of dermatomyositis. Cutaneous changes and multiple subcutaneous nodules of both breasts and axillae were described in one 49-year-old woman with long-standing dermatomyositis (138). Mammography revealed numerous coarse branching calcifications, similar to those formed in periductal mastitis with duct stasis, and a cluster of punctate calcifications suggestive of carcinoma. With tangential views, it was possible to demonstrate that both types of calcification were situated in

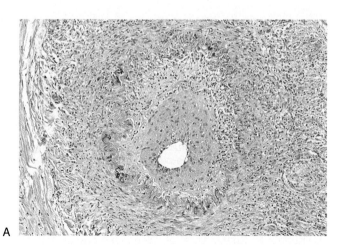
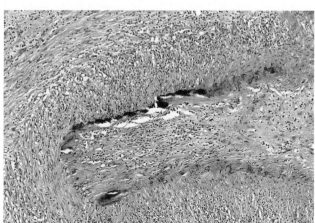

A
B

**FIG. 3.25.** *Polyarteritis.* Fragmentation of the internal elastica and calcification in vessels cut transversely **(A)** and in the long axis **(B)**. Blood vessel lumens are occluded by reactive tissue.

the skin and subcutaneous tissue rather than in the breast, as it appeared in conventional views. No biopsy was performed.

Several survey studies of patients with dermatomyositis documented an association with malignant neoplasms (139–142). Breast carcinoma has been among the more common neoplasms in some series (139,141), but a study of Japanese patients reported more frequent association with gastric, thyroid, and ovarian carcinomas (142). Patients often experience remission of their dermatomyositis after treatment for their neoplasm. In one exceptional case, fulminant dermatomyositis became apparent clinically shortly after surgical treatment for a T1N0M0 breast carcinoma (143).

### Other Collagen-Vascular Diseases

Involvement of the breast in *rheumatoid disease* is extremely unusual. One case report described a 32-year-old woman with clinically active rheumatoid disease who had a microscopic rheumatoid nodule detected in a breast biopsy performed for clinical symptoms of duct stasis and mastitis (89).

*Weber-Christian disease* presents as recurrent subcutaneous nodules accompanied by fever, arthralgias, and malaise. The lesions may or may not be tender. The typical distribution is on the lower extremities and trunk, but mammary involvement has been reported (144). The excised nodule consists of fat necrosis with a granulomatous reaction. The lesion usually is subcutaneous, but superficial involvement of mammary parenchyma may occur.

*Granulomatous angiopanniculitis* presents as a superficial mass in the breast, fixed to indurated red skin (145). The age range of the cases reported by Wargotz and Lefkowitz (145) was 36 to 64 years, and all but one patient was female. Two patients had diabetes mellitus. No other systemic conditions were described. The lesions consisted of multiple nonnecrotizing histiocytic granulomas in subcutaneous fat and superficial breast parenchyma with Langhans-type giant cells (Fig. 3.26). Fat necrosis was present. Small blood vessels and capillaries were infiltrated and rimmed by lymphocytes without necrosis. Inflammatory changes were not found in larger vessels. Ductal and lobular structures were largely uninvolved by the granulomatous process. Several patients had recurrences in the breast or at other subcutaneous sites. No patient was known to have developed systemic symptoms.

*Lupus mastopathy* is a rare complication of lupus erythematosus (146). In some cases, this is manifested by lymphocytic mastopathy distributed mainly in and around lobules, but a perivascular component may be detected (Fig. 3.27). Lupus mastitis is a form of lupus panniculitis characterized

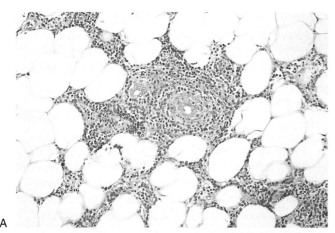

A

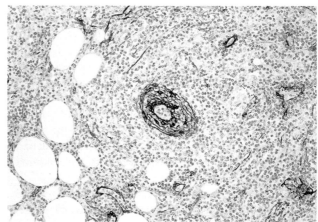

B

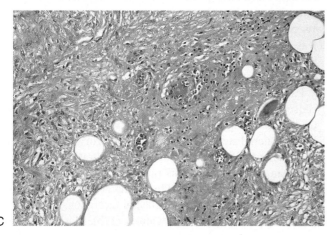

C

**FIG. 3.26.** *Angiopanniculitis.* **A:** Small artery surrounded by lymphocytes in fat necrosis. Inflammatory cells are present in the vessel wall, but the lumen is patent. **B:** Separation of mural smooth muscle layers by inflammatory cells is demonstrated by an antiactin immunostain (avidin-biotin). **C:** Secondary necrosis of a small artery in the center of an area of advanced fat necrosis.

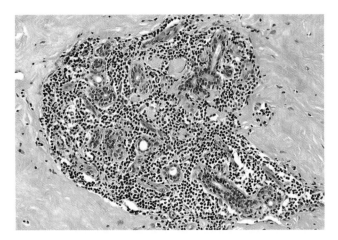

**FIG. 3.27.** *Lupus mastopathy.* Lymphocytic lobulitis in a breast biopsy performed for an ill-defined mass in a 39-year-old woman with arthritis and a positive antinuclear antibody test.

clinically by nodular lesions and histologically by fat necrosis in various stages of evolution (147). Advanced lesions may have considerable calcification. Immunoglobulin deposits can be demonstrated around blood vessels in the lesional tissue, and serum antinuclear antibodies are present. Clinical findings in the skin may mimic inflammatory carcinoma.

### Phlebitis

Inflammatory lesions of veins within the breast have rarely been encountered. The most common form of phlebitis affecting the mammary region is *superficial thrombophlebitis* or *Mondor's disease.* The first modern clinical description of superficial thrombophlebitis of the chest wall and breast often has been attributed to the report by Henri Mondor (148) in 1939. Kaufman (149) reviewed the literature in 1956 and noted descriptions of the syndrome dating to 1922 (150–152). Despite the earlier reports, the condition usually is referred to as Mondor's disease.

About 25% of patients with Mondor's disease have been men. Onset of the lesion has been noted after trauma, physical exertion, and operations performed on the breast or chest wall (153,154). A chronic heroin addict who frequently injected her breasts with the drug reportedly developed Mondor's disease (155). Two patients with Mondor's disease attributed to a jellyfish sting have been reported (156). Coexistent mammary carcinoma and Mondor's disease has been described (157–159). In one series, 12.7% of patients with Mondor's disease had breast carcinoma (160). No association with other malignant tumors has been described, but in one case report, Mondor's disease was found shortly before diagnosis of oat cell carcinoma of the lung that metastasized to the affected breast (161).

Most patients are between 20 and 40 years of age. Despite the youth of female patients with Mondor's disease, only rarely has it been reported as a complication of pregnancy (162). In one series, however, a substantial number of women were multiparous (154). The left and right breast are equally affected; rarely, both breasts may be involved (163). Physical examination reveals a subcutaneous cord that may be painless or painful and tender. When the area is stretched, as upon elevation of the ipsilateral arm, a groove may be formed along the distribution of the cord. Mondor's disease most often involves the upper outer or inframammary portions of the breast and adjacent chest wall. Rarely, various other patterns of extension have been described, including the cervical region, upper arm, abdomen, and even the groin. These unusual distributions reflect anastomoses in the subcutaneous venous plexus.

The diagnosis of Mondor's disease usually is established clinically. The mammographic features of Mondor's disease confirm the superficial nature of the process (164). The typical finding is a linear density, sometimes appearing beaded, that proves to be superficial on tangential films (165). A biopsy reveals thrombophlebitis of subcutaneous veins characterized by thrombosis with varying stages of organization and recanalization (163,166). Inflammation of the vein and surrounding tissue tends to be mild in contrast to a relatively brisk fibroblastic proliferation throughout the vessel wall. Abundant stromal mucin, presumably hyaluronic acid, has been observed in the vessel wall during the acute phase of the process.

Subcutaneous thrombophlebitis of the breast and chest wall is a self-limiting condition that resolves over a period of weeks to months after symptomatic treatment. There is no evidence that Mondor's disease heralds a malignant visceral neoplasm, and only rarely is it associated with deep venous thrombosis. Antibiotic and anticoagulant therapy rarely are necessary.

## PARAFFINOMA

Paraffin injection for cosmetic purposes was first attempted at the turn of the twentieth century when testicular prostheses were fashioned by this method in a patient who had undergone orchiectomy for tuberculosis (167). A variety of other clinical applications were subsequently reported, including breast augmentation (168). Although paraffin injection was abandoned after a relatively short time in most Western nations, it continued to be used in the Orient until it was supplanted by the introduction of liquid silicone (169,170). The use of beeswax and other waxes for breast augmentation has been described (171).

Paraffin induces a foreign body reaction similar to that caused by other irritating substances injected into the breasts. Within weeks to months following injection, the injected material and consequent reaction form a hard, nodular mass that is likely to distort the breast. Infiltration of the skin has been described, and this may be associated with sinus tract formation accompanied by discharge of paraffin (172). One male patient developed bilateral ulcerations caused by paraffin injected 35 years previously (173). Mammography reveals a variety of patterns, including a homogeneous mass, a honeycomb appearance (169), or dense fibrosis with "bizarre" architectural distortion (170). Calcifications are flocculent or ring shaped. One patient developed bilateral carcinoma 30 years after injection of both breasts with paraffin (170).

## SILICONE MASTITIS AND OTHER PATHOLOGY ASSOCIATED WITH BREAST AUGMENTATION

Injection of liquid silicone composed of long-chain polymers of dimethylsiloxane into the breasts for cosmetic augmentation was a fairly widespread practice in the 1960s and 1970s. This illicit procedure, not approved by government agencies, was carried out without control in many locations abroad as well as in the United States. The foreign body inflammatory reaction induced by this material may cause a diffuse process throughout the breast, referred to as silicone mastitis, or nodular lesions, so-called silicone granulomas (174).

Leakage of silicone gel contained in prostheses causes an inflammatory reaction that usually is less severe than the response to direct silicone injection. The changes tend to be limited to the immediate vicinity of the implant, resulting in the formation of a capsule (175). Quantitative measurements of silicone in tissues surrounding such implants have not shown a consistent correlation between silicone concentrations and the overall appearance of the inflammatory reaction (176,177). The amount of silicone was significantly associated with the intensity of histiocytic reaction but not with calcification or giant cell reaction (177). Silicone levels are higher in the capsule than in breast tissue surrounding the capsule, regardless of whether the implant contains saline or silicone (178). This finding indicates that some of the silicone in tissues derives from the implant itself even if it is filled with saline.

Capsule formation is due not only to the foreign body effect of the implant but also to seepage of material that it contains. Capsule formation may cause distortion and excess firmness of the breast. Migration of silicone from a silicone gel mammary implant into the soft tissue of the ipsilateral upper arm with secondary neurologic changes has been described (179). In this case, the distribution of silicone was determined by MRI. Ultrasound reportedly is not as effective for detecting leakage of silicone gel within the periprosthetic capsule (180).

### Clinical Presentation

Numerous complications have been observed as a result of liquid silicone injections (181). These include induration of the skin, draining sinuses, deformity, and development of firm or hard masses in the breast. The masses may be visible as well as palpable. Migration of injected silicone from a ruptured implant to the chest wall and as far as the groin has been described (182,183). Addition of oils and other sclerosing agents to the silicone to minimize migration increases the

intensity of the reaction in the breast, often causing fixation to the skin and/or pectoral muscle. Expression of silicone from the nipple after rupture of a silicone implant has been reported (184,185).

Tissue alterations attributable to silicone are detected in the breast and at other sites by many techniques, including mammography, MRI, computed tomography, and gallium-67 scintigraphy (179,186,187). Screening mammography of 350 women revealed fibrous encapsulation in 257 (73%) patients, periprosthetic calcification in 90 (26%), and silicone leakage in 16 (5%) (187). One study of 300 consecutive patients found disruption in 214 (71.3%) (188). In this series, mammography and MRI had low sensitivity for detecting implant disruption and silicone leakage, but other authors found MRI to be superior to mammography and sonography for detected implant failure (189,190).

The reaction attributable to silicone mastitis makes it very difficult to detect carcinoma in the breast (191,192). Clinical examination is complicated by nodularity, skin retraction, hard masses, nipple inversion, and other alterations that may simulate or obscure a carcinoma (193,194). Axillary lymph node changes have been described as a result of leakage from silicone gel-filled prostheses as well as after injection of liquid silicone into the mammary parenchyma. Axillary lymph node enlargement secondary to migration of silicone can suggest metastatic nodal carcinoma or disguise metastatic involvement (195). FNA of silicone lymphadenitis reveals vacuolated histiocytes that contain refractile particles (196). The pathologic changes of silicone lymphadenitis are discussed in Chapter 45.

The ability to detect carcinoma by mammography is impaired because injected silicone and the associated reaction cause numerous opaque nodules. When an implant is present, special imaging techniques with four or more views may be required to examine the entire breast (187,197). Calcifications in silicone mastitis generally are irregular and coarse, but fine calcifications resembling those of carcinoma also have been found in silicone mastitis (198,199); when present, they should be biopsied (194). Ultrasonography has not proven to be particularly effective for detecting carcinoma in a breast altered by silicone mastitis (200).

### Gross Pathology

A specimen of silicone mastitis consists of firm-to-hard nodular tissue. When bisected, a gritty sensation is noted when there is extensive calcification (Fig. 3.28). Numerous cystic spaces that contain pale yellow or white viscous material are seen on the cut surface after injection of liquid silicone.

### Microscopic Pathology

Liquid silicone by itself or with adulterants causes fat necrosis and elicits a foreign body giant cell reaction (Fig. 3.28). The microscopic features of these processes are not

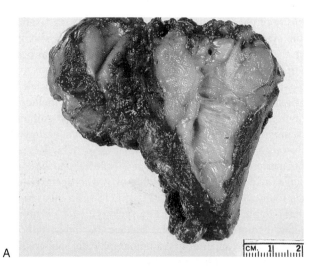

A

FIG. 3.28. *Silicone granuloma.* **A:** Gross specimen containing a nodular silicone granuloma formed after injections of silicone for breast augmentation. **B:** Diffuse granulomatous reaction to silicone. Spaces contained silicone. **C:** Asteroid bodies are present on either side of the *arrow,* which points to a crystalline fragment in giant cell.

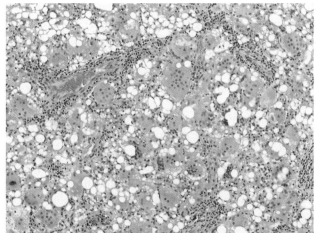

B

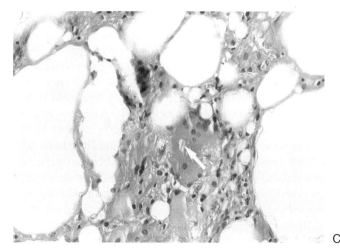

C

specific for silicone injection. Silicone also may enter the lumens of ducts and lobular glands. During the processing of histologic sections, some of the silicone is lost from the tissue, leaving clear spaces of varying size. The spaces and histiocytes may contain fine particles or crystals of birefringent material, but these are not seen in all cases (Fig. 3.29) (176,192). The presence of silicone can be confirmed by electron microscopy, infrared spectroscopy, atomic absorption spectrophotometry, and other procedures. The accompanying chronic inflammatory reaction and fibrosis vary in intensity. The reactive changes may be mistakenly interpreted as liposarcoma when a history of prior silicone injection is not provided (199).

The capsule or bursa formed in reaction to silicone-containing implants consists largely of a relatively well-defined band of collagenized fibrous tissue that contains fibroblasts, myofibroblasts, and variable amounts of elastic tissue. The latter components are largely responsible for capsular contracture. Calcification is more likely to occur in the capsule of an implant in place for a decade or longer than in the capsule around a more recent implant (201). Calcification is found more often in the capsules formed around silicone implants with a thicker wall and Dacron patches typically used in earlier generation implants (202). Calcification occurs in

two forms: "globular aggregates" and true bone formation. Ultrastructural analysis and other studies confirmed that both types of calcification were composed of hydroxyapatite crystals. The crystals were deposited in an orderly fashion on collagen fibers at sites of bone formation, whereas in globu-

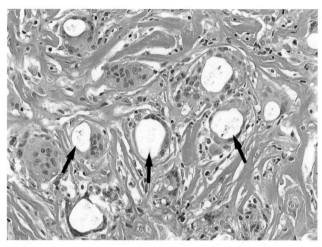

FIG. 3.29. *Silicone granuloma.* Birefringent crystalline material *(arrows)* in vacuolated histiocytes in giant cells in a silicone granuloma.

lar aggregates they were larger and not related to collagen fibers.

The fine microscopic structure of the capsule is influenced by the surface configuration and composition of the implant (203). The inflammatory reaction tends to be concentrated on the inner and outer surfaces of the capsule formed around the implant. The outer reaction consists of lymphocytes, plasma cells, histiocytes, and occasional foreign body giant cells. Fibrohistiocytic cells and multinucleated giant cells are more conspicuous at the interface between the capsule and prosthesis. A largely fibrous type of capsule consists of layered bands of collagen with a mixed inflammatory cell infiltrate composed mainly of lymphocytes and histiocytes. Fibroblasts are distributed in the collagenous tissue and calcification is found in some instances. No synovial differentiation is present, but fibrin may be deposited on the inner surface. Other capsules are thicker with a more complex mural structure, and a primitive synovial-like membrane is formed on the surface in contact with the implant. A distinct zone of capillaries develops in a region composed of loosely organized polygonal histiocytic cells incompletely invested by reticulin fibers beneath the synovial-like membrane.

Analysis of tissue removed from capsules formed around silicone breast implants revealed increased amounts of hyaluronic acid when compared to normal breast tissue removed during reconstructive surgery (204). The inflammatory cells were predominantly T cells and macrophages. Large amounts of interleukin-2 were found in association with the infiltrating lymphocytes. There was no increase in serum levels of hyaluronic acid or interleukin-2 (204).

In up to 50% of cases, the surface of the inner reaction develops a more organized structure composed of fibrohistiocytic cells polarized perpendicular to the surface (Figs. 3.30 and 3.31). There is a well-developed reticulin network among these cells. This synovial-like reaction in the bursa

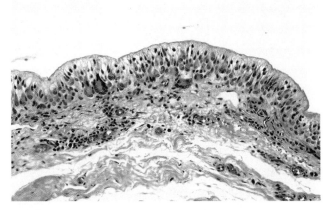

**FIG. 3.31.** *Synovial metaplasia around a breast implant.* Reactive cells are polarized perpendicular to the surface of the membrane. Giant cells are present.

has been referred to as synovial metaplasia (205–207). Synovial metaplasia was most pronounced in capsules examined after the shortest interval between initial placement and removal, an observation suggesting that the occurrence of this change was not dependent on long-term implantation (208,209). Synovial metaplasia occurs in the capsules formed around smooth and textured implants (209). The synovial membrane has a flat surface in specimens around smooth implants. An irregular, knob-like surface develops in the capsule around a textured implant (Fig. 3.32) (203).

The lining cells have immunohistochemical properties similar to those of synovial cells, including staining for vimentin, $\alpha_1$-antichymotrypsin, lysozyme, and CD68 (205,206,210). Stains for cytokeratins and factor VIII are negative (208). Reactivity for CD44 was present in macrophages and foreign body giant cells of implant capsules studies by immunohistochemistry (211).

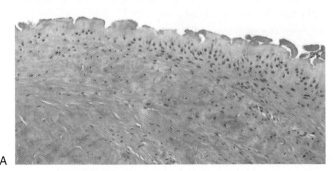
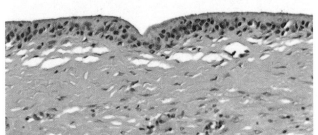

**FIG. 3.30.** *Synovial metaplasia around a breast implant.* **A:** Early phase in which histiocytes with basally oriented nuclei are present at the interface between the fibrous capsule and a space around an implant that has a smooth surface. An irregular layer of fibrin is present over the synovial metaplasia. **B:** Later phase in which histiocytic cells have formed a synovial-like membrane over the fibrous capsule.

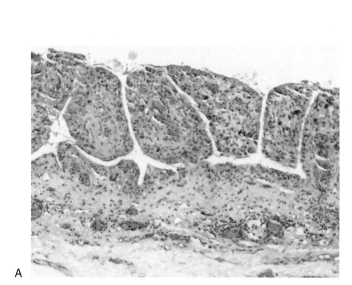
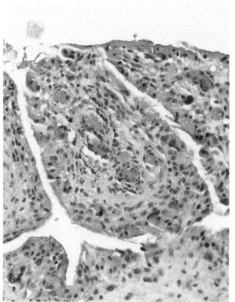

A

B

**FIG. 3.32.** *Papillary synovial metaplasia.* **A:** Polypoid reaction on the surface of the capsule formed around a textured implant. **B:** Multinucleated giant cells and chronic inflammation are apparent.

A variety of foreign substances can be found histologically in implant capsules. Liquid silicone droplets form smooth-surfaced refractile, translucent, or clear vacuoles in histiocytes and in the chronic inflammatory reaction (212). Fragments of the implant bag, referred to as silicone elastomer, are seen as irregular, nonbirefringent particles, often encompassed by multinucleated foreign body giant cells. Polyhedral polyurethane crystals will be found in the capsule formed around polyurethane-covered textured implants (Fig. 3.33), and this material may become mixed with silicone from within the implant (213). These crystals with varied geometric shapes induce a strong granulomatous reaction. Talc also has been detected in tissues associated with breast implant capsules (214).

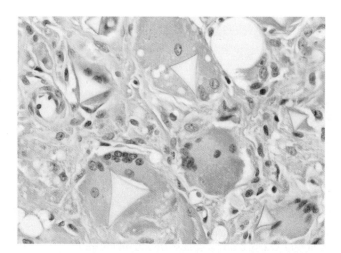

**FIG. 3.33.** *Polyurethane-covered implant.* Triangular polyurethane crystals are present in the granulomatous reaction.

Ultrastructural features of the cells forming the metaplastic synovial membrane have been described (205,207). Studies in experimental animals and in human specimens suggest that the capsular reaction has the functional capacity to transport foreign particulate matter in a manner similar to true synovial membranes (210). Scanning electron microscopy reveals that the layer of synovial metaplasia has a bosselated surface, with fine cellular processes directed toward the lumen (215).

Silicone particles have been identified by light microscopy and other procedures in all layers of the capsule formed around silicone gel implants (205,216,217). Definitive identification can be made by scanning electron microscopy, backscattered electron imaging with x-ray spectroscopy, or electron probe microanalysis (217,218). Laser-Raman microspectroscopy has been shown to provide rapid, accurate, and sensitive analysis of silicone and other particulate material associated with breast implants (219,220).

The mononuclear cell reaction in and around the silicone implant capsule consists largely of T cells (211,221,222), which are distributed diffusely throughout the capsule (207) and in fluid surrounding the implant (221). In one study, the majority of the T cells were CD4$^+$, CD29$^+$ helper/inducer cells (221). These investigators also found human leukocyte antigen (HLA)-DR immunoreactivity in foamy macrophages. HLA-DR$^+$ and CD4$^+$, CD29$^+$ T lymphocytes were present in significantly greater numbers in capsular tissue than in the peripheral blood. These observations suggested the presence of an active cellular immune response in the periprosthetic capsular tissue (221). Germinal centers were positive for CD20, and plasma cells in the capsule exhibited polyclonal immunoglobulin light-chain reactivity (211).

Most investigators found no evidence of epithelial differentiation in the synovial metaplasia with immunohistochemical stains. However, rare instances of squamous metaplasia and squamous carcinoma arising from the surface of implant capsules have been reported (223). Squamous cells lining a breast implant bursa presumably arise from the mammary ductal epithelium damaged during insertion of the implant. Squamous metaplasia is not unusual in breast tissue at the site of a healing surgical site after excisional biopsy; rarely, the metaplastic epithelium is observed to grow on the surface of granulation tissue around a biopsy cavity.

### Treatment and Prognosis

It may become necessary to perform a total mastectomy to control significant inflammatory or cosmetic complications of injected liquid silicone. Cosmetic results of reconstruction have been unsatisfactory when patients had cutaneous infiltration by silicone. Usually, the effects of leakage from silicone filled prostheses have been managed by replacing the prosthesis and removing the surrounding contracture. Masses caused by migration of silicone out of the breast are treated by resection when necessary.

There have been reports of mammary carcinoma arising after injection of liquid silicone into the breast (193,194,196,224) or following leakage from prostheses containing silicone gel (194). The interval between silicone injection or prosthesis placement and the diagnosis of carcinoma has been 5 to 20 years (191,194). One patient who developed silicone mastitis as a result of the migration of silicone injected over her sternum to treat pectus excavatum was unexpectedly found to have an invasive duct carcinoma in one breast when bilateral mastectomy was performed for cosmetic reasons (225). Histologically, carcinomas found in breasts with silicone mastitis have been of the ductal variety, usually poorly differentiated. Most of the patients had axillary lymph node metastases reflecting relatively advanced lesions.

Epidemiologic studies of women with silicone breast implants have not detected evidence of increased frequency of breast carcinoma (226,227,227a). In one study, the risk for breast carcinoma among women with silicone implants proved to be significantly lower than expected (226). This observation suggested that women who underwent augmentation were "drawn from a population already at low risk and that the implants do not substantially increase the risk." The reduced risk was found even in the group with the longest follow-up ranging from 10 to 18 years and at all ages. Rare instances of mammary fibromatosis have been described in women with implanted breast prostheses. This observation probably reflects the association between mammary fibromatosis and any type of prior surgical procedure (228). Some of the implants contained saline rather than sil-

icone. At present, the relationship of injected or leaked silicone and/or additives to the development of breast carcinoma or other breast neoplasms appears to be coincidental.

Isolated case reports have documented the occurrence of systemic scleroderma in women who had silicon-containing breast implants (229–231). The average interval between implantation and the onset of symptoms is about 8 years (232). The reported observed frequency of scleroderma associated with silicone breast implants is less than would be by chance alone. A case-control study of a large group of patients failed to detect a significant relationship between silicone breast implants and the risk for developing systemic lupus erythematosus (233). In 1994, Edelman et al. (234) reviewed all currently available case reports, totaling 40 patients in case series, case-control studies, surveys of plastic surgeons, and cohort studies. They found no evidence of an association between silicone breast implants and connective tissue diseases (234). This conclusion was supported by another review of the subject published in 1997 (235). Weinzweig et al. (178) found no correlation between capsular or breast tissue levels of silicone in patients with and without connective tissue disorders who had either saline or silicone breast implants.

Because small carcinomas are difficult to detect in the presence of silicone mastitis, patients with this condition should have careful clinical follow-up. Women with a strong family history for breast carcinoma or other predisposing factors are candidates for "prophylactic" mastectomy if they have significant silicone mastitis. Slight clinical changes in the breast should be evaluated by mammography and biopsy.

## DIABETIC MASTOPATHY

The occurrence of fibrous tumor-forming stromal proliferations in patients with diabetes mellitus was first noted in 1984 (236) and subsequently described as mastopathy in insulin-dependent diabetics (237) and diabetic mastopathy (238). It has been reported that glycosylation and an increase in intermolecular cross linkages observed in diabetics render collagen resistant to degradation in these patients (239,240). This process could be responsible for the accumulation of fibrous tissue characteristic of some connective tissue disorders in diabetics, including mastopathy (236).

The pathologic changes that characterize diabetic mastopathy appear to be relatively specific for insulin-dependent diabetes mellitus. A review of breast biopsies from patients with diabetes revealed diabetic mastopathy only in those with insulin-dependent disease (241). However, other authors have reported the characteristic constellation of pathologic changes in a small number of patients who did not have diabetes (242). In the latter study, one patient had hypothyroidism and another had systemic lupus erythematosus. The remaining 11 women and one man had insulin-dependent diabetes.

## Clinical Presentation

With rare exceptions in men (238,242–244), reported examples of diabetic mastopathy have been in females (Table 3.1). Most patients were younger than 30 years, and the majority were 20 years or less in age when type I insulin-dependent diabetes mellitus was diagnosed. A few patients with type II diabetes have been described (238,241). The mean ages at onset of diabetes in two studies were 12 and 13 years (236,245). Almost all patients were premenopausal when the breast lesions were biopsied. In six studies, age at biopsy ranged from 19 to 63 years, with a mean of 34 to 47 years. The interval between onset of diabetes and detection of the breast lesion has averaged about 20 years. Bilateral lesions have been diagnosed in 19 (45%) of 42 cases. The majority of the patients had complications of juvenile-onset diabetes, with severe diabetic retinopathy reported in 51% of cases. In one series, five of 12 patients had thyroiditis with elevated serum levels of thyroid microsomal antibodies and enlarged thyroid glands (236). One woman was thyrotoxic, whereas 11 were euthyroid. None of the patients had antibodies to thyroglobulin. These authors found neuropathy in four patients, and 11 of 12 patients had limited joint mobility indicative of cheiroarthropathy. Hypothyroidism has been reported in some cases (242,244–246).

It has been suggested that diabetic mastopathy is one of the manifestations of HLA-associated autoimmune disease. In a series of 13 patients with lymphocytic lobulitis studied by Lammie et al. (247), only three had juvenile-onset diabetes. In individual cases, circulating autoantibodies were detected to smooth muscle, parietal cells, thyroid microsomes, and thyroid epithelium. No autoantibodies were detected with the panel used in three cases. HLA typing of DR3,4 and DR1,4 was found in two patients with type I diabetes. Others reported that HLA histocompatibility typing did not reveal a distinct subtype (236).

The initial clinical symptom is a palpable, firm-to-hard tumor detected in one or both breasts. The lesions tend to be ill defined and nontender, and they may suggest carcinoma to the examiner. The mammogram reveals localized increased density, but no changes have been specifically associated with this condition. In some cases, the mammographic appearance of the mass resembles carcinoma or a fibroadenoma (237,245,248). Spontaneous regression and clinical disappearance of diabetic mastopathy have been reported (248).

## Gross Pathology

The tumors have measured 2.0 to 6.0 cm. Most specimens do not contain a visible tumor, but a distinct firm or hard mass is palpable and the area of involvement has a firm edge when bisected. The cut surface of the tumor discloses homogeneous white to pale gray tissue that may be trabeculated but often is visibly indistinguishable from the surrounding fibrous breast parenchyma (Fig. 3.34). Cysts and other gross alterations of proliferative breast disease are not an integral part of diabetic mastopathy.

## Microscopic Pathology

The lesional tissue consists of collagenous stroma with keloidal features and a slightly increased concentration of stromal spindle cells when compared to the surrounding breast tissue (Fig. 3.35). Polygonal epithelioid cells are found dispersed in the collagen among spindly cells (Fig. 3.36) (241). Tomaszewski et al. (238) concluded that these cells were specifically associated with diabetic mastopathy and that they are absent from nondiabetic lobulitis, but this distinction has not been emphasized by other authors (247,249). Multinucleated stromal giant cells and mitotic activity are not part of this proliferative process (Fig. 3.37). Mature lymphocytes are clustered circumferentially around small blood vessels throughout the lesion, as well as in and around lobules and ducts (Fig. 3.38). In most instances,

**TABLE 3.1.** *Clinical findings in diabetic mastopathy*

| Reference | No. cases | Age at onset of diabetes (yr) | Age at breast biopsy (yr) | Bilaterality [no. patients (%)] | Retinopathy [no. patients (%)] | Thyroid disease |
|---|---|---|---|---|---|---|
| Soler and Khardori (236) | 12 | 4–32 (mean 13) | 25–40 (mean 34) | 10 (83) | 11 (92) | 5 thyroiditis |
| Gump and McDermmott (245) | 11 | 8–15 (mean 12) | 27–41 (mean 35) | 5 (45) | — | 3 hypothyroid |
| Byrd et al. (237) | 8 | 4–19 (mean 34) | 19–41 | — | 5 (63) | — |
| Tomaszewski et al. (238) | 8 | 12–33 | 32–63 (mean 40) | 3 (38) | 4 (50) | 1 hypothyroid |
| Lammie et al. (247) | 3 | — | 31–41 (mean 36) | 1 (33) | — | 1 thyroid microsomal antibodies |
| Seidman et al. (241) | 5 | — | 34–59 (mean 47) | 0 | 4 | 0 |
| Total | 47 | 4–33 | 19–63 | 19 (40) | 24 (51) | |

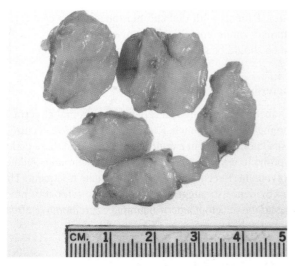

**FIG. 3.34.** *Diabetic mastopathy.* Gross specimen transected to reveal ill-defined fibrous stroma in diabetic mastopathy.

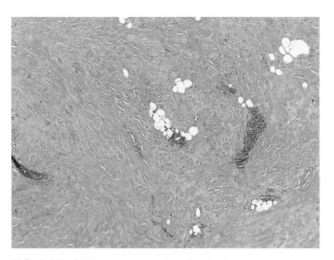

**FIG. 3.35.** *Diabetic mastopathy.* Histologic section showing typical expansion of the collagenous stroma, which contains prominent myofibroblasts and perivascular lymphocytic infiltrates.

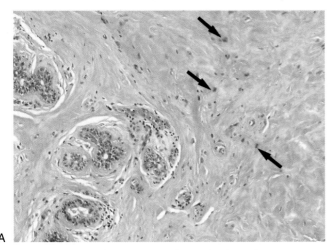

A

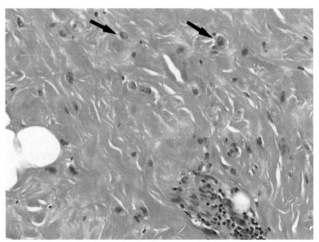

B

**FIG. 3.36.** *Diabetic mastopathy.* **A:** Prominent myofibroblasts *(arrows)* in keloid-like stroma. **B:** Myofibroblasts with a characteristic epithelioid appearance *(arrows).*

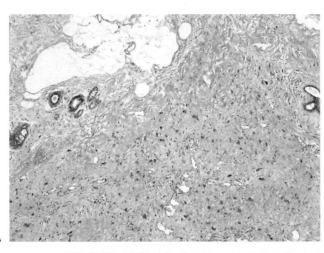

A

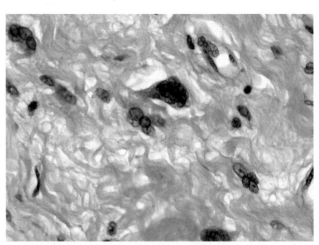

B

**FIG. 3.37.** *Multinucleated stromal giant cells.* **A:** Localized groups of these cells are an incidental finding unrelated to diabetic mastopathy. **B:** Multinucleated stromal giant cells.

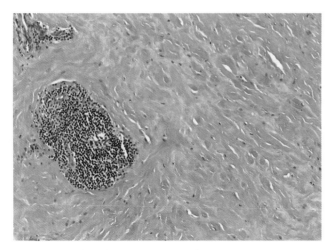

**FIG. 3.38.** *Diabetic mastopathy.* Perivascular infiltrate of mature lymphocytes and myofibroblasts in surrounding stroma.

diabetic mastopathy has all of the foregoing histologic features, but occasionally one or more of the typical findings may be absent (250).

Very few plasma cells or other leukocytes are present in the perivascular infiltrates. Germinal centers are rarely formed. Infarcts, fat necrosis, duct stasis, arteritis, and other inflammatory lesions are not a feature of diabetic mastopathy. Stromal collagen fibers may appear prominent, but they do not have a keloidal appearance. Stains for amyloid were negative in two cases, and mast cells have not been present in increased numbers (237).

The lymphocytic infiltrate is composed predominantly of B cells (238,247). It has been suggested that the lymphocytic infiltrate composed predominantly of B cells is a feature associated with diabetic mastitis and that nondiabetic mastitis features higher proportions of T cells (238). However, Schwartz and Strauchen (249) studied eight patients with a lesion they characterized as lymphocytic mastopathy, including only one patient with diabetes mellitus. They reported that the lymphocytic infiltrate in all cases had a B-cell phenotype (249). Similar results were obtained by Lammie et al. (247). Hunfeld and Bässler (244) compared the stromal and lymphocytic features of diabetic mastopathy and nondiabetic lymphocytic mastitis. Diabetic mastopathy was characterized by greater stromal fibrosis with lobular atrophy and the presence of epithelioid myofibroblasts in each case; fibrosis tended to be less pronounced and there were epithelioid myofibroblasts in only one case of lymphocytic mastitis. There was also a more intense B-cell lymphocyte reaction with relatively fewer T cells and macrophages in diabetic mastopathy.

Needle core biopsy is a reliable method for establishig a diagnosis of diabetic mastopathy in the proper clinical setting (250a). FNA cytology may be helpful in monitoring patients with recurrent lesions after a diagnosis of diabetic mastopathy has been established by surgical biopsy (251). The FNA specimen is usually sparse, consisting of ductal epithelial cells in clusters, lymphocytes, and epithelioid fibroblasts, which are identified most readily in fragments of connective tissues. Patients with diabetic mastopathy also can develop mammary carcinoma; therefore any mass that occurs in these women should be subjected to diagnostic assessment.

### Prognosis and Treatment

Diabetic mastopathy is a self-limited stromal abnormality of premenopausal women. Recurrent tumors have occurred in the ipsilateral breast in a minority of cases, and these patients are prone to asynchronous, as well as synchronous, bilateral involvement. Excisional biopsy is adequate treatment. There is no evidence to suggest that diabetic mastopathy predisposes to the development of mammary carcinoma or stromal neoplastic diseases such as fibromatosis.

### CYSTIC FIBROSIS

The breast tissue in these patients exhibits normal duct and lobular development (252). Stromal fibrosis with lobular atrophy and ductal sclerosis has been described. There does not appear to be a specific inflammatory lesion. Various epithelial proliferative changes including carcinoma can occur in patients with cystic fibrosis.

### AMYLOID TUMOR

Amyloid deposits in the breast have been described in patients with predisposing systemic diseases such as primary amyloidosis (253,254), rheumatoid arthritis (255–257), multiple myeloma (258), and Waldenstrom's macroglobulinemia (259). Some of these patients had concurrent pulmonary and mammary lesions (253,258). The underlying disease is well documented in these cases, and breast involvement, when clinically evident, is invariably a late development. Amyloid has been detected in the stroma of mammary carcinomas. Primary amyloid tumors clinically limited to the breast are uncommon (260–264). Concurrent pulmonary and mammary amyloid tumors in the absence of an underlying systemic disease are rare (265).

### Clinical Presentation

With the exception of men studied at autopsy (266), reported patients with amyloid tumor of the breast have been women. Age at diagnosis ranged from 45 to 79 years (median 56 years). Bilateral involvement has been described clinically in patients who presented with discrete tumors in both breasts (257,263,267,268). Eighty percent of unilateral tumors have been located in the right breast. The tumors usually have been solitary. They may be located in any part of the breast, including the axillary tail (255,264) and subareolar region (256). Involvement of the nipple was described in one case (266). Most patients report the recent detection of a painless mass.

Examination usually reveals a discrete, firm or hard tumor that occasionally is tender (265,269). Retraction or dimpling of the overlying skin has been described in patients with lesions located near the skin. Rarely, axillary lymph node enlargement may indicate involvement of one or more lymph nodes by amyloidosis (256). The physical findings may lead to a clinical diagnosis of mammary carcinoma (256). This impression is strengthened if mammographic examination reveals calcifications in the lesion (254,260,263,267,268).

### Gross Pathology

Amyloid tumors of the breast usually have measured 2 to 3 cm in diameter. The largest lesion reported was 5 cm (263). Grossly, the lesion is firm, gray or white, and opalescent. If calcification is present, there may be a gritty sensation when the lesion is incised. Fat and small cysts may be present in breast parenchyma incorporated in the lesion.

### Microscopic Pathology

Histologic examination reveals eosinophilic, amorphous, homogeneous deposits of amyloid. This material is distributed not only in fat, fibrocollagenous stroma, and blood vessels, but also around ducts and within lobules (Fig. 3.39). Deposits of amyloid around ducts and in lobules are associated with atrophy and obliteration of these glandular components (Fig. 3.40). In adipose tissue, thin ribbons of amyloid may be formed around individual fat cells. These so-called amyloid rings are accentuated when sections stained with Congo red are examined with polarized light (253,270,271). Varying numbers of plasma cells and lymphocytes are present in association with the amyloid deposits, which also can have punctate or irregular calcifications. Multinucleated giant cells appear to be a manifestation of a foreign-body–like reaction to the amyloid, which may have prominent granulomatous features (Fig. 3.41). Amyloid deposits in the breast may develop focal calcification, and rarely osseous metaplasia is encountered in an amyloid tumor (272).

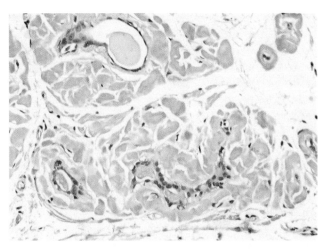

**FIG. 3.40.** *Amyloidosis.* Amyloid is deposited in the basement membranes and collagen surrounding lobular glands and ductules.

Amyloid is stained red-orange with alkaline Congo red, and it exhibits apple-green birefringence when the section stained with Congo red is examined with polarized light. Staining with crystal violet results in a strong metachromatic reaction. In most cases, apple-green birefringence has been preserved after incubation of Congo red-stained sections with potassium permanganate, indicating the presence of immunoglobulin light chains characteristic of AL amyloid (Fig. 3.42). In one study, direct immunofluorescence revealed weak staining for immunoglobulin G (IgG), immunoglobulin M, and kappa and lambda light chains, with prominent staining for immunoglobulin A in bilateral amyloid tumors in one case and strong focal staining for IgG and lambda chains in the amyloid and plasma cells in another lesion (263). Other authors reported staining for kappa light chains in one case (262) and for IgG and kappa chains in another (258).

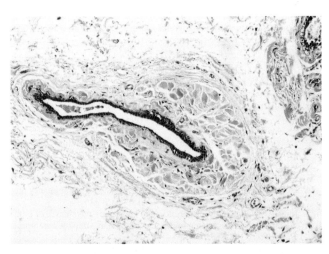

**FIG. 3.39.** *Amyloidosis.* Nodular deposits of amyloid are present in the periductal collagen.

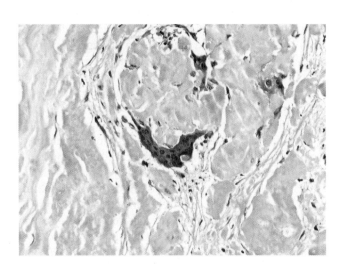

**FIG. 3.41.** *Amyloid tumor.* The lesion is composed of masses of amyloid not associated with epithelial structures and multinucleated giant cells.

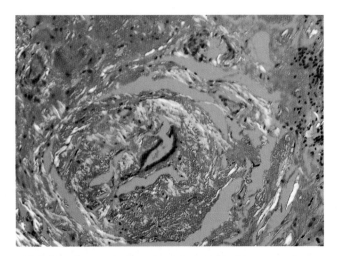

**FIG. 3.42.** *Amyloid tumor.* Apple-green birefringence of amyloid is present in the periductal tissue (Congo red stain with polarized light).

Electron microscopy reveals the presence of straight, non-branching haphazardly arranged amyloid fibrils measuring 5 to 10 mm (255,260,263). The amyloid fibrils are enmeshed to some extent with bands of collagen fibers.

Amyloid obtained by FNA appears as refractile or glassy amorphous material in Papanicolaou-stained smears. Metachromasia is evident with a modified Wright's stain, and the amyloid appears purple with the May-Grünwald-Giemsa stain (263). The sparsely cellular smears reveal scattered plasma cells, lymphocytes, spindly stromal cells, epithelial cells, and occasional multinucleated giant cells.

**Prognosis and Treatment**

Excisional biopsy or needle core biopsy are necessary for the diagnosis of amyloid tumor of the breast. The distinction between a primary amyloid tumor and secondary amyloidosis can only be made by careful clinical evaluation to rule out a systemic condition. This evaluation should include a thorough clinical history and physical examination, bone marrow examination, as well as appropriate studies of serum proteins and blood.

When limited to the breast, amyloid tumor has proven to be a benign condition that has been treated by excisional biopsy. This is in contrast to patients with tumoral amyloidosis of the soft tissues, usually in the retroperitoneum or mediastinum, which frequently is associated with lymphoma (273). One woman had bilateral amyloid tumors detected asynchronously over an interval of 10 months (263). Most patients have remained well following excisional biopsy in the limited follow-up thus far reported. However, one woman who presented with bilateral mammary amyloid tumors developed systemic amyloidosis 1 year later (267). The prognosis of patients with systemic amyloidosis depends on the clinical course of the underlying condition.

# REFERENCES

## Fat Necrosis

1. Haagensen CD. Traumatic fat necrosis. In: *Diseases of the breast,* 2nd ed. Philadelphia: WB Saunders, 1971:202–211.
2. Adair FE, Munger JT. Fat necrosis of the female breast: report of 110 cases. *Am J Surg* 1947;74:117–128.
3. Lee BJ, Adair F. Traumatic fat necrosis of the female breast and its differentiation from carcinoma. *Ann Surg* 1920;72:188–195.
4. Leborgne R. Esteato necrosis quistica calcificada de la mama. *Torax* 1967;16:172–175.
5. Clarke D, Curtis JL, Martinez A, et al. Fat necrosis of the breast simulating recurrent carcinoma after primary radiotherapy in the management of early breast cancer. *Cancer* 1983;52:442–445.
6. Rostom AY, el-Sayed ME. Fat necrosis of the breast: an unusual complication of lumpectomy and radiotherapy in breast cancer. *Clin Radiol* 1987;38:31.
7. Girling AC, Hanby AM, Millis RR. Radiation and other pathological changes in breast tissue after conservation treatment for carcinoma. *J Clin Pathol* 1990;43:152–156.
8. Ilkani R, Gardezi S, Hedayati H, et al. Necrotizing mastopathy caused by calciphylaxis: a case report. *Surgery* 1997;122:967–968.
9. Hogge JP, Robinson RE, Magnant CM, et al. The mammographic spectrum of fat necrosis of the breast. *Radiographics* 1995; 15:1347–1356.
10. Bassett LW, Gold RH, Cove HC. Mammographic spectrum of traumatic fat necrosis: the fallibility of "pathognomonic" signs of carcinoma. *AJR Am J Roentgenol* 1978;130:119–122.
11. Bargum K, Moller Nielsen S. Case report: fat necrosis of the breast appearing as oil cysts with fat-fluid levels. *Br J Radiol* 1993; 66:718–720.
12. Hooley R, Lee C, Tocino I, et al. Calcifications in axillary lymph nodes caused by fat necrosis. *AJR Am J Roentgenol* 1996; 167:627–628.
13. Soo MS, Kornguth PJ, Hertzberg BS. Fat necrosis in the breast: sonographic features. *Radiology* 1998;206:261–269.

## Hemorrhagic Necrosis and Anticoagulant Therapy

14. Verhagen H. Local hemorrhage and necrosis of the skin and underlying tissues, during anticoagulant therapy with dicumarol or dicumacyl. *Acta Med Scand* 1954;148:453–467.
15. Flood PE, Redish MH, Bocie SJ, et al. Thrombophlebitis migrans disseminata. Report of a case in which gangrene of the breast occurred. *N Y J Med* 1943;43:1121–1124.
16. Isenberg JS, Tu Q, Rainey W. Mammary gangrene associated with warfarin ingestion. *Ann Plast Surg* 1996;37:553–555.
17. Rick ME. Protein C and protein S. *JAMA* 1990;263:701–703.
18. Martin BF, Phillips JD. Gangrene of the female breast with anticoagulant therapy: report of two cases. *Am J Clin Pathol* 1970;53:622–626.
19. Nadelman HL, Kempson RL. Necrosis of the breast: a rare complication of anticoagulant therapy. *Am J Surg* 1966;111:728–737.
20. Ekeh AP, Marti JR. Spontaneous necrosis of an accessory breast during pregnancy. *Breast Dis* 1996;9:291–293.

## Breast Infarct

21. Robitaille Y, Seemayer TA, Thelmo WL, et al. Infarction of the mammary region mimicking carcinoma of the breast. *Cancer* 1974;33:1183–1189.
22. Lucey JJ. Spontaneous infarction of the breast. *J Clin Pathol* 1975;28:937–943.
23. Newman J, Kahn LB. Infarction of fibro-adenoma of the breast. *Br J Surg* 1973;60:738–740.
24. Hasson J, Pope CH. Mammary infarcts associated with pregnancy presenting as breast tumors. *Surgery* 1961;49:313–316.
25. Flint A, Oberman HA. Infarction and squamous metaplasia of intraductal papilloma: a benign breast lesion that may simulate carcinoma. *Hum Pathol* 1984;15:764–767.
26. Walker AN, Betsill WL. Infarction of intraductal papilloma associated with hyperprolactinemia. *Arch Pathol Lab Med* 1980;104:280.

27. Jones EL, Codling BW, Oates GD. Necrotic intraduct breast carcinomas simulating inflammatory lesions. *J Pathol* 1973;110:101–103.

## Inflammatory Lesions in Pregnancy and Lactation

28. Eschenbach DA. Acute postpartum infections. *Emerg Med Clin North Am* 1985;3:87–115.
29. Rickert RR, Rajan S. Localized breast infarcts associated with pregnancy. *Arch Pathol* 1974;97:159–161.
30. Boyle M, Lakhoo K, Ramani P. Galactocele in a male infant: case report and review of literature. *Pediatr Pathol* 1993;13:305–308.
31. Golden GT, Wangensteen SL. Galactocele of the breast. *Am J Surg* 1972;123:271–273.
32. Salvador R, Salvador M, Jimenez JA, et al. Galactocele of the breast: radiologic and ultrasonographic findings. *Br J Radiol* 1990;63:140–142.
33. Gómez A, Mata JM, Donoso L, et al. Galactocele: three distinctive radiographic appearances. *Radiology* 1986;158:43–44.
34. Novotny DB, Maygarden SJ, Shermer RW, et al. Fine needle aspiration of benign and malignant breast masses associated with pregnancy. *Acta Cytol* 1991;35:676–686.
35. Raso DS, Greene WB, Silverman JF. Crystallizing galactocele. A case report. *Acta Cytol* 1997;41:863–870.
36. Lawlor-Smith L, Lawlor-Smith C. Vasospasm of the nipple—a manifestation of Raynaud's phenomenon: case reports. *BMJ* 1997;314:644–645.

## Plasma Cell Mastitis

37. Adair FE. Plasma cell mastitis—a lesion simulating mammary carcinoma. *Arch Surg* 1933;735–749.
38. Wilhelmus JL, Schrodt GR, Mahaffey LM. Cholesterol granulomas of the breast. A lesion which clinically mimics carcinoma. *Am J Clin Pathol* 1982;77:592–597.
39. Parsons WH, Henthorne JC, Clark RL Jr. Plasma cell mastitis. Report of five additional cases. *Arch Surg* 1944;49:86–89.

## Mammary Duct Ectasia

40. Haagensen CD. Mammary duct ectasia. A disease that may simulate carcinoma. *Cancer* 1951;4:749–761.
41. Bloodgood JC. The pathology of chronic cystic mastitis of the female breast with special consideration of the blue-domed cyst. *Arch Surg* 1921;3:445–542.
42. Bloodgood JC. The clinical picture of dilated ducts beneath the nipple frequently to be palpated as a doughy worm-like mass—the varicocele tumor of the breast. *Surg Gynecol Obstet* 1923;36:486–495.
43. Tice GI, Dockerty MB, Harrington SW. Comedo mastitis: a clinical and pathologic study of data in 172 cases. *Surg Gynecol Obstet* 1948;87:525–540.
44. Frantz VK, Pickren JW, Melcher GW, et al. Incidence of chronic cystic disease in so-called "normal breasts": a study based on 225 postmortem examinations. *Cancer* 1951;4:762–783.
45. Davies JD. Inflammatory damage to ducts in mammary dysplasia: a cause of duct dilatation. *J Pathol* 1975;117:47–54.
46. Payne RI, Strauss AF, Glasser RD. Mastitis obliterans. *Surgery* 1943;14:719–727.
47. Dixon JM, Anderson TJ, Lumsden AB, et al. Mammary duct ectasia. *Br J Surg* 1983;70:601–603.
48. Habif DV, Perzin KH, Lipton R, et al. Subareolar abscess associated with squamous metaplasia of lactiferous ducts. *Am J Surg* 1970;119:523–526.
49. Passaro ME, Broughan TA, Sebek BA, et al. Lactiferous fistula. *J Am Coll Surg* 1994;178:29–32.
50. Furlong AJ, Al-Nakib L, Knox WF, et al. Periductal inflammation and cigarette smoke. *J Am Coll Surg* 1994;179:417–420.
51. Bundred NJ, Dover MS, Coley S, et al. Breast abscesses and cigarette smoking. *Br J Surg* 1992;79:58–59.
52. Hunter-Craig ID, Tuddenham EGD, Earle JHO. Lipogranuloma of the breast due to phenothiazine therapy. *Br J Surg* 1970;57:76–79.
53. Shousha S, Backhouse CM, Dawson PM, et al. Mammary duct ectasia and pituitary adenomas. *Am J Surg Pathol* 1988;12:130–133.

54. Stringel G, Perelman A, Jimenez C. Infantile mammary duct ectasia: a cause of blood nipple discharge. *J Pediatr Surg* 1986;21:671–674.
55. Rees BI, Gravelle IH, Hughes LE. Nipple retraction in duct ectasia. *Br J Surg* 1977;64:577–580.
56. Khoda J, Lantsberg L, Yegev Y, et al. Management of periareolar abscess and mamillary fistula. *Surg Gynecol Obstet* 1992;175:306–308.
57. Walker JC, Sandison AT. Mammary duct ectasia. *Br J Surg* 1964;51:350–355.
58. Tedeschi LG, McCarthy PE. Involutional mammary duct ectasia and periductal mastitis in a male. *Hum Pathol* 1974;5:232–236.
59. Sweeney DJ, Wylie EJ. Mammographic appearances of mammary duct ectasia that mimic carcinoma in a screening programme. *Australas Radiol* 1995;39:18–23.
60. Davies JD. Human colostrum cells: their relation to periductal mononuclear inflammation. *J Pathol* 1974;112:153–160.
61. Davies JD. Periductal foam cells in benign mammary dysplasia. *J Pathol* 1975;117:39–45.
62. Hamperl H. The myothelia (myoepithelial cells). Normal state, regressive changes, hyperplasia, tumors. *Curr Top Pathol* 1970;53:161–220.
63. Dabbs DJ. Mammary ductal foam cells: macrophage immunophenotype. *Hum Pathol* 1993;24:977–981.
64. Damiani S, Cattani MG, Buonamici L, et al. Mammary foam cells. Characterization by immunohistochemistry and in situ hybridization. *Virchows Arch* 1998;432:433–440.
65. Davies JD. Pigmented periductal cells (ochrocytes) in mammary dysplasias: their nature and significance. *J Pathol* 1974;114:205–216.
66. Dabbs DJ. Mammary ductal foam cells: macrophage immunophenotype for further cells? *Hum Pathol* 1994;25:214–215.
67. Reynolds HE, Cramer HM. Cholesterol granuloma of the breast: a mimic of carcinoma. *Radiology* 1994;191:249–250.
68. Davies JD. Hyperelastosis, obliteration and fibrous plaques in major ducts of the human breast. *J Pathol* 1973;110:13–26.

## Granulomatous Lobular Mastitis

69. Fitzgibbons PL. Granulomatous mastitis. *N Y State J Med* 1990;90:287.
70. Cohen C. Granulomatous mastitis: a review of 5 cases. *S Afr Med J* 1977;52:15–16.
71. Fletcher A, Magrath IM, Riddell RH, et al. Granulomatous mastitis: a report of seven cases. *J Clin Pathol* 1982;35:941–945.
72. Going JJ, Anderson TJ, Wilkinson S, et al. Granulomatous lobular mastitis. *J Clin Pathol* 1987;40:535–540.
73. Davies JD, Burton PA. Post-partum lobular granulomatous mastitis. *J Clin Pathol* 1983;36:363.
74. Kessler E, Wolloch Y. Granulomatous mastitis: a lesion clinically simulating carcinoma. *Am J Clin Pathol* 1972;58:642–646.
75. Brown KL, Tang PHL. Postlactational tumoral granulomatous mastitis: a localized immune phenomenon. *Am J Surg* 1979;138:326–329.
76. Murthy MSN. Granulomatous mastitis and lipogranuloma of the breast. *Am J Clin Pathol* 1973;60:432–433.
77. Donn W, Rebbeck P, Wilson C, et al. Idiopathic granulomatous mastitis. A report of three cases and review of the literature. *Arch Pathol Lab Med* 1994;118:822–825.
78. Han B-K, Choe YH, Park JM, et al. Granulomatous mastitis: mammographic and sonographic appearances. *AJR Am J Roentgenol* 1999;173:317–320.
79. Kumarasinghe MP. Cytology of granulomatous mastitis. *Acta Cytol* 1997;41:727–730.
80. Kobayashi TK, Sugihara H, Kato M, et al. Cytologic features of granulomatous mastitis. Report of a case with fine needle aspiration cytology and immunocytochemical findings. *Acta Cytol* 1998;42:716–720.
81. Oberman HA. Invasive carcinoma of the breast with granulomatous response. *Am J Clin Pathol* 1987;88:718–721.
82. De Hertogh DA, Rossof AH, Harris AA, et al. Prednisone management of granulomatous mastitis. *N Engl J Med* 1980;308:799–800.
83. Jorgensen MB, Nielsen DM. Diagnosis and treatment of granulomatous mastitis. *Am J Med* 1992;93:97–101.

## Sarcoidosis

84. Fitzgibbons PL, Smiley DF, Kern WH. Sarcoidosis presenting initially as breast mass: report of two cases. *Hum Pathol* 1985; 16:851–852.
85. Banik S, Bishop PW, Ormerod LP, et al. Sarcoidosis of the breast. *J Clin Pathol* 1986;39:446–448.
86. Reitz ME, Seidman I, Roses DF. Sarcoidosis of the breast. *N Y State J Med* 1985;85:262–263.
87. Kenzel PP, Hadijuana J, Hosten N, et al. Boeck sarcoidosis of the breast: mammographic, ultrasound, and MR findings. *J Comp Assist Tomogr* 1997;21:439–441.
88. Kirshy D, Gluck B, Brancaccio W. Sarcoidosis of the breast presenting as a spiculated lesion. *AJR Am J Roentgenol* 1999;172:554–555.
89. Cooper NE. Rheumatoid nodule of the breast. *Histopathology* 1991;19:193–194.
90. Gorton G, Linell F. Malignant tumors and sarcoid reactions in regional lymph nodes. *Acta Radiol* 1957;47:381–392.
91. Bässler R, Birke F. Histopathology of tumour associated sarcoid-like stromal reaction in breast cancer. An analysis of 5 cases with immunohistochemical investigations. *Virchows Arch [A]* 1988; 412:231–239.
92. Symmers WStC. Localized tuberculoid granulomas associated with carcinoma, their relationship to sarcoidosis. *Am J Pathol* 1951;27:493–521.
93. Oberman HA. Invasive carcinoma of the breast with granulomatous response. *Am J Clin Pathol* 1987;88:718–721.
94. Voravud N, Sneige N, Theriault R, et al. Sarcoidosis and breast cancer. *Breast Dis* 1992;5:191–197.
95. Gansler TS, Wheeler JE. Mammary sarcoidosis. Two cases and literature review. *Arch Pathol Lab Med* 1984;108:673–675.
96. Shah AY, Solomon L, Gumbs MA. Sarcoidosis of the breast coexisting with mammary carcinoma. *N Y State J Med* 1990;90:331–333.
97. Santini D, Pasquinelli G, Alberghini M, et al. Invasive breast carcinoma with granulomatous response and deposition of unusual amyloid. *J Clin Pathol* 1992;45:885–888.
98. Bodo M, Döbrössy L, Sugar J. Boeck's sarcoidosis of the breast: cytologic findings with aspiration biopsy cytology. A case clinically mimicking carcinoma. *Acta Cytol* 1978;22:1–2.
99. Brincker H, Wilbek E. The incidence of malignant tumours in patients with respiratory sarcoidosis. *Br J Cancer* 1974;29:247–251.

## Inflammatory Pseudotumor

100. Yip CH, Wong KT, Samuel D. Bilateral plasma cell granuloma (inflammatory pseudotumour) of the breast. *Aust N Z J Surg* 1997;67:300–303.
101. Pettinato G, Manivel JC, Insabato L, et al. Plasma cell granuloma (inflammatory pseudotumour) of the breast. *Am J Clin Pathol* 1988;90:627–632.
102. Chetty R, Govender D. Inflammatory pseudotumor of the breast. *Pathology* 1997;29:270–271.

## Vasculitis

103. Waugh TR. Bilateral mammary arteritis. Report of a case. *Am J Pathol* 1950;26:851–861.
104. Clement PB, Senges H, How AR. Giant cell arteritis of the breast: case report and literature review. *Hum Pathol* 1987;18:1186–1189.
105. Cook DJ, Benson WG, Carroll JJ, et al. Giant cell arteritis of the breast. *Can Med Assoc J* 1988;139:513–515.
106. Horne D, Crabtree TS, Lewkonia RM. Breast arteritis in polymyalgia rheumatica. *J Rheumatol* 1987;14:613–615.
107. McKendry RJR, Guindi M, Hill DP. Giant cell arteritis (temporal arteritis) affecting the breast: report of two cases and review of published reports. *Ann Rheum Dis* 1990;49:1001–1004.
108. Polter BT, Housley E, Thomson D. Giant-cell arteritis mimicking carcinoma of the breast. *Br Med J* 1981;282:665–666.
109. Susmano A, Roseman D, Haber MH. Giant cell arteritis of the breast. A unique syndrome. *Arch Intern Med* 1990;150:900–904.
110. Lau Y, Mak YF, Hui PK, et al. Giant cell arteritis of the breast. *Aust N Z J Surg* 1996;66:259–261.
111. Pappo I, Beglaibter N, Amir G. Mammary arteritis mimicking cancer. *Eur J Surg* 1992;158:191–193.
112. Dega FJ, Hunder GG. Vasculitis of the breast. An unusual manifestation of polyarteritis. *Arthritis Rheum* 1974;17:973–976.
113. Stephenson TJ, Underwood JCE. Giant cell arteritis: an unusual cause of palpable masses in the breast. *Br J Surg* 1986;73:105.
114. Codman GC, Churg J. Wegener's granulomatosis: pathology and review of the literature. *Arch Pathol* 1954;58:533–553.
115. Fauci AS, Haynes BF, Katz P, et al. Wegener's granulomatosis: prospective clinical and therapeutic experience with 85 patients in 21 years. *Ann Intern Med* 1983;98:76–85.
116. Elsner B, Harper FB. Disseminated Wegener's granulomatosis with breast involvement. *Arch Pathol* 1969;87:544–547.
117. Deininger HZ. Wegener's granulomatosis of the breast. *Radiology* 1985;154:59–60.
118. Jordan JM, Manning M, Allen NB. Multiple unusual manifestations of Wegener's granulomatosis: breast mass, microangiopathic hemolytic anemia, consumptive coagulopathy, and low erythrocyte sedimentation rate. *Arthritis Rheum* 1986;29:1527–1531.
119. Jordan JM, Rowe TW, Allen NB. Wegener's granulomatosis involving the breast. Report of three cases and review of the literature. *Am J Med* 1987;83:159–164.
120. Oimoni M, Suehiro I, Mizuno N, et al. Wegener's granulomatosis with intracerebral granuloma and mammary manifestation. *Arch Intern Med* 1980;140:853–854.
121. Pambakian H, Tighe JR. Breast involvement in Wegener's granulomatosis. *J Clin Pathol* 1971;24:343–347.
122. Goulart RA, Mark EJ, Rosen S. Tumefactions as an extravascular manifestation of Wegener's granulomatosis. *Am J Surg Pathol* 1995;19:145–153.
123. Trüeb RM, Pericin M, Kohler E, et al. Necrotizing granulomatosis of the breast. *Br J Dermatol* 1997;137:799–803.
124. Göbel U, Kettritz R, Kettritz U, et al. Wegener's granulomatosis masquerading as breast cancer. *Arch Intern Med* 1995;155:205–207.
125. Matsuoka Y, Yoshino K, Kohno M, et al. Necrotizing angiitis localized to the breasts. *Rynmachi* 1982;22:234–239.
126. McCarty DJ, Imbrigia J, Hung JK. Vasculitis of the breasts. *Arthritis Rheum* 1968;11:796–803.
127. Nishizawa T, Enomoto H, Hino T, et al. Vasculitis of the breast with thrombocytopenia. *J Rheumatol* 1979;5:595–597.
128. Yamashina M, Wilson TK. A mammographic finding in focal polyarteritis nodosa. *Br J Radiol* 1985;58:91–92.
128a. Trueb RM, Scheidegger EP, Pericin M, et al. Periarteritis nodosa presenting as a breast lesion: report of a case and review of the literature. *Br J Dermatol* 1999;41:1117–1121.
129. Harrison GO, Elliott RL. Scleroderma of the breast: light and electron microscopy study. *Am Surg* 1987;53:526–531.
130. Forbes AM, Woodrow JC, Verbov JL, et al. Carcinoma of the breast and scleroderma: four further cases and a literature review. *Br J Rheumatol* 1989;28:65–69.
131. Papasavvas G, Goodwill CJ. Scleroderma and breast carcinoma. *Br J Rheumatol* 1989;28:366–367.
132. Roumm AD, Medsger TA. Cancer and systemic sclerosis. An epidemiologic study. *Arthritis Rheum* 1985;28:1336–1340.
133. Peters-Golden M, Wise RA, Hochberg M, et al. Incidence of lung cancer in systemic sclerosis *J Rheumatol* 1985;12:1136–1139.
134. Byron MA, Venning VA, Mowat AG. Postmammoplasty human adjuvant disease. *Br J Rheumatol* 1984;12:227–229.
135. Sahn EE, Garen PD, Silver RM, et al. Scleroderma following augmentation mammoplasty. Report of a case and review of the literature. *Arch Dermatol* 1990;126:1198–1202.
136. Van Nunen SA, Gatenby PA, Basten A. Postmammoplasty connective tissue disease. *Arthritis Rheum* 1982;25:694–697.
137. Sappino A-P, Masouye I, Saurat J-H, et al. Smooth muscle differentiation in scleroderma fibroblastic cells. *Am J Pathol* 1990;137:585–591.
138. Gyves-Ray KM, Adler DD. Dermatomyositis: an unusual cause of breast calcifications. *Breast Dis* 1989;2:195–201.
139. Bonnetblanc JM, Bernard P, Fayol J. Dermatomyositis and malignancy. A multicenter cooperative study. *Dermatologica* 1990;180:212–216.
140. Hidano A, Kaneko A, Arai Y, et al. Survey of the prognosis of DM with special reference to its association with malignancy and pulmonary fibrosis. *J Dermatol (Tokyo)* 1986;13:233–241.

141. Sigurgeirsson B, Lindelöf B, Edhag O, et al. Risk of cancer in patients with dermatomyositis or polymyositis. A population-based study. *N Engl J Med* 1992;326:363–367.

142. Hatada T, Aoki I, Ikeda H, et al. Dermatomyositis and malignancy: case report and review of the Japanese literature. *Tumori* 1996; 82:273–275.

143. Abraham Z, Rozenbaum M, Gläck Z, et al. Fulminant dermatomyositis after removal of a cancer. *J Dermatol* 1992;19:424–427.

144. Markopoulos CJ, Gogas HJ, Anastassiades OT. Weber-Christian disease with breast involvement. A case report. *Breast Dis* 1994;7: 273–276.

145. Wargotz ES, Lefkowitz M. Granulomatous angiopanniculitis of the breast. *Hum Pathol* 1989;20:1084–1088.

146. Cernea SS, Kihara SM, Sotto MN, et al. Lupus mastitis. *J Am Acad Dermatol* 1993;29:343–346.

147. Holland NW, McKnight K, Challa VR, et al. Lupus panniculitis (Profundus) involving the breast: report of 2 cases and review of the literature. *J Rheumatol* 1995;22:344–346.

148. Mondor H. Tronculite sous-cutanée subaigné de la paroi thoracique antéro-latérale. *Mem Acad Chir* 1939;65:1271–1278.

149. Kaufman PA. Subcutaneous phlebitis of the breast and chest wall. *Ann Surg* 1956;144:847–853.

150. Daniels WB. Superficial thrombophlebitis: new cause of chest pain. *Am J Med Sci* 1932;183:398–401.

151. Fleissinger N, Mathieu P. Thrombophlébitis des veins de la paroi thoraco-abdominale. *Bull Soc Med Hop Paris* 1922;46:352–354.

152. Williams GA. Thoraco-epigastric phlebitis producing dyspnea. *JAMA* 1931;96:2196–2197.

153. Bejanga BI. Mondor's disease: analysis of 30 cases. *J R Coll Surg Edinb* 1992;37:322–324.

154. Green RA, Dowden RV. Mondor's disease in plastic surgery patients. *Ann Plast Surg* 1988;20:231–235.

155. Cooper RA. Mondor's disease secondary to intravenous drug abuse. *Arch Surg* 1990;125:807–808.

156. Ingram DM, Sheiner HJ, Ginsberg AM. Mondor's disease of the breast resulting from jellyfish sting. *Med J Aust* 1992;157:836–837.

157. Chiedozi LC, Aghahowa JA. Mondor's disease associated with breast cancer. *Surgery* 1988;103:438–439.

158. Miller DR, Cesario TC, Slater LM. Mondor's disease associated with metastatic axillary node. *Cancer* 1985;56:903–904.

159. Vieta JO. Mondor's disease with carcinoma of the breast. *N Y State J Med* 1977;77:120–121.

160. Catania S, Zurrida S, Veronesi P, et al. Mondor's disease and breast cancer. *Cancer* 1992;69:2267–2270.

161. Courtney SP, Polacarz S, Raftery AT. Mondor's disease associated with metastatic lung cancer in the breast. *Postgrad Med J* 1989;65:779–780.

162. Terada S, Suzuki N, Uchide K, et al. Imaging study of Mondor's disease in the lactating breast. *Breast Dis* 1996;9:211–216.

163. Skipworth GB, Morris JB, Goldstein N. Bilateral Mondor's disease. *Arch Dermatol* 1967;95:95–97.

164. Tabar L, Dean PB. Mondor's disease: clinical, mammographic and pathologic features. *Breast* 1981;7:18–20.

165. Conant EF, Wilkes AN, Mendelson EB, et al. Superficial thrombophlebitis of the breast (Mondor's disease): mammographic findings. *AJR Am J Roentgenol* 1993;160:1201–1203.

166. Duff P. Mondor disease in pregnancy. *Obstet Gynecol* 1981;58:117–119.

## Paraffinoma

167. Gersuny R. Veber eine subcutane prosthese. *Ztschr F Heilkund* 1900;1:199.

168. Boo-Chai K. Paraffinoma. *Plast Reconstr Surg* 1965;36:101–110.

169. Alagaratnam TT, Ng WF. Paraffinomas of the breast: an Oriental curiosity. *Aust N Z Surg* 1996;66:138–140.

170. Yang WT, Suen M, Ho WS, et al. Paraffinomas of the breast: mammographic, ultrasonographic and radiographic appearances with clinical and histopathological correlation. *Clin Radiol* 1996;51:130–133.

171. Symmers WStC. Silicone mastitis in "topless" waitresses and some other varieties of foreign-body mastitis. *Br Med J* 1968;3:19–22.

172. Tinckler LF, Stock FE. Paraffinoma of the breast. *Aust N Z J Surg* 1955;25:142–147.

173. Merckx L, Lamote J, Sacre R. Bilaterial ulcerating paraffinoma of the breast in a man. *Breast Dis* 1993;6:41–44.

## Silicone Mastitis and Other Pathology Associated with Breast Augmentation

174. Nosanchuk JS. Silicone granuloma in breast. *Arch Surg* 1968; 97:583–585.

175. Barker DE, Retsky MI, Shultz S. "Bleeding" of silicone from bag-gel breast implants, and its clinical relation to fibrous capsule reaction. *Plast Reconstr Surg* 1978;61:836–841.

176. Thomsen JL, Christensen L, Nielsen M, et al. Histologic changes and silicone concentrations in human breast tissue surrounding silicone breast prostheses. *Plast Reconstr Surg* 1990;85:38–41.

177. McConnell JP, Moyer TP, Nixon DE, et al. Determination of silicon in breast and capsular tissue from patients with breast implants performed by inductively coupled plasma emission spectroscopy. Comparison with tissue histology. *Am J Clin Pathol* 1997;107:236–246.

178. Weinzweig J, Schnur PL, McConnell JP, et al. Silicon analysis of breast and capsular tissue from patients with saline or silicone gel breast implants: II. Correlation with connective-tissue disease. *Plast Reconstr Surg* 1998;101:1836–1841.

179. Persellin ST, Vogler JB III, Brazis PW, et al. Detection of migratory silicone pseudotumor with use of magnetic resonance imaging. *Mayo Clin Proc* 1992;67:891–895.

180. Chilcote WA, Dowden RV, Paushter DM, et al. Ultrasound detection of silicone gel breast implant failure: a prospective analysis. *Breast Dis* 1994;7:307–316.

181. Ellenbogen R, Ellenbogen R, Rubin L. Injectable fluid silicone therapy: human morbidity and mortality. *JAMA* 1975;234:308–309.

182. Capozzi A, DuBou R, Pennisi VR. Distant migration of silicone gel from a ruptured breast implant. *Plast Reconstr Surg* 1978;62: 302–303.

183. Travis WE, Balogh K, Abraham JL. Silicone granulomas: report of three cases and review of the literature. *Hum Pathol* 1985;16:19–27.

184. Leibman AJ, Kossoff MB, Kruse BD. Intraductal extension of silicone from a ruptured breast implant. *Plast Reconstr Surg* 1992;89: 546–547.

185. Shermis RB, Adler DD, Smith DJ, et al. Intraductal silicone secondary to breast implant rupture. *Breast Dis* 1990;3:17–20.

186. Palestro CJ, Chau P, Goldsmith SJ. Gallium-67 uptake after breast and hip augmentation with silicone. *Clin Nucl Med* 1992;17:897–898.

187. Destouet JM, Monsees BS, Oser RF, et al. Screening mammography in 350 women with breast implants: prevalence and findings of implant complications. *AJR Am J Roentgenol* 1992;159:973–978.

188. Robinson OG Jr, Bradley EL, Wilson DS. Analysis of explanted silicone implants: a report of 300 patients. *Ann Plast Surg* 1995;34:1–7.

189. Gorczyca DP, Sinha S, Ahn CY, et al. Silicone breast implants in vivo: MR imaging. *Radiology* 1992;185:407–410.

190. Morris EA, Dershaw DD. Breast MRI: ready for general use? *Breast J* 1999;5:219–220.

191. Maddox A, Schoenfeld A, Sinnett HD, et al. Breast carcinoma occurring in association with silicone augmentation. *Histopathology* 1993;23:379–382.

192. Winer LH, Sternberg TH, Lehman R, et al. Tissue reactions to injected silicone liquids. *Arch Dermatol* 1964;90:588–593.

193. Lewis CM. Inflammatory carcinoma of the breast following silicone injections. *Plast Reconstr Surg* 1980;66:134–136.

194. Morgenstern L, Gleischman SH, Michel SL, et al. Relation of free silicone to human breast carcinoma. *Arch Surg* 1986;120:573–577.

195. Truong LD, Cartwright J Jr, Goodman MD, et al. Silicone lymphadenopathy associated with augmentation mammoplasty. *Am J Surg Pathol* 1988;12:484–491.

196. Tabatowski K, Elson CE, Johnston WW. Silicone lymphadenopathy in a patient with a mammary prosthesis. Fine needle aspiration cytology, histology and analytical electron microscopy. *Acta Cytol* 1990;34:10–14.

197. Eklund GW, Busby RC, Miller SH, et al. Improved imaging of the augmented breast. *AJR Am J Roentgenol* 1988;151:469–473.

198. Koide T, Katayama H. Calcification in augmentation mammoplasty. *Radiology* 1979;130:337–340.

199. Warner E, Lipa H, Pearson D, et al. Silicone mastopathy mimicking malignant disease of the breast in Southeast Asian patients. *Can Med Assoc J* 1991;144:569–571.

200. Rosenbaum JL, Bernardino ME, Thomas JC, et al. Ultrasonic findings in silicone-augmented breasts. *South Med J* 1981;74:455–458.

201. Peters W, Smith D. Calcification of breast implant capsules: incidence, diagnosis, and contributing factors. *Ann Plast Surg* 1995;34:8–11.

202. Peters W, Pritzker K, Smith D, et al. Capsular calcification associated with silicone breast implants: incidence, determinants, and characterization. *Ann Plast Surg* 1998;41:348–360.

203. Kasper CS. Histologic features of breast capsules reflect surface configuration and composition of silicone bag implants. *Am J Clin Pathol* 1994;102:655–659.

204. Wells AF, Daniels S, Gunasekaran S, et al. Local increase in hyaluronic acid and interleukin-2 in the capsules surrounding silicone breast implants. *Ann Plast Surg* 1994;33:1–5.

205. del Rosario AD, Bui HX, Singh J, et al. True synovial metaplasia of breast implant capsules: a light and electron microscopic study. *Lab Invest* 1994;70:14A.

206. Hameed MR, Erlandson R, Rosen PP. Capsular synovial-like hyperplasia (CSH) around mammary implants similar to detritic synovitis: a morphologic and immunohistochemical study of 15 cases. *Am J Surg Pathol* 1995;19:433–438.

207. Raso DS, Greene WB, Metcalf JS. Synovial metaplasia of a periprosthetic breast capsule. *Arch Pathol Lab Med* 1994;118:249–251.

208. Chase DR, Oberg KC, Chase RL, et al. Pseudoepithelialization of breast implant capsules. *Int J Surg Pathol* 1994;1:151–154.

209. Ko CY, Ahn CY, Ko J, et al. Capsular synovial metaplasia as a common response to both textured and smooth implants. *Plast Reconstr Surg* 1996;97:1427–1435.

210. Emery JA, Hardt NS, Caffee H, et al. Breast implant capsules share synovial transporting capabilities. *Lab Invest* 1994;70:15A.

211. Abbondanzo SL, Young VL, Wei MQ, et al. Silicone gel-filled breast and testicular implant capsules: a histologic and immunophenotypic study. *Mod Pathol* 1999;12:706–713.

212. Emery JA, Spanier SS, Kasnic G Jr, et al. The synovial structure of breast-implant-associated bursae. *Mod Pathol* 1994;7:728–733.

213. Cook PD, Osborne BM, Connor RL, et al. Follicular lymphoma adjacent to foreign body granulomatous inflammation and fibrosis surrounding silicone breast prosthesis. *Am J Surg Pathol* 1995;19:712–717.

214. Kasper CS, Chandler PJ. Talc deposition in skin and tissues surrounding gel-containing prosthetic devices. *Arch Dermatol* 1994;130:48–53.

215. Raso DS, Crymes LW, Metcalf JS. Histological assessment of fifty breast capsules from smooth and textured augmentation and reconstruction mammoplasty prostheses with emphasis on the role of synovial metaplasia. *Mod Pathol* 1994;7:310–316.

216. Domanskis EJ, Owsley JQ. Histological investigation of the etiology of capsule contracture following augmentation mammaplasty. *Plast Reconstr Surg* 1976;58:689–693.

217. Raso DS, Greene WB. Silicone identification by electron probe microanalysis in periprosthetic breast capsules and distant sites in women with silicone breast implants. *Lab Invest* 1994;70:20A.

218. Hardt NS, Yu LT, La Torre G, et al. Fourier transform infrared microspectroscopy used to identify foreign materials related to breast implants. *Mod Pathol* 1994;7:669–676.

219. Centeno JA, Mullick FG, Panos RG, et al. Laser-Raman microprobe identification of inclusions in capsules associated with silicone gel breast implants. *Mod Pathol* 1999;12:714–721.

220. Pasteris JD, Wopenka B, Freeman JJ, et al. Analysis of breast implant capsular tissue for crystalline silica and other refractile phases. *Plast Reconstr Surg* 1999;103:1273–1276.

221. Katzin WE, Feng LJ. Phenotype of lymphocytes associated with the inflammatory reaction to silicone-gel breast implants. *Lab Invest* 1994;70:17A.

222. Raso DS. B and T lymphocytes in periprosthetic breast capsules. *Lab Invest* 1994;70:20A.

223. Kitchen SB, Paletta CE, Shehadi SI, et al. Epithelialization of the lining of a breast implant capsule. *Cancer* 1994;73:1449–1452.

224. Timberlake GA, Looney GR. Adenocarcinoma of the breast associated with silicone injections. *J Surg Oncol* 1986;32:79–81.

225. Pennisi VR. Obscure carcinoma encountered in subcutaneous mastectomy in silicone- and paraffin-injected breasts: two patients. *Plast Reconstr Surg* 1984;74:535–538.

226. Berkel H, Birdsell DC, Jenkins H. Breast augmentation: a risk factor for breast cancer? *N Engl J Med* 1992;326:1649–1653.

227. Deapen DM, Pike MC, Casagrande JT, et al. The relationship between breast cancer and augmentation mammaplasty: an epidemiologic study. *Plast Reconstr Surg* 1986;77:361–368.

227a. Mellemkjaer L, Kjoller K, Friis S, et al. Cancer occurrence after cosmetic breast implantation in Denmark. *Int J Cancer* 2000;88:301–306.

228. Rosen PP, Ernsberger D. Mammary fibromatosis. A benign spindle-cell tumor with significant risk for local recurrence. *Cancer* 1989;63:1363–1369.

229. Gutierrez FJ, Espinoza LR. Progressive systemic sclerosis complicated by severe hypertension: reversal after silicone implant removal. *Am J Med* 1990;89:390–392.

230. Spiera H. Scleroderma after silicone augmentation mammoplasty. *JAMA* 1988;260:236–238.

231. Varga J, Schumacher NA, Jimenez SE. Systemic sclerosis after augmentation mammoplasty with silicone implants. *Ann Intern Med* 1989;111:377–383.

232. Englert HJ, Howe GB, Penny R, et al. Scleroderma and silicone breast implants. *Br J Rheumatol* 1994;33:397–399.

233. Strom BL, Reidenberg MM, Freundlich B, et al. Breast silicone and risk of systemic lupus erythematosus. *J Clin Epidemiol* 1994;47:1211–1214.

234. Edelman DA, Grant S, van Os WAA. Autoimmune disease following the use of silicone gel-filled breast implants: a review of the clinical literature. *Semin Arthritis Rheum* 1994;24:183–189.

235. Noone RB. A review of the possible health implications of silicone breast implants. *Cancer* 1997;79:1747–1756.

## Diabetic Mastopathy

236. Soler NG, Khardori R. Fibrous disease of the breast, thyroiditis, and cheiroarthropathy in Type I diabetes mellitus. *Lancet* 1984;1:193–195.

237. Byrd BF Jr, Hartmann WH, Graham LS, et al. Mastopathy in insulin-dependent diabetics. *Ann Surg* 1987;205:529–532.

238. Tomaszewski JE, Brooks JSJ, Hicks D, et al. Diabetic mastopathy: a distinctive clinicopathologic entity. *Hum Pathol* 1992;23:780–786.

239. Chang K, Uitto EA, Rowald EA, et al. Increased collagen cross-linkages in experimental diabetes: reversal by beta aminopropionitrile and D-penicillamine. *Diabetes* 1980;29:778–781.

240. Golub LM, Greenwald RA, Zebrowski EJ, et al. The effect of experimental diabetes mellitus on molecular characterization of soluble rat tendon collagen. *Biochem Biophys Acta* 1978;534:73–81.

241. Seidman JD, Schnaper LA, Phillips LE. Mastopathy in insulin-requiring diabetes mellitus. *Hum Pathol* 1994;25:819–824.

242. Ashton MA, Lefkowitz M, Tavassoli FA. Epithelioid stromal cells in lymphocytic mastitis—a source of confusion with invasive carcinoma. *Mod Pathol* 1994;7:49–54.

243. Lee AHS, Zafrani B, Kafiri G, et al. Sclerosing lymphocytic lobulitis in the male breast. *J Clin Pathol* 1996;49:609–611.

244. Hunfeld KP, Bässler R. Lymphocytic mastitis and fibrosis of the breast in long-standing insulin-dependent diabetics. A histopathologic study on diabetic mastopathy and report of ten cases. *Gen Diagn Pathol* 1997;143:49–58.

245. Gump FE, McDermmott J. Fibrous disease of the breast in juvenile diabetes. *N Y State J Med* 1990;90:356–357.

246. Pluchinotta AM, Talenti E, Lodovichetti G, et al. Diabetic fibrous breast disease: a clinical entity that mimics cancer. *Eur J Surg Oncol* 1995;21:207–209.

247. Lammie GA, Bobrow LG, Staunton MDM, et al. Sclerosing lymphocytic lobulitis of the breast—evidence for an autoimmune pathogenesis. *Histopathology* 1991;19:13–20.

248. Bayer U, Horn LC, Schulz HG. Bilateral, tumorlike diabetic mastopathy—progression and regression of the disease during 5-year follow up. Case report. *Eur J Radiol* 1998;26:248–253.

249. Schwartz IS, Strauchen JA. Lymphocytic mastopathy. An autoimmune disease of the breast? *Am J Clin Pathol* 1990;93:725–730.

250. Morgan MC, Weaver MG, Crowe JP, et al. Diabetic mastopathy: a clinicopathologic study of palpable and nonpalpable breast lesions. *Mod Pathol* 1995;8:349–354.

250a. Andrews-Tang D, Diamond AB, Rogers L, et al. Diabetic mastopathy: adjunctive use of ultrasound and utility of core biopsy in diagnosis. *Breast J* 2000;6:183–188.

251. Peppoloni L, Buttaro FM, Cristallini EG. Diabetic mastopathy. A report of two cases diagnosed by aspiration cytology. *Acta Cytol* 1997;41:1349–1352.

## Cystic Fibrosis

252. Garcia FU, Galindo LM, Holsclaw DSJ. Breast abnormalities in patients with cystic fibrosis: previously unrecognized changes. *Ann Diagn Pathol* 1998;2:281–285.

## Amyloid Tumor

253. O'Connor CR, Rubinow A, Cohen AS. Primary (AL) amyloidosis as a cause of breast masses. *Am J Med* 1984;77:981–986.
254. Symonds DA, Eichelberger MF, Sager GL. Calcifying amyloidoma of the breast. *South Med J* 1995;88:1169–1172.
255. Cetti R, Reuther K, Hansen JPH, et al. Amyloid tumor of the breast. *Dan Med Bull* 1983;30:34–35.
256. Goonatillake HD, Allsop JR. Amyloid tumour of the breast simulating carcinoma. *Aust N Z J Surg* 1988;58:589–590.
257. Sedeghee SA, Moore SW. Rheumatoid arthritis, bilateral amyloid tumors of the breast and multiple cutaneous nodules. *Am J Clin Pathol* 1974;62:472–476.
258. Hardy TJ, Myerowitz RL, Bender BL. Diffuse parenchymal amyloidosis of lungs and breast. *Arch Pathol Lab Med* 1979;103:583–585.
259. McLellan GL, Steward JH, Balachandran S. Localization of Tc-99m-MDP in amyloidosis of the breast. *Clin Nucl Med* 1981;6:579–580.
260. Fernandez BB, Hernandez FJ. Amyloid tumor of the breast. *Arch Pathol* 1973;95:102–105.
261. Luo J-H, Rotterdam H. Primary amyloid tumor of the breast: a case report and review of the literature. *Mod Pathol* 1997;10:735–738.
262. McMahon RF, Connolly CE. Amyloid breast tumor. *Am J Surg Pathol* 1987;11:488.
263. Silverman JF, Dabbs DJ, Norris HT, et al. Localized primary (AL) amyloid tumor of the breast. Cytologic, histologic, immunocytochemical and ultrastructural observations. *Am J Surg Pathol* 1986;10:539–545.
264. Walker AN, Fechner RE, Callicott JH Jr. Amyloid tumor of the breast. *Diagn Gynecol Obstet* 1982;4:339–341.
265. Liaw Y-S, Kuo S-H, Yang P-C, et al. Nodular amyloidosis of the lung and the breast mimicking breast carcinoma with pulmonary metastasis. *Eur Respir J* 1995;5:871–873.
266. Ganor S, Dollberg L. Amyloidosis of the nipple presenting as pruritus. *Cutis* 1983;31:318.
267. Hecht AH, Tan A, Shen JF. Case report: primary systemic amyloidosis presenting as breast masses, mammographically simulating carcinoma. *Clin Radiol* 1991;44:123–124.
268. Lynch LA, Moriarty AT. Localized primary amyloid tumor associated with osseous metaplasia presenting as bilateral breast masses: cytologic and radiologic features. *Diagn Cytopathol* 1993;9:570–575.
269. Lipper S, Kahn LB. Amyloid tumor. *Am J Surg Pathol* 1978;2:141–145.
270. Pearson B, Rice MM, Dickens KL. Primary systemic amyloidosis. *Arch Pathol* 1941;32:1–10.
271. Libbey CA, Skinner M, Cohen AS. The abdominal fat aspirate for the diagnosis of systemic amyloid. *Arch Intern Med* 1983;143:1549–1552.
272. Yokoo H, Nakazato Y. Primary localized amyloid tumor of the breast with osseous metaplasia. *Pathol Int* 1998;48:545–548.
273. Krishnan J, Chu W-S, Elrod JP, et al. Tumoral presentation of amyloidosis (amyloidomas) in soft tissues. A report of 14 cases. *Am J Clin Pathol* 1993;100:135–144.

# CHAPTER 4

# Specific Infections

## FUNGAL INFECTIONS

Clinically apparent mycotic infections of the breast are uncommon, even in patients who are severely immunocompromised as a consequence of an underlying illness or therapy.

### Actinomycosis

The route of infection usually is via the nipple (1). One patient was infected by a grain of corn that became lodged in her nipple during harvesting (2). The infecting organism was identified as *Actinomyces bovis* in one case (1). A breast abscess attributed to *Actinomyces meyerii* has been associated with chronic periodontal disease (3). *Paecilomyces variotii* was recovered from the lumen of a saline-filled breast implant removed because of capsular contracture. The organisms did not infect the implant bursa and capsule (4).

Actinomycotic infection of the breast typically presents as an abscess beneath or near the nipple and areola (5). The mammographic appearance of the parenchymal mass and skin thickening suggested inflammatory carcinoma in a 66-year-old diabetic woman with a breast abscess due to *A. israeli* (5a). Sinus tracts develop following incision and drainage, when the specific diagnosis is unsuspected clinically or with progression of the untreated lesion. When a sinus tract does not appear, a chronic abscess may form, creating a hard mass that simulates carcinoma. Axillary nodal enlargement reflects reaction to the inflammatory process more often than spread of actinomycosis to the lymph nodes, but actinomycotic axillary lymphadenitis has been reported (6). In advanced cases, the infection can spread to the chest wall (2). Extension of pulmonary actinomycosis to the breast also has been reported (7).

The diagnosis of mammary actinomycosis is made by demonstrating the gram-positive organism as filaments or colonies (sulfur granules) in tissue sections, a fine needle aspirate, or sinus tract drainage. *Actinomyces* can be isolated under anaerobic culture conditions, but positive cultures are obtained in less than 50% of cases (6). Treatment with penicillin reportedly has been effective (6), but recurrent or advanced infections may require mastectomy.

### Nocardia

Cutaneous and subcutaneous abscesses due to *Nocardia asteroides* occur most frequently as a result of direct percutaneous inoculation from an environmental source. A single case report described a parenchymal mammary abscess due to *N. asteroides* confirmed by culture and surgical excision in a 58-year-old woman with systemic lupus who was receiving immunosuppressive therapy (8). The source of infection was not determined in this patient.

### Histoplasmosis

Infection with *Histoplasma capsulatum* is endemic in some regions of the United States and other nations where many individuals have evidence of healed granulomatous lesions in the lungs, liver, spleen, and other organs. Calcified granulomas have not been described in the breast, and there have been rare instances of localized mammary *Histoplasma* infection (9,10). All were women 21, 34, and 35 years old. Each patient presented with a single, unilateral mass that suggested a neoplasm clinically. Two lesions were painful, and inflammatory changes involved the skin in one of these cases, raising a question of inflammatory carcinoma (9). Clinical evaluation in two cases failed to demonstrate evidence of systemic *H. capsulatum* infection, but one patient had an elevated complement fixation test. The excised tumors proved grossly to be multinodular abscesses up to 3 cm in diameter that contained necrotic material. Histologically, the lesions consisted of confluent necrotizing granulomas in which *H. capsulatum* was demonstrated by a methamine silver reaction. The granulomatous reaction was histologically similar to that of nonspecific granulomatous lobular mastitis (9). A fourth 55-year-old woman presented with a mass in the lateral mammary region that proved to be enlarged lymph nodes. *H. capsulatum* was isolated in culture and seen in tissue sections. Involvement of breast parenchyma was not described in this case.

The diagnosis of mammary histoplasmosis in a needle

core biopsy of the breast that revealed granulomatous mastitis has been reported (11).

## Blastomycosis

A 4-cm unilateral breast abscess that contained organisms histologically consistent with *Blastomyces dermatitidis* was excised from the paraareolar region of a 30-year-old woman (10). She had no other evidence of infection and remained well 8 years later. Mammography revealed well-demarcated lesions (12,13). Large nodules may become cavitary with an air–fluid level (12). The diagnosis usually is made when *Blastomyces* sp is cultured from skin lesions or from fine needle aspiration biopsy specimens of the breast (11). One patient also had a tumorous pulmonary lesion and another had a pleural effusion (12,13). The breast and lung lesions may resolve completely with amphotericin treatment (12,13).

## Cryptococcosis

One unusual example of cryptococcal mastitis was described by Symmers (14). The patient underwent mastectomy for a mistaken diagnosis of mucinous mammary carcinoma. The specimen was preserved in a museum and studied microscopically 61 years after surgery, at which time there was no evidence of carcinoma, but the breast was found to be infected with *Cryptococcus*. Follow-up of the patient revealed that, 37 years after mastectomy, she died of an unrelated cause with no evidence of recurrent cryptococcosis. In another case, disseminated cryptococcal infection including the breasts was detected at autopsy in a patient with systemic lupus erythematosus (10).

## Aspergillosis

Mammary aspergillosis has been reported at the site of prosthetic augmentation implants, affecting both breasts in one case (15). Involvement of the nipple by *Aspergillus flavus* in a 51-year-old woman apparently followed traumatic rupture of a superficial keratotic cyst (16).

## Chromomycosis

Cutaneous infection of the nipple by *Fonsecaea pedrosoi* has been described (17). The lesion was a circumscribed oval erythematous plaque with crusting. Biopsy revealed epidermal hyperplasia and "granulomatous infiltration of the upper and middle dermis" containing characteristic fungal hyphae that also may be seen in a fine needle aspiration specimen (Fig. 4.1).

## Coccidioidomycosis

A single example of isolated breast involvement by *Coccidioides immitis* has been reported (18). The patient was a

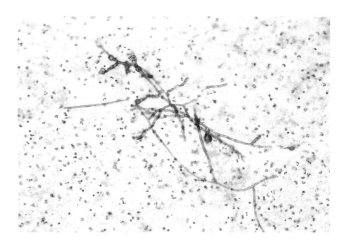

**FIG. 4.1.** *Chromomycosis.* Sample obtained by fine needle aspiration. (Courtesy of Kusum Kapila, M.D. and Kusum Verma, M.D.)

60-year-old woman being treated with prednisone for temporal arteritis. Clinical examination revealed a circumscribed 1.0-cm breast tumor that had sharply defined borders on mammography. The excised mass consisted of a rim of granulation tissue around a necrotic center that contained spherules characteristic of *C. immitis*. No pulmonary lesions were identified.

## PARASITIC INFECTIONS

### Filariasis

Mammary filariasis caused most frequently by *Wuchereria bancrofti* has been reported from tropical and semitropical regions in South America, China, and the Indian subcontinent, where infection with this organism is endemic (19,20). Involvement of the breast occurs in the chronic phase of infection. The appearance of breast lesions may be a late manifestation of low-grade, clinically inapparent infection as evidenced by emigrants and travelers found to have mammary filariasis as late as 3 (21) and 6 (22) years after last exposure to infection. Microfilariae sometimes are demonstrable in thick blood smear samples taken around midnight, but some investigators failed to detect microfilaremia in patients with breast lesions (21,22). Microfilariae have been detected in nipple secretions, suggesting that communication may become established between ducts and dilated, ruptured lymphatics (lymphovarix) (23).

The patient usually presents with a solitary, nontender, painless unilateral breast mass. Multiple lesions occur in a minority of cases. The upper outer quadrant is the most common site, but central or periareolar nodules occur with notable frequency (19,22). Many of the lesions involve subcutaneous tissue, and they may be fixed to the skin. The resultant hard mass with cutaneous attachment, sometimes accompanied by inflammatory changes including edema of the skin, may be clinically indistinguishable from carcinoma (24). In this setting, axillary nodal enlargement caused by fi-

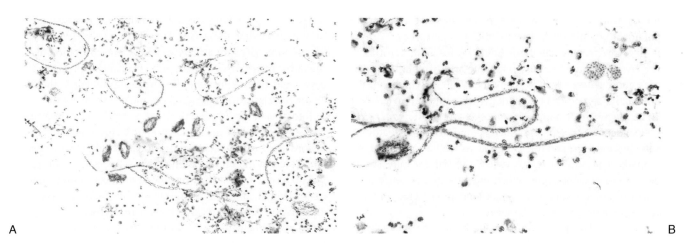

A    B

**FIG. 4.2.** *Filariasis.* **A,B:** Microfilariae in the fine needle aspiration specimen from a breast lesion. (Courtesy of Kusum Kapila, M.D. and Kusum Verma, M.D.)

larial lymphadenitis further complicates the differential diagnosis. In endemic areas, mammary filariasis may be detected coincidentally in patients whose primary breast lesion is carcinoma (20). Viable microfilariae can be detected in the breast by ultrasound examination if they produce a distinctive pattern of movement referred to as the "filaria dance sign"(25). Mammographically detected calcifications attributed to *W. bancrofti* and *Loa loa* infection have been described as having a spiral or serpiginous configuration (24,26,27).

Microfilariae and gravid adult worms can be detected in fine needle aspirates from breast lesions (Fig. 4.2) (28–30). The aspirate usually contains numerous eosinophils as well as other inflammatory cells. Features of a granulomatous reaction may be evident.

Grossly, the majority of the tumors measure between 1 and 3 cm in diameter. They are composed of firm, gray or white tissue that tends to merge with the breast parenchyma. A softer, degenerated region may be noted centrally, and rarely an abscess can develop. Thread-like white worms sometimes are evident grossly in the lesion (19).

Microscopic examination of the excised mass typically reveals adult filarial worms that may be well preserved or in varying stages of degeneration (Fig. 4.3). Granulomatous reaction is most pronounced in areas of degenerating organisms. Eosinophils are a prominent feature. Degenerative changes may lead to the formation of eosinophilic abscesses (Fig. 4.4). Chronic inflammation also affects lymphatic channels of the surrounding breast tissue and overlying skin.

Female worms are about three times the size of male worms. Eggs in varying stages of maturation are identifiable in the gravid uterus of adult females. Microfilariae may be seen within the uterus and in inflammatory tissue surrounding the worms. They are very difficult to find in tissue, but they can be detected by finding nuclei arranged in a linear

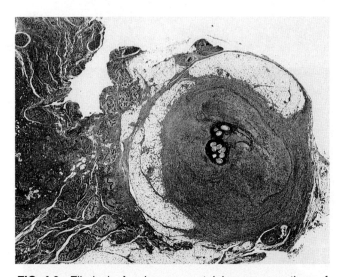

**FIG. 4.3.** *Filariasis.* An abscess containing cross sections of gravid female *Wuchereria bancrofti* in the subcutaneous tissue adjacent to mammary parenchyma. (Courtesy of R.C. Naefie.) (From Rosen PP, Oberman HA. Tumors of the mammary gland. In: *Atlas of tumor pathology.* Washington, DC: Armed Forces Institute of Pathology, 1993, with permission.)

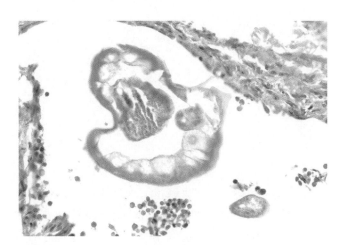

**FIG. 4.4.** *Filariasis.* A degenerated filarial worm in a breast abscess. (Courtesy of Kusum Kapila, M.D. and Kusum Verma, M.D.)

pattern. Rarely, granulomatous lesions in the breast have contained only microfilariae (19). Fully degenerated worms are likely to become calcified. Adult worms and microfilariae may be found in axillary lymph nodes (19), but in some cases nodal enlargement is solely the result of lymphangitis and reactive hyperplasia without parasitic infestation (21).

The diagnosis of mammary involvement by *W. bancrofti* is dependent on the specific microscopic structural features of the worm, eggs, and microfilariae, as well as information about the geographic region where the patient may have been exposed to infection. When the parasites are very degenerated and microfilariae cannot be demonstrated, only a presumptive diagnosis can be made.

Zoonotic filarial infections of the breast are much less common than those caused by *W. bancrofti.* The microfilariae are transmitted to humans by mosquito vectors, including *Aedes* and *Anopheles* species. Infections of the breast have been reported most often from North America, Europe, and Asia (31–35). Lesions caused by zoonotic filariasis occur predominantly in the subcutaneous tissue, conjunctiva, and

lungs (31,36). The organism responsible for most examples of mammary dirofilariasis is *Dirofilaria repens* (31–35,37), which ordinarily infects cats and dogs, but infestation of humans by *Dirofilaria tenuis,* which primarily infects raccoons, has been reported (33). The lesions occur in the subcutaneous tissue or superficial mammary parenchyma.

Infection of the breast typically presents as a discrete firm-to-hard nodule that measures around 1 cm in diameter. The lesions tend to be superficially located rather than deeply embedded in the breast parenchyma. The excised specimen usually consists of a firm fibrous tissue mass with a central cavity (Fig. 4.5). It may be limited to subcutaneous tissue or also involve the underlying breast parenchyma.

Microscopically, cross sections of the adult worm are found in the central necrotic area, accompanied by an intense inflammatory reaction that includes many eosinophils. A fibrous capsule with lymphocytes, plasma cells, and eosinophils encompasses the necrotic zone.

The diagnosis of mammary dirofilariasis usually is not suspected until the excised lesion has been examined microscop-

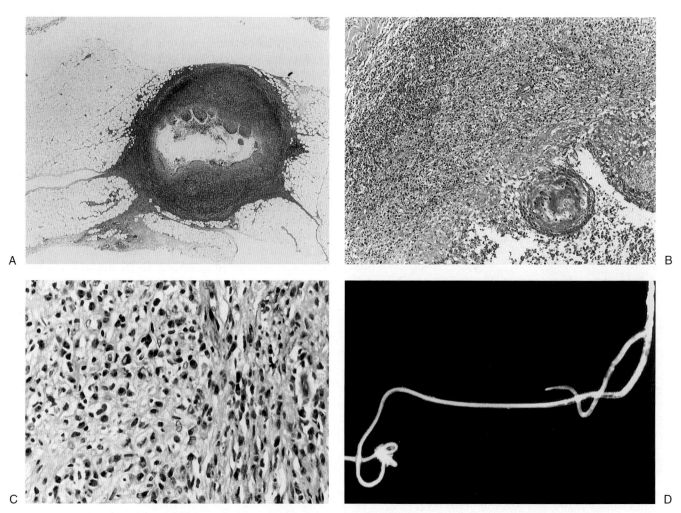

**FIG. 4.5.** *Filariasis.* **A:** An abscess caused by *Dirofilaria repens* in subcutaneous fat. Mammary lobules are present at the lower edge of the tissue. **B:** The wall of the abscess from the inside out consists of an inner layer of fibrin, the granulomatous reaction, a lymphocytic zone, and peripheral fibrosis. **C:** Granulomatous area in the abscess wall. **D:** Worm removed from the abscess cavity. (Courtesy of J. Searle, M.D.)

ically. However, in one case, ". . . a thread-like object was seen projecting from the puncture site" after an attempt at needle aspiration and a 2-cm organism was pulled out by forceps (32). Microfilariae of *W. bancrofti* were identified in fluid aspirated from a 2-cm cystic lesion in a 35-year-old woman (28). Excisional biopsy revealed lymphangiectasia in structurally normal breast tissue with edema and eosinophilia. No adult worm was found, and microfilariae were not present in peripheral blood samples. A similar experience was reported in another case (29). Both patients were in regions of India where *W. bancrofti* infection is endemic.

## Other Parasites

Infection of the breast by *Shistosoma japonicum* has been reported in two women 35 years old (38,39) and in a third who was 50 years old (40). Calcifications detected by mammography proved to be calcified ova embedded in breast parenchyma in each case. The 50-year-old woman had a painless mass at the site of the mammographic abnormality, which consisted of "branching microcalcifications suggestive of carcinoma in situ" (40). The calcified ova found in a biopsy specimen were identified as *S. japonicum.* Similar lesions have been described in the subcutaneous tissue (41).

Several examples of mammary coenurosis and cysticercosis, infections caused by the larval stages of tapeworms, have been described. Coenurosis results from infestation by tapeworms related to *Taenia* sp, which is responsible for cysticercosis. In one case, a 38-year-old Canadian woman developed a 6-cm mass in the upper inner quadrant of her left breast (42). At surgery, the lesion, which also involved the pectoral muscle, contained gelatinous material and cysts with scolices typical for tapeworms. An axillary mass that clinically resembled metastatic carcinoma in another patient proved to be cystic coenurus infection caused by *Taenia multiceps* (43). No source of infection was identified in either case.

Mammary cysticercosis caused by *Taenia solium* has been reported (Fig. 4.6) (44,45). In a 25-year-old woman, the

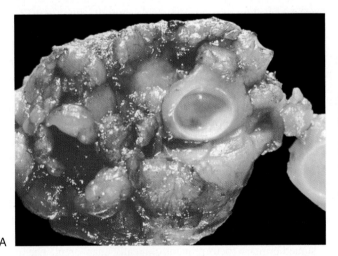

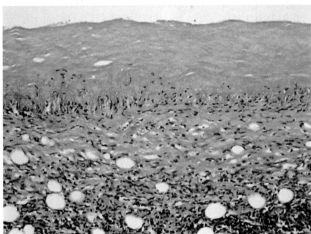

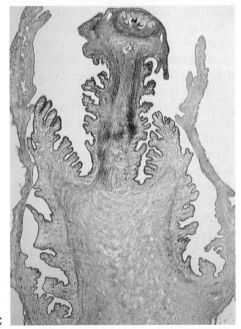

**FIG. 4.6.** *Cysticercosis:* **A:** Cyst of *Taenia solium* in the breast. **B:** The wall of the cyst resembles the reaction to a breast implant. Fat necrosis is present outside the cyst wall. **C:** Head of the tapeworm with everted scolex found in the cyst. (Courtesy of J. Searle, M.D.)

infestation resulted in the formation of a circumscribed nodule near the areola (45). Another patient was a 43-year-old woman with a 5-mm nodule in the upper outer quadrant (44). Both lesions were cystic and contained diagnostic scolices within protruding mural nodules. Clinical examination revealed no other evidence of parasitic infestation in either case. Mammary hydatid disease in another case presented as a ruptured infected cyst with cutaneous drainage (46). The breast contained numerous cysts, and hydatid infection of the spleen was detected by ultrasound examination.

The breast is a very infrequent site of hydatid cyst formation caused by *Echinococcus granulosus* (47). A review of breast tumors in 915 Saudi Arabian females reported one (0.1%) instance of mammary hydatid cyst (48). Analysis of 306 surgically resected hydatid cysts in Jordan revealed one (0.35%) female patient with a breast lesion (49). The lesion typically presents as a firm, discrete mobile mass that may be adherent to the pectoral fascia (50). Mammography reveals a dense well-circumscribed tumor, within which internal ring structures representing air–fluid levels may be seen in an overpenetrated view. Air–fluid levels and multiple cysts are seen to better advantage by ultrasound (51). On magnetic resonance imaging, the hydatid cyst presents as a well-circumscribed cystic lesion with capsular enhancement (52). The diagnosis of cystic mammary hydatid disease can be made by finding fragments of hydatid membranes and hooklets in the aspirated cyst contents (51,53,54). Treatment consists of excision of the intact cyst.

Sparganosis, an infection cased by larvae of tapeworms of the genus *Spirometra,* has been reported in the breast (55). The usual host for this parasite is the cat. Human infection typically results from ingestion of water containing *Cyclops,* a microscopic crustacean that harbors the procercoid larval form that migrates to the subcutaneous tissue. The excised mass typically consists of hemorrhagic, necrotic, and sometimes cystic tissue containing larval worms. In one instance, ultrasonography revealed "folded band-like hypoechoic structure in an ill-defined heterogeneous hypoechoic mass" (56).

*Dracunculus medinensis,* the guinea worm, forms tumorous granulomatous lesions in the subcutaneous tissue. In one case report, the lesion presented clinically as a breast mass (57). The excised specimen consisted of a cystic lesion containing four worms 5 to 25 cm in length, surrounded by granulomatous inflammation with eosinophils.

Calcifications in the pectoral muscle that were attributed to *Trichinella* infection have been found by mammography (58,59). Although the diagnosis was not confirmed by biopsy, serologic study in one case revealed antibodies for *Trichinella* (58).

Liesegang's rings are spherical deposits similar to corpora amylacea, which occur in the lungs and prostate gland. The characteristic structure consists of a double-layer outer wall that is separated from an amorphous central nidus by a striated zone. Liesegang's rings occur in breast cysts, and similar calcifications sometimes are present in pregnancy-like hyperplasia. They may be mistaken for parasitic ova in a fine needle aspiration specimen (60).

## MYCOBACTERIAL INFECTION

Almost all reported cases of mammary mycobacterial infection have been caused by *Mycobacterium tuberculosis.* The earliest modern clinical report of tuberculosis of the breast is attributed to Sir Astley Cooper in 1829 (61). Halstead and LeCount (62) reviewed the published history of scrofulous mastitis in 1898 and provided a detailed description of the histopathologic appearance of the lesions. As the disease has come under better medical control in many parts of the world, tuberculosis of the breast has been mentioned less frequently as a clinical problem in developed countries (63) but it remains a serious condition in less well developed regions. Tuberculous mastitis has been reported as a manifestation of acquired immunodeficiency syndrome (AIDS), and this presentation may be encountered with increasing frequency in human immunodeficiency virus (HIV)-positive individuals (64).

### Clinical Presentation

Tuberculous mastitis is primarily a disease of premenopausal women that may have a predilection for the lactating breast (65–68), but it may affect the adult female breast at any age and occurs rarely in the male breast (69). In younger patients, the lesion is more likely to have signs and symptoms of an abscess, whereas in older women tuberculous infection tends to cause a mass that simulates carcinoma. Unilateral tuberculous mastitis is much more common than involvement of both breasts (70). Mammary tuberculosis was found in 6 (0.52%) of 1,152 consecutive mammographic examinations performed at a university hospital in Saudi Arabia (71).

Infection of the breast may be the primary manifestation of tuberculosis, but this probably is not the most common pattern of involvement. It is considered more likely that the breasts are infected secondarily in most patients even when the presumed primary focus remains clinically unapparent. The majority of patients also have ipsilateral axillary granulomatous lymphadenitis, which may be the source of mammary infection. The occasional presence of anthracotic pigment in axillary lymph nodes is evidence that retrograde lymphatic flow from the thorax to the axilla could be the mechanism for spread from an inconspicuous primary thoracic focus of mycobacterial infection. Another route of spread from the lungs is via tracheobronchial and paratracheal lymph nodes to internal mammary lymph nodes and then to the subareolar lymphatic plexus. Retrograde spread from infected cervical lymph nodes also is possible. Hematogenous dissemination is another cause of primary infection of the breast and/or axillary lymph nodes. This manner of spread has been observed in patients with AIDS who develop disseminated tuberculosis that includes the breast (72). Finally, the breast may be involved by extension from primary lesions in the lungs that involve the chest wall or from tuberculous infection originating in bone, cartilage, or the retromammary region of the chest wall (73–75). Direct inoculation of the nipple via the lactiferous ducts, which are particularly dilated during lactation, may account for some pregnancy-associated infections.

The diagnosis of tuberculous mastitis is difficult because the disease has multiple patterns of clinical presentation (62). The most common form is nodular mastitis, in which the patient develops a slowly growing, solitary mass. The lesion generally is painless, but it may be tender. The mammographic appearance of such lesions resembles carcinoma (65,67,76). Microcalcifications typically are absent. Ultrasound and magnetic resonance imaging typically reveal a solid, heterogeneous mass, but cystic encapsulated lesions have been described (75). Advanced nodular lesions become fixed to the skin and may develop draining sinuses. The combination of a mass in the breast with a sinus tract extending to superficial bulge and thickened skin was noted as a distinctive feature of mammary tuberculosis in one study (71). When located near the nipple, such lesions can be mistaken for abscesses related to periductal mastitis or lactation. A diffuse type of tuberculous mastitis is characterized by the acute development of multiple painful nodules throughout the breast, producing a pattern that can be mistaken for inflammatory carcinoma clinically and mammographically (67,77). The third, sclerosing variety of infection occurs predominantly in elderly women, resulting in diffuse induration of the breast and diffuse increased density on mammography (67). Nipple discharge occurs in all forms of mammary tuberculosis. It is most common in the nodular and diffuse forms of the disease.

The clinical distinction between tuberculous mastitis and mammary carcinoma is complicated further by the occasional coexistence of the lesions in the same breast or in opposite breasts (67,78–80). This association probably is coincidental. Some of these cases may be examples of carcinoma with sarcoid-like granulomas, because tubercle bacilli were not identified in sections or cultured (78,79). Mammary involvement by tuberculosis and Hodgkin's disease has been described in one patient (81), and another report documents a patient with dermatomyositis treated with adrenal cortical steroids who developed large cell lymphoma and tuberculo-

sis of the breast (82). Mammary tuberculosis is rarely the presenting manifestation of AIDS (83).

A few examples of atypical mycobacterial infection associated with mammary prosthetic implants have been described. A number of patients with silicone gel implants have developed infections with *Mycobacterium fortuitum* (84,85). Smears of exudate around the implants usually have been positive for acid-fast bacilli. No common source of infection was identified. There have been fewer examples of implant associated mastitis attributed to *Mycobacterium avium-intracellulare* infection (86,87). One HIV-negative patient being treated with prednisone for systemic lupus developed a breast abscess due to *M. avium-intracellulare* caused by hematogenous spread from a paraspinal abscess (88). In another instance, a patient who became HIV positive 4 years after bilateral subglandular silicone breast implantation developed *M. avium-intracellulare* infection of one breast (89). Ten years elapsed between the onset of HIV positivity and clinical evidence of the breast infection.

## Gross Pathology

The specimen consists of nodular, indurated gray or tan tissue with yellow-to-white foci of caseous necrosis. Confluent nodular lesions with central necrotic cavitation grossly resemble necrotic carcinoma or a suppurative abscess.

## Microscopic Pathology

Granulomatous lesions in tuberculous mastitis feature caseous necrosis. In chronic cases, fibrosis may be prominent. The granulomas tend to be associated with ducts more than with lobules (Figs. 4.7 and 4.8). Acid-fast bacteria are not detected histologically in most cases (62,65).

The diagnosis of granulomatous infection of the breast may be suggested by the findings in a fine needle aspirate (76,90–92). In one series from New Delhi, India, 14 (3.4%) of

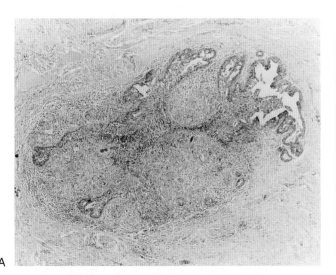
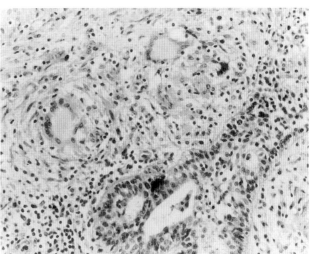

A                                                                 B

**FIG. 4.7.** *Tuberculosis.* **A:** Granulomas form multiple nodules that distort the wall of this duct, resulting in necrosis of the epithelium. **B:** Langhans-type giant cells and granulomatous inflammation.

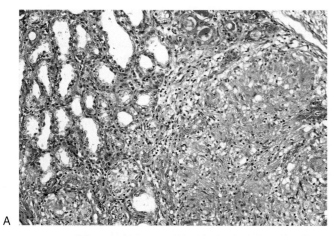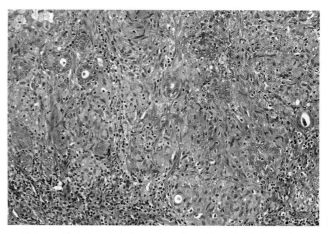

**FIG. 4.8.** *Tuberculosis.* Both images are from the same postpartum lactating breast. **A:** Granulomas and lactating glands. **B:** Confluent granulomas have destroyed the glandular tissue. *Mycobacterium tuberculosis* was isolated from the specimen.

410 breast aspiration specimens were consistent with tuberculous mastitis (91). Tuberculosis was suspected clinically in only two of these cases, whereas in three cases the clinical diagnosis was carcinoma. The aspiration cytology specimen consists of epithelioid histiocytes, polygonal or elongated Langhans giant cells, and varying numbers of neutrophils, lymphocytes, and plasma cells. Neutrophils may obscure the granulomatous character of the process in specimens from patients with necrotizing abscesses or sinus tracts. Calcifications are uncommon. Duct epithelial cells may be present. In one study, acid fast organisms were found in only 39% of fine needle aspiration specimens from mammary tuberculosis (92a).

Cytologic examination of nipple discharge shows a nonspecific mixture of foamy histiocytes, neutrophils, and necrotic debris. If tuberculous mastitis is suspected, the material should be submitted for culture as well as acid-fast stain (91).

### Treatment and Prognosis

Surgical biopsy may be necessary to establish a diagnosis of tuberculous mastitis, even if the diagnosis is suggested by the clinical presentation and the findings on fine needle aspiration biopsy. Often, the diagnosis is one of exclusion after bacteriologic and histochemical studies have been completed, because cultures and the acid-fast stain are negative in most cases. Molecular analysis of material obtained by needle or surgical biopsy can be used for the detection of *M. avium* DNA (75). Mastectomy may be necessary for advanced lesions with extensive sinus formation, but most patients respond to antibiotic management after excisional biopsy (66). Failure to control the lesion has been reported in patients who received antibiotic therapy without excision of the lesion (93).

### VIRAL INFECTIONS

#### Herpes Simplex

Two examples of unilateral *Herpes simplex* infection of the breast diagnosed cytologically and confirmed by *in situ*

hybridization have been reported (94). Neither patient had a documented underlying immunosuppressive disorder. In one case, herpetic gingivostomatitis was known to be present prior to the onset of bloody nipple discharge and crusting vesicles on the nipple surface. The second patient presented with a nipple lesion and no other evidence of infection.

### MISCELLANEOUS INFECTIONS

#### Typhoid Mastitis

Few cases of typhoid mastitis have been reported. *Salmonella typhi* was isolated from a biopsy specimen obtained from a 32-year-old patient who had a painful breast tumor (95). She had no gastrointestinal or other symptoms suggestive of typhoid infection. Blood, urine, and stool cultures were negative for *S. typhi.* Radiologic study of the gallbladder was not performed. Histologically, the tissue exhibited nonnecrotizing granulomatous inflammation with no detectable acid-fast bacteria. Gram stain examination of the tissue was not described, other possible causes of granulomatous mastitis were not evaluated, and the patient was lost to follow-up. Another patient was a 43-year-old woman who presented with fever and a 5-cm painful breast mass (96). Needle biopsy revealed acute inflammation in the breast, and *S. typhi* was isolated from the wound. *Salmonella choleraesuis* was isolated from the site of a saline-filled silicone implant removed from a patient 1 month after an episode of diarrhea and vomiting (97).

#### Cat Scratch Disease

Granulomatous lesions of cat scratch disease have been described in intramammary lymph nodes (98–100). All were women 21 to 60 years of age who had 1- to 3-cm tumors. Most lesions were in the axillary tail of the breast; one was in the 4 o'clock radius of the left breast. Clinically, these appeared to be intrinsic mammary lesions, and only one of the women also had axillary adenopathy. A well-defined hypoechoic mass was described by ultrasound in one case (98). Microscopic examination of the excised tumors reveals necrotizing granulomas. Filamentous and branching gram-negative Warthin-Starr–positive bacilli may be detected in the necrotic centers. The surrounding breast tissue has a lymphoplasmacytic infiltrate, but no granulomas have been described outside the lymph nodes. Aspiration cytology yields a cellular specimen composed of acute and chronic inflammatory cells with benign epithelial cells (98).

## Human Immunodeficiency Virus Infection

The breast does not appear to be predisposed to any particular pattern of microbial disease in HIV-infected individuals. Roca et al. (101) described a 21-year-old woman with HIV who developed a breast abscess caused by *Pseudomonas aeruginosa*. A review of mammograms obtained from 67 HIV-infected women compared with age-matched controls revealed significantly larger and more dense axillary lymph nodes in the former group (102). There was no difference in the frequency with which lymph nodes were detected in the axillary region or in the frequency of benign-appearing nodules or calcifications. See the section on Mycobacterial Infection earlier in this chapter for a discussion of these infections associated with HIV and AIDS.

## Breast Abscesses

Lactational mastitis and abscess formation develop as a result of obstruction to the flow in one or more major lactiferous ducts. The initial phases of stasis and mastitis caused by extruded milk usually are sterile. At this stage, the secreted milk has low leukocyte and bacterial counts (103). Infected lactational mastitis has been characterized by a leukocyte count of more than $10^6$ and a bacterial count of more than $10^3$ per milliliter. Fever in addition to increased pain and tenderness heralds infected lactational mastitis. Bacteria isolated from nipple discharge usually are skin inhabitants such as streptococci, *Staphylococcus aureus,* and coagulase-negative staphylococci (103). If drainage by needle aspiration and antibiotic therapy are unsuccessful, surgical drainage may be required. Specimens removed in such operations show a mixed acute and chronic inflammatory reaction that may include fat necrosis (Fig. 4.9).

A breast abscess caused by *Aeromonas hydrophilia* in an immunocompetent 12-year-old girl with no known predisposing factors was reported by Vine et al. (104). Chagla et al. (105) reported a breast abscess due to *Helcococcus kunzii* in an immunocompetent 57-year-old woman.

## Subareolar Abscesses

These abscesses usually occur in nonlactating premenopausal women (106). The condition is characterized by repeated episodes of abscess formation in the subareolar region. The lesions evolve slowly, eventually rupturing and draining through periareolar sinus tracts. Secondary infection with common skin organisms occurs occasionally, but in some cases the abscesses are sterile (106). Subareolar abscesses are the result of duct obstruction caused by squamous metaplasia in the terminal portion of one or more lactiferous ducts (107). Excision of the affected duct, sinus tract, and abscess is successful in most cases, but recurrences may occur when the process develops in another duct (108,109).

Breast abscesses have been described as a delayed complication in women treated for breast carcinoma by lumpectomy and radiotherapy (110). Factors predisposing to infection were the excision of relatively large volumes of tissue and the addition of a boost. Cultures revealed staphylococci and other bacteria of cutaneous origin.

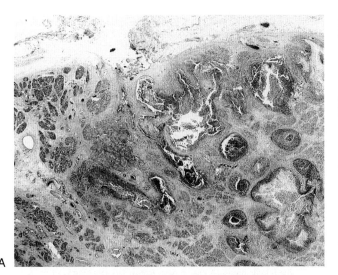
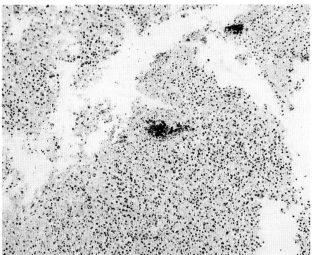

A B

**FIG. 4.9.** *Staphylococcal abscess.* **A:** Lactational mastitis with multiple abscesses from which *Staphylococcus aureus* was cultured. **B:** Exudate in an abscess containing a cluster of gram-positive cocci. (Courtesy of R.C. Naefie.) (From Rosen PP, Oberman HA. Tumors of the mammary gland. In: *Atlas of tumor pathology.* Washington, DC: Armed Forces Institute of Pathology, 1993, with permission.)

Infection of a polyurethane-coated silicone gel breast implant site caused by *Clostridium perfringens* has been reported (111). The cause probably was hematogenous contamination initiated by multiple dental procedures. The origin of *Enterococcus avium* infection of a silicone gel implant site in another patient was not found (112).

## REFERENCES

### Fungal Infections

1. Davies JAL. Primary actinomycosis of the breast. *Br J Surg* 1951;38:378–381.
2. Pemberton M. A case of primary actinomycosis of the breast. *Br J Surg* 1942;29:362–363.
3. Allen JN. *Actinomyces meyerii* breast abscess. *Am J Med* 1987;83:186–187.
4. Young VL, Hertl C, Murray PR, et al. *Paecilomyces variotii* contamination in the lumen of a saline-filled breast implant. *Plast Reconstr Surg* 1995;96:1430–1434.
5. Gogas J, Sechas M, Diamantis S, et al. Actinomycosis of the breast. *Int Surg* 1972;57:664–665.
5a. DeBarros N, Issa FKK, Barros A, et al. Imaging of primary actinomycosis of the breast. *AJR Am J Roentgenol* 2000;174:1784–1786.
6. Jain BK, Sehgal VN, Jagdish S, et al. Primary actinomycosis of the breast: a clinical review and a case report. *J Dermatol* 1994;21:497–500.
7. Pinto MM, Longstreth GB, Khoury GM. Fine needle aspiration of *Actinomyces* infection of the breast. A novel presentation of thoracopleural actinomycosis. *Acta Cytol* 1991;35:409–411.
8. Simpson AJH, Jumaa PA, Das SS. Breast abscess caused by *Nocardia asteroides*. *J Infect* 1995;30:266–267.
9. Osborne BM. Granulomatous mastitis caused by histoplasma and mimicking inflammatory breast carcinoma. *Hum Pathol* 1989;20:47–52.
10. Salfelder K, Schwarz J. Mycotic "pseudotumors" of the breast. *Arch Surg* 1975;110:751–754.
11. Farmer C, Stanley MW, Bardales RH, et al. Mycoses of the breast: diagnosis by fine-needle aspiration. *Diagn Cytopathol* 1995;12:51–55.
12. Seymour EQ. Blastomycosis of the breast. *AJR Am J Roentgenol* 1982;139:822–823.
13. Propeck PA, Scanlan KA. Blastomycosis of the breast. *AJR Am J Roentgenol* 1996;166:726.
14. Symmers WStC. Deep-seated fungal infections currently seen in the histopathologic service of a medical school laboratory in Britain. *Am J Clin Pathol* 1966;46:515–537.
15. Williams K, Walton RL, Bunkis I. Aspergillus colonization associated with bilateral silicone mammary implants. *J Surg Pathol* 1982;71:260–261.
16. Govindarajan M, Verghese S, Kuruvilla S. Primary aspergillus of the breast. Report of a case with fine needle aspiration cytology diagnosis. *Acta Cytol* 1993;37:234–236.
17. Hiruma M, Ohnishi Y, Ohata H, et al. Chromomycosis of the breast. *Int J Dermatol* 1992;31:184–185.
18. Bocian JJ, Fahmy RN, Michas CA. A rare case of "coccidioidoma" of the breast. *Arch Pathol Lab Med* 1991;115:1064–1067.

### Parasitic Infections

19. Chen YH, Qun X. Filarial granuloma of the female breast: a histopathologic study of 131 cases. *Am J Trop Med Hyg* 1981;30:1206–1210.
20. Rangabashyam N, Gnananprakasam D, Krishnaraj B. Spectrum of benign breast lesions in Madras. *J R Coll Surg Edinb* 1983;28:369–373.
21. Lang AP, Luchsinger IS, Rawling EG. Filariasis of the breast. *Arch Pathol Lab Med* 1987;111:757–759.
22. Miller JJ, Moore S. Nodular breast lesion caused by Bancroft's filariasis. *Can Med Assoc J* 1965;93:771–774.
23. Lahiri VL. Microfilariae in nipple secretion. *Acta Cytol* 1975;19:154.
24. Choudhury M. Bancroftian microfilaria in the breast clinically mimicking malignancy. *Cytopathology* 1995;6:132–133.
25. Dreyer G, Brandão AC, Amaral F, et al. Detection by ultrasound of living adult *Wuchereria bancrofti* in the female breast. *Mem Inst Oswaldo Cruz* 1996;91:95–96.

26. Novak R. Calcifications in the breast in filaria loa infection. *Acta Radiol* 1989;30:507–508.
27. Chow CK, McCarthy JS, Neafie R, et al. Mammography of lymphatic filariasis. *AJR Am J Roentgenol* 1996;167:1425–1426.
28. Bapat KC, Pandit AA. Filarial infection of the breast. Report of a case with diagnosis by fine needle aspiration cytology. *Acta Cytol* 1992;36:505–506.
29. Sodhani P, Murty DA, Pant CS. Microfilaria in a fine needle aspirate from a breast lump: a case report. *Cytopathology* 1993;4:59–62.
30. Kapila K, Verma K. Diagnosis of parasites in fine needle breast aspirates. *Acta Cytol* 1996;40:653–656.
31. Beaver PC, Orihel TC. Human infection with filariae of animals in the United States. *Am J Trop Med Hyg* 1980;29:1018–1019.
32. Bennett IC, Furnival CM, Searle J. Dirofilariasis in Australia: unusual cause of a breast lump. *Aust N Z J Surg* 1989;59:671–673.
33. Gutierrez Y, Paul GM. Breast nodule produced by *Dirofilaria tenuis*. *Am J Surg Pathol* 1984;8:463–465.
34. Pampiglione S, Franco F, Canestri Trotti G. Human subcutaneous dirofilariasis I: two new cases in Venice: identification of the causal agent as *Dirofilaria repens. Parassitologia* 1982;24:155–165.
35. Pinon JM, Dousset H, Ologoudou L, et al. Dirofilariasis of the breast in France. *Am J Trop Med Hyg* 1980;29:1018–1019.
36. Beaver PC, Jung RC, Cup EW. *Clinical parasitology,* 9th ed. Philadelphia: Lea & Febiger, 1984:390–391.
37. MacDougall LT, Magoon CC, Fritsche TR. *Dirofilaria repens* manifesting as a breast nodule. Diagnostic problems and epidemiologic considerations. *Am J Clin Pathol* 1992;97:625–630.
38. Gorman JD, Champaign JL, Sumida FK, et al. Schistosomiasis involving the breast. *Radiology* 1992;185:423–424.
39. Varin CR, Eisenberg BL, Ladd WA. Mammographic microcalcifications associated with Schistosomiasis. *South Med J* 1989;82:1060–1061.
40. Sloan BS, Rickman LS, Blau EM, et al. Schistosomiasis masquerading as carcinoma of the breast. *South Med J* 1996;89:345–347.
41. Fishbon H. A case in which eggs of *Shistosoma japonicum* were demonstrated in multiple skin lesions. *Am J Trop Med Hyg* 1946;26:319–326.
42. Benger A, Rennie RP, Roberts JT, et al. A human coenurus infection in Canada. *Am J Trop Med Hyg* 1981;30:638–644.
43. Kurtycz DFI, Alt B, Mack E. Incidental coenurosis: larval cestode presenting as an axillary mass. *Am J Clin Pathol* 1983;80:735–738.
44. Alagaratnam TT, Wing YK, Tuen H. Cysticercosis of the breast. *Am J Trop Med Hyg* 1988;38:601–602.
45. Kunkel JM, Hawksley CZ. Cysticercosis presenting as a solitary dominant breast mass. *Hum Pathol* 1987;18:1190–1191.
46. Thurairatnam TP. Echinococcus breast abscess. *Trop Doct* 1992;22:192.
47. Abi F, El Fares I, Khaiz D, et al. Les localisations inhabituelles de kyste hydatique: a propos de 40 cases. *J Chir (Paris)* 1989;126:307–312.
48. Amr SS, Sa'di ARM, Ilahi F, et al. The spectrum of breast diseases in Saudi Arab females: a 26 year pathological survey at Dhahran Health Center. *Ann Saudi Med* 1995;15:125–132.
49. Amr SS, Amr ZS, Jitawi S, et al. Hydatidosis in Jordan: an epidemiological study of 306 cases. *Ann Trop Med Parasitol* 1994;88:623–627.
50. Günay K, Müslümanoglu M, Taviloglu K, et al. Hydatid cyst of the breast—a rare form of hydatid disease. *Breast Dis* 1996;9:295–298.
51. Vega A, Ortega E, Cavada A, et al. Hydatid cyst of the breast: mammographic findings. *AJR Am J Roentgenol* 1994;162:825–826.
52. Tükel S. Hyatid cyst of the breast: MR imaging findings. *AJR Am J Roentgenol* 1997;168:1386–1387.
53. Epstein NA. Hydatid cyst of the breast: diagnosis by using cytological techniques. *Acta Cytol* 1969;13:420–421.
54. Sagin HB, Kiroglu Y, Aksoy F. Hydatid cyst of the breast diagnosed by fine needle aspiration biopsy. A case report. *Acta Cytol* 1994;38:965–967.
55. Norma SH, Kreutner A Jr. Sparganosis: clinical and pathologic observations in 10 cases. *South Med J* 1980;73:297–300.
56. Chung SY, Park KS, Lee Y, et al. Breast sparganosis: mammographic and ultrasound features. *J Clin Ultrasound* 1995;23:447–451.
57. Booth T, Schepps B, Scola FH. *Dracunculus medinensis* infestation of the female breast. A case report. *Breast Dis* 1992;5:45–49.
58. Helvie MA, Elson BC, Billi JE, et al. Pectoral muscle microcalcifications shown by mammography in a patient with trichinosis. *Breast Dis* 1995;8:111–113.

59. Ikeda DM, Sickles EA. Mammographic demonstration of pectoral muscle microcalcifications. *AJR Am J Roentgenol* 1988;151:475–476.

60. Gupta RK. Ringlike structures in fine needle aspirates from the breast. *Cytopathology* 1996;7:352–356.

## Mycobacterial Infections

61. Cooper AP. *Illustrations of the diseases of the breast.* London: Longman, Rees Co., 1829.

62. Halstead AC, LeCount ER. Tuberculosis of the mammary gland. *Ann Surg* 1898;28:685–707.

63. Hamit HF, Ragsdale TH. Mammary tuberculosis. *J R Soc Med* 1982;75:764–765.

64. Hartstein M, Leaf HL. Tuberculosis of the breast as a presenting manifestation of AIDS. *Clin Infect Dis* 1992;15:692–693.

65. Alagaratnam TT, Ong GB. Tuberculosis of the breast. *Br J Surg* 1980;67:125–126.

66. McKeown KC, Wilkinson KW. Tuberculous disease of the breast. *Br J Surg* 1952;39:420–429.

67. Tabar L, Kelt K, Nemeth A. Tuberculosis of the breast. *Radiology* 1976;118:587–589.

68. Wilson TS, MacGregor JW. The diagnosis and treatment of tuberculosis of the breast. *Can Med Assoc J* 1963;89:1118–1124.

69. Atiq OT, Reyes CV, Zvetina JR. Male tuberculous mastitis. *Breast Dis* 1992;5:273–275.

70. Ducroz B, Nael LM, Gautier G, Tubreculose mammaire bilatérale: un cas. Révue de la literature. *J Gynécol Obstét Biol Réprod (Paris)* 1992;21:484–488.

71. Makanjuola D, Murshid K, Sulaimani A, et al. Mammographic features of breast tuberculosis: the skin bulge and sinus tract sign. *Clin Radiol* 1996;51:354–358.

72. Aguirrezabalaga J, Sogo C, Parajó A, et al. Mammary tuberculosis. Three case reports. *Breast Dis* 1994;7:377–382.

73. Kappas AM, Bourantas KL, Batsis CP, et al. Chest tuberculosis mimicking breast cancer. *Breast Dis* 1995;8:85–89.

74. Chung SY, Yang I, Bae SH, et al. Tuberculous abscess in retromammary region: CT findings. *J Comp Assist Tomogr* 1996;20:766–769.

75. Greenberg D, Hingston G, Harman J. Chest wall tuberculosis. *Breast J* 1999;5:60–62.

76. Oh KK, Kim JH, Kook SH. Imaging of tuberculous disease involving breast. *Eur Radiol* 1998;8:1475–1480.

77. Sopeña B, Arnillas E, Garcia-Vila LM, et al. Tuberculosis of the breast: unusual clinical presentation of extrapulmonary tuberculosis. *Infection* 1996;24:57–58.

78. Grausman RI, Goldman ML. Tuberculosis of the breast. Report of nine cases including two cases of co-existing carcinoma and tuberculosis. *Am J Surg* 1945;67:48–56.

79. Miller RE, Salomon PF, West JP. The coexistence of carcinoma and tuberculosis of the breast and axillary lymph nodes. *Am J Surg* 1971;121:338–340.

80. Rothman GM, Kolkov Z, Meroz A, et al. Breast tuberculosis and carcinoma. *Isr J Med Sci* 1989;25:339–340.

81. Graeme-Cook F, O'Briain S, Daly PA. Unusual breast masses. The sequential development of mammary tuberculosis and Hodgkin's disease of a young woman. *Cancer* 1988;61:1457–1459.

82. Cheng W, Alagaratnam TT, Leung CY, et al. Tuberculosis and lymphoma of the breast in a patient with dermatomyositis. *Aust N Z J Surg* 1993;63:660–661.

83. Hartstein M, Leaf HL. Tuberculosis of the breast as a presenting manifestation of AIDS. *Clin Infect Dis* 1992;15:692–693.

84. Clegg HW, Foster MT, Sanders WE Jr, et al. Infection due to organisms of the *Mycobacterium fortuitum* complex after augmentation mammaplasty: clinical and epidemiologic features. *J Infect Dis* 1983;147:427–433.

85. Toranto IR, Malow JB. Atypical mycobacteria periprosthetic infections—diagnosis and treatment. *Plast Reconstr Surg* 1980;66:226–228.

86. Lee D, Goldstein EJC, Zarem HA. Localized *Mycobacterium avium-intracellulare* mastitis in an immunocompetent woman with silicone breast implants. *Plast Reconstr Surg* 1995;95:142–144.

87. Perry RR, Jacques DP, Lesar MSL, et al. *Mycobacterium avium* infection in a silicone-injected breast. *Plast Reconstr Surg* 1985;75:104–106.

88. Brodkin H. Paraspinous abscess with *Mycobacterium avium-intracellulare* in a patient without AIDS. *South Med J* 1991;84:1385–1386.

89. Eliopoulos DA, Lyle G. *Mycobacterium avium* infection in a patient with the acquired immunodeficiency syndrome and silicone breast implants. *South Med J* 1999;92:80–83.

90. Das DK, Sodhani P, Kashyap V, et al. Inflammatory lesions of the breast: diagnosis by fine needle aspiration. *Cytopathology* 1992;3:281–289.

91. Nayar M, Saxena HMK. Tuberculosis of the breast. A cytomorphologic study of needle aspirates and nipple discharges. *Acta Cytol* 1984;28:325–328.

92. Gupta D, Rajwanshi A, Gupta SK, et al. Fine needle aspiration cytology in the diagnosis of tuberculous mastitis. *Acta Cytol* 1999;43:191–194.

92a. Kakkar S, Kapila K, Singh MK, et al. Tuberculosis of the breast. A cytomorphologic study. *Acta Cytol* 2000;44:292–296.

93. McMeeking AA, Gonzalez R, Hanna B. Mammary tuberculosis. *N Y State J Med* 1989;89:288–289.

## Viral Infections

94. Kobayashi TK, Okamoto H, Yakushiji M. Cytologic detection of herpes simplex virus DNA in nipple discharge by in situ hybridization: report of two cases. *Diagn Cytopathol* 1993;9:296–299.

## Miscellaneous Infections

95. Campbell FC, Eriksson BL, Angorn IB. Localized granulomatous mastitis—an unusual presentation of typhoid. A case report. *S Afr Med J* 1980;57:793–795.

96. Barrett GS, MacDermot J. Breast abscess: a rare presentation of typhoid. *Br Med J* 1972;2:628–629.

97. Asaadi M, Suh EDW. Salmonella infection following breast reconstruction. *Plast Reconstr Surg* 1995;96:1749–1750.

98. Chess Q, Santarsieri V, Kostroff K, et al. Aspiration cytology of cat scratch disease of the breast. *Acta Cytol* 1990;34:761–762.

99. Lefkowitz M, Wear DJ. Cat-scratch disease masquerading as a solitary tumor of the breast. *Arch Pathol Lab Med* 1989;113:473–475.

100. Lobrano ME, Clayton MJ, Levine EA, et al. Cat scratch disease of the breast. *Breast J* 1999;5:59.

101. Roca B, Vilar C, Peréz EV, et al. Breast abscess with lethal septicemia due to *Pseudomonas aeruginosa* in a patient with AIDS. *Presse Med* 1996;25:803–804.

102. Solomon SB, Gatewood OMB, Brem RF. HIV infection: analysis of mammographic findings. *Breast J* 1999;5:112–115.

103. Thomsen AC, Esperson T, Maigaard S. Course and treatment of milk stasis, non-infectious inflammation of the breast and infectious mastitis in nursing women. *Am J Obstet Gynecol* 1984;149:492–495.

104. Vine AJ, Bleiweiss IJ, Mizrachy B. *Aeromonas hydrophila* breast abscess. *Breast J* 1994;7:387–391.

105. Chagla AH, Borczyk AA, Facklam RR, et al. Breast abscess associated with *Helcococcus kunzii*. *J Clin Microbiol* 1998;36:2377–2379.

106. Golinger RC, O'Neal BJ. Mastitis and mammary duct disease. *Arch Surg* 1982;1182:1027–1029.

107. Habif DV, Perzin KH, Lipton R, et al. Subareolar abscess associated with squamous metaplasia of lactiferous ducts. *Am J Surg* 1970;119:523–526.

108. Abramson DJ. Mammary duct ectasia, mamillary fistula and subareolar sinuses. *Ann Surg* 1969;169:217–226.

109. Urban JA. Excision of the major ductal system of the breast. *Cancer* 1963;16:516–520.

110. Bowers GJ, Prestidge B, Getz JB, et al. Infectious complications in irradiated breasts following conservative breast therapy. *Breast J* 1995;1:295–299.

111. Hunter JG, Padilla M, Cooper-Vastola S. Late *Clostridium perfringens* breast implant infection after dental treatment. *Ann Plast Surg* 1996;36:309–312.

112. Ablaza VJ, La Trenta GS. Late infection of a breast prosthesis with *Enterococcus avium*. *Plast Reconstr Surg* 1998;102:227–230.

# CHAPTER 5

# Papilloma and Related Benign Tumors

This chapter includes a heterogeneous group of lesions. Some are fundamentally papillary (intraductal papilloma and subareolar sclerosing papilloma), prominently papillary (florid papillomatosis and radial sclerosing lesion [RSL]), or partly papillary (cystic and papillary apocrine metaplasia). Syringomatous adenoma is discussed in this chapter because it is clinically and histologically part of the differential diagnosis of florid papillomatosis. Collagenous spherulosis is a stromal component seen in various papillary lesions, including papilloma and duct hyperplasia, and rarely in adenosis.

## PAPILLOMA

Papillomas are discrete benign tumors of the epithelium of mammary ducts. They arise more often in the central part of the breast from lactiferous ducts, but they can occur peripherally in any quadrant. *Intracystic papilloma* is the designation applied to a papilloma in a cystically dilated duct. Large complex papillomas that have a cystic component sometimes have been referred to as *papillary cystadenomas*, whereas solid, noncystic papillomas have been variously classified as *ductal adenoma* and *adenomyoepithelioma*. A *solitary papilloma* is a single discrete papillary tumor in one duct. *Multiple papillomas* usually occur in contiguous branches of the ductal system. Solitary papillomas are more common than multiple papillomas. A distinction must be made between intraductal papilloma and papillomatosis (epitheliosis). The latter terms are used to describe microscopic duct hyperplasia. Papillomatosis may coexist with solitary or multiple papillomas.

### Clinical Presentation

In 1951, Haagensen et al. (1) reviewed a series of 367 patients with benign intraductal papillary breast lesions who had been treated at Presbyterian Hospital between 1916 and 1941. After excluding 243 patients with "microscopic papillomas," 14 with incomplete data, and two with a gross intraductal papilloma and unrelated nonpapillary carcinoma, they concentrated on describing 108 patients treated for gross, be-

nign intraductal papillomas. Microscopic papillomas were characterized as "small multiple papillary projections, with or without fibrous cores, which project into the ducts and cysts of chronic cystic mastitis." By contrast, gross papilloma was defined as a "definite disease entity in which one or more papillomas grow within a relatively localized portion of a duct, or in several adjacent ducts, and attain sufficient size to fill up the duct and become evident grossly."

The study confirmed some now well-established features of duct papilloma. The majority (75%) of lesions were located in the central part of the breast. Discharge, bloody or nonbloody, was the primary symptom in 72% of cases, but was less commonly seen with peripheral lesions (29%) than with those in a central duct (86%). Bloody discharge occurred from 71% of central papillomas. Lesions that caused nipple discharge, whether central or peripheral, tended to have a frond-forming papillary configuration, whereas a more solid growth pattern was observed in tumors not associated with discharge.

A subareolar mass may be palpable in patients with a central solitary papilloma, and a palpable tumor may be the first clinical manifestation of a papilloma in one of the quadrants. Cystic solitary papillary tumors may appear to be well circumscribed on mammography. The presence of a cystic component is best appreciated by ultrasonography or pneumocystography. Solitary papillomas may occur at any age from infancy to the ninth decade, but they are most frequent in the sixth decade of life.

Multiple papillomas develop more often peripherally than centrally and typically present as a palpable lesion. These patients tend to be younger on average than women with solitary papillomas, most often presenting in their 40s and early 50s.

Cardenosa and Eklund (2) compared the clinical and mammographic findings in patients with solitary and multiple papillomas. The latter group was subdivided into peripheral and central lesions. Nipple discharge occurred more often in women with central lesions, whether solitary or multiple, and these patients were more likely to have a positive ductogram. Most lesions consisting of multiple peripheral papillomas were asymptomatic clinically and were detected as a result of mam-

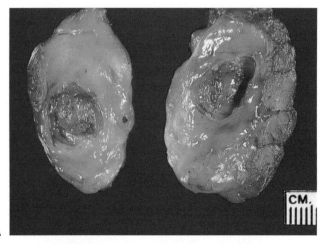

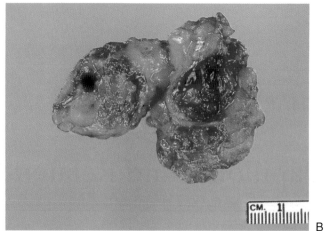

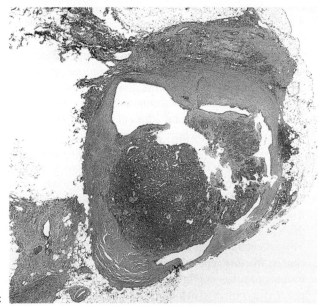

**FIG. 5.1.** *Papilloma.* Gross appearance of two lesions. **A:** Intracystic papilloma. **B:** Solid intracystic papilloma virtually filling the cyst lumen. **C:** Histologic whole mount of a tumor similar to the tumor shown in **(B)**.

mographic abnormalities, including calcifications, nodules, masses, or various opacities. Magnetic resonance imaging in women with solitary intraductal papillomas and nipple discharge revealed duct dilation and well-circumscribed enhancing intraductal lesions (3). Fiberoptic ductoscopy is a diagnostic procedure for locating and sampling single or multiple papillomas in women who present with nipple discharge (3a).

### Gross Pathology

A part of the mass associated with some solitary papillomas is a cyst formed by the dilated duct in which the papilloma arose (Fig. 5.1). The cyst may contain clear fluid, bloody fluid, or clotted blood. The papilloma usually forms a single mural nodule protruding into the lumen, but occasionally multiple, separate, or aggregated nodules are present. Some papillomas grow as soft friable masses that obliterate the cystic space. The underlying papillary nature of these lesions becomes apparent when the tissue fragments during gross sampling.

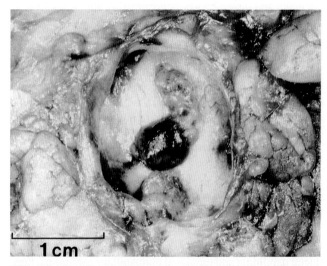

**FIG. 5.2.** *Papilloma.* Gross appearance of an intracystic papilloma consisting of two mural nodules. The cyst wall is a distinct fibrous membrane with a smooth inner surface.

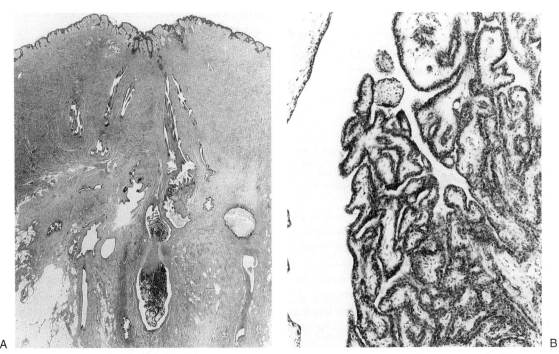

**FIG. 5.3.** *Papilloma of lactiferous duct.* **A:** A dumbbell-shaped papilloma with a central zone of fibrosis. **B:** The papillary fronds are composed of somewhat edematous fibrovascular stroma with a thin layer of epithelium on the surface. Similar epithelium lines the lumen of the dilated duct. (From Rosen PP. Arthur Purdy Stout and papilloma of the breast. Comments on the occasion of his 100th birthday. *Am J Surg Pathol* 1986;10[Suppl 1]:100, with permission.)

Solitary papillomas typically are bosselated, soft-to-firm tumors that are gray to reddish-brown when examined grossly in the fresh state. The lesions are well circumscribed and appear to be enclosed in a capsule formed by the duct wall and accompanying reactive changes (Figs. 5.2 and 5.3). Multiple associated papillomas sometimes can be appreciated grossly when they form nodules in contiguous dilated ducts (Fig. 5.4).

Solitary papillomas may form clinically symptomatic tumors 1 cm or less in diameter in a major lactiferous duct, but the average size is 2 to 3 cm. Benign cystic papillomas may be larger than 10 cm. Tumors formed by multiple papillomas typically are larger than 2 cm (1,4).

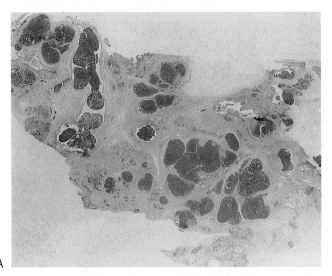

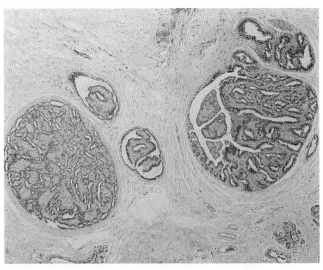

**FIG. 5.4.** *Multiple intraductal papillomas.* **A:** Macroscopic view of a histologic section with multiple papillomas, many of which completely fill ducts. **B:** Intraductal papillomas.

## Microscopic Pathology

The basic microscopic structure of a papilloma consists of the proliferation of ductal epithelium supported by frond-forming fibrovascular stroma. The most orderly form of papilloma consists of branching fronds of stroma supporting a layer of epithelium composed of epithelial and myoepithelial cells (Fig. 5.5). The epithelial cells are cuboidal to columnar without pleomorphism, nuclear hyperchromasia, or mitotic activity. The supporting stroma may arise from a single base or from several foci in the duct wall. Epithelium lining the nonpapillary portion of the duct usually exhibits little or no hyperplasia in such lesions.

Many benign papillomas have more complex structures caused by stromal overgrowth and hyperplasia of the epithelium that results in distortion and fusion of papillary fronds (Figs. 5.6 and 5.7). The most exaggerated form of this process is the solid intraductal papilloma, in which virtually all space between fibrovascular stalks is filled by proliferative duct epithelium. More often, secondary lumens are formed within the hyperplastic epithelium, resulting in irregular microlumens, micropapillary fronds, focal solid areas, or heterogeneous combinations of these patterns.

Foci of apocrine metaplasia are not uncommon in papillomas, and rarely, most or all of the epithelium is of the apocrine type (Fig. 5.8). When present in the conventional papillary configuration, apocrine metaplasia usually is cytologically bland, but apocrine atypia manifested by nuclear pleomorphism and cytoplasmic clearing is likely to be encountered in sclerosing papillary tumors. This is especially common when sclerosing adenosis is incorporated into a papilloma (5).

The appearance of the fibrovascular stroma varies considerably among papillomas. In some lesions, the stroma is limited to slender inconspicuous bands consisting of thin-walled capillaries accompanied by sparse fibroblasts, collagen, and mononuclear cells forming a network to support the voluminous epithelium. The distribution of this stroma can be seen more clearly in sections stained for reticulin, vimentin, basement membrane proteins, or vascular markers such as CD34 or CD31. Expansion of the fibrovascular stroma by accumulated histiocytes is an infrequent finding (Fig. 5.9).

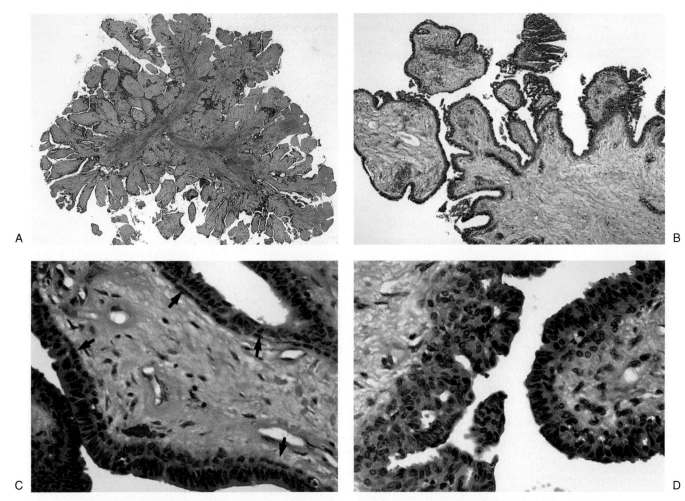

**FIG. 5.5.** *Papilloma.* **A:** This papilloma has dense collagenized stroma. **B:** Epithelium on the surfaces of the fronds is thin. **C:** A thin layer of cuboidal and columnar epithelial cells overlies a continuous layer of myoepithelial cells *(arrows).* **D:** Slight epithelial hyperplasia at the surface of one papillary frond.

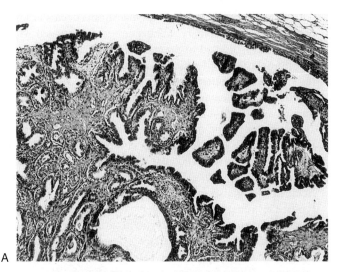

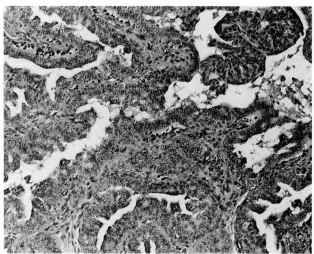

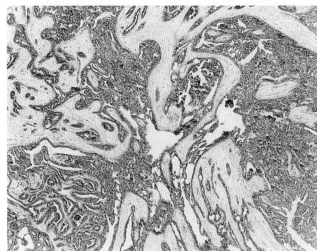

**FIG. 5.6.** *Papillomas.* Histologic appearances of three different tumors. **A:** Papilloma with simple epithelium and an area of adenosis. **B:** Papilloma with prominent epithelial hyperplasia. **C:** Papilloma with complex anastomosing epithelial hyperplasia and sclerosis, which distorts the underlying papillary architecture.

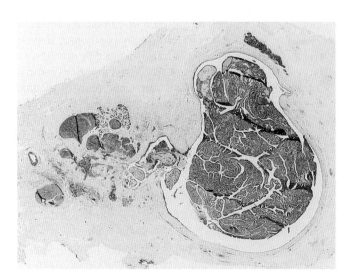

**FIG. 5.7.** *Papilloma.* Part of the papilloma inhabits a cystically dilated duct, while an adjacent portion has the configuration of a radial scar. (From Rosen PP. Arthur Purdy Stout and papilloma of the breast. Comments on the occasion of his 100th birthday. *Am J Surg Pathol* 1986;10[Suppl 1]:100, with permission.)

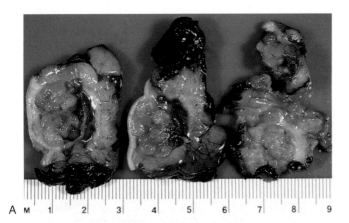

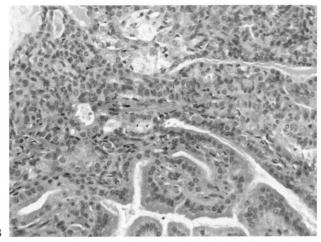

**FIG. 5.8.** *Papilloma with apocrine metaplasia.* **A:** The light-brown color of this cystic papillary lesion is typical of tumors with apocrine metaplasia. **B:** Columnar apocrine epithelium on the surface of a papillary frond.

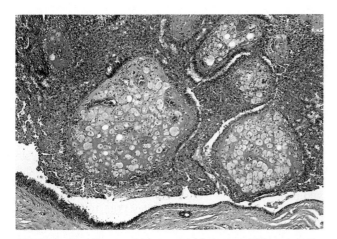

**FIG. 5.9.** *Papilloma with stromal histiocytes.* Fibrovascular stroma is prominent as a result of accumulated histiocytes in a papilloma that nearly fills a cystically dilated duct. Part of the duct wall is seen at the *bottom* of the image.

Collagenization of the fibrovascular stroma occurs in some papillomas. The papillary architecture is accentuated when this process is limited to the intrinsic papillary structure. If myofibroblastic proliferation accompanies collagenization of the stroma, the papillary arrangement is likely to become distorted. Epithelial elements entrapped in this stroma may simulate invasive carcinoma within or at the periphery of the lesion (Figs. 5.10 and 5.11). In the most extreme situations, fibrous sclerosis is so severe as to virtually obliterate the papilloma, reducing it to a nodular scar containing scattered benign glandular elements (Fig. 5.12). Such a lesion may be difficult to distinguish from a fibroadenoma. This problem is typified by a case report purported to represent an infarcted fibroadenoma in which the illustrations are highly suggestive of a fibrotic and partially infarcted cystic papilloma (6). The epithelial cells in papillomas typically exhibit strong nuclear immunoreactivity for estrogen receptors (Fig. 5.13).

The epithelium of intraductal papillomas contains a myoepithelial cell layer (7). Elongated myoepithelial cells with nuclei that are flattened along the basement membrane are inconspicuous. Hyperplastic myoepithelial cells typically form a prominent layer of cuboidal cells that tend to have relatively clear cytoplasm (Fig. 5.14). Myoepithelial cells in papillomas can be demonstrated with immunostains for S-100 and actin (7). The smooth muscle myosin heavy-chain and calponin stains are particularly helpful for specifically highlighting myoepithelial cells in a sclerosing papillary lesion with prominent stromal myofibroblasts (8). Myoepithelial cells are not equally apparent in all portions of a sclerosing papilloma. In such lesions they can be very attenuated and focally not detectable, especially when there is florid epithelial hyperplasia with atypia. Papillomas in which there is marked hyperplasia of myoepithelial cells represent a variant of adenomyoepithelioma.

Infarction occurs in solitary and in multiple papillomas (Figs. 5.15 and 5.16). No specific cause for the necrosis is evident in most cases. The presence of chronic inflammation and hemosiderin in and around many papillomas suggests that these lesions are prone to transient bleeding secondary to ischemia or incidental trauma. Needling procedures can contribute to infarction and cause fresh hemorrhage, sometimes associated with displaced epithelium. Spontaneous infarction usually involves superficial portions of a papilloma. Rarely, the entire lesion is destroyed. The underlying structure of a fully infarcted papilloma can be demonstrated with a reticulin stain. In some infarcted lesions where degeneration is not too advanced, the structure of the epithelium can be displayed more clearly with a cytokeratin immunostain. However, there is no procedure for reliably distinguishing between the completely infarcted epithelium of a papilloma and a papillary carcinoma. Cytologic atypia is commonly found in the partially degenerated epithelium of a papilloma in the vicinity of infarcts, usually manifested by nuclear hyperchromasia and pleomorphism. These cytologic abnormalities may lead to an erroneous diagnosis of carcinoma in the fine needle aspiration (FNA) specimen from an infarcted papilloma (9).

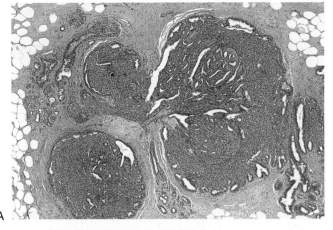

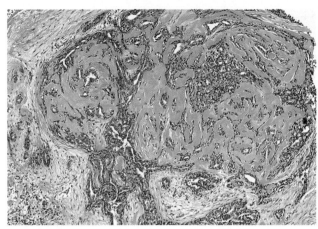

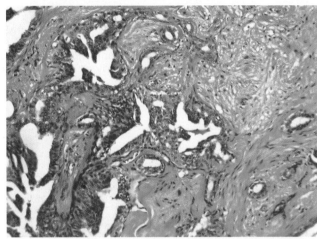

FIG. 5.10. *Papilloma with stromal sclerosis.* **A:** A trilobate solid papilloma showing early central sclerosis. **B:** Well-developed sclerosis is present throughout this papilloma. **C:** Epithelium in the collagenized myofibroblastic stroma resembles invasive carcinoma. Needle core biopsy of such a lesion may present a difficult diagnostic problem.

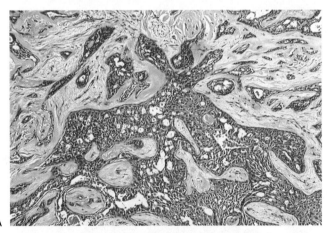

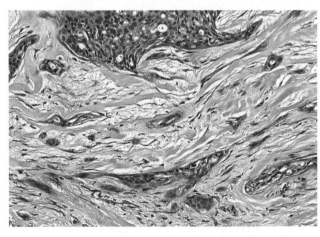

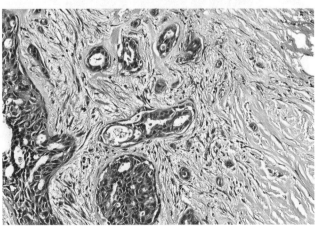

FIG. 5.11. *Papilloma with stromal sclerosis.* Images from one tumor similar to the lesion shown in Fig. 5.10B. **A:** An area near the center of the lesion showing residual papilloma with fenestrated epithelium. **B:** Attenuated epithelium is distributed between layers of myofibroblasts and collagen within the tumor. **C:** Image from the periphery of the lesion shows rounded groups of cells and isolated cells, a characteristic finding at the edges of a papilloma with sclerosis.

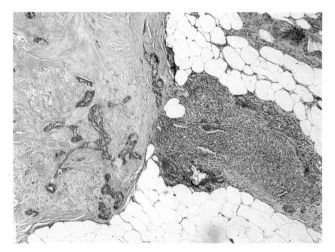

**FIG. 5.12.** *Papilloma with extreme stromal sclerosis.* The main tumor is almost entirely effaced by collagenized stroma. An intraductal papilloma persists in a peripheral duct.

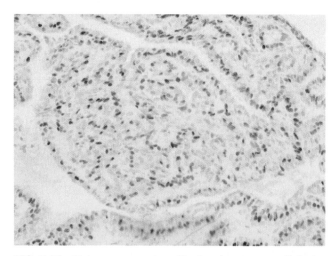

**FIG. 5.13.** *Estrogen receptors.* Nuclear immunoreactivity for estrogen receptors is present in virtually all of the epithelial cells (avidin-biotin).

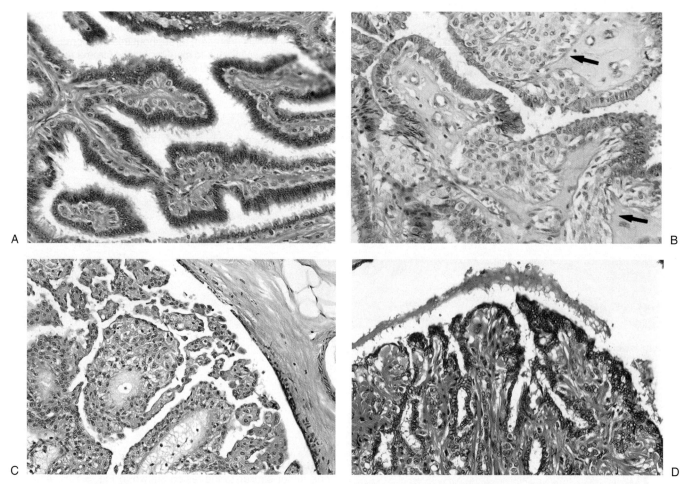

**FIG. 5.14.** *Myoepithelial cell hyperplasia.* **A:** Hyperplastic myoepithelial cells forming an expanded zone beneath the thin epithelium. **B:** The myoepithelial cells have an epithelioid phenotype *(arrows).* **C:** Myoepithelial cells with an epithelial phenotype are markedly hyperplastic in this papilloma. The epithelium is reduced to a thin layer of flat cells overlying the multilayered myoepithelium. **D:** A papilloma in which the myoepithelial cells have a striking myoid phenotype and resemble smooth muscle.

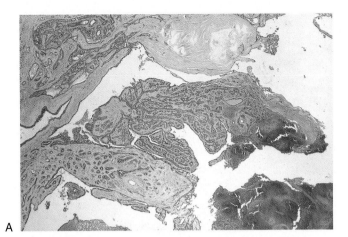

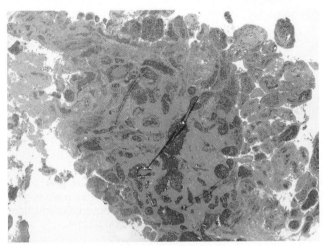

**FIG. 5.15.** *Infarcted papilloma.* **A:** Low-magnification view of infarction in the apical portion of a papilloma. **B:** This papillary lesion is entirely infarcted.

Squamous metaplasia can develop in the epithelium of a papilloma (Fig. 5.17). This is more likely to occur when there is infarction, probably as a reactive or reparative process (10). Rarely, squamous metaplasia constitutes a con-spicuous component of the papilloma or of the epithelium lining the cystic portion of the lesion. Extension of squamous metaplasia to the epithelium of adjacent ducts is an uncommon finding (11). Entrapped metaplastic epithelium in the stromal reaction may simulate metaplastic or squamous carcinoma. In some instances, the distinction between these processes is very difficult (10). Electron microscopy and immunohistochemistry suggest that some examples of squamous metaplasia derive from myoepithelial cells (12).

The diagnosis of an intraductal papilloma may be suggested by the cytologic findings in an FNA specimen (13,14). The smear typically has cohesive three-dimensional groups of cytologically benign-appearing cells accompanied by variable amounts of stromal cells, apocrine cells, inflammatory cells, and histiocytes. FNA is not a reliable procedure for identifying focal carcinoma in a papilloma (14). Immunostains may help in the diagnosis of FNA specimens of papillary breast tumors. Chang et al. (15) reported that the percentage of Ki67-positive cells was significantly higher in papillary carcinomas (21.0% ±19.23%) than in papillomas (6.23% ±7.25%). These investigators did not find cyclin D1 reactivity to be a useful differential feature.

Intraductal papillomas can be recognized by frozen section, but in most circumstances, it is preferable to rely on paraffin sections for diagnosis of papillary tumors. Sometimes it is difficult to prepare satisfactory frozen sections from these fragile lesions or to identify foci of carcinoma that have developed in a papilloma.

**Treatment and Prognosis**

Surgical excision is recommended for papillomas. Reexcision of the biopsy site may be performed in patients with multiple papillomas, especially if the lesion exhibits atypia.

Management of a papilloma diagnosed by needle core biopsy currently is problematic. Excisional biopsy is recommended for patients who have an atypical component in the

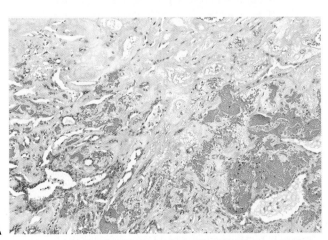

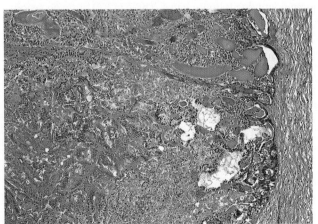

**FIG. 5.16.** *Infarcted papillary tumors.* **A:** Hemorrhage is present at the border of the infarcted zone *(above)* in a sclerosing papilloma. **B:** The ghost architecture of this papillary lesion is visible *(left)* and a thin zone of residual viable epithelium is present at the periphery *(right)*. This was probably an infarcted solid papilloma.

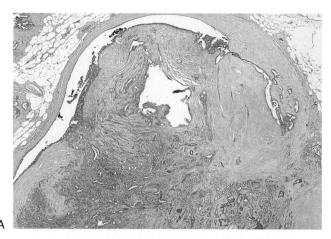

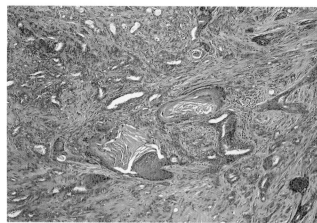

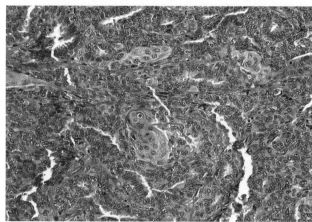

**FIG. 5.17.** *Papilloma with squamous metaplasia.* **A,B:** Intracystic sclerosing papilloma with focal squamous metaplasia. **C:** A small cluster of cells exhibiting squamous differentiation is present in the epithelium of this florid papilloma.

papillary lesion or in the surrounding tissue because the surgical specimens disclose carcinoma in an appreciable number of cases. Data from several studies suggest that excision of papillary lesions diagnosed by core biopsy would be prudent even in the absence of atypia. Liberman et al. (16) studied 26 patients with papillary lesions diagnosed by core biopsy, followed by excision in 22 and at least 2 years of mammographic follow-up in 4. Three (43%) of seven lesions initially diagnosed as papillary carcinoma had invasive carcinoma in the excisional specimen, and three (30%) of 10 with atypical hyperplasia in a papilloma on core biopsy had intraductal carcinoma in the excision specimen. No carcinomas were diagnosed in excision specimens or during the published follow-up of seven benign papillomas. However, after publication, one patient with a papilloma that had not been excised later developed invasive metaplasia that originated in the cystic papilloma (17).

Berg et al. (18) studied a series of patients with benign papillary lesions diagnosed by needle core biopsy. Excisional biopsy of 10 papillomas revealed adjacent intraductal carcinoma in one case (10%) and atypical hyperplasia in 3 (30%). Six papillomas with atypia diagnosed by needle core biopsy also were excised. Two contained carcinoma, two showed further atypia, and two were RSLs. Excisional surgery was performed during follow-up of 22 other papillo-

mas because the lesions enlarged or developed additional calcifications. None of the four lesions excised subsequently had carcinoma. The authors concluded that "a result of 'benign papilloma' on core biopsy should be viewed in the same context as a high-risk lesion; excision may be warranted."

Mastectomy was considered appropriate therapy for intraductal papilloma in the first half of the twentieth century because of the widespread belief that the lesion was "precancerous" and that the breast that harbored a papilloma was cancer prone even if the papilloma itself was not malignant.

> Every surgeon hesitates to mutilate a woman, and particularly this organ, but every surgeon with a conscience will attack that which is or may become cancer. Benign means "born good," but all tumors of the breast which have this title are apt to go bad and are not to be trusted. . . . Bleeding from the nipple we see associated with them at all times . . . for tumors only "born good" we have not as yet a definite plan of attack. Some surgeons resect in part; some do a complete plastic subcutaneous resection, and others a radical removal. Can we today say who does wisely? (19)

Bloodgood recommended that papillomas be treated by excision in 1922 (20), but it was not until 1951 that a follow-up study by Haagensen et al. (1) documented the low risk for subsequent carcinoma in women following excision of a papilloma. This study reported the follow-up of 72 women, none of whom developed ipsilateral carcinoma after excision of a papilloma. Four women had additional papillomas in the same breast, including three in the area of prior excision. A fifth woman was treated for a contralateral papilloma. Thirty-two patients had been treated initially by mastectomy. In four of these cases, an erroneous pathologic diagnosis of carcinoma was reported on paraffin sections, and in five an error was made in the interpretation of a frozen section. From this experience, it was determined that it was not advisable

> . . . to rely upon frozen sections in distinguishing benign from malignant papillary tumors of the breast. . . . Following removal of a satisfactory piece of the lesion the wound is closed and we wait for paraffin sections. . . . We believe that the disadvantage of having to delay and carry out our definitive treatment at a second stage is more than compensated for by the avoidance of the risk of subjecting the patient to the unnecessary radical mastectomy for a benign papilloma. (1)

The precancerous significance of papillomas has been the subject of many studies (5,21–25). Carter (26) reviewed the subject and concluded that

> . . . any of the intraductal papillary tumors may precede invasive carcinoma of the breast. The risk of developing invasive carcinoma increases progressively from those patients with a solitary papilloma with only minor associated changes to those patients with solitary papilloma and associated hyperplastic changes to those patients with multiple papillomas to those patients with intraductal papillary carcinoma.

Sometimes the close proximity of mammary carcinoma to a papilloma is such that it is difficult to regard them as arising separately. Although this is not a frequent occurrence, in such cases it is appropriate to conclude that the carcinomatous portion of the lesion arose from the coexisting papilloma. It is generally recognized today that the diagnosis of orderly papillary carcinoma often is complicated by coexisting areas of papilloma. This combination was observed in seven of 41 papillary carcinomas studied by Papotti et al. (7).

**TABLE 5.1.** *Intraductal papilloma and carcinoma: a selected literature review*

| Reference | No. cases biopsied | Follow-up |
|---|---|---|
| Kilgore et al. (23) | 57 | 8 Ca: 6 ipsi, 2 contra |
| Lewison and Lyons (25) | 23 | No Ca |
| Haagensen et al. (1) | 76 | No Ca |
| Snyder and Chaffin (27) | 30 | No Ca |
| Hendrick (22) | 207 | 2 Ca: 2 contra |
| Kraus and Neubecker (24) | 19 | No Ca |
| Buhl-Jorgensen et al. (21) | 53 | 7 Ca: 3 ipsi, 3 contra, 1 bilat |
| Carter (26) | 64 | 6 Ca: 2 ipsi, 3 contra, 1 bilat |
| Total | 529 | 11 ipsi (2%) 10 contra (2%) 2 bilat (0.3%) |

*bilat*, bilateral; *Ca*, carcinoma; *contra*, contralateral; *ipsi*, ipsilateral.

Most follow-up studies of papillomas document the low "precancerous" potential of these lesions, but it must be emphasized that there are significant limitations in many of the reports. A substantial number of patients in earlier studies had their papillomas treated by mastectomy. In some papers, the distinction between papilloma and carcinoma may not have been reliable, and sometimes patients with multiple and solitary papillomas were grouped together. As can be seen in Table 5.1, the reported frequency of carcinoma subsequent to the excision of a papilloma has been less than 5%. Nearly half of the subsequent carcinomas were detected in the opposite breast. A substantially greater risk for subsequent carcinoma has been demonstrated in women with multiple papillomas (26,28,29).

## RADIAL SCLEROSING LESIONS

Attention has been focused in the past two decades on proliferative lesions that have a stellate configuration radiologically and histologically. This interest derives from the realization that these abnormalities may be difficult to distinguish from carcinoma by mammography and concern that they are precursors for the development of carcinoma.

The existence of these lesions has been recognized throughout most of the century. In 1928, Semb (30) referred to RSLs as *rosettes* or *proliferation centers* that might give rise to carcinoma. Bloodgood (31) drew attention to these lesions in a study of "borderline breast tumors," emphasizing the diagnostic problems they present and uncertainty about their precancerous potential. RSLs have been described by a variety of names introduced since the 1970s. The investigators who proposed these terms generally addressed three issues that still are central concerns with regard to RSLs: histogenesis, differential diagnosis, and precancerous potential.

Fenoglio and Lattes (32) described 30 examples they termed *sclerosing papillary proliferations* because the lesions had a prominent papillary component. This name has not been met with general acceptance because some of the lesions in this category have little or no papillary element. Fisher et al. (33) suggested the term *nonencapsulated sclerosing lesion,* which has the advantage of avoiding issues related to histogenesis. *Infiltrating epitheliosis* has not been widely accepted because it could be misconstrued as indicating an invasive malignant neoplasm (34). The unpopularity of *indurative mastopathy* probably is attributed to the fact that most of the lesions are too small to be palpable as indurated foci and the vague meaning of the term *mastopathy* (35).

*Radial scar,* presently the most widely used name for these lesions, is a translation of *strahlige Narben,* the term Hamperl (36) introduced in 1975. This designation refers to the stellate configuration of most of these lesions; it is short and it avoids terminology that suggests particular association with proliferative duct lesions. However, use of the word *scar* implies that there is a reparative process in the stroma. Although the stellate configuration has a cicatrix-like appearance, it is equally likely that the stromal change is an integral part of the overall proliferative lesion, perhaps enhanced by paracrine growth factors, rather than being a reactive process. The term *radial sclerosing lesion* used here is preferable because it describes the mammographic and histopathologic appearance of the process without implying histogenesis, and it is sufficiently nonspecific to encompass the many histologic variants included in this category. RSLs are discussed in this chapter devoted to benign papillary tumors because a substantial proportion have a component of papillary ductal proliferation.

## Clinical Presentation

Most RSLs are microscopic in size and not detectable by palpation or mammography. The frequency of these subclinical lesions varies in different reports, depending on the groups of patients studied and the diagnostic criteria. Multiple microscopic RSLs are not uncommon in one breast (37),

and both breasts can be affected (38). The frequency of RSLs in mastectomy specimens from patients with carcinoma has been 4% (33), 16% (37), and 26% (39). RSLs have been detected in 1.7% (40), 1.8% (41), 5.3% (36), 7.1% (42), 14% (39), and 28% (43) of benign breast specimens. The broad and overlapping ranges of the frequency of RSL associated with benign and carcinomatous breasts suggest that RSLs occur with similar frequency in both circumstances. The amount of tissue available for study and the thoroughness with which it is examined are important factors affecting frequency. The age distribution of patients from whom specimens are obtained also is important because RSLs are uncommon before age 30 years and they are most frequent between 40 and 60 years of age.

RSLs diagnosed clinically usually are detected by mammography because they rarely are large enough to be palpable. Most RSLs are larger than 5 mm when radiologically detected, forming stellate or spiculated structures with a central dense or lucent core (Fig. 5.18). In one study of lesions sub-

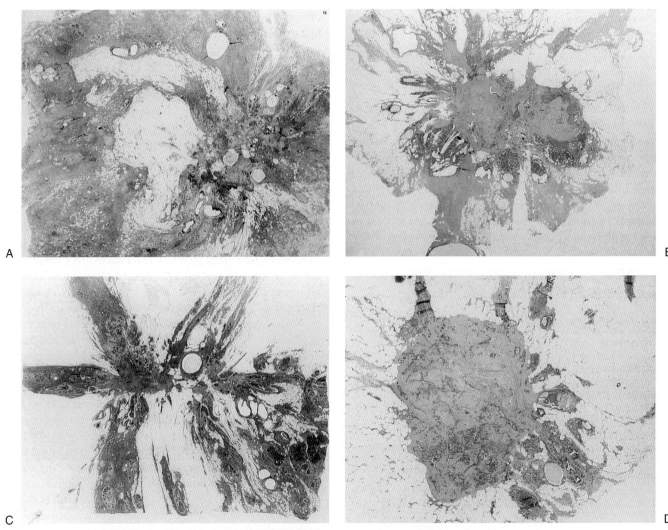

**FIG. 5.18.** *Radial sclerosing lesion.* Whole-mount histologic sections of different structural patterns. **A:** Relatively ill-defined lesion with multiple cysts. **B:** Asymmetric, oval lesion with dense central fibrosis. A proliferative component and cysts are present around half of the circumference. **C:** Lesion with a stellate pattern. **D:** Ovoid tumor with a contour that is partly smooth and partly stellate.

jected to stereotactic aspiration biopsy, the average size was 8 mm (44); in another report, lesional size averaged 1.3 cm (45). Microcalcifications are not detected in the majority of RSLs studied by mammography (44,46).

Some mammographic features favor the radiologic diagnosis of a benign RSL over a stellate carcinoma, but these are not distinct enough to be the basis for a specific diagnosis in many cases. Several authors emphasized the unreliability of radiologic criteria for distinguishing between a benign RSL and a stellate carcinoma (45–48). The ability to visualize an RSL mammographically is enhanced if the lesion is situated in predominantly fatty tissue, which provides contrast for the core and radial strands of fibrous stroma containing proliferating epithelium and cysts.

### Gross Pathology

Most RSLs excised after mammographic localization have a gross appearance similar to that of small invasive carcinomas. The tumor is firm and, when bisected, reveals a pale, retracted center in which there may be white streaks. Slender bands of pale stroma extend radially into the fat from the core. Small cysts can be appreciated in some lesions. A minority of RSLs lack a distinct stellate gross configuration, presenting instead as ill-defined areas of firmness or as circumscribed nodules.

### Microscopic Pathology

Linell defined the histologic appearance of the RSL or, in his terminology, the *radial scar* as "a distinct histologic structure, characterized by a sclerotic center with a central core containing obliterated duct(s), elastin deposits, and mostly infiltrating tubules and the center is surrounded by a corona of contracted ducts and lobules, which may show different types of proliferative lesions" (Fig. 5.19) (49).

The proliferative components that most commonly contribute in differing proportions to an RSL are duct hyperplasia, sclerosing adenosis, and cysts (Figs. 5.20 and 5.21).

There is a common architectural or structural configuration to RSLs despite the various components. The central nidus is a relatively sclerotic zone composed of fibrosis and elastosis. Abundant elastin in the walls of ducts and throughout the stroma appears as a dense, sometimes granular, eosinophilic or weakly basophilic deposit that can be highlighted by an elastic tissue stain such as Verhoeff or van Gieson. One or more ductal structures within the core appear to be partially or completely obliterated. Sections of an RSL in a relatively early phase of development reveal branching and budding ductal structures in the central core. At this stage, the stroma appears to be relatively cellular, with spindle cells distributed around the ductal units, extending along radiating fibrous bands toward the periphery. A light scattered infiltrate of lymphocytes and plasma cells is found in the stroma. Conspicuous lymphocytic aggregates are unusual in the usual RSL, and their presence may indicate a low-grade adenosquamous carcinoma (see Chapter 18). In later stages, the stromal cells are less conspicuous by light microscopy. Electron microscopy reveals that many of the stromal cells are myofibroblasts (50).

Small ductules and distorted lobules are distributed between bands of sclerotic tissue radiating from the core into the surrounding stroma. A "corona" of ducts, lobules, and cysts is variably present at the periphery of the lesion, resulting from incorporation of these structures from the surrounding tissue (Fig. 5.20). This peripheral zone is not evident around every RSL. It may appear to be incomplete or asymmetric due to intrinsic differences among lesions, or it may be a consequence of asymmetric sectioning. The peripheral zone can include nonproliferative ducts and lobules that appear to be drawn toward the core. In some lesions, the "corona" consists mainly or entirely of cysts (Fig. 5.20).

Small ductules trapped in the fibrous reaction may be mistaken for invasive carcinoma (Fig. 5.21). This is an important consideration when examining needle core biopsy samples (Fig. 5.22). Nests of epithelium trapped in the stroma at the periphery of a sclerosing papilloma or an RSL simulate

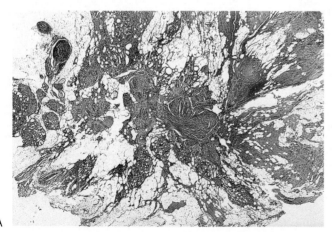

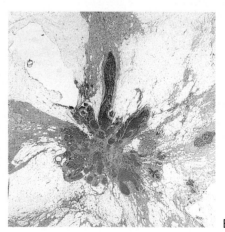

A

B

**FIG. 5.19.** *Radial sclerosing lesions, elastosis.* **A:** Foci of sclerosing adenosis radiate from the elastotic core. **B:** Florid duct hyperplasia around an elastotic core.

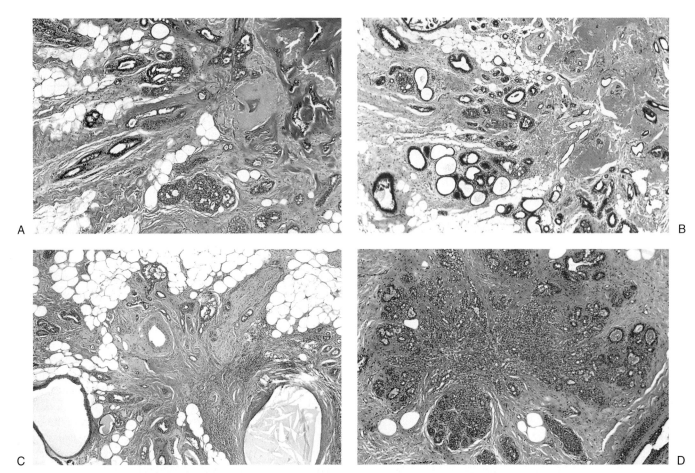

**FIG. 5.20.** *Radial sclerosing lesions.* **A:** The elastotic center is in the *upper right* corner. Mild duct hyperplasia is present at the periphery. **B:** The elastotic center is in the *upper right* corner. The lesion features adenosis with microcystic dilation of glands. **C:** Radial sclerosing lesion with peripheral apocrine cysts and a larger nerve *(upper right)*. **D:** Radial sclerosing lesion composed of sclerosing adenosis.

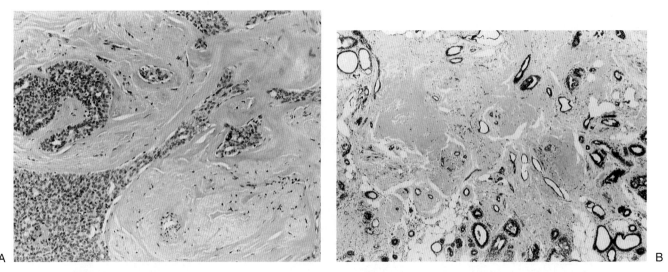

**FIG. 5.21.** *Radial sclerosing lesion.* **A:** Duct hyperplasia with sclerotic stroma. **B:** Adenosis with a pattern that simulates tubular carcinoma.

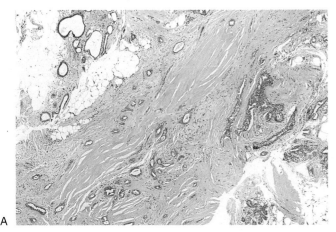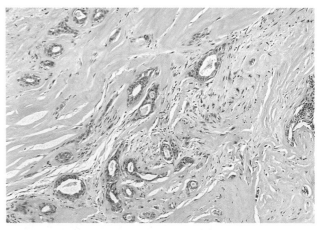

A                                                                                                          B

**FIG. 5.22.** *Radial sclerosing lesion, needle core biopsy.* **A:** Low-magnification view of the biopsy sample shows angular glands in the fibroelastotic stroma. A focus of duct hyperplasia is present near the right border. This specimen was misinterpreted as tubular carcinoma. **B:** Angular glands in the myofibroblastic stromal proliferation.

invasive carcinoma (Figs. 5.11 and 5.23). The presence of a myoepithelial cell layer that often is hyperplastic, demonstrated with an actin immunostain (preferably smooth muscle myosin heavy chain), and basement membrane components, demonstrated with immunostains for laminin and collagen type IV, characterize epithelial entrapment.

Apocrine metaplasia frequently is observed in the cystic component of RSLs. Occasionally it may be present more widely in the proliferative component, especially in areas of sclerosing adenosis. Clear cell change and nuclear atypia are not uncommon in this apocrine epithelium. Squamous metaplasia is relatively infrequent in RSLs (Fig. 5.24). Focal necrosis occurs in the hyperplastic duct epithelium of about 10% of RSLs (Fig. 5.25). The presence of these comedo-like foci may suggest intraductal carcinoma, but the epithelium

usually is indistinguishable from the epithelium of hyperplastic ducts lacking necrosis. Entrapped nerves apparently are incorporated into RSLs by the same mechanism that is responsible for this phenomenon in other sclerosing lesions (Figs. 5.20 and 5.26) (51).

RSLs usually occur as isolated, separate lesions, but on occasion contiguous foci may be joined to form a larger complex proliferative lesion in a fashion analogous to the formation of an adenosis tumor.

The major consideration in the differential diagnosis of RSLs is tubular carcinoma (Fig. 5.22). The epithelium in tubular carcinoma lacks the myoepithelial layer characteristically present in hyperplastic component in RSLs. The glands in tubular carcinoma have round or distinctive angular shapes not ordinarily found in RSLs. The cystic

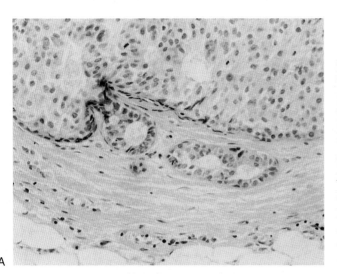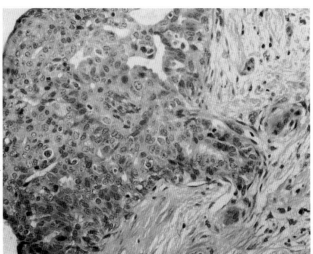

A                                                                                                          B

**FIG. 5.23.** *Radial sclerosing lesion.* Epithelium at the periphery that simulates invasive carcinoma. **A:** Ductule in continuity with the central nodule of hyperplastic epithelium. Seeming discontinuity is an artifact of sectioning. **B:** Ductule protruding into peripheral myofibroblastic stroma where the distinction between epithelial and stromal cells is obscured.

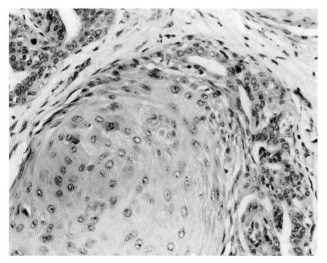

**FIG. 5.24.** *Squamous metaplasia in a radial sclerosing lesion.*

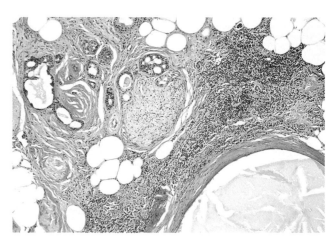

**FIG. 5.26.** *Nerve entrapment in a radial sclerosing lesion.* A nerve is shown in the upper center at the periphery of a radial sclerosing lesion. Small glands at the perimeter of the perineurium indent the nerve.

component of RSLs is absent from most tubular carcinomas, and RSLs lack micropapillary or cribriform intraductal carcinoma, which characterizes tubular carcinoma.

RSLs with squamous metaplasia may resemble metaplastic carcinoma, especially the low-grade adenosquamous variant. Rarely, low-grade adenosquamous carcinoma arises in an RSL (see Chapter 18). Ductal elements in RSL can exhibit florid and atypical hyperplasia (Figs. 5.25 and 5.27), as well as intraductal carcinoma. Rarely, tubular carcinoma can be traced to an RSL, and lobular structures may give rise to atypical lobular hyperplasia or lobular carcinoma *in situ* (Fig. 5.28).

FNA cytology provides a sampling of the cellular constituents of an RSL. The finding of benign proliferative epithelium and spindle-shaped stromal cells in conjunction with a characteristic mammographic appearance is presump-

tive evidence for a diagnosis of RSL. In some instances, it may be difficult to distinguish between the FNA aspirate from a fibroepithelial tumor with epithelial hyperplasia and the aspirate from an RSL. Atypical epithelium and carcinoma can be found in such samples (52). Cells obtained from foci of atypical apocrine metaplasia present a particularly challenging diagnostic problem in an aspiration cytology specimen (53). Because of the heterogeneous structure of many of these lesions, the FNA sample may not be representative in all cases, and this is not a reliable method for detecting focal carcinoma in RSLs (54). Orell (55) reported a false-positive rate of 4.3% in RSL diagnosed by FNA in a mammography screening program.

Stereotactic needle core biopsy provides a tissue sample that is a more reliable basis for the specific diagnosis of an RSL than FNA. However, nests of hyperplastic epithelium

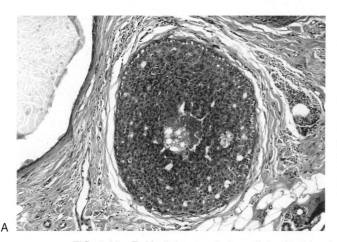

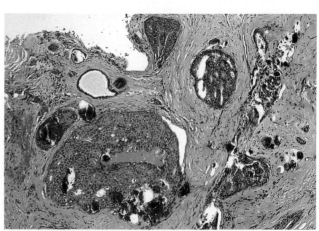

A

B

**FIG. 5.25.** *Epithelial necrosis in radial sclerosing lesions.* **A:** Small area of necrosis in the center of a duct with florid hyperplasia at the periphery of a radial sclerosing lesion. **B:** Needle core biopsy sample of a radial sclerosing lesion with multiple calcifications. Atypical duct hyperplasia is present in the ducts. Necrosis is evident in the center of the largest duct.

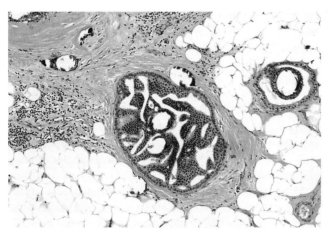

**FIG. 5.27.** *Radial sclerosing lesion with atypical duct hyperplasia.* A duct at the periphery of a radial sclerosing lesion showing atypical micropapillary hyperplasia. Note the presence of orderly, cuboidal epithelium at the periphery of the duct and nuclear condensation in central epithelium. Calcifications are present in the epithelium and stroma.

or sclerosing adenosis trapped in the stroma of an RSL can be misinterpreted as invasive carcinoma in a needle core biopsy sample (Fig. 5.22). Ultimately, complete excision is necessary to fully evaluate these lesions, especially to rule out focal carcinoma. Jackman et al. (56) reported that two of five lesions diagnosed as "radial scars" on "large-core needle biopsy" contained carcinoma when surgically excised, representing a false-negative rate of 40%. Specimen radiography should be performed to confirm the excision of an RSL detected by mammography. Frozen section is not appropriate for diagnosis of an excised RSL (49).

**Treatment and Prognosis**

The presence of carcinoma in RSLs has been well documented. In one series, 28% of mammographically detected RSLs larger than 1 cm had foci of carcinoma (54). In this context, it is important to distinguish between carcinomas with a stellate configuration and RSL with foci of carcinoma. In the absence of residual RSL, it is not possible to prove that an entirely stellate carcinoma arose in an RSL. Carcinoma is found more frequently in RSLs larger than 2 cm and occurs more often in RSLs from women older than 50 years (57). The most common form of carcinoma arising in an RSL is lobular carcinoma *in situ*. Intraductal carcinoma and tubular carcinoma are less frequent. The treatment and prognosis of a carcinoma arising in an RSL depends on the stage of the carcinoma.

The presence of carcinoma or atypical hyperplasia in some RSLs has been an important factor in the concern over the precancerous potential of these lesions. This association was most strongly championed by Linell et al. (37) and supported by Fisher et al. (33). Wellings and Alpers (39) reported finding radial scars significantly more often in the breasts of women with carcinoma than in the breasts of women without carcinoma. Other authors found no significant differences in the number or frequency of RSLs in the breasts of women with and without carcinoma (43,58). RSLs from the breast of women with carcinoma do not appear appreciably different from comparable lesions not associated with carcinoma (58).

One retrospective follow-up study of patients after excision of RSL failed to disclose an increased risk for subsequent development of carcinoma. Andersen and Gram (40) reported one patient with subsequent carcinoma among 32 women followed for a mean of 19.5 years.

A prospective cohort study of 1,396 women with a median follow-up of 12 years after biopsy of a benign breast lesion revealed that "radial scars" were an independent risk factor for breast carcinoma (42). In this study, "radial scar" was defined by a "fibroelastotic core from which ducts and lobules radiate. These ducts and lobules exhibit various alternations, including cysts and proliferative lesions." As so defined, radial scars were found in 99 women (7.1%). These radial scars were solitary in 60.6% of affected women and had a median size of 4 mm. During follow-up, 255 women developed breast carcinoma. The relative risk (RR) for carcinoma

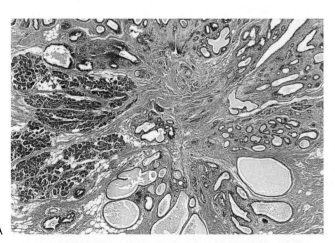

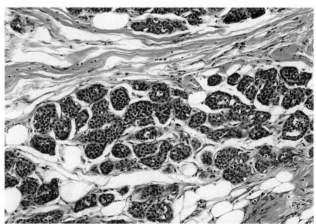

A

B

**FIG. 5.28.** *Radial sclerosing lesion with lobular carcinoma in situ.* **A:** Lobular carcinoma *in situ* occupies adenosis glands in the left half of this lesion. **B:** Magnified view of the lobular carcinoma *in situ.*

in women with a radial scar when compared to those not having a radial scar was 1.8 (95% confidence interval [CI] 1.1 to 2.9). RR was increased by concurrent proliferative changes and was greatest when the radial scar coexisted with atypical hyperplasia (RR 5.8, 95% CI 2.7 to 12.7) when compared to women with nonproliferative breast specimens. The mean and median size and distribution of size among radial scars were not significantly different between women who did or did not develop carcinoma, and the risk was not influenced by the number of radial scars.

## SUBAREOLAR SCLEROSING DUCT HYPERPLASIA

Sclerosing papillary hyperplasia of ducts within the nipple is a sclerosing papillary variant of an RSL in the subareolar region (59). Sclerosing duct hyperplasia also can produce a tumor of the central or subareolar breast parenchyma with-out involving the substance of the nipple. The term *subareolar sclerosing duct hyperplasia* should be reserved for those lesions that constitute a clinicopathologic entity distinct from florid papillomatosis of the nipple (60).

### Clinical Presentation

The age at diagnosis ranges from 26 to 73 years, averaging about 50 years. The left and right breasts are affected with equal frequency; there have been no examples of bilateral involvement reported.

The presenting symptom is a mass located beneath the nipple and/or areola or in the breast close to the areola. None of the lesions has been within the nipple. Erosion or ulceration of the nipple surface are absent. Nipple retraction may occur, and several patients had bloody discharge. The mammographic findings have not been specific for this lesion and can suggest carcinoma.

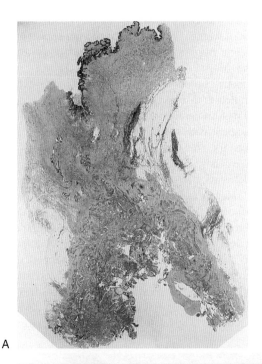

A

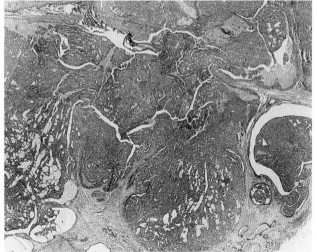

B

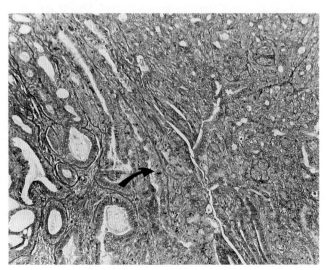

C

**FIG. 5.29.** *Subareolar sclerosing papilloma.* **A:** Whole-mount histologic section of nipple and subareolar tissue with a sclerosing papilloma below rather than in the nipple. **B:** Typical solid growth pattern with focal papillary areas. **C:** The lesion is cellular with occasional mitotic figures (*arrow*). (From Rosen PP. Subareolar sclerosing duct hyperplasia of the breast. *Cancer* 1987; 59:1927–1930, with permission.)

## Gross Pathology

The excised lesion is a firm-to-hard round or oval tumor with indistinct borders measuring up to 2.0 cm (average 1.2 cm). Yellow streaks may be noted in some lesions. Excisions generally have been achieved without removing the nipple, because the lesion is located in the underlying mammary parenchyma. This difference in surgical approach is a useful adjunct in the differential diagnosis of florid papillomatosis and subareolar sclerosing duct hyperplasia.

## Microscopic Pathology

The histologic structure of subareolar sclerosing duct hyperplasia is similar to that of radial sclerosing papillary lesions in other parts of the breast. Sclerosis and elastosis are more marked toward the center of the tumor, whereas duct hyperplasia is most prominent at the periphery. Cartilaginous metaplasia, a rare occurrence in these lesions, typically occurs in the sclerotic core. In some cases, small hyperplastic ducts are seen at the margin, resulting in irregular borders. More often, much of the tumor has a rounded border created by the nodular expansion of confluent large ducts (Figs. 5.29 and 5.30). Scattered mitotic figures may be encountered in the florid hyperplastic epithelium or in hyperplastic myoepithelial cells, which are found throughout much of the lesion. Rarely, focal comedonecrosis is found in the hyperplastic duct epithelium. In contrast to radial sclerosing proliferative lesions that occur elsewhere in the breast, subareolar sclerosing duct hyperplasia generally lacks cysts, cystic and papillary apocrine change, and squamous metaplasia. Carcinoma may arise in subareolar sclerosing duct hyperplasia.

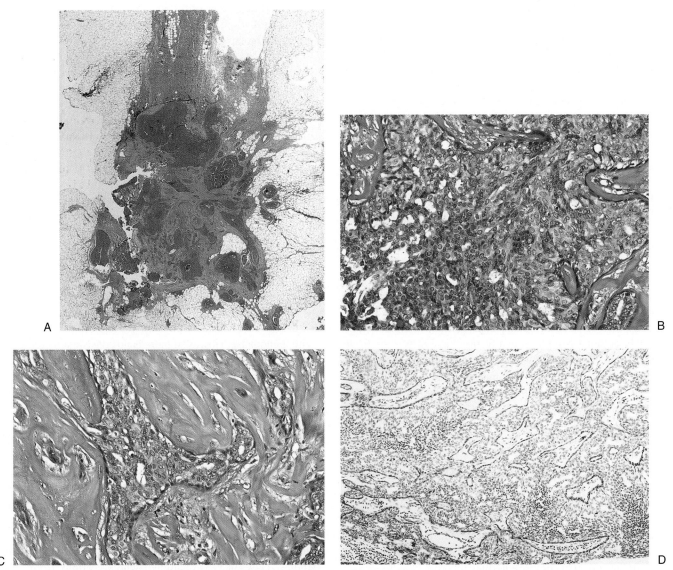

**FIG. 5.30.** *Subareolar sclerosing papilloma.* **A:** Whole-mount histologic section. The nipple is above the *upper border* of the image. **B:** Florid hyperplasia in the lesion. **C:** Focus of stromal sclerosis. **D:** Intact myoepithelial cell layer, highlighted with the smooth muscle myosin heavy chain immunostain, outlines the epithelium (avidin-biotin).

## Treatment and Prognosis

The tumors should be treated by excisional biopsy, which usually can be performed through a circumareolar incision, sparing the nipple. Recurrence may occur after incomplete excision, but in most cases the patients have remained well for up to 4 years after initial treatment. Total mastectomy has been performed when intraductal carcinoma was present in subareolar sclerosing duct hyperplasia or because the lesion was mistakenly diagnosed as carcinoma. At present, there is no evidence that this condition is precancerous, but longer follow-up will be necessary to fully evaluate the question.

## CYSTIC AND PAPILLARY APOCRINE METAPLASIA

Apocrine glands are part of the odoriferous or accessory sex gland system. They normally are present in the skin, particularly in the groin, axilla, and anogenital region. Modified apocrine glands occur in the ears (ceruminous glands) and eyelids (Moll's glands). Apocrine glands are morphologically and functionally different from the cutaneous sebaceous and sweat glands. Several observations suggest that cutaneous apocrine glands are responsive to hormonal stimulation in a fashion analogous to the mammary gland. The development of normal apocrine glands is largely delayed until puberty in both sexes. In women, apocrine gland function waxes and wanes somewhat with the phases of the menstrual cycle. Axillary apocrine gland hyperplasia during pregnancy occasionally may produce palpable glandular enlargement, which can be mistaken for a neoplasm or ectopic breast tissue. Increased secretory activity of the axillary apocrine glands has been reported during pregnancy. At present, there is no evidence to indicate that exogenous estrogens contribute to apocrine metaplasia in humans. Comparison of breast tissue of women receiving exogenous estrogen and untreated women revealed no increase in the frequency of apocrine metaplasia in the treated group (61).

Cutaneous apocrine gland cells contain abundant pink finely granular cytoplasm that forms apical tufts or blebs at the luminal surface typical of merocrine secretion. Round, regular nuclei with a punctate nucleolus are located near the base of the cell. At the ultrastructural level, the cytoplasm contains abundant endoplasmic reticulum, mitochondria, intermediate filaments, and secretory vesicles that are responsible for the granularity observed in hematoxylin and eosin sections (62).

Embryologically, the breasts develop from the anlage that gives rise to apocrine glands, but apocrine glands are not a constituent of the normal microscopic anatomy of the mammary gland. Any benign proliferative lesion may contain cells with apocrine cytologic features. In their most banal form, these metaplastic apocrine cells are indistinguishable from the cells that comprise normal apocrine glands.

The proliferative capacity of ordinary apocrine metaplasia is uncertain. The flat apocrine cells lining cysts may be an end stage of cellular differentiation, but studies of the cyst fluid indicate metabolic activity. The fluid in apocrine cysts contains high concentrations of the androgen conjugate dehydroepiandrosterone sulfate (63), a steroid that also is concentrated in sweat from axillary glands (64). This finding suggests that accumulation of the hormone occurs as a result of active transport or synthesis by the cyst epithelium. Mitoses are almost never seen in ordinary apocrine metaplasia, and a low proportion of cells are in S-phase (65).

## Clinical Presentation

Grossly palpable cysts frequently are lined by apocrine epithelium, which can be recognized cytologically in fluid aspirated from the cyst. The fluid tends to have a $K^+/Na^+$ ratio greater than 1.5, a characteristic of the type I cyst described by Naldoni et al. (66). Type I cysts were significantly associated with low parity and recurrence of cysts, but not with a family history of breast carcinoma. There are no clinical features specifically attributable to apocrine cysts. Apocrine metaplasia frequently is present in the epithelial lining of cysts in gross cystic disease described clinically by Haagensen et al. (67), who reported finding apocrine metaplasia in 78% of 1,169 biopsies performed for gross cystic disease.

Other palpable benign tumors composed of apocrine epithelium are generally divided into two groups: adenomas and papillomas. The distinction between these diagnostic categories is not clear, because illustrations of some lesions reported to be apocrine adenomas have shown a conspicuous papillary component (68,69). These lesions present as firm, mobile circumscribed tumors that are clinically indistinguishable from nonapocrine counterparts.

Microscopic apocrine metaplasia is common in the female breast after age 30 years; occasionally it may be found in younger women (70,71). The frequency of microscopic apocrine change is highest in the fifth decade and continues to be greater after age 50 years than in younger women, which probably reflects physiologic alterations associated with menopause. However, there is no consistent increase or decrease in the occurrence of apocrine metaplasia with advancing age beyond 50 years (70,71). One group of investigators reported that apocrine cysts were significantly more numerous and more frequent in lower than in upper quadrants of breasts with and without carcinoma (70). Apocrine cysts and hyperplasia with apocrine metaplasia were more common in the breasts of American women in New York than in Japanese women from Tokyo (72).

The relationship of apocrine metaplasia, especially apocrine cysts, to breast carcinoma remains uncertain. Several investigators reported finding no significant difference in the frequency of apocrine metaplasia when breasts with and without carcinoma were compared. In one of the earliest studies, Dawson (73) examined whole sections from 120 carcinomatous breasts and 48 breasts without carcinoma. Apocrine metaplasia was detected in all but four of the 168 specimens, leading to the conclusion that apocrine change was not associated with the development of carcinoma. A similar study of "cancerous and noncancerous breasts" was described in 1945 by Foote and Stewart (74). They observed that apocrine metaplasia often was present in breasts with other "noncancerous proliferative lesions," but they found no significant difference in the frequency of apocrine metaplasia between "cancerous and noncancerous breasts." Tóth et al. (75) reported that atypical duct hyperplasia was present more frequently in breasts with apocrine metaplasia than when apocrine change was absent. This effect was seen with simple cysts alone, but it was strongest in association with papillary apocrine cysts.

Although the foregoing anatomic studies of apocrine metaplasia did not show an association between the frequency of apocrine metaplasia and concurrent carcinoma, some follow-up studies suggested that apocrine metaplasia may be a predictor for the subsequent development of carcinoma. Haagensen et al. (67) reported a 10-fold greater frequency of carcinoma in women who had apocrine metaplasia in a prior biopsy than when apocrine change was absent. The majority of the subsequent carcinomas had "apocrine features," but the origin was rarely traceable to apocrine metaplasia. When compared to Connecticut state incidence figures, patients with apocrine metaplasia had 3.5 times the expected frequency of carcinoma, whereas the risk was only 0.3 times expected when apocrine metaplasia was absent.

A slight overall increase in the number of subsequent carcinomas was observed by Page et al. (76) in women with papillary apocrine change in an antecedent biopsy when compared to the expected number of carcinomas based on an age-matched comparison with the Third National Cancer Survey. The difference was statistically significant only in women who were older than 45 years when the apocrine lesion was detected. There also was an increased risk in this age group when apocrine metaplasia occurred in duct hyperplasia, but the difference was not statistically significant. A subsequent study by Page et al. (77) confirmed the latter observation. They concluded that "when characteristic apocrine-type nuclei are present in fairly complex patterns of hyperplasia, they do not represent a worrisome lesion or a reliable risk indicator, particularly if confined to small clusters of cysts or glands" (77).

Histologic evidence of transitions from apocrine metaplasia to apocrine carcinoma have been described. Yates and Ahmed (78) reported a case in which a biopsy showing "florid apocrine metaplasia intermingled with atypical apocrine cells" was followed 19 months later by the finding of a 2.5-cm tumor composed of apocrine carcinoma. Haagensen et al. (67) reported that they had "traced the transformation of benign apocrine metaplasia into apocrine carcinoma in a considerable number of cases." Florid apocrine metaplasia with atypia often is coexistent with apocrine carcinoma (79), but follow-up of patients with atypical lesions has not revealed a predisposition to the early onset of carcinoma of apocrine or nonapocrine type (5). When carcinoma arises in the opposite breast of a patient with apocrine atypia or apocrine carcinoma in the ipsilateral breast, the contralateral carcinoma is not necessarily apocrine.

## Gross Pathology

There are no specific gross features associated with apocrine metaplasia. Apocrine foci sometimes have a brown color in the fresh state (Fig. 5.8).

## Microscopic Pathology

Mammary apocrine metaplasia is encountered most frequently in the epithelium of simple cysts. Cystic apocrine metaplasia is composed of flat and cuboidal cells that may form a single layer or exhibit proliferative change resulting in isolated blunt papillae (Fig. 5.31). The cells usually are evenly spaced, and they contain round nuclei with homogeneous moderately dense chromatin (Fig. 5.32). There typically is a single central small nucleolus. A myoepithelial cell layer usually is readily apparent in cystic and papillary apocrine epithelium. A slight degree of cellular crowding often results in a palisaded organization of the epithelium that may be more than one cell in depth, whereas florid papillary proliferation can produce more elaborate patterns of hyperplasia with a micropapillary or a branching, true papillary architecture. In extreme cases, this results in the formation of a papilloma composed entirely of apocrine epithelium (Fig. 5.33). Apocrine metaplasia also can be found focally in sclerosing adenosis, fibroadenomas (80), papillomas (81), and other benign proliferative abnormalities. Nielsen (82) reported finding apocrine metaplasia in 63% of palpable adenosis tumors.

In its proliferative phase, apocrine metaplasia consists of cuboidal to tall columnar cells with eosinophilic cytoplasm. The nuclei are uniform in size, round, and basally oriented. "Tufts" or "snouts" of epithelium protrude from the apical surface of the cell into the glandular lumen. The cytoplasm typically is finely granular and uniformly stained, but in rare instances associated with inflammation, coarse granules are conspicuous, possibly as a degenerative change. Metaplastic apocrine epithelium in cysts is prone to regressive changes that may lead to complete disappearance of these cells. This transition is marked by conversion of columnar and cuboidal apocrine epithelium to a flattened layer of cells that ultimately may be shed into the cyst, leaving only a fibrous shell.

Papillary apocrine change is found most often in cystic apocrine metaplasia, associated with other fibrocystic proliferative alterations. The apocrine epithelium usually is arranged in a micropapillary pattern composed of regularly spaced cytologically benign cells (Figs. 5.31 and 5.32). Fibrovascular stroma is absent from or minimally present in these epithelial fronds. Page et al. (83) described three patterns of papillary apocrine change. The simple form was characterized by independent mounds or fronds, three or

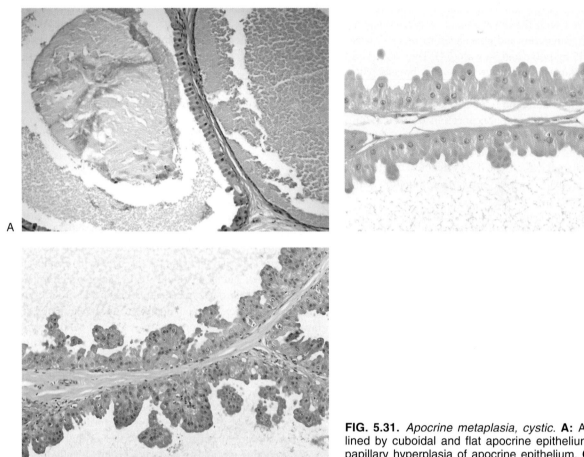

FIG. 5.31. *Apocrine metaplasia, cystic.* **A:** Adjacent cysts lined by cuboidal and flat apocrine epithelium. **B:** Minimal papillary hyperplasia of apocrine epithelium. **C:** Micropapillary apocrine hyperplasia in a cyst.

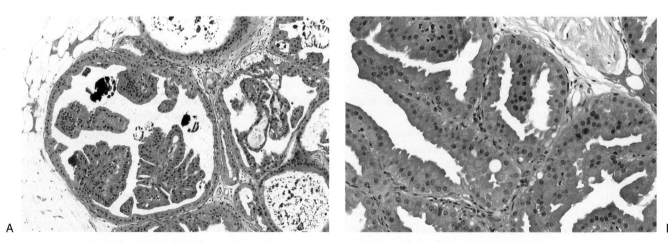

FIG. 5.32. *Apocrine metaplasia, papillary.* **A:** Part of a complex cystic and papillary apocrine lesion with calcifications. The nuclei are uniform, small, and evenly spaced. They are generally equidistant from the basement membrane. **B:** Another complex benign papillary apocrine lesion with slight nuclear heterogeneity. *(continued)*

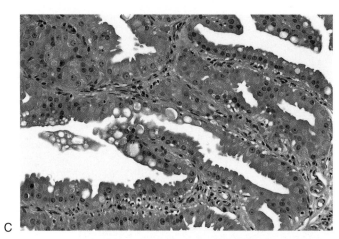

C

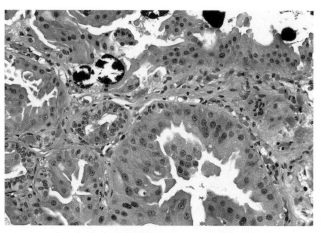

D

**FIG. 5.32.** *Continued.* **C:** Part of the lesion where there is greater nuclear heterogeneity and cytoplasmic vacuoles are present. Nuclei are distributed uniformly and in a single layer. **D:** Focus of apocrine hyperplasia with calcifications. Note slight nuclear heterogeneity, micropapillary growth, multilayered epithelium, and loss of cell polarity with respect to the basement membrane. Images **B–D** are from a single lesion.

more cells thick. A second complex pattern had a broader, thicker base surmounted by more slender fronds that may approximate each other. In the third highly complex arrangement, the slender papillae were two or three cells thick and formed arcades, some of which are entwined within the lumen. The authors noted mild cytologic variability in less than 10% of cells within highly complex papillary apocrine change, consisting mainly of prominent nucleoli and nuclear enlargement.

Atypical changes may be encountered in apocrine metaplasia in virtually any proliferative configuration (5). Architectural atypia consists of irregular papillary fronds with little or no stromal support in which the metaplastic apocrine cells are arranged in a disordered fashion (Fig. 5.34). Epithelial bridges and cribriform areas may be present. Cytologic atypia tends to be more severe in sclerosing lesions

such as sclerosing adenosis and RSLs, but it may be found in apocrine foci in fibroadenomas, cysts, and papillomas. Atypical cytologic features were present in 71% of adenosis tumors with apocrine metaplasia reported by Nielsen (82).

Apocrine cells with mild cytologic atypia retain abundant granular eosinophilic cytoplasm and exhibit characteristic "decapitation secretion." Small clear vacuoles may be found, especially in the nonbasal cytoplasm. In comparison with regular apocrine metaplasia, the nuclei in mild apocrine atypia are not spaced at regular intervals, and they may not be basally oriented. Nucleoli are less uniform, they may be eccentric, and an occasional nucleus has more than one nucleolus. With progressively more severe atypia, the cytoplasm of individual cells becomes increasingly vacuolated or clear, and "decapitation" of cytoplasm at the luminal border is lost. Nuclear pleomorphism and hyperchromasia may

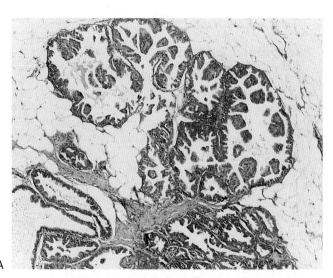

A

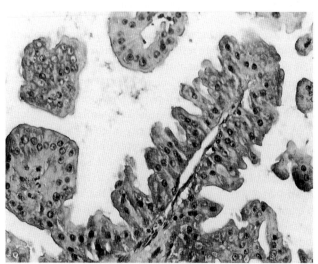

B

**FIG. 5.33.** *Apocrine papilloma.* **A:** Multiloculated focus of papillary apocrine metaplasia. **B:** Papillary frond with a fibrovascular core and surface epithelium composed of bland apocrine cells.

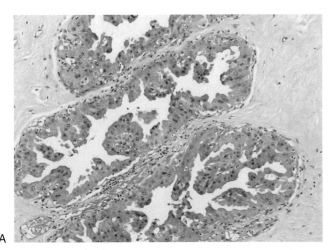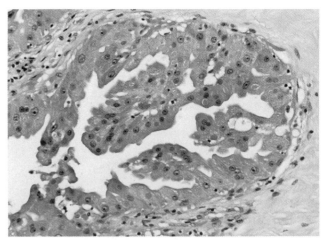

**FIG. 5.34.** *Papillary apocrine metaplasia with mild atypia.* **A:** Papillary and micropapillary duct hyperplasia. **B:** Magnified view of **A**, with atypia manifested by irregular positioning of large nuclei with prominent nucleoli.

become striking. Prominent pleomorphic nucleoli characterize the most atypical lesions. The nuclear-to-cytoplasmic ratio increases as apocrine metaplasia becomes more atypical, but the cells generally retain relatively abundant cytoplasm when compared with those of nonapocrine epithelium.

When atypical apocrine metaplasia is present, the severity of the change usually is not homogeneous in a given lesion. Cysts and papillary duct hyperplasia, partly or entirely occupied by bland metaplastic apocrine epithelium, usually are found in the vicinity of atypical apocrine metaplasia. The distinction between atypical apocrine metaplasia and apocrine carcinoma ordinarily is not difficult, but this may be a challenging diagnostic problem when extreme atypia is present or in the limited sample of a needle core biopsy. In the latter situation, cytologic features may be less important than the growth pattern, especially in sclerosing lesions. In this setting, a diagnosis of carcinoma is warranted when the atypical apocrine proliferation has the configuration of one of the conventional forms of intraductal carcinoma (see Chapter 21) (5).

The cytologic changes observed in apocrine metaplasia and apocrine atypia are reflected in the altered deoxyribonucleic acid (DNA) content of these cells. Izuo et al. (84) studied apocrine metaplasia by microspectrophotometric measurement of Feulgen-stained paraffin sections. Cutaneous apocrine glands from the vulva used as controls had a diploid DNA content. Although the majority of cells in samples of mammary apocrine metaplasia were diploid, a subset of tetraploid nuclei was found in all of these specimens. The proportion of tetraploid cells was related to the amount and severity of atypia in the apocrine lesion. One lesion reported to exhibit high-grade atypia, which proved to be aneuploid, appears to be an orderly papillary apocrine carcinoma in the authors' illustration. This patient was found to have an invasive mammary carcinoma of unspecified histologic type 2.5 years after the lesion described as apocrine atypia was biopsied.

### Immunohistochemistry and Electron Microscopy

When studied by histochemistry or electron microscopy, cells in cystic and papillary apocrine metaplasia have been found to be similar to the cells of normal apocrine glands (62,65,75,81,85). Refractile golden-brown supranuclear granules, sometimes in vacuoles, may be seen in the cytoplasm. These glycolipid granules stain positively with periodic acid-Schiff (PAS), Sudan black, and in the Prussian blue reaction for iron. The apical cytoplasm is immunoreactive for epithelial membrane antigen, and the cytoplasm stains diffusely with the antibody to gross cystic disease fluid protein 15 (GCDFP-15). Strong cytoplasmic immunohistochemical staining in apocrine cells with the antibody to prolactin has been reported (86). Ultrastructural study reveals numerous mitochondria with sparse, thin incomplete cristae, abundant endoplasmic reticulum, complex folding of the plasma membrane, and membrane-bound dense lysosomal granules. There is a well-developed Golgi region typically located between the nucleus and the apex of the cell.

### Prognosis and Treatment

As indicated previously in this chapter, the relationship of apocrine metaplasia to the development of mammary carcinoma is uncertain. In most instances, apocrine metaplasia appears to be part of the fibrocystic complex manifested in cysts with simple or papillary epithelium or as a component of ordinary duct hyperplasia. Cytologic and architectural atypia are uncommon in apocrine metaplasia and usually occur in sclerosing proliferative lesions such as adenosis or papilloma, often with a radial scar or adenosis tumor configuration. Very few examples of apocrine carcinoma have been traced to atypical apocrine lesions, and most patients with atypical apocrine hyperplasia have remained well during short-term follow-up (5).

The precancerous risk of papillary apocrine change depends largely on its association with other proliferative lesions (83). When compared to a control population, RR for carcinoma in women who had any type of papillary apocrine change unassociated with atypical hyperplasia was 1.2; for those with the highly complex type, RR was 2.4. Neither RR was statistically significant (83).

No specific treatment is indicated for proliferative lesions with apocrine metaplasia. Most cysts with metaplastic apocrine epithelium collapse and do not reform after aspiration. The shed epithelium is readily recognized in a cytologic preparation of the fluid. Surgical excision of apocrine cysts is not indicated unless the fluid is bloody, the cysts reform, or there is atypia in the cytologic specimen. Follow-up of women with breast biopsies that exhibit apocrine metaplasia depends on the overall findings in the specimen and clinical circumstances. Patients with atypical apocrine metaplasia require clinical evaluation comparable to that of women with other atypical proliferative lesions. The precancerous significance of this abnormality remains uncertain.

## FLORID PAPILLOMATOSIS OF THE NIPPLE

Florid papillomatosis of the nipple may have been described as early as 1923 by Miller and Lewis (87), but the authors only provided a photograph of the gross specimen, which is not diagnostic without histopathologic confirmation. Stowers (88) illustrated an example of florid papillomatosis in 1935. An excellent low-magnification photograph was published in a paper about papillary tumors by Haagensen et al. (1) in 1951. They offered the following commentary:

> In rare cases the papilloma is situated within the portion of a duct traversing the nipple. In this location it may be palpable as a thickening within the nipple, or it may present through the dilated orifice of the duct as a friable granulating lesion. . . . In the intraductal papillary tumor involving the orifice of a nipple duct . . . the original duct wall has almost disappeared, leaving the epithelial proliferations in a mass of scar tissue suggesting the infiltrative growth of cancer. (1)

It was not until 1955, when Jones (89) reported a series of five cases, that the lesion was established as a distinct clinicopathologic entity. Jones reported that "Frank W. Foote has seen three of the most exuberant of these cases and states, 'I think all your cases show a lesion that for many years has been designated in the laboratory as terminal duct papillomatosis.'"

> As Jones observed, the growth patterns seen in florid papillomatosis are not specific for this condition. Similar or identical proliferative lesions can be found elsewhere in the breast. However, growth within the nipple produces an unusual clinicopathologic constellation which may include any or all of the following: erosion of the nipple surface with replacement of the epidermis by glandular epithelium, inflammatory changes, and enlargement of the nipple by a firm tumor mass.

The literature is replete with alternative names that can be divided into two groups. Before the lesion was well characterized, Stewart used the terms *adenoma* or *papillomatosis* at various times. Handley and Thackray (90) preferred designating the tumor *adenoma of the nipple*. They pointed to the absence of papillary components in some lesions and observed that "the lesion does not in the least resemble either macroscopically or microscopically a typical duct papilloma." They concluded that the lesion resembles an adenoma of sweat gland origin and suggested that it arises as a result of a developmental abnormality of the nipple. Gros et al. (91) reached a similar conclusion and recommended the name *l'adenomatose erosive*.

Perzin and Lattes (92) concluded that the main feature of the lesion is a papillary proliferation when they commented that ". . . in reality, they are essentially composed of an adenomatous proliferation of ductal epithelium with more or less conspicuous papillary foci." They urged that the name *papillary adenoma* be adopted.

None of these other terms is an improvement on the name proposed by Jones, and in some respects the alternatives may be misleading. The term *adenoma* has been applied to a lesion resembling syringoma of the skin (93–95). Foci of syringomatous differentiation may be associated with florid papillomatosis, but syringomatous adenomas lack the papillary features seen in most examples of florid papillomatosis. Seizing upon the adenomatous feature of a minority of the lesions to justify the term *adenoma* for all cases is no more satisfactory than the original term *florid papillomatosis,* which recognizes duct hyperplasia as the dominant feature in most cases.

### Clinical Features

The majority of patients are 40 to 50 years old when florid papillomatosis of the nipple is diagnosed (89–92,96,97), but age at diagnosis ranges from birth (59) to 89 years (59,98). Approximately 15% of patients are younger than 35 years, and an equal proportion are older than 65 years. There has been no predilection for either breast, and bilateral florid papillomatosis is extremely uncommon (90,99).

Most of these tumors are present for no more than a few months before the patient seeks medical attention. However, there are instances on record in which the lesion was reportedly present for 10 (59,96,98), 11 (90), 14 (97), 15 (59), and 20 (92) years. The most frequent presenting symptom is discharge that often is bloody. Pain, itching, or burning sensations are not unusual. Symptoms may worsen late in the menstrual cycle (90). Small lesions may not cause nipple enlargement; in these cases, palpation usually reveals thickening of the nipple but no discrete mass. In many instances, the nipple appears enlarged, and a mass can be palpated. The surface of the nipple may appear granular, ulcerated, reddened, warty, or crusted. Often these symptoms and clinical findings are mistaken for Paget's disease, or the patient is thought to have a papilloma. In most series, florid papillomatosis was rarely considered clinically in the differential diagnosis. The mammographic and sonographic findings may suggest carcinoma (100). There presently is no evidence to indicate that florid papillomatosis is associated with a positive family history or other risk factors for breast carcinoma. However, data on this subject have been incomplete in most studies.

Fewer than 5% of the reported examples of florid papillomatosis of the nipple were in men (59,87,97,101). The age at diagnosis in men ranged from 43 to 83 years, with all but one patient older than 65 years. Three of the 10 male patients with florid papillomatosis had carcinoma in the breast (59,102). One man developed florid papillomatosis of the nipple after receiving diethylstilbestrol to treat prostatic carcinoma over a 10-year period (103). The lesion described as "an adenoma of the nipple in a male" in one case report appears in retrospect to have been entirely a carcinoma (104). The 74-year-old patient was treated by simple mastectomy described by the authors as follows: "The nipple was present and adjacent to it was a slightly raised fairly firm nodule approximately 2.5 cm in diameter. . . on being cut, the nodule was seen to measure 3 cm in diameter. It lay directly beneath the nipple. . . ." Hence, there does not seem to have been a lesion in the nipple grossly. The illustrations show areas that appear to be solid carcinoma with an alveolar pattern and foci best interpreted as papillary carcinoma. No follow-up was given.

**Gross and Microscopic Pathology**

Most pathologists who studied this condition have commented on the heterogeneous histologic features that may be present. However, the lesions can be grouped according to growth pattern into four categories. In three subtypes, one particular structural feature dominates the lesion or is present exclusively; the fourth group consists of tumors with mixed patterns. No prognostic significance can be attached to these subtypes, nor is there evidence that they differ in pathogenesis. Some clinicopathologic correlations have been noted with these categories, and it may be helpful to bear them in mind when faced with a proliferative lesion of the nipple.

1. *Sclerosing papillomatosis pattern.* This lesion typically presents as a discrete tumor. Scaling of the nipple skin may occur, but redness, ulceration, and inflammation are rarely present. About 50% of the patients have nipple discharge that is serous rather than bloody. The preoperative diagnosis usually is papilloma rather than Paget's disease or carcinoma.

Grossly, the nipple contains a firm tumor on palpation, although the margins may not appear well defined. The epidermis may look thickened, white, and scaly. Histologically, the lesion is indistinguishable in many respects from a sclerosing papilloma elsewhere in the breast (Figs. 5.35 and 5.36). Exuberant papillary hyperplasia of ductal epithelium is distorted by an accompanying stromal proliferation within and around the affected ducts. The complex proliferative process is arranged in papillary, solid, tubular, and glandular structures. Foci of myoepithelial cell hyperplasia usually can be identified, but as is generally the case with sclerosing pap-

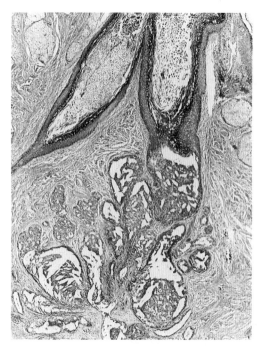

**FIG. 5.35.** *Florid papillomatosis of the nipple.* An early lesion at the squamocolumnar junction of a lactiferous duct and the epidermis. An early phase in the formation of a sclerotic center is evident near the lower border. (From Rosen PP, Oberman HA. Tumors of the mammary gland. In: *Atlas of tumor pathology.* Washington, DC: Armed Forces Institute of Pathology, 1993; and Rosen PP, Caicco JA. Florid papillomatosis of the nipple: a study of 51 patients, including nine having mammary carcinoma. *Am J Surg Pathol* 1986; 10:87–101, with permission.)

illary lesions, myoepithelial cells may be inconspicuous or absent in parts of the tumor (Fig. 5.37).

These lesions exhibit some qualitative and quantitative microscopic differences from the other subtypes of florid papillomatosis. The overlying cutaneous squamous epithelium usually is intact and hyperplastic. Squamous cysts are commonly formed in the terminal portions of lactiferous ducts. Focal comedo-type necrosis may be found in the hyperplastic duct epithelium, sometimes associated with infrequent mitoses in epithelial cells (Fig. 5.37). Apocrine metaplasia and extension of glandular epithelium to the nipple surface are uncommon and not prominent when present.

2. *Papilloma pattern.* Many of these patients complain of bleeding from the nipple. Although examination reveals a palpable lesion, this often is described as induration rather than as a discrete mass. The nipple often appears ulcerated or inflamed, and the clinical diagnosis is likely to be Paget's disease or carcinoma.

A discrete, firm nodule is evident grossly within the nipple, often extending to the skin surface. Microscopic examination reveals florid papillary hyperplasia of ductal epithelium causing expansion and crowding of the affected ducts (Fig. 5.38). Focal epithelial necrosis and scattered mitotic figures may be found, but these tumors lack the stromal proliferation that characterizes the sclerosing papillomatosis

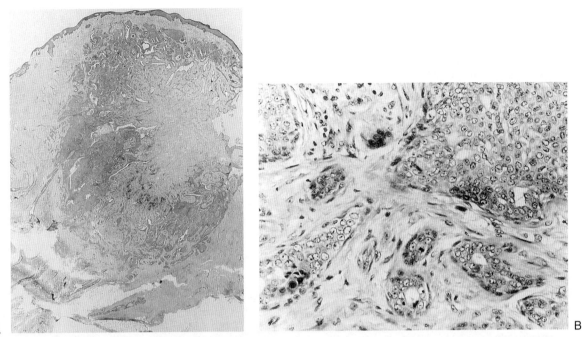

**FIG. 5.36.** *Florid papillomatosis, sclerosing papilloma pattern.* **A:** Whole-mount histologic section of the nipple lesion with a central area of fibrosis. The irregular border on the *right* is the site of erosion and a prior biopsy. **B:** Duct hyperplasia and proliferative stroma. (From Rosen PP, Oberman HA. Tumors of the mammary gland. In: *Atlas of tumor pathology.* Washington, DC: Armed Forces Institute of Pathology, 1993; and Rosen PP, Caicco JA. Florid papillomatosis of the nipple: a study of 51 patients, including nine having mammary carcinoma. *Am J Surg Pathol* 1986;10:87–101, with permission.)

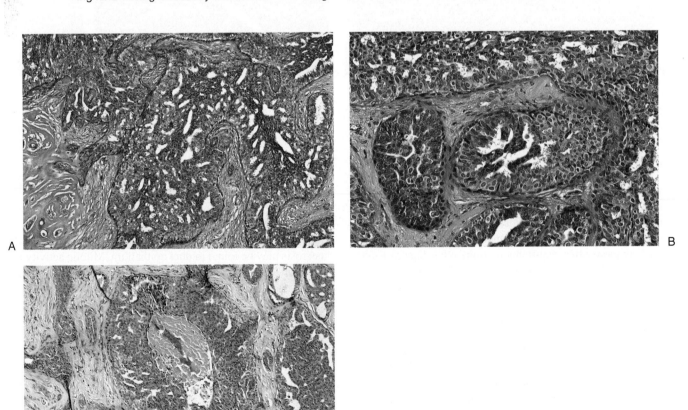

**FIG. 5.37.** *Florid papillomatosis, sclerosing papilloma pattern.* **A,B:** Two foci of florid epithelial hyperplasia with a prominent myoepithelial layer. **A:** The sclerotic core is near the *left* border. **B:** Micropapillary hyperplasia. **C:** Another lesion with epithelial necrosis.

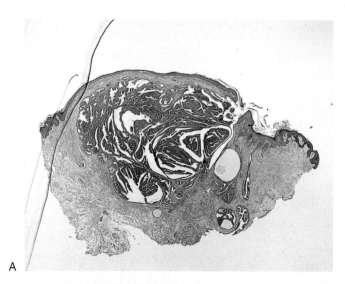

A

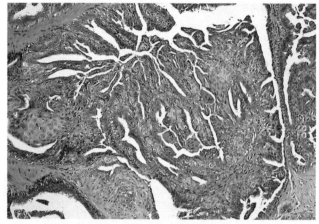

B

**FIG. 5.38.** *Florid papillomatosis, papilloma pattern.* **A:** Complex papilloma arising from lactiferous ducts in the nipple shown in an excisional biopsy specimen. **B:** Foci of squamous metaplasia are present in papillary epithelium. **C:** Florid hyperplasia of epithelial and myoepithelial cells.

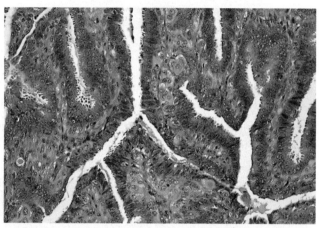

C

type of lesion. Hyperplastic glandular tissue may replace the overlying squamous epithelium over part or all of the surface. Squamous-lined cysts and apocrine metaplasia are not prominent in these lesions.

3. *Adenosis pattern.* These patients may have bloody or serous discharge. One patient had nipple retraction. The lesion produces a discrete nodule within the nipple. The nipple may appear ulcerated, inflamed, and swollen, and the epidermis usually is hyperplastic and intact. The clinical diagnosis is more often papilloma or some other benign lesion rather than Paget's disease. Microscopically, the lesion consists of crowded, orderly glandular structures arranged in a pattern that resembles an adenosis tumor in the breast parenchyma (Fig. 5.39). Myoepithelial hyperplasia accompanies the epithelial proliferation. Prominent apocrine metaplasia, hyperplasia of the squamous epithelium, and superficial squamous cysts may be encountered. Mitotic figures and focal necrosis are uncommon.

4. *Mixed proliferative pattern.* Patients with this type of florid papillomatosis may report a variety of symptoms, including scaling, bleeding pain, or burning and ulceration. Examination usually reveals a mass or nodule in the nipple, and the surface typically appears eroded. The clinical diagnosis often is carcinoma or Paget's disease.

Microscopic examination reveals varying combinations of the other three patterns (Fig. 5.40). Prominent features that are present in most cases include superficial squamous metaplasia of ducts with cysts, apocrine metaplasia, and acanthosis of the overlying epithelium. Hyperplastic duct epithelium may extend to the nipple surface, accounting for the impression of ulceration. Cystic dilation of ducts is not uncommon near the deep margin of the lesion, where this feature is interspersed with foci of duct hyperplasia. Focal necrosis may be found in duct epithelium. Mitotic activity is minimal. Adenosis occurs in about one-third of these lesions. Rarely, foci with a syringomatous pattern may be found at the edge of the lesion.

## Florid Papillomatosis and Mammary Carcinoma

A review of the literature revealed that 37 (16.5%) of 224 patients with florid papillomatosis also had mammary carcinoma (59). Nineteen of the 37 patients had carcinoma that arose coincidentally but separately in the same breast. This association is not surprising, because florid papillomatosis of the nipple was reportedly found in 1.2% (12 of 967) of the nipples studied in a review of mastectomy specimens from patients with breast carcinoma (105). To the extent that they

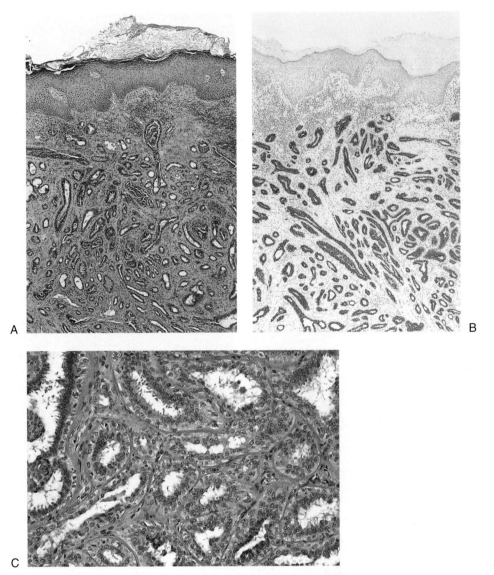

**FIG. 5.39.** *Florid papillomatosis, adenosis pattern.* **A:** Glandular proliferation has an adenosis pattern composed of tubular and oval glands. **B:** The architecture is highlighted by a CAM5.2 cytokeratin immunostain (avidin-biotin). **C:** Glandular elements in the lesion with epithelial and myoepithelial hyperplasia.

have been described, these coincidental carcinomas have largely been of the ductal variety. One patient had a separate invasive lobular carcinoma (106).

There were three other reported patients who developed carcinoma in a breast from which florid papillomatosis had been excised previously. One woman was found to have intraductal carcinoma 10 years later. At mastectomy, she had no residual florid papillomatosis of the nipple and the axillary lymph nodes were negative (98). She remained well 2 years later. In another patient, infiltrating duct carcinoma with metastases in axillary lymph nodes developed 17 years after resection of a "papillary adenoma" (92). The nipple had no residual papillomatosis. Four years later, she had pulmonary metastases. The third patient was 44 years old when she developed invasive duct carcinoma with axillary metas-

tases, 3 years after excision of florid papillomatosis from the ipsilateral nipple (59).

Carcinoma arose directly from florid papillomatosis in eight patients; three were men (59,102). Two of these men, 43 and 53 years old, had intraductal carcinoma arising in florid papillomatosis that was confined to the nipple. Both exhibited nipple enlargement and bloody discharge. Hyperpigmentation of the nipple was evident in one case. Paget's disease was seen in the overlying epidermis, and neither patient had evidence of invasive carcinoma (Fig. 5.41). Melanin pigment was present in Paget's cells in the patient with hyperpigmentation. Both mastectomy specimens contained no residual carcinoma, and the axillary lymph nodes were free of metastatic tumor. One of these men had concurrent contralateral intraductal carcinoma also treated by

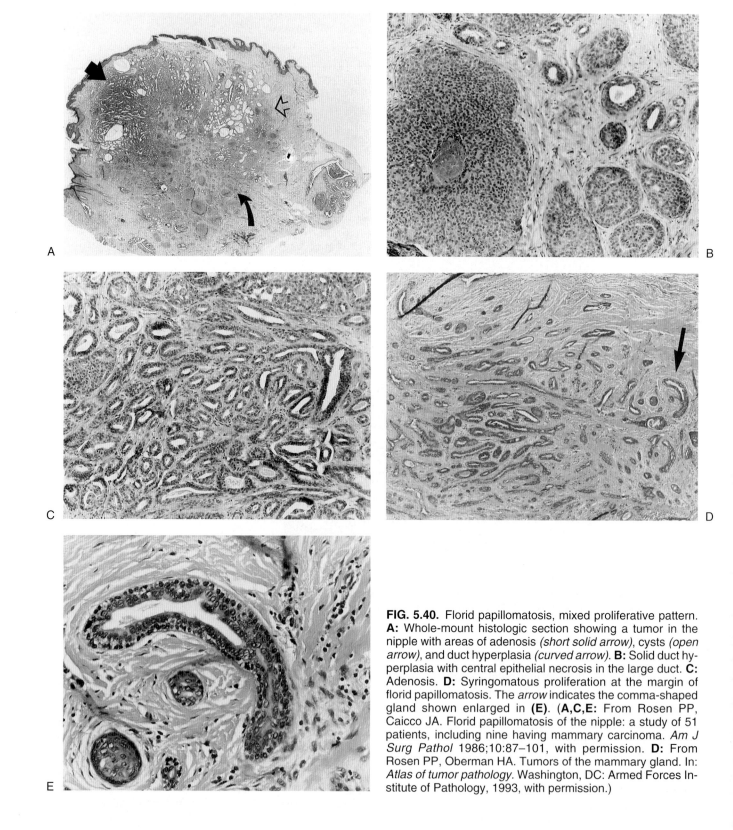

**FIG. 5.40.** Florid papillomatosis, mixed proliferative pattern. **A:** Whole-mount histologic section showing a tumor in the nipple with areas of adenosis *(short solid arrow)*, cysts *(open arrow)*, and duct hyperplasia *(curved arrow)*. **B:** Solid duct hyperplasia with central epithelial necrosis in the large duct. **C:** Adenosis. **D:** Syringomatous proliferation at the margin of florid papillomatosis. The *arrow* indicates the comma-shaped gland shown enlarged in **(E)**. (**A,C,E:** From Rosen PP, Caicco JA. Florid papillomatosis of the nipple: a study of 51 patients, including nine having mammary carcinoma. *Am J Surg Pathol* 1986;10:87–101, with permission. **D:** From Rosen PP, Oberman HA. Tumors of the mammary gland. In: *Atlas of tumor pathology.* Washington, DC: Armed Forces Institute of Pathology, 1993, with permission.)

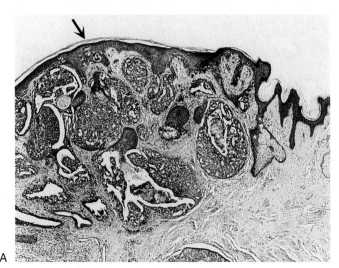
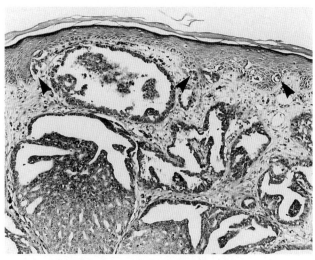

**FIG. 5.41.** *Intraductal carcinoma arising in florid papillomatosis.* **A:** Part of the nipple tumor that contains intraductal carcinoma as well as duct hyperplasia. Paget's disease in the epidermis can be been seen (*arrow*). **B:** *Arrows* indicate Paget's disease in the epidermis overlying duct hyperplasia in another section of the lesion. (From Rosen PP, Oberman HA. Tumors of the mammary gland. In: *Atlas of tumor pathology.* Washington, DC: Armed Forces Institute of Pathology, 1993, with permission.)

mastectomy. The third man, 66 years old, presented with scaling and itching of an enlarged nipple that contained a mass. Examination revealed bilateral gynecomastia. Biopsy yielded a 1.8-cm invasive duct carcinoma arising from florid papillomatosis in the nipple. The overlying nipple epidermis exhibited Paget's disease. The remainder of the breast had only gynecomastia, and the axillary lymph nodes were free of metastases. The patient was well 136 months later.

Five women reportedly had carcinoma arising directly in florid papillomatosis. Two patients, 43 and 67 years old, had intraductal carcinoma, with separate coexistent lobular carcinoma *in situ* in one of these cases (106). No comment was made about Paget's disease in either case, no invasion was seen, the patients had negative axillary lymph nodes, and no follow-up was given. Two other women, 52 and 63 years old, had invasive duct carcinoma arising in florid papillomatosis (Fig. 5.42) (59). The younger of these patients had no Paget's disease or other lesion of the breast, had negative lymph nodes, and remained well 2 years later. The older patient had Paget's disease of the nipple, a separate focus of intraductal and invasive duct carcinoma in the lower outer quadrant, and metastatic carcinoma in a single axillary lymph node.

The fifth woman, 43 years old, developed systemic metastases from invasive duct carcinoma that arose in florid papillomatosis (107). She had been aware of a tumor in her right nipple for 2 to 3 years prior to seeking medical attention. When she was examined, there was a 2-cm mass in the nipple and the ipsilateral axillary lymph nodes were enlarged. The patient had evidence of systemic metastases, which were confirmed at autopsy 5 weeks later. The nipple of the right breast contained a lesion that appeared microscopically to be florid papillomatosis. Paget's disease was noted in the overlying epidermis, and "in some small areas there was a

more florid type of epithelium with a larger nucleoli." Neither breast contained any other evidence of carcinoma, and as no primary lesions were found in other organs it seems likely that the patient had systemic dissemination of carcinoma that arose in florid papillomatosis. The experience with this patient is reminiscent of another patient with florid papillomatosis who had axillary lymph node metastases, although no definite evidence of carcinoma could be found histologically in the nipple lesion (Fig. 5.43) (59).

Carcinoma of the contralateral breast was described in seven women. Three had bilateral breast carcinoma with florid papillomatosis as a separate coincidental lesion in one breast. The other four patients had florid papillomatosis in the nipple of one breast and carcinoma only in the contralateral breast.

Subsequent to the review of 224 cases of florid papillomatosis that revealed 37 associated carcinomas (59), nine additional patients have been described (108,109). Five were women who had duct carcinomas, four of which were invasive, present concurrently but clinically and pathologically separate from florid papillomatosis in the same breast. In a sixth case, the patient reportedly had invasive duct carcinoma in the lower outer quadrant and invasive duct carcinoma that arose separately in the florid papillomatosis (108). A seventh patient was reported to have intraductal carcinoma in florid papillomatosis, but the diagnosis is doubtful because Paget's disease was not present (108). Two patients had invasive duct carcinoma in the nipple adjacent to, and possibly arising from, florid papillomatosis (109).

Carcinoma and florid papillomatosis of the nipple are each uncommon lesions of the male breast. Their coexistence in nearly 50% of male patients reported to have florid papillomatosis suggests this may be a precancerous lesion in men, especially because the carcinomas seem to have arisen in the

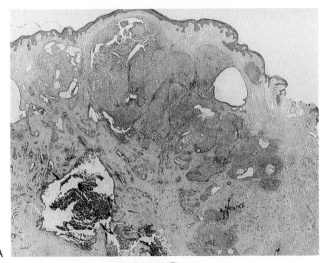

A

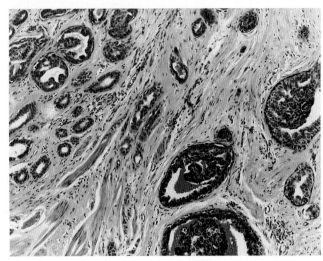

B

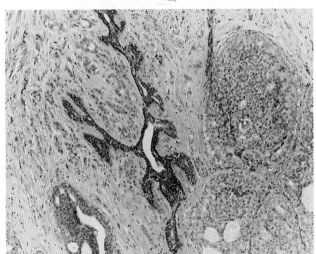

C

**FIG. 5.42.** *Invasive carcinoma in florid papillomatosis.* **A:** Whole-mount histologic section of a nipple with carcinoma in the right half of the lesion. A blood-filled recent biopsy site is evident on the left. The area of carcinoma was not sampled in the biopsy and the lesion was diagnosed as florid papillomatosis. **B:** Papillary epithelial proliferation in the lesion. **C:** Intraductal and infiltrating duct carcinoma around a lactiferous duct in the lesion. (**A,C:** From Rosen PP, Caicco JA. Florid papillomatosis of the nipple: a study of 51 patients, including nine having mammary carcinoma. *Am J Surg Pathol* 1986;10:87–101, with permission. **B:** From Rosen PP, Oberman HA. Tumors of the mammary gland. In: *Atlas of tumor pathology.* Washington, DC: Armed Forces Institute of Pathology, 1993, with permission.)

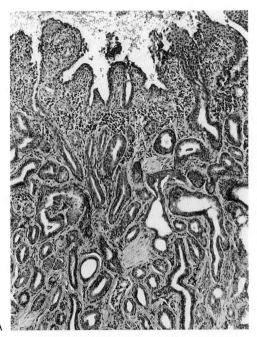

A

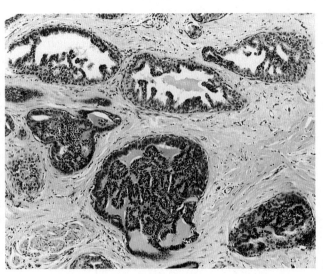

B

**FIG. 5.43.** *Occult carcinoma with lymph node metastases associated with florid papillomatosis.* **A:** Superficial portion of the lesion with erosion at the surface of the nipple. **B:** The most florid and atypical ductal proliferation found in the tumor. *(continued)*

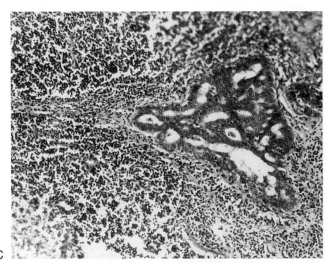
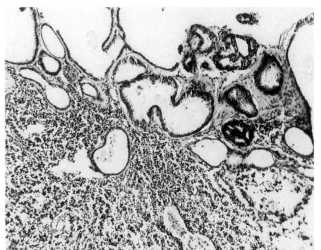

C

D

**FIG. 5.43.** *Continued.* **C,D:** Metastatic carcinoma was found in the two lymph nodes illustrated here. (**A,B:** From Rosen PP, Caicco JA. Florid papillomatosis of the nipple: a study of 51 patients, including nine having mammary carcinoma. *Am J Surg Pathol* 1986;10:87–101; and Rosen PP, Oberman HA. Tumors of the mammary gland. In: *Atlas of tumor pathology.* Washington, DC: Armed Forces Institute of Pathology, 1993, with permission.)

nipple lesion. This association may be a reflection of the fact that male breast carcinoma typically arises in the subareolar region.

The evidence indicating that florid papillomatosis is precancerous in women is less substantial. Nonetheless, a woman with florid papillomatosis should have both breasts carefully examined clinically and radiologically to exclude an independent concurrent coincidental carcinoma. If the florid papillomatosis lesion is completely excised and found not to harbor carcinoma, the risk for subsequently developing carcinoma in the same breast seems to be relatively low.

As indicated by some of the foregoing case reports, it may be difficult to detect carcinoma arising in florid papillomatosis of the nipple. Hyperplastic areas in the lesions often exhibit atypical features that may include foci with comedonecrosis as well as cribriform and micropapillary growth patterns, mitoses, and cytologic atypia. In the absence of definitive evidence of invasion, Paget's disease of the nipple epidermis is the most reliable evidence for a diagnosis of carcinoma arising in florid papillomatosis. The CAM5.2 immunostain for cytokeratin is helpful for detecting Paget's cells, which are immunoreactive for this marker (Fig. 5.44). Paget's cells were not present in any of the larger series of cases of florid papillomatosis regarded as benign, but these studies were published before current immunostains were generally available. When Paget's disease is found, there usually are underlying areas of intraductal carcinoma that differ from the rest of the tumor in their growth pattern. The differential diagnosis also includes primary invasive duct carcinoma arising from lactiferous ducts in the nipple without associated florid papillomatosis (Fig. 5.45).

In the absence of Paget's disease or invasive carcinoma, a diagnosis of intraductal carcinoma arising in florid papillo-

matosis is extremely difficult to substantiate with routine sections. In all forms of florid papillomatosis glandular cells are uniformly immunoreactive for cytokeratin and focally for carcinoembryonic antigen (110). Well-formed basement membrane is demonstrated by reactivity for collagen type IV. Myoepithelial cells exhibit immunoreactivity for actin, myosin, and calponin. It remains to be determined whether the focal absence of this pattern is by itself sufficient evidence for a diagnosis of carcinoma arising in florid papillomatosis.

Two examples of florid papillomatosis studied by flow cytometry (111) proved to be diploid with relatively high S-phase fractions (10.9% and 34.4%), similar to a series of intraductal carcinomas (6.4% to 15.8%). Neither of the lesions was immunoreactive for the c-*erb*B-2 oncogene product or for the tumor-associated glycoprotein-72 (TAG-72). Epithelial S-100 protein immunoreactivity was detected in both florid papillomatosis tumors. Analysis of many more lesions will be necessary to determine whether these procedures can reliably detect carcinoma in florid papillomatosis. Regardless of the degree of atypia, a conservative approach to the histologic diagnosis of these lesions is recommended when Paget's disease and/or invasive carcinoma is not present.

**Treatment and Follow-up**

The diagnosis of florid papillomatosis may be suggested by the cytologic findings in a scraping from the nipple surface (100,112,113). FNA yields a cellular specimen containing variable proportions of glandular and myoepithelial cells (112). If there is marked atypia, the cytologic specimen can be misinterpreted as carcinoma (100,114). Incisional biopsy or needle biopsy is not satisfactory to exclude the

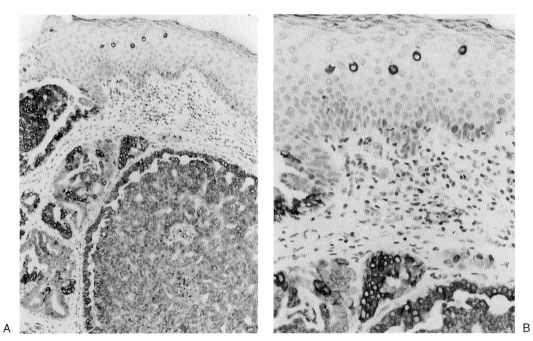

**FIG. 5.44.** *Paget's disease in florid papillomatosis.* **A,B:** Five cells are highlighted in the epidermis with the immunostain for CAM 5.2. Similar immunoreactive cells representing pagetoid spread of carcinoma are evident focally in the underlying papillary proliferation (avidin-biotin).

possibility of carcinoma arising in the lesion. In one case seen by the author, an incisional biopsy revealed only florid papillomatosis. When excised, the lesion contained an area of invasive carcinoma. Complete excision, which is recommended as definitive treatment, usually requires removal of the nipple. Resection by Mohs microsurgery has been reported (115). Local recurrence of florid papillomatosis may occur following subtotal excision (59,92,97), but a substantial number of patients have reportedly remained asymptomatic after incomplete excision. Mastectomy is not indicated as primary treatment of florid papillomatosis unassociated with carcinoma.

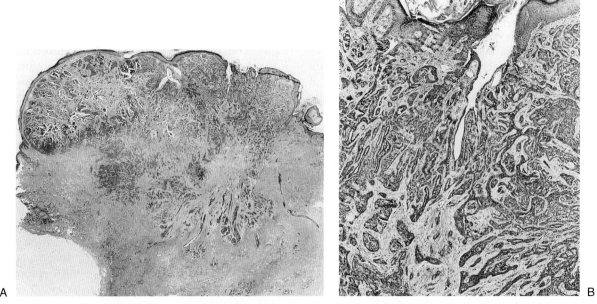

**FIG. 5.45.** *Infiltrating carcinoma in the nipple.* **A:** Whole-mount microscopic section of the nipple containing a tumor composed entirely of carcinoma. **B:** Superficial portion of the carcinoma with papillary features. No Paget's disease was present. *(continued)*

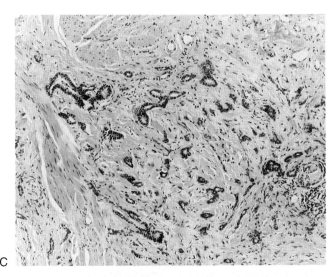 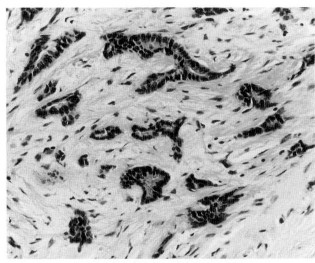

C       D

**FIG. 5.45.** *Continued.* **C,D:** Invasive duct carcinoma involving smooth muscle of the nipple growing as tubular carcinoma. (From Rosen PP, Caicco JA. Florid papillomatosis of the nipple: a study of 51 patients, including nine having mammary carcinoma. *Am J Surg Pathol* 1986;10:87–101, with permission.)

## SYRINGOMATOUS ADENOMA OF THE NIPPLE

This is a benign locally infiltrating neoplasm of the nipple. Syringomatous adenoma of the breast has a close histopathologic resemblance to syringomatous tumors that commonly arise in the skin of the face and other anatomic sites. Included in this category are locally infiltrating syringomatous tumors of minor salivary gland arising in the lip (116), microcystic adnexal carcinoma of the skin of the face (117), and sclerosing sweat gland duct (syringomatous) carcinoma (118).

The precise anatomic source of the breast lesions is uncertain. The absence of epithelial proliferation in the mammary ducts and the lack of connection with the epidermis in most cases suggest origin from other structures. Because random sections of nipples taken from breasts removed for mammary carcinoma sometimes reveal sweat gland ducts, these may give rise to syringomatous adenomas.

Early descriptions of this lesion were included in studies of florid papillomatosis of the nipple. Handley and Thackray (90) described an example of syringomatous adenoma in a 39-year-old woman whose biopsy revealed an "adenoma, suggesting a sweat gland origin." Doctor and Sirsat (93) found five syringomatous adenomas in a series of epithelial tumors of the nipple. They concluded that ". . . the lesion designated as florid papillomatosis or adenoma of the nipple does not seem to be one entity, but two distinct lesions . . . the term florid papillomatosis is applicable to lesions showing a papillomatous pattern and is linked with fibrocystic disease and intracystic papilloma of the breast. The term adenoma of the nipple should be reserved for lesions showing an adenomatous pattern and is related more to the sweat gland tumours."

Rosen (95) described six additional cases in 1983 and proposed the term *syringomatous adenoma.* At least 15 cases have since been described (94,119,120).

### Clinical Presentation

The patients reported since 1983 (94,95,119–121) ranged from 11 to 74 years of age at diagnosis. The median age was 36 and the average age was 39 years. One man was 76 years old (95). Onset within a year of diagnosis was usually reported, but a duration of several years has been described.

Syringomatous adenomas have been unilateral lesions affecting either breast with approximately equal frequency. The initial symptom is a mass in the nipple and/or subareolar region. Pain, tenderness, redness, itching, discharge, or nipple inversion have been noted in isolated cases. Crusting of the nipple surface, which proves microscopically to be due to hyperkeratosis, has been reported, but ulceration or erosion are not features of syringomatous adenoma. Mammography reveals a dense stellate subareolar lesion (121).

Except for one patient who later developed and died of colonic carcinoma (95), syringomatous adenomas have not been associated with other neoplasms.

### Gross Pathology

The excised tumors have measured 1.0 to 3.5 cm, with a mean of 1.7 and median of 1.5 cm. Most consist of ill-defined, firm-to-hard gray, tan, or white tissue. Discrete nodules and microcystic areas have been noted infrequently.

### Microscopic Pathology

The lesion consists of tubules, ductules, and strands composed of small, uniform generally basophilic cells infiltrating the dermis of the skin and the stroma of the nipple (Fig. 5.46). Hyperplasia of the epidermis is slight in most cases, but occasionally pseudoepitheliomatous hyperplasia may be encountered. Neoplastic glands that proliferate throughout

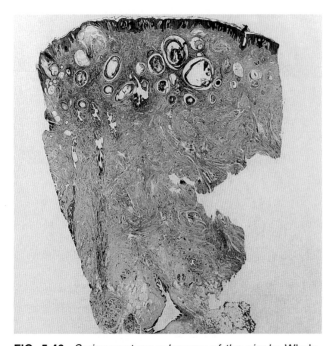

**FIG. 5.46.** *Syringomatous adenoma of the nipple.* Whole-mount microscopic section of the lesion. Keratotic cysts are prominent at this magnification. (From Rosen PP, Oberman HA. Tumors of the mammary gland. In: *Atlas of tumor pathology.* Washington, DC: Armed Forces Institute of Pathology, 1993, with permission.)

the dermis sometimes appear to be connected with the basal layer of the epidermis.

The ducts, lined by one or more layers of cells, have teardrop, comma-like, and branching shapes, with lumens that usually are open and round (Fig. 5.47). Cords of small uniform cells appear to be tangentially sectioned ducts. Although some cells may exhibit cytoplasmic clearing, a distinct layer of myoepithelial cells is not apparent. Mitoses are virtually absent, and nuclei lack prominent nucleoli and pleomorphism.

The lumens are empty, or they contain deeply eosinophilic, retracted secretion. Flattening of cells around the lumens is early evidence of squamous differentiation, which in a fully developed form results in keratotic cysts (Fig. 5.48). A foreign body giant cell reaction may be elicited in the vicinity of ruptured squamous cysts. Calcification is rarely seen in the keratinized epithelium.

The secretion in tubular lumens is PAS positive and weakly mucicarmine positive (Fig. 5.49) (95). Carcinoembryonic antigen has been found in the secretion and in the cytoplasm of periluminal cells. One report stated that "sparse tumor cells contained S-100 protein" (120). Other authors noted that some cells in the neoplastic tubules were reactive for actin, suggesting the presence of a myoepithelial cell component, but these cells were not reactive for S-100 protein, and electron microscopic findings were inconclusive (120).

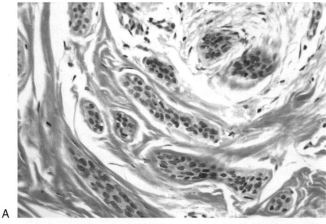

A

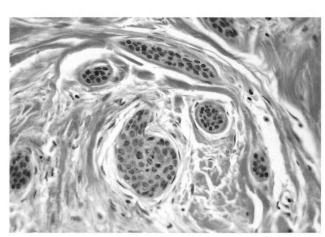

B

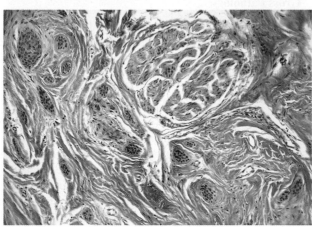

C

**FIG. 5.47.** *Syringomatous adenoma.* **A:** Elongated ductular structures. **B:** Squamous differentiation and a teardrop shape. **C:** Infiltration of smooth muscle in the nipple.

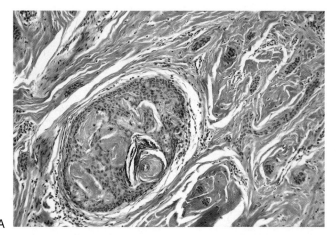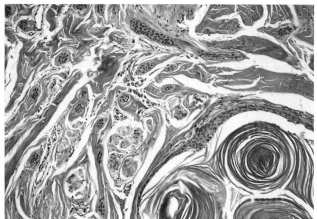

A
B

**FIG. 5.48.** *Syringomatous adenoma.* **A:** Solid focus of squamous differentiation. **B:** Cystic squamous differentiation.

The adenomatous tubules diffusely infiltrate the periductal stroma of the nipple and, in larger lesions, may extend into the subareolar breast parenchyma. Invasion into the smooth muscle bundles of the nipple is very common, and occasionally perineural invasion is observed (Fig. 5.47). The stroma appears to be altered in the vicinity of the infiltrating tubules, because the collagen and fibroblasts tend to be concentrically oriented around the epithelial structures (Fig. 5.47).

Syringomatous adenomas probably arise from sweat gland ducts in the nipple or areola. Syringomatous glands may be found in close proximity to, and rarely in direct contact with, the epithelium of nipple ducts or ductules and lobules of the breast parenchyma and the epidermis of the nipple. This appears to be a result of the infiltrative growth pattern of the neoplasm and should not be interpreted as evidence of origin from any of these structures. Coincidental epithelial hyperplasia of lactiferous ducts or the underlying breast tissue occasionally may be seen, but this is not an intrinsic component of syringomatous adenoma. Paget's disease, a manifestation of duct carcinoma, also is not a feature of syringomatous adenoma.

Several lesions should be considered in the differential di-

agnosis of syringomatous adenoma of the nipple. Florid papillomatosis is predominantly a hyperplastic epithelial proliferation of the major lactiferous ducts (59). Patients with florid papillomatosis tend to be older, they are more likely to have erosion of the nipple with bleeding, and the duration usually is brief compared to syringomatous adenoma. Syringomatous foci occasionally are encountered as a minor component of the proliferative complex that forms florid papillomatosis.

Tubular carcinoma sometimes arises in the subareolar region and nipple, where it has an infiltrative growth pattern that may be difficult to distinguish from syringomatous adenoma. Both invade smooth muscle and around nerves. Features of tubular carcinoma that are not seen in syringomatous adenoma include intraductal carcinoma, Paget's disease of the epidermis, and angular glands. Squamous metaplasia and round glands formed by ductules that often have a branching pattern are not features of tubular carcinoma.

Despite some structural similarities between the two lesions, syringomatous adenoma and some variants of low-grade adenosquamous carcinoma (122) are not, as has been suggested (89), part of a single neoplastic process. Syringomatous adenoma arises in the nipple and secondarily involves the breast parenchyma underlying the nipple in almost all cases. Low-grade adenosquamous carcinoma usually develops peripherally, sparing the nipple, although very infrequently it can arise in the subareolar region and involve the nipple.

Squamous cysts may develop in syringocystadenoma papilliferum, a lesion that usually arises in the skin of the head and neck area. In the breast, this tumor has been reported arising from major lactiferous ducts (123). Papillary proliferation of the epithelium distinguishes this lesion from syringomatous adenoma.

**Treatment and Prognosis**

Most patients have been treated by local excision, which in some instances has required removing the entire nipple. Reexcision is recommended if the margins appear involved

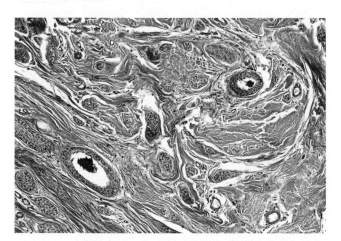

**FIG. 5.49.** *Syringomatous adenoma.* Secretion in two glands is stained magenta with the periodic acid-Schiff reaction.

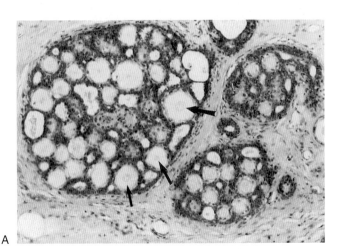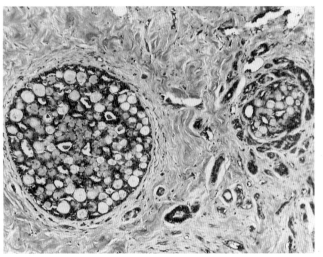

A                                                B

**FIG. 5.50.** *Collagenous spherulosis.* **A:** Hyperplasia in three duct cross sections exhibiting collagenous spherulosis. *Arrows* indicate central nidi in the spherules. The combination of spherules and glandular lumens simulates cribriform growth. **B:** One of two ducts with collagenous spherulosis is centered in sclerosing adenosis on the *right.*

(89). Total mastectomy is not indicated as primary treatment, although this operation has been performed in a few cases when the diagnosis was uncertain because the lesion was not recognized as syringomatous adenoma. Recurrence after incomplete excision has occurred in approximately 30% of cases reported since 1983 (94,95,121). The time to recurrence has varied from less than 1 year to 8 years. In one case, the lesion was known to have persisted and slowly enlarged for 22 years after initial biopsy, at which time a partial mastectomy was performed for a 3-cm tumor that invaded the breast parenchyma (95). One patient experienced three recurrences over a 4-year period (94). None of the patients has developed metastases in regional lymph nodes or at distant sites, and there is no evidence of an association with mammary adenocarcinoma.

## COLLAGENOUS SPHERULOSIS

This unusual structural alteration, more frequently encountered in ducts than in lobules, is typically an incidental microscopic finding in 1% to 2% of biopsies that contain hyperplastic duct lesions. Calcification in collagenous spherulosis may lead to its identification by mammography and diagnosis by needle core biopsy. Because of a superficial resemblance to adenoid cystic carcinoma, adenoid cystic hyperplasia is an alternative name for this condition (124). Collagenous spherulosis may be found in association with other benign proliferative lesions, including papilloma, papillary duct hyperplasia, atypical duct hyperplasia, and sclerosing adenosis (Figs. 5.50 and 5.51) (125). When these proliferative lesions produce a palpable mass, collagenous spherulosis remains a microscopic com-

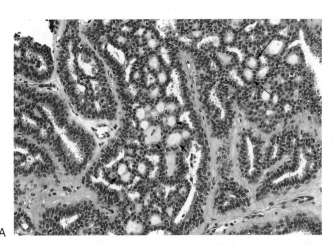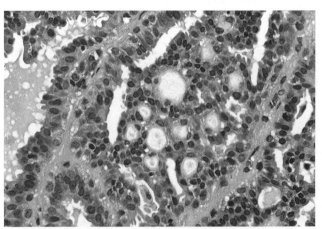

A                                                B

**FIG. 5.51.** *Collagenous spherulosis in a papilloma.* **A:** Two appearances are seen in this papilloma. Some spherules are in the form of opaque eosinophilic nodules *(short arrows),* whereas others appear to be open spaces surrounded by a dense border *(long arrows).* A small nidus is seen in some open spherules. **B:** The open spherules shown here have dense borders of basement membrane material. The lumens contain fibrillar material. Myoepithelial cells are difficult to identify.

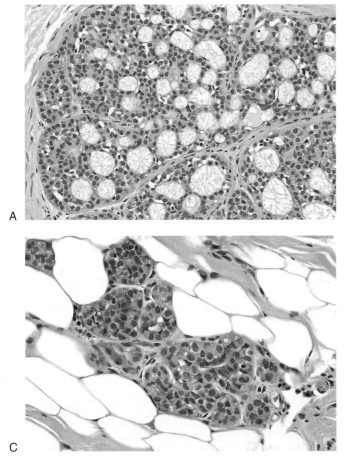

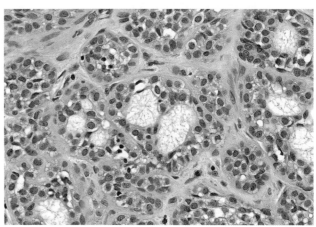

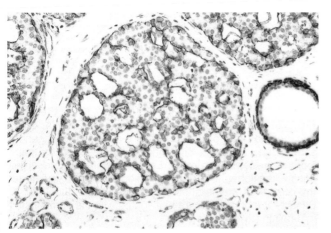

**FIG. 5.52.** *Collagenous spherulosis with lobular carcinoma* in situ. **A,B:** Radial fibrillar deposits in spherules surrounded by *in situ* lobular carcinoma. E-cadherin immunoreactivity was absent. **C:** Lobule involved by lobular carcinoma *in situ* in the surrounding tissue.

ponent that is not responsible for the clinical presentation (125a).

Carcinoma may be present coincidentally in the same specimen, but these usually are independent processes (126). Rarely, carcinoma *in situ* is found "colonizing" and replacing the epithelium of collagenous spherulosis (Fig. 5.52). E-cadherin reactivity is present when collagenous spherulosis occurs in ductal hyperplasia or intraductal carcinoma, but it is absent when lobular carcinoma *in situ* involves collagenous spherulosis. There is no evidence to indicate that the presence of collagenous spherulosis is associated with precancerous lesions (124,127), or that it is associated with adenoid cystic carcinoma.

In lesions with collagenous spherulosis, the hyperplastic epithelium forms true glands and acellular spherules, creating an adenoid cystic structural arrangement. The lumens of

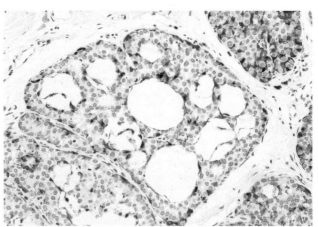

**FIG. 5.53.** *Collagenous spherulosis, myoepithelial cells.* **A:** Spherules are outlined by myoepithelial cells stained for smooth muscle actin. **B:** Myoepithelial cells are S-100 immunoreactive (both avidin-biotin).

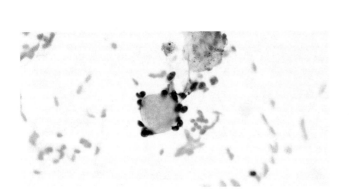

**FIG. 5.54.** *Collagenous spherulosis, cytology specimen.* Spherule in a fine needle aspiration sample. Myoepithelial cells are adherent to the surface.

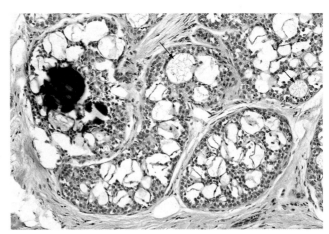

**FIG. 5.55.** *Collagenous spherulosis, calcification.* A large basophilic calcification is shown on the *left*. Fibrillar material is evident in two spherules *(arrows)*. Filaments that traverse many empty spherules are basement membranes with adherent myoepithelial cells that have collapsed into the spherules. Note myoepithelial cell nuclei associated with the basement membrane filaments.

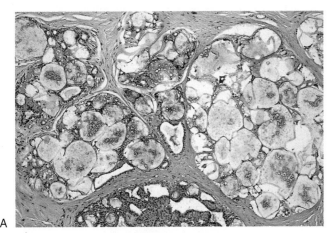

A

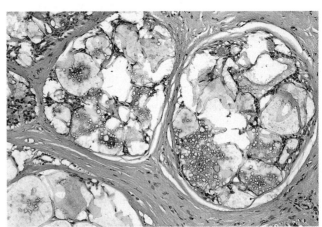

B

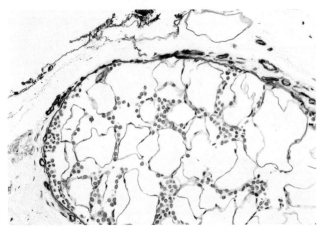

C

**FIG. 5.56.** *Collagenous spherulosis, degenerative.* **A:** Cystic degeneration has occurred in this example of collagenous spherulosis. Traces of this condition are seen in the papilloma at the lower border. **B:** Epithelial elements are largely absent, the spherule material is basophilic and vesicular, and the basement membranes appear as flaccid filaments. **C:** Basement membranes are highlighted with the immunostain for laminin (avidin-biotin).

the glandular spaces tend to have a more irregular shape than in adenoid cystic carcinoma. The attenuated myoepithelial cells are difficult to identify in hematoxylin and eosin sections. Immunostains for actin and S-100 protein highlight these cells (Fig. 5.53).

Collagenous spherulosis may be suggested by the findings in an aspiration cytology specimen (128,129). The typical features are a moderately cellular specimen consisting of epithelial clusters as well as dispersed epithelial and myoepithelial cells. The spherules stain light green with the Papanicolaou stain and pink with the Diff-Quik stain. They are surrounded by crescentic myoepithelial cells or papillary clusters of epithelial cells (Fig. 5.54). A fibrillary quality may be detected in the spherules with the Diff-Quik stain (130).

The stromal component of the lesion consists of spherules measuring 20 to 100 μm in diameter. The spherules have various staining patterns and may be eosinophilic, amphophilic, or nearly transparent. They consist of ground substance and basement membrane material that may calcify (Fig. 5.55). Fibrillar deposits within spherules rarely have a laminar concentric distribution. More often, stellate fibrils radiate from a central nidus toward the periphery of the spherule (Fig. 5.52). Degenerative changes can occur in the spherule material, creating a myxoid appearance sometimes accompanied by shrinkage of the outer basement membrane layer, which collapses into the spherule (Figs. 5.55 and 5.56). Immunohistochemical studies and electron microscopy have identified several constituents in spherules, including elastin, PAS-positive polysaccharides, and other components of basement membrane including type IV collagen and laminin (Figs. 5.53 and 5.56) (131,132).

## REFERENCES

1. Haagensen CD, Stout AP, Phillips JS. The papillary neoplasms of the breast. I. Benign intraductal papilloma. *Ann Surg* 1951;133:18–36.
2. Cardenosa G, Eklund GW. Benign papillary neoplasms of the breast: mammographic findings. *Radiology* 1991;181:751–755.
3. Rovno HD, Siegelman ES, Reynolds C, et al. Solitary intraductal papilloma: findings at MR imaging and MR galactography. *AJR Am J Roentgenol* 1999;172:151–155.
3a. Shen K-W, Wu J, Lu J-S, et al. Fiberoptic ductoscopy for patients with nipple discharge. *Cancer* 2000;89:1912–1919.
4. Roy I, Meakins JL, Tremblay G. Giant intraductal papilloma of the breast: a case report. *J Surg Oncol* 1985;28:281–283.
5. Carter DJ, Rosen PP. Atypical apocrine metaplasia in sclerosing lesions of the breast. A study of 51 patients. *Mod Pathol* 1991;4:1–5.
6. Ichihara S, Matsuyama T, Kubo K, et al. Infarction of breast fibroadenoma in a postmenopausal woman. *Pathol Int* 1994;44:398–400.
7. Papotti M, Gugliotta P, Eusebi V, et al. Immunohistochemical analysis of benign and malignant papillary lesions of the breast. *Am J Surg Pathol* 1983;7:451–461.
8. Dabbs DJ, Gown AM. Distribution of calponin and smooth muscle myosin heavy chain in fine-needle aspiration biopsies of the breast. *Diagn Cytopathol* 1999;20:203–207.
9. Kobayashi TK, Ueda M, Nishino T, et al. Spontaneous infarction of an intraductal papilloma of the breast: cytological presentation on fine needle aspiration. *Cytopathology* 1992;3:379–384.
10. Flint A, Oberman HA. Infarction and squamous metaplasia of intraductal papilloma: a benign breast lesion that may simulate carcinoma. *Hum Pathol* 1984;15:764–767.
11. Soderstrom KO, Toikkanen S. Extensive squamous metaplasia simulating squamous cell carcinoma in benign breast papillomatosis. *Hum Pathol* 1983;14:1081–1082.
12. Reddick RL, Jennette JC, Askin FB. Squamous metaplasia of the breast. An ultrastructural and immunologic evaluation. *Am J Clin Pathol* 1985;84:530–533.
13. Dawson AE, Mulford DK. Benign versus malignant papillary neoplasms of the breast. Diagnostic clues in fine needle aspiration cytology. *Acta Cytol* 1994;38:23–28.
14. Jeffrey PB, Ljung B-M. Benign and malignant papillary lesions of the breast. A cytomorphologic study. *Am J Clin Pathol* 1994;101:500–507.
15. Chang JH, Lawson D, Mosunjac MB. Use of proliferation (Ki-67) and G1-cell cycle (cyclin D1) marker in evaluating breast papillary lesions in FNA cell block preparations. *Mod Pathol* 2000;13:31A.
16. Liberman L, Bracero N, Vuolo MA, et al. Percutaneous large-core biopsy of papillary breast lesions. *AJR Am J Roentgenol* 1999;172:331–337.
17. Liberman L. Personal communication, 1999.
18. Berg WA, Gill HK, Philpotts LE, et al. Should a result of benign papilloma on core biopsy be viewed as a high risk lesion? *Radiol Suppl* 1999;213:288.
19. Dickinson GK. The breast physiologically and pathologically considered with relation to bleeding from the nipple. *Am J Obstet Gynecol* 1922;3:31–34.
20. Bloodgood JC. Benign lesions of the female breast for which operation is not indicated. *JAMA* 1922;78:859–863.
21. Buhl-Jorgensen SE, Fischermann K, Johansen H, et al. Cancer risk in intraductal papilloma and papillomatosis. *Surg Gynecol Obstet* 1968;127:307–313.
22. Hendrick JW. Intraductal papilloma of the breast. *Surg Gynecol Obstet* 1957;105:215–223.
23. Kilgore AR, Fleming R, Ramos N. The incidence of cancer with nipple discharge and the risk of cancer in the presence of papillary disease of the breast. *Surg Gynecol Obstet* 1953;96:649–660.
24. Kraus FT, Neubecker RD. The differential diagnosis of papillary tumors of the breast. *Cancer* 1962;15:444–455.
25. Lewison EF, Lyons JG Jr. Relationship between benign breast disease and cancer. *Arch Surg* 1953;66:94–114.
26. Carter D. Intraductal papillary tumors of the breast. A study of 76 cases. *Cancer* 1977;39:1689–1692.
27. Snyder WH, Chaffin L. Main duct papilloma of the breast. *Arch Surg* 1955;70:680–685.
28. Estabrook A. Are patients with solitary or multiple intraductal papillomas at a higher risk of developing breast cancer? *Surg Oncol Clin North Am* 1993;2:45–56.
29. Haagensen CD, Bodian C, Haagensen DE. *Breast carcinoma: risk and detection*. Philadelphia: WB Saunders, 1981:146–237.

## Radial Sclerosing Lesions

30. Semb C. Pathologico-anatomical and clinical investigations of fibro-adenomatosis cystica mammae and its relation to other pathological conditions in mamma, especially cancer. *Acta Chir Scand (Suppl)* 1928;64:1–484.
31. Bloodgood JC. Borderline breast tumors; encapsulated and non-encapsulated cystic adenomata, observed from 1890–1931. *Am J Cancer* 1932;16:103–176.
32. Fenoglio C, Lattes R. Sclerosing papillary proliferations in the female breast. A benign lesion often mistaken for carcinoma. *Cancer* 1974;33:691–700.
33. Fisher ER, Palekar AS, Kotwal N, et al. A nonencapsulated sclerosing lesion of the breast. *Am J Clin Pathol* 1979;71:240–246.
34. Azzopardi JG. Overdiagnosis of malignancy. In: Azzopardi JG. *Problems in breast pathology*. London: Saunders, 1979:174.
35. Rickert RR, Kalisher L, Hutter RVP. Indurative mastopathy: a benign sclerosing lesion of breast with elastosis which may simulate carcinoma. *Cancer* 1981;47:561–571.
36. Hamperl H. Strahlige Narben und obliterierende Mastopathie Beitrage zur pathologischen histologie der Mamma. *Virchows Arch [A]* 1975;369:55–68.
37. Linell F, Ljungberg O, Anderson I. Breast carcinoma: aspects of early stage, progression and related problems. *Acta Pathol Microbiol Scand (Suppl)* 1980;272:1–233.
38. Nielsen M, Jensen J, Andersen JA. An autopsy study of radial scar in the female breast. *Histopathology* 1985;9:287–295.
39. Wellings SR, Alpers CE. An atlas of subgross pathology of the human breast with special reference to possible precancerous lesions. *J Natl Cancer Inst* 1975;55:231–273.

40. Andersen JA, Gram JB. Radial scar in the female breast: a long-term follow-up study of 32 cases. *Cancer* 1984;53:2557–2560.
41. Bondeson L, Linell F, Ringberg A. Breast reductions: what to do with all the tissue specimens? *Histopathology* 1985;9:281–285.
42. Jacobs TW, Byrne C, Colditz G, et al. Radial scars in benign breast-biopsy specimens and the risk of breast cancer. *N Engl J Med* 1999;340:430–436.
43. Nielsen M, Christensen L, Andersen J. Radial scars in women with breast cancer. *Cancer* 1987;59:1019–1025.
44. Vazquez MF, Mitnick JS, Pressman P, et al. Radial scar: cytologic evaluation by stereotactic aspiration. *Breast Dis* 1994;7:299–306.
45. Adler DD, Helvie MA, Oberman HA, et al. Radial sclerosing lesion of the breast: mammographic features. *Radiology* 1990;176:737–740.
46. Ciatto S, Morrone D, Catarzi S, et al. Radial scars of the breast: review of 38 consecutive mammographic diagnoses. *Radiology* 1993;187:757–760.
47. Mitnick JS, Vazquez MF, Harris MN, et al. Differentiation of radial scar from scirrhous carcinoma of the breast: mammographic-pathologic correlation. *Radiology* 1989;173:697–700.
48. Orel SG, Evers K, Yeh IT, et al. Radial scar with microcalcification: radiologic-pathologic correlation. *Radiology* 1992;183:479–484.
49. Andersen JA, Carter D, Linell F. A symposium of sclerosing duct lesions of the breast. *Pathol Annu* 1986;21[Pt 2]:145–179.
50. Battersby S, Anderson TJ. Myofibroblast activity of radial scars. *J Pathol* 1985;147:33–40.
51. Taylor HB, Norris HJ. Epithelial invasion of nerves in benign diseases of the breast. *Cancer* 1967;20:2245–2249.
52. Mitnick JS, Vazquez MF, Roses DF, et al. Stereotactic localization for fine needle aspiration breast biopsy: initial experience with 300 patients. *Arch Surg* 1991;126:1137–1140.
53. Makunura CN, Curling OM, Yeomans P, et al. Apocrine adenosis within a radial scar: a case of false positive breast cytodiagnosis. *Cytopathology* 1994;5:123–128.
54. Caneva A, Bonetti F, Manfrin E, et al. Is radial scar of the breast a premalignant lesion? *Mod Pathol* 1997;10:17A.
55. Orell SR. Radial scar/complex sclerosing lesion—a problem in the diagnostic work-up of screen-detected breast lesions. *Cytopathology* 1999;10:250–258.
56. Jackman RJ, Nowels KW, Rodriguez-Soto J, et al. Stereotactic, automated, large-core needle biopsy of nonpalpable breast lesions: false-negative and histologic underestimation rates after longer-term follow-up. *Radiology* 1999;210:799–805.
57. Sloane JP, Mayers MM. Carcinoma and atypical hyperplasia in radial scars and complex sclerosing lesions: importance of lesion size and patient age. *Histopathology* 1993;23:225–231.
58. Anderson TJ, Battersby S. Radial scars of benign and malignant breasts: comparative features and significance. *J Pathol* 1985;147:23–32.

## Subareolar Sclerosing Duct Hyperplasia

59. Rosen PP, Caicco JA. Florid papillomatosis of the nipple: a study of 51 patients, including nine having mammary carcinoma. *Am J Surg Pathol* 1986;10:87–101.
60. Rosen PP. Subareolar sclerosing duct hyperplasia of the breast. *Cancer* 1987;59:1927–1930.

## Cystic and Papillary Apocrine Metaplasia

61. Fechner RE. Benign breast disease in women on estrogen therapy. A pathologic study. *Cancer* 1972;29:273–279.
62. Charles A. An electron microscopic study of the human axillary apocrine gland. *J Anat* 1959;93:226–232.
63. Miller WR, Dixon JM, Forrest PM. Hormonal correlates of apocrine secretion in the breast. *Ann N Y Acad Sci* 1986;464:275–287.
64. Labows JN, Preti G, Hoelzle E, et al. Steroid analysis of human apocrine secretion. *Steroids* 1979;34:249–258.
65. Bussolati G, Cattani MG, Gugliotta P, et al. Morphologic and functional aspects of apocrine metaplasia in dysplastic and neoplastic breast tissue. *Ann N Y Acad Sci* 1986;464:262–274.
66. Naldoni C, Massimo C, Dogliotti L, et al. Association of cyst type with risk factors for breast cancer and relapse rate in women with gross cystic disease of the breast. *Cancer Res* 1992;52:1791–1795.
67. Haagensen CD, Bodian C, Haagensen DE Jr. Apocrine epithelium. In: Haagensen CD, Bodian C, Haagensen DE Jr., eds. *Breast carcinoma. Risk and detection.* Philadelphia: WB Saunders, 1981:83–105.
68. De Potter CR, Cuvelier CA, Roels HJ. Apocrine adenoma presenting as gynaecomastia in a 14-year-old boy. *Histopathology* 1988;13:697–699.
69. Tesluk H, Amott T, Goodnight JE. Apocrine adenoma of the breast. *Arch Pathol Lab Med* 1986;110:351–352.
70. Benigni G, Squartini F. Uneven distribution and significant concentration of apocrine metaplasia in lower breast quadrants. *Tumori* 1986;72:179–182.
71. Wellings SR, Alpers CE. Apocrine cystic metaplasia: subgross pathology and prevalence in cancer-associated versus random autopsy breasts. *Hum Pathol* 1987;18:381–386.
72. Schuerch C III, Rosen PP, Hirota T, et al. A pathologic study of benign breast diseases in Tokyo and New York. *Cancer* 1982;50:1899–1903.
73. Dawson EK. Sweat carcinoma of the breast. *Edinb Med J* 1932;39:409–438.
74. Foote FW Jr, Stewart FW. Comparative studies of cancerous versus non-cancerous breasts. *Ann Surg* 1945;12:6–79.
75. Tóth J, Számel I, Svastics E, Significance of apocrine metaplasia in mammary carcinogenesis. A preliminary morphological and immunohistochemical study. *Ann N Y Acad Sci* 1990;586:238–251.
76. Page DL, Van der Zwaag R, Rogers LW, et al. Relation between component parts of fibrocystic disease complex and breast cancer. *J Natl Cancer Inst* 1978;61:1055–1063.
77. Page DL, Jensen RA, Dupont WD. Papillary apocrine change of the breast—cancer risk indicator? *Lab Invest* 1994;70:26A.
78. Yates AJ, Ahmed A. Apocrine carcinoma and apocrine metaplasia. *Histopathology* 1988;13:228–231.
79. Abati AD, Kimmel M, Rosen PP. Apocrine mammary carcinoma: a clinicopathologic study of 72 cases. *Am J Clin Pathol* 1990;94:371–377.
80. Archer F, Omar M. Pink cell (oncocytic) metaplasia in a fibroadenoma of the human breast: electron microscopic observations. *J Pathol* 1969;99:119–124.
81. Pier WJ Jr, Garancis JC, Kuzma JF. The ultrastructure of apocrine cells in intracystic papilloma and fibrocystic disease of the breast. *Arch Pathol* 1970;89:446–452.
82. Nielsen BB. Adenosis tumour of the breast—a clinicopathological investigation of 27 cases. *Histopathology* 1987;11:1259–1275.
83. Page DL, Dupont WD, Jensen RA. Papillary apocrine change of the breast: associations with atypical hyperplasia and risk of breast cancer. *Cancer Epidemiol Biomarkers Prev* 1996;5:29–32.
84. Izuo M, Okagari T, Tichart RM, Lattes R. DNA content in "apocrine metaplasia" of fibrocystic disease of the breast. *Cancer* 1971;27:643–650.
85. Ahmed A. Apocrine metaplasia in cystic hyperplastic mastopathy. Histochemical and ultrastructural observations. *J Pathol* 1975;115:211–214.
86. Kumar S, Mansel RE, Jasani B. Presence and possible significant of immunohistochemically demonstrable prolactin in breast apocrine metaplasia. *Br J Cancer* 1987;55:307–309.

## Florid Papillomatosis of the Nipple

87. Miller EM, Lewis D. The significance of serohemorrhagic or hemorrhagic discharge from the nipple. *JAMA* 1923;81:1651–1657.
88. Stowers JE. The significance of bleeding or discharge from the nipple. *Surg Gynecol Obstet* 1935;61:537–545.
89. Jones DB. Florid papillomatosis of the nipple ducts. *Cancer* 1955;8:315–319.
90. Handley RS, Thackray AC. Adenoma of the nipple. *Br J Cancer* 1962;16:187–194.
91. Gros C-M, LeGal Y, Bader P. L'adenomatose erosive de mamelon. *Ann Anat Pathol* 1959;4:292–304.
92. Perzin KH, Lattes R. Papillary adenoma of the nipple (florid papillomatosis adenoma, adenomatosis). A clinicopathologic study. *Cancer* 1972;29:996–1009.

93. Doctor VM, Sirsat MV. Florid papillomatosis (adenoma) and other benign tumors of the nipple and areola. *Br J Cancer* 1971;25:1–9.

94. Jones MW, Norris HJ, Snyder RC. Infiltrating syringomatous adenoma of the nipple. *Am J Surg Pathol* 1989;13:197–201.

95. Rosen PP. Syringomatous adenoma of the nipple. *Am J Surg Pathol* 1984;7:739–745.

96. Nichols FC, Dockerty MD, Judd ES. Florid papillomatosis of the nipple. *Surg Gynecol Obstet* 1958;107:474–480.

97. Taylor HB, Robertson AG. Adenomas of the nipple. *Cancer* 1965;18:995–1002.

98. Brownstein MH, Phelps RG, Magnin PH. Papillary adenoma of the nipple: analysis of fifteen new cases. *J Am Acad Dermatol* 1985;12:707–715.

99. Bergdahl L, Bergman F, Rais O, et al. Bilateral adenoma of nipple. Report of a case. *Acta Chir Scand* 1971;137:583–586.

100. Fornage BD, Faroux MJ, Pluot M, et al. Nipple adenoma simulating carcinoma. Misleading clinical, mammographic, sonographic and cytologic findings. *J Ultrasound Med* 1991;10:55–57.

101. Shapiro L, Karpas CM. Florid papillomatosis of the nipple. First reported case in a male. *Am J Clin Pathol* 1965;49:155–159.

102. Burdick C, Rinhart RM, Matsumoto T, et al. Nipple adenoma and Paget's disease in a man. *Arch Surg* 1965;91:835–838.

103. Waldo ED, Sidhu GS, Hu AW. Florid papillomatosis of the male nipple after diethystilbestrol therapy. *Arch Pathol* 1975;99:364–366.

104. Richards AT, Jaffe A, Hunt JA. Adenoma of the nipple in a male. *S Afr Med J* 1973;47:581–583.

105. Fisher ER, Gregorio RM, Fisher B, et al. The pathology of invasive breast cancer. A syllabus derived from findings of the National Surgical Adjuvant Breast Project (Protocol No. 4). *Cancer* 1975;36:1–85.

106. Bhagavan BS, Patchefsky A, Koss LG. Florid subareolar duct papillomatosis (nipple adenoma) and mammary carcinoma: report of three cases. *Hum Pathol* 1973;4:289–295.

107. Gudjonsdottir A, Hagerstrand I, Ostberg G. Adenoma of the nipple with carcinomatous development. *Acta Path Microbiol Scand (A)* 1971;79:676–680.

108. Santini D, Taffurelli M, Carolina M, et al. Adenoma of the nipple. A clinico-pathologic study and its relation with carcinoma. *Breast Dis* 1990;3:153–163.

109. Jones MW, Tavassoli FA. Coexistence of nipple duct adenoma and breast carcinoma: a clinicopathologic study of five cases and review of the literature. *Mod Pathol* 1995;8:633–636.

110. Diaz NM, Palmer JO, Wick MR. Erosive adenomatosis of the nipple: histology, immunohistology, and differential diagnosis. *Mod Pathol* 1992;5:179–184.

111. Myers JL, Mazur MT, Urist MM, et al. Florid papillomatosis of the nipple: immunohistochemical and flow cytometric analysis of two cases. *Mod Pathol* 1990;3:288–293.

112. Stormby N, Bondeson L. Adenoma of the nipple. An unusual diagnosis in aspiration cytology. *Acta Cytol* 1984;28:729–732.

113. Pinto RGW, Mandreker S. Fine needle aspiration cytology of adenoma of the nipple. A case report. *Acta Cytol* 1996;40:789–791.

114. Scott P, Kissin MW, Collins C, et al. Florid papillomatosis of the nipple: a clinico-pathologic surgical problem. *Eur J Surg Oncol* 1991;17:211–213.

115. Van Mierlo PL, Geelen GM, Neumann HA. Mohs micrographic surgery for an erosive adenomatosis of the nipple. *Dermatol Surg* 1998;24:681–683.

## Syringomatous Adenoma of the Nipple

116. Johnston CA, Toker C. Syringomatous tumors of minor salivary gland origin. *Hum Pathol* 1982;13:182–184.

117. Goldstein DJ, Barr RJ, Santa Cruz DJ. Microcystic adnexal carcinoma: a distinct clinicopathologic entity. *Cancer* 1982;50:566–572.

118. Cooper PH, Mills SE, Leonard DD, et al. Sclerosing sweat duct (syringomatous) carcinoma. *Am J Surg Pathol* 1985;9:422–433.

119. Ferrari A, Roncalli M. Adenoma siringomatoso della mammella. *Istocitopatologia* 1984;6:231–234.

120. Ward BE, Cooper PH, Subramony C. Syringomatous tumor of the nipple. *Am J Clin Pathol* 1989;92:692–696.

121. Slaughter MS, Pomerantz RA, Murad T, et al. Infiltrating syringomatous adenoma of the nipple. *Surgery* 1992;111:711–713.

122. Rosen PP, Ernsberger D. Low grade adenosquamous carcinoma. A variant of metaplastic mammary carcinoma. *Am J Surg Pathol* 1987;11:351–358.

123. Subramony C. Bilateral breast tumors resembling syringocystadenoma papilliferum. *Am J Clin Pathol* 1987;87:656–659.

## Collagenous Spherulosis

124. Rosen PP. Adenoid cystic carcinoma of the breast. A morphologically heterogeneous neoplasm. *Pathol Annu* 1989;24[Pt 2]:237–254.

125. Guarino M, Tricomi P, Cristofori E. Collagenous spherulosis of the breast with atypical epithelial hyperplasia. *Pathologica* 1993;85:123–127.

125a. Divaris DXG, Smith S, Leask D, et al. Complex collagenous spherulosis of the breast presenting as a palpable mass. *Breast J* 2000;6:199–203.

126. Stephenson TJ, Hird PM, Laing RW, et al. Nodular basement membrane deposits in breast carcinoma and atypical ductal hyperplasia: mimics of collagenous spherulosis. *Pathologica* 1994;86:234–239.

127. Clement PB. Collagenous spherulosis [Letter]. *Am J Surg Pathol* 1987;11:907.

128. Highland KE, Finley JL, Neill JSA, et al. Collagenous spherulosis. Report of a case with diagnosis by fine needle aspiration biopsy with immunocytochemical and ultrastructural observations. *Acta Cytol* 1993;37:3–9.

129. Pérez JS, Pérez-Guillermo M, Bernal AB, et al. Diagnosis of collagenous spherulosis of the breast by fine needle aspiration cytology. A report of two cases. *Acta Cytol* 1993;37:725–728.

130. Rey A, Redondo E, Servent R. Collagenous spherulosis of the breast diagnosed by fine needle aspiration biopsy. *Acta Cytol* 1995;39:1701–1703.

131. Clement PB, Young RH, Azzopardi JG. Collagenous spherulosis of the breast. *Am J Surg Pathol* 1987;11:411–417.

132. Grignon DJ, Ro JY, MacKay BN, et al. Collagenous spherulosis of the breast. Immunohistochemical and ultrastructural studies. *Am J Clin Pathol* 1989;91:386–392.

# CHAPTER 6

# Myoepithelial Neoplasms

Myoepithelial cells are widely present in the breast where they comprise part of the normal microscopic anatomy of lobules and ducts (1). They participate in many benign proliferative processes, most notably sclerosing adenosis and papillary proliferative lesions of ducts. Myoepithelial hyperplasia may be found in association with intraductal and invasive duct carcinoma (2–6).

Mammary neoplasms composed in part or entirely of myoepithelial cells are uncommon. Cameron et al. (7) commented that "purely myoepithelial benign tumours are called *myoepitheliomas* or even *myomas;* if epithelial cells participate in their structure the term *adenomyoepithelioma* seems appropriate. . . (and) . . . if we are left with a purely myothelial malignant tumour, the term *myothelial sarcoma* or even *leiomyosarcoma* seems suitable." Benign tumors composed of myoepithelial cells are termed *myoepitheliomas*. Occasional lesions may have separate areas of adenomyoepithelial and myoepithelial proliferation, especially when the latter element has prominent spindle cell myoid features. Classification is complicated further by uncommon tumors that exhibit combined adenomyoepithelial and microglandular adenosis growth patterns (8,9). Most of these neoplasms are benign, but very unusual malignant variants occur.

Evidence for the concept that myoepithelial cells are derived from ectoderm rather than mesoderm has come from studies of mammary and salivary gland tissues (10,11). Differentiation of epithelial and myoepithelial cells has been observed in the terminal end buds of the developing pubertal breast (12). Cytologic and immunocytologic characteristics of the two types of cells have been documented in histologic preparations and by examining *in vitro* preparations of cells isolated by flow cytometry from fresh tissue (13).

The presence of myoepithelial cells in the salivary gland epithelium has been well documented. These cells contribute to the histogenesis of pleomorphic adenomas (mixed tumors) and carcinomas that arise in these glands (14,15). Morphologic similarities between certain tumors of the breast, salivary glands, and skin appendage glands reflect the contribution of myoepithelial cells to these lesions.

## ADENOMYOEPITHELIOMA

The first full description of adenomyoepithelioma of the breast was published in 1970 by Hamperl (5). With the exception of four studies consisting respectively of 6, 13, 18, and 27 cases (16–19), reports of these lesions have been case studies (9,20–28).

### Clinical Presentation

Virtually all patients have been women ranging in age from 27 to 80 years (average 58 years) in one series of 18 cases (18), and from 26 to 82 years (average 63 years) among patients in the other series and in various case reports. Most patients present with a solitary unilateral painless mass located in a peripheral portion of the breast. Occasionally, the lesions have been found centrally or near the areola (Fig. 6.1) (19,20,23). Nipple discharge, pain, and tenderness are infrequent (19). The tumor reportedly has been palpable for a year or more (18,19,25) before excision, but most patients describe recent onset. The lesion was observed by mammography 2 years before excision in one case (18), and the mammographic findings were considered to be suspicious in some patients (18,22). Nonpalpable adenomyoepitheliomas measuring 1 to 2 cm can present as well-circumscribed mass lesions on mammography and may be the target of needle core biopsy sampling. The compact glandular structure may be mistaken for invasive carcinoma in a core biopsy. Calcifications, although not typically present, have been described in an adenomyoepithelioma (29). One malignant adenomyoepithelioma appeared to be cystic on mammography (26).

Berna et al. (30) described a partially cystic 2.5-cm circumscribed adenomyoepithelioma that arose in an 84-year-old man. The tumor was histologically benign, with immunoreactivity for actin and cytokeratin.

Adenomyoepithelioma does not have a predilection for either breast. Data on family history of breast carcinoma or of other significant diseases are rarely mentioned in published

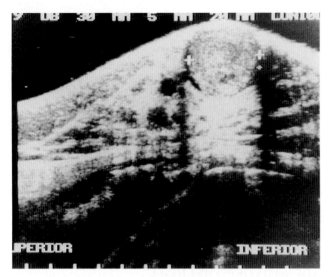

**FIG. 6.1.** *Adenomyoepithelioma.* Ultrasound image showing a well-circumscribed, slightly inhomogeneous mass in the subareolar region.

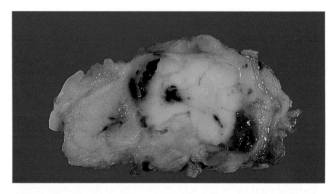

**FIG. 6.2.** *Adenomyoepithelioma.* This bisected tumor is circumscribed and has a nodular architecture. The tumor measures about 2 cm.

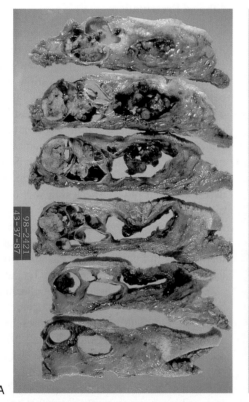

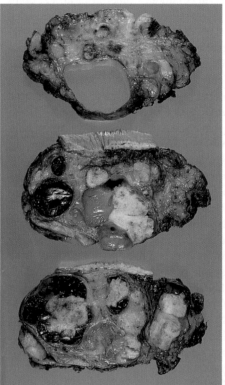

A

B

**FIG. 6.3.** *Adenomyoepithelioma.* Two different gross specimens. **A:** Multiple transverse sections of a mastectomy extensively involved by a multicystic adenomyoepithelioma with papillary areas. **B:** Solid and cystic multinodular adenomyoepithelioma measuring about 7 cm in greatest diameter shown in transverse sections. Skin is present on the *upper border* of the specimen.

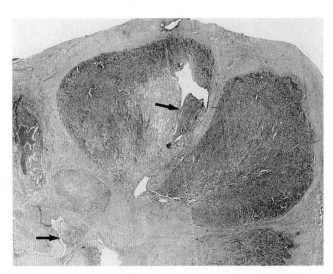

**FIG. 6.4.** *Adenomyoepithelioma.* Whole-mount histologic section in which multiple nodules surround a sclerotic core. There are remnants of ducts with papillary elements *(arrows).*

case reports, and the information available does not suggest any associated condition. Biochemical estrogen receptor (ER) and progesterone receptor (PR) analysis performed on some tumors (18,31) yielded the following results: ER+ (171 fmol); ER+ (44.7 fmol), PR−; ER+ (23 fmol), PR−; ER+ (13 fmol), PR−; ER−, PR− (three cases). Another lesion also had positive ERs (37 fmol) (27). When studied by immunohistochemistry, hormone receptor activity is limited to the nuclei of epithelial cells.

### Gross Pathology

The reported grossly measured size of adenomyoepitheliomas varied from 0.5 to 7.0 cm, with an average and median size of about 2.5 cm. With rare exceptions, the tumors

have been described as solid, well circumscribed, and firm or hard. Lobulation often is noted (Fig. 6.2). Several lesions were described as translucent. Tan, gray, white, yellow, and pink coloration have been mentioned. Small cysts were observed in a minority of cases (18,19,22). Very large grossly cystic tumors can occupy a substantial part of the breast (Fig. 6.3). There does not appear to be a good correlation between the gross appearance of the tumor and its microscopic composition.

### Microscopic Pathology

A spectrum of histologic patterns is encountered among these tumors and even within different portions of a given lesion. Factors that influence these variations include the proportions of proliferating glandular and myoepithelial cells, the degree to which myoepithelial cells have a spindle or polygonal configuration, the prominence of papillary components, and the extent of fibrosis.

Microscopically, most adenomyoepitheliomas are circumscribed and composed of aggregated nodules (Fig. 6.4). The majority of adenomyoepitheliomas are variants of intraductal papilloma, but a small number of these tumors appear to arise from a lobular proliferation or adenosis (Figs. 6.5 and 6.6). Some nodules consist of a single compact proliferation of epithelial and myoepithelial cells, but most lesions have one or more nodules in which there is a focal papillary growth pattern. Sometimes the papillary intraductal component extends into ducts outside the gross tumorous lesion. This characteristic may be responsible for recurrence after seemingly adequate excision. A minority of adenomyoepitheliomatous tumors consist largely or entirely of intraductal papillary elements, an observation that supports the conclusion that these lesions are variants of intraductal papilloma. In this respect, adenomyoepithelioma is closely related to ductal adenoma (22,32,33) and pleomorphic

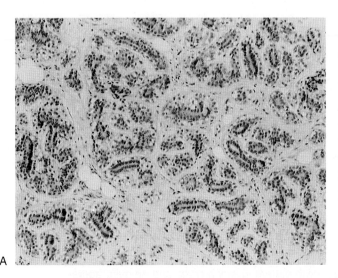

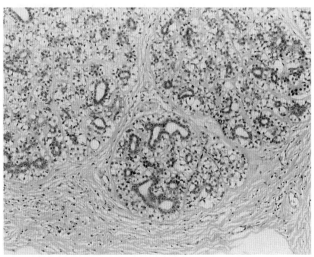

A          B

**FIG. 6.5.** *Adenomyoepithelial hyperplasia of lobules.* **A:** Group of lobules in which hyperplastic myoepithelial cells surround the lobular glands, duplicating the pattern found in an adenomyoepithelioma. **B:** Aggregated lobules with very prominent myoepithelial hyperplasia forming a tumor.

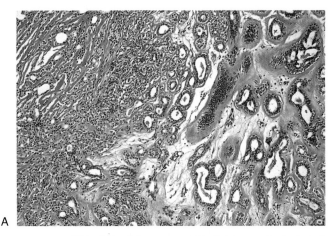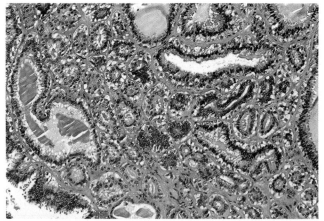

A B

**FIG. 6.6.** *Adenomyoepithelial hyperplasia in adenosis.* **A:** Myoepithelial hyperplasia and sclerosing adenosis composed of small cells with clear cytoplasm *(left)*. Sclerosing adenosis without myoepithelial hyperplasia *(right)*. **B:** Florid adenosis with myoepithelial hyperplasia composed of epithelioid cells with clear cytoplasm around the perimeter of adenosis glands.

adenoma (34,35). Foci of adenomyoepithelioma can be detected frequently in tubular adenomas. They are less apparent in mammary pleomorphic adenomas in which an associated papilloma usually is evident.

The basic structural unit of the adenomyoepithelioma is a small round or oval glandular lumen encompassed by cuboidal epithelial cells. At the periphery of the glands are polygonal or spindle-shaped myoepithelial cells with clear cytoplasm and a basement membrane (Fig. 6.7). The most common microscopic pattern, referred to as the tubular type of adenomyoepithelioma, features a balanced proliferation of round, oval, or tubular glandular elements with islands and bands of polygonal myoepithelial cells that have clear cytoplasm. In some tumors, myoepithelial cells with clear cytoplasm are more numerous than epithelial cells, resulting

in zones virtually devoid of glands (Figs. 6.8 and 6.9). Other lesions feature myoepithelial cells that proliferate in broad bands and trabeculae separated by strands of fibrovascular stroma (Figs. 6.10 and 6.11). The contrast between the dark-staining cytoplasm of glandular cells and the pale cytoplasm of myoepithelial cells is striking (Fig. 6.12). Small glandular lumens formed within the epithelial areas have a pattern reminiscent of an endocrine neoplasm. In papillary regions, distinct polygonal myoepithelial cells accompany the epithelium in its various branches and ramifications (Fig. 6.13).

The epithelial cells tend to have sparse darkly stained cytoplasm and hyperchromatic nuclei. In some cases, this produces a plasmacytoid appearance. Apocrine metaplasia may be encountered in the glandular epithelium, particularly in papillary areas (Fig. 6.14). The apocrine epithelium can be

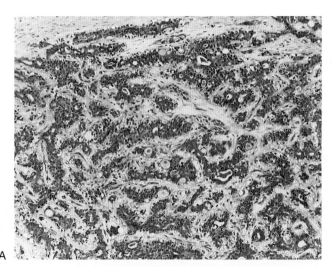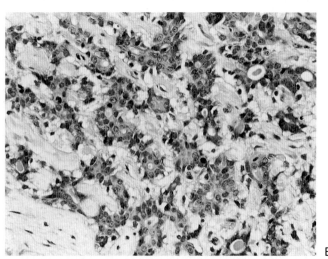

A B

**FIG. 6.7.** *Adenomyoepithelioma.* **A:** Characteristic growth pattern in which cords and irregular aggregates of epithelial cells are separated by bands of fibrovascular stroma. Some glandular lumens contain secretion. **B:** Myoepithelial cells with clear cytoplasm aligned along the serrated outer edges of epithelial cords.

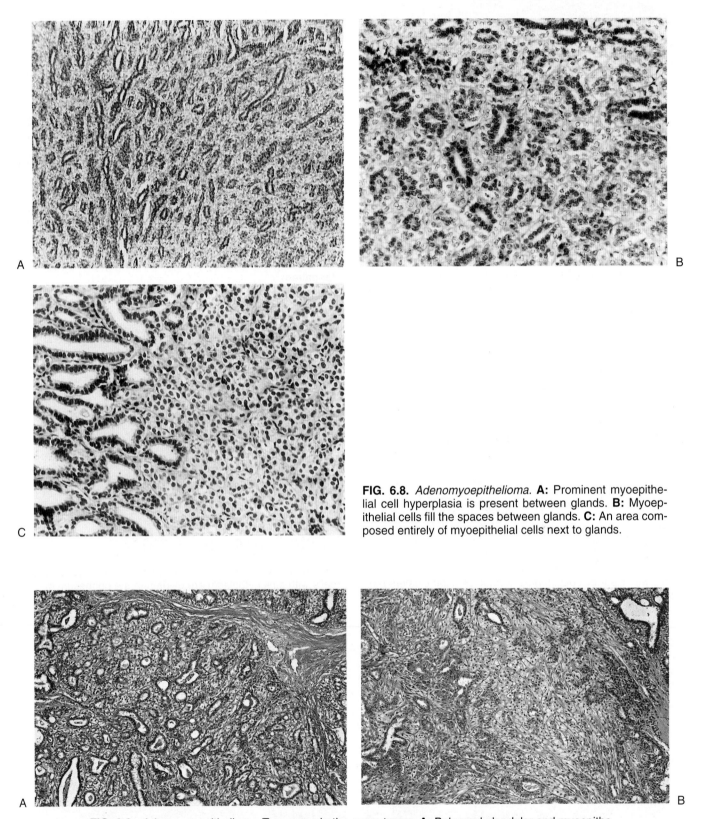

**FIG. 6.8.** *Adenomyoepithelioma.* **A:** Prominent myoepithelial cell hyperplasia is present between glands. **B:** Myoepithelial cells fill the spaces between glands. **C:** An area composed entirely of myoepithelial cells next to glands.

**FIG. 6.9.** *Adenomyoepithelioma.* Two areas in the same tumor. **A:** Balanced glandular and myoepithelial proliferation. **B:** Epithelioid clear cell myoepithelial hyperplasia has displaced glandular structures.

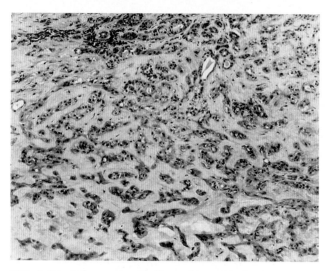

**FIG. 6.10.** *Adenomyoepithelioma.* Myoepithelial cells with a trabecular pattern have arisen from glandular units such as those located at the upper border of this microscopic field.

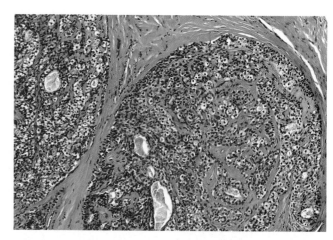

**FIG. 6.11.** *Adenomyoepithelioma.* Epithelioid myoepithelial cells, many with clear cytoplasm, are arranged in a trabecular pattern.

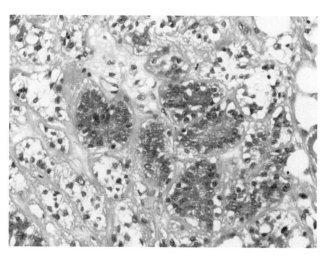

**FIG. 6.12.** *Adenomyoepithelioma.* In this view, myoepithelial cells with clear cytoplasm have formed alveolar clusters between glands.

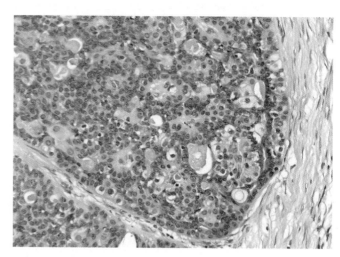

**FIG. 6.13.** *Adenomyoepithelioma.* Clusters of myoepithelial cells with pink cytoplasm are evident in the epithelium of the solid papillary hyperplasia in a duct at the margin of an adenomyoepithelioma.

A
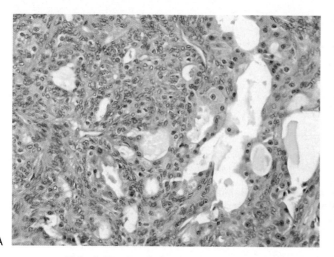

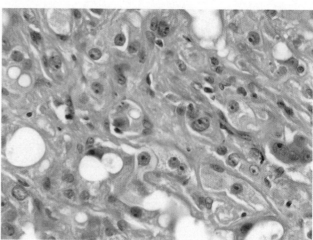
B

**FIG. 6.14.** *Apocrine metaplasia in an adenomyoepithelioma.* **A:** Apocrine epithelium is evident in the glands. Spindly myoepithelial cells are present. **B:** Apocrine metaplasia with nuclear atypia.

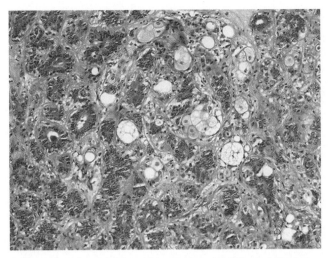

**FIG. 6.15.** *Sebaceous metaplasia in an adenomyoepithelioma.*

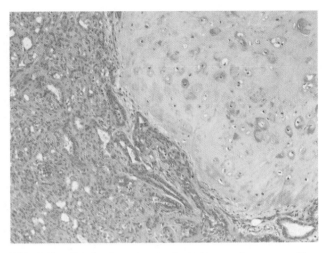

**FIG. 6.17.** *Cartilaginous metaplasia in an adenomyoepithelioma.*

cytologically atypical. Glands exhibiting sebaceous metaplasia are variably present (Fig. 6.15), and focal squamous metaplasia (Fig. 6.16) occurs in a minority of cases. Cartilaginous and osseous metaplasia are rarely seen (Fig. 6.17). A previously undescribed adenomyoepithelioma with mucoepidermoid differentiation has been encountered (Fig. 6.18). Cytologic atypia and mitotic activity are very infrequent or absent from lesions in which the myoepithelial cells retain a polygonal configuration and there are conspicuous papillary areas. Stromal and myoepithelial elements may have an adenoid cystic pattern. Calcifications occasionally are present. Some tumors develop central fibrosis or necrosis leading to calcification (Fig. 6.19). The cystic papillary type of adenomyoepithelioma is very uncommon (Fig. 6.20).

The extent to which myoepithelial cells assume a spindly, myoid shape varies greatly. Tumors composed entirely of such elements with no identifiable epithelial cells are classi-

fied as myoepitheliomas and are discussed separately. However, many adenomyoepitheliomas have foci of spindle cell myoid growth (Fig. 6.21). Usually, the myoid areas have a mixture of spindle and polygonal cells. The glandular component may be intermixed with myoid areas, or it may appear to be largely independent (Fig. 6.22). Palisading of spindle cells and alveolar clustering of polygonal myoepithelial cells are common myoid patterns. The latter configuration has been referred to as the lobulated type of adenomyoepithelioma (19). A myoepithelial tumor of the male breast composed of spindle cells arranged in a storiform pattern was described by Tamura et al. (36). Despite the spindle cell phenotype, the neoplasm was most strongly reactive for cytokeratin and S-100, with little staining for actin and no vimentin reactivity.

Cytologic atypia of myoepithelial cell nuclei may be encountered in lesions where there is a tendency to form spindle cells resulting in a distinctly myoid appearance (Fig. 6.23). In these foci, atypical features include scattered mitotic figures, nuclear pleomorphism, hyperchromasia, and occasional multinucleated cells. Myoid hyperplasia may give rise to areas with leiomyomatous features (5,28), and rarely this process produces leiomyosarcoma (5). Cytologic atypia and mitotic activity also have been described in the lobulated type of adenomyoepithelioma (19).

Origin of a malignant neoplasm in an adenomyoepithelioma resulting in a *malignant adenomyoepithelioma* has only very rarely been documented. Malignant transformation may be limited to the epithelial or myoepithelial component, or both elements may be involved. Histologic evidence of malignant growth includes mitotic activity, necrosis, and cellular pleomorphism, and frequently there is invasion at the periphery of the tumor. Many of the lesions purported to be malignant adenomyoepitheliomas have featured a spindle cell component; in some instances, the distinction from metaplastic carcinoma is not clear (37). Some lesions were reported to have local recurrence (17,38–40), whereas others resulted in metastases and a fatal outcome (39–42). In one

*text continues on p. 130*

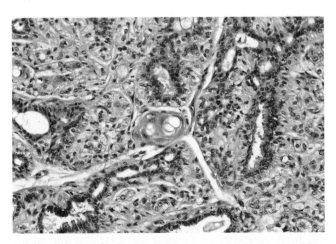

**FIG. 6.16.** *Squamous metaplasia in an adenomyoepithelioma.* Squamous metaplasia in the form of a keratin pearl is seen in the midst of myoepithelial cells with clear cytoplasm. Squamous and sebaceous metaplasia appear to originate in the myoepithelial cells.

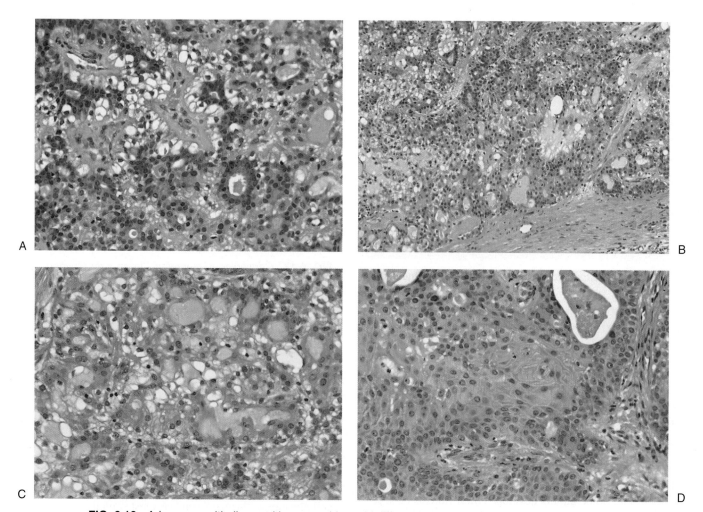

**FIG. 6.18.** *Adenomyoepithelioma with mucoepidermoid differentiation.* **A:** Part of a tumor with the typical adenomyoepithelioma growth pattern. **B,C:** Mucinous secretion in glands. **D:** Squamous metaplasia with glandular elements.

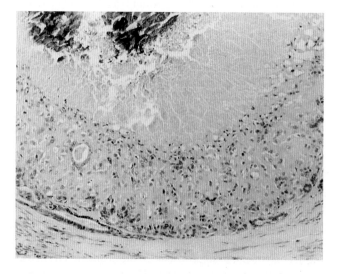

**FIG. 6.19.** *Adenomyoepithelioma with infarction and calcification.*

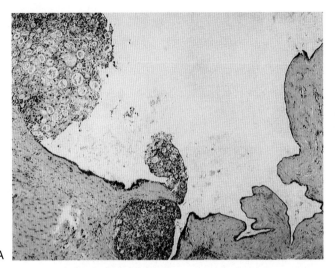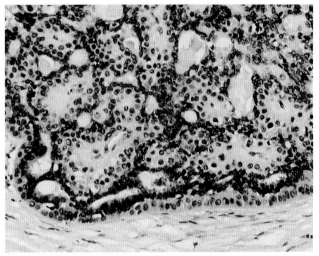

A                       B

**FIG. 6.20.** *Cystic adenomyoepithelioma.* **A:** At low magnification, nodules of adenomyoepitheliomatous growth protrude from the surface of the cyst, which is otherwise lined by ordinary duct epithelium. **B:** Adenomyoepitheliomatous nodule at the periphery of a duct.

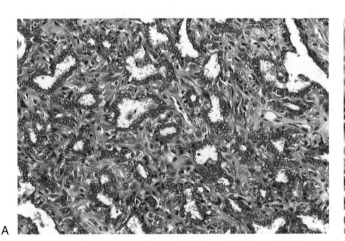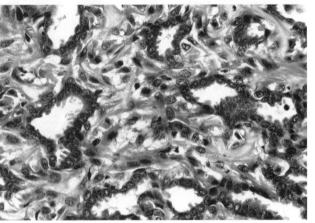

A                       B

**FIG. 6.21.** *Adenomyoepithelioma.* **A,B:** Lesion showing a conspicuous myoid component composed of spindle cells with deeply eosinophilic cytoplasm between the glands.

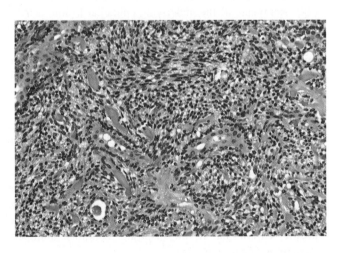

**FIG. 6.22.** *Adenomyoepithelioma.* Two oval glands in the *center* and one round gland *(lower left)* are surrounded by a spindly myoepithelial proliferation.

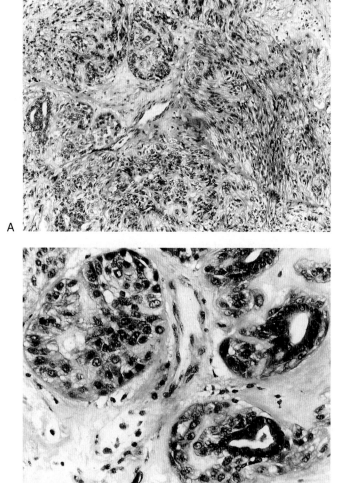

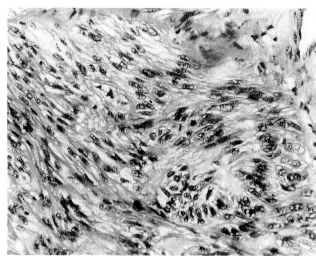

**FIG. 6.23.** *Adenomyoepithelioma.* **A:** Spindle-shaped myoid myoepithelial cells in a palisade arrangement. **B:** Nuclear atypia in myoid myoepithelial cells. **C:** Nuclear atypia in epithelioid myoepithelial cells.

fatal case, the malignant component, described as "undifferentiated," lacked reactivity for cytokeratin and actin (42), but in other tumors, these cytoskeletal components were immunohistochemically detectable (39,41). Malignant adenomyoepitheliomas with a biphasic growth pattern at the primary site and in metastases have been reported (Fig. 6.24) (26). Myoepithelial carcinoma with an epithelial phenotype can arise in an adenomyoepithelioma (Fig. 6.25). These neoplasms are characterized by overgrowth of the epithelial component exhibiting mitotic activity and cytologic evidence of carcinoma, often with foci of necrosis (39). Simpson et al. (40) described a malignant adenomyoepithelioma with carcinomatous and osteogenic elements.

The group of tumors sometimes referred to as *mixed tumors* or *pleomorphic adenomas* of the breast are variants of intraductal papilloma and adenomyoepithelioma. These tumors are located more frequently in the subareolar region than in the periphery of the breast and probably arise from

large lactiferous ducts (43,44). Most are solid, circumscribed tumors, but an intracystic mural lesion has been described (44). Remnants of the underlying epithelial lesion, usually with myoepithelial cell hyperplasia, can be found in almost all of these lesions (43). A characteristic feature of many mixed tumors in the breast is the formation of collagenized matrix that frequently is converted into cartilage (Fig. 6.26). Calcification and ossification occurs in some mixed tumors as well. Various proliferative patterns are found in the lesions, including foci that resemble cellular mixed tumor and a distinct papillary component (Fig. 6.27). The epithelium may develop squamous and sebaceous metaplasia similar to the metaplastic changes that occur in conventional adenomyoepitheliomas (Fig. 6.26). The cytologic findings in a fine needle aspiration specimen may suggest phyllodes tumor when numerous bipolar spindle cells are present, or metaplastic carcinoma if the aspirate contains abundant metachromatic stroma (45).

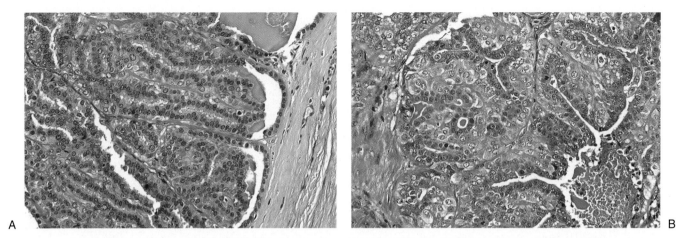

**FIG. 6.24.** *Malignant adenomyoepithelioma with epithelial and myoepithelial carcinoma.* **A:** Neoplastic proliferation of epithelial and myoepithelial cells with mitotic activity. **B:** Comedonecrosis is present in the epithelial component *(right)*. Mitotic activity is present.

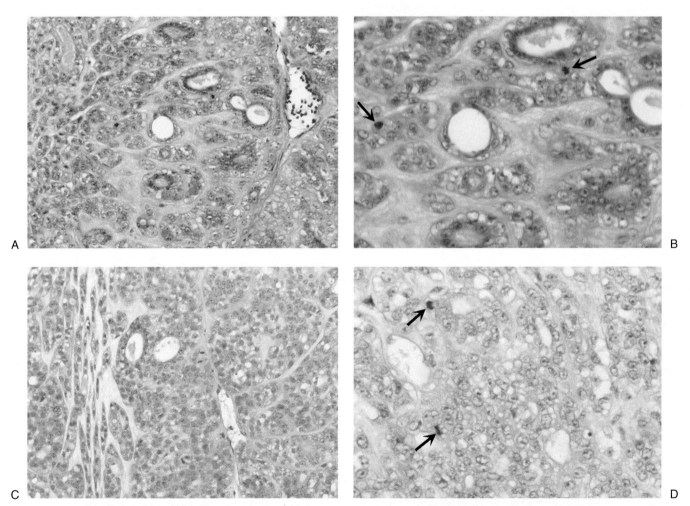

**FIG. 6.25.** *Myoepithelial carcinoma arising in adenomyoepithelioma.* **A:** Overgrowth of myoepithelial cells in the primary tumor. **B:** Area in **A** with mitotic activity in myoepithelial cells that have prominent nucleoli and mitoses *(arrows)*. **C:** Part of the primary tumor composed almost entirely of atypical myoepithelial cells with an epithelial phenotype. **D:** Recurrent tumor growing as myoepithelial carcinoma. The carcinoma cells have prominent nucleoli and mitoses *(arrows)*.

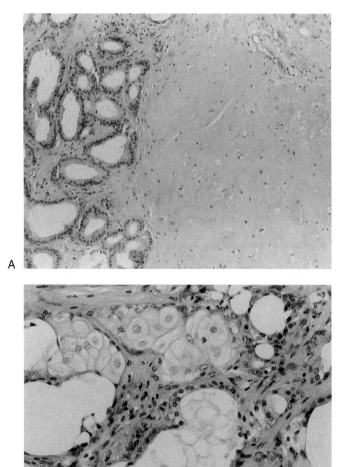

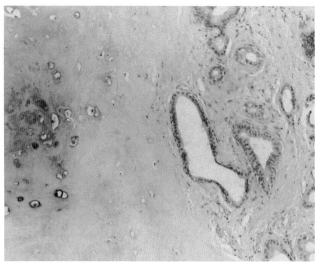

A

B

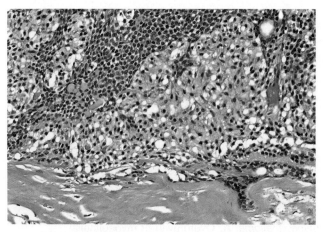

C

**FIG. 6.26.** *Mixed tumor.* **A:** Collagenized matrix adjacent to glandular elements with an adenosis pattern. **B:** Cartilaginous differentiation in the stroma. **C:** Sebaceous metaplasia of the epithelium.

**FIG. 6.27.** *Mixed tumor.* Part of the tumor is composed of a myoepithelial proliferation in a myxoid matrix that resembles a cellular mixed tumor.

### Histochemistry

By and large, the diverse cellular components exhibit expected histochemical properties. Glands may contain periodic acid-Schiff or mucicarmine-positive secretion, but intracytoplasmic secretion is rarely detectable. In most cases, the secretion also is positive for carcinoembryonic antigen. The cytoplasm of glandular cells tends to be strongly reactive with antibodies to cytokeratin, and the luminal surfaces of these cells are positive for epithelial membrane antigen (Fig. 6.28). Although most of the epithelial cells are S-100 negative, small groups may be strongly reactive for this antigen.

Polygonal and spindle myoepithelial cells are not reactive for epithelial membrane antigen or carcinoembryonic antigen and variably reactive for cytokeratin. The distribution and intensity of staining obtained with antiactin antibodies is heterogeneous. Reactivity is most pronounced for smooth muscle myosin heavy chain. Antiactin staining tends to be

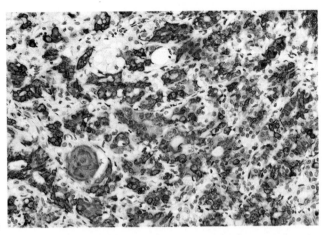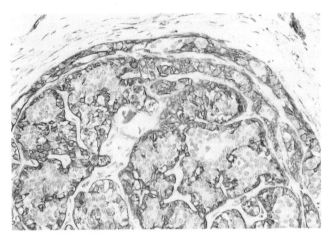

A                                                                                                          B

**FIG. 6.28.** *Adenomyoepithelioma.* **A:** Epithelial cells including a keratin pearl in the *lower left* corner are stained with antikeratin antibody. The myoepithelial cells are not immunoreactive (anti-AE1/AE3, avidin-biotin). **B:** Myoepithelial cells are immunoreactive for actin, which does not stain the epithelial cells (anti-smooth muscle actin, avidin-biotin).

more conspicuous in spindle than in clear polygonal cells, and no reactivity is seen in epithelial cells (Figs. 6.28 and 6.29). Some myoepithelial cells are S-100 positive in virtually all tumors, but the intensity and uniformity of reactivity varies considerably. There does not appear to be a consistent relationship between staining with antiactin and anti–S-100 antibodies in myoepithelial cells. Because S-100 reactivity is expressed by glandular and myoepithelial cells, it is not a specific marker for the latter cell type in adenomyoepitheliomas (46).

### Electron Microscopy

Several papers have described the ultrastructural features of individual lesions classified as adenomyoepitheliomas (8,16,20,27,28,31,47). In general, these case reports documented the presence of epithelial and myoepithelial compo-nents in the lesions. Short microvilli are present at the luminal surfaces of glandular cells, which are joined at the luminal edges by tight cell junctions. The cytoplasm contains scattered mitochondria as well as smooth and rough endoplasmic retic-ulum. Polygonal and spindle myoepithelial cells have desmo-somes that may be well or poorly formed, and interdigitating cell processes. Keratin and actin cytofilaments are prominent in the cytoplasm of myoepithelial cells, sometimes arranged in perinuclear bundles or peripheral arrays. Fusiform densities or condensation zones are commonly found along these arrays of cytofilaments. Distinct basal lamina material is found around and among the myoepithelial cells.

### Cytology

Aspiration cytology of a typical adenomyoepithelioma yields a cellular specimen composed of relatively large

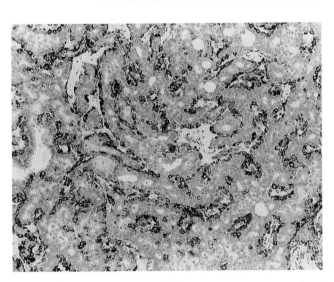

**FIG. 6.29.** *Adenomyoepithelioma.* Immunoreactivity for actin is present in myoepithelial cells bordering on the glandular proliferation (anti-smooth muscle actin, avidin-biotin).

epithelial cells distributed in clusters or separately (31,48). The epithelial cells tend to have deeply staining cytoplasm and prominent round-to-oval nuclei that may be eccentrically placed. Spindle cells and myoid fibrillary material are variably present in the background (48). The cytologic features may suggest a diagnosis of carcinoma (49,50).

**Prognosis and Treatment**

The majority of adenomyoepitheliomas are benign tumors that can be treated by local excision (18). Local recurrence has been reported usually more than 2 years after the initial excision (9,17,19). In two cases, two (18) and three (9) episodes of recurrence, respectively, may be attributed to incomplete excision. The multinodular character of the lesion and peripheral intraductal extension in one of these patients were probably contributory factors (18). There is no evidence that cytologic atypia or the proportions of spindle and polygonal myoepithelial cells are related to the risk for local recurrence. Carcinoma may be detected as a separate lesion coincidentally or subsequent to excision of an adenomyoepithelioma (19). Adenocarcinoma reportedly was found in one recurrent adenomyoepithelioma (19).

Reexcision may be performed when the tumor is incompletely excised, especially for multinodular lesions with peripheral intraductal extension. Mastectomy, breast irradiation, and axillary dissection are not appropriate treatment for benign adenomyoepitheliomas, but may be indicated for exceptional patients who have malignant or recurrent tumors.

## MYOEPITHELIOMA

Myoid transformation of myoepithelial cells is commonly observed as an incidental finding in breast tissue from premenopausal and postmenopausal women. When this occurs, the myoepithelial cells acquire the cytologic and histochemical features of smooth muscle cells, including a spindle shape and eosinophilic cytoplasm. They stain bright red with Masson's trichrome, and they are strongly reactive immunohistochemically with antiactin.

Myoid transformation is encountered most frequently around terminal ducts and lobules in the absence of appreciable epithelial proliferation (see Chapter 1). These changes are not associated with any particular types of tumor and may be found in specimens from patients undergoing biopsy for benign or malignant lesions. Myoid transformation often is present in foci of sclerosing adenosis, and occasionally it may dominate the process leading to a leiomyomatous appearance (Fig. 6.30). A smooth muscle tumor of the breast that may have arisen in this fashion was described by Eusebi et al. (51). The patient was a 55-year-old woman who had a 10-cm nodular circumscribed tumor present for 8 years. Histologically, the lesion was found to be composed largely of smooth muscle cells when studied by light and electron microscopy.

Neoplasms composed entirely of myoepithelial cells represent one end of a spectrum of differentiation that includes tumors with adenomyoepithelial differentiation. Myoepithelial neoplasms of the breast are extremely uncommon, and reports are limited to case studies. The review of the subject by Hamperl (5) in 1970 described lesions composed of epithelioid and spindle myoepithelial cells. Leiomyomatous proliferation in these neoplasms may be coordinated with glandular components, thus retaining adenomyoepitheliomatous features. Toth (52) described such a lesion, which presented as a painful hard breast tumor. The specimen was grossly nodular and consisted microscopically of dilated ducts "filled with cellular adenomatous intraductal papillomas" in which "the proliferating myoepithelial elements almost filled the ducts. . . with leiomyoma-like tumors the spindle cells of which formed either bundles or whorl-like patterns." The myoepithelial nature of the spindle cells was confirmed by electron microscopy. After treatment that evidently was limited to the diagnostic excision, the patient was well for approximately 3 years.

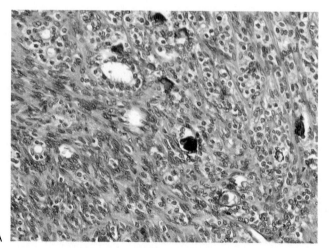
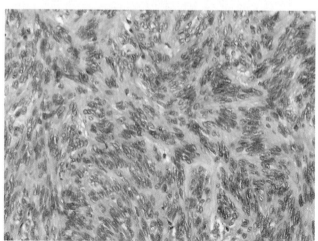

**FIG. 6.30.** *Myoid differentiation in sclerosing adenosis.* **A:** Spindle cells surround glands with calcifications. **B:** Palisading of spindly myoepithelial cells in nodular sclerosing adenosis.

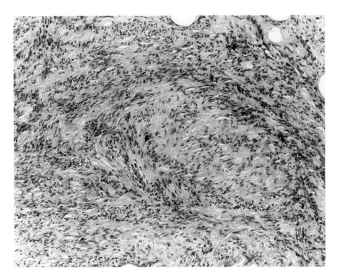

**FIG. 6.31.** *Myoid hamartoma.* Myomatous nodule with palisading of spindle cells. The tumor infiltrates fat at the edges of the photograph.

Tumors referred to as muscular (53) and myoid (54) hamartomas probably arise from myoepithelial hyperplasia. Davies and Riddell (53) noted "the intimate relationship of the smooth muscle to the lobular epithelium" in one of their cases and suggested that "the smooth muscle is of myoepithelial origin." Three patients, 38, 39, and 61 years of age, were described by Daroca et al. (54). The well-circumscribed tumors that measured 2.5 to 3.5 cm and appeared grossly encapsulated consisted of grossly mottled areas of fat and fibrous stroma. Microscopically, interlacing fascicles of plump spindle cells were distributed in the fibrofatty tissue (Fig. 6.31). The myoid character of these cells was confirmed by demonstrating strong fuchsinophilia with Masson's trichrome and immunohistochemical reactivity for actin. Electron microscopy in two cases revealed myoid and myoepithelial features. In one tumor, areas of sclerosing adenosis were apparent within the lesion merging with the myoid component. The patients remained well with follow-up of 5 to 13 months after excisional biopsy of these benign tumors.

Cameron et al. (7) reported the case of a 40-year-old woman with a 5 × 7 cm adenomyoepitheliomatous tumor in which a portion of the lesion was a highly cellular spindle cell neoplasm. One year after treatment by mastectomy, the patient developed a local recurrence involving fat and skeletal muscle consisting entirely of spindle cells with no epithelial structures. The authors stated that "if confronted exclusively with this picture, one would come to the diagnosis 'leiomyosarcoma'." No further follow-up was given.

Spindle cell neoplasms composed entirely of myoepithelial cells have been described (47,55–58). The histogenesis of these lesions was confirmed by electron microscopy and in most instances by immunohistochemistry (55–58). Light microscopy reveals interlacing bundles of spindle cells sometimes arranged in a storiform pattern (Fig. 6.32). The cytoplasm tends to be eosinophilic or sometimes clear. An infiltrative growth pattern may be present at the periphery of the tumor (Fig. 6.33). The spindle cells are immunoreactive for actin. In three women, 53, 54, and 60 years old, three tumors measuring 2.4, 0.9, and 2.8 cm, respectively, had few or no mitotic figures and all had a benign clinical course after relatively short follow-up (47,55,56). Negative axillary nodes were described in one case, and one specimen had negative ERs and PRs (47). Numerous mitoses were seen in a 21-cm tumor from an 81-year-old woman (58) and in a 7-cm tumor from a 53-year-old patient (57). Metastatic tumor was found in an axillary lymph node from the former patient, and the latter patient died of pulmonary metastases 6 months after diagnosis. ER and PR analyses were negative in both of these examples of malignant myoepithelial neoplasms.

An unusual spindle cell neoplasm of the male breast was described by Lucas et al. (59). The 72-year-old patient was

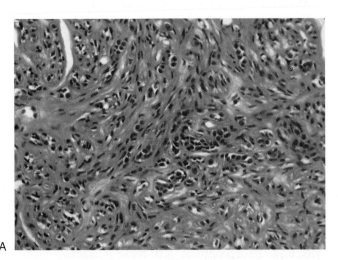
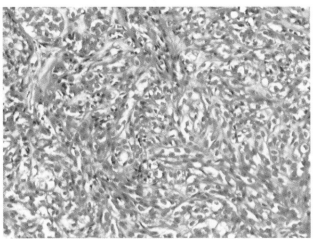

**FIG. 6.32.** *Myoepithelioma.* **A:** Interlacing spindle cells. **B:** Interspersed epithelioid myoepithelial cells having clear cytoplasm are present in the tumor and are arranged in a storiform pattern.

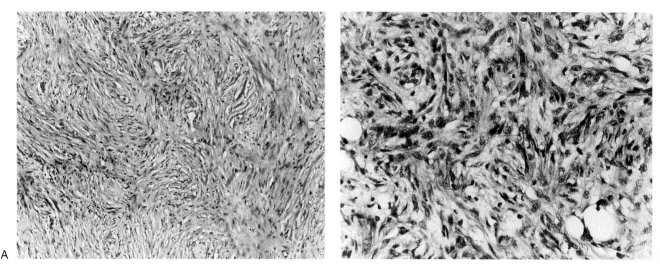

**FIG. 6.33.** *Myoepithelioma.* **A:** Tumor with collagenous stroma and a storiform structure. **B:** Invasion of fat.

treated by radical mastectomy for an 8.5-cm tumor that superficially invaded the pectoralis major muscle. Microscopically, the lesion was a highly cellular infiltrating spindle cell neoplasm with a high mitotic rate. Numerous benign-appearing foreign body-type giant cells were distributed throughout the tumor. The axillary lymph nodes were free of metastases. When examined by electron microscopy, the spindle cells had features of myofibroblastic and myoepithelial cells. No basal lamina material was found, and the authors concluded that the tumor might be "composed of a transitional type of cell expressing features of both myoepithelial and myofibroblastic cells."

Pure spindle cell myoepithelial tumors may be difficult to distinguish from other spindle cell mammary neoplasms by light microscopy. The differential diagnosis includes metaplastic carcinoma, primary spindle cell sarcomas, especially leiomyosarcoma or fibrous histiocytoma, myofibroblastoma, and metastatic tumor such as metastatic malignant melanoma. In most cases, the issue can be resolved by considering the clinical history, as well as careful histologic and immunohistochemical analysis, but sometimes electron microscopy is required. Cytologic findings in a myoepithelioma have been reported (60).

Myoepithelial neoplasms composed of polygonal cells have received less attention than spindle cell myoepithelial tumors. This is remarkable, because myoepithelial cells frequently have an epithelial configuration within adenomyoepithelial neoplasms of the breast. These lesions typically have an alveolar or nodular growth pattern, and they resemble clear cell myoepithelial tumors arising in the salivary glands (61). These uncommon breast tumors usually are not recognized, and most probably are misclassified as examples of clear cell or adenoid cystic carcinoma (Fig. 6.34). An invasive clear cell myoepithelial neoplasm that occurred in a 77-year-old woman was documented by electron microscopy and immunohistochemistry (62). The 3.5-cm tumor was treated only by excisional biopsy, and no follow-up information was provided. Remarkably high levels of ER

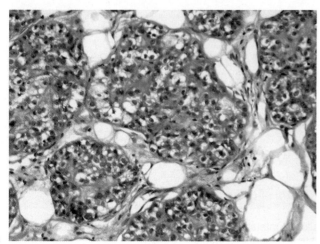

**FIG. 6.34.** *Myoepithelioma.* **A,B:** Alveolar structure characteristic of a myoepithelioma with an epithelioid phenotype. No epithelial elements are present. *(continued)*

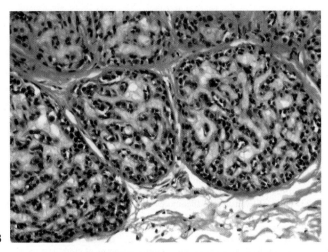
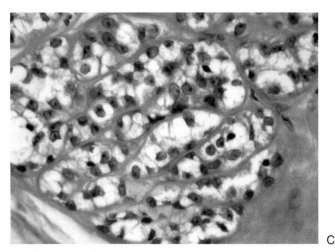

**FIG. 6.34.** *Continued.* **C:** Myoepithelial cells with clear cytoplasm are similar to myoepithelial cells in an adenomyoepithelioma.

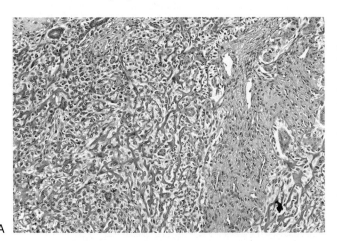
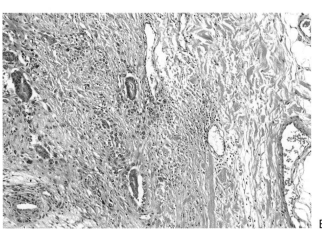

**FIG. 6.35.** *Myoepithelial carcinoma.* Both images are from a single tumor. **A:** Most of this portion of the lesion consists of polygonal cells with pale or clear cytoplasm in a reticular stroma. A few glandular structures in the tumor suggest an underlying adenomyoepithelial neoplasm. **B:** This region at the periphery of the tumor illustrates invasive plasmacytoid myoepithelial carcinoma cells. The same cells, seen encircling a gland in the *lower center*, appear to be *in situ* myoepithelial carcinoma.

(470 fmol/mg protein) were detected in the lesion. Two examples of intralobular myoepithelial carcinoma have been described (63).

Prasad et al. (64) studied 18 patients with *myoepithelial carcinomas.* The patients were 31 to 72 years old (mean 50 years). Tumor size ranged from 1.4 to 17 cm (mean 3.5 cm). The lesions typically were multinodular and had central necrosis. Cytologic appearances included epithelial, clear, plasmacytoid, and spindle cells (Fig. 6.35). All tumors were mitotically active and lacked receptors for estrogen or progesterone. Three patients had axillary nodal metastases. Median follow-up of 50 months in 17 cases revealed two recurrences, one of which was fatal.

## REFERENCES

1. Gusterson BA, Warburton MJ, Mitchell D, et al. Distribution of myoepithelial cells and basement membrane proteins in the normal breast and in benign and malignant breast diseases. *Cancer Res* 1982;42:763–770.

2. Ahmed A. The myoepithelium in human breast carcinoma. *J Pathol* 1974;112:129–135.

3. Goldenberg VE, Goldenberg NS, Sommers SC. Comparative ultrastructure of atypical duct hyperplasia, intraductal carcinoma and infiltrating duct carcinoma of the breast. *Cancer* 1969;24:1152–1168.

4. Gould VE, Jao W, Battifora H. Ultrastructural analysis in the differential diagnosis of breast tumors: the significance of myoepithelial cells, basal lamina, intracytoplasmic lumina and secretory granules. *Pathol Res Pract* 1980;167:45–70.

5. Hamperl H. The myoepithelia (myoepithelial cells): normal state; regressive changes; hyperplasia; tumors. *Curr Top Pathol* 1970;53:161–213.

6. Ohtani H, Sanso N. Myofibroblasts and myoepithelial cells in human breast carcinoma. *Virchows Arch [A]* 1980;385:247–261.

7. Cameron NM, Hamperl H, Warambo W. Leiomyosarcoma of the breast originating from myoepithelium (myoepithelioma). *J Pathol* 1974;114:89–92.

8. Eusebi V, Casadei GP, Bussolati G, et al. Adenomyoepithelioma of the breast with a distinctive type of apocrine adenosis. *Histopathology* 1987;11:305–315.

9. Young RH, Clement PB. Adenomyoepithelioma of the breast. A report of three cases and review of the literature. *Am J Clin Pathol* 1988;89:308–314.

10. Franke WW, Schmid E, Freudenstein C, et al. Intermediate sized

filaments of the prekeratin type in myoepithelial cells. *J Cell Biol* 1980;36:633–654.

11. Joshi K, Smith JA, Perusingle N, et al. Cell proliferation in human mammary epithelium. Differential contribution of epithelial and myoepithelial cells. *Am J Pathol* 1986;124:199–206.

12. Rudland PS. Histochemical organization and cellular composition of ductal buds in developing human breast: evidence of cytochemical intermediates between epithelial and myoepithelial cells. *J Histochem Cytochem* 1991;39:1471–1484.

13. O'Hare MJ, Ormerod MO, Monaghan P, et al. Characterization in vitro of luminal and myoepithelial cells isolated from the human mammary gland by cell sorting. *Differentiation* 1991;46:209–221.

14. Dardick I, Van Nostrand AWP. Myoepithelial cells in salivary gland tumors revisited. *Head Neck Surg* 1985;7:395–408.

15. Kahn HJ, Baumol R, Marks A, et al. Myoepithelial cells in salivary gland tumors: an immunohistochemical study. *Arch Pathol Lab Med* 1985;109:190–195.

16. Decorsiere JB, Thibaut I, Bouissou H. Les proliférations àdeno-myoepithéliales du sein. *Ann Pathol* 1988;8:311–316.

17. Loose JH, Patchefsky AS, Hollander IJ, et al. Adenomyoepithelioma of the breast. A spectrum of biologic behavior. *Am J Surg Pathol* 1992;16:868–876.

18. Rosen PP. Adenomyoepithelioma of the breast. *Hum Pathol* 1987;18:1232–1237.

19. Tavassoli FA. Myoepithelial lesions of the breast. Myoepitheliosis, adenomyoepithelioma, and myoepithelial carcinoma. *Am J Surg Pathol* 1991;15:554–568.

20. Decorsiere JB, Bouissou H, Becue J. Problèmes posés par l'adénomyoépithéliome du sein. *Gynecologie* 1985;36:221–227.

21. Betta PG, Spinoglio G. Benign mixed salivary type tumour of the breast. *Eur J Surg Oncol* 1992;18:304–306.

22. Gusterson BA, Sloane JP, Middwood C, et al. Ductal adenoma of the breast—a lesion exhibiting a myoepithelial/epithelial phenotype. *Histopathology* 1987;11:103–110.

23. Jabi M, Dardick I, Cardigos N. Adenomyoepithelioma of the breast. *Arch Pathol Lab Med* 1988;112:73–76.

24. Saez A, Serrano T, Azpeitia D, et al. Adenomyoepithelioma of the breast. A report of two cases. *Arch Pathol Lab Med* 1992;116:36–38.

25. Tamura S, Enjoji M, Toyoshima S, et al. Adenomyoepithelioma of the breast. A case report with an immunohistochemical study. *Acta Pathol Jpn* 1988;38:659–665.

26. Trojani M, Guiu M, Trouette H, et al. Malignant adenomyoepithelioma of the breast. An immunohistochemical, cytophotometric and ultrastructural study of a case with lung metastases. *Am J Clin Pathol* 1992;98:598–602.

27. Weidner N, Levine JD. Spindle-cell adenomyoepithelioma of the breast. A microscopic ultrastructural and immunocytochemical study. *Cancer* 1988;62:1561–1567.

28. Zarbo RJ, Oberman HA. Cellular adenomyoepithelioma of the breast. *Am J Surg Pathol* 1983;7:863–870.

29. Rubin E, Dempsey PJ, Listinsky CM, et al. Adenomyoepithelioma of the breast: a case report. *Breast Dis* 1995;8:103–109.

30. Berna JD, Arcas I, Ballester A, et al. Adenomyoepithelioma of the breast in a male [Letter]. *AJR Am J Roentgenol* 1997;169:917–918.

31. Vielh P, Theiry JP, Validire P, et al. Adenomyoepithelioma of the breast: fine-needle sampling with histologic, immunohistologic and electron microscopic analysis. *Diagn Cytol* 1993;9:188–193.

32. Guarino M, Reale D, Squillaci S, et al. Ductal adenoma of the breast. An immunohistochemical study of five cases. *Pathol Res Pract* 1993;189:515–520.

33. Jensen ML, Johansen P, Noer H, et al. Ductal adenoma of the breast: the cytological features of six cases. *Diagn Cytopathol* 1994;10:143–145.

34. Chen KTK. Pleomorphic adenoma of the breast. *Am J Clin Pathol* 1990;93:792–794.

35. Diaz NM, McDivitt RW, Wick MR. Pleomorphic adenoma of the breast: a clinicopathologic and immunohistochemical study of 10 cases. *Hum Pathol* 1991;22:1206–1214.

36. Tamura G, Monma N, Suzuki Y, et al. Adenomyoepithelioma of the breast in a male. *Hum Pathol* 1993;24:678–681.

37. Van Dorpe J, De Weer F, Bekaert J, et al. Malignant myoepithelioma of the breast. Case report with immunohistochemical study. *Arch Anat Cytol Pathol* 1996;44:193–198.

38. Pauwels C, de Potter C. Adenomyoepithelioma of the breast with features of malignancy. *Histopathology* 1994;24:94–96.

39. Rasbridge SA, Millis RR. Adenomyoepithelioma of the breast with malignant features. *Virchows Arch* 1998;432:123–130.

40. Simpson RH, Cope N, Skáová A, et al. Malignant adenomyoepithelioma of the breast with mixed osteogenic, spindle cell, and carcinomatous differentiation. *Am J Surg Pathol* 1998;22:631–636.

41. Chen PC, Chen C-K, Nicastri AD, et al. Myoepithelial carcinoma of the breast with distant metastasis and accompanied by adenomyoepitheliomas. *Histopathology* 1994;24:543–548.

42. Michal M, Baumruk L, Burger J, et al. Adenomyoepithelioma of the breast with undifferentiated carcinoma component. *Histopathology* 1994;24:274–276.

43. Narita T, Matsuda K. Pleomorphic adenoma of the breast: case report and review of the literature. *Pathol Int* 1995;45:441–447.

44. Nevado M, Lopez JI, Dominguez MP, et al. Pleomorphic adenoma of the breast. *APMIS* 1991;99:866–868.

45. Kanter MH, Sedeghi M. Pleomorphic adenoma of the breast: cytology of fine-needle aspiration and its differential diagnosis. *Diagn Cytopathol* 1993;9:555–558.

46. Gillett CE, Bobrow LG, Millis RR. S100 protein in human mammary tissue—immunoreactivity in breast carcinoma including Paget's disease of the nipple, and value as a marker of myoepithelial cells. *J Pathol* 1990;160:19–24.

47. Erlandson RA, Rosen PP. Infiltrating myoepithelioma of the breast. *Am J Surg Pathol* 1982;6:785–793.

48. Hock Y-L, Chan S-Y. Adenomyoepithelioma of the breast. A case report correlating cytologic and histologic features. *Acta Cytol* 1994;38:953–956.

49. Plaza JA, Lopez JL, Garcia S, et al. Adenomyoepithelioma of the breast. Report of two cases. *Arch Anat Cytol Pathol* 1993;41:99–101.

50. Niemann TH, Benda JA, Cohen MB. Adenomyoepithelioma of the breast: fine-needle aspiration biopsy and histologic findings. *Diagn Cytopathol* 1995;12:245–250.

51. Eusebi V, Cunsolo A, Fedeli F, et al. Benign smooth muscle metaplasia in breast. *Tumori* 1980;66:643–653.

52. Toth J. Benign human mammary myoepithelioma. *Virchows Arch [A]* 1977;374:263–269.

53. Davies JD, Riddell RH. Muscular hamartomas of the breast. *J Pathol* 1973;111:209–211.

54. Daroca PJ Jr, Reed RJ, Love GL, et al. Myoid hamartomas of the breast. *Hum Pathol* 1985;16:212–219.

55. Bigotti G, DiGiorgio G. Myoepithelioma of the breast: histologic, immunologic and electron microscopic appearance. *J Surg Oncol* 1986;32:58–64.

56. Rode L, Nesland JM, Johannessen JV. A spindle cell breast lesion in a 54-year-old woman. *Ultrastruct Pathol* 1986;10:421–425.

57. Schürch W, Potvin C, Seemayer TA. Malignant myoepitheliomas (myoepithelial carcinoma) of the breast: an ultrastructural and immunocytochemical study. *Ultrastruct Pathol* 1985;8:1–11.

58. Thorner PS, Kahn HJ, Baumal R, et al. Malignant myoepithelioma of the breast: an immunohistochemical study by light and electron microscopy. *Cancer* 1986;57:745–750.

59. Lucas JG, Sharma HM, O'Toole RV. Unusual giant cell tumor arising in a male breast. *Hum Pathol* 1981;12:360–364.

60. Nguyen G-K, Shnitka TK, Jewell LD. Aspiration cytology of mammary myoepithelioma. *Diagn Cytopathol* 1987;3:335–338.

61. Saksela E, Tarkkanen J, Wartiovaara J. Parotid clear-cell adenoma of possible myoepithelial origin. *Cancer* 1972;30:742–748.

62. Cartagena N, Cabello-Inchausti B, Willis I, et al. Clear cell myoepithelial neoplasm of the breast. *Hum Pathol* 1988;10:1239–1243.

63. Soares J, Tomasic G, Bucciarelli M, et al. Intralobular growth of myoepithelial cell carcinoma of the breast. *Virchows Arch [A]* 1994;425:205–210.

64. Prasad AR, Zarbo RJ. Myoepithelial carcinoma of the breast: a clinicopathologic study of 18 cases. *Mod Pathol* 2000;13:46A.

# CHAPTER 7

# Adenosis and Microglandular Adenosis

## ADENOSIS

Adenosis is a proliferative lesion largely derived from the terminal duct-lobular unit. Larger duct structures sometimes are incorporated into the lesion, but they are involved in the lobulocentric proliferative process to a lesser degree than lobules. Epithelial and myoepithelial cells participate in adenosis. Ewing (1) referred to adenosis as "fibrosing adenomatosis." Foote and Stewart (2) subsequently described the lesion as "sclerosing adenomatosis" and "sclerosing adenosis." The earliest clinicopathologic studies of sclerosing adenosis were published in 1949 and 1950 (3,4).

### Clinical Presentation

Adenosis occurs most often as part of a spectrum of proliferative abnormalities commonly referred to as *fibrocystic changes.* The entire complex may produce a palpable mass that usually is not attributable only to the adenosis component. When limited to isolated lobules that are not part of fibrocystic change, adenosis is a microscopic lesion that comes to attention clinically if it contains calcifications that are detected by mammography (Fig. 7.1). Microcalcifications frequently are formed in the sclerosing type of adenosis.

Adenosis by itself forms a distinct clinically palpable or radiographically detectable mass when there is confluence or fusion of the affected lobules to create an *adenosis tumor.* Patients with adenosis tumor almost always are premenopausal, averaging about 30 years of age at diagnosis (3). An adenosis tumor usually is smaller than 2 cm. It is rarely attached to the skin, and the lesion usually is a firm, clinically discrete, or ill-defined mass easily mistaken for a fibroadenoma (3,5,6). A few patients report pain or tenderness. Nonpalpable adenosis tumors that contain calcifications may be detected by mammography. The mammographic appearance of nodular adenosis is usually that of an oval or lobular mass, but the imaging findings are not specific, and biopsy is necessary to rule out carcinoma (6a).

### Gross Pathology

Excised adenosis tumors vary in gross appearance, depending on their microscopic composition (Figs. 7.2 and 7.3). Lesions consisting of florid adenosis with a prominent glandular component typically are well-circumscribed nodules composed of gray or pale tan, firm, homogeneous tissue. With increasing sclerosis, adenosis tumors are likely to be grossly less well defined at the borders, multinodular, and more fibrous in appearance. Lesions with abundant calcifications may seem gritty when cut. Gross cyst formation is infrequent. Necrosis or infarction occasionally is encountered in adenosis, usually during pregnancy or lactation.

Nontumorous adenosis in isolated lobules is difficult to detect grossly, and it usually mingles with other proliferative lesions. Rarely, minute discrete foci of sclerosing adenosis may be palpated in unfixed breast tissue as fine granules by brushing a finger gently over the cut surface. With tangential light, these foci sometimes are visible as pale tan dots in white breast stroma (Fig. 7.4).

### Microscopic Pathology

The microscopic structural features described here may be encountered in individual microscopic foci of adenosis and in adenosis tumors. Adenosis tends to have a more prominent glandular pattern in premenopausal women, whereas sclerosis and diminished gland formation are conspicuous after menopause. In some patients, there is very little variability in the spectrum of adenosis, whereas others exhibit diverse patterns.

The most cellular type of adenosis, often referred to as *florid adenosis,* is characterized by hyperplasia of epithelial and myoepithelial cells. Proliferation of ductules and lobular glands severely distorts and usually effaces the architecture of the underlying lobules. The hyperplastic structures appear to elongate, becoming tortuous and entwined in a fashion that results in many more ductular cross sections than are present in an anatomically normal lobule (Fig. 7.5). In the plane of section, the complex proliferative structure has a swirling pattern, punctuated by glands cut transversely.

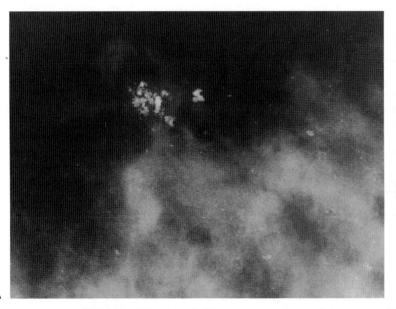
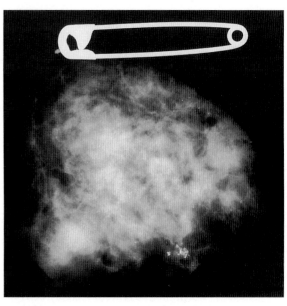

A

**FIG. 7.1.** *Adenosis.* **A:** Mammogram showing clustered calcifications that proved to be in sclerosing adenosis. **B:** Specimen radiograph confirming excision of the calcifications. The safety pin was used for orientation.

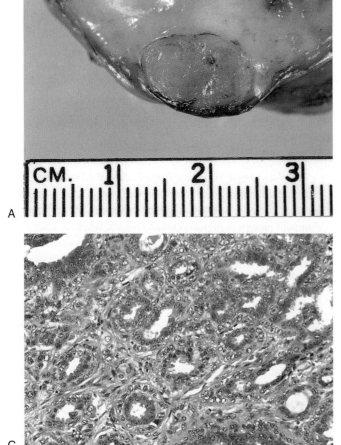

A

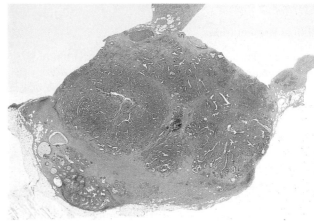

B

**FIG. 7.2.** *Adenosis tumor.* **A:** Gross specimen with an adenosis tumor composed of beige homogeneous tissue forming an oval 1-cm nodule. **B:** Same tumor in a whole-mount histologic section showing internal nodular architecture. **C:** Florid adenosis with epithelial and myoepithelial hyperplasia in this adenosis tumor.

C

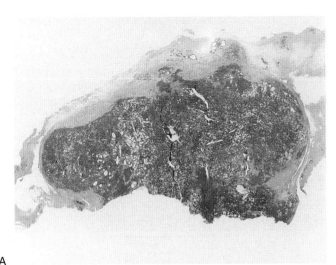

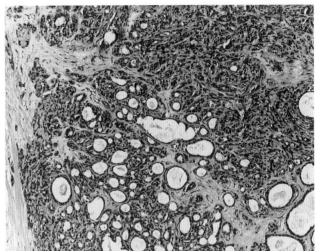

A

B

**FIG. 7.3.** *Adenosis tumor.* **A:** Whole-mount histologic section showing the well-circumscribed tumor. **B:** Confluent sclerosing adenosis.

Some glands have round, open lumens, but the majority of the ductular structures cut tangentially or longitudinally have elongated lumens, sometimes with angular contours. The caliber of the lumens is relatively constant regardless of the plane of section. Cystic dilation of ductules or glands is not prominent in florid adenosis.

Epithelial cells lining the tubules and glands most often are flattened, cuboidal, or slightly columnar, and they are arranged in one or two orderly layers surrounded by myoepithelial cells. Increase in cell size and nuclear pleomorphism are found in florid adenosis, especially during pregnancy or lactation. Hyperplastic change in the epithelial component of florid adenosis is mirrored in hyperplasia of the myoepithelium (Fig. 7.6). Mitoses in epithelial and myoepithelial cells are very infrequent. They are more numerous during pregnancy. Degeneration of individual cells, manifested by nu-

clear debris, nuclear pyknosis, apoptosis, and rarely geographic areas of necrosis can be found in pregnancy-associated tumoral florid adenosis (Fig. 7.7). Apocrine metaplasia is uncommon in florid adenosis. Florid adenosis may surround nerves in adjacent breast parenchyma, and invasion of blood vessel walls was found in 10% of the cases in one study (7).

Eosinophilic secretion deposited in the lumens of ductules is typically periodic acid-Schiff (PAS) and mucicarmine positive. Intracytoplasmic mucin vacuoles and signet-ring cells are not present in the glandular epithelium in florid adenosis. Luminal secretion may undergo calcification, but this is less common and less extensive in florid than in sclerosing adenosis.

Fine needle aspiration of an adenosis tumor yields a cellular specimen composed of clusters of epithelial cells, spindly, bipolar, "naked" nuclei of myoepithelial cells, and stromal fragments (8). The findings resemble the cytologic specimen that may be obtained from a fibroadenoma but usually lack larger, flat sheets of epithelial cells. Immunohistochemical examination of the cytologic specimen reveals reactivity for actin and S-100 in the sparse cytoplasm associated with bipolar nuclei.

The ultrastructural features of adenosis tumor are similar to those of sclerosing adenosis (8,9). Glandular epithelial cells surrounded by myoepithelial cells are supported by a basement membrane that may be thickened by reduplication (10).

In *sclerosing adenosis,* there is preferential preservation of myoepithelial cells with variable atrophy of epithelial cells, accompanied by lobular fibrosis (Fig. 7.8). The swirling lobulocentric pattern encountered in florid adenosis is retained, but epithelial cells are less conspicuous and the ductular structures are largely attenuated (Fig. 7.9). In some instances, sclerosing adenosis is not limited to a lobulocentric pattern. When this occurs, the proliferating benign glands have an infiltrative pattern in the stroma and fat that can be mistaken for invasive carcinoma (Fig. 7.10). Epithelial cells may be markedly reduced in number or even absent, leaving compressed elon-

*text continues on p. 145*

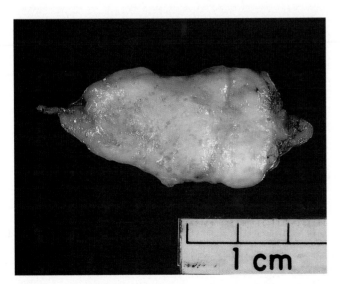

**FIG. 7.4.** *Florid adenosis, gross specimen.* Multiple tan nodules of florid adenosis are visible on the surface of a breast biopsy.

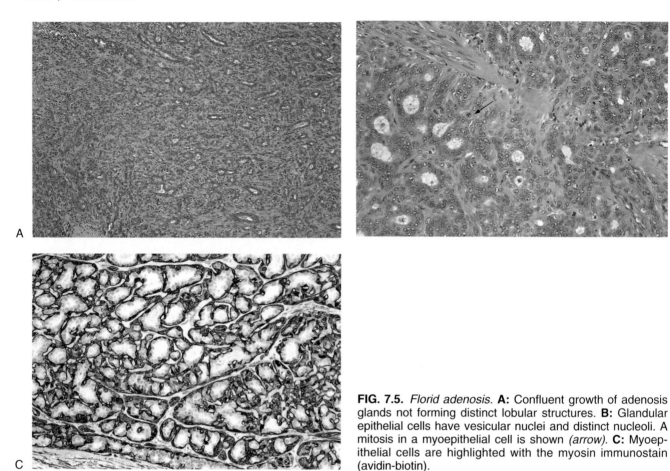

**FIG. 7.5.** *Florid adenosis.* **A:** Confluent growth of adenosis glands not forming distinct lobular structures. **B:** Glandular epithelial cells have vesicular nuclei and distinct nucleoli. A mitosis in a myoepithelial cell is shown *(arrow).* **C:** Myoepithelial cells are highlighted with the myosin immunostain (avidin-biotin).

**FIG. 7.6.** *Florid adenosis.* **A:** Adenosis with a prominent glandular pattern and a microcalcification *(arrow).* **B:** Glandular structures are partially effaced by florid epithelial and myoepithelial hyperplasia. *(continued)*

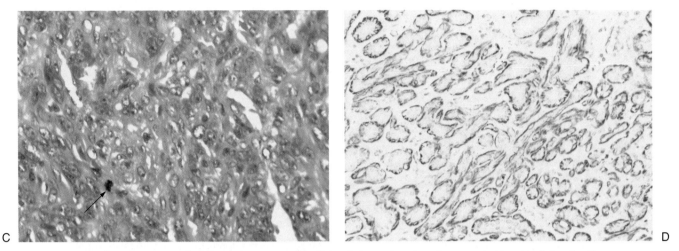

**FIG. 7.6.** *Continued.* **C:** Mitosis in a myoepithelial cell *(arrow)* and nuclear atypia in epithelial cells. **D:** Myoepithelial cells are stained for actin (anti-smooth muscle actin, avidin-biotin).

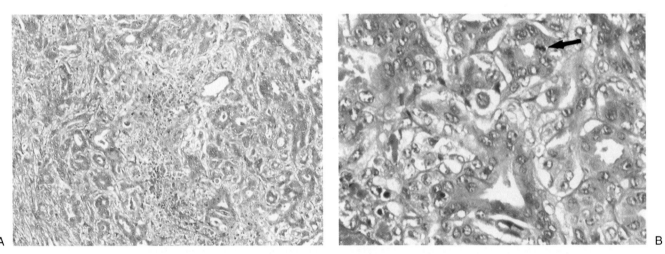

**FIG. 7.7.** *Florid adenosis in pregnancy.* **A:** Florid adenosis with central necrosis in a pregnant woman. **B:** A mitotic figure *(arrow)* and nuclear atypia are present.

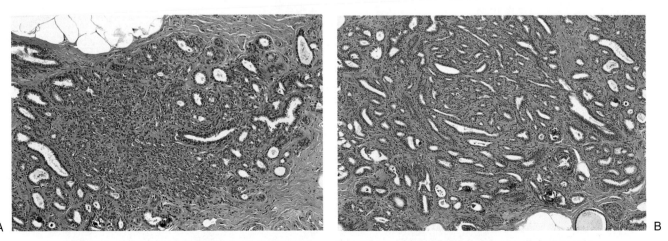

**FIG. 7.8.** *Sclerosing adenosis.* **A:** Swirling pattern with a lobulocentric distribution composed of dilated glands and spindly myoepithelial cells. **B:** Numerous microcalcifications near the lower border and a tubular growth pattern.

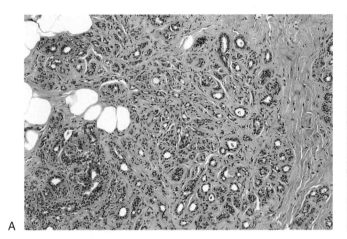

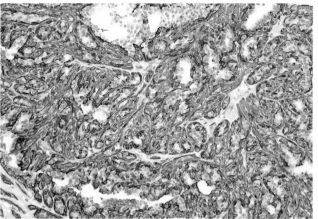

**FIG. 7.9.** *Sclerosing adenosis.* **A:** Well-developed lobular sclerosis that tends to merge with fat in a post-menopausal woman. **B:** Myoepithelial cell overgrowth is highlighted with the myosin immunostain (avidin-biotin).

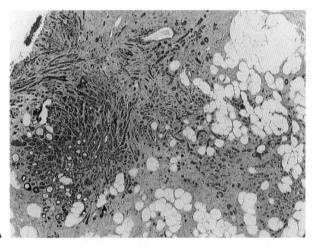

**FIG. 7.10.** *Sclerosing adenosis involving fat.* **A:** Lobulocentric growth on the *left* is accompanied by diffuse spread into the fibrous stroma and fat on the *right*. **B:** Sclerosing adenosis mingling with fat. **C:** Sclerosing adenosis that resembles invasive lobular carcinoma in fat. The cell groups are evenly spaced, they appear to be "packaged" by the stroma, and signet-ring cells are absent. Myoepithelial cells are present and would be highlighted with an antiactin stain to rule out lobular carcinoma.

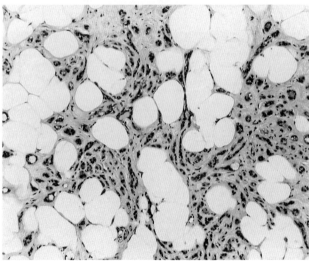

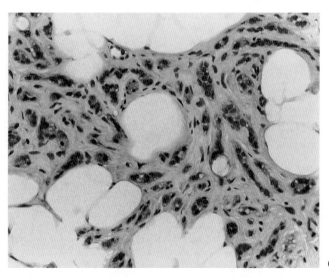

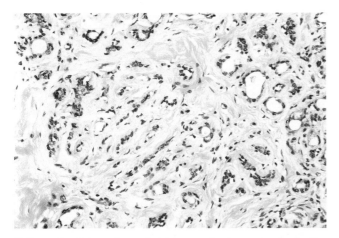

**FIG. 7.11.** *Sclerosing adenosis, marked atrophy.* Note the linear distribution of myoepithelial cells, simulating infiltrating lobular carcinoma.

gated strands of myoepithelial cells (Fig. 7.11). With increasing sclerosis, ductular lumens are progressively obliterated to the point where they may not be recognizable (Fig. 7.12). The persisting myoepithelial cells with a pronounced spindle shape (myoid phenotype) are strongly immunoreactive with markers of smooth muscle differentiation. Cystically dilated ductule cross sections are variably present in sclerosing adenosis. Papilloma-like nodular foci of proliferating ductules may protrude into such cysts. These have been referred to as "glomeruloid structures" (6). Calcifications become progressively more numerous with increasing sclerosis.

Apocrine metaplasia is relatively more common in sclerosing than in florid adenosis (Fig. 7.13) (6). When apocrine change is extensive, the condition has been referred to as *apocrine adenosis* (11). The cytologic appearance of apocrine metaplasia in adenosis is quite varied (12). In some cases, the cells have conventional, pink, finely granular apocrine cytoplasm and round regular nuclei. When compared

with ordinary apocrine metaplasia, atypical features include cytoplasmic clearing or vacuolization, nuclear enlargement, irregular nuclear membranes, and nuclear pleomorphism (Figs. 7.14 and 7.15). Mitotic figures are not a feature of atypical apocrine metaplasia in sclerosing adenosis, and they are more likely to be present when apocrine carcinoma arises in or involves adenosis. Hyperchromasia of nuclei and prominent nucleoli are found in the most extreme examples of apocrine atypia. Florid proliferation of atypical apocrine elements in sclerosing adenosis produces lesions that may be difficult to distinguish from intraductal apocrine carcinoma (12,13). Extreme cytologic atypia with readily identifiable mitotic activity and/or a proliferative pattern characteristic of intraductal carcinoma are necessary to make a diagnosis of carcinoma in this setting. Membrane expression of c-erbB2 oncoprotein has been detected in lesions described as benign apocrine adenosis (13a). In this study, a gene amplification was not detected in samples studied by the FISH method. A diagnosis of carcinoma arising in apocrine adenosis should not be based solely on the presence of c-erbB2 immunoreactivity.

Extremely unusual variants of sclerosing adenosis show clear cell change (Fig. 7.16) and collagenous spherulosis (Fig. 7.17).

The first systematic study of perineural invasion in sclerosing adenosis was reported by Taylor and Norris (14). Perineural invasion was found in 20 (2%) of 1,000 biopsies with sclerosing adenosis. The median age of the 20 patients who were biopsied, 32 years, did not differ significantly from the median age of women with sclerosing adenosis that lacked perineural invasion. Only two of the women had prior surgery. Four women were pregnant. The proliferative lesions most frequently associated with perineural invasion were sclerosing adenosis and papillomatosis. Histologically benign structures were found around nerves, involving the perineurium and rarely within nerve fibers (Fig. 7.18). After a median follow-up of 7 years, no patient with perineural invasion manifested clinical evidence of carcinoma. The authors found no evidence that the glandular epithelium was in lymphatic or other vascular spaces.

Davies (15) found neural invasion in four (1.3%) of 316 cases of mammary "dysplasia." Overall, sclerosing adenosis was present in 25% of the specimens. In three of the four cases, neural invasion had concurrent sclerosing adenosis, and the fourth patient had sclerosing adenosis in a prior biopsy. Nerves were found in 53.5% of biopsies, but not more frequently when there was sclerosing adenosis. Neural invasion was not attributable to prior surgery, because only one of the four patients had been operated on previously. Sclerosing adenosis penetrated into and focally through the perineurium of affected nerves. Myoepithelial cells were evident in most, but not all, foci of perineural invasion. The glandular elements appeared histologically benign, lacking cytologic atypia or mitotic activity. The patients remained disease free 8 to 38 months after biopsy. Perivascular invasion that simulated the perineural pattern was found in two specimens that did not exhibit perineural invasion.

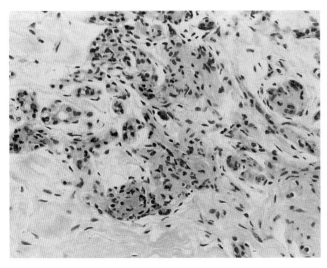

**FIG. 7.12.** *Sclerosing adenosis.* Glandular atrophy with preservation of myoid myoepithelial cells.

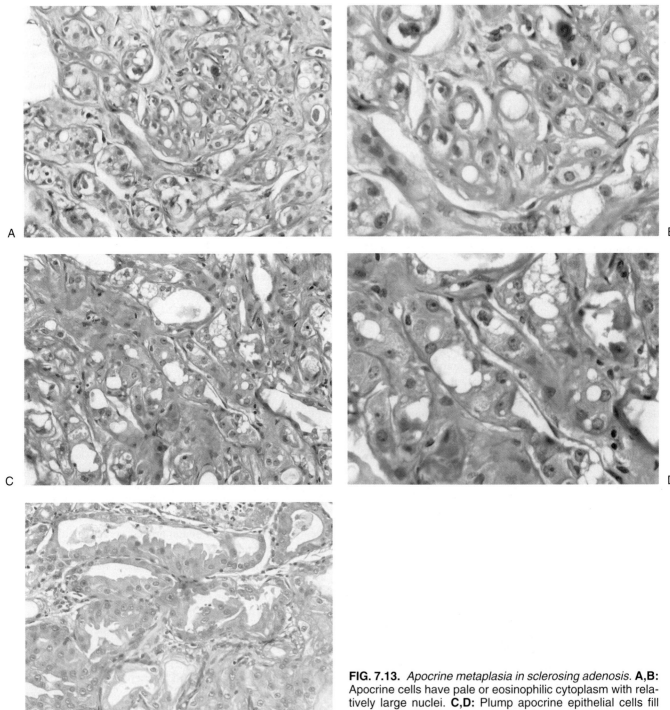

**FIG. 7.13.** *Apocrine metaplasia in sclerosing adenosis.* **A,B:** Apocrine cells have pale or eosinophilic cytoplasm with relatively large nuclei. **C,D:** Plump apocrine epithelial cells fill many of the glands. Note cytoplasmic clearing in some cells. **E:** Florid apocrine hyperplasia in adenosis.

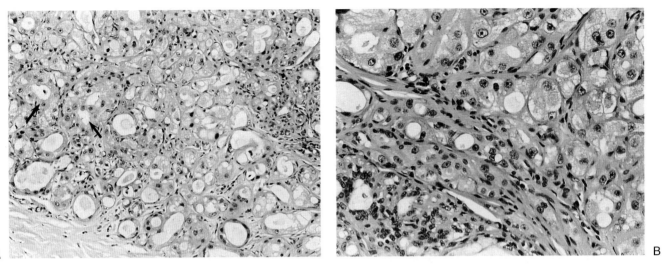

**FIG. 7.14.** *Atypical apocrine metaplasia in sclerosing adenosis.* **A:** Lobular glands are expanded by plump apocrine cells. Some glands are filled by this cellular accumulation, and there are foci of secondary lumen formation (*arrows*). **B:** Ordinary sclerosing adenosis with apocrine metaplasia is present below an area of atypical apocrine hyperplasia in adenosis.

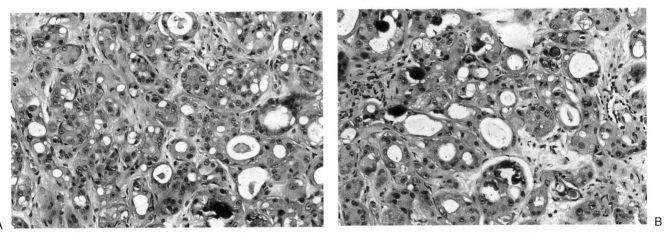

**FIG. 7.15.** *Atypical apocrine metaplasia in sclerosing adenosis.* **A,B:** Numerous calcifications are present. Note nuclear pleomorphism.

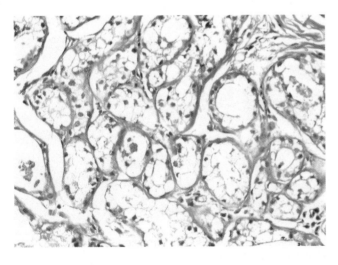

**FIG. 7.16.** *Clear cell apocrine metaplasia in sclerosing adenosis.* The dilated glands contain voluminous cells with clear cytoplasm.

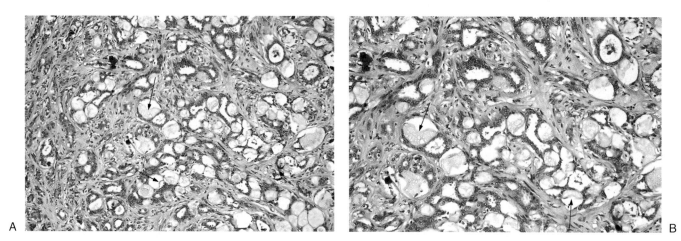

**FIG. 7.17.** *Collagenous spherulosis in sclerosing adenosis.* **A,B:** Degenerative changes are present in the spherules. Detached basement membranes are present in some glandular lumens *(arrows).*

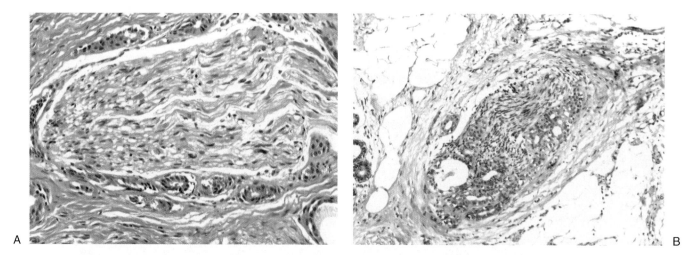

**FIG. 7.18.** *Neural invasion.* **A:** Adenosis glands are wrapped around a nerve. **B:** Adenosis glands are present around and within this nerve.

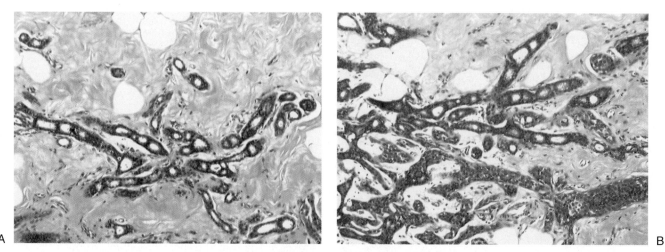

**FIG. 7.19.** *Tubular adenosis.* **A:** Uncomplicated example illustrating stellate tubule formation. **B:** Complex example with interlacing tubules and florid epithelial hyperplasia below.

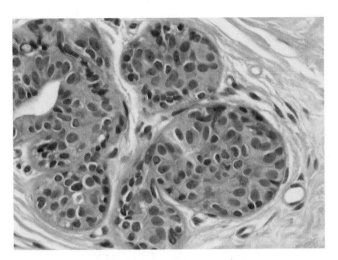

**FIG. 7.20.** *Blunt duct adenosis.*

*Tubular adenosis* is characterized by the formation of ductules arranged so that most are cut longitudinally in the plane of the histologic section (Fig. 7.19). The proliferation lacks the lobulocentric distribution of florid or sclerosing adenosis, because the ductules extend in a seemly haphazard pattern into fibrous mammary stroma and fat. In some instances, there is a dense proliferation of tubular structures that appear to be woven or interdigitated like a ball of twine. Bifurcating tubules and mild cystic dilation of ductules sometimes are observed. Secretion that may calcify is variably present in the ductules. Although the proliferation appears to be largely epithelial, virtually all of the tubular structures have basement membranes and an outer myoepithelial cell layer (16). These features are important in the distinction between tubular carcinoma and tubular adenosis.

*Blunt duct adenosis* is a form of terminal duct hyperplasia with abortive lobule formation (2). The proliferating ductular epithelium forms aggregates of lobule-like nodules that appear to be the ends of the ductules (Fig. 7.20). Myoepithelial hyperplasia may be conspicuous in these nodules. Lumens are present in some of these lobule-like structures,

which occasionally are cystically dilated. Blunt duct adenosis sometimes exhibits apocrine metaplasia. Blunt duct adenosis may be mistakenly diagnosed as atypical lobular hyperplasia or lobular carcinoma *in situ.*

*Adenosis in fibroadenomas* usually is readily distinguished from carcinoma. Fibroadenomas are likely to develop adenosis, because both lesions arise from the terminal duct-lobular unit. All forms of adenosis occur in fibroadenomas, sometimes accompanied by other proliferative changes such as cystic and papillary apocrine metaplasia. Adenosis may be localized to one part of a fibroadenoma, or it may be diffuse, obscuring the underlying fibroepithelial structure. A needle core biopsy of adenosis in a fibroadenoma may simulate the appearance of invasive carcinoma (Fig. 7.21). A fibroadenoma with sclerosing adenosis or other components of fibrocystic change is termed a "complex fibroadenoma" (see Chapter 8).

**Differential Diagnosis**

The major consideration in the differential diagnosis of adenosis and its variant forms is the distinction between these lesions and carcinoma, especially the tubular type. A discussion of features distinguishing tubular carcinoma from adenosis can be found in Chapter 15, which is devoted to tubular carcinoma.

*In situ* carcinoma can arise in adenosis, or adenosis can be secondarily involved by carcinoma established in the surrounding tissue. Nielsen (6) reported finding carcinoma in adenosis tumors as well as in other forms of adenosis. *In situ* lobular and intraductal carcinoma occur in sclerosing adenosis and in tubular adenosis. The majority of carcinomas that develop in adenosis are of the lobular type (Fig. 7.22) (17). Lobular carcinoma *in situ* usually causes expansion of the epithelial component in adenosis, but in some foci of sclerosing adenosis, the neoplastic process is manifested by sparsely distributed dyscohesive pagetoid cells (18). Lobular carcinoma *in situ* in adenosis often has signet-ring cells that are demonstrated with the mucicarmine stain. Signet-ring cells and stainable intracytoplasmic mucin are not a feature of

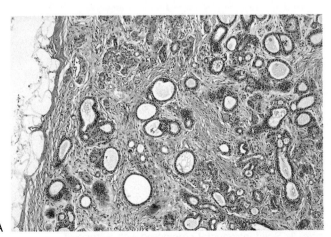

A

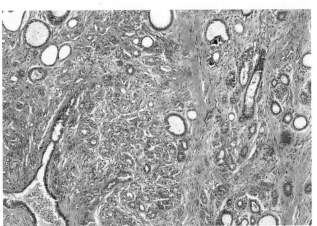

B

**FIG. 7.21.** *Sclerosing adenosis in a fibroadenoma.* **A:** Photograph from a needle core biopsy sample that was interpreted as invasive duct carcinoma. **B:** The excised tumor was a fibroadenoma extensively involved by sclerosing adenosis. Cleft-forming fibroadenomatous epithelium is shown on the *lower left.*

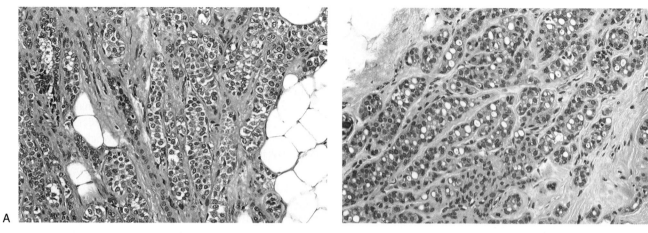

**FIG. 7.22.** *Lobular carcinoma* in situ *in sclerosing adenosis.* **A:** Loss of cohesion. **B:** Signet-ring cells.

benign epithelium in adenosis. A mucin stain should be performed in most cases to confirm that cytoplasmic mucin is present when cytoplasmic vacuoles are seen in hematoxylin and eosin sections. Lobular carcinoma *in situ* in sclerosing adenosis is characterized by absence of E-cadherin reactivity. It is not unusual to find lobular carcinoma *in situ* in surrounding lobules not affected by sclerosing adenosis.

Intraductal carcinoma arises less often in adenosis than does lobular carcinoma *in situ*. In this setting, intraductal carcinoma can be identified most readily when there is comedonecrosis or if the proliferation has cribriform or papillary features (Fig. 7.23) (6,17). Apocrine differentiation, which is relatively frequent in intraductal carcinoma in adenosis, usually is of the cribriform, solid, or comedo type. As noted earlier, the distinction between atypical apocrine metaplasia and apocrine carcinoma in adenosis can be extremely difficult (12,13,19). Despite considerable cytologic atypia, apocrine metaplasia in adenosis should not be interpreted as carcinoma until there is sufficient epithelial proliferation to form one of the conventional structural patterns of intraductal carcinoma and/or there is extreme cytologic atypia with readily identified mitotic activity. Cytoplasmic clearing or vacuolization

occurs in atypical sclerosing apocrine lesions as well as in apocrine carcinoma (see Chapter 21). Pleomorphic lobular carcinoma *in situ* in adenosis can be distinguished from apocrine ductal carcinoma by absence of E-cadherin reactivity in the former, and its presence in the latter.

The underlying architecture of adenosis is preserved when *in situ* lobular and intraductal carcinoma arise in this setting. The integrity of individual glands, sometimes difficult to ascertain in these complex proliferative lesions, may be confirmed with a reticulin stain and immunohistochemical studies for basement membrane or myoepithelial cells (16,20).

Even when basement membranes and a myoepithelial layer appear discontinuous, it is difficult to diagnose invasion with confidence within foci of adenosis. It is possible to perform immunostains for actin and cytokeratin on the same tissue section when assessing carcinoma in adenosis for microinvasion (21). The results obtained with a conventional actin antibody, such as one directed at smooth muscle actin (SMA), can be confusing because it stains myofibroblasts as well as myoepithelial cells. Immunostaining should be done with a reagent more specific for myoepithelial cells, such as anti-smooth muscle myosin heavy chain, maspin or calponin (Figs. 7.23 and 7.24).

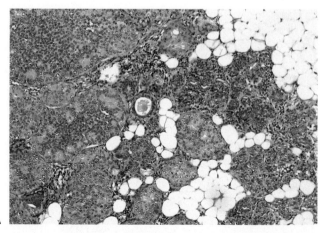
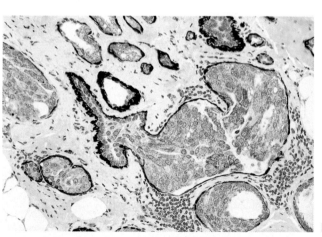

**FIG. 7.23.** *Intraductal carcinoma in sclerosing adenosis.* **A:** Solid intraductal carcinoma with a trace of cribriform growth in adenosis glands. **B:** Basement membranes are attenuated in the adenosis gland occupied by intraductal carcinoma. Myofibroblasts are not stained (anti-smooth muscle myosin heavy chain, avidin-biotin).

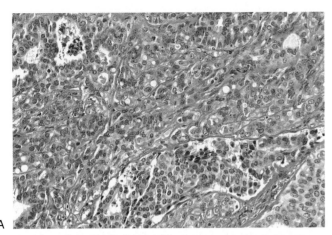
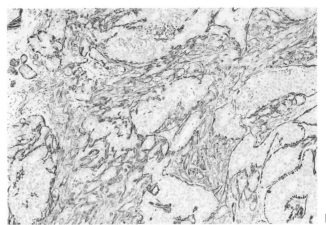

A      B

**FIG. 7.24.** *Intraductal carcinoma in sclerosing adenosis.* **A:** Enlarged gland contains intraductal carcinoma in the midst of florid adenosis that resembles invasive carcinoma. **B:** Antiactin immunostain highlights myoepithelial cells around all glandular structures and intervening areas of myofibroblastic cells. Note the serrated appearance produced by myoepithelial cells protruding into larger glandular spaces occupied by intraductal carcinoma (anti-smooth muscle actin; avidin-biotin).

The most convincing evidence for a diagnosis of invasive carcinoma arising in adenosis is the presence of invasive foci extending beyond the adenosis lesion. The invasive carcinoma should have cytologic features duplicating those of the *in situ* carcinoma in the adenosis. The glands or cells interpreted as invasive carcinoma should not be accompanied by myoepithelial cells, and basement membrane should be largely or completely absent. Finally, the invasive elements should have a distribution and pattern that differ from the adenosis.

**Treatment and Prognosis**

Excisional biopsy is adequate treatment for adenosis. When adenosis occurs as part of fibrocystic change, microscopic foci may extend beyond the region of palpable clinical involvement. Further excision is not recommended in such cases. If adenosis is suggested by a fine needle aspiration cytology specimen or a needle core biopsy, surgical excision of the lesional area may be required to rule out an associated carcinoma. With respect to needle core biopsies, it is important to correlate the clinical and radiologic findings with the biopsy specimen to determine if surgical excision should be performed. The treatment of carcinoma arising in adenosis depends on the stage and extent of the lesion. In many of these cases, carcinoma also is present in breast tissue outside the area of adenosis (17,18).

Foote and Stewart (2) studied the frequency of various fibrocystic changes in patients with and without breast carcinoma. They reported that adenosis, especially sclerosing adenosis, was not found more often in breasts with carcinoma, and they concluded that adenosis is not a precursor lesion or risk factor for carcinoma. A retrospective review of breast specimens from patients with and without carcinoma by Kern and Brooks (22) revealed that sclerosing adenosis was present more frequently in patients who did not have carcinoma (22). Page et al. (23) did not detect a significantly increased risk associated with sclerosing adenosis in a follow-up study of women with fibrocystic changes published in 1978. Later investigations by Page and his associates identified women with sclerosing adenosis as having an increased relative risk for breast carcinoma (24,25). Jensen et al. (25) found an overall relative risk of 2.1 in women with "sclerosing adenosis." This decreased to 1.7 in women without concomitant atypical hyperplasia and was not significantly changed by the presence or absence of a family history of breast carcinoma. When sclerosing adenosis was accompanied by atypical hyperplasia, often of the lobular type, the relative risk was 6.7. Other investigators also reported an increased risk of subsequent carcinoma after a diagnosis of sclerosing adenosis (26–30). Krieger and Hiatt (30) reported that the overall relative risk when compared to control populations for women with adenosis was 2.5. Bodian et al. (26) reported a relative risk of 2.2 for "adenosis" in women without other proliferative changes and no family history of breast carcinoma. Neither of these studies defined "adenosis" or indicated that the data referred to sclerosing adenosis in contrast to florid adenosis.

The precancerous significance of atypical apocrine metaplasia in sclerosing adenosis was assessed in two studies. Carter and Rosen (12) evaluated 51 patients with sclerosing proliferative lesions that included adenosis with apocrine atypia. After a mean follow-up of 35 months, no subsequent carcinomas were detected. Seidman et al. (13) described 37 patients with a mean follow-up of 8.7 years and reported that four (11%) developed invasive ductal carcinoma subsequently (three ipsilateral and one contralateral). The histologic appearance of the carcinomas (apocrine vs. nonapocrine) was not stated. The relative risk for developing carcinoma was 5.5 (95% confidence interval [CI] 1.9 to 16) when compared to age-specific incidence rates. All patients who developed carcinoma were over 60 years of age when adenosis with apocrine atypia was diagnosed, and the 11 patients in this age group had a relative risk for carcinoma of 14 (95% CI 4.1 to 48). All carcinomas were diagnosed more than 3 years after the initial adenosis diagnosis (mean interval 5.6 years), an observation that may explain the absence of subsequent carcinoma in the study by Carter and Rosen (12), which had a mean follow-up of 35 months, which is slightly less than 3 years.

## MICROGLANDULAR ADENOSIS

Microglandular adenosis (MGA) is a proliferative glandular lesion that may mimic carcinoma clinically and pathologically. Although it had been described previously (31–33), MGA was not well characterized as a clinicopathologic entity until the publication in 1983 of three series totaling 29 patients (34–36). One patient probably was included in two of these reports (34,35). This entity differs substantially in its structural features from lesions conventionally termed "adenosis." It is included in this chapter because no more suitable placement is readily evident, and the word "adenosis" is used to name the lesion.

### Clinical Presentation

All patients with MGA have been women, ranging in age from 28 to 82 years. The majority of the patients were 45 to 55 years old. The presenting symptom in most instances has been a mass or "thickening" in the breast. Occasionally, MGA has been one of several lesions responsible for the mass. MGA can be accompanied by cysts and various benign proliferative changes. The mass sometimes is painful. In one case, the lesion changed in size during the menstrual cycle. Duration prior to biopsy has varied from a few weeks to as long as 5 years. A positive family history of breast carcinoma has rarely been mentioned.

Mammography may reveal increased density and sometimes is reported to be "suspicious," but there are no specific radiologic changes. Rarely, nonpalpable MGA is detected mammographically at the site of an ill-defined density with calcifications. Such a lesion may be sampled by needle core biopsy.

### Gross Pathology

MGA forms an ill-defined infiltrative lesion. As a consequence, the size is rarely accurately measured, but it has been estimated to be 3 to 4 cm in most cases and possibly as large as 20 cm. In some specimens, the process has been described as multifocal or as composed of confluent multifocal lesions. Cysts and other microscopically detectable proliferative changes often contribute to the grossly evident mass. In some instances, they obscure the true extent of the MGA component.

### Microscopic Pathology

The basic histologic pattern of MGA is an infiltrative proliferation of small glands in fibrous or fatty mammary stroma (Fig. 7.25). When examined at low magnification,

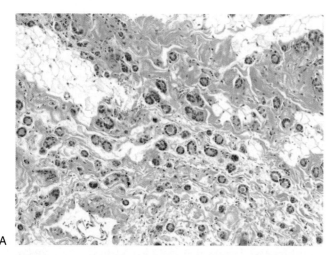
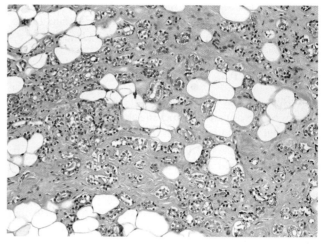
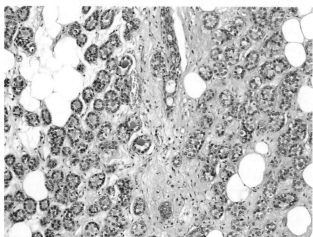

**FIG. 7.25.** *Microglandular adenosis.* **A:** Regular round glands are diffusely distributed in fibrofatty stroma. **B:** Cells in this variant have clear cytoplasm. **C:** Lesion infiltrates fat *(left)* and fibrous stroma *(right)*.

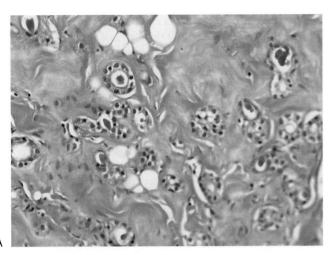
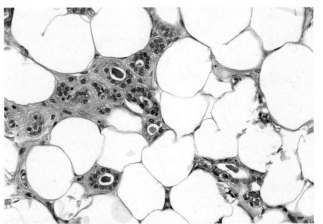

**FIG. 7.26.** *Microglandular adenosis.* **A:** Typical glands composed of uniform cuboidal cells regularly spaced around a lumen containing eosinophilic secretion. Slight cytoplasmic clearing is evident. **B:** Microglandular adenosis in fat.

there sometimes appears to be clustering by the glands, forming lobule-like aggregates, but most often the distribution seems disorderly.

In its most characteristic form, MGA is composed of round glands lined by a single layer of flat to cuboidal epithelial cells (Fig. 7.26). Each cell has a single round nucleus with an inconspicuous or inapparent nucleolus. The cytoplasm tends to be clear or amphophilic, but pronounced eosinophilia may be encountered, sometimes with cytoplasmic granularity. Inspissated secretion forms distinct deeply stained globules in the glands. This material usually is PAS and mucicarmine positive, and it may calcify (Fig. 7.27). The PAS-positive secretion is diastase resistant.

Cells forming MGA are strongly immunoreactive for cytokeratin, S-100, and cathepsin D (Fig. 7.28). They have proven to be negative for nuclear estrogen and progesterone receptor, nuclear p53 oncogene expression, and for HER2/*neu* membrane immunoreactivity (37). Eusebi et al.

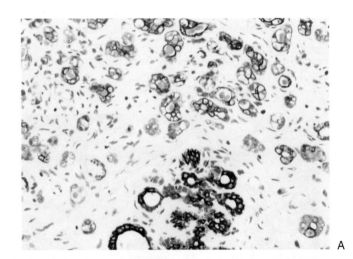

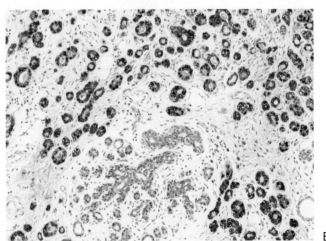

**FIG. 7.28.** *Microglandular adenosis.* **A:** Epithelial cells of a lobule in the *lower center* are more strongly immunoreactive for cytokeratin than are the surrounding microglandular adenosis glands (anti-AE1, avidin-biotin). **B:** Strong immunoreactivity for S-100 protein is present in microglandular adenosis around a nonreactive normal lobule (avidin-biotin).

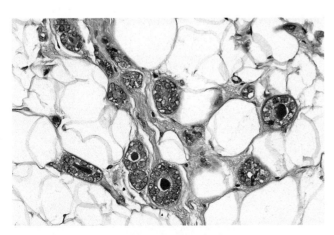

**FIG. 7.27.** *Microglandular adenosis.* Secretion in the lumens reacts positively with the periodic acid-Schiff (PAS) stain, which also highlights the intact basement membranes around glands (PAS reaction).

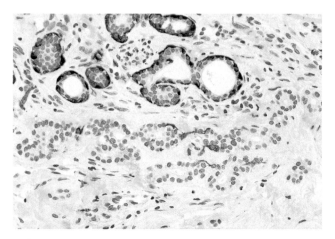

**FIG. 7.29.** *Microglandular adenosis.* Myoepithelial cells are immunoreactive for myosin in adenosis *(above)*. No reactivity is seen in microglandular adenosis *(below)* (anti-smooth muscle myosin heavy chain, avidin-biotin).

(38) reported that MGA lacks immunoreactivity for gross cystic disease fluid protein 15 (GCDFP-15) and for epithelial membrane antigen (EMA). The absence of EMA was helpful in distinguishing MGA from tubular carcinoma, which was consistently EMA positive.

Myoepithelial cells are not evident in sections stained with hematoxylin and eosin, and they are not demonstrable with immunohistochemical stains for actin (Fig. 7.29). A basement membrane is manifested by immunoreactivity for laminin and type IV collagen, and the glands typically are invested by a reticulin ring that can be highlighted by silver impregnation and PAS stains (Fig. 7.30) (37,38). In some cases, the glands are surrounded by a thick collar of collagen and reticulin.

Substantial variation in the growth pattern and cytologic appearance of the glands can be encountered in MGA. When elongated, the glands acquire a tubular rather than round configuration. This appearance sometimes merges with elements of sclerosing adenosis (Fig. 7.31). In these more proliferative patterns, the cells lining the glands tend to be pleomorphic, with varying amounts of cytoplasm that is clear or exhibits eosinophilia. Prominent, coarse, deeply eosinophilic oncocytic cytoplasmic granules are present in a minority of cases. The latter cytoplasmic appearance sometimes is accompanied by a lymphoplasmacytic reaction that is otherwise not a feature of ordinary MGA (Fig. 7.32).

Lesions classified as "atypical" MGA have elements of MGA in its ordinary form as well as foci with a more complex structure and cytologic atypia. Atypical lesions have a heterogeneous mixture of connected microacini and larger

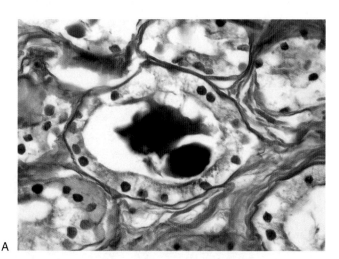

A

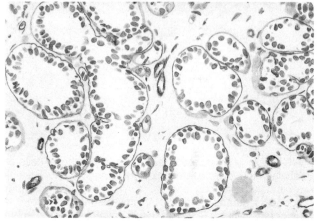

B

**FIG. 7.30.** *Microglandular adenosis.* **A:** Basement membrane is highlighted by the silver reticulin stain in this example of clear cell microglandular adenosis. **B:** Laminin reactivity outlines each gland in microglandular adenosis. **C:** Laminin immunoreactivity in sclerosing adenosis shown for comparison (avidin-biotin).

C

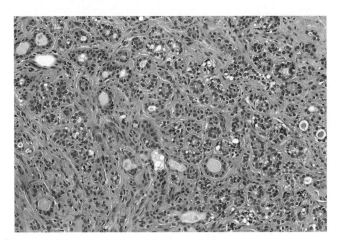

FIG. 7.31. *Microglandular adenosis and sclerosing adenosis.* Microglandular adenosis occupying most of this image merges with sclerosing adenosis *(lower left)*.

glands (Fig. 7.33). Ordinary MGA may have crowded, "back-to-back" glands, but each acinus remains separate. The more florid epithelial proliferation of the atypical lesion produces interconnected budding glandular units with microcribriform nests. When luminal bridging occurs, the monolayered epithelium is replaced by a stratified proliferation that evolves into solid nests of cells.

Three studies have described carcinoma arising in MGA (36,37,39). Structural transitions from atypical MGA to intraductal carcinoma are observed in these cases. With extensive sampling, it may be possible to find residual ordinary MGA without atypia. The carcinomatous areas have the acinar pattern of MGA, but they are enlarged and filled by cells with a high mitotic rate, substantial cytologic abnormalities, and necrosis. A chronic inflammatory infiltrate and a desmoplastic stromal reaction often accompany the development of carcinoma in MGA. The carcinomatous epithelium may exhibit cytoplasmic features found in MGA, such as secretory activity, cytoplasmic clearing, and prominent oncocytic granulation (Fig. 7.34). Acinic cell differentiation manifested by reactivity for amylase, lysozyme, and alpha-1-antichymotrypsin has been described in some examples of carcinoma arising in MGA (39a). These tumors tend to have clear or granular cytoplasm. Benign chondromyxoid metaplasia of the stroma has been described in a minority of cases (39), and one example of carcinoma with matrix-forming chondroid metaplasia arising in MGA was studied by the author (Fig. 7.35).

Intraductal carcinomas arising in MGA can be readily identified because they tend to retain the underlying alveolar growth pattern of the adenosis. In most cases, the fully developed lesion is composed of malignant cells growing in solid nests. The pattern differs somewhat from any of the structural configurations encountered in most ordinary types

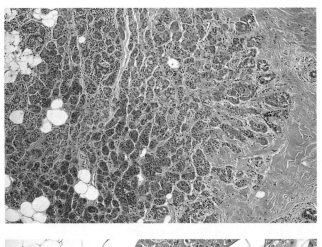

A

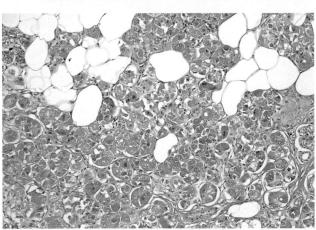

C

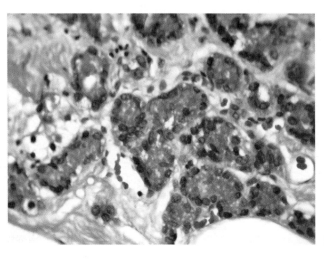

B

FIG. 7.32. *Microglandular adenosis.* **A:** Microglandular adenosis surrounds a normal lobule *(upper center).* Oncocytic change is evident on the *left.* Glandular enlargement on the *right* is an atypical feature. **B:** Cytoplasmic granularity and eosinophilia. **C:** Marked oncocytic change obscures glandular lumens.

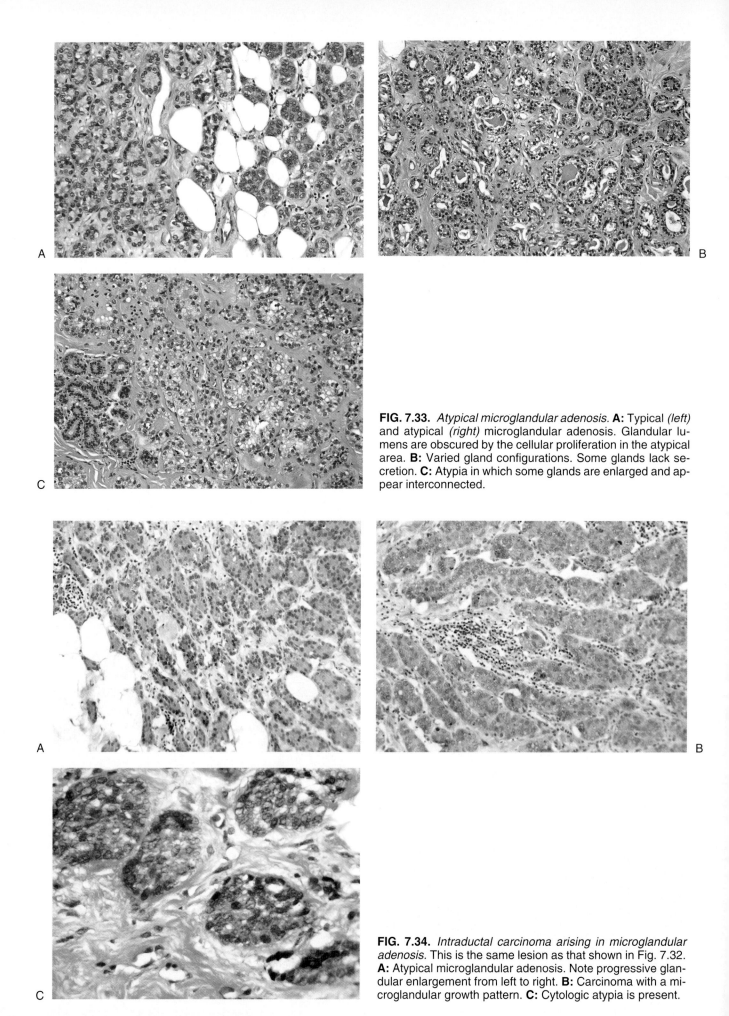

**FIG. 7.33.** *Atypical microglandular adenosis.* **A:** Typical *(left)* and atypical *(right)* microglandular adenosis. Glandular lumens are obscured by the cellular proliferation in the atypical area. **B:** Varied gland configurations. Some glands lack secretion. **C:** Atypia in which some glands are enlarged and appear interconnected.

**FIG. 7.34.** *Intraductal carcinoma arising in microglandular adenosis.* This is the same lesion as that shown in Fig. 7.32. **A:** Atypical microglandular adenosis. Note progressive glandular enlargement from left to right. **B:** Carcinoma with a microglandular growth pattern. **C:** Cytologic atypia is present.

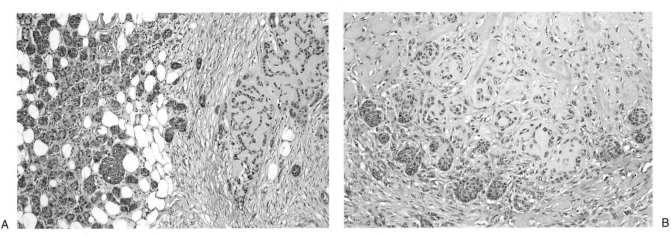

**FIG. 7.35.** *Carcinoma arising in microglandular adenosis with matrix-forming chondroid metaplasia.* **A:** Microglandular adenosis on the *left* showing atypia and transition to *in situ* carcinoma. Invasive carcinoma, matrix-forming type, is on the *right.* **B:** Matrix-forming carcinoma is shown arising in carcinoma in microglandular adenosis.

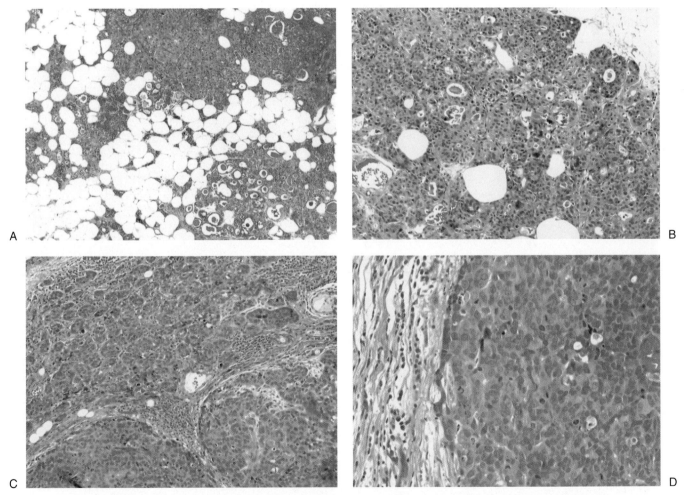

**FIG. 7.36.** *Carcinoma arising in microglandular adenosis.* All images are from a single specimen. **A:** Atypical microglandular adenosis is present in the *lower part* of this picture; the *upper area* depicts carcinoma in microglandular adenosis. **B:** Atypical microglandular adenosis. **C:** Carcinoma with adenosis pattern *(upper left)* forming invasive solid nodules *(below).* A lymphoid reaction, seen focally here, is commonly present in this type of carcinoma. **D:** High-grade invasive carcinoma that typifies these lesions.

of duct or lobular carcinoma (Fig. 7.36). The carcinomas frequently have some clear cells, and a few tumors are entirely composed of such cells or of cells with prominent eosinophilic oncocytic cytoplasmic granularity.

Invasive carcinoma that arises in MGA usually forms microscopic solid tumor masses that are appreciably larger than the surrounding alveolar MGA glands filled by *in situ* carcinoma (Fig. 7.36). The invasive foci typically are enveloped by a conspicuous lymphocytic reaction, necrosis may be present, and these are usually regions with conspicuous mitotic activity. It often appears that invasive foci are formed by the coalescent growth of expanding alveolar *in situ* carcinoma elements.

Unusual forms of carcinoma, other than the aforementioned high-grade type, are rarely found in association with MGA. These include carcinoma with secretory differentiation (Fig. 7.37), carcinoma with squamous metaplasia, and basaloid carcinoma (Fig. 7.38). Paget's disease was found associated with carcinoma that involved MGA throughout the breast, including the axillary tail adjacent to axillary lymph nodes.

Tsuda et al. (40) described an example of carcinoma in MGA that they interpreted as "malignant progression of ade-

nomyoepithelial adenosis." Five foci of carcinoma were identified in the 5.5-cm tumor, three with invasion. No axillary nodal metastases were found. Restriction fragment length polymorphism analysis of tissue containing MGA did not reveal clonal DNA, a finding interpreted by the authors to indicate that this region was not neoplastic. Carcinomatous areas exhibited a high mitotic rate, whereas mitoses were rare in the MGA. Both portions had widespread nuclear staining for proliferating cell nuclear antigen. Samples from the MGA revealed 14.8 fmol/mg and 38.3 fmol/mg of estrogen and progesterone receptor, respectively.

Two ultrastructural studies of MGA have been published. The authors of both reports described finding basement membranes surrounded by a loose collagenous layer around the glands (36,41). Infrequent myoepithelial cells were found in less than 5% of glands by Tavassoli and Norris (36). The lesion studied by Kay (41), an example of carcinoma arising in MGA, had glands lined by stratified cells with numerous lysosomal granules.

The histologic differential diagnosis of MGA includes tubular carcinoma and sclerosing adenosis. Tubular carcinoma usually is composed of angular glands of varying size,

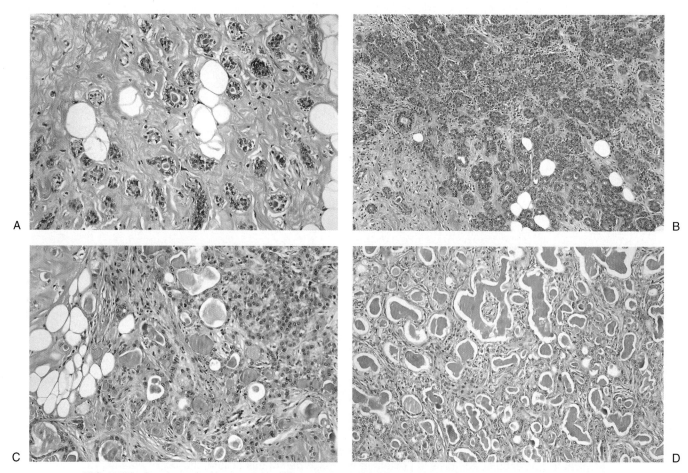

**FIG. 7.37.** *Carcinoma with secretory differentiation arising in microglandular adenosis.* All images are from the same specimen. **A:** Usual microglandular adenosis. **B:** Atypical microglandular adenosis. **C:** Carcinoma glands contain varying amounts of secretion. **D:** Marked glandular proliferation with secretion. This appearance is reminiscent of a cystic hypersecretory lesion.

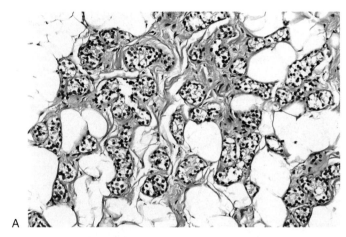
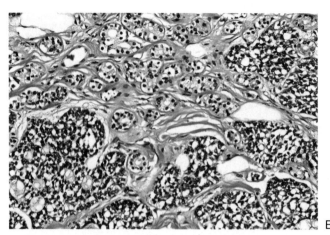

**FIG. 7.38.** *Carcinoma with basaloid differentiation arising in microglandular adenosis.* **A:** Atypical microglandular adenosis with cytoplasmic clearing. **B:** Carcinoma with basaloid growth in microglandular adenosis.

and usually it has a stellate or radial configuration. Intraductal carcinoma is present in many tubular carcinomas, typically with micropapillary or cribriform patterns. Tubular carcinoma glands lack myoepithelial cells and a basement membrane. Although the foregoing features of tubular carcinoma serve to distinguish it from MGA in most instances, there are situations where the distinction is difficult. Occasionally, the glands in tubular carcinoma are rounded and the cells have clear or apocrine cytoplasm, making it difficult to distinguish them from MGA (Fig. 7.26). A thorough search for intraductal carcinoma and stains for basement membrane components may be helpful in this circumstance.

Sclerosing or florid adenosis, which may merge with MGA, typically features myoepithelial proliferation that often has a spindle cell configuration. The process usually is distinctly lobulocentric, and the compressed glands tend to be arranged in a whorled or laminated fashion within the lobular nodules. Myoepithelial cells in sclerosing or florid adenosis are highlighted with immunostains for actin. Small areas of round glands growing in a disorderly manner in association with otherwise typical sclerosing adenosis usually have a myoepithelial cell layer and, therefore, should be considered part of the sclerosing adenosis process rather than as associated MGA.

### Prognosis and Treatment

Ordinary MGA is a benign proliferative lesion that is properly treated by local excision. Recurrences in the breast have rarely been encountered after incomplete excision, and none of the lesions has given rise to regional or systemic metastases. Reexcision should be considered if the margins are found to be microscopically involved, because little is known about the long-term course of incompletely excised MGA. Excisional biopsy is indicated when a needle core biopsy sample suggests MGA.

The term *atypical* has been introduced to describe some examples of MGA with uncertain biologic potential. These lesions exhibit substantially more proliferative activity than ordinary MGA, but they lack the mitoses, necrosis, and the desmoplastic stromal reaction of carcinoma arising in this setting. Patients with atypical MGA should undergo wide excision with histologically documented negative margins. Reexcision is strongly recommended if the margins of the initial excision are involved, and careful clinical follow-up should be instituted so that treatment can be started promptly should carcinoma develop.

Carcinoma has been found in 22% of patients with MGA (37,39). In almost all cases, carcinoma is within the MGA. This proportion of cases of MGA associated with carcinoma may be biased by the fact that some instances were identified because of the distinctive growth pattern of carcinoma that arises in MGA. One unusual patient had coincidental but separate MGA and carcinoma in one breast (36). Another exceptional situation involved a patient with benign MGA in one breast who developed infiltrating duct carcinoma not associated with MGA in the other breast (37). The median age of patients with MGA and carcinoma was 47 years, ranging from 26 to 68 years. All patients presented with a mass. Six (43%) had a family history of breast carcinoma.

When carcinoma arose in MGA, *in situ* carcinoma was found in expanded MGA glands composed of cells with vesicular poorly differentiated nuclei. Basement membranes were present in benign MGA and *in situ* carcinoma, but they were disrupted in invasive foci that appeared to be formed by coalescent alveolar masses of *in situ* carcinoma in MGA. Strong immunoreactivity for cytokeratin, S-100, and cathepsin D was detected in the carcinomas. Two carcinomas had nuclear progesterone receptor, and one of these had estrogen receptor. One carcinoma exhibited membrane staining for HER2/*neu*, and four had nuclear immunoreactivity for p53 protein.

Lymph node metastases were found in three of 11 axillary dissections (Fig. 7.39). Ten patients treated by mastectomy were recurrence free with a median follow-up of 57 months (range 3 to 108 months). Two of three patients treated by excisional surgery were recurrence free 12 and 105 months

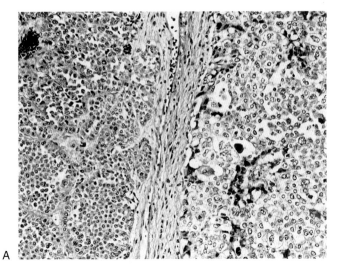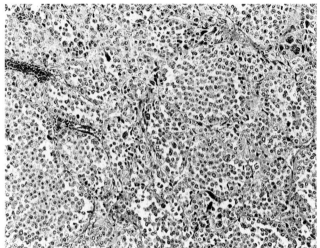

A

B

**FIG. 7.39.** *Metastatic carcinoma.* **A:** Invasive carcinoma with two cytologic appearances that arose in microglandular adenosis. **B:** Carcinoma metastatic from the tumor shown in **A** in an axillary lymph node. (From Rosen PP. Microglandular adenosis. *Am J Surg Pathol* 1983;7:137–144, with permission.)

later. The third woman had bone metastases at 51 months and was alive 98 months after treatment.

Carcinomas arising in MGA have a distinctive histopathologic pattern. They are composed of epithelial cells (cytokeratin positive, actin negative) that are strongly immunoreactive for S-100 protein and cathepsin D. After a median follow-up of nearly 5 years, patients with these carcinomas appear to have a relatively favorable outcome despite histopathologic and immunohistochemical features usually associated with a poor prognosis, but conclusive data are lacking.

It would be prudent to predicate the treatment of carcinoma arising in MGA on the stage of disease in the individual patient. Because of the insidiously invasive character of MGA, carcinoma arising in this condition is likely to extend microscopically well beyond the grossly apparent tumor. Therefore, it may be difficult to achieve negative margins in some instances. When breast conservation is selected, radiotherapy should be added. Adjuvant chemotherapy is recommended for patients with axillary lymph node metastases or with invasive tumors larger than 1 cm in the absence of nodal metastases.

## REFERENCES

### Adenosis

1. Ewing J. Epithelial tumors of the breast. In: Ewing J. *Neoplastic diseases,* 4th ed. Philadelphia: WB Saunders, 1919:780.
2. Foote FW Jr, Stewart FW. Comparative studies of cancerous versus non-cancerous breasts. *Ann Surg* 1945;12:6–53.
3. Urban JA, Adair FE. Sclerosing adenosis. *Cancer* 1949;2:625–634.
4. Heller EL, Fleming JC. Fibrosing adenomatosis of the breast. *Am J Clin Pathol* 1950;20:141–146.
5. Haagensen CD. Adenosis tumor. In: Haagensen CD. *Diseases of the breast,* 2nd ed. Philadelphia: WB Saunders, 1971:177–184.
6. Nielsen BB. Adenosis tumour of the breast—a clinicopathological investigation of 27 cases. *Histopathology* 1987;11:1259–1275.
6a. DiPiro PJ, Gulizia JA, Lester SC, et al. Mammographic and sonographic appearances of nodular adenosis. *AJR Am J Roentgenol* 2000;175:31–34.

7. Eusebi V, Azzopardi JG. Vascular infiltration in benign breast disease. *J Pathol* 1976;118:9–16.
8. Silverman JF, Dabbs DJ, Gilbert CF. Fine needle aspiration cytology of adenosis tumor of the breast with immunocytochemical and ultrastructural observations. *Acta Cytol* 1989;33:181–187.
9. Wellings SR, Roberts P. Electron microscopy of sclerosing adenosis and infiltrating duct carcinoma of the human mammary gland. *J Natl Cancer Inst* 1963;30:267–287.
10. Jao W, Recant W, Swerdlow MA. Comparative ultrastructure of tubular carcinoma and sclerosing adenosis of the breast. *Cancer* 1976;38:180–186.
11. Simpson JF, Page DL, Dupont WD. Apocrine adenosis—a mimic of mammary carcinoma. *Surg Pathol* 1990;3:289–299.
12. Carter DJ, Rosen PP. Atypical apocrine metaplasia in sclerosing lesions of the breast. A study of 51 patients. *Mod Pathol* 1991;4:1–5.
13. Seidman JD, Aston M, Lefkowitz M. Atypical apocrine adenosis of the breast. A clinicopathologic study of 37 patients with 8.7-year follow-up. *Cancer* 1996;77:2529–2537.
13a. Selim A-GA, El-Ayat G, Wells CA. c-erbB2 oncoprotein expression, gene amplification and chromosome 17 aneusomy in apocrine adenosis of the breast. *J Pathol* 2000;191:138–142.
14. Taylor HB, Norris HJ. Epithelial invasion of nerves in benign diseases of the breast. *Cancer* 1967;20:2245–2249.
15. Davies JD. Neural invasion in benign mammary dysplasia. *J Pathol* 1973;109:225–231.
16. Lee K-C, Chan JKC, Gwi E. Tubular adenosis of the breast. A distinctive benign lesion mimicking invasive carcinoma. *Am J Surg Pathol* 1996;20:46–54.
17. Oberman HA, Markey BA. Non-invasive carcinoma of the breast presenting in adenosis. *Mod Pathol* 1991;4:31–35.
18. Fechner RE. Lobular carcinoma *in situ* in sclerosing adenosis. A potential source of confusion with invasive carcinoma. *Am J Surg Pathol* 1981;5:233–239.
19. Abati AD, Kimmel M, Rosen PP. Apocrine mammary carcinoma: a clinicopathologic study of 72 cases. *Am J Clin Pathol* 1990;94:371–377.
20. Eusebi V, Collina G, Bussolati G. Carcinoma *in situ* in sclerosing adenosis of the breast: an immunocytochemical study. *Semin Diagn Pathol* 1989;6:146–152.
21. Prasad ML, Osborne MP, Hoda SA. Observations on the histopathologic diagnosis of microinvasive carcinoma of the breast. *Anat Pathol* 1998;3:209–232.
22. Kern WH, Brooks RN. Atypical epithelial hyperplasia associated with breast cancer and fibrocystic disease. *Cancer* 1969;24:668–675.
23. Page DL, Van der Zwaag R, Rogers LW, et al. Relation between component parts of fibrocystic disease complex and breast cancer. *J Natl Cancer Inst* 1978;61:1055–1063.

24. Dupont WD, Page DL. Risk factors for breast cancer in women with proliferative breast disease. *N Engl J Med* 1985;312:146–151.
25. Jensen RA, Page DL, DuPont WD, et al. Invasive breast cancer risk in women with sclerosing adenosis. *Cancer* 1989;64:1977–1983.
26. Bodian CA, Perzin KH, Lattes R, et al. Prognostic significance of benign proliferative breast disease. *Cancer* 1993;71:3896–3907.
27. Carter CL, Corle DK, Micozzi MS, et al. A prospective study of the development of breast cancer in 16,692 women with benign breast disease. *Am J Epidemiol* 1988;128:467–477.
28. Hutchinson WB, Thomas DB, Hamlin WB, et al. Risk of breast cancer in women with benign breast disease. *J Natl Cancer Inst* 1980;65:13–20.
29. Kodlin D, Winger EE, Morgenstern NL, et al. Chronic mastopathy and breast cancer. *Cancer* 1977;39:2603–2607.
30. Krieger N, Hiatt RA. Risk of breast cancer after benign breast diseases, variation by histologic type, degree of atypia, age at biopsy, and length of follow-up. *Am J Epidemiol* 1992;136:619–631.

## Microglandular Adenosis

31. Linell F. Breast carcinoma: aspects of early stages, progression and related problems. *Acta Path Microbiol Scand (A)* 1980;272[Suppl]: 123–128.
32. McDivitt RW, Stewart FW, Berg JW. *Tumors of the breast. Atlas of tumor pathology, 2nd series, fascicle 2*. Bethesda, MD: Armed Forces Institute of Pathology, 1968:91.
33. Rosen PP. *Microglandular adenosis*. Anatomic Pathology Check Sample. No. AP11-12 (1977). Chicago: American Society of Clinical Pathologists, 1978.
34. Clement PB, Azzopardi JG. Microglandular adenosis of the breast. A lesion simulating tubular carcinoma. *Histopathology* 1983;7:169–180.
35. Rosen PP. Microglandular adenosis. *Am J Surg Pathol* 1983;7: 137–144.
36. Tavassoli FA, Norris HJ. Microglandular adenosis of the breast. *Am J Surg Pathol* 1983;7:731–737.
37. James BA, Cranor ML, Rosen PP. Carcinoma of the breast arising in microglandular adenosis. *Am J Clin Pathol* 1993;100:507–513.
38. Eusebi V, Faschini MP, Betts CM, et al. Microglandular adenosis, apocrine adenosis and tubular carcinoma of the breast. An immunohistochemical comparison. *Am J Surg Pathol* 1993;17:99–109.
39. Rosenblum MK, Purrazzella R, Rosen PP. Is microglandular adenosis a precancerous disease? A study of carcinoma arising therein. *Am J Surg Pathol* 1986;10:237–245.
39a. Damiani S, Pasquinelli G, Lamovec J, et al. Acinic cell carcinoma of the breast: an immunohistochemical and ultrastructural study. *Virchows Arch* 2000;437:74–81.
40. Tsuda H, Mukai K, Fukutomi T, et al. Malignant progression of adenomyoepithelial adenosis of the breast. *Pathol Int* 1994;44: 475–479.
41. Kay S. Microglandular adenosis of the female mammary gland: study of a case with ultrastructural observations. *Hum Pathol* 1985; 16:637–640.

# CHAPTER 8

# Fibroepithelial Neoplasms

## SCLEROSING LOBULAR HYPERPLASIA (FIBROADENOMATOID MASTOPATHY)

### Clinical Presentation

This benign proliferative lesion is noted initially as a localized tumor that is up to 8 cm in diameter (mean, about 4 cm), usually in the upper outer quadrant of the breast (1,2). Skin retraction and pain are absent, but the tumor may be tender. Asymptomatic lesions have been detected by mammography (2). The most frequent mammographic finding is a well-defined mass. Microcalcifications may be present (3). The imaging characteristics are not sufficiently specific to distinguish sclerosing lobular hyperplasia from a fibroadenoma. Patients range in age from 14 to 46 years (mean age, about 32 years) (1,2). There is no significant association with oral contraceptive use. Sclerosing lobular hyperplasia occurs in black and in white women (2).

### Gross and Microscopic Pathology

The excised specimen is composed of firm, nodular, tan tissue with a granular appearance on the cut surface. Microscopic examination reveals enlarged lobules composed of an increased number of intralobular glands. The intralobular stroma is collagenized with loss of stromal mucopolysaccharide, and there is variable sclerosis of the interlobular stroma (Fig. 8.1). Individual lobules and groups of lobules have the appearance of miniature fibroadenomas. The lobular glands have distinct epithelial and myoepithelial components, each composed of a single layer of cells. Secretory activity is minimal or absent.

Sclerosing lobular hyperplasia or fibroadenomatoid mastopathy is found in breast tissue surrounding about 50% of fibroadenomas (1). This association suggests that the same or related factors contribute to the pathogenesis of both lesions. The ratio of sclerosing lobular hyperplasia to fibroadenoma in one series was 9.3:1, a relationship consistent with the hypothesis that some fibroadenomas arise as localized foci of accelerated proliferation in a background of sclerosing lobular hyperplasia (1). Because the initial clinical sign of fibroadenoma is a dominant tumor, its association

with sclerosing lobular hyperplasia may be overlooked clinically and pathologically.

### Treatment and Prognosis

A diagnosis of sclerosing lobular hyperplasia usually is not made preoperatively, and most patients have a clinical diagnosis of fibroadenoma or fibrocystic change. Excisional biopsy of the palpable lesion is adequate therapy. No systematic follow-up study has documented the frequency of recurrence. Anecdotal experience suggests that recurrence as a fibroadenoma occurs infrequently but that this condition may contribute to the syndrome of multiple recurrent fibroadenomas.

## FIBROADENOMA

This benign tumor arises from the epithelium and stroma of the terminal duct–lobular unit. It is the most common breast tumor clinically and pathologically in adolescent and young women. In one consecutive series of patients, 44% of fibroadenomas occurred in postmenopausal women (4), accounting for 20% of benign masses and 12% of all masses in postmenopausal patients. A study of fibroadenomas from premenopausal women found no difference in mitotic index or nuclear volume in fibroadenomas obtained in the luteal and secretory menstrual phases (5). These researchers concluded that fibroadenomatous epithelium is independent of the cyclic action of circulating hormones and is influenced mainly by paracrine factors.

Risk factors for developing fibroadenomas have not been extensively investigated. In Connecticut, Canny et al. carried out a case-control study of 251 women with fibroadenomas (6). Women younger than 45 years of age with fibroadenomas were less likely than controls to have taken contraceptives. This difference was not observed in women older than 45 years when a fibroadenoma was diagnosed, and no significant association was found between reduced fibroadenoma risk and oral contraceptive use in black women, regardless of age. On the other hand, a significant, positive

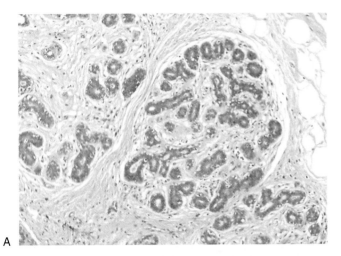

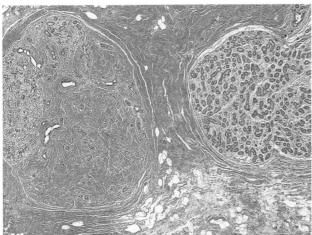

**FIG. 8.1.** *Fibroadenomatoid mastopathy (sclerosing lobular hyperplasia).* **A:** The tumor is composed of enlarged lobules. **B:** In this case, one lobule with sclerotic stroma has the appearance of a small fibroadenoma.

correlation was found between fibroadenomas and exogenous estrogen-replacement therapy, regardless of the patient's age. The reduced risk for developing a fibroadenoma among users of oral contraceptives is not related to the extent of epithelial atypia in the fibroadenoma (7). A case-control study of Australian women reported a direct association between contraceptive use before age 20 and the risk of developing a fibroadenoma (8). Risk was inversely related to the Quetelet index and the number of full-term pregnancies. In this series, the use of estrogen-replacement therapy was not significantly related to the presence of fibroadenomas.

Cytogenetic abnormalities have been detected in 20% to 30% of fibroadenomas (9–13). These abnormalities usually involved translocations, but no consistent pattern with respect to specific chromosomes or breakpoints was identified. In one report, cells in three fibroadenomas from a single patient exhibited the same chromosomal abnormality (9). Kobayashi et al. used the polymerase chain reaction for clonal analysis of the stroma in multiple fibroadenomas from a single patient and determined that all lesions were poly-

clonal (14). Immunoreactivity for alpha estrogen receptor was present only in epithelial cells. Using a technique similar to that of Kobayashi et al. (14), Kasami et al. detected stromal monoclonality in 1 of 20 (5%) complex fibroadenomas and 1 of 25 (4%) simple fibroadenomas (15). The microdissected epithelium was polyclonal in all tumors, including the two with monoclonal stroma. These researchers commented that "the one monoclonal simple fibroadenoma was also the only one with mixed features to contain a phyllodes component," an observation that suggests that the sample analyzed as a "simple fibroadenoma" might have been a fibroadenoma-like part of a heterogeneous phyllodes tumor (PT). Multiple bilateral fibroadenomas diagnosed simultaneously in two identical female twins have been described, but the lesions were not subjected to cytogenetic analysis (16).

Epidemiologic studies suggest that the risk of developing breast carcinoma is increased in women who have had a fibroadenoma compared with various control groups. The relative risk has been reported to be 1.6 (17), 1.7 (18,19), 2.2 (20), and 2.6 (21). Some investigators have not excluded patients with synchronous tumors, and others have limited their analysis to patients who developed invasive carcinoma. In two reports, the relative risk was significantly higher for patients with a concurrent fibroadenoma and benign proliferative changes (20,22). Dupont et al. found that increased risk of breast carcinoma was dependent on the presence of proliferative changes in the fibroadenoma itself or in the surrounding breast and a family history of breast carcinoma (20). The relative risk for women who had a fibroadenoma with cysts, sclerosing adenosis, calcifications, or papillary apocrine metaplasia (complex fibroadenoma) was 3.1. When benign proliferative changes were present in the nonfibroadenomatous breast, the relative risk was 3.88; for women with a complex fibroadenoma and a family history of breast carcinoma, the risk was 3.72. No significant increase in risk was found among women with noncomplex fibroadenomas and no family history of breast carcinoma.

## Clinical Presentation

The age distribution ranges from the early teens to more than 70 years of age (mean age, about 30; median age, around 25 years) (23). Fewer than 5% of women with a fibroadenoma as their presenting tumor are older than 50 years or postmenopausal.

In most cases, the initial symptom is a painless, firm, well-circumscribed solitary tumor found by the patient. A small percentage of fibroadenomas are nonpalpable tumors that are detected by mammography (Fig. 8.2). The left breast is affected slightly more often than the right, and the single most frequent location is the upper outer quadrant (23). Multiple fibroadenomas occur in about 15% of patients, with equal proportions detected synchronously and metachronously in the same or opposite breast. Foster et al. found that 36% of metachronous fibroadenomas developed in the same quadrant as the first fibroadenoma after a mean interval of about 4 years (23).

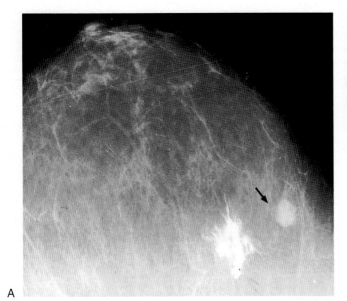
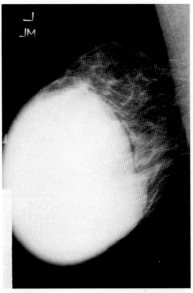

**FIG. 8.2.** *Fibroadenoma.* **A:** The nonpalpable tumor was detected as a homogeneous, oval, circumscribed mass on this mammogram *(arrow).* The stellate white focus is the site of dye injected for localization of the lesion at surgery. **B:** This fibroadenoma nearly fills the right breast of an 18-year-old girl in a mediolateral view.

Fibroadenomas and cysts may be indistinguishable on palpation and by mammography. Aspiration with a needle typically causes cysts to collapse. Solid and cystic lesions are readily differentiated by ultrasound examination. Most fibroadenomas have ultrasound features of a benign tumor. A minority of fibroadenomas, including lactating adenomas, have irregular margins, heterogeneous appearance, and posterior shadowing, which may suggest a malignant tumor (24). The magnetic resonance imaging (MRI) characteristics of a large fibroadenoma containing fluid-filled epithelial-lined clefts may suggest a diagnosis of PT (25). The MRI appearance of fibroadenomas is variable and influenced by the structure and relative proportions of epithelial and stromal components (26). Large, coarse calcifications are not uncommon in fibroadenomas after menopause.

Estrogen receptors have been demonstrated by biochemical analysis in fibroadenomas. Estrogen receptor activity is largely in the epithelium of fibroadenomas examined by immunohistochemistry (27,28), whereas progesterone receptor reportedly is also localized in the stroma (29).

Most fibroadenomas are not larger than 3 cm. In one series, only 10% of the tumors were larger than 4.0 cm (23). Tumors larger than 4 cm are significantly more frequent in patients 20 years of age or younger than in older patients (23). An occasional tumor may grow to involve most or all of the breast. These tumors, often referred to as *adolescent giant fibroadenomas,* develop as solitary or multiple tumors shortly after puberty (30,31) (Figs. 8.2 and 8.3). One or both breasts can be affected.

Another uncommon syndrome occurring in adolescence is

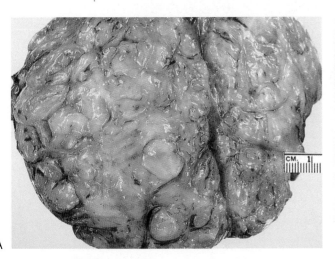
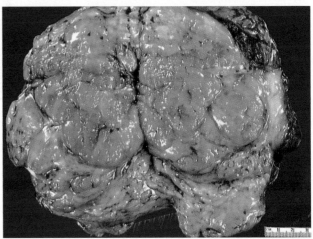

**FIG. 8.3.** *Fibroadenomas in young girls.* **A,B:** The tumors measured over 10 cm. The patients were 11 and 14 years old.

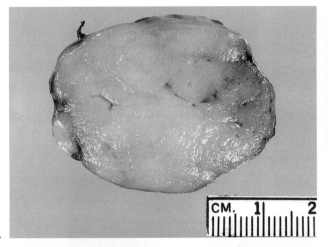

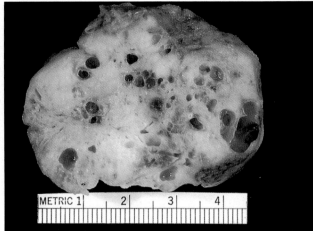

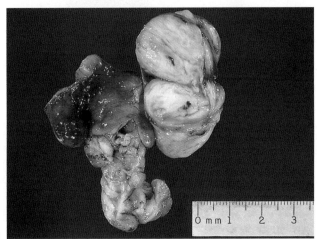

**FIG. 8.4.** *Fibroadenomas.* **A:** Relatively homogeneous cut surface. **B:** Multiple cysts are present. **C:** Two adjacent fibroadenomas, the larger of which *(above)* is solid, in contrast to the smaller, partly cystic tumor near the center of the picture.

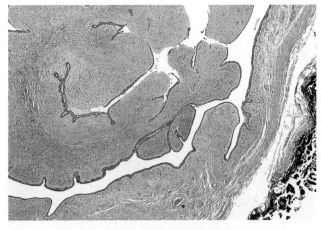

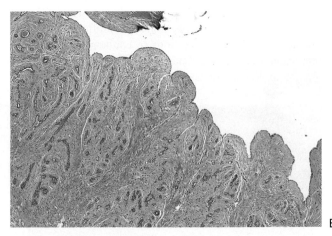

**FIG. 8.5.** *Fibroadenomas, cystic.* Whole-mount sections of cystic fibroadenomas. The tumor in **A** has fibrotic stroma, and adenosis is shown in **B**.

the metachronous and synchronous development of multiple fibroadenomas, usually in both breasts. This condition occurs more often in adolescent black girls than in white or Asian girls (31). Despite repeated excision, new tumors are formed in the remaining breast tissue, probably because the breast tissue exhibits diffuse fibroadenomatoid hyperplasia. The familial occurrence of multiple successive fibroadenomas has been observed.

## Gross Pathology

Fibroadenomas often are excised by using blunt dissection to peel away the surrounding tissue. The outer surface of a "shelled-out" fibroadenoma has a smooth bosselated contour. The cut surface of the bisected tumor is composed of bulging, firm, and gray, white, or tan tissue (Fig. 8.4). A minority of fibroadenomas have a myxoid or gelatinous appearance. Some tumors appear to be composed of multiple aggregated nodules divided by septae.

Fine clefts in the tissue can be identified in the cut surface of many tumors examined with a magnifying glass. Infrequently, these elongated spaces are pronounced. Discrete round cysts are sometimes present, usually measuring 1 mm to 1.0 cm or more in diameter, and rarely the tumor is so cystic that it grossly resembles a cystic papilloma (Figs. 8.4 and 8.5).

## Microscopic Pathology

Several terms have been used to subclassify fibroadenomas. Large or giant fibroadenomas are histologically indistinguishable from counterparts of average size. Tumors described by this term have included benign PT and hamartoma, and therefore this term is best reserved to designate a clinical presentation rather than a specific pathologic diagnosis. More than 90% of fibroadenomas are of the adult type, with the remainder fulfilling criteria for a diagnosis of juvenile fibroadenoma or other unusual variants of fibroadenoma.

Some tumors referred to as *adenomas* are unusual types of fibroadenomas. The so-called *tubular adenoma* (32) or *pure adenoma* (33) is a variant of pericanalicular fibroadenoma with an exceptionally prominent or florid adenosis-like epithelial proliferation (Figs. 8.6 and 8.7). The clinical presentation as a mobile, circumscribed, painless mass is indistinguishable from a typical fibroadenoma. These tumors are not associated with pregnancy or oral contraceptive use (34). They tend to be softer than the average fibroadenoma and tan rather than white. Microscopic examination reveals closely approximated round or oval glandular structures composed of a single layer of epithelium supported by a layer of myoepithelial cells. A small amount of secretion is frequently present in the glandular lumens, even in tumors from patients who are not pregnant or who are taking oral contraceptives (35). This secretion is not immunoreactive for alpha-lactalbumin (36). Foci of florid adenosis can be encountered within an otherwise ordinary fibroadenoma.

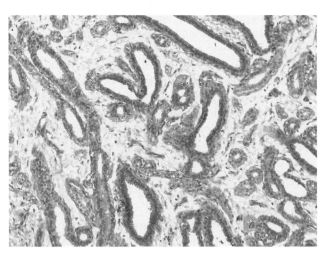

**FIG. 8.6.** *Tubular adenoma.* The glandular proliferation has a pattern that resembles tubular adenosis.

Other so-called adenomas are unrelated to the fibroadenoma category. *Apocrine adenoma* is a localized nodular focus of prominent papillary and cystic apocrine metaplasia (37,38). Nodular foci of sclerosing adenosis with apocrine metaplasia have been variously termed *apocrine adenoma* and *apocrine adenosis*. *Ductal adenoma* (39,40) and *pleomorphic adenoma* (41–43) are variants of intraductal papilloma or adenomyoepithelioma, and are discussed in Chapter 6 relating to the latter group of tumors.

The origin of a fibroadenoma from the terminal duct–lobular unit was elegantly demonstrated by Demetrakopoulos, who used a serial section reconstruction technique (44). The stroma caused numerous invaginations in the walls of branches of the duct within the tumor corresponding to the intracanalicular pattern seen in histologic sections. The significance of specialized stroma in the growth of fibroadenomas was emphasized by Koerner and O'Connell (45). These

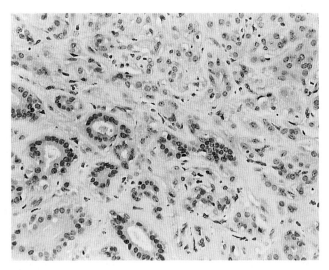

**FIG. 8.7.** *Tubular adenoma.* The growth pattern resembles florid adenosis.

observations confirmed the long-held view that fibroadenomas are formed as a result of proliferation of stroma around the terminal duct and within the lobule (46).

The histologic hallmark of all fibroadenomas is concurrent proliferation of glandular or stromal elements. Most adult fibroadenomas have growth patterns that can be divided into categories referred to as *intracanalicular* and *pericanalicular*. The former pattern is produced when the stroma is abundant enough to compress ducts into elongated linear branching structures with slit-like lumens. When the ducts are not compressed by the stroma, the architecture is described as having a pericanalicular pattern. These structural features are of no known prognostic or clinical significance, and many tumors have both components. Fibroadenomas with a prominent intracanalicular pattern may be mistaken for benign PTs, especially in needle core biopsy samples.

In most instances, the microscopic diagnosis of a fibroadenoma is accomplished without difficulty when the tumor has a sharply defined border and the pericanalicular or intracanalicular growth pattern. The distinction between some variants of fibroadenoma, especially those with cellular stroma, and benign PTs, however, is sometimes problematic and unclear. In these situations, it may be helpful to review the characteristic cytologic features of fibroadenomas in formulating the diagnosis. Unfortunately, neoplasms that ultimately recur with the histologic and clinical features of a PT may present in a form that is histologically not distinguishable from a fibroadenoma.

Microscopic characteristics of fibroadenomatous stroma are especially important diagnostic features. The appearance of the stroma varies from one fibroadenoma to another, but it is usually homogeneous in any given lesion. This is an important distinction from PTs, which can exhibit considerable stromal heterogeneity, including regions indistinguishable from a fibroadenoma. In the average adult fibroadenoma, the relative proportions of epithelium and stroma are evenly balanced throughout the tumor (Figs. 8.8 and 8.9); the density of stromal cellularity is not related to tumor size. Fibroadenomas from women younger than 20 years of age, however, tend to have more cellular stroma as a group than tumors from older women, and this effect is seen in fibroadenomas stratified by size in these age categories (15). Mitotic figures are extremely unusual in fibroadenomatous stroma. Elastic tissue is virtually absent from the stroma of fibroadenomas. The fibroblastic stromal cells are variably CD34 positive, and immunoreactivity for actin is seen when there is myofibroblastic proliferation. Estrogen and progesterone receptors are usually present in the epithelium of a fibroadenoma. Stromal cells are variably reactive for progesterone receptor and at most weakly positive for estrogen receptor.

Numerous electron microscopic studies of fibroadenomas have characterized the stromal cells as fibroblastic, although a few investigators noted myoid or myofibroblastic differentiation (47–50). Ohtani and Sasano classified fibroadenomas into three groups on the basis of their stromal patterns: myxoid, fibrous-cellular, and sclerotic (49). Ultrastructural study of myxoid and fibrocellular stroma revealed that the cells were fibroblasts containing actin-type microfilaments that lacked the dense bodies characteristic of smooth-muscle cells.

Reddick et al. reported that stromal cells in most fibroadenomas studied, including one tumor characterized as a cellular fibroadenoma (juvenile giant fibroadenoma), actually were fibroblasts (50). The cytoplasm of individual cells contained small numbers of lysosomes, a Golgi complex, and abundant rough endoplasmic reticulum. Junctional complexes were found between fibroblasts in most tumors. Myoid cells, characterized by numerous filaments with dense body condensations, were present in the stroma of one fibroadenoma. This finding was not unexpected because myoid differentiation of myofibroblasts is sometimes present in a fibroadenoma.

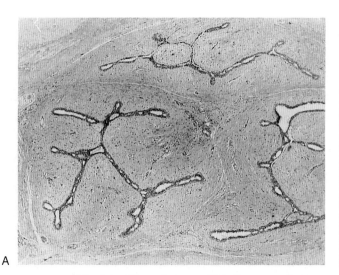

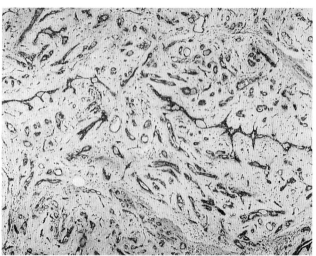

A

B

**FIG. 8.8.** *Fibroadenoma.* **A,B:** Two growth patterns in which the underlying lobular structure is preserved. Sclerosing adenosis is present in **B**.

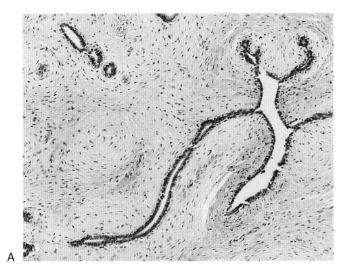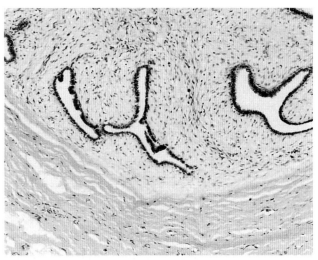

A                                                                          B

**FIG. 8.9.** *Fibroadenoma.* Homogeneous stroma within **A** and at the border **B** of the tumor.

Unusual forms of stromal differentiation are encountered in a minority of fibroadenomas, including smooth muscle (myoid) metaplasia (51) (Fig. 8.10) and adipose differentiation. Most fibroepithelial tumors with adipose differentiation are PTs (52). Giant cells, sometimes with multiple nuclei, are found in the stroma of fibroadenomas (53,54) as well as in PTs (54). The nuclei of multinucleated stromal giant cells may be pleomorphic and hyperchromatic (Fig. 8.11). In some tumors, these cells have a florette pattern. These multinucleated cells have ultrastructural features consistent with fibroblasts. In some cases, the giant cells were reactive for CD68, a histiocytic marker, and only a minority of these cells were immunoreactive for actin or CD34. Despite their

atypical cytologic appearance, the presence of these cells does not influence the clinical course of the lesion. A tumor that has the structural features of a fibroadenoma should not be classified as a PT because it contains multinucleated stromal giant cells. Osteochondroid metaplasia in a fibroadenoma is uncommon and almost always occurs in postmenopausal women (55,56). Small fibroadenomas with calcification and ossification detected by mammography may be sampled by needle core biopsy.

The stroma of fibroadenomas can undergo marked myxoid change (Fig. 8.12). Specimens from such lesions examined by frozen section, by imprint cytology, by fine needle aspiration, or by needle core biopsy may be mistaken for

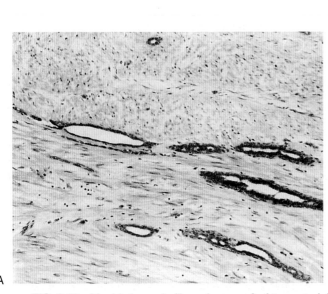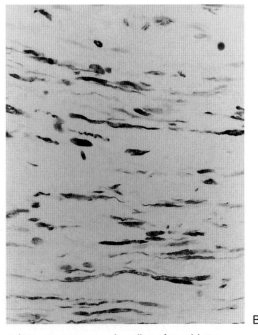

A                                                                               B

**FIG. 8.10.** *Myoid stroma in fibroadenoma.* **A:** Attenuated ductal structures among bundles of myoid stromal cells. **B:** Immunoreactivity of actin in the stroma (anti-HHF35, avidin-biotin).

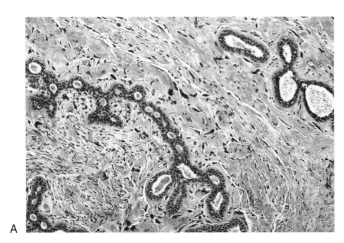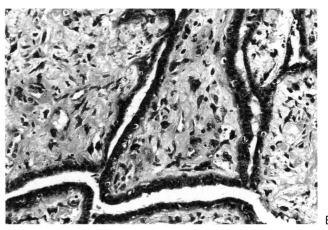

**FIG. 8.11.** *Fibroadenoma with stromal giant cells.* **A:** Cells with hyperchromatic nuclei are present in pseudoangiomatous stromal hyperplasia in a fibroadenoma. **B:** Multinucleated stromal giant cells in another tumor.

mucinous carcinoma. Myxoid fibroadenomas and myxomatous stromal masses have been encountered in the familial condition of cutaneous and cardiac myxomas, spotty cutaneous pigmentation, endocrine overactivity, and melanotic schwannomas referred to as *Carney's syndrome* (57). In this condition, myxoid change is more conspicuous in the intralobular than in the interlobular stroma; however, most patients with a myxoid fibroadenoma do not have a known systemic abnormality.

The epithelial component of fibroadenomas is also prone to various alterations, including foci of squamous metaplasia (58), cyst formation, and the spectrum of proliferation termed *fibrocystic change,* including apocrine metaplasia. Fibroadenomas with sclerosing adenosis, papillary apocrine hyperplasia, cysts, or epithelial calcifications have been designated as complex (20) (Figs. 8.13–8.15). At least one of these features must be present for the lesion to be classified as complex. Compared with controls, patients with complex fibroadenomas had a higher relative risk for developing breast carcinoma than women who had noncomplex fibroadenomas (20). Prominent myoid metaplasia arising in sclerosing adenosis within a complex fibroadenoma is a source of smooth-muscle differentiation in fibroadenomatous stroma. Marked epithelial hyperplasia can be encountered in a complex fibroadenoma or in the absence of a background of fibrocystic changes. Generally, these proliferative foci have the same features as hyperplastic lesions outside a fibroadenoma. Although once attributed to oral contraceptive use (59), these changes occur independent of exogenous hormones (60,61). Excessive fibrocystic changes, especially papillary epithelial hyperplasia and sclerosing adenosis, can mask the basic fibroadenomatous nature of a tumor, espe-

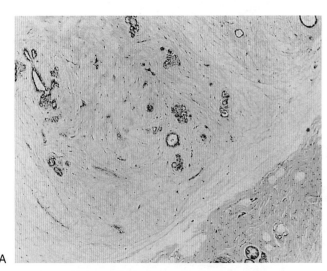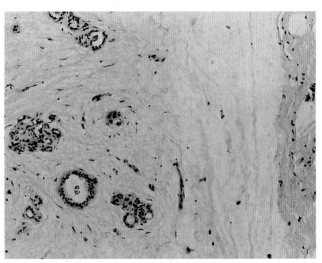

**FIG. 8.12.** *Fibroadenoma with myxoid stroma.* **A:** Sparse ductal and lobular units in the tumor. **B:** A sharp border between the myxoid stroma of the tumor and the breast parenchyma is evident on the *right.*

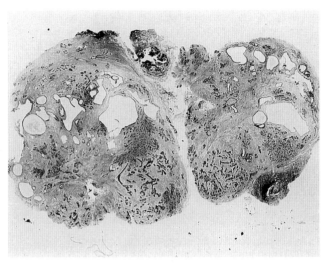

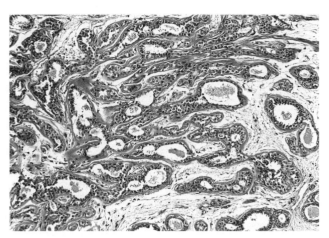

**FIG. 8.15.** *Fibroadenoma with sclerosing adenosis.* Thickened basement membranes are not unusual when sclerosing adenosis occurs in a fibroadenoma.

**FIG. 8.13.** *Complex fibroadenoma.* Whole mount histologic section showing cysts and dark, irregular foci of sclerosing adenosis.

cially in the limited sample of a needle core biopsy. Lobular and ductal carcinomas can arise in fibroadenomas (Figs. 8.16–8.18). For a discussion of carcinoma arising in fibroadenomas, see Chapter 35.

Secretory hyperplasia sometimes occurs diffusely in fibroadenomas during pregnancy (35), or a preexisting fibroadenoma may be unaltered (36). Fibroadenomas with secretory hyperplasia should be distinguished from the tumor commonly referred to as *lactating adenoma,* which is a compact aggregate of lobules exhibiting secretory hyperplasia (Fig. 8.19). Most tumors characterized as lactating adenomas actually are diagnosed and excised during pregnancy and do not have lactational secretion. Secretory hyperplasia in the lesional tissue is histologically and ultrastructurally similar to the physiologic changes of pregnancy in the surrounding breast (36,62) (Fig. 8.20). If the tumor is allowed to remain in

the breast or it is not detected until after delivery, it will be classified as a fibroadenoma with lactational change. Alpha-lactalbumin is detectable in the epithelium of lactating adenomas (36). Involutional change in a lactating adenoma after treatment with bromocriptine has been reported (62). Tumors with the histologic appearance of lactating adenomas can arise in ectopic breast tissue during pregnancy (35). One of the most unusual instances of this phenomenon is lactational change in breast tissue present in an ovarian cystic teratoma removed from a 20-year-old woman at the time of cesarean section for a full-term pregnancy (63). Fibroadenomas and "tubular adenomas" with focal lactational change are encountered rarely in women who are neither pregnant nor postpartum (35).

Fibroadenomas and lactating adenomas are prone to develop foci of infarction during pregnancy (64), but infarction can occur in tumors removed from patients who were neither pregnant nor lactating (65,66). The tumor may be tender or painful. Recent onset of discomfort in a previously painless tumor is suggestive of infarction in a fibroadenoma (65,66). The area of the infarct can be appreciated grossly as a relatively well demarcated, pale yellow or white zone of coagulation necrosis. Microscopic examination of the necrotic region reveals the ghostly outline of the underlying structure of the fibroadenoma in hematoxylin and eosin (H&E)-stained sections (Fig. 8.21). The architecture of the tissue can be seen to better advantage by using a reticulin stain (65) and, if the tissue is not too degenerated, by using a cytokeratin stain. Thrombosed vessels have been detected in some infarcted lesions (66).

*Juvenile fibroadenomas* account for about 4% of all fibroadenomas (67). These patients tend to be younger than the average age for adult fibroadenomas, with most younger than 20 years of age (67,68) (Fig. 8.22). Tumors with the histologic features of juvenile fibroadenoma have been found in adult women up to 72 years of age (69). Most patients initially have a single, painless, discrete mass that may grow

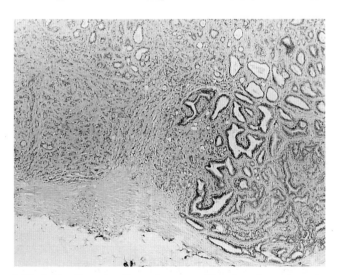

**FIG. 8.14.** *Complex fibroadenoma with sclerosing adenosis.* Sclerosis is shown on the *left* and dilated gland on the *right.*

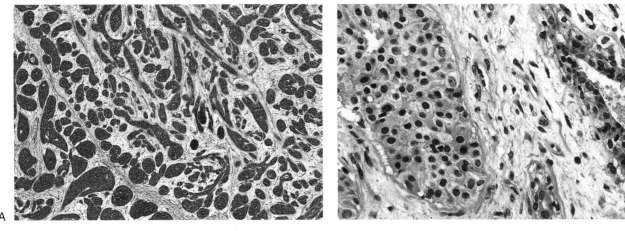

**FIG. 8.16.** *Fibroadenoma with lobular carcinoma* in situ. **A:** Lobular carcinoma *in situ* fills the sclerosing adenosis glands of a fibroadenoma. **B:** *In situ* carcinoma *(left)* and uninvolved gland *(right)*. Figure 8.15 is from the same tumor in a 54-year-old woman.

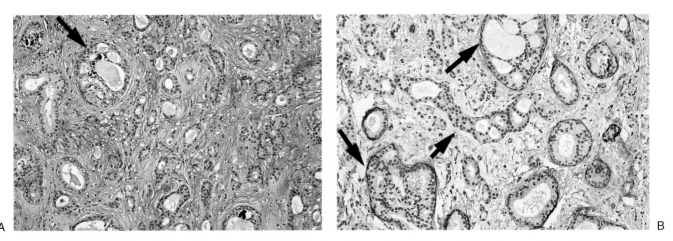

**FIG. 8.17.** *Myxoid fibroadenoma with invasive duct carcinoma.* **A:** This myxoid fibroadenoma from a 30-year-old woman contains cribriform intraductal carcinoma *(arrow)* and invasive duct carcinoma composed of small well-differentiated glands. **B:** Myoepithelial cells are present around ducts with intraductal carcinoma *(long arrows)*, and absent around invasive carcinoma glands *(short arrow)* in this myosin heavy-chain immunostain (avidin-biotin).

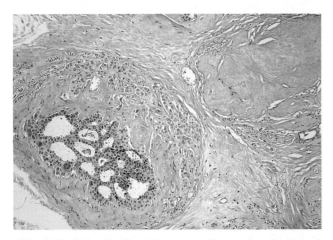

**FIG. 8.18.** *Sclerotic fibroadenoma with invasive duct carcinoma.* Cribriform intraductal carcinoma is surrounded by invasive duct carcinoma at the edge of a sclerotic fibroadenoma.

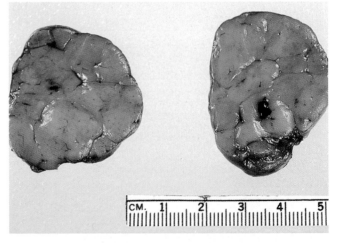

**FIG. 8.19.** *Lactating adenoma.*

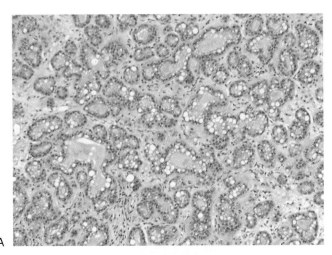
A

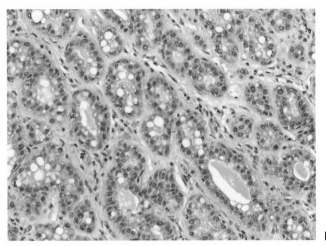
B

**FIG. 8.20.** *Lactating adenoma.* **A:** The glandular elements diffusely distributed in sparsely cellular stroma. **B:** These glandular cells have vacuolated cytoplasm.

rapidly, sometimes becoming large enough to cause marked asymmetry. Multiple and recurrent tumors occur more often in black patients (68). In one study consisting only of black women, eight patients had multiple lesions; in 13 patients, the tumors were solitary (67). The age distribution and median age of women with single and multiple tumors were similar at the time of first operation. The frequency of recurrences decreases in early adulthood and lesions that are not excised may stop growing in adulthood, remaining stable even during pregnancy (68).

Juvenile fibroadenomas are grossly indistinguishable from the adult variety of the tumor (67). In one series, the mean sizes of solitary and multiple tumors were 2.8 and 2.2 cm, respectively, with the largest measuring 13 cm in a patient with multiple tumors. Other investigators have reported solitary lesions up to 22 cm in diameter (68).

Juvenile fibroadenomas are characterized microscopically by stromal cellularity and epithelial hyperplasia. The architecture is more often pericanalicular than intracanalicular or a mixture of these patterns with no appreciable overall differences between tumors in patients with solitary and multiple fibroadenomas (68). Heterogeneity may be seen in the histologic appearance of different tumors from a patient with multiple lesions. The tumor border is usually well defined microscopically, sometimes by a pseudocapsule of compressed parenchyma (Fig. 8.23). Secondary peripheral nodules of fibroadenomatous growth outside the main tumor are encountered in a minority of cases, usually in patients who develop multiple tumors.

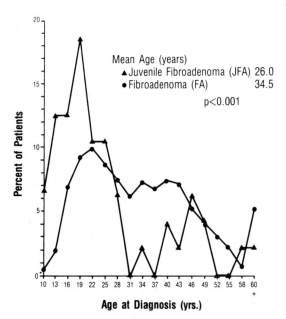

**FIG. 8.22.** *Age distribution of typical and juvenile fibroadenomas.* Juvenile fibroadenomas have a lower mean age and biphasic age distribution. (From Mies C, Rosen PP. Juvenile fibroadenoma with atypical epithelial hyperplasia. *Am J Surg Pathol* 1987;11:184–190, with permission.)

**FIG. 8.21.** *Infarcted lactating adenoma.* Degenerating glands in an infarcted tumor.

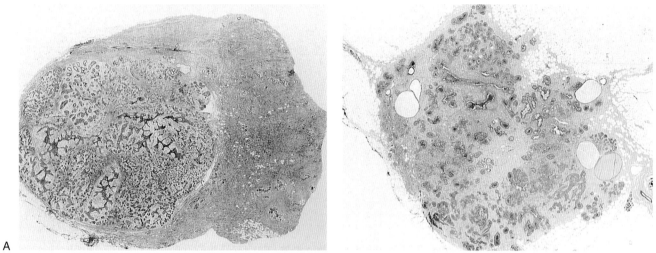

**FIG. 8.23.** *Juvenile fibroadenoma.* Whole-mount histologic sections of two tumors. **A:** The lesion has a circumscribed border and the typical architecture of a fibroadenoma. **B:** The tumor has a slightly irregular border, a patchy distribution of epithelium, and a few cysts.

The myxoid mucopolysaccharide is largely absent from juvenile fibroadenomas. Mitoses rarely are detected in the stroma. Little or no atypia and pleomorphism are encountered in the bipolar fibroblastic stromal cells (Fig. 8.24). The fibroblastic histogenesis of stroma has been confirmed by electron microscopy (50).

Epithelial elements usually are distributed homogeneously in the tumor without the stromal overgrowth that characterizes a PT. It is exceptional to find a ×40 microscopic field occupied entirely by stroma. Most juvenile fibroadenomas feature conspicuous epithelial hyperplasia that may have a ductal, lobular, or combined ductal–lobular configuration. Several patterns of epithelial proliferation can be found, including laciform, papillary, solid, lobular–terminal ductal and cribriform (69) (Fig. 8.25). Usually, more than one pattern is present in a given tumor. The laciform pattern features a fenestrated proliferation of ductal epithelial that

resembles cribriform intraductal carcinoma; however, in contrast to this form of carcinoma, the epithelium in laciform hyperplasia contains a hyperplastic myoepithelial zone and has the cytologic features of micropapillary hyperplasia, including overlapping, streaming, nuclear condensation, and pyknosis of apical nuclei. The papillary type of hyperplasia typically arises in tumors with an intracanalicular architecture and may coexist with laciform hyperplasia to create complex branching fronds in dilated duct lumens. A hyperplastic myoepithelial cell layer is typically present. In solid hyperplasia, the epithelium fills expanded duct structures that have a largely pericanalicular distribution. Rather than the columnar cytology observed in laciform and papillary hyperplasia, solid hyperplasia features round to ovoid cells. The lobular–terminal duct pattern is present when the solid epithelial proliferation branches into lobular radicles.

Cellular pleomorphism and cytologic atypia are seen in all

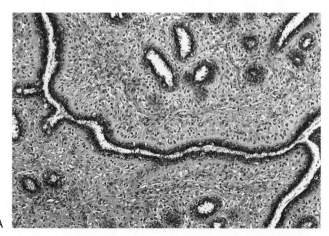
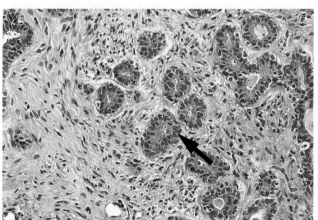

**FIG. 8.24.** *Juvenile fibroadenoma.* **A:** The stroma is moderately cellular. **B:** Mitotic activity is present in the epithelium (*arrow*).

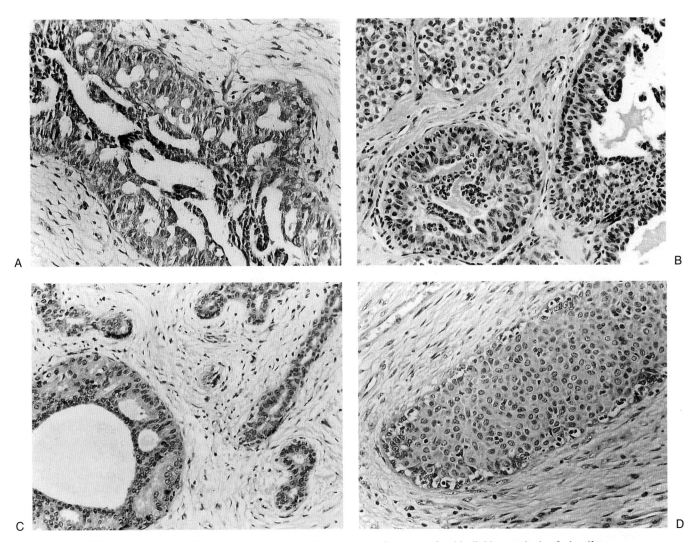

**FIG. 8.25.** *Juvenile fibroadenoma, epithelial hyperplasia.* Patterns of epithelial hyperplasia. **A:** Laciform and micropapillary. **B:** Micropapillary and solid. **C:** Cribriform. **D:** Solid.

histologic patterns of epithelial hyperplasia in juvenile fibroadenomas, but they tend to be more extreme in solid hyperplasia. Epithelial necrosis is not a feature of the hyperplasia in juvenile fibroadenomas, and the tumors ordinarily do not develop epithelial calcifications. Hyperplastic changes are rarely found in the surrounding breast tissue. It is unusual to find carcinoma in a juvenile fibroadenoma (Fig. 8.26).

**Cytology**

The fine needle aspiration (FNA) cytology specimen obtained from a fibroadenoma typically presents a characteristic combination of epithelial and stromal features (70–72). The findings considered to be diagnostic are abundant bipolar stromal cells, usually seen as bare nuclei, irregular flat sheets of epithelium composed of uniform evenly spaced polygonal cells, so-called antler horn clusters, and fenestrated or honeycomb sheets composed of similar cells. These features are especially useful in distinguishing be-

tween the aspirate from a fibroadenoma and that from benign proliferative (fibrocystic) changes. Making this distinction can be difficult if the fibroadenoma contains a substantial component of proliferative change. From 30% to 50% of aspirates from fibroadenomas contain foam cells and apocrine cells (72). Prominent nucleoli are encountered in the epithelium of at least 80% of fibroadenomas and pleomorphic nuclei in 25% (72). Failure to appreciate the cytologic variability that may be found in FNA specimens from fibroadenomas can lead to a false suspicion of or a false diagnosis of carcinoma (73). Conversely, careful attention must be paid to atypical cytologic features because fibroadenomas may contain carcinoma. FNA may induce hemorrhagic infarction in a fibroadenoma in nonpregnant patients (74).

The aspirate from a lactating adenoma is cellular (70). It differs from that of a typical fibroadenoma in lacking antler horn and honeycomb flat sheets of epithelium. The epithelium is distributed in three-dimensional acinar clusters, and there is a tendency to discohesion, resulting in many single

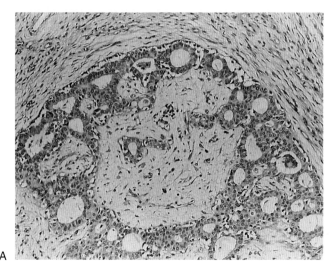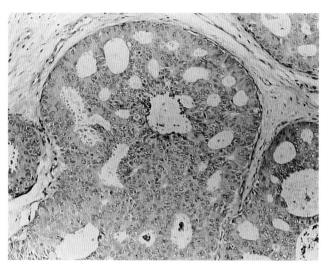

**FIG. 8.26.** *Carcinoma in a juvenile fibroadenoma.* The patient was 21 years of age. **A:** Cribriform hyperplasia. **B:** Cribriform intraductal carcinoma.

cells (75,76). The uniform nuclei have prominent nucleoli, and they often appear to be stripped of cytoplasm. The background may appear foamy, and the cytoplasm of intact cells is vacuolated.

### Treatment and Prognosis

Many solitary fibroadenomas are treated by local excision. When the preoperative clinical findings suggest this diagnosis, the tumor can be "shelled out" from the breast, but it is preferable to include at least a thin rim of surrounding normal breast to minimize the need for reexcision in rare instances when the lesion proves to be a PT. There is no evidence that ordinary adult fibroadenomas are susceptible to local recurrence or that they predispose to the development of PT if shelled out or incompletely excised.

Because fibroadenomas can be diagnosed reliably by FNA or needle core biopsy, there has been interest in conservative management consisting of clinical follow-up rather than excision (77,78). In one study, most tumors diagnosed clinically as fibroadenomas by FNA continued to grow before excision during a predetermined 12-month follow-up (78). A survey of patient preferences revealed that most women chose excisional biopsy, even if they were assured that the lesion was benign by FNA (77). Clinical and mammographic follow-up is recommended for women who do not undergo surgical excision after a needle core biopsy diagnosis of a fibroadenoma. If the needle core biopsy findings suggest a complex fibroadenoma or if atypical features are noted in the fibroadenomatous epithelium, excision of the tumor with sampling of the surrounding tissue should be performed to assess the epithelial component for evidence of occult carcinoma.

The distinction between a fibroadenoma and a benign PT is sometimes difficult in a FNA or needle core biopsy specimen. Because of the histologic heterogeneity of many PTs, small samples can be unrepresentative of the entire lesion

and indistinguishable from a fibroadenoma. If the sample obtained by needle core biopsy contains part of the border of the tumor, invasive growth is a clue to the presence of a PT.

Despite substantial epithelial proliferation, sometimes with considerable atypia and stromal cellularity, follow-up of patients with juvenile fibroadenomas has not revealed a predisposition to develop PT or carcinoma subsequently in either breast (67–69). Excision should be carried out to preserve as much breast tissue as possible because near-normal breast development may occur, even if removal of large or multiple tumors leaves a minimal amount of residual uninvolved tissue in young patients (68).

### PHYLLODES TUMOR

Although PTs may have been described as early as 1774, the lesion was first fully characterized in 1838 by Johannes Müller (79). The term *cystosarcoma phyllodes* was chosen to emphasize the leaf-like pattern and fleshy appearance of the lesion. Among the many other names subsequently applied to the tumor, the only other terms currently widely used are *periductal stromal tumor* and *phyllodes tumor*. The former term has been put forth to emphasize putative origin from specialized periductal stroma. Use of the term *phyllodes tumor* is considered preferable to avoid a diagnosis of sarcoma for benign variants. The diagnosis of PT always should include subclassification as benign, low-grade malignant (borderline), or high-grade malignant. The distinction between these three subgroups is based on the histologic characteristics of the tumor and is predictive of the probable clinical course.

### Clinical Presentation

The patient presents with a firm to hard, discrete, palpable tumor. There are no specific clinical features that reliably distinguish between a fibroadenoma, a benign PT, and a malignant PT (80). A diagnosis of PT may be favored if the tumor is larger than 4 cm or if there is a history of rapid growth. Origin in a preexisting fibroadenoma or malignant transformation of a benign PT is suggested when the patient reports enlargement of a preexisting tumor that was previously stable for a number of years. Further evidence suggesting that a fibroadenoma sometimes may evolve into a PT was obtained from clonal analysis of three tumors initially diagnosed as fibroadenomas that recurred as PTs (81). The tumors were studied for evidence of trinucleotide repeat polymorphism of the X chromosome–linked androgen receptor (AR) gene and random inactivation of the gene by methylation. The same allele of the AR gene was inactivated in the fibroadenoma and PT samples from each patient, a result unlikely to occur in three separate cases by chance alone.

Phyllodes tumors usually occur as solitary unilateral tumors. Rarely, multifocal PT has been detected in a single breast (82,83), or both breasts may be affected (82–86). Co-existent fibroadenomas, which are found histologically in nearly 40% of cases, are less frequently apparent clinically (82).

Phyllodes tumors have been reported in patients ranging in age from 10 to 86 years (80,87–90). The median and mean age is about 45 years, about 15 years older than the median age of patients with fibroadenomas. Isolated examples of PT in men have been described (91–93). These tumors are uncommon in patients younger than 30 years of age. A review of Swedish Cancer Registry data revealed eight histologically documented PTs and 29 breast carcinomas in women younger than 25 years of age diagnosed from 1960 to 1969 (94). There are few reports of PT in adolescent girls

(88,94–100). Most have been classified as benign, but a few examples of malignant PT have been described in this age group (96,97,100). Aspiration of cyst fluid from a benign PT in one 15-year-old patient yielded an elevated carcinoembryonic antigen level (95). This lesion proved to be diploid, progesterone receptor positive, and negative for estrogen receptor. Another benign PT obtained from a 13-year-old girl had a low estrogen receptor content and no progesterone receptor. Successful treatment by surgical excision of a 5-cm benign PT diagnosed during pregnancy was reported (101). The tumor did not recur during a second pregnancy.

A population-based study conducted in Los Angeles County, California, revealed an annual age-adjusted incidence of PT of 2.1 per 1 million women (102). The highest incidence was in women aged 45 to 49 years. Analysis by ethnicity revealed significantly younger Asian and Latino patients than non-Latino whites. Foreign-born Latino women from Mexico or the Americas had a threefold to fourfold higher risk for PT than Latino women born in the United States.

The reported average size of PT is 4 to 5 cm, ranging from 1 cm to larger than 20 cm (80,87,89,90). Although malignant PTs tend to be larger than benign variants, there are many exceptions, with high-grade malignant lesions smaller than 2 cm and some of the largest lesions histologically benign. Large tumors may invade and ulcerate the skin or extend into the chest wall (103).

Mammography reveals a rounded or lobulated, sharply defined, opaque mass in most cases (Fig. 8.27). Indistinct borders are seen in a minority of cases. The tumor also appears to be well circumscribed by ultrasound, but it may be

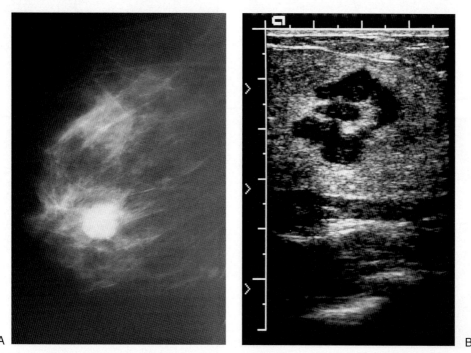

A                                                                                          B

**FIG. 8.27.** *Phyllodes tumor, mammography, and ultrasound.* **A:** This mammogram shows a well-circumscribed tumor that proved to be a malignant phyllodes tumor with leiomyosarcomatous differentiation. **B:** Inhomogeneous ultrasound transmission in a partly cystic tumor is illustrated.

inhomogeneous because of cysts and epithelium-lined clefts (Fig. 8.27) (104). Cystic components were evident by ultrasound slightly more frequently in malignant tumors in one study (105). Calcifications are uncommon and occur with equal frequency in benign and malignant lesions (105,106). It is not possible to distinguish reliably between benign and malignant PTs by mammography or ultrasonography (104–106). MRI of benign PTs revealed an oval or lobulated shape with internal septations (107,108). Dynamic enhancement was observed after the administration of contrast material (107).

The role of flow cytometry analysis of ploidy and S-phase as a predictor of recurrence in PT remains controversial. Layfield et al. reported finding aneuploidy in 75% of benign and in 50% of malignant PTs (109). Keelan et al. found that 12 of 16 (76%) PTs did not recur, and all five tumors that recurred were diploid (91). Low S-phase was observed in 70% of tumors that did not recur and in 80% that were followed for recurrence. Among samples of metastatic or recurrent PT, three (38%) were diploid, three (38%) were aneuploid,

and two (25%) were tetraploid. Intermediate to high S-phase was found in 88% of the samples of recurrent PT that were analyzed. The results obtained for recurrent PT are consistent with the observation that these tumors tend to become less differentiated when recurrent. No association between ploidy and histologic features of eight PTs was evident in another study (82). Tumors classified as borderline or malignant tend to have a higher S-phase (82). Other investigators observed a trend to a higher recurrence rate in tumors with an S-phase greater than 5% (110,111) and in aneuploid tumors (110).

Cytogenetic studies have uncovered karyotypic changes in benign and malignant PTs (112). The abnormalities are more complex in the malignant lesions. Karyotypic changes also have been found in a lesion described as a *recurrent fibroadenoma* (113). The data indicated clonal origin in the tumors evaluated (114,115). Others reported finding that a recurrent tumor had the same genomic imbalances as the primary tumor and that the genetic alterations detected in PT were similar to those found in breast carcinoma (116).

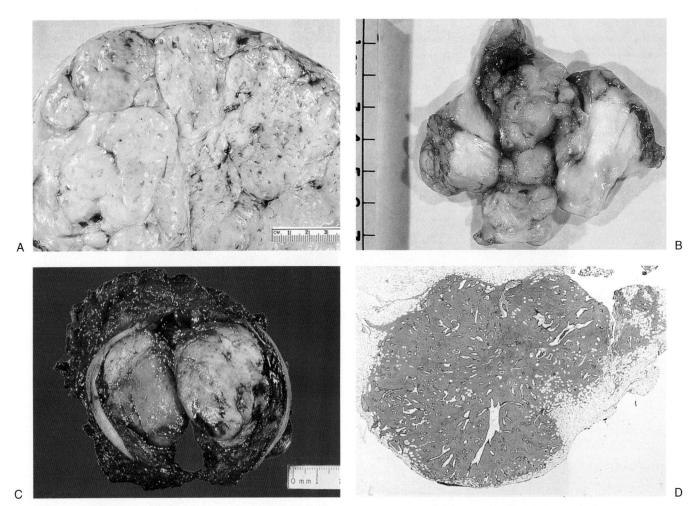

**FIG. 8.28.** *Phyllodes tumor. Gross appearances of transected benign tumors.* **A**: Classic phyllodes architecture consisting of dense stroma and interlacing clefts. **B**: A lobulated tumor. **C**: A relatively homogeneous tumor with dark foci of infarction. **D**: Whole-mount histologic section of a small benign phyllodes tumor. The tumor margin is slightly ragged in areas of invasion into fat.

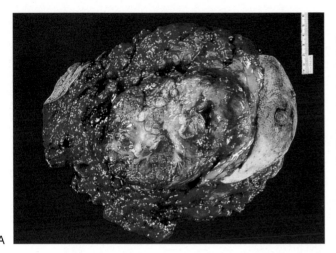 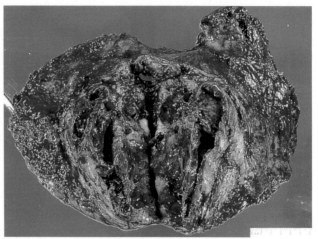

A
B

**FIG. 8.29.** *Phyllodes tumor, gross.* Gross appearances of transected malignant tumors in mastectomy specimens. **A:** The cut surface has a variegated appearance with cysts and clefts. The border appears to be well circumscribed. **B:** Extensive necrosis with cysts containing clotted blood.

Biochemical analysis reportedly has detected proges-terone receptor in the stromal of many PTs, whereas only a minority of the tumors show stromal expression of estrogen receptor (117). Insulin-like growth factor II (IGF-II) pro-duced by a malignant PT was associated with hypoglycemia in one case (118). The patient had elevated levels of plasma IGF-II, which fell when the 30-cm tumor was removed by mastectomy and her blood glucose returned to normal. IGF-II was detected immunohistochemically in tumor stromal cells.

### Gross Pathology

The external surface of a PT is well circumscribed but not encapsulated. It may be a single mass or multinodular. PTs with microscopically invasive borders usually appear to be well circumscribed grossly.

The bisected tumor is composed of firm, bulging gray to tan tissue (Figs. 8.28 and 8.29). Foci of degeneration, necro-sis, and infarction may appear gelatinous or hemorrhagic. These alterations are more common in malignant PTs but may occur in large benign lesions. Cysts that may contain keratotic debris are rarely present. An unusual variant of PT has an exaggerated cystic component, resulting in a gross ap-pearance that is difficult to distinguish from cystic papilloma (119,120) (Fig. 8.30).

### Microscopic Pathology

The tumors arise from periductal rather than from in-tralobular stroma and usually contain sparse lobular ele-ments. Most PTs have a heterogeneous histologic appear-ance, and only a minority of the lesions actually resemble the tumor conventionally described as having the exaggerated structure of an intracanalicular fibroadenoma with increased stromal cellularity. In numerous cases, the intracanalicular

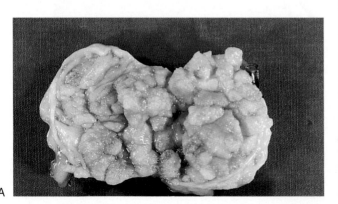 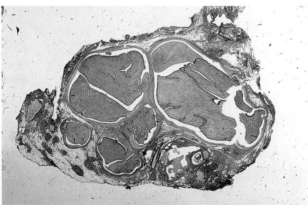

A
B

**FIG. 8.30.** *Phyllodes tumor, cystic.* **A:** Grossly, the incised tumor consists of numerous papillary nod-ules. **B:** A whole-mount histologic section of a cystic benign phyllodes tumor demonstrating the papillary structure.

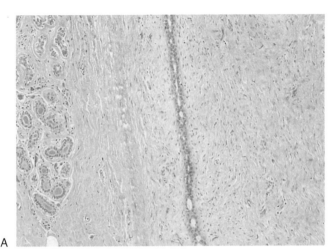 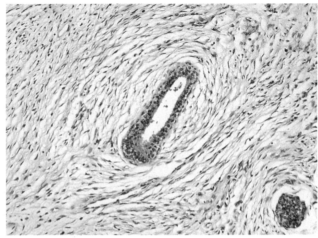

**FIG. 8.31.** *Phyllodes tumor, benign.* **A:** Border of a benign tumor showing the well-defined interface with the surrounding normal stroma *(left)*. Note the contrasting stromal cellularity and an epithelial-lined cleft in the tumor. **B:** A transversely cut epithelial unit surrounded by homogeneous stroma.

pattern of clefts is obscured by hyperplasia of the ductal epithelium, or there may be conspicuous lobular component.

Several features must be taken into consideration in making a distinction between a fibroadenoma and benign PT. PTs are characterized in most cases by expansion and increased cellularity of the stromal component compared with fibroadenoma. In some PTs, stromal cellularity is more dense in zones adjacent to epithelial components, the so-called periductal stroma. Mitotic activity also may be accentuated in this distribution, whereas mitoses are virtually absent from fibroadenomas; however, a substantial group of PTs exhibit little or none of this zonal stromal distribution.

The presence of elongated epithelial-lined clefts is a feature associated with PTs (Figs. 8.31 and 8.32). Occasionally, these spaces are dilated, and condensation of the immediately adjacent stroma may be found. Epithelial clefts also can

occur in fibroadenomas. The intracanalicular structure of some fibroadenomas bears a superficial resemblance to the clefted architecture of benign PTs, and occasionally the distinction between the two tumor types may be difficult. This problem is encountered, particularly in large or so-called giant fibroadenomas, when tumor size by itself suggests PT, and clefts may be apparent on the cut surface of the tumor. Histologically, the stroma in intracanalicular fibroadenomas tends to be hypocellular and uniform.

Myxoid change occurs in the stroma of fibroadenomas and PTs. It tends to be homogeneously distributed in fibroadenomas but may be patchy and undergo degenerative changes in PTs. Pseudoangiomatous stromal hyperplasia (PASH) occurs in PT; in some instances, PASH is a prominent feature of the lesion (Fig. 8.32). Rarely, multinucleated stromal giant cells are found in a PT with PASH stroma

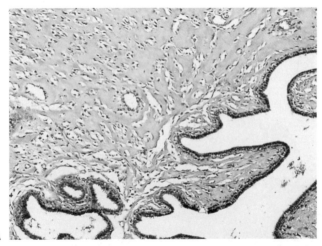 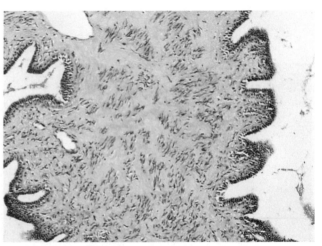

**FIG. 8.32.** *Benign phyllodes tumor with pseudoangiomatous stroma.* **A:** Stroma in a benign tumor with a pseudoangiomatous pattern. **B:** Pseudoangiomatous stroma with myofibroblasts in fascicular arrangement. The fibroepithelial structure has a pseudopapillary configuration. (*continued*)

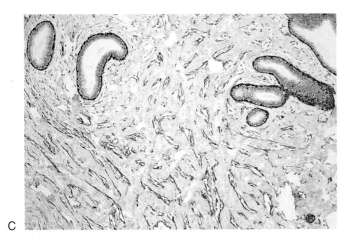

C

**FIG. 8.32.** *Continued.* **C:** The pseudoangiomatous structure is highlighted with the smooth muscle actin immunostain (avidin-biotin).

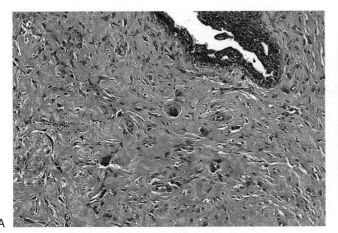

A

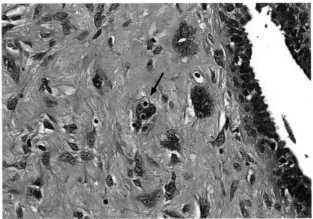

B

**FIG. 8.33.** *Benign phyllodes tumor with pseudoangiomatous stromal hyperplasia and stromal giant cells.* **A:** Multinucleated cells are present in the stroma. **B:** Lymphophagocytosis is shown in a giant cell (*arrow*).

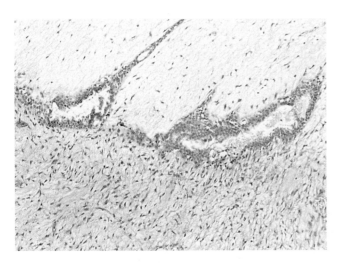

**FIG. 8.34.** *Benign phyllodes tumor.* An example of heterogeneity in the stroma of a benign tumor.

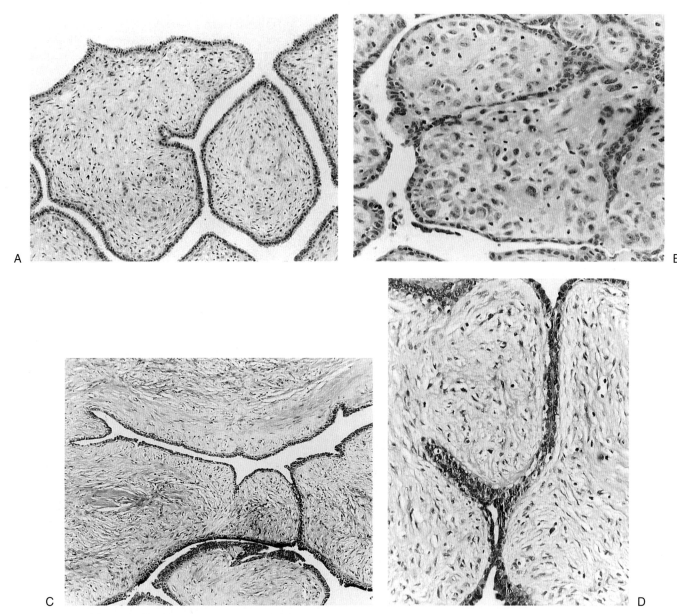

**FIG. 8.35.** *Benign phyllodes tumor.* **A,B:** A tumor with polygonal stromal cells in the subepithelial zone. Note the pseudopapillary structure. **C,D:** A tumor with bipolar stromal cells.

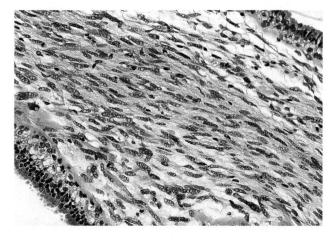

**FIG. 8.36.** *Benign phyllodes tumor.* Characteristic nuclear cytology with intranuclear vacuoles ("popcorn" nuclei).

(Fig. 8.33). These cells can exhibit lymphophagocytosis. They may express histiocytic immunomarkers, suggesting histiocytic rather than myofibroblastic histogenesis.

Stromal cellularity is often heterogeneous in PT with foci that are indistinguishable from fibroadenomas that abut sharply on more cellular regions (Fig. 8.34). Such areas can lead to the conclusion that the PT arose from a fibroadenoma, when in fact this is an intrinsic feature of some PTs. This structural variability also creates substantial difficulty in the accurate classification of some lesions sampled by FNA or needle core biopsy. Reported cases of malignant clinical behavior or metastases from a "benign" PT are probably a reflection of inaccurate classification of the tumor because of incomplete sampling. Ultimately, excisional biopsy is required to grade a PT, a determination based on stromal cellularity, mitotic activity, and the microscopic character of the tumor border.

The subclassification of PT encompasses three groups of lesions. It is important to distinguish benign from low-grade malignant PTs because the former do not metastasize; they have less risk for local recurrence; the interval to recurrence tends to be longer; most importantly, when they occur, initial local recurrences are histologically benign in almost all instances. Low-grade malignant PTs have earlier local recurrences, and the recurrences are likely to be histologically high grade more often.

Benign PT is characterized by few, if any, mitoses, rarely numbering one to two per 10 high-power fields (hpf). Modest to marked cellular overgrowth with slight to moderate cytologic pleomorphism is present in most tumors (Figs. 8.35 and 8.36). The stromal expansion is typically uniform throughout the lesion, but, as noted, it can be heterogeneous. The degree of epithelial proliferation usually corresponds to the appearance of the stroma. Epithelial hyperplasia is not conspicuous in the average benign PT, but it can be quite pronounced, as discussed later. The border of the tumor is usually well defined (Fig. 8.31), but invasion may be present, sometimes in the form of secondary fibroepithelial nodules (Fig. 8.37). Lipomatous and osseous metaplasia can occur in the stroma of a benign PT (Figs. 8.38 and 8.39). An

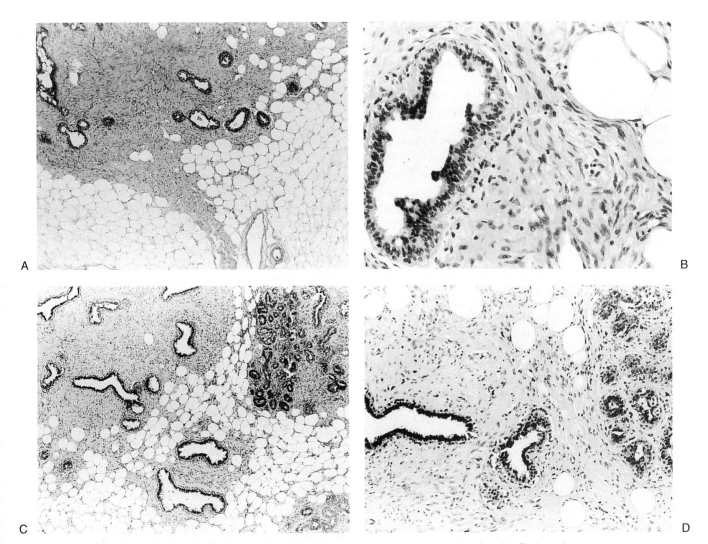

**FIG. 8.37.** *Benign phyllodes tumor.* **A:** The tumor has an irregular invasive border. **B:** Invasive component composed of epithelium and stroma in fat. **C:** Invasion with secondary nodules reaching to the lower right corner. **D:** Tumor extending into fat around a lobule (*right*).

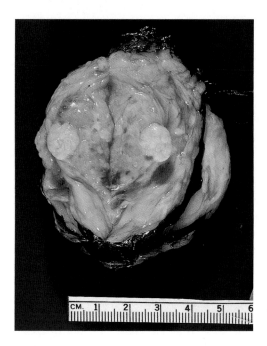

**FIG. 8.38.** *Benign phyllodes tumor with lipomatous metaplasia.* The bright yellow nodule in this bisected tumor is an area of lipomatous stromal metaplasia.

extremely unusual example of a benign PT with adipose stromal differentiation that arose in a lipomatous hamartoma has been reported (121) (Fig. 8.40). Multinucleated stromal cells with hyperchromatic nuclei may be present (Figs. 8.33 and 8.41). Focal myxoid stroma is not uncommon in a benign PT, but a tumor with a composition entirely of this tissue is unusual.

At the other extreme, a fully malignant PT features a marked degree of hypercellular stromal overgrowth, in most cases resulting in substantial separation of epithelial elements with proliferative activity in the stroma, typically greater than 5 mitoses per 10 hpf, and usually an invasive tumor border (Figs. 8.42 and 8.43). Stromal cellular pleomorphism is com-

mon in these lesions. Rarely, the stroma contains heterologous sarcomatous elements, such as angiosarcoma (Fig. 8.44), liposarcoma (Fig. 8.45), chondrosarcoma, myosarcoma, or osteosarcoma (122–125) (Fig. 8.46).

Low-grade malignant or borderline PTs usually have a microscopically invasive border, an average of 2 to 5 mitoses per 10 hpf, and moderate stromal cellularity that is often heterogeneously distributed in the midst of hypocellular areas (Fig. 8.47). The spindle cell stroma in many of these lesions resembles fibromatosis or low-grade fibrosarcoma (Fig. 8.48). Infrequent cases of cartilaginous, osseous, and lipomatous metaplasia have been encountered in low-grade malignant PTs.

*Text continues on page 188*

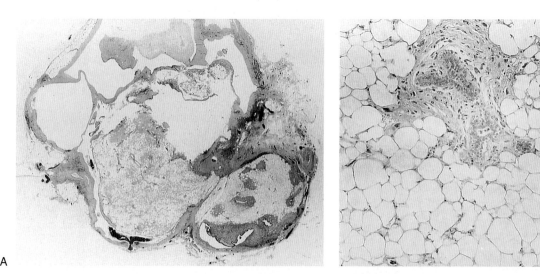

A

B

**FIG. 8.39.** *Benign phyllodes tumor with lipomatous metaplasia (lipophyllodes tumor).* **A:** Whole-mount histologic section showing extensive lipomatous transformation of the stroma and cystic areas. **B:** Lipomatous stroma.

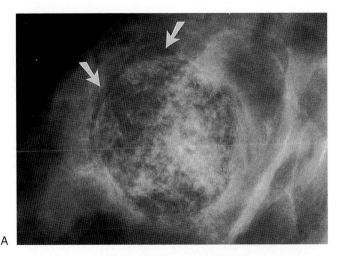

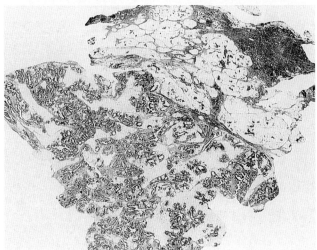

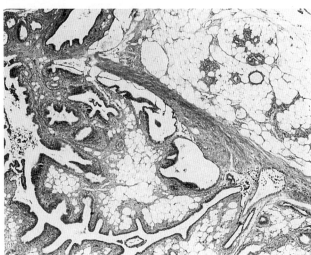

**FIG. 8.40.** *Benign phyllodes tumor associated with a lipomatous hamartoma.* **A:** Magnified view of the mammogram revealing an inhomogeneous tumor with a well-defined border in part demarcated by a zone of decreased density *(arrows)* in the region of the lipomatous hamartoma. **B:** Whole-mount histologic section showing the lipomatous hamartoma *above* and the lipophyllodes tumor *below.* **C:** Lipomatous hamartoma *(above)* and lipophyllodes tumor *(below).* (From Rosen PP, Romain K, Liberman L. Mammary cytosarcoma with adipose differentiation (lipophyllodes tumor) arising in a lipomatous hamartoma. *Arch Pathol Lab Med* 1994; 118:91–94, with permission.)

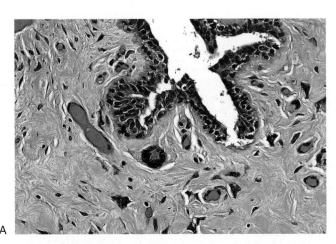

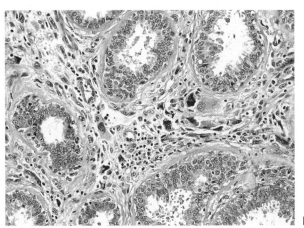

**FIG. 8.41.** *Benign phyllodes tumor with stromal giant cells.* **A:** A florette cell. **B:** Numerous multinucleated stromal cells in a tumor with prominent adenosis proliferation of the epithelium.

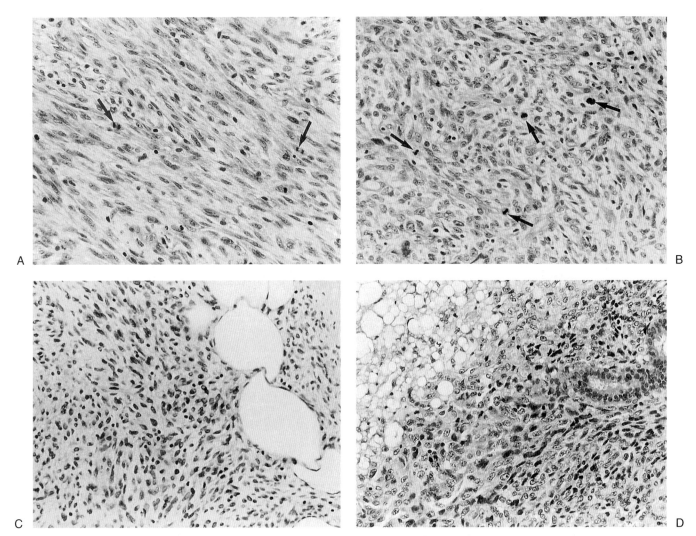

**FIG. 8.42.** *High-grade malignant phyllodes tumor.* Varied appearances of the stroma. **A:** Bipolar spindle cells. There are two mitotic figures *(arrows).* **B:** Plump bipolar cells and polygonal cells with multiple mitotic figures *(arrows).* **C:** Small round cells and bipolar cells. **D:** Liposarcoma with a solid component.

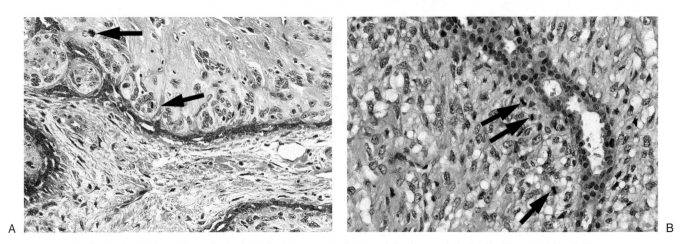

**FIG. 8.43.** *High-grade malignant phyllodes tumor.* Mitotic activity (*arrows*) limited to the subepithelial region in cells with epithelioid **(A)** and spindle cell **(B)** phenotypes.

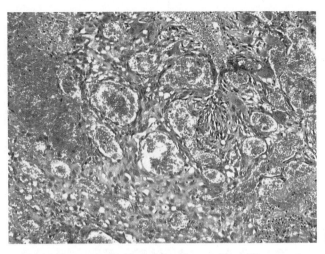

**FIG. 8.44.** *Angiosarcoma in high-grade malignant phyllodes tumor.* **A:** Vasoformative pattern. **B:** Telangiectatic pattern.

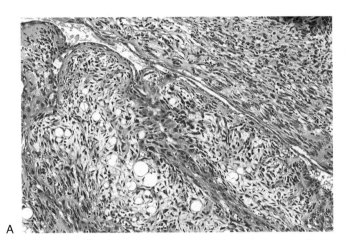
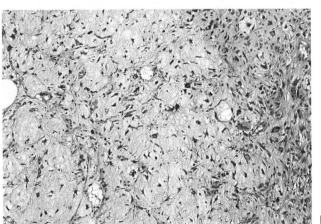

**FIG. 8.45.** *Liposarcoma in malignant phyllodes tumor.* **A:** Pleomorphic liposarcoma. **B:** Myxoid liposarcoma.

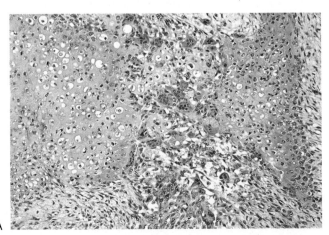
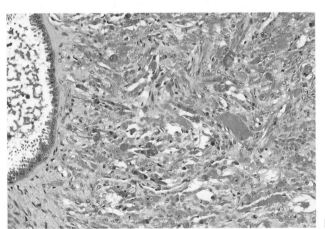

**FIG. 8.46.** *Chondrosarcoma and myosarcoma in malignant phyllodes tumors.* **A:** Malignant phyllodes tumor with chondrosarcoma and osteoid. *(continued)*

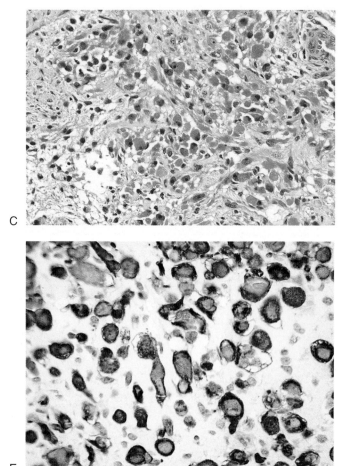

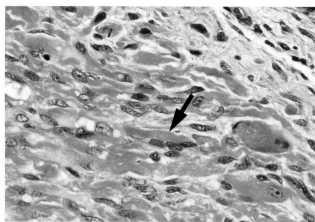

**FIG. 8.46.** *Continued.* **B,C:** Rhabdomyosarcoma in phyllodes tumor. **D:** Cross striations in rhabdomyosarcoma (*arrow*). **E:** Immunoreactivity for myoglobin (avidin-biotin). The rhabdoid tumor cells were also immunoreactive for desmin.

Many PTs exhibit epithelial hyperplasia, often represented by a variable increase in the thickness of the cuboidal or columnar epithelium lining the glandular spaces. Increased thickness resulting from several layers of cells, including hyperplasia of myoepithelial cells, is common and may progress focally or diffusely to papillary or cribriform hyperplasia (Fig. 8.49). There is a general tendency for the severity of epithelial hyperplasia to parallel the intensity of stromal proliferation, but many exceptions to this rule are encountered. Grimes found "marked epithelial hyperplasia" in one-third of benign PTs, including four (13%) with atypia, and in 26% of malignant PTs (82). Two of the 13 (15%) hyperplasias in malignant PTs were described as atypical. Atypical epithelial hyperplasia is sometimes extreme, leading to consideration of the diagnosis of intraductal carcinoma (Fig. 8.50). The PT character of the lesion may be overlooked if the stromal component is interpreted as reactive rather than as an intrinsic part of the neoplasm. Tumors in which the fundamental phyllodes growth pattern is obscured, usually by an unusual epithelial distribution (PT variants), often masquerade as papillary neoplasms or as adenosis tumors (Figs. 8.41B, 8.51, and 8.52).

The epithelial abnormality rarely reaches a level acceptable as intraductal carcinoma, and the diagnosis of intraduc-

tal carcinoma in PT is infrequent (126,127). Invasive duct and lobular carcinoma *in situ* also have been described in PTs. The subject of carcinoma in fibroadenoma and PT is discussed further in Chapter 35.

Squamous metaplasia of ductal epithelium, which occurs in benign and malignant tumors, is found in about 10% of PTs (82,87) (Fig. 8.53). Aspiration of a cystic area of squamous metaplasia may lead to a mistaken diagnosis of a squamous cyst (128). Apocrine metaplasia has been reported in the epithelium of PTs (Fig. 8.54) (82,129,130). Lobules occasionally are included in or formed in PTs, and they may exhibit proliferative changes, including sclerosing adenosis. The presence of lobules can lead to an erroneous diagnosis of fibroadenoma, especially when there is lobular hyperplasia and stromal cellularity is not greatly increased. In rare cases, the epithelial proliferation in the form of adenosis or papillary hyperplasia can be so extreme that it obscures the underlying PT, which may not be recognized until the tumor recurs (Figs. 8.51 and 8.52).

An unusual benign PT in a 42-year-old woman had stromal cells that contained intracytoplasmic inclusion bodies of the type found in infantile digital fibromatosis (131) (Fig. 8.55). Electron microscopy revealed a mixture of fibroblasts

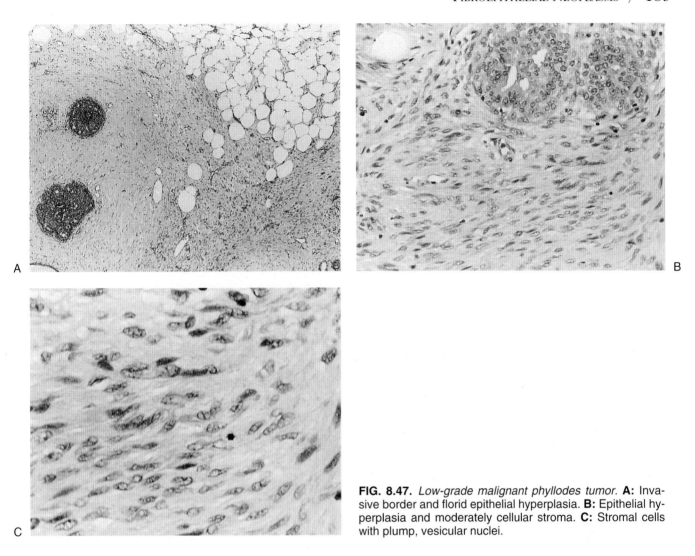

**FIG. 8.47.** *Low-grade malignant phyllodes tumor.* **A:** Invasive border and florid epithelial hyperplasia. **B:** Epithelial hyperplasia and moderately cellular stroma. **C:** Stromal cells with plump, vesicular nuclei.

**FIG. 8.48.** *Low-grade malignant phyllodes tumor.* **A:** Cellular stroma with a storiform pattern. **B:** Palisaded stromal cells.

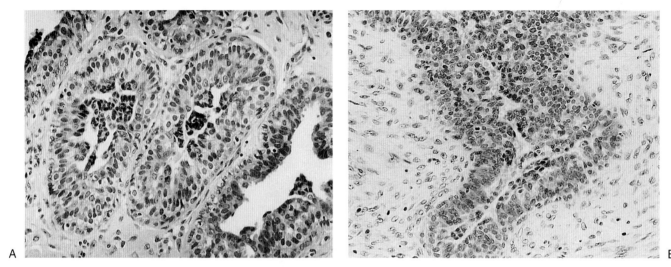

**FIG. 8.49.** *Florid epithelial hyperplasia in phyllodes tumors.* **A:** The proliferative epithelium has a micropapillary architecture. **B:** Atypical hyperplasia.

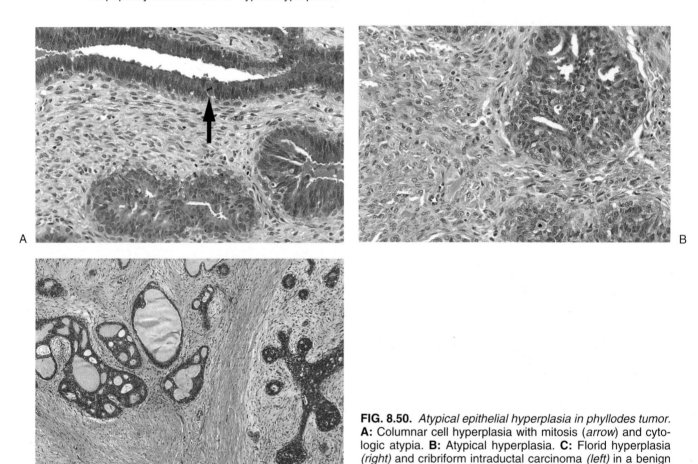

**FIG. 8.50.** *Atypical epithelial hyperplasia in phyllodes tumor.* **A:** Columnar cell hyperplasia with mitosis *(arrow)* and cytologic atypia. **B:** Atypical hyperplasia. **C:** Florid hyperplasia *(right)* and cribriform intraductal carcinoma *(left)* in a benign phyllodes tumor.

and myofibroblasts. The intracytoplasmic inclusions were associated closely with cytoplasmic microfilaments, forming tadpole-like structures. These cells weakly stained for actin by routine immunohistochemistry, with no reactivity in the inclusion bodies. After pretreatment with potassium hydroxide in 70% ethanol and 0.1% trypsin, the cells and inclusions were strongly actin positive.

Ductal elements may be present in locally recurrent PT in the breast or chest wall, and, with rare exception, metastatic PT at distant sites consists entirely of the stromal component. Two case reports claimed to demonstrate an epithelial component in lung metastases (132,133). One of these represented the inclusion of pulmonary alveolar tissue in the metastatic lesion (133). In the other case, the primary

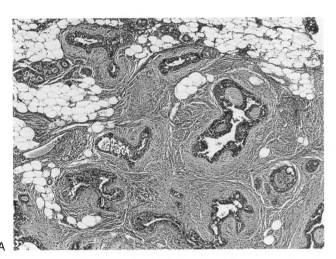
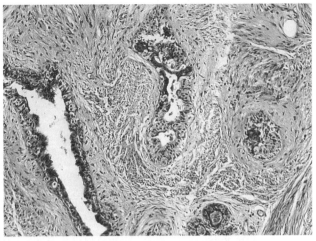

**FIG. 8.51.** *Phyllodes tumor variant.* **A:** The structure of the tumor resembles a radial scar with periductal stromal proliferation, chronic inflammation, and ductal epithelial hyperplasia. These tumors are susceptible to recurrence. One patient with this lesion had three recurrences with progressive stromal overgrowth over 10 years. **B:** The stromal proliferation is largely periductal.

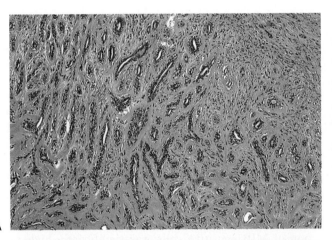
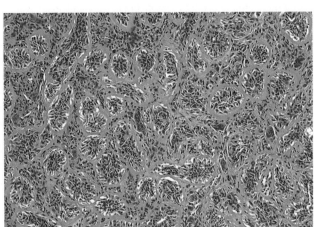
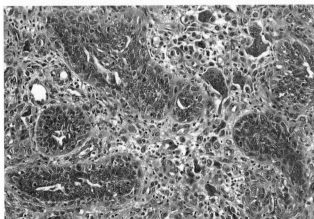

**FIG. 8.52.** *Phyllodes tumor variant.* The three images are from different regions in a single tumor. **A:** Part of the lesion resembles sclerosing adenosis. **B:** Glandular hyperplasia accompanied more prominent stroma with osteoclast-like giant cells. **C:** The fully developed lesion with atypical epithelial hyperplasia and malignant stroma with osteoclast-like giant cells.

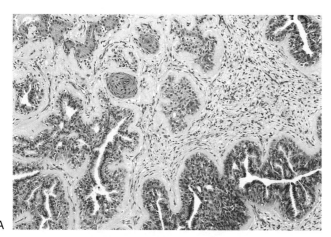
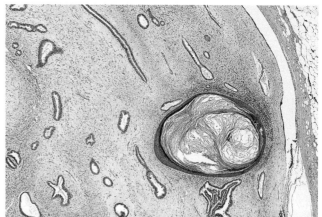

A                                                                    B

**FIG. 8.53.** *Squamous metaplasia in a benign phyllodes tumor.* **A:** Focal squamous metaplasia associated with florid epithelial hyperplasia. **B:** Cystic squamous metaplasia (both stained with hematoxylin–phloxine–safranin).

malignant PT exhibited liposarcomatous differentiation with an adenosis-like glandular component (133). These features were duplicated in lung metastases (Fig. 8.56). The adenosis-like elements in the primary lesion and in the metastases were immunoreactive for gross cystic disease fluid protein 15. The glandular cells in these structures were surrounded by actin-positive myoepithelial cells.

Because most malignant PTs are high-grade spindle cell tumors with a fibrosarcomatous pattern, this is the most common appearance encountered in metastatic lesions. Rarely, locally recurrent or metastatic lesions exhibit heterologous differentiation that was not apparent in the primary tumor (134). Uncommon heterologous sarcomatous elements in the primary tumor, such as liposarcoma (82,123), chondrosarcoma (82,135), osteosarcoma (82,136), and leiomyosarcoma (82), can be expressed in metastases. In one exceptional case, metastatic malignant PT in the lung exhibited osseous, cartilaginous, and angiosarcomatous elements that had been present in the primary tumor 5 years earlier (137). Rhabdomyosarcoma was present in the lung metastases from a

malignant PT that contained rhabdomyosarcoma (122). Metastases from a liposarcomatous PT consisted mainly of immature lipoblasts with few adipocytes (138).

### Immunohistochemistry and Molecular Analysis

The stroma of PTs is vimentin positive. Actin, CD34, and desmin reactivity are present in a variable proportion of cases that exhibit myoid or pseudoangiomatous stromal differentiation of myofibroblasts (139,140). Stromal cells are not S-100 positive. Excess perivascular deposition of type IV collagen was observed in the stroma of malignant PTs compared with benign tumors, and a similar pattern was found in noncystosarcomatous sarcomas (141). The immunohistochemical distribution of Ki67 antigen detected with the MIB1 antibody correlates with the distinction between benign and malignant PT (142). An MIB1 index derived from the stromal cellularity of tumors and the proportion of MIB1-positive cells was significantly higher in malignant than in benign PTs. Much less difference was seen between the MIB1 indices of benign PTs and fibroadenomas. Differential expression of p53 also has been observed in fibroepithelial tumors; the greatest activity was in malignant PTs, especially in the periepithelial stroma (143).

Phyllodes tumors contain much higher concentrations of endothelin-1 than fibroadenomas (144). This vasoconstrictive peptide stimulates DNA synthesis in vascular smooth-muscle cells and in breast stromal cells (145). Immunohistochemical study revealed that endothelin-1 was localized to the epithelium of PTs and that it was absent from stromal cells in these tumors (144). This observation suggests that endothelin-1 elaborated by the epithelial component of PTs may have a paracrine function in stimulating proliferation of stromal cells in PTs. Conventional histologic observations and morphometric studies have shown that mitoses tend to be more frequent in stroma close to epithelium in PT rather than in more distant stroma are also consistent with a paracrine function in phyllodes tumor epithelium (146). Further evidence of paracrine interaction between epithelial and

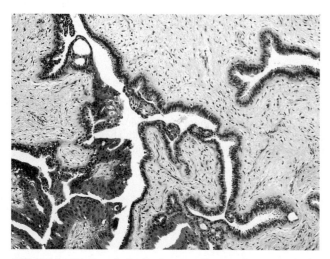

**FIG. 8.54.** *Benign phyllodes tumor with apocrine metaplasia.*

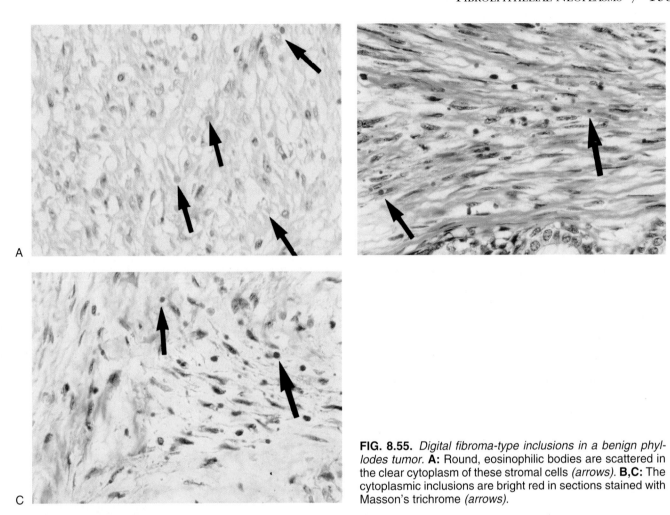

**FIG. 8.55.** *Digital fibroma-type inclusions in a benign phyllodes tumor.* **A:** Round, eosinophilic bodies are scattered in the clear cytoplasm of these stromal cells *(arrows).* **B,C:** The cytoplasmic inclusions are bright red in sections stained with Masson's trichrome *(arrows).*

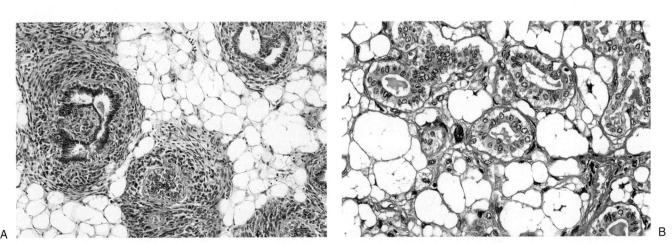

**FIG. 8.56.** *Malignant phyllodes tumor with metastases of stromal and epithelial components.* **A:** The primary tumor displayed periglandular malignant spindle cell elements with intervening zones of mature adipose tissue. **B:** Glandular and adipose components were present in the lung metastasis illustrated here. (Courtesy of Drs. Kracht, Sapino, and Bussolati.)

stromal components in PTs comes from the observed coexpression of platelet-derived growth factor (PDGF) and a PDGF beta receptor in both tissue compartments (146a). Allelic imbalance has been detected in epithelial and stromal samples of PT, suggesting that both components may contribute to the neoplastic process in some instances (146b).

Tenascin is an extracellular matrix glycoprotein that inhibits interactions of cells with other cells and stroma. Immunohistochemical study reveals tenascin to be distributed in a limited subepithelial zone of stroma in the normal breast and in fibroadenomas, but it is reportedly present more diffusely in the stroma of PTs (147).

### Electron Microscopy

At the ultrastructural level, the stroma of a PT is composed of cells with features of fibroblasts and myofibroblasts that resemble the normal cellular constituents of the mammary stroma (140). Electron-dense cytoplasmic bodies, sometimes with a crescent shape, were described as a distinctive feature by Harris and Khan (148). These structures appeared to be lysosomal in origin, and they were more numerous in malignant tumors. Various types of cytoplasmic inclusions were described in other reports (149,150). Toker also observed a "distorted resemblance to the morphology of

normal fibroblasts" (150). The cells have occasional tight junctions. Normal fibroblasts have been found among neoplastic cells ultrastructurally (149). Intermediate filaments and dense bodies are observed in myofibroblastic cells (140). Electron microscopy has not revealed unusual features in the epithelial components of PTs (140).

### Cytology

The cytologic diagnosis of a PT may be suggested by an aspirate that has an epithelial component typical of a fibroepithelial neoplasm, with excess bipolar stromal cells in the background (Fig. 8.57). Stromal cells with cytoplasm rather than naked bipolar nuclei typify PTs (151). Cellular stromal fragments are helpful in distinguishing PT from fibroadenoma (152,153). Aspiration cytology is an unreliable procedure for the diagnosis of PT in some situations, as pointed out by McDivitt et al. in 1967 (129) and also by other investigators (154). Lesions with marked epithelial hyperplasia may yield an aspirate or needle core biopsy in which the stromal element is obscured, and this situation can lead to misdiagnosis of carcinoma (155) or of a fibroadenoma if the sample obtained from a heterogeneous tumor has bland epithelium and sparse stromal cells. Scarcity of single epithelial cells, epithelial cohesion, and polarity and the

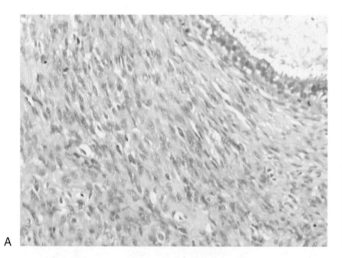

A

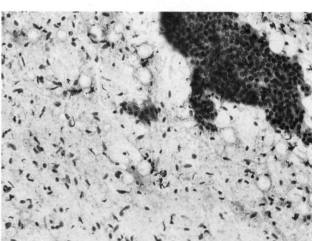

B

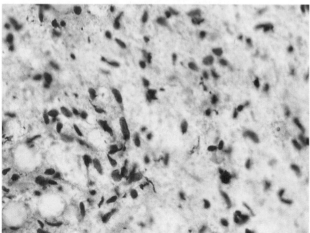

C

**FIG. 8.57.** *Phyllodes tumor, fine needle aspiration.* **A:** Histologic section of the low-grade malignant tumor. **B:** Aspiration smear showing numerous bipolar stromal cells and an irregular cluster of epithelial cells. **C:** Stromal cells with hyperchromatic, pleomorphic nuclei.

frequent presence of foam cells are features associated with PT rather than carcinoma in such specimens (155). The aspirate from a malignant PT is likely to contain cellular stromal fragments composed of atypical cells and possibly mitotic figures. Fragments of stroma with adipose differentiation may be present in the cytologic specimen from a PT with liposarcomatous differentiation (156).

**Treatment and Prognosis**

The classification of PT as benign and low- or high-grade malignant tumor reflects an estimate of the probable clinical course based on the histologic appearance of the tumor. A benign PT will not metastasize and has a low probability (about 20%) for local recurrence after excision (157). Low-grade malignant PT has a low probability (<5%) of metastasis, but such a tumor is more likely than a benign PT (>25%) to recur locally. Metastases occur in about 25% of high-grade malignant PTs, and these lesions are also susceptible to local recurrence. Recurrences occur earlier with high-grade malignant PT than after initial treatment of be-

nign or low-grade malignant tumors. Fewer than 1% of high-grade PTs give rise to axillary lymph node metastases (82,83,87,158) (Fig. 8.58). Metastatic PT in a Rotter lymph node also has been reported (159).

Barth summarized breast recurrence data based on an extensive literature review (160). Classification of PT as benign, low-grade malignant (borderline) and high-grade malignant proved to be correlated with local breast recurrence in women who did not undergo mastectomy. Twenty published studies provided information about patients treated by local excision or lumpectomy. Breast recurrences were reported in 111 of 540 (21%), 18 of 39 (46%), and 26 of 40 (65%) patients who had benign, low-grade malignant and high-grade malignant tumors, respectively. Thirteen studies had data for women treated by "wide local excision" with "at least 1 to 2 cm of normal tissue around the tumor." Overall, breast recurrences were reported in 17 of 212 (8%), 20 of 68 (29%), and 16 of 45 (36%) patients with benign, low-grade, and high-grade malignant tumors, respectively. Combined survival data from the published studies indicated deaths from disease in 2 of 600 (0.3%), 7 of 107 (6.6%), and 48 of

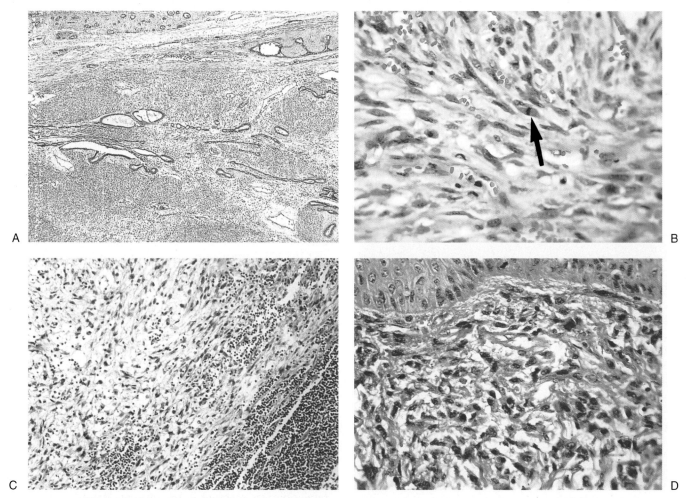

**FIG. 8.58.** *Malignant phyllodes tumor with metastases.* **A:** The primary tumor had a circumscribed border and cellular stroma. **B:** Cellular pleomorphism and a mitotic figure in the primary tumor (*arrow*). **C:** Metastatic phyllodes tumor in an axillary lymph node at the time of mastectomy. **D:** A subsequent metastasis in the skin of a finger.

240 (20%) patients with benign, low-grade, and high-grade malignant tumors.

The fundamental principle of therapy is complete excision to prevent local recurrence (157,161–164). Features that predispose to local recurrence are incomplete excision, an invasive tumor border, and secondary tumor nodules at the periphery. Primary tumor size may be a factor in the success of local excision because a more generous margin may be possible when tumors are small (161). Local recurrence is deleterious, especially because of the tendency of PTs to have a higher grade in recurrent lesions than in corresponding primary tumors and the risk of chest wall invasion (Fig. 8.59).

Patterns of recurrence were well documented in a series reported by Grimes (82). Follow-up of 51 benign PTs revealed local recurrence in 14 (27%). Six recurrences occurred within a year of diagnosis; in the remaining cases, the interval was 3 to 17 years. Fibroadenomas or fibroadenomatous areas were present at the site of breast recurrence in five cases. Twelve of the 14 recurrences (86%) had a fibroepithelial structure, and two were entirely stromal. Recurrences were of a higher grade in 10 cases (71%), including five that were histologically malignant. Local recurrences also were detected in 7 of 22 low-grade malignant (borderline) PTs (32%), including four recurrences in the first year; the longest interval was 15 years. Fibroadenomatous foci were not found at sites of recurrence following low-grade malignant PTs. Several patients had multiple recurrences in the breast. Four initial recurrences were fibroepithelial, and three were purely stromal. Five of seven recurrences (71%) had a higher grade than the primary tumor, and four of these were considered fully malignant. Local recurrence also occurred in 7 of 27 (26%) cases of high-grade malignant PT, almost always within a year of diagnosis. Initial recurrences were fibroepithelial or entirely stromal, whereas subsequent recurrences were only stromal. All local recurrences duplicated features of the original malignant PT.

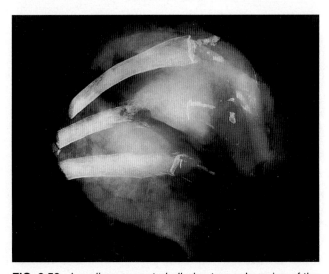

**FIG. 8.59.** *Locally recurrent phyllodes tumor.* Invasion of the chest wall and destruction of ribs by recurrent phyllodes tumor are evident in this x-ray of a surgical specimen.

Local recurrence is not a necessary antecedent event to the development of systemic metastases in patients with malignant PT; however, rare cases of benign or low-grade malignant PT that result in metastases almost always have had local recurrences with higher-grade malignant features before the appearance of systemic lesions. About 40% of patients with a malignant PT who develop metastases do not experience a local recurrence before systemic spread (87,89, 165,166).

Because the diagnosis of PT is not anticipated clinically, in many cases, surgical excision is initially incomplete, and reexcision is required. The primary excision and reexcision specimens should be inked and margins thoroughly examined histologically. Mastectomy is indicated as primary therapy if a malignant PT cannot be encompassed with a cosmetically acceptable excision. Axillary dissection is appropriate only if the lymph nodes appear clinically involved or if there is concurrent carcinoma in the same breast.

There appear to be differences in prognosis for tumors with different types of stromal differentiation. Several patients with osteogenic or chondrosarcoma have developed systemic metastases (135,136), but most patients with liposarcomatous PT have remained disease-free (123,138, 167,168).

The most common sites of distant metastases are the lungs, bone, and heart (169). One report described an unusual case of surgically resected metastatic PT in the lung with intravascular dumbbell extension through the pulmonary vein into the left atrium (170). Virtually any organ may have metastases, but many of these sites are not apparent antemortem. Exceptional sites of clinically detected metastases include the mandible (171), the maxilla (172), and the central nervous system (173,174).

The overall 5-year survival rate for PT is about 90% (82). Local recurrences, which occur in about 30% of cases, and metastases that develop in about 10% of cases, usually are detected within 3 years of primary treatment (82,90,103, 162,163,175), although occasional cases of late recurrence have been reported (82,129). Most deaths from metastatic PT occur within 5 years of diagnosis (82,176). Virtually all fatalities occur in patients who have high-grade tumors primarily or who develop recurrences that are high grade. These neoplasms typically are characterized by stromal overgrowth, invasive borders, cellular pleomorphism, and frequent mitoses (177,178). Grimes reported that all PTs that resulted in metastases in her series (8 of 100 tumors) had mitotic rates of at least 15 per 50 hpf in the primary tumors or in a recurrence (82). Other investigators reported mitotic counts of 11 to 52 (176) and 3 to 30 (87) per hpf in tumors that developed metastases.

Metastatic PT is not responsive to most currently available chemotherapy regimens or to radiotherapy (178). Prolonged remission was reported in two patients treated with ifosfamide (177), and palliation reportedly was achieved with combination chemotherapy and radiation in other cases

(179). Among patients with high-grade PT, the 5-year survival rate is about 65% (90,132).

## REFERENCES

### Sclerosing Lobular Hyperplasia (Fibroadenomatoid Mastopathy)

1. Kovi J, Chu HB, Leffall Jr L. Sclerosing lobular hyperplasia manifesting as a palpable mass of the breast in young black women. *Hum Pathol* 1984;15:336–340.
2. Poulton TB, Shaw de Paredes E, Baldwin M. Sclerosing lobular hyperplasia of the breast: imaging features in 15 cases. *AJR Am J Roentgenol* 1995;165:291–294.
3. Kamal M, Evans AJ, Denley H, et al. Fibroadenomatoid hyperplasia: a cause of suspicious microcalcification on mammographic screening. *AJR Am J Roentgenol* 1998;171:1331–1334.

### Fibroadenoma

4. Hunter TB, Roberts CC, Hunt KR, et al. Occurrence of fibroadenomas in postmenopausal women referred for breast biopsy. *J Am Geriatr Soc* 1996;44:61–64.
5. Simomoto MM, Nazário ACP, Gebrim LH, et al. Morphometric analysis of the epithelium of mammary fibroadenomas during the proliferative and secretory phases of the menstrual cycle. *Breast J* 1999;5:256–261.
6. Canny PF, Berkowitz GS, Kelsey JL, et al. Fibroadenoma and the use of exogenous hormones. *Am J Epidemiol* 1988;127:454–461.
7. Li Volsi V, Stadel BV, Kelsey JL, et al. Fibroadenoma in oral contraceptive users: a histopathologic evaluation of epithelial atypia. *Cancer* 1979;44:1778–1781.
8. Yu H, Rohan TE, Cook MG, et al. Risk factors for fibroadenoma: a case–control study in Australia. *Am J Epidemiol* 1992;135:247–258.
9. Calabrese G, Di Virgilio C, Cianchetti E, et al. Chromosome abnormalities in breast fibroadenomas. *Genes Chromosomes Cancer* 1991;3:202–204.
10. Fletcher JA, Pinkus GS, Weidner N, et al. Lineage-restricted clonality in biphasic solid tumors. *Am J Pathol* 1991;138:1119–1207.
11. Stephenson CF, Davis RI, Moore GE, et al. Cytogenetic and fluorescence *in situ* hybridization analysis of breast fibroadenomas. *Cancer Genet Cytogenet* 1992;63:32–36.
12. Rohen C, Staats B, Bonk U, et al. Significance of clonal chromosome aberrations in breast fibroadenomas. *Cancer Genet Cytogenet* 1996;87:152–155.
13. Petersson C, Pandis N, Rizou H, et al. Karyotypic abnormalities in fibroadenomas of the breast. *Int J Cancer* 1997;70:282–286.
14. Kobayashi S, Iwase H, Kuzushima T, et al. Consecutively occurring multiple fibroadenomas of the breast distinguished from phyllodes tumors by clonality analysis of stromal tissue. *Breast Cancer* 1999;6:201–206.
15. Kasami M, Vnencak-Jones CL, Manning S, et al. Monoclonality in fibroadenomas with complex histology and phyllodal features. *Breast Cancer Res Treat* 1998;50:185–191.
16. Morris JA, Kelly JF. Multiple bilateral breast adenomata in identical adolescent negro twins. *Histopathology* 1982;6:539–547.
17. Levi F, Randimbison L, Te V-C, et al. Incidence of breast cancer in women with fibroadenoma. *Cancer* 1994;57:681–683.
18. Carter CL, Corle DK, Micozzi MS, et al. A prospective study of the development of breast cancer in 16,692 women with benign breast disease. *Am J Epidemiol* 1988;128:467–477.
19. McDivitt RW, Stephens JA, Lee NC, et al. Histologic types of benign breast disease and the risk of breast cancer. *Cancer* 1992;69:1408–1414.
20. Dupont WD, Page DL, Parl FF, et al. Long-term risk of breast cancer in women with fibroadenoma. *N Engl J Med* 1994;331:10–15.
21. Krieger N, Hiatt RA. Risk of breast cancer after benign breast diseases, variation by histologic type, degree of atypia, age at biopsy, and length of follow-up. *Am J Epidemiol* 1992;136:619–631.
22. Hutchinson WB, Thomas DB, Hamlin WB, et al. Risk of breast cancer in women with benign breast disease. *J Natl Cancer Inst* 1980;65:13–20.
23. Foster ME, Garrahan N, Williams S. Fibroadenoma of the breast: a clinical and pathological study. *J R Coll Surg Edinb* 1988;33:16–19.
24. Sumkin JH, Perrone AM, Harris KM, et al. Lactating adenoma: US features and literature review. *Radiology* 1998;206:271–274.
25. Stomper PC, Mazurchuk RV, Tsangaris TN. MRI appearance of giant fibroadenoma of the breast: overlap with phyllodes tumor. *Breast Dis* 1996;9:37–43.
26. Hochman MG, Orel SG, Powell CM, et al. Fibroadenomas: MR imaging appearances with radiologic-histopathologic correlation. *Radiology* 1997;204:123–129.
27. Giani C, D'Amore E, Delarue JC, et al. Estrogen and progesterone receptors in benign breast tumors and lesions: relationship with histological and cytological features. *Int J Cancer* 1986;37:7–10.
28. Mechtersheimer G, Kruger KH, Born IA, et al. Antigenic profile of mammary fibroadenoma and cystosarcoma phyllodes: a study using antibodies to estrogen and progesterone receptors and to a panel of cell surface molecules. *Pathol Res Pract* 1990;186:427–438.
29. Rao BR, Meyer JS, Fry CG. Most cystosarcoma phyllodes and fibroadenomas have progesterone receptor but lack estrogen receptor: a stromal localization of progesterone receptor. *Cancer* 1981;47:2016–2021.
30. Farrow JH, Ashikari H. Breast lesions in young girls. *Surg Clin North Am* 1969;49:261–269.
31. Oberman HA. Breast lesions in the adolescent female. *Pathol Annu* 1979;14:175–201.
32. Moross T, Lang AP, Mahoney L. Tubular adenoma of breast. *Arch Pathol Lab Med* 1983;107:84–86.
33. Persaud V, Talerman A, Jordan R. Pure adenoma of the breast. *Arch Pathol Lab Med* 1968;86:481–483.
34. Hertel BF, Zaloudek C, Kempson RL. Breast adenomas. *Cancer* 1976;37:2891–2905.
35. O'Hara MF, Page DL. Adenomas of the breast and ectopic breast under lactational influences. *Hum Pathol* 1985;16:707–712.
36. James K, Bridger J, Anthony PP. Breast tumour of pregnancy ("lactating" adenoma). *J Pathol* 1988;156:37–44.
37. Baddoura FK, Judd RL. Apocrine adenoma of the breast: a report of a case with investigation of lectin binding patterns in apocrine breast lesions. *Mod Pathol* 1990;3:373–376.
38. Tesluk H, Amott T, Goodnight JE. Apocrine adenoma of the breast. *Arch Pathol Lab Med* 1986;110:351–352.
39. Azzopardi JG, Salm R. Ductal adenoma of the breast: a lesion which can mimic carcinoma. *J Pathol* 1984;144:15–23.
40. Gusterson BA, Sloane JP, Middwood C, et al. Ductal adenoma of the breast—a lesion exhibiting a myoepithelial/epithelial phenotype. *Histopathology* 1987;11:103–110.
41. Ballance WA, Ro JY, El-Naggar AK, et al. Pleomorphic adenoma (benign mixed tumor) of the breast. *Am J Clin Pathol* 1990;93:795–801.
42. Chen KTK. Pleomorphic adenoma of the breast. *Am J Clin Pathol* 1990;93:792–794.
43. Søreide JA, Anda O, Eriksen L, et al. Pleomorphic adenoma of the human breast with local recurrence. *Cancer* 1988;61:997–1001.
44. Demetrakopoulos NJ. Three-dimentional reconstruction of a human mammary fiboadenoma. *Quarterly Bulletin of Northwestern University Medical School* 1958;32:221–228.
45. Koerner FC, O'Connell JX. Fibroadenoma: a theory of pathogenesis. *Pathol Annu* 1994;29:1–20.
46. Cheatle GL. Hyperplasia of epithelial and connective tissues in the breast: its relation to fibroadenoma and other pathological conditions. *Br J Surg* 1923;10:436–455.
47. Carstens PHB. Ultrastructure of human fibroadenoma. *Arch Pathol* 1974;98:23–32.
48. Yeh I-T, Francis DJ, Orenstein JM, et al. Ultrastructure of cystosarcoma phyllodes and fibroadenoma. A comparative study. *Am J Clin Pathol* 1985;84:131–136.
49. Ohtani H, Sasano N. Stromal cells of the fibroadenoma of the human breast: an immunohistochemical and ultrastructural study. *Virchows Arch* 1984;404:7–16.
50. Reddick RL, Shin TK, Sawhney D, et al. Stromal proliferations of the breast: an ultrastructural and immunohistochemcial evaluation of cystosarcoma phyllodes, juvenile fibroadenoma, and fibroadenoma. *Hum Pathol* 1987;18:45–49.
51. Goodman ZD, Taxy JB. Fibroadenomas of the breast with prominent smooth muscle. *Am J Surg Pathol* 1981;5:99–101.
52. Powell CM, Rosen PP. Adipose differentiation in cystosarcoma phyllodes. *Am J Surg Pathol* 1994;18:720–727.

53. Berean K, Tron VA, Churg A, et al. Mammary fibroadenoma with multinucleated stromal giant cells. *Am J Surg Pathol* 1986;10:823–827.

54. Powell CM, Cranor ML, Rosen PP. Multinucleated stromal giant cells in mammary fibroepithelial neoplasms: a study of 11 patients. *Arch Pathol Lab Med* 1994;118:912–916.

55. Meyer JE, Lester SC, DiPiro PJ, et al. Occult calcified fibroadenomas. *Breast Dis* 1995;8:29–38.

56. Spagnolo DV, Shilkin KB. Breast neoplasms containing bone and cartilage. *Virchows Arch* 1983;400:287–295.

57. Carney JA, Toorkey BC. Myxoid fibroadenoma and allied conditions (myxomatosis) of the breast: a heritable disorder with special associations including cardiac and cutaneous myxomas. *Am J Surg Pathol* 1991;15:713–721.

58. Salm R. Epidermoid metaplasia in mammary fibro-adenoma with formation of keratin cysts. *J Pathol Bacteriol* 1957;74:221–223.

59. Goldenberg VE, Wiegenstein L, Mottet NK. Florid breast fibroadenomas in patients taking hormonal oral contraceptives. *Am J Clin Pathol* 1968;49:52–59.

60. Fechner RE. Fibroadenomas in patients receiving oral contraceptives: a clinical and pathologic study. *Am J Clin Pathol* 1970;53:857–864.

61. Oberman HA. Hormonal contraceptives and fibroadenomas of the breast. *N Engl J Med* 1971;284:984.

62. Terada S, Uchide K, Suzuki N, et al. A lactating adenoma of the breast. *Gynecol Obstet Invest* 1992;34:126–128.

63. Oi RH, Dobbs M. Lactating breast tissue in benign cystic teratoma. *Am J Obstet Gynecol* 1978;130:729–731.

64. Majmudar B, Rosales-Quintana S. Infarction of breast fibroadenomas during pregnancy. *JAMA* 1975;231:963–964.

65. Delarue J, Redon H. Les infarctus des fibro-adénomes mammaire: probleme clinique et pathogénique. *Semin Hôp Paris* 1949;73:2901–2906.

66. Newman J, Kahn LB. Infarction of fibro-adenoma of the breast. *Br J Surg* 1973;60:738–740.

67. Fekete P, Petrek J, Majmudar B, et al. Fibroadenomas with stromal cellularity: a clinicopathologic study of 21 patients. *Arch Pathol Lab Med* 1987;111:427–432.

68. Pike A, Oberman HA. Juvenile (cellular) adenofibromas: a clincopatholgic study. *Am J Surg Pathol* 1985;9:730–736.

69. Mies C, Rosen PP. Juvenile fibroadenoma with atypical epithelial hyperplasia. *Am J Surg Pathol* 1987;11:184–190.

70. Bottles K, Taylor RN. Diagnosis of breast masses in pregnant and lactating women by aspiration cytology. *Obstet Gynecol* 1985;66:76S–78S.

71. Dejmek A, Lindholm K. Frequency of cytologic features in fine needle aspirates from histologically and cytologically diagnosed fibroadenomas. *Acta Cytol* 1991;35:695–699.

72. Bottles K, Chan JS, Holly EA, et al. Cytologic criteria for fibroadenoma: a step-wise logistic regression analysis. *Am J Clin Pathol* 1988;89:707–713.

73. Benoit JL, Kara R, McGregor SE, et al. Fibroadenoma of the breast: diagnostic pitfalls of fine-needle aspiration. *Diagn Cytopathol* 1992;8:643–648.

74. McCutcheon JM, Lipa M. Infarction of a fibroadenoma of breast following fine needle aspiration. *Cytopathology* 1993;4:247–250.

75. Finley JL, Silverman JF, Lannin DR. Fine needle aspiration cytology of lactating adenoma. *Acta Cytol* 1987;31:666.

76. Grenko RT, Lee KP, Lee KR. Fine needle aspiration cytology of lactating adenoma of the breast: a comparative light microscopic and morphometric study. *Acta Cytol* 1990;34:21–26.

77. Cant PJ, Madden MV, Close PM, et al. Case for conservative management of selected fibro-adenomas of the breast. *Br J Surg* 1987;74:857–859.

78. Wilkinson S, Anderson TJ, Rifkin E, et al. Fibroadenoma of the breast: a follow-up of conservative management. *Br J Surg* 1989;76:390–391.

## Phyllodes Tumor

79. Fiks A. Cystosarcoma phyllodes of the mammary gland—Müller's tumor. *Virchows Arch* 1981;392:1–6.

80. Cohn-Cedermark G, Rutqvist LE, Rosendahl I, et al. Prognostic factors in cystosarcoma phyllodes: a clinicopathologic study of 77 patients. *Cancer* 1991;68:2017–2022.

81. Noguchi S, Yokouchi H, Aihora T, et al. Progression of fibroadenoma to phyllodes tumor demonstrated by clonal analysis. *Cancer* 1995;76:1779–1785.

82. Grimes MM. Cystosarcoma phyllodes of the breast: histologic features, flow cytometry analysis, and clinical correlations. *Mod Pathol* 1992;5:232–239.

83. Minkowitz S, Zeichner M, Di Maio V, et al. Cystosarcoma phyllodes: a unique case with multiple unilateral lesions and ipsilateral axillary metastasis. *J Pathol Bacteriol* 1968;96:514–517.

84. Bader E, Isaacson C. Bilateral malignant cystosarcoma phyllodes. *Br J Surg* 1961;48:519–521.

85. Notley RG, Griffiths HJL. Bilateral malignant cystosarcoma phyllodes. *Br J Surg* 1965;52:360–362.

86. Reich T, Solomon C. Bilateral cystosarcoma phyllodes, malignant variant, with 14-year follow-up. *Ann Surg* 1958;147:39–43.

87. Norris HJ, Taylor HB. Relationship of histologic features to behavior of cystosarcoma phyllodes: analysis of ninety-four cases. *Cancer* 1967;20:2090–2099.

88. Amerson JR. Cystosarcoma phyllodes in adolescent females. A report of seven patients. *Ann Surg* 1970;171:849–853.

89. Hart WR, Bauer RC, Oberman HA. Cystosarcoma phyllodes: a clinicopathologic study of twenty-six hypercellular periductal stromal tumors of the breast. *Am J Clin Pathol* 1978;70:211–216.

90. Reinfuss M, Mitus J, Smolak K, et al. Malignant phyllodes tumours of the breast: a clinical and pathological analysis of 55 cases. *Eur J Cancer* 1993;29A:1252–1256.

91. Keelan PA, Myers J, Wold LE, et al. Phyllodes tumor: clinicopathologic review of 60 patients and flow cytometric analysis in 30 patients. *Hum Pathol* 1992;23:1048–1054.

92. Nielsen VT, Andreasen C. Phyllodes tumour of the male breast. *Histopathology* 1987;11:761–765.

93. Reingold IM, Ascher GS. Cystosarcoma phyllodes in a man with gynecomastia. *Am J Clin Pathol* 1970;53:852–856.

94. Andersson A, Bergdahl L. Cystosarcoma in young women. *Arch Surg* 1978;113:742–744.

95. Adachi Y, Matsushima T, Kido A, et al. Phyllodes tumor in adolescents: report of two cases and review of the literature. *Breast Dis* 1993;6:285–293.

96. Briggs RM, Walters M, Rosenthal D. Cystosarcoma phylloides in adolescent female patients. *Am J Surg* 1983;146:712–714.

97. Hoover HC, Trestioreanu A, Ketcham AS. Metastatic cystosarcoma phylloides in an adolescent girl: an unusually malignant tumor. *Ann Surg* 1975;181:279–282.

98. Roisman I, Barak V, Okon E, et al. Benign cystosarcoma phyllodes of breast in an adolescent female. *Breast Dis* 1991;4:299–305.

99. Senocak ME, Gögüs S, Hiçsönmez A, et al. Cystosarcoma phylloides in an adolescent female. *Z Kinder* 1989;44:253–254.

100. Rajan PB, Cranor ML, Rosen PP. Cystosarcoma phyllodes in adolescent girls and young women: a study of 45 patients. *Am J Surg Pathol* 1998;22:64–69.

101. Way JC, Culham BA. Phyllodes tumour in pregnancy: a case report. *Can J Surg* 1998;41:407–409.

102. Bernstein L, Deapen D, Koss RK. The descriptive epidemiology of malignant cystosarcoma phyllodes tumors of the breast. *Cancer* 1993;71:3020–3024.

103. Browder W, McQuitty Jr JT, McDonald JC. Malignant cystosarcoma phylloides. Treatment and prognosis. *Am J Surg* 1978;136:239–241.

104. Buchberger W, Strasser K, Heim K, et al. Phylloides tumor: findings on mammography, sonography, and aspiration cytology in 10 cases. *AJR Am J Roentgenol* 1991;157:715–719.

105. Cosmacini P, Zurrida S, Veronesi P, et al. Phyllode tumor of the breast: mammographic experience in 99 cases. *Eur J Radiol* 1992;15:11–14.

106. Liberman L, Bonaccio E, Hamele-Bena D, et al. Benign and malignant phyllodes tumors: mammographic and sonographic findings. *Radiology* 1996;198:121–124.

107. Farria DM, Gorczyca DP, Barsky SH, et al. Benign phyllodes tumor of the breast: MR imaging features. *AJR Am J Roentgenol* 1996;167:187–189.

108. Grebe P, Wilhelm K, Brunier A, et al. MR tomography of cystosarcoma phyllodes: a case report. *Aktuelle Radiol* 1992;2:376–378(abst).

109. Layfield LJ, Hart J, Neuwirth H, et al. Relation between DNA ploidy and the clinical behavior of phyllodes tumors. *Cancer* 1989;64:1486–1489.

110. El-Naggar AK, Ro JY, McLemore D, et al. DNA content and proliferative activity of cystosarcoma phyllodes of the breast: potential prognostic significance. *Am J Clin Pathol* 1990;93:480–485.

111. Palko MJ, Wang SE, Shackney SE, et al. Flow cytometric S fraction as a predictor of clinical outcome in cystosarcoma phyllodes. *Arch Pathol Lab Med* 1990;114:949–952.

112. Dietrich CU, Pandis N, Bardi G, et al. Karyotypic changes in phyllodes tumors of the brest. *Cancer Genet Cytogenet* 1994;76:200–206.

113. Leuschner E, Meyer-Bolte K, Caselitz J, et al. Fibroadenoma of the breast showing a translocation (6;14), a ring chromosome and two markers involving parts of chromosome 11. *Cancer Genet Cytogenet* 1994;76:145–147.

114. Birdsall SH, Summersgill BM, Egan M, et al. Additional copies of 1q in sequential samples from a phyllodes tumor of the breast. *Cancer Genet Cytogenet* 1995;83:111–114.

115. Noguchi S, Motomura K, Inaji H, et al. Clonal analysis of fibroadenoma and phyllodes tumor of the breast. *Cancer Res* 1993;53: 4071–4074.

116. Lu Y-J, Birdsall S, Osin P, et al. Phyllodes tumors of the breast analyzed by comparative genomic hybridization and association of increased 1q copy number with stromal overgrowth and recurrence. *Genes Chromosomes Cancer* 1997;20:275–281.

117. Rao BR, Meyer JS, Fry CG. Most cystosarcoma phyllodes and fibroadenomas have progesterone receptor but lack estrogen receptor: a stromal localization of progesterone receptor. *Cancer* 1981;47: 2016–2021.

118. Kataoka T, Haruta R, Goto T, et al. Malignant phyllodes tumor of the breast with hypoglycemia: report of a case. *Jpn J Clin Oncol* 1998;28:276–280.

119. Shet T, Rege J. Cystic degeneration in phyllodes tumor. A source of error in cytologic interpretation. *Acta Cytologica* 2000;44:163–168.

120. Horiguchi J, Iino Y, Aiba S, et al. Phyllodes tumor showing intracystic growth: a case report. *Jpn J Clin Oncol* 1998;28:705–708.

121. Rosen PP, Romain K, Liberman L. Mammary cystosarcoma with adipose differentiation (lipophyllodes tumor) arising in a lipomatous hamartoma. *Arch Pathol Lab Med* 1994;118:91–94.

122. Barnes L, Pietruszka M. Rhabdomyosarcoma arising within a breast and its mimic: an immunohistochemical and cystosarcoma phyllodes. *Am J Surg Pathol* 1978;2:423–429.

123. Powell CM, Rosen PP. Adipose differentiation in cystosarcoma phyllodes. *Am J Surg Pathol* 1994;18:720–727.

124. Iihara K, Machinami R, Kubota S, et al. Malignant cystosarcoma phyllodes tumor of the breast mainly composed of chondrosarcoma: a case report. *Diagn Pathol* 1997;142:241–245.

125. Silver SA, Tavassoli FA. Osteosarcomatous differentiation in phyllodes tumors. *Am J Surg Pathol* 1999;23:815–821.

126. Grove A, Deibjerg Kristensen L. Intraductal carcinoma within a phyllodes tumor of the breast: a case report. *Tumori* 1986;72:187–190.

127. Knudsen PJ, Ostergaard J. Cystosarcoma phyllodes with lobular and ductal carcinoma *in situ. Arch Pathol Lab Med* 1987;111:873–875.

128. Agarwal J, Kapila K, Verma K. Phyllodes tumor with keratin cysts: a diagnostic problem in fine needle aspiration of the breast. *Acta Cytol* 1991;35:255–256.

129. McDivitt RW, Urban JA, Farrow JH. Cystosarcoma phyllodes. *Johns Hopkins Med J* 1967;120:33–45.

130. Salisbury JR, Singh LN. Apocrine metaplasia in phyllodes tumours of the breast. *Histopathology* 1986;10:1211–1215.

131. Hiraoka N, Mukai M, Hosoda Y, et al. Phyllodes tumor of the breast containing the intracytoplasmic inclusion bodies identical with infantile digital fibromatosis. *Am J Surg Pathol* 1994;18:506–511.

132. West TL, Weiland LH, Clagett OT. Cystosarcoma phyllodes. *Ann Surg* 1971;173:520–528.

133. Kracht J, Sapino A, Bussolati G. Malignant phyllodes tumor of breast with lung metastases mimicking the primary. *Am J Surg Pathol* 1998;22:1284–1290.

134. Graadt van Roggen JF, Zonderland HM, Welvaart K, et al. Local recurrence of a phyllodes tumour of the breast presenting with widespread differentiation to a telangiectatic osteosarcoma. *J Clin Pathol* 1998;51:706–708.

135. Gisser SD, Toker C. Chondroblastic sarcoma of the breast. *Mt Sinai J Med* 1975;42:232–235.

136. Anani PA, Baumann RP. Osteosarcoma of the breast. *Virchows Arch* 1972;357:213–218.

137. Lubin J, Rywlin AM. Cystosarcoma phyllodes metastasizing as a mixed mesenchymal sarcoma. *South Med J* 1972;65:636–637.

138. Jackson AV. Metastasising liposarcoma of the breast arising in a fibro-adenoma. *J Pathol Bacteriol* 1962;83:582–584.

139. Aranda FI, Laforga JB, Lopez JI. Phyllodes tumor of the breast: an immunohistochemical study of 28 cases with special attention to the role of myofibroblasts. *Pathol Res Pract* 1994;190:474–481.

140. Auger M, Hanna W, Kahn HJ. Cystosarcoma phylloides of the breast and its mimics. An immunohistochemical and ultrastructural study. *Arch Pathol Lab Med* 1989;113:1231–1235.

141. Kim WH, Kim CW, Noh D-Y, et al. Differential pattern of perivascular type IV collagen deposits in phyllodes tumors of the breast. *J Korean Med Sci* 1992;7:360–363.

142. Kocová L, Skálová A, Fakan F, et al. Phyllodes tumour of the breast: immunohistochemical study of 37 tumours using MIB1 antibody. *Pathol Res Pract* 1998;194:97–104.

143. Millar EK, Beretov J, Marr P, et al. Malignant phyllodes tumours of the breast display increased stromal p53 protein expression. *Histopathology* 1999;34:491–496.

144. Yamashita J-I, Ogawa M, Egami H, et al. Abundant expression of immunoreactive endothelin 1 in mammary phyllodes tumor: possible paracrine role of endothelin 1 in the growth of stromal cells in phyllodes tumor. *Cancer Res* 1992;52:4046–4049.

145. Schrey MP, Patel KV, Tezapsidis N. Bombesin and glucocorticoids stimulate human breast cancer cells to produce endothelin, a paracrine mitogen for breast stromal cells. *Cancer Res* 1992;52:1786–1790.

146. Sawhney N, Garrahan N, Douglas-Jones AG, et al. Epithelial-stromal interactions in tumors. *Cancer* 1992;70:2115–2120.

146a. Feakins RM, Wells CA, Young KA, et al. Platelet-derived growth factor expression in phyllodes tumors and fibroadenomas of the breast. *Hum Pathol* 2000;31:1214–1222.

146b. Sawyer EJ, Hanby AM, Ellis P, et al. Molecular analysis of phyllodes tumors reveals distinct changes in the epithelial and stromal components. *Am J Pathol* 2000;156:1093–1098.

147. McCune B, Kopp J. Tenascin distribution in phyllodes tumor is distinctly different than in fibroadenoma of the breast. *Lab Invest* 1994;70:18A.

148. Harris M, Khan MK. Phyllodes tumour and stromal sarcoma of the breast: an ultrastructural comparison. *Histopathology* 1984;8: 315–330.

149. Fernandez BB, Hernandez FJ, Spindler W. Metastatic cystosarcoma phyllodes. A light and electron microscopic study. *Cancer* 1976; 37:1737–1746.

150. Toker C. Cystosarcoma phyllodes: an ultrastructural study. *Cancer* 1968;21:1171–1179.

151. Shimizu K, Masawa N, Yamada T, et al. Cytolgoic evaluation of phyllodes tumors as compared to fibroadenomas of the breast. *Acta Cytol* 1994;38:891–897.

152. Mottot C, Pouliquen X, Bastien H, et al. Fibroadenomes et tumeurs phyllodes: approche cytopatholgoique. *Ann Anat Pathol* 1978;23: 233–240.

153. Simi U, Moretti D, Iacconi P, et al. Fine needle aspiration cytopathology of phyllodes tumor: differential diagnosis with fibroadenoma. *Acta Cytol* 1988;32:63–66.

154. Ciatto S, Bonardi R, Cataliotti L, et al. Members of the Coordinating Center and Writing Committee of FONCAM. Phyllodes tumor of the breast: a multicenter series of 59 cases. *Eur J Surg Oncol* 1992; 18:545–549.

155. Dusenbery D, Frable WL. Fine needle aspiration cytology of phyllodes tumor. Potential diagnostic pitfalls. *Acta Cytol* 1992;36: 215–221.

156. Lee W-Y, Cheng L, Chang T-W. Fine needle aspiration cytology of malignant phyllodes tumor with liposarcomatous stroma of the breast. A case report. *Acta Cytol* 1998;42:391–395.

157. Reinfuss M, Mitus J, Duda K, et al. The treatment and prognosis of patients with phyllodes tumor of the breast: an analysis of 170 cases. *Cancer* 1996;77:910–916.

158. Treves N, Sunderland DA. Cystosarcoma phyllodes of the breast: a malignant and a benign tumor: a clinicopathological study of seventy-seven cases. *Cancer* 1951;4:1286–1332.

159. Harada S, Fujiwara H, Hisatsugu T, et al. Malignant cystosarcoma phyllodes with lymph nodes metastasis: a case report. *Jpn J Surg* 1987;17:174–177.

160. Barth RJ Jr. Histologic features predict local recurrence after breast conserving therapy of phyllodes tumors. *Breast Cancer Res Treat* 1999;57:291–295.

161. Bartoli C, Zurrida S, Veronesi P, et al. Small sized phyllodes tumor of the breast. *Eur J Surg Oncol* 1990;16:215–219.

162. Hart J, Layfield LJ, Trumbull WE, et al. Practical aspects in the diagnosis and management of cystosarcoma phyllodes. *Arch Surg* 1988;123:1079–1083.

163. McGregor GI, Knowling MA, Este FA. Sarcoma and cystosarcoma phyllodes tumors of the breast—a retrospective review of 58 cases. *Am J Surg* 1994;167:477–480.

164. Salvadori B, Cusumano F, Del Bo R, et al. Surgical treatment of phyllodes tumors of the breast. *Cancer* 1989;63:2532–2536.

165. Blichert-Toft M, Hart Hansen JP, Hart Hansen O, et al. Clinical course of cystosarcoma phyllodes related to histologic appearance. *Surg Gynecol Obstet* 1975;140:1929–1932.

166. Oberman HA. Cystosarcoma phyllodes: a clinicopathologic study of hypercellular periductal stromal neoplasms of breast. *Cancer* 1965;18:697–710.

167. Oberman HA, Nosanchuk JS, Finger JE. Periductal stromal tumors of breast with adipose metaplasia. *Arch Surg* 1969;98:384–387.

168. Qizilbash AH. Cystosarcoma phyllodes with liposarcomatous stroma. *Am J Clin Pathol* 1976;65:321–327.

169. Kessinger A, Foley JF, Lemon HM, et al. Metastatic cystosarcoma phyllodes: a case report and review of the literature. *J Surg Oncol* 1972;4:131–136.

170. Fleisher AG, Tyers FO, Hu D, et al. Dumbbell metastatic cystosarcoma phyllodes of the heart and lung. *Ann Thorac Surg* 1990;49:309–311.

171. Abemayor E, Nast CC, Kessler DJ. Cystosarcoma phyllodes metastatic to the mandible. *J Surg Oncol* 1988;39:235–240.

172. Tenzer JA, Rypins RD, Jakowatz JG. Malignant cystosarcoma phyllodes metastatic to the maxilla. *J Oral Maxillofac Surg* 1988;46:80–82.

173. Grimes MM, Lattes R, Jaretzki A III. Cystosarcoma phyllodes. Report of an unusual case, with death due to intraneural extension to the central nervous system. *Cancer* 1985;56:1691–1695.

174. Hlavin ML, Kaminski HJ, Cohen M, et al. Central nervous system complications of cystosarcoma phyllodes. *Cancer* 1993;72:126–130.

175. Hines JR, Murad TM, Beal JM. Prognostic indicators in cystosarcoma phylloides. *Am J Surg* 1987;153:276–280.

176. Pietruszka M, Barnes L. Cystosarcoma phyllodes: a clinicopathologic analysis of 42 cases. *Cancer* 1978;41:1974–1983.

177. Hawkins RE, Schofield JB, Fisher C, et al. The clinical and histologic criteria that predict metastases from cystosarcoma phyllodes. *Cancer* 1992;69:141–147.

178. Lindquist KD, van Heerden JA, Weiland LH, et al. Recurrent and metastatic cystosarcoma phyllodes. *Am J Surg* 1982;144:341–343.

179. Burton GV, Hart LL, Leight GS, et al. Cystosarcoma phyllodes: effective therapy with cisplatin and etoposide chemotherapy. *Cancer* 1989;63:2088–2092.

# CHAPTER 9

# Ductal Hyperplasia

## Ordinary and Atypical

## INVESTIGATIONAL STUDIES

This chapter is concerned primarily with the histopathology of ductal hyperplasia. Chapter 10 deals in greater detail with the concept of hyperplasia as a precancerous condition. Issues related to *in situ* carcinoma are addressed in Chapter 11. Chapter 12 is devoted to intraductal carcinoma. Because these topics are intimately interrelated, some subject matter may be covered in more than one chapter. The discussions of ductal hyperplasia and intraductal carcinoma are presented in separate chapters to emphasize the importance of distinguishing pathologically between these entities in the clinical setting.

Ellis et al. proposed that epithelial hyperplasia of the breast be defined and "identified by a mixture of cell types demonstrated principally by morphology but that could be supported by immunophenotypic diversity and by lack of a dominant epithelial population" (1). It was further suggested that "the distinction of the boundary between hyperplasia and neoplasia in the breast should be recognized . . . [and] . . . is practicable at present . . ." with *in situ* carcinoma "identified by presence of a dominant clonal epithelial cell population that can be identified morphologically by a single cell population having distinctive morphological, immunophenotypic and molecular genetic characteristics."

For research purposes, it may be useful to view the spectrum of intraductal proliferation as a continuum with no subdivisions. This concept is embodied in the terms *mammary intraepithelial neoplasia* (MIN) (2) and *ductal intraepithelial neoplasia* (DIN) (3). Although these alternative classifications replace the word *carcinoma* with *neoplasia*, they retain diagnostic groupings intended to distinguish lesions equivalent to hyperplasia, atypical hyperplasia, and intraductal carcinoma of low and high grade. Boundaries are suggested for these groupings with no compelling evidence that they are more meaningful biologically or clinically than the

existing classification or that they improve diagnostic reproducibility. Using the term *neoplasia* for lesions that are generally agreed to be hyperplasia of the usual type (hyperplasia without atypia) is contradictory.

If ductal carcinoma in the breast evolves in a stepwise fashion comparable to that proposed for other organs, such as the colon (4), then it is likely that some stages in this progression are manifested in the histologic phenotype of intraductal proliferations. On the other hand, some significant genotypic alterations may not be manifested in the histologic appearance of lesions. Proliferative foci grouped together under a diagnosis of hyperplasia might consist of genotypically diverse abnormalities with differing risks for carcinoma. The unraveling of this puzzle will be the main focus of research in the realm of "precancerous" breast pathology for decades to come. Immunohistochemistry and molecular analysis of microdissected samples will be necessary to identify relevant markers, and it is likely that these tests eventually will be incorporated into diagnostic procedures when the information becomes clinically useful and simplified technology becomes available.

Research to date on molecular correlates of usual hyperplasia, atypical hyperplasia, and "precancerous" breast pathology suggests that this is a complex undertaking fraught with difficulty. Genetic abnormalities have been detected by chromosomal analysis and by molecular techniques in lesions considered to be benign proliferative breast disease (5–7). These investigations have used microdissection to isolate individual ductal lesions for molecular analysis. The results of studies that report loss of heterozygosity (LOH) (6) or monoclonality (8) in atypical duct hyperplasia must be interpreted cautiously. Images purported by the investigators to show atypical ductal hyperplasia in these two studies would be interpreted by this investigator as intraductal carcinoma. One may reasonably question whether the molecular data should guide the interpretation of the histologic phenotype or if the reverse interpretation should apply. Nonetheless, it is apparent that molecular analysis will not soon resolve the diagnostic issues of interpreting "borderline" lesions in routine histologic sections. As long as the primary method for diagnosis is histologic examination, the information gained from molecular studies will become applicable to routine diagnosis only if it results in the identification of one or more specific cancer-associated immunohistochemical markers and procedures are developed for studying LOH or other genetic alterations directly *in situ* in tissues, or conveniently in microdissected samples.

Ultimately, correlation of molecular alterations in proliferative lesions with clinical outcome will be necessary to determine which phenotypic and genotypic changes are meaningful. Presently, these studies must be retrospective in the sense that the histologic samples to be analyzed were obtained sometime in the past and patient outcome is determined subsequently without standardized interval follow-up procedures. Prospective studies of the "natural history" of atypical proliferative lesions subjected to molecular analysis are likely to be difficult because of the introduction of breast cancer prevention with tamoxifen and other medications presently being developed.

The complexity of the task in retrospective analysis is illustrated by several recent investigations. Kasami et al. studied microdissected samples of proliferative breast lesions from eight women (9). Follow-up ranging from 8 to 25 years was available for four patients. The samples were analyzed for LOH and microsatellite instability at 10 loci. In one patient, five loci with microsatelite instability and two loci with LOH were found in a lesion described as a papilloma with florid hyperplasia and atypia, whereas 10 other proliferative lesions from this patient showed no genetic alterations or atypia. Three loci of microsatellite instability were detected in a proliferative lesion without atypia from another patient. For both patients, more than 20 years had passed since the biopsies were performed that produced these samples. These investigators concluded "that several genetic alterations in proliferative breast disease lesions may not indicate clinically meaningful premalignancy for remaining breast."

It is likely that large-scale studies of multiple proliferative lesions from substantial numbers of patients with well-defined follow-up will be needed to detect significant associations between genetic alterations and cancer risk.

One prospective investigation examined the relationship between HER2/*neu* and p53 expression in benign breast lesions and breast cancer risk in a nested case-control study (10). The patients were part of the Canadian National Breast Screening Study. P53 protein detected by immunohistochemistry in benign proliferative lesions was associated with an increased risk of developing carcinoma [adjusted odds ratio (OR) = 2.5; 95% confidence interval (CI) = 1.01–6.40). There was no increased risk associated with HER2/*neu* overexpression (adjusted OR = 0.65; 95% CI = 0.27–1.53). In two other studies, the frequency of detecting p53 overexpression by immunohistochemistry in duct hyperplasia was

low. Mommers et al. studied the expression of several proliferation and apoptosis-related proteins in foci of usual hyperplasia (11). HER2/*neu* and p53 were found in 2% and 8%, respectively, and decreased expression of *bcl*-2 was detected in 16%. Other markers with abnormal expression in some examples of usual hyperplasia were cyclin D1, Ki67, p21, and p27. Of 91 lesions, 23 (25%) had more than one abnormal proliferation or apoptosis-related protein expression.

Studies that report p53 accumulation detected by immunohistochemistry in hyperplastic lesions do not appear well supported by molecular analysis of p53 mutations in these lesions. Done et al. used microdissection to isolate foci of epithelial hyperplasia and intraductal carcinoma associated with invasive carcinomas with known p53 mutations (12). The samples of intraductal carcinoma had the same p53 mutations as the corresponding invasive carcinomas but none of the hyperplasias exhibited any p53 mutations. These researchers did not report immunohistochemical data for these specimens, but the results suggest that p53 mutations are not a frequent occurrence in hyperplastic lesions, even in a breast that harbors carcinoma with this genetic alteration.

Another complicating factor lies in the reported detection of genetic changes in histologically normal appearing breast tissues. LOH has been described in cells obtained from microdissected histologically normal lobules obtained from tissue adjacent to breast carcinomas (13). Gobbi et al. studied the immunohistochemical expression of transforming growth factor-β receptor II (TGF-β RII) as a marker of breast cancer risk in hyperplastic breast lesions without atypia and in the normal breast (14). Reduced expression of TGF-β RII in nonatypical hyperplasia and in adjacent lobules was associated with an increased risk of developing invasive carcinoma in this retrospective study. Expression of HER2/*neu* also been detected in histologically normal breast tissue associated with breast carcinoma. Ratcliffe et al. used a combined *in situ* hybridization and immunohistochemical technique to assess this oncogene and its protein expression (15). Membrane staining was generally weak when present in normal breast tissue, corresponding to the level of expression in carcinomas lacking HER2/*neu* amplification. The presence of a signal detected by *in situ* hybridization in scattered nuclei in histologically normal cells, however, may indicate an early stage of amplification preceding histologic evidence of transformation in isolated cells.

These findings raise concern about the specificity of associations between molecular markers and particular types of proliferative lesions. Some alterations may occur in tissues exhibiting little or no proliferative change. Were this to be a widespread phenomenon, the criteria for selecting samples for analysis, which currently concentrate on proliferative abnormalities, might need to be revised.

Ultimately, a combination of histology, immunohistochemistry, and molecular analysis will be needed to arrive at a more meaningful, clinically relevant classification of proliferative ductal lesions than the existing system based entirely on histologic criteria.

Presently, the distinction between intraductal hyperplasia and intraductal carcinoma is important for management of the disease (16). In most cases, intraductal proliferations are readily classified by pathologists on the basis of generally accepted histopathologic features as either ductal hyperplasia or *in situ* ductal carcinoma (17). A subset exists for which assignment to either of these categories is less certain and most of these abnormalities qualify as atypical hyperplasia. The existence of *borderline lesions*, which may be diagnosed as hyperplasia or *in situ* carcinoma, depending on which criteria are used, is not a compelling reason for abandoning the existing practice of distinguishing pathologically and clinically between ductal hyperplasia of usual type, atypical ductal hyperplasia, and *in situ* ductal carcinoma. Studies of interobserver reproducibility in the diagnosis of highly selected examples of these lesions have focused undue attention on the troublesome diagnostic problem of borderline abnormalities, which applies to only a small percentage of proliferative breast changes (2,18,19).

## CLINICAL PRESENTATION

There are no clinical features specifically associated with ductal hyperplasia. The alterations caused by epithelial proliferation in individual ducts or in multiple branches of a ductal system are microscopic in dimension and usually not palpable. A mass lesion that incorporates elements of ductal hyperplasia may develop if other coexisting tissue alterations, such as pseudoangiomatous stromal hyperplasia, are present, or if the process has the complexity of a radial sclerosing lesion or multiple papillomas. For example, ductal hyperplasia in various forms is a frequent constituent of "fibrocystic changes" that can be detected by mammography or as a palpable tumor. In addition to ductal hyperplasia, the lesion complex can include one or more of the following pathologic changes, which are discussed individually elsewhere in this volume: sclerosing adenosis, cystic and papillary apocrine metaplasia, duct stasis and inflammation, fibrosis and pseudoangiomatous stromal hyperplasia, and lobular hyperplasia.

An important corollary to the lack of clinical indicators of ductal hyperplasia is an inability to determine the duration of these lesions. The date on which ductal hyperplasia was biopsied customarily is used as though it were the date of "onset" in follow-up studies. This practice, a consequence of an inability to determine the preclinical duration of hyperplastic ductal lesions, could be a source of bias in assessing the precancerous significance of proliferative lesions in individual patients.

When clinically evident, ductal hyperplasia most often occurs in an ill-defined palpable area that is described as breast thickening. The nonspecific mammographic manifestations of these changes include altered duct patterns, parenchymal distortion, nonpalpable mass lesions, calcification and asymmetry when both breasts are compared. Calcifications are the most frequent mammographic indication of atypical ductal hyperplasia in the absence of a palpable abnormality (20–22). Radial sclerosing lesions described on mammography as "radial scars" often have a component of ductal hyperplasia. Some but not all radial sclerosing lesions contain microcalcifications. One of the most distinctive clinical forms of fibrocystic change with a prominent component of duct hyperplasia is juvenile papillomatosis, which typically presents as a single, discrete, unilateral tumor in women in their teens and early twenties (23).

In the era that preceded the widespread use of mammography, when the indication for biopsy was a palpable abnormality, ductal hyperplasia was found in 25% or fewer of the specimens obtained (24,25). Not more than 5% of these biopsies had atypical ductal hyperplasia. The frequency of atypical abnormalities is higher among mammographically directed biopsies, including surgical excisions and needle core biopsies (26,27). Issues associated with the diagnosis of atypical duct hyperplasia in needle core biopsies are discussed later in this chapter.

Ductal hyperplasia can be found in female patients at virtually any age. In patients younger than 30 years, most examples of ductal hyperplasia occur either as juvenile papillomatosis (23) or as one of the group of lesions referred to as papillary duct hyperplasia in children and young women (28). Most women with ductal hyperplasia are between 35 and 60 years of age. A significant subset of these patients have hyperplasia of the columnar cell type, a lesion that is often multifocal and associated with microcalcifications (29,30). In women older than 60, ductal hyperplasia becomes less frequent; when it is present, the growth pattern is usually less florid than in younger women. Occasionally, however, a woman older than 60 years may have extensive proliferative changes with florid ductal hyperplasia. This finding is likely to be accompanied by disproportionately less lobular atrophy than would be expected at this age, or there may be lobular hyperplasia with secretion in lobular glands. The use of exogenous estrogens can be documented in many but not all of these cases.

## GROSS PATHOLOGY

There are no grossly apparent pathologic features specifically associated with intraductal hyperplasia. It is often present in specimens containing cysts and other fibrocystic changes.

## MICROSCOPIC PATHOLOGY

Ductal hyperplasia describes a proliferative condition that is manifested histologically as an increase in the cellularity of ductal epithelium. Because the normal resting epithelium consists of a continuous monolayer of cuboidal to columnar epithelial cells supported by myoepithelial cells, an increase in the cellularity of this two-layer configuration constitutes hyperplasia. Physiologic hyperplasia during pregnancy is manifested by an increase in the number of glandular structures as well as growth in the thickness of the epithelial layer, especially in lobular glands and ductules. Concurrent but usually less extreme expansion of the myoepithelium may be present.

Hyperplasia not attributable to normal physiologic conditions also causes an increase in the thickness of the epithelial layer, resulting in partial or complete obstruction of the duct lumen at the site of the proliferative abnormality. If intraductal hyperplasia is traced in serial sections, it is often possible to observe the discontinuous, multifocal nature of the condition along the course of a single duct. Enlargement of the entire affected glandular structure is also frequently observed, both in terms of increased diameter and greater length, resulting in a sinuous structure. Various distortions of the basic ductal architecture occur when hyperplastic ducts become more sinuous or when they are incorporated into complex proliferative abnormalities, such as papillomas or radial sclerosing lesions. Hyperplasia can extend into branches of a ductal system and frequently involves terminal duct–lobular units.

Ductal hyperplasia has been described by terms such as *epitheliosis* (31) and *papillomatosis* (32). The former term was applied to ". . . the solid and quasi-solid benign epithelial proliferation which is found predominantly in small ducts, ductules and lobules" (31). Because it refers to epithelium in general, epitheliosis could be construed to include lobular hyperplasia. Because intraductal hyperplasia includes a variable component of proliferative elements that contain some fibrovascular stroma, the distinction between epitheliosis and papillary hyperplasia is not always clear. Consequently, there is no apparent advantage to replacing the term *ductal hyperplasia* with *epitheliosis*. *Papillomatosis,* often used interchangeably with duct hyperplasia, is a term more appropriately applied to hyperplastic lesions in which a distinct fibrovascular structure supports papillary epithelial hyperplasia. Ductal hyperplasia that is not atypical is referred to as "usual," "regular," or "ordinary" to distinguish it from atypical duct hyperplasia.

Instances of proliferative lesions originating in major lactiferous ducts or in larger terminal ducts can be readily found to document the capacity of the epithelium of these structures to undergo hyperplastic or carcinomatous change. The term *intraductal*, as it applies to hyperplasia or *in situ* carcinoma, relates to a pattern of epithelial proliferation. Studies of breast tissue by subgross dissection suggest that many of the proliferative changes commonly described as ductal hyperplasia arise from ductular structures of the lobules (33). The specific histologic features of hyperplasia arising in a major duct or in the components of an unfolded lobule are not readily distinguishable in conventional histologic sections, although the overall structure of the lesion and its microscopic distribution in the breast may suggest the anatomic level of origin.

When subgross dissection is performed, the breast tissue is fixed and processed by a method that makes it possible to study the specimen by using a dissecting microscope. The tissue thus can be examined to visualize its three-dimensional structure and abnormalities in the duct-lobular architecture. Foci of interest can be excised from subgross samples as small tissue blocks and embedded for histologic examination. Microscopic study of these selected specimens has shown that lobular unfolding occurs as a result of dilatation and stretching of terminal duct-lobular structures. The dilated structures are termed *ducts* if they are more than three to four times the diameter of a lobular ductule. In some instances, the dilated structures remain clustered together, and there may be remnants of one or more lobules that participated either partially or not at all in the process of unfolding. The ducts formed in some unfolded lobules appear to drift apart so that their origin in a terminal duct-lobular structure may no longer be apparent in two-dimensional histologic sections.

Whereas many of these dilated structures arising from unfolded terminal ducts and lobules maintain continuity with the duct system, others appear to become isolated and cystic. Some cysts are formed from dilated acinar glands, representing the terminal portions of the intralobular duct system. Others seem to develop in segments of the duct system, possibly caused by internal duct obstruction resulting from hyperplasia or as a result of compression resulting from periductal fibrosis or proliferative changes. It appears that a frequent fate of unfolded lobular-duct structures is to form cysts or to be the site of hyperplastic changes (Fig. 9.1). This morphogenetic relationship is the probable explanation for the frequent coexistence of the pathologic alterations that constitute fibrocystic changes, including ductal hyperplasia.

Ductal hyperplasia may be limited to one or more isolated foci, or it may involve multiple contiguous foci in a segmental region of the breast. Occasionally, it appears to arise in more than one segmental duct system. Quantitatively, the amount of hyperplasia in any one duct varies from a minimal increase in the number of cells to complete filling of the duct, with occlusion of the lumen. The size or degree of distention of a duct is not a direct function of the amount of epithelial hyperplasia at that site. Segments of ducts occluded by hyperplastic epithelium may have a relatively small diameter, and ducts that are dilated sometimes exhibit slight hyperplasia.

## Ordinary (Usual) Ductal Hyperplasia

The amount, growth patterns, and anatomic distribution of ductal hyperplasia vary greatly from one patient to another. The structural spectrum of ductal hyperplasia is quite heterogeneous. Nonetheless, these lesions have certain features in common that are the basis for diagnosis.

The cytologic characteristics of ordinary ductal hyperplasia are similar regardless of the amount of hyperplasia present. The cellular proliferation in ductal hyperplasia often

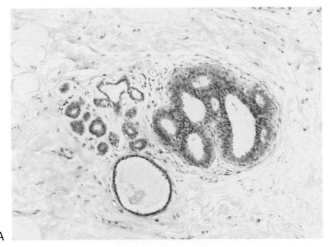

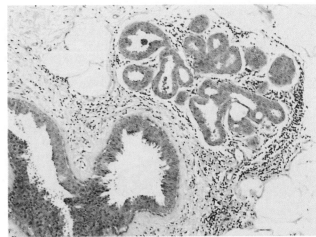

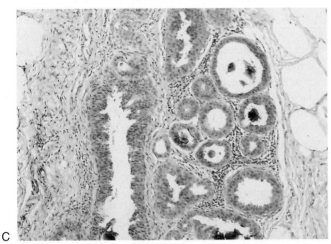

**FIG. 9.1.** *Ductal hyperplasia, mild, in terminal duct-lobular unit.* **A:** Columnar cell change in a terminal duct-lobular structure with cystic dilatation of a lobular gland. **B:** Mild columnar cell hyperplasia in a terminal duct and in the epithelium of an adjacent lobule. **C:** Mild columnar cell hyperplasia in an intralobular ductule and lobular glands with calcification.

has a syncytial appearance because individual cell borders are inconspicuous (Fig. 9.2). The cytoplasm is amphophilic or weakly eosinophilic and homogeneous. Cytoplasmic vacuolization is uncommon. True cytoplasmic microlumens that contain secretion stained positively with the mucicarmine or Alcian blue–periodic acid-Schiff (PAS) stains are exceedingly unusual. The presence of intracytoplasmic mucin-containing microlumens is an atypical feature that should

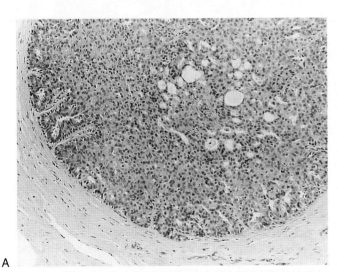

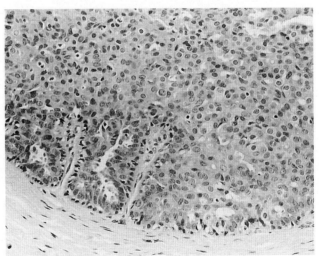

**FIG. 9.2.** *Ductal hyperplasia, florid.* **A:** Florid hyperplasia that fills the duct. Microlumens in the hyperplastic epithelium are unevenly distributed and vary in shape from slit-like to round. **B:** The cells with indistinct borders have overlapping nuclei. Persisting original ductal epithelium is evident on the *lower left*.

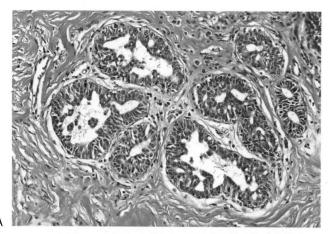

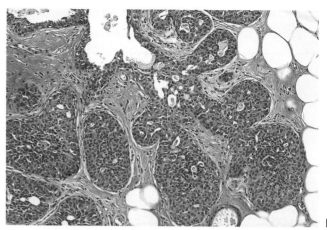

**FIG. 9.3.** *Ductal hyperplasia, mild.* **A:** Minimal micropapillary growth is present. **B:** Solid growth mainly involves expanded terminal duct–lobular units.

occasion careful consideration of a diagnosis of intraductal carcinoma. In making this determination, it is critical to distinguish between intracytoplasmic vacuoles and small spaces that are remnants of the central duct lumen caught between cells.

The cytoplasmic volume of hyperplastic ductal cells tends to be reduced by comparison with normal ductal cells, causing the nuclear: cytoplasmic ratio to be elevated; however, there is little increase, if any, in nuclear size in ordinary ductal hyperplasia. Nuclei are round, ovoid to spindly, or reniform, depending in part on the plane of section. Nuclear spacing is uneven, resulting in areas where the cells appear crowded and nuclei overlap.

Nuclear membranes are delicate and the chromatin pattern is typically uniform. Clear nuclear vesicles that occur in some examples of ductal hyperplasia are intranuclear inclu-

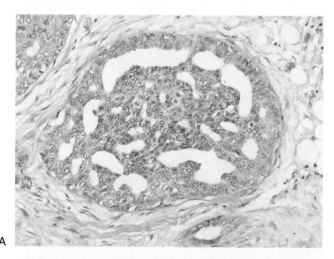

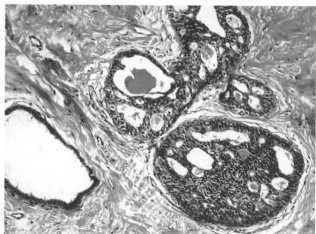

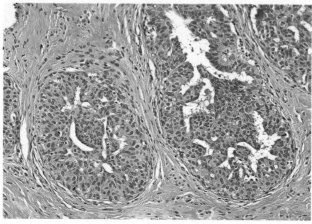

**FIG. 9.4.** *Ductal hyperplasia, moderate.* **A:** Hyperplasia forming a fenestrated mass connected to the hyperplastic ductal epithelium by strands of cells. **B:** A fenestrated growth pattern. Note that the cells forming the center of the lesion have sparse cytoplasm and small hyperchromatic nuclei. **C:** The original duct lumens are subdivided into crescentic and stellate spaces.

sions of cytoplasm. Nucleoli are inapparent or inconspicuous unless there is apocrine metaplasia in the hyperplastic epithelium. Mitotic figures are infrequent and, when present, have a regular configuration.

Ductal hyperplasia of the usual type has been subdivided on the basis of quantitative criteria into the categories of mild, moderate, and severe or florid. Application of this classification is limited by the fact that disordered epithelial growth with varied structural patterns is a characteristic feature of ductal hyperplasia. As a consequence, hyperplastic epithelium is not uniformly distributed in a stratified fashion that permits easy determination of the number of cell layers. Epithelial thickness is also difficult to judge in tangentially sectioned ducts. The criteria for making these distinctions, which are based largely on the thickness of the epithelium, are difficult to apply to small ductules and terminal ducts. In these structures, the lumen is relatively small and can be filled when there is relatively little increase in epithelial thickness. These levels or degrees of hyperplasia are meaningful only when applied to selected nontangential sections of duct structures of sufficient diameter to manifest diagnostic features. Consequently, the classification of ductal hyperplasia based on epithelial thickness has significant limitations and may not be applicable in all instances.

Ductal hyperplasia is considered mild if the epithelium is 3 to 4 cell layers thick, exclusive of the myoepithelium (Figs. 9.1 and 9.3). Mild hyperplasia may affect the entire epithelium circumferentially in a duct cross section or in only a segment of the duct. It usually occurs as a simple flat or slightly papillary increase in epithelial thickness. Mild hyperplasia is often considered a nonproliferative component of fibrocystic change, as discussed in Chapter 10.

In moderate hyperplasia, the epithelium has a thickness of five or more cell layers. As in mild hyperplasia, the thickened epithelium may be distributed as a flat or papillary layer at the periphery of the duct. In some instances, strands of epithelium extend across or bridge the lumen, resulting in the formation of secondary glandular spaces in the hyperplastic epithelium (Fig. 9.4).

Micropapillary hyperplasia is part of the spectrum of moderate ductal hyperplasia (Figs. 9.5 and 9.6). The papillae are blunt or slender, unevenly shaped fronds of hyperplastic epithelium in which cells at the tip are smaller and have more condensed nuclei than those at the base or in the intervening nonpapillary basal epithelium (Fig. 9.7). Micropapillary hyperplasia should be distinguished from micropapillary intraductal carcinoma (see Chapter 13).

The distinction between moderate and severe or florid

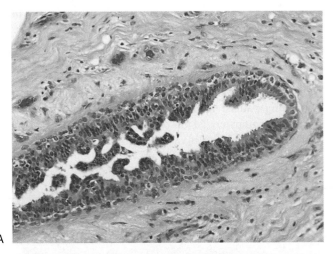

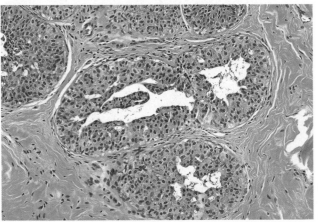

FIG. 9.5. *Ductal hyperplasia, micropapillary.* **A:** Moderate hyperplasia. Ductal epithelium and hyperplastic myoepithelial cells support micropapillary fronds of hyperplastic ductal epithelium. **B:** Micropapillary hyperplasia traverses the duct lumen. **C:** A complex example of micropapillary hyperplasia in which fusion of the epithelial fronds is creating a fenestrated structure.

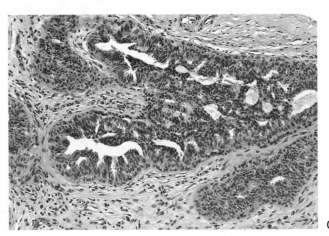

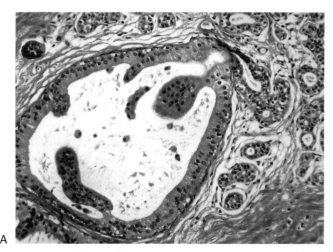
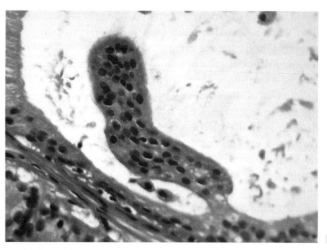

**FIG. 9.6.** *Ductal hyperplasia, micropapillary.* **A:** Moderate micropapillary hyperplasia of apocrine epithelium. Association of the hyperplastic duct with a lobule is evident on the *right*. **B:** Micropapillary apocrine hyperplasia shown in **A**. Note the small, dark nuclei in the apical region.

hyperplasia is not sharp, but lesions generally are placed in the latter category when the affected ducts are appreciably enlarged compared with nonhyperplastic counterparts and the lumina are nearly or completely filled by the proliferative epithelium. Squamous metaplasia sometimes develops in moderate and florid hyperplasia (Fig. 9.8). Moderate and severe ductal hyperplasia together constitute the category of ductal hyperplasia without atypia (*ordinary* or *usual* ductal hyperplasia) in the classification of proliferative breast changes used in the assessment of breast cancer risk (discussed in Chapter 10).

The nuclei in ductal hyperplasia are often overlapping and may be distributed in a "streaming" fashion. *Streaming* refers to a growth pattern in which hyperplastic epithelial cells are oriented parallel to their long axes, an appearance most readily manifested by the distribution of nuclei (Fig.

9.9). Because the cytoplasmic borders of these cells are indistinct, streaming usually is detected as a parallel orientation of oval or spindle-shaped nuclei. The spectrum of streaming is broad, ranging from subtle foci composed of only a few cells to conspicuous swirling patterns. Streaming occurs in all types of intraductal hyperplasia.

Florid hyperplasia has papillary and bridging growth patterns that are encountered in moderate hyperplasia, but the overall proliferation tends to be more cellular and complex than in moderate hyperplasia. Foci of florid hyperplasia are more likely to fill the entire duct lumen in a solid or fenestrated fashion. Often the cells are distributed in a streaming pattern in solid or in fenestrated areas. The association of the streaming pattern with ductal hyperplasia has been confirmed by computerized morphometric analysis of the orientation of nuclei in proliferative duct lesions (34). A part of

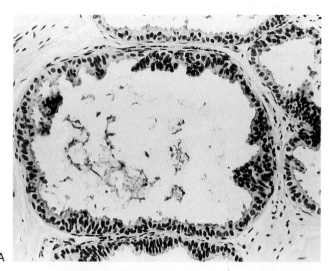
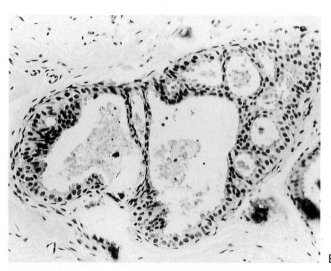

**FIG. 9.7.** *Ductal hyperplasia, micropapillary.* **A:** Moderate hyperplasia forming small epithelial tufts and mounds on low columnar ductal epithelium. **B:** Epithelial tufts are evident on the *left*, a transluminal epithelial bridge in the *center*, and fenestrated epithelium is on the *right*.

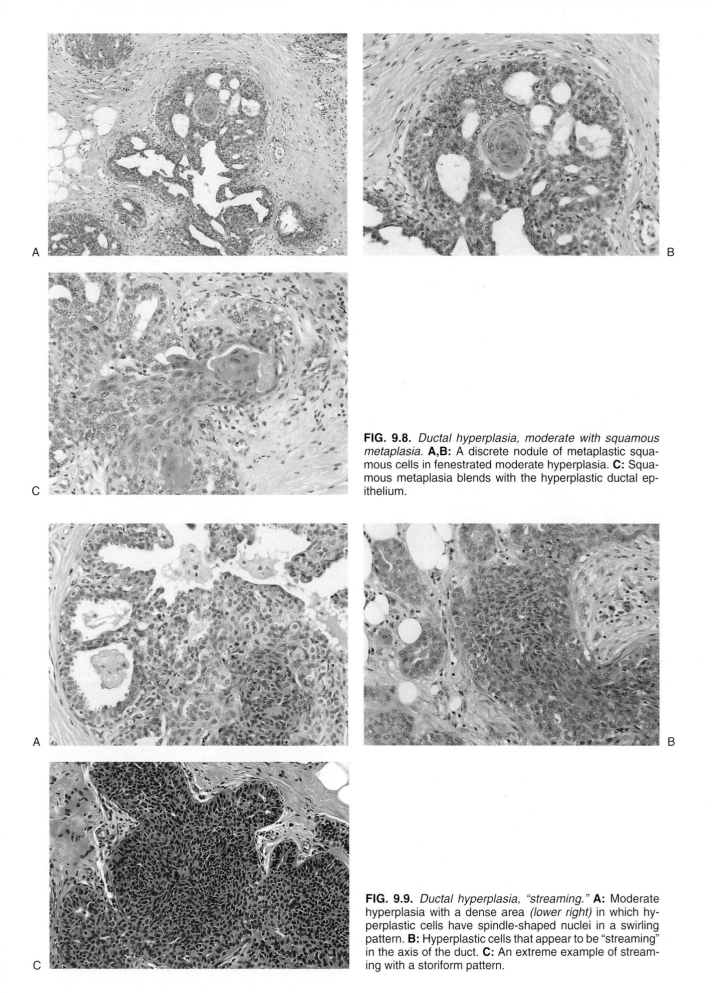

**FIG. 9.8.** *Ductal hyperplasia, moderate with squamous metaplasia.* **A,B:** A discrete nodule of metaplastic squamous cells in fenestrated moderate hyperplasia. **C:** Squamous metaplasia blends with the hyperplastic ductal epithelium.

**FIG. 9.9.** *Ductal hyperplasia, "streaming."* **A:** Moderate hyperplasia with a dense area *(lower right)* in which hyperplastic cells have spindle-shaped nuclei in a swirling pattern. **B:** Hyperplastic cells that appear to be "streaming" in the axis of the duct. **C:** An extreme example of streaming with a storiform pattern.

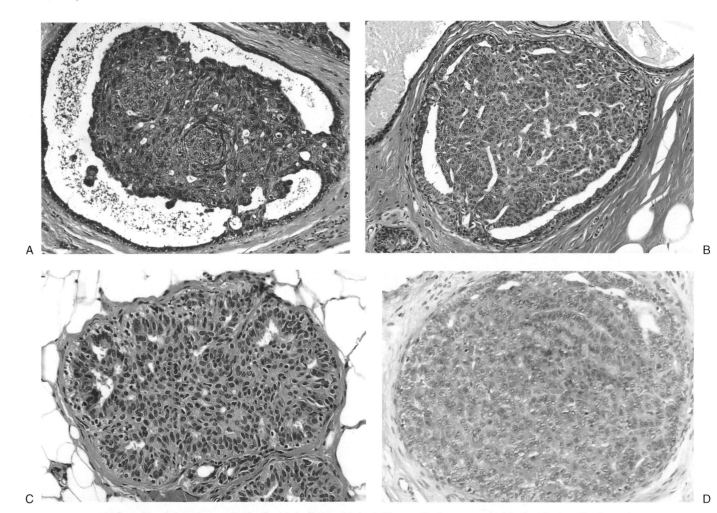

A

B

C

D

**FIG. 9.10.** *Ductal hyperplasia, florid.* **A:** Polypoid ductal hyperplasia connected to the duct epithelium at only two points. Note swirling and streaming of the hyperplastic epithelium. **B:** Solid mass of hyperplastic epithelium with several peripheral connections. **C:** Persisting cuboidal ductal cells define the outer borders of slits that remain between points at which hyperplastic epithelium is in contact with the perimeter of the duct. **D:** Peripheral slits remain at only part of the circumference of the duct.

the duct lumen may remain as a crescentic space or spaces at the edge of the duct (Figs. 9.10–9.13). The predominantly peripheral distribution of microlumens that characterizes hyperplasia is an important difference from cribriform intraductal carcinoma, wherein microlumens tend to be distributed more evenly across the entire duct cross section.

Necrotic cellular debris is rarely present in hyperplastic ducts and, when found, usually is associated with sclerosing papillary foci. This phenomenon is illustrated in Chapter 5. A distinction should be made between necrotic debris resulting from degeneration of epithelial cells that constitutes a form of comedonecrosis and accumulation of inflammatory cells, mainly histocytes (Figs. 9.13 and 9.14), which frequently occurs at sites of duct hyperplasia. Histiocytes or foam cells are found relatively often in hyperplastic duct epithelium that lacks necrosis. Hyperplastic ducts with necrosis are indistinguishable cytologically and structurally from

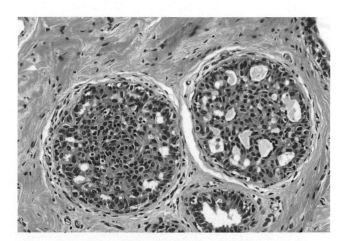

**FIG. 9.11.** *Ductal hyperplasia, florid.* Fenestrations are distributed mainly at the periphery of these ducts. Note the swirling pattern in the center of the duct on the *left.*

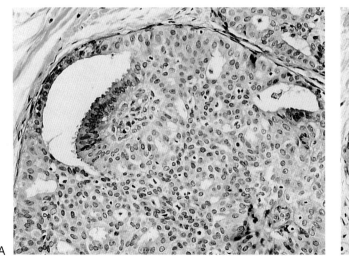
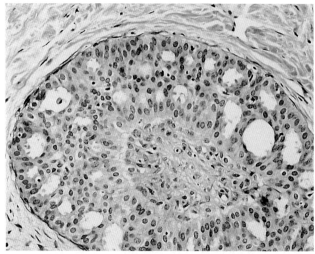

**FIG. 9.12.** *Ductal hyperplasia, florid.* **A:** Columnar ductal epithelium outlines part of a crescentic space next to a fibrovascular core in papillary hyperplasia. **B:** Two rows of fenestrations, one at the periphery and the second centrally around a fibrovascular core.

adjacent ducts with nonnecrotic hyperplastic epithelium. The epithelium in florid sclerosing papillary duct hyperplasia may have isolated mitotic figures as well as focal necrosis, but this combination is not by itself diagnostic of carcinoma in this setting.

The fenestrated growth pattern that occurs in moderate and florid ductal hyperplasia results from the joining of epithelial bridges as they traverse the duct lumen. The fenestrations represent residual portions of the original lumen that has been passively subdivided by the complex arborizing

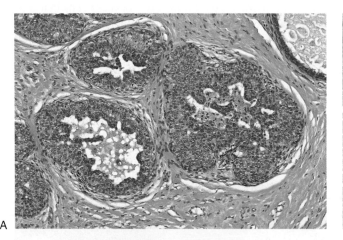
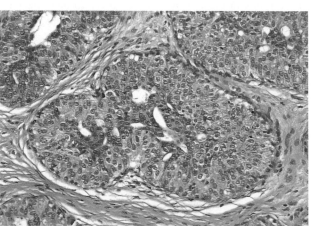
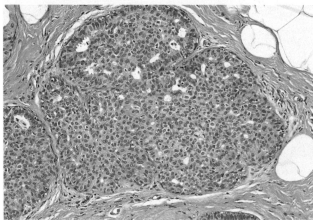

**FIG. 9.13.** *Ductal hyperplasia, florid.* **A:** Moderate hyperplasia. The duct on the *right* has luminal histiocytes. **B:** Florid hyperplasia in which preexisting ductal epithelium outlines crescentic central spaces. **C:** Florid hyperplasia with a substantial solid component.

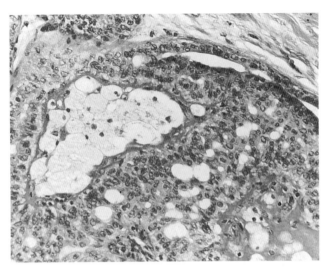

**FIG. 9.14.** *Ductal hyperplasia, histocytes.* A group of histiocytes in florid hyperplasia.

epithelial proliferation. Using a serial-section three-dimensional reconstruction method, Ohuchi et al. demonstrated that the lumens that appeared to be separated from each other in a two-dimensional histologic section of intraductal hyperplasia are part of a network of channels surrounded by the proliferating epithelium (35). By contrast, three-dimensional reconstruction of intraductal carcinoma revealed that the fenestrations in these lesions were newly formed disconnected spaces bordered by polarized neoplastic cells.

The spaces found in histologic sections of fenestrated intraductal hyperplasia have distinctive features. The secondary lumens tend to be larger and more numerous at the periphery of the duct than centrally (Figs. 9.4, 9.8, 9.11, and 9.12). Cells outlining these spaces are distributed in a haphazard fashion except at the edge of the duct, where residual columnar or cuboidal duct epithelium sometimes persists, composed of cells with oriented nuclei (Figs. 9.10 and 9.13).

The spaces in a given hyperplastic duct usually have varied shapes rather than being uniformly rounded as in cribriform carcinoma. In hyperplasia, the spaces may be ovoid, crescentic, irregular, or serpiginous, although in exceptional cases, the lumens may be round and larger toward the center of the duct (Fig. 9.15). Cell membranes bordering on the spaces tend to be smooth, or they may present an uneven, finely serrated surface that results from cytoplasmic blebs formed by complex folding of the cell membrane and microvilli (36) (Fig. 9.16). Apical blebs that result in a fluffy cytoplasmic border resemble the "snouts" that characterize apocrine cells. In the absence of other apocrine cytologic features, apical cytoplasmic blebs should not be interpreted as a manifestation of apocrine change.

The spaces formed in intraductal hyperplasia usually appear to be devoid of cells and secretion. Occasionally, there may be histiocytes or lymphocytes present, sometimes with wisps of secretion. Calcification in the form of coarse granular concretions, calcospherites, or crystalline deposits is uncommon in usual ductal hyperplasia unless there is an associated sclerosing component such as adenosis or a radial scar configuration. Columnar cell hyperplastic lesions are an exception to this generalization because they are prone to form multifocal calcifications with distinctive histologic characteristics described later.

It is usually difficult to detect myoepithelial cells in ductal hyperplasia except for the layer of these cells that is present at the edge of the duct. Myoepithelial cells may accompany the proliferation into the duct lumen when the fibrovascular stromal framework of papillary hyperplasia is present. Because myoepithelial cells may persist at the periphery of ducts with intraductal carcinoma or with intraductal hyperplasia, the presence of these cells is not a useful criterion for distinguishing these lesions. In most situations, absence of myoepithelial cells documented by immunohistochemistry indicates intraductal carcinoma.

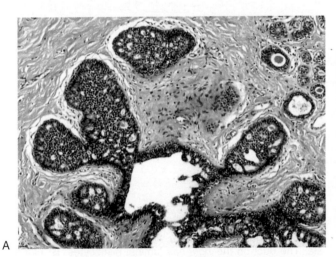

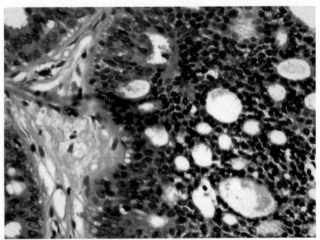

A                                                                                                              B

**FIG. 9.15.** *Ductal hyperplasia, fenestrated.* **A:** Branches of a large duct showing fenestrated hyperplasia. **B:** Uneven pattern of microlumens of varying sizes among cells with overlapping nuclei. There is no cellular orientation around the microlumens. Peripheral ductal epithelium has been cut tangentially along the left border of the large duct. Myoepithelial hyperplasia is evident in the upper left corner.

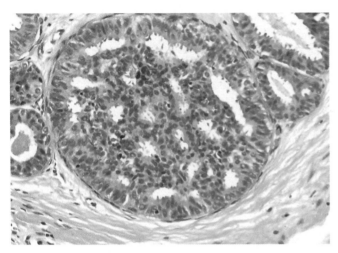

**FIG. 9.16.** *Ductal hyperplasia.* Epithelial tufting produces fuzzy edges around microlumens at the periphery and center of the duct.

## Atypical Ductal Hyperplasia

There is broad agreement on the general description of atypical ductal hyperplasia as a proliferative lesion that fulfills some but not all criteria for a diagnosis of intraductal carcinoma. By extension, it can be stated that atypical ductal hyperplasia has features of ordinary hyperplasia and of intraductal carcinoma. The difficulty in arriving at a "crisper" definition lies in the specifics. In general, these can be considered under two headings: *quantitative* and *qualitative*. The former refers to the amount of a proliferative abnormality, and the latter is concerned with microscopic structural and cytologic details.

Quantitative criteria for distinguishing between ductal hyperplasia and intraductal carcinoma have been based on the number of ductal cross sections that exhibit the abnormality or the dimension of the affected area. Some investigators have classified as atypical ductal hyperplasia proliferative lesions limited to a single duct, even if the abnormality is qualitatively consistent with intraductal carcinoma (25). This scheme requires at least two fully involved duct cross sections to make a diagnosis of intraductal carcinoma and arbitrarily assigns cases with one qualitatively similar duct to the category of atypical hyperplasia.

Tavassoli and Norris emphasized the concept of microscopic dimensions as a fundamental criterion for a diagnosis of atypical ductal hyperplasia (37). They chose to classify foci measuring less than 2 mm as atypical ductal hyperplasia, regardless of the number of affected duct cross sections, even if the individual ducts qualified as intraductal carcinoma. These investigators stated that they arrived at the 2-mm criterion because ". . . it was at the level of one or more small ducts or ductules measuring around 2 mm in aggregate cross-sectional diameter that most pathologists felt hesitant in diagnosing a lesion as intraductal carcinoma" (38). Elsewhere, Tavassoli and Norris commented that "questions about quantity are raised generally when dispersed lesions

add up to from 1.6 to 2.7 mm in aggregate size. Therefore, we arbitrarily chose 2 mm as a cutoff point" (37).

The foregoing quantitative criteria are clearly arbitrary and lack biologic validation. There is no *a priori* reason for choosing two ductal cross sections or 2 mm as critical decision points in relation to risk. No published scientific studies have compared the clinical significance of different quantitative criteria. For example, no data exist for the risk of developing subsequent carcinoma in patients whose biopsies contained proliferative lesions qualitatively consistent with intraductal carcinoma limited to one, two, or three ductal cross sections. Regarding the dimensions of the lesion, no analysis comparing foci measuring 1.5 mm, 2.0 mm, 2.5 mm, or larger has been reported.

Technical issues hamper the application of quantitative criteria. What appear to be two contiguous cross sections may prove in serial sections to be part of a single duct, or deeper sections of a single duct lesion may uncover more involved ductal cross sections. How close do two ductal cross sections need to be to be considered contiguous? Quantitative criteria assume that the ducts in question have been sectioned transversely, that is, perpendicular to their long axis. Assessing ducts cut longitudinally has not been adequately considered. For example, if the longitudinal dimension of a duct in a section exceeds 2 mm, but the transverse diameter is 1 mm, should this focus be considered intraductal carcinoma when using the criteria of Tavassoli and Norris? How is the "aggregate size" of "dispersed lesions" determined to fulfill the Tavassoli and Norris criteria?

Despite an imaginative effort to address some of these issues through the elaboration of an increasingly complex classification scheme for DIN, a scientific basis for quantitative criteria remains elusive (39). In an era of evolving studies that can assess the molecular alterations in the proliferative epithelium of single ducts or even subsets of cells in these structures, the concept of using the size of a proliferative lesion in a histologic section as a fundamental diagnostic criterion is likely to become less meaningful, but lesional size will remain a consideration in therapeutic decision making.

Others have rejected quantitative factors in the diagnosis of atypical ductal hyperplasia. This position was elaborated by Fisher et al., who stated that "our definition of atypical ductal hyperplasia consists of a ductal epithelial alteration approximating but not unequivocally satisfying the criteria for a diagnosis of ductal carcinoma *in situ* (DCIS). It does not include arbitrarily established quantities of unequivocal DCIS (< 2.0 mm or 2 'spaces')" (40). In their study of the prognostic significance of proliferative breast "disease," Bodian et al. reported that ". . . during the course of many years, intraductal carcinoma has been diagnosed if the characteristic features are present in only one ductal space" (24).

The role of quantitative factors in the diagnosis of proliferative ductal lesions seems to lie between these extremes. The use of rigid criteria such as two ductal cross sections or

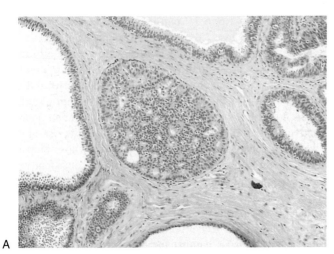
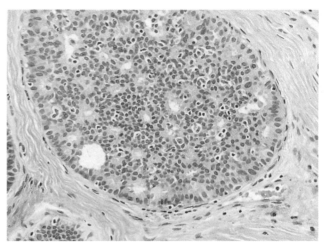

A

B

**FIG. 9.17.** *Atypical ductal hyperplasia.* **A:** Columnar cell change and mild columnar cell hyperplasia are evident in dilated ducts around a focus of atypical ductal hyperplasia. **B:** Magnified view showing residual ductal epithelium around much of the duct perimeter. Centrally, the epithelium in the duct is composed of cells with relatively scant cytoplasm and dark nuclei that are oriented radially around microlumens, most of which are round.

2 mm can be justified in a research setting to ensure a homogeneous study group or to assess a particular criterion, but the strict application of these arbitrary rules in a clinical setting is difficult for technical reasons and poorly substantiated by existing data. Nonetheless, given the limitations of current methods for diagnosing intraductal lesions, lesion size sometimes is taken into consideration, along with other features, in assessing a particular lesion. Other aspects considered include nuclear cytology, mitotic activity, structure, the presence of necrosis and calcifications, and the appearance of associated proliferative lesions. Atypia is diagnosed if a pattern of growth consistent with intraductal carcinoma is present in part of one duct structure in association with otherwise usual hyperplastic changes. If a carcinoma-like element associated with usual hyperplasia is more widespread in a duct or partially involves multiple ducts in this or other foci, severe atypia is diagnosed.

A diagnosis of atypical hyperplasia depends on the presence of structural or cytologic features of intraductal carcinoma mingling with hyperplasia. Architecturally, this may be manifested by a cribriform pattern involving a duct (Figs. 9.17–9.19). These foci feature sharply defined, round to ovoid spaces outlined by cells with distinct borders and a rigid arrangement. Atypical hyperplasia can have a solid growth pattern (Figs. 9.20–9.22), and atypical hyperplasia occurs in ducts exhibiting apocrine metaplasia (Figs. 9.23–9.25).

Cytologic atypia may involve individual cells, focal groups of cells, or the entire population of a proliferative le-

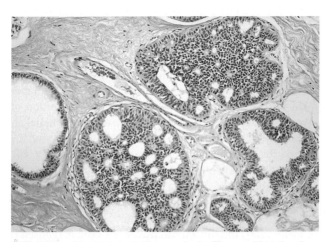

**FIG. 9.18.** *Atypical ductal hyperplasia.* The proliferation has a cribriform growth pattern in which microlumens are relatively round. Cells tend to be polarized around the microlumens. Nuclei are smaller centrally than at the periphery, and central nuclei are hyperchromatic. Microlumens are larger at the periphery.

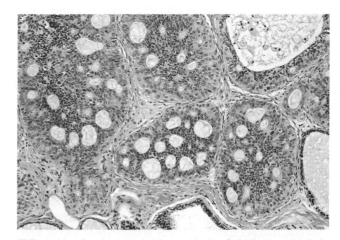

**FIG. 9.19.** *Atypical ductal hyperplasia.* Cribriform growth in four contiguous duct cross sections. The centers of the ducts consist of small, crowded cells with overlapping hyperchromatic nuclei. Cells are not oriented around the circular microlumens. Hyperplastic cells at the periphery of ducts are largely not oriented with respect to the basement membrane.

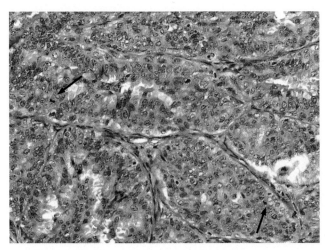

**FIG. 9.20.** *Atypical ductal hyperplasia.* Mitotic activity (*arrows*) and cellular pleomorphism are depicted.

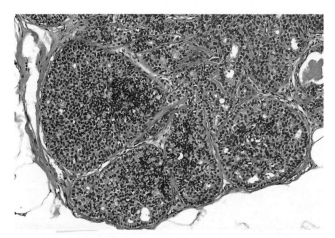

**FIG. 9.22.** *Atypical ductal hyperplasia.* These duct cross sections display variable amounts of growth consisting of nearly solid patches in which there are monomorphic small cells. Areas within the same ducts display streaming and cells with overlapping hyperchromatic nuclei.

sion. Atypical features include nuclear enlargement resulting in an increased nuclear:cytoplasmic ratio, nuclear hyperchromasia, an irregular chromatin pattern, or nucleoli. Atypical cells may have distinct cell borders, a feature that is especially noticeable when these cells occur singly or in small groups in an otherwise typical hyperplastic focus.

Mitotic activity is extremely low in hyperplasia of the usual type. The presence of readily identified mitotic figures is an atypical feature. Prosser et al. reported that the proliferative index of hyperplastic lesions was greater than in normal breast when measured by MIB1 immunoreactivity, whereas an apoptotic index determined by the terminal deoxynucleotidyl transferase-mediated dUTP-biotin end labeling (TUNEL) assay tended to be lower in proliferative lesions (41).

Intracytoplasmic lumens containing mucinous secretion, typically associated with lobular carcinoma in the form of signet ring cells, also may occur in intraductal carcinoma cells (42). A minute dot of secretion is often evident in hema-

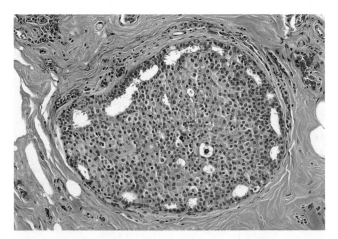

**FIG. 9.21.** *Atypical ductal hyperplasia.* A solid growth of monomorphic cells fills the duct lumen. Oval microlumens have formed at the periphery. Two small round calcifications are present centrally.

toxylin and eosin (H&E)-stained sections in these tiny, sharply defined cytoplasmic lumens. Intracytoplasmic mucin vacuoles can be found in the cells of nonapocrine and apocrine types of intraductal carcinoma and in papillary and nonpapillary intraductal carcinomas. The mucinous secretion is highlighted with the Alcian blue and mucicarmine stains. Intracytoplasmic mucin is only very rarely present in the cells of ductal hyperplasia. The finding of any cells with this feature should be regarded as indicative of an atypical lesion or intraductal carcinoma, depending on the overall appearance of the proliferation.

Azzopardi, who referred to ductal hyperplasia as *epitheliosis,* limited the term *atypical ductal hyperplasia* to describe a particular proliferative lesion of lobules that has a ductal pattern (43). This type of hyperplasia is composed of crowded, tall, columnar or cuboidal cells arranged in a pseudostratified pattern with hyperchromatic nuclei. The cells at the periphery of the dilated lobular glands maintain polarity with respect to the ductal lumen. Secondary lumens may be formed by the hyperplastic epithelium. These lesions are examples of ductal hyperplasia in unfolding lobules or *columnar cell hyperplasia* (CCH). Many do not exhibit atypical features and consequently qualify as ordinary duct hyperplasia.

## Columnar Cell Hyperplasia

Proliferative lesions of the duct–lobular complex termed *ductal hyperplasia* by Azzopardi, have become the subject of closer scrutiny as a result of the widespread use of a needle core biopsy to sample mammographically detected lesions. These abnormalities now are recognized as being part of a complex spectrum of lesions described by the terms *columnar cell change* and *columnar cell hyperplasia* (29,30). Other more cumbersome names that have been offered include atypical cystic lobules (44), cancerization of

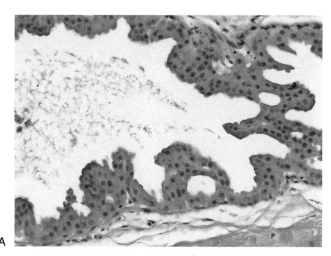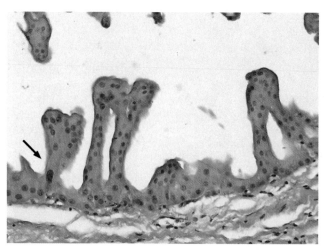

A                                                                                                    B

**FIG. 9.23.** *Atypical ductal hyperplasia,* apocrine. **A:** Blunt micropapillary structures composed of cells with small regular nuclei. Atypical features are the pattern and uneven distribution of nuclei. **B:** Elongated micropapillary structures. One large hyperchromatic nucleus is present *(arrow).*

lobules, atypical ductal hyperplasia adjacent to ductal carcinoma *in situ* (45), and columnar alteration with prominent apical snouts and secretions, or CAPSS (46).

Columnar cell hyperplasia was previously described as *pretubular hyperplasia* (47). This name was derived from the observation that patients with tubular carcinoma of the breast often had foci of these lesions distributed in surrounding tissue or sometimes even merging with the carcinomatous lesions. This association suggested that tubular carcinoma sometimes might arise when the hyperplastic lesions transformed to intraductal carcinoma, hence the term *pretubular hyperplasia.* Lobular carcinoma *in situ* is sometimes also present, an association that was noted by Azzopardi. Thus, lobular carcinoma *in situ* is associated with pretubular hyperplasia and with tubular carcinoma.

I have become less enthusiastic regarding the term *pretubular.* Foremost is the growing frequency with which these

lesions are being encountered in needle core and surgical biopsies performed for microcalcifications. In this circumstance, the ductal lesion itself prompts the procedure. Although we should be aware of the possibility of coincidental tubular carcinoma, it is not demonstrated in most of these women, and the risk for subsequent tubular carcinoma is poorly documented. Because cells with a columnar configuration are a conspicuous feature of these lesions (often with apocrine snouts), the term *columnar cell hyperplasia* has been adopted as a simple name for the spectrum of these abnormalities (47).

Columnar cell hyperplasia is a multifocal process that also may be bilateral. It is most often encountered in women 35 to 50 years of age, but CCH can be present after menopause. CCH rarely produces a palpable abnormality, and it usually is detected mammographically because calcifications are frequently formed, becoming the target of needle core biopsy sampling. The fundamental lesion is localized in ter-

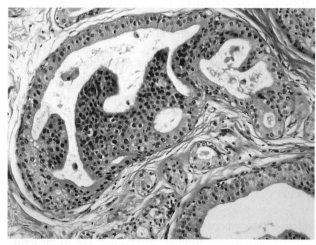

**FIG. 9.24.** *Atypical ductal hyperplasia,* apocrine. Micropapillary fronds arise from part of the circumference of a duct. The remainder of the duct is lined by regular cuboidal apocrine cells.

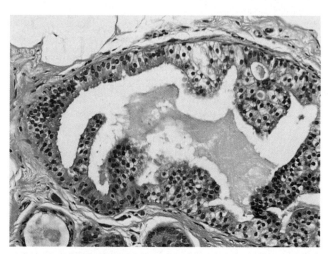

**FIG. 9.25.** *Atypical ductal hyperplasia,* apocrine. Some cells exhibit cytoplasmic clearing.

minal duct–lobular units, which become enlarged as a result of epithelial proliferation and cystic dilatation.

The simplest form of this process features a thin, flat epithelial layer composed of predominantly cuboidal to tall columnar cells distributed in a relatively uniform pattern. Because the nuclei tend to be relatively large, the cells appear crowded and dark. The apical cell surface usually has an apocrine-type cytoplasmic protrusion ("snout"), and, in some cases, this feature is prominent. In the most banal columnar cell lesion, which is best termed *columnar cell change,* the epithelium is one to two cells deep, and there is little nuclear pleomorphism. Nucleoli and mitotic figures are rarely found or are absent (Fig. 9.26). Calcification is infrequent and usually consists of amorphous granular material (Fig. 9.27). Discrete basophilic calcifications are uncommon in columnar cell change.

The cytologic features of columnar cell lesions suggest apocrine differentiation. The cells express gross cystic disease fluid protein 15, an apocrine marker; however, they are immunoreactive for *bcl*-2 and estrogen receptor protein, which are typically absent in benign apocrine change (48). CCH is present when the cellular distribution is more than two cells thick. This is most readily apparent when cellular crowding becomes pronounced and nuclei are not distributed in a single plane relative to the basement membrane. This tendency to "stacking" of nuclei usually is accompanied by

increased nuclear chromasia, and small mounds may be formed in the most cellular regions (Figs. 9.28 and 9.29).

More complex columnar cell proliferative foci comprise lesions described as CCH with atypia. Mild atypia usually manifests by the presence of small and often isolated foci of micropapillary growth in a background of otherwise usual CCH (Fig. 9.30). The presence of more elaborate growth patterns as well as cytologic atypia characterize CCH with moderate to marked atypia, which in its most severe form approaches the appearance of intraductal carcinoma (Figs. 9.31–9.33). In some instances, cytologic atypia is more pronounced than the structural abnormalities (Fig. 9.34). When carcinoma arises in CCH, the growth pattern is usually one of the characteristic patterns of intraductal carcinoma (Figs. 9.35 and 9.36), but rarely so-called flat micropapillary carcinoma with relatively little epithelial complexity is encountered (Fig. 9.37). Atypical lobular hyperplasia and lobular carcinoma *in situ* frequently accompany columnar cell abnormalities, and tubular carcinoma may also be present (Fig. 9.38) (see Chapter 15).

Columnar cell lesions develop calcifications that are formed in multiple glands in many of the proliferative sites. Two types of calcification are encountered: *crystalline* and *ossifying.* The more frequent crystalline type, usually associated with lesions with less atypia, is deeply basophilic; opaque, round, or angular; and prone to fragmentation in the

*Text continues on page 222*

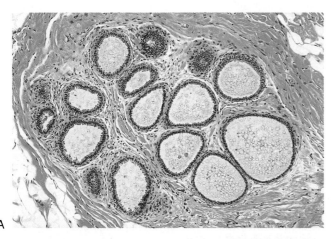

A

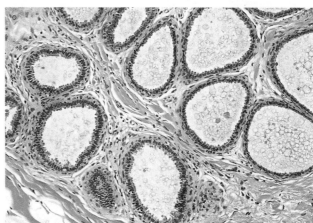

B

C

**FIG. 9.26.** *Columnar cell change.* **A,B:** Cystic dilatation of lobular ductules lined by cuboidal and columnar cells characterized by closely approximated, basally oriented nuclei and luminal cytoplasmic "snouts." The structures are encircled by relatively loose, vascularized intralobular stroma. **C:** A magnified view of the crowded epithelium, indistinct myoepithelium, and surrounding stroma.

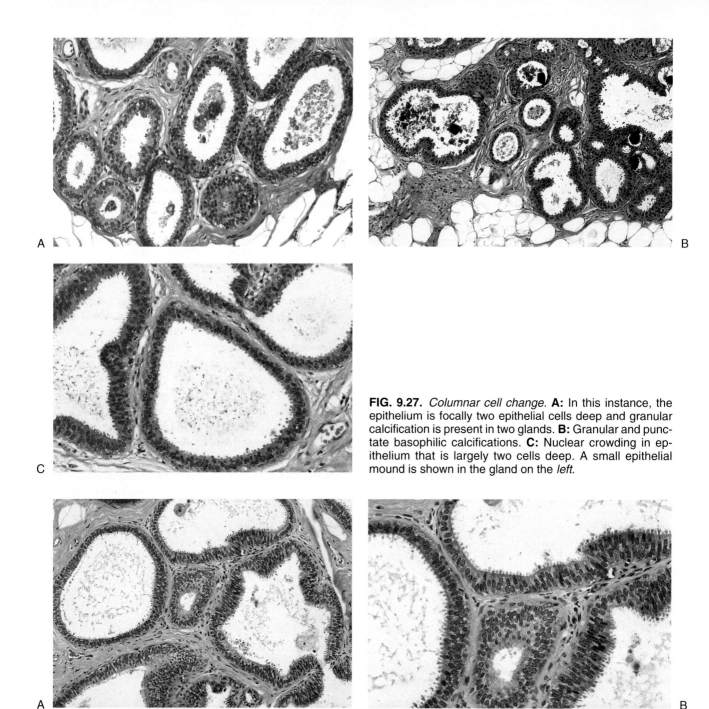

**FIG. 9.27.** *Columnar cell change.* **A:** In this instance, the epithelium is focally two epithelial cells deep and granular calcification is present in two glands. **B:** Granular and punctate basophilic calcifications. **C:** Nuclear crowding in epithelium that is largely two cells deep. A small epithelial mound is shown in the gland on the *left*.

**FIG. 9.28.** *Columnar cell hyperplasia.* **A,B:** Plaque-like areas of epithelium in which overlapping nuclei of columnar cells are several cells deep. The myoepithelium is indistinct.

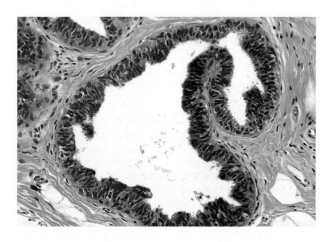

**FIG. 9.29.** *Columnar cell hyperplasia.* The thickened epithelium composed of crowded columnar cells forms small mounds. The myoepithelium is inconspicuous.

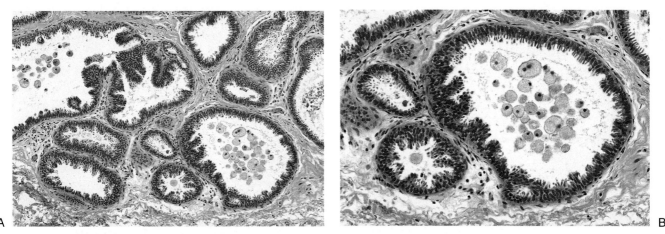

**FIG. 9.30.** *Columnar cell hyperplasia, mild atypia.* **A,B:** Focal blunt micropapillary proliferation of the hyperplastic columnar cell epithelium. Note the marked nuclear hyperchromasia and the high nuclear:cytoplasmic ratio. Histiocytes are present in the lumen.

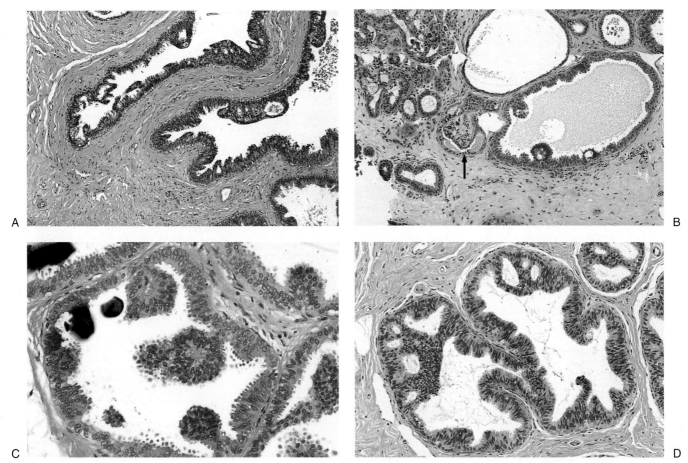

**FIG. 9.31.** *Columnar cell hyperplasia, moderate atypia.* **A–C:** Three examples of moderate atypia with micropapillary architecture. An "ossifying" calcification is shown in **B** (*arrow*), a section stained with hematoxylin–phloxine–safranin. Dense basophilic calcifications are shown in **C.** **D:** Fenestrated moderately atypical micropapillary hyperplasia.

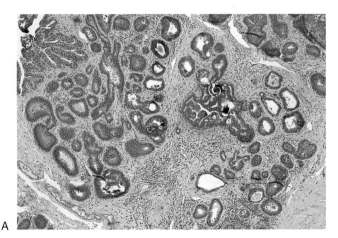
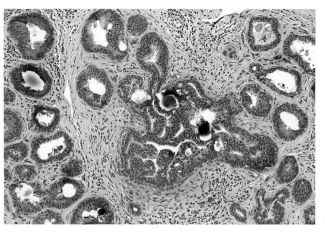

A

B

**FIG. 9.32.** *Columnar cell hyperplasia, severe atypia.* **A:** At low magnification, the lesion consists of confluent lobular units with a central focus of papillary proliferation. **B:** The severely atypical epithelium is composed of monomorphic cells uniformly distributed in the micropapillae. Columnar cell change is evident in surrounding glandular structures, and calcifications are present.

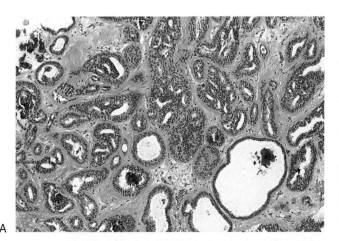
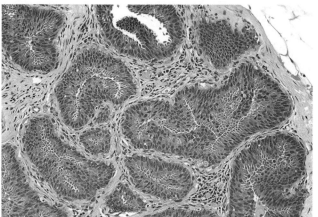

A

B

**FIG. 9.33.** *Columnar cell hyperplasia, severe atypia.* **A:** The cribriform growth is composed of monomorphic cells. Microlumens are oval and crescentic rather than round. Columnar cell change is also evident. **B:** No mitotic activity is present in this columnar cell proliferation where hyperplastic epithelium fills gland lumens.

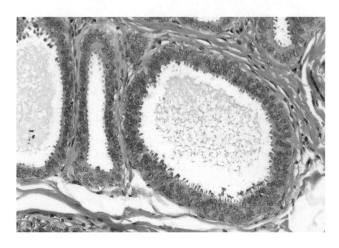

**FIG. 9.34.** *Columnar cell hyperplasia, mild cytologic atypia.*

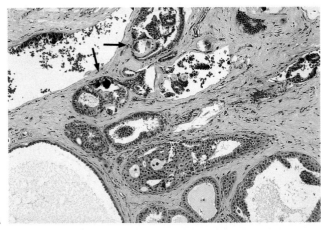 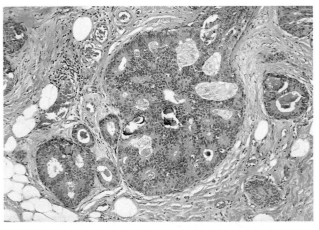

A                                              B

**FIG. 9.35.** *Intraductal carcinoma associated with atypical columnar cell hyperplasia.* **A:** This needle core biopsy was obtained from a focus of nonpalpable mammographically detected calcifications. Basophilic and ossifying-type calcifications are present *(arrows)*. Atypical hyperplasia with micropapillary and fenestrated structure is apparent in the *lower center*. Hematoxylin–phloxine–safranin. **B:** Cribriform intraductal carcinoma that was present in the excisional biopsy performed after the core biopsy shown in **A**.

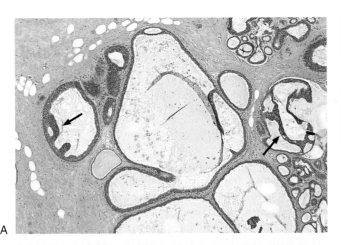 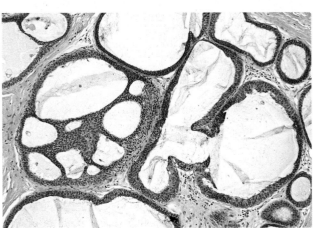

A                                              B

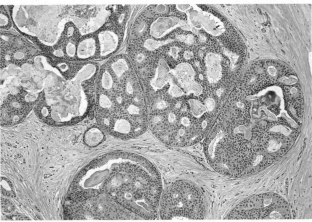

**FIG. 9.36.** *Intraductal carcinoma associated with atypical columnar cell hyperplasia.* **A:** Excisional biopsy revealed multifocal, predominantly cystic columnar cell hyperplasia with focal atypia, shown here with micropapillary architecture *(arrows)*. **B:** Four years later, repeat biopsy of the same breast performed for calcifications revealed columnar cell hyperplasia with severe atypia. **C:** Also present in the biopsy shown in **B** was cribriform intraductal carcinoma illustrated here.

C

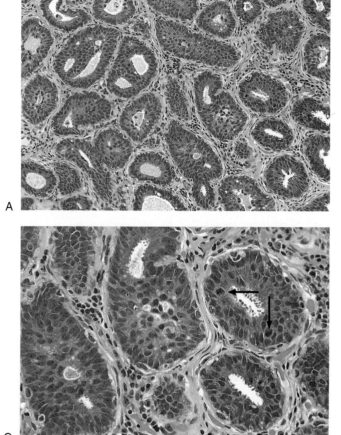

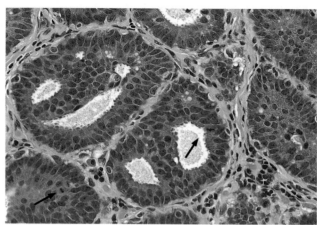

**FIG. 9.37.** *Intraductal carcinoma associated with atypical columnar cell hyperplasia.* The sample shown here is from the same biopsy as in Fig. 9.33B, which displayed atypical columnar cell hyperplasia. **A:** Low magnification view showing cribriform and flat micropapillary intraductal carcinoma. **B,C:** Intraductal carcinoma with cribriform and flat growth. *Arrows* indicate mitoses.

process of histologic sectioning (Figs. 9.27, 9.31–9.33, and 9.35). A second type of calcification usually has a rounded, well-defined contour and an internal structure that resembles an ossifying nodule in which basophilic granular calcific deposits are embedded in lacunar-like spaces with an orangophilic or eosinophilic matrix (Figs. 9.31, 9.35, and 9.39). Ossifying-type calcifications occur throughout the range of

CCHs, and they appear to develop in proliferative epithelium, whereas basophilic crystalline deposits are predominantly intraluminal. Both types of calcification can be found in one specimen, and they may occur together in a single proliferative focus. The finding of ossifying-type calcifications is an indication of proliferative activity in CCH; and if they are present in a needle core biopsy, excisional biopsy of the

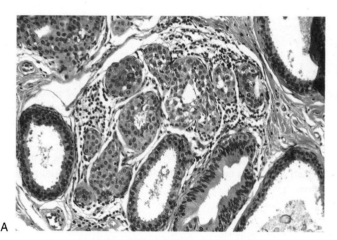

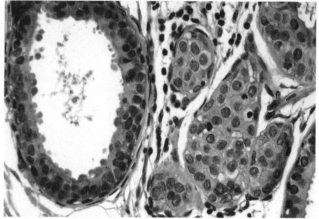

**FIG. 9.38.** *Lobular carcinoma* in situ *associated with columnar cell change.* **A:** Lobular carcinoma *in situ* is surrounded by cystic ducts with columnar cell change. **B:** Magnified view of **A** showing the mosaic pattern of cells in the lobular carcinoma *in situ.* Note the different nuclear appearances of the columnar cell and lobular lesions.

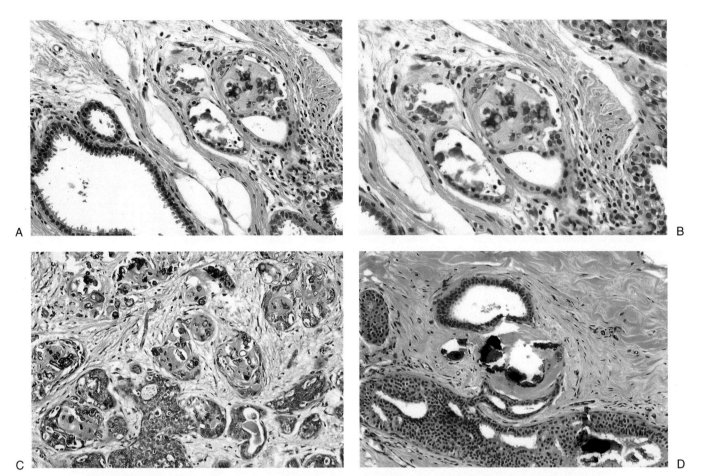

**FIG. 9.39.** *Ossifying calcifications in columnar cell hyperplasia.* **A,B:** Fine granules of basophilic calcification are present in the discrete eosinophilic intraepithelial nodule. **C:** Multiple ossifying calcifications in a single proliferative focus. This is an unusual finding. **D:** A basophilic calcification in ossifying matrix arising in atypical columnar cell hyperplasia.

lesional area would be prudent. Excisional biopsy also is recommended when a needle core biopsy contains CCH with atypia or if a columnar cell lesion is associated with lobular carcinoma *in situ* or atypical lobular hyperplasia.

### Borderline Lesions

The most challenging atypical ductal proliferations that constitute the majority of borderline lesions subject to varied interpretation feature marked cytologic and architectural atypia (Figs. 9.40–9.42). Some of these foci retain a minor characteristic of hyperplasia, exemplified by the presence of nuclear overlap or streaming in an otherwise typical cribriform structure formed by rigid epithelial bridges (Fig. 9.35). These slight variations will be disregarded by observers who classify the lesions as intraductal carcinoma, whereas others may diagnose atypical hyperplasia. Similarly, those who place credence in quantitative criteria will diagnose atypical hyperplasia because the extent of a lesion is not sufficient, whereas others not adhering to these arbitrary rules will diagnose intraductal carcinoma in the same lesion.

Insufficient emphasis has been placed on diagnosing specific proliferative lesions in the context of the overall spectrum of histologic changes in a biopsy specimen. In a research setting, a pathologist can be required to make a diagnosis that is based only on a focus circled on a single slide (2,18). This artificial setting differs from the circumstances under which the various diagnostic criteria originally were refined by reviewing multiple histologic sections (25,27). In clinical practice, the pathologist has an opportunity to examine a case extensively, including recourse to serial sections. As a rule, it is helpful to prepare multiple sections (*recuts*) of a tissue sample that contains a borderline focus of ductal proliferation. In most instances of intraductal carcinoma, the lesion will persist, and it may enlarge or exhibit features considered to be diagnostic. On the other hand, atypical hyperplasia can be diagnosed with greater confidence if the lesion is diminished or does not evolve into intraductal carcinoma in recut sections. In exceptional cases, features diagnostic of intraductal carcinoma are present in few or in only one of a series of sections containing recuts of a problematic focus.

A review of slides from previous biopsies is often helpful. The primary pathologist should attempt to assemble prior

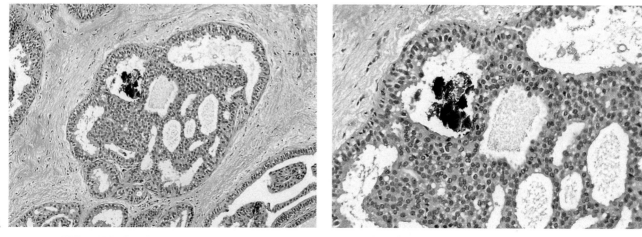

**FIG. 9.40.** *Atypical ductal hyperplasia.* **A:** The proliferation in the duct suggests carcinoma. The fragmented calcification is a type found in intraductal carcinoma. **B:** Bands of cells with overlapping nuclei encircling the lumens appear rigid. Ductal epithelium persists focally at the periphery.

material if faced with a diagnostic problem, although the mobility of patients who are sometimes treated in multiple facilities makes this goal difficult to achieve. Whenever possible, the diagnosis of borderline intraductal proliferations is best made in the context of the spectrum of pathologic changes

present in current and prior specimens. A focus of concern may be substantially more atypical and different qualitatively from the overall proliferative level in a given case, or it may prove to be part of a spectrum of changes lacking distinct histologic boundaries. The former situation would tend to sup-

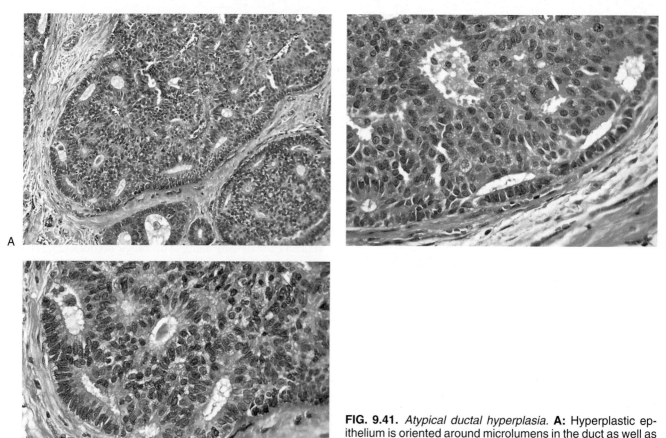

**FIG. 9.41.** *Atypical ductal hyperplasia.* **A:** Hyperplastic epithelium is oriented around microlumens in the duct as well as at the periphery. **B:** Cells are oriented around part of a central microlumen and at the outer borders of peripheral slits. **C:** Microlumens with circumferentially oriented cells and residual columnar ductal epithelium.

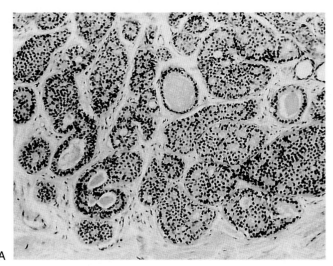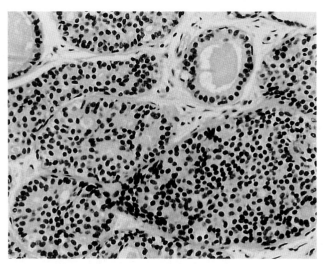

**FIG. 9.42.** *Severely atypical ductal hyperplasia.* **A:** Solid and fenestrated proliferation in an adenosis configuration. Some unaffected glands are evident. **B:** The lesion is composed of small uniform cells. There is little nuclear overlapping.

port a diagnosis of intraductal carcinoma in the lesional area, whereas the latter suggests atypical hyperplasia.

## NEEDLE CORE BIOPSY

The increasing use of mammography combined with needle biopsy procedures is presenting pathologists with a growing number of small, limited tissue and cytologic samples from proliferative lesions to interpret. Given the diagnostic difficulties sometimes encountered when such lesions are examined in their entirety in histologic sections, it is not surprising that the fragmentary material obtained by needling procedures presents a challenging problem.

Atypical ductal hyperplasia has been diagnosed in fewer than 10% of patients subjected to needle core biopsy (21,22,49). In four studies consisting of 323 to 900 patients who underwent needle core biopsy of mammographically detected lesions, the frequencies of atypical ductal hyperplasia were 6.7%, 4.7%, 4.5%, and 4.3% (50–53). Follow-up surgical biopsy was performed on most of the women with atypical hyperplasia in these reports. Among women who underwent biopsy, the reported frequencies of intraductal carcinoma in the surgical specimen were 27%, 12.5%, 33%, and 36%. Invasive carcinoma was found in 14%, 12.5%, 0%, and 11% of patients. In these reports, about 25% of surgical biopsies revealed atypical duct hyperplasia. The high frequency of carcinoma detected after a diagnosis of atypical ductal hyperplasia in a needle core biopsy sample indicates that surgical excision should be performed promptly in this setting (21,22).

The reliability of needle core biopsy to provide a fully diagnostic sample of atypical duct hyperplasia may depend on the biopsy method used. Burbank compared the findings at surgery in 18 women who had atypical duct hyperplasia diagnosed in a sample obtained by "automated needle biopsy" with those in eight other women who underwent a "directional vacuum-assisted biopsy" (53). Intraductal or invasive carcinoma was found in eight (44%) of the first group and in none of the latter group. The importance of quantitative criteria and adequate sampling was documented by Jackman et al., who ". . . progressively increased the average number of core samples obtained per lesion and have found a decrease in both the number of ADH (atypical duct hyperplasia) lesions and the discordance of ADH lesion" (21). The greater success in diagnosis in the needle core biopsy material was attributable to more lesions being diagnosed as intraductal carcinoma rather than as atypical ductal hyperplasia as a result of more extensive sampling (21).

Other investigators have studied needle core biopsy samples with molecular markers in an effort to predict the likelihood of finding carcinoma in a subsequent excisional biopsy. Tocino et al. evaluated p53 expression in the needle core biopsies from 34 women with atypical ductal hyperplasia (54). Subsequent surgical biopsy revealed carcinoma in eight (23.5%), including five cases of intraductal carcinoma and three of invasive carcinoma. Mutations in p53 were detected in microdissected samples from seven of the eight (88%) needle core biopsies that were followed by carcinoma at surgery and in 35% of atypical hyperplasias without carcinoma in the subsequent surgical biopsy, a difference that was statistically significant.

Some needle core biopsies contain samples of lesions that constitute atypical hyperplasia on the basis of histologic criteria. In other instances, the diagnosis of atypical ductal hyperplasia in needle biopsies is arrived at in a manner that differs somewhat from the interpretation of histologic sections. Atypical ductal hyperplasia may be diagnosed if there are detached fragments of abnormal epithelium that suggest carcinoma or if only part of a duct with features of carcinoma is contained in the sample. The limited and often fragmented nature of needle core biopsies leads to greater emphasis on quantitative criteria. There is a temptation to overinterpret small biopsy samples because of the expectation that more lesional tissue remains at the biopsy site, a tendency embodied in the statement that"what you see may not be all there is." In the proper clinical context, this approach has merit. In the evaluation of needle core biopsies of breast lesions, however, especially those from abnormalities that are evident only by mammography, it must be assumed that the material seen in the needle biopsy sample may be the most extreme and potentially the only abnormality present, expressed as "what you see may be all there is." A comprehensive discussion of the pathologic diagnosis of atypical ductal hyperplasia in needle core biopsy specimens can be found in *Breast Pathology: Diagnosis by Needle Core Biopsy* (30).

## PROGNOSIS AND TREATMENT

The prognoses for ordinary and atypical intraductal hyperplasia are also discussed in Chapter 10. The major concern attributable to these lesions is the risk for subsequently developing carcinoma. This risk is greater when there is atypia than when hyperplasia is in the ordinary category. The risk for developing carcinoma subsequently is equal in either breast, even if hyperplasia was documented in only one breast.

Patients with hyperplasia, especially when there is atypia, are encouraged to participate in a regular follow-up program that includes physician examination, self-examination, and mammography. The goal of this approach is to detect carcinoma at a stage when it would be most amenable to cure. Examinations may be scheduled more frequently for women with atypia, especially if there are associated risk factors, such as a family history of breast carcinoma (55).

Prophylactic bilateral mastectomy may be considered in selected cases but should be "reserved only for those patients with an extraordinarily high risk, as defined by genetic pedigree analysis demonstrating a hereditary trait or those with severe atypia who find surveillance an unacceptable method of management" (55). If bilateral mastectomy is performed, the operation should be a total mastectomy that includes the axillary tail and preferably a sampling of contiguous lymph nodes in the low axilla to ensure the most complete removal of breast tissue. It is unlikely that a subcutaneous mastectomy will accomplish this goal. The development of carcinoma in residual breast tissue after a prophylactic mastectomy, although uncommon, is a discouraging event (56).

Tamoxifen, a competitive inhibitor of estrogen, has proven effective in the primary treatment of breast carcinoma and as an agent for adjuvant therapy. The possibility that tamoxifen could be used for primary prevention was strongly suggested by the observation that the frequency of contralateral breast carcinoma was reduced by about 35% in women receiving adjuvant tamoxifen therapy for carcinoma in one breast (57–59). It is believed that the preventive action of tamoxifen is accomplished mainly by interfering with the promoting action of estrogen on proliferative lesions. An effect at the level of initiation is also possible.

The estrogen dependence of ductal proliferative lesions is suggested by several observations. Failure to suppress the growth of estrogen receptor-positive cells may contribute to the progression of hyperplastic foci in some cases. Visscher et al. reported that nuclear estrogen receptor (ER) reactivity was present in significantly more cells in hyperplasias than in normal terminal duct–lobular units and that nuclear reactivity was even more pronounced in receptor-positive intraductal carcinomas (60). Shoker et al. also reported increased ER expression in hyperplastic ductal foci and correlated these findings with proliferative activity represented by Ki67 reactivity (61). The mean percentages of ER-positive cells in lobules from both premenopausal and postmenopausal women were 6.8 and 42, respectively. The percentages of Ki67-positive cells were 2.6 and 0.34, respectively. The mean percentages of cells with nuclear expression of ER and Ki67 in hyperplasia of the usual type were 45 and 2.4, respectively, and in atypical hyperplasia the respective mean percentages of reactivity were 91 and 3.6. The mean percentages of cells with dual expression of ER and Ki67 in usual and atypical hyperplasia were 0.42 and 2.8, respectively. On the other hand, data from several studies reviewed by Dupont et al. indicated that breast carcinoma risk was not increased significantly by the administration of estrogen replacement therapy to women with a history of benign breast disease or of atypical hyperplasia (62).

A clinical trial of the preventive effects of tamoxifen sponsored by the National Surgical Adjuvant Breast Project enrolled more than 13,000 women at high risk of developing breast carcinoma (63). This randomized study compared women receiving tamoxifen with women given a placebo. There was an 86% reduction in subsequent invasive carcinoma in the treated women with atypical hyperplasia compared with controls.

## REFERENCES

1. Ellis IO, Pinder SE, Lee AH, et al. A critical appraisal of existing classification systems of epithelial hyperplasia and *in situ* neoplasia of the breast with proposals for future methods of categorization: where are we going? *Semin Diagn Pathol* 1999;16:202–208.
2. Rosai J. Borderline epithelial lesions of the breast. *Am J Surg Pathol* 1991;15:209–221.
3. Tavassoli FA. Ductal carcinoma *in situ:* introduction of the concept of ductal intraepithelial neoplasia. *Mod Pathol* 1998;11:140–154.
4. Vogelstein B, Fearon ER, Hamilton SR, et al. Genetic alterations during colorectal-tumor development. *N Engl J Med* 1988;319:525–532.
5. Dietrich CU, Pandis N, Teixeira MR, et al. Chromosome abnormalities in benign hyperproliferative disorders of epithelial and stromal breast tissue. *Int J Cancer* 1995;60:49–53.
6. Lakhani SR, Collins N, Stratton MR, et al. Atypical ductal hyperplasia of the breast: clonal proliferation with loss of heterozygosity on chromosomes 16q and 17p. *J Clin Pathol* 1995;48:611–615.
7. Lakhani SR, Slack DN, Hamoudi RA, et al. Detection of allelic imbalance indicates that a proportion of mammary hyperplasia of usual type are clonal neoplastic proliferations. *Lab Invest* 1996;74:129–135.
8. Rosenberg CL, Larson PS, Romo JD, et al. Microsatellite alterations indicating monoclonality in atypical hyperplasias associated with breast cancer. *Hum Pathol* 1997;28:214–219.
9. Kasami M, Vnencak-Jones CL, Manning S, et al. Loss of heterozygosity and microsatellite instability in breast hyperplasia: no obligate cor-

relation of these genetic alterations with subsequent malignancy. *Am J Pathol* 1997;150:1925–1932.

10. Rohan TE, Hartwick W, Miller AB, et al. Immunohistochemical detection of c-*erb*B-2 and p53 in benign breast disease and breast cancer risk. *J Natl Cancer Inst* 1998;90:1262–1269.

11. Mommers EC, van Diest PJ, Leonhart AM, et al. Expression of proliferation and apoptosis-related proteins in usual ductal hyperplasia of the breast. *Hum Pathol* 1998;29:1539–1545.

12. Done SJ, Arneson NC, Ozcelik H, et al. p53 mutations in mammary ductal carcinoma *in situ* but not in epithelial hyperplasias. *Cancer Res* 1998;58:785–789.

13. Deng G, Lu Y, Zlotnikov G, et al. Loss of heterozygosity in normal tissue adjacent to breast carcinomas. *Science* 1996;274:2057–2059.

14. Gobbi H, Dupont WD, Simpson JF, et al. Transforming growth factor-β and breast cancer risk in women with mammary epithelial hyperplasia. *J Natl Cancer Inst* 1999;91:2096–2101.

15. Ratcliffe N, Wells W, Wheeler K, et al. The combination of *in situ* hybridization and immunohistochemical analysis: an evaluation of Her2/*neu* expression in paraffin-embedded breast carcinomas and adjacent normal-appearing breast epithelium. *Mod Pathol* 1997;10:1247–1252.

16. Connolly JL, Schnitt SJ. Benign breast disease: resolved and unresolved issues. *Cancer* 1993;71:1187–1189.

17. Bodian CA, Perzin KH, Lattes R, et al. Reproducibility and validity of pathologic classifications of benign breast disease and implications for clinical applications. *Cancer* 1993;71:3908–3913.

18. Schnitt SJ, Connolly JL, Tavassoli FA, et al. Interobserver reproducibility in the diagnosis of ductal proliferative breast lesions using standardized criteria. *Am J Surg Pathol* 1992;16:1133–1143.

19. Palli D, Galli M, Bianchi S, et al. Reproducibility of histological diagnosis of breast lesions: results of a panel in Italy. *Eur J Cancer* 1996;32A:603–607.

20. Helvie MA, Hessler C, Frank TS, et al. Atypical hyperplasia of the breast: mammographic appearance and histologic correlation. *Radiology* 1991;179:759–764.

21. Jackman RJ, Nowels KW, Shepard MJ, et al. Stereotaxic large-core needle biopsy of 450 nonpalpable breast lesions with surgical correlation in lesions with cancer or atypical hyperplasia. *Radiology* 1994;193:91–95.

22. Liberman L, Cohen MA, Abramson AF, et al. Atypical ductal hyperplasia diagnosed at stereotaxic core biopsy of breast lesions: an indication for surgical biopsy. *AJR Am J Roentgenol* 1995;164:1111–1113.

23. Rosen PP, Cantrell B, Mullen DL, et al. Juvenile papillomatosis (Swiss cheese disease) of the breast. *Am J Surg Pathol* 1980;4:3–12.

24. Bodian CA, Perzin KH, Lattes R, et al. Prognostic significance of benign proliferative breast disease. *Cancer* 1993;71:3896–3907.

25. Page DL, Rogers LW. Combined histologic and cytologic criteria for the diagnosis of mammary atypical ductal hyperplasia. *Hum Pathol* 1992;23:1095–1097.

26. Rubin E, Visscher DW, Alexander RW, et al. Proliferative disease and atypia in biopsies performed for nonpalpable lesions detected mammographically. *Cancer* 1988;61:2077–2082.

27. Stomper PC, Cholewinski SP, Penetrante RB, et al. Atypical hyperplasia, frequency and mammographic and pathologic relationships in excisional biopsies guided by mammography and clinical examination. *Radiology* 1993;189:667–671.

28. Wilson M, Cranor ML, Rosen PP. Papillary duct hyperplasia of the breast in children and young women. *Mod Pathol* 1993;6:570–574.

29. Rosen PP. Columnar cell hyperplasia is associated with lobular carcinoma *in situ* and tubular carcinoma. *Am J Surg Pathol* 1999;23:1561.

30. Rosen PP. Ductal hyperplasia and intraductal hyperplasia. In: *Breast pathology: diagnosis by needle core biopsy*. Philadelphia: Lippincott Williams & Wilkins, 1999:89–92.

31. Azzopardi JG. In: *Problems in breast pathology*. Philadelphia: WB Saunders, 1979:25.

32. Haagensen CD. In: *Diseases of the breast*, 3rd ed. Philadelphia: WB Saunders, 1986:118–124.

33. Wellings SR, Jensen HM, Marcum RG. An atlas of subgross pathology of the human breast with special reference to possible precancerous lesions. *J Natl Cancer Inst* 1975;55:231–273.

34. Ozaki D, Kondo Y. Comparative morphometric studies of benign and malignant intraductal proliferative lesions of the breast by computerized image analysis. *Hum Pathol* 1995;26:1109–1113.

35. Ohuchi N, Abe R, Takahashi T, et al. Three-dimensional atypical structure in intraductal carcinoma differentiating from papilloma and papillomatosis of the breast. *Breast Cancer Res Treat* 1985;5:57–65.

36. Ozzello L. Ultrastructure of the human mammary gland. *Pathol Annu* 1971;6:1–59.

37. Tavassoli FA, Norris HJ. A comparison of the results of long-term follow-up for atypical intraductal carcinoma of the breast. *Cancer* 1990;65:518–529.

38. Tavassoli FA. Intraductal hyperplasias, ordinary and atypical. In: *Pathology of the breast*. New York: Elsevier Science, 1992:155–191.

39. Tavassoli FA. In: *Pathology of the breast*. 2nd ed. Stamford, CT: Appleton & Lange, 1999:205–260.

40. Fisher ER, Costantino J, Fisher B, et al. for the National Surgical Adjuvant Breast and Bowel Project Collaborating Investigators. Pathologic findings from the National Surgical Adjuvant Breast Project (NSABP) Protocol B-17: intraductal carcinoma (ductal carcinoma *in situ*). *Cancer* 1995;75:1310–1319.

41. Prosser J, Hilsenbeck SG, Fuqua SAW, et al. Cell turnover (proliferation and apoptosis) in normal epithelium and premalignant lesions in the same breast. *Mod Pathol* 1997;10:38.

42. Arapantoni-Dadioti P, Panayiotides J, Georgakila H, et al. Significance of intracytoplasmic lumina in the differential diagnosis between epithelial hyperplasia and carcinoma *in situ* of the breast. *Breast Dis* 1996;9:277–282.

43. Azzopardi JG. In: *Problems in breast pathology*. Philadelphia: WB Saunders, 1979:213–214.

44. Oyama T, Maluf H, Koerner F. Atypical cystic lobules: an early stage in the formation of low-grade ductal carcinoma *in situ*. *Virchows Arch* 1999;435:413–421.

45. Goldstein NS, Lacerna M, Vicini F. Cancerization of lobules and atypical ductal hyperplasia adjacent to ductal carcinoma *in situ* of the breast. *Am J Clin Pathol* 1998;110:357–367.

46. Fraser JL, Raza S, Chorny K, et al. Columnar alteration with prominent apical snouts and secretions: a spectrum of changes frequently present in breast biopsies performed for microcalcifications. *Am J Surg Pathol* 1998;22:1521–1527.

47. Green I, McCormick B, Cranor M, et al. A comparative study of tubular and tubulo-lobular carcinoma of the breast. *Am J Surg Pathol* 1997;21:653–657.

48. Fraser JL, Pliss N, Connolly JL, et al. Immunophenotype of columnar alteration with prominent apical snouts and secretions (CAPSS). *Mod Pathol* 2000;13:21A.

49. Tocino I, Garcia BM, Carter D. Surgical biopsy findings in patients with atypical hyperplasia diagnosed by stereotaxic core needle biopsy. *Ann Surg Oncol* 1996;3:483–488.

50. Brem RF, Behrndt VS, Sanow L, et al. Atypical ductal hyperplasia: histologic underestimation of carcinoma in tissue harvested from impalpable breast lesions using 11-gauge stereotactically guided directional vacuum-assisted biopsy. *AJR Am J Roentgenol* 1999;172:1405–1407.

51. Moore MM, Hargett CW, Hanks JB, et al. Association of breast cancer with the finding of atypical ductal hyperplasia at core breast biopsy. *Ann Surg* 1997;225:726–731.

52. Gadzala DE, Cederbom GJ, Bolton JS, et al. Appropriate management of atypical ductal hyperplasia diagnosed by stereotactic core needle breast biopsy. *Ann Surg Oncol* 1997;4:283–286.

53. Burbank F. Stereotactic breast biopsy of atypical ductal hyperplasia and ductal carcinoma *in situ* lesions: improved accuracy with directional, vacuum-assisted biopsy. *Radiology* 1997;202:843–847.

54. Tocino I, Dillon D, Costa J, et al. Atypical hyperplasia of the breast diagnosed by stereotactic core needle biopsy: correlation of molecular markers with surgical outcome. *Radiology* 1999;213(Suppl):289.

55. Osborne MP, Borgen PI. Atypical ductal and lobular hyperplasia and breast cancer risk. *Surg Oncol Clin N Am* 1993;2:1–11.

56. Hughes KS, Papa MZ, Whitney T, et al. Prophylactic mastectomy and inherited predisposition to breast carcinoma. *Cancer* 1999;86:1682–1696.

57. Cancer Research Campaign Adjuvant Breast Trial Working Party. Cyclophosphamide and tamoxifen as adjuvant therapies in the management of breast cancer. *Br J Cancer* 1988;57:604–607.

58. Nayfield SG, Karp JE, Ford LG, et al. Potential role of tamoxifen in prevention of breast cancer. *J Natl Cancer Inst* 1991;83:1450–1459.

59. Rutqvist LE, Cedermark B, Glas U, et al. Contralateral primary tumors in breast cancer patients in a randomized trial of adjuvant tamoxifen therapy. *J Natl Cancer Inst* 1991;83:1299–1306.

60. Visscher DW, Padiyar N, Long D, et al. Immunohistologic analysis of estrogen receptor expression in breast carcinoma precursor lesions. *Breast J* 1998;4:447–451.

61. Shoker BS, Jarvis C, Clarke RB, et al. Estrogen receptor-positive proliferating cells in the normal and precancerous breast. *Am J Pathol* 1999;155:1811–1815.

62. Dupont WD, Page DL, Parl FF, et al. Estrogen replacement therapy in women with a history of proliferative breast disease. *Cancer* 1999;85:1277–1283.

63. Fisher B, Costantino JP, Wickerham DL, et al. Tamoxifen for prevention of breast cancer: report of the National Surgical Adjuvant Breast and Bowel Project P-1 Study. *J Natl Cancer Inst* 1998;90:1371–1388.

# CHAPTER 10

# Precancerous Breast Disease

## Epidemiologic, Pathologic, and Clinical Considerations

As advances have been made in the diagnosis and treatment of mammary carcinoma, more recently attention has been directed toward prevention strategies and to markers of increased risk for developing the disease. The strongest risk factors have proven to be genetic predisposition to breast carcinoma and antecedent proliferative breast changes documented by biopsy. These factors may be interactive in their effect on breast cancer risk.

### GENETIC PREDISPOSITION TO BREAST CARCINOMA

Genetic susceptibility is manifested clinically by a history of breast carcinoma in one or more female relatives. The risk associated with a positive family history increases when a maternal first-degree relative is affected, if the relative has premenopausal bilateral breast carcinoma, and if multiple relatives are affected. Other indications of possible hereditary susceptibility include early onset of breast carcinoma, multiple site-specific cancers (e.g., breast and ovarian), and the presence of rare cancers or cancer-associated syndromes.

Specific chromosomal alterations have been related to breast carcinoma risk as a result of the identification of mutations in the BRCA1 gene on the long arm of chromosome 17 (1–3) and the BRCA2 gene located on chromosome 13 (4). Various types of mutations in different segments of these genes have been identified (4–7). The lifetime risk for developing breast carcinoma as a result of a BRCA1 mutation has been reported in various studies to be 56% to nearly 90% (8,9). A slightly lower risk of breast carcinoma has been associated with BRCA2 mutations, reported to be 37% to 84% (9,10). BRCA1 may account for up to 45% of cases of hereditary breast carcinoma as well as nearly 90% of patients with combined breast and ovarian carcinoma (11,12). The life-

time risk for ovarian carcinoma attributed to BRCA1 mutations is about 45% (13).

The risks associated with BRCA1 and BRCA2 mutations appear to be modified by other genes or genetic alterations, as suggested by a study of genotypes of the androgen receptor (14). Reproductive factors such as parity and age of first live birth, well-established epidemiologic indicators of breast carcinoma risk, interact with familial risk to a slight degree (15). Parity may influence BRCA1-associated breast carcinoma risk (16). Exogenous factors such as cigarette smoking and oral contraceptive hormones also have been identified as factors that might modify BRCA1 or BRCA2 penetrance (17–19). Dietary, environmental, and other as yet undefined factors appear to influence the penetrance of BRCA1 and BRCA2 in individual women. This is illustrated by data from a study of 403 BRCA1 mutation carriers summarized by Rebbeck (20). Breast carcinoma alone had been diagnosed in 209 patients (52%) whose mean age at diagnosis was 42.6 years, but there was a broad range of ages (19–96 years). Among the other women, 40 (10%) developed ovarian carcinoma, and 22 (5%) had a history of ovarian and breast carcinoma. Nine (7%) of the remaining 132 women who had not developed breast or ovarian carcinoma were older than 70 years. The relationship between particular BRCA1 and BRCA2 mutations and susceptibility to breast or ovarian carcinoma or to specific types of carcinoma has not been well defined (21,22).

In the clinical screening situation, 16% of women who had breast carcinoma and reported a family history of breast or ovarian carcinoma were found to have detectable BRCA1 mutations (23). BRCA1 mutations were found in 7% of women with breast carcinoma and a positive family history. No association was detected between bilateral breast carcinoma in the patient or the number of breast carcinomas in a family and the presence of a BRCA1 mutation. These data add further support to the notion that BRCA mutations have variable penetrance and also suggest that alterations of other BRCA gene sites or entirely different genes are responsible for breast carcinoma in some women who have a positive family history.

Various reports have indicated that BRCA1-associated breast carcinomas have distinctive pathologic features, although they are not unique to these patients (24–27). The intraductal and infiltrating duct carcinomas are typically poorly differentiated histologically (grade 3) and have a poorly differentiated nuclear grade. A relatively high frequency of medullary carcinomas and of duct carcinomas with medullary features has been reported in these patients. These tumors also are characterized by high proliferative rates when studied by flow cytometry or by MIB1 immunohistochemistry (24,26). BRCA1-associated breast carcinomas typically do not express estrogen receptors (24,28) or HER2/neu (24,28), but they exhibit p53 nuclear reactivity (24,28,29). Angiogenesis also may be enhanced in BRCA1-associated carcinomas (24).

Breast carcinomas associated with BRCA2 mutations tend to have biologic and pathologic features that are generally similar to non-BRCA-related breast carcinomas when compared with BRCA1-associated controls and nonhereditary controls (24). One review found carcinomas with lobular features and lobular carcinoma in situ to be significantly more frequent in women with BRCA2 mutations than in those with BRCA1-associated carcinoma (25).

Several major genes that are less commonly identified than BRCA1 and BRCA2 also have been linked to a strong degree of breast carcinoma susceptibility. These typically are involved in cancer syndromes, such as TP53 in the Li-Fraumeni syndrome (30,31), PTEN in Cowden syndrome (32), and STK11 in Peutz-Jeghers syndrome (33).

Another group of genes that appear to confer an increased risk for breast carcinoma has been referred to as *low-penetrance genes*. These genes may account for some instances of nonfamilial or sporadic breast carcinoma. Their influence on breast cancer risk probably is mediated through interaction with other factors, such as the metabolism of environmental carcinogens or hormone metabolism. Examples of low-penetrance genes are GSTM1, a glutathione-S-transferase, which is involved in carcinogen metabolism (34,35), and AIB1, the amplified in breast cancer gene, which is involved in estrogen signal transduction in breast cells (36).

The BRCA genes also might play a role in the development of breast carcinoma through mechanisms other than gene mutations. These alternative pathways may be the consequence of other genetic alterations that might have a negative effect on the tumor-suppression function of the BRCA gene (37).

The relationship of BRCA1 and BRCA2 mutations to breast carcinoma prognosis has been reported by a number of investigators. Some studies found no significant difference in disease-free and overall survival when patients with

BRCA1-associated and sporadic carcinoma were compared (27,38,39). Using a different method of analysis, Foulkes et al. reported a statistically significant adverse prognosis among Ashkenazi Jewish women with BRCA1 mutations compared with women from the same ethnic background whose tumors did not exhibit BRCA1 mutations (40).

Breast-conservation therapy is a concern among women with BRCA1 and BRCA2 mutations because of the presumed high degree or risk in all breast tissue. Robson et al. compared the outcome of breast-conserving therapy in Ashkenazi Jewish women with and without BRCA1 or BRCA2 mutations (41). Patients with BRCA mutations were younger at diagnosis, they tended to develop ipsilateral breast recurrences more often, and they experienced substantially more frequent contralateral carcinomas. Mutation status was not predictive of distant disease-free survival in multivariate analysis.

Because the risk for developing breast carcinoma associated with BRCA1 and BRCA2 most likely involves all tissue in both breasts, surgical treatment to reduce substantially or to eliminate the risk requires bilateral prophylactic mastectomy (42). Most reports of breast carcinoma occurring at the site of prophylactic mastectomy refer to patients treated by subcutaneous mastectomy. Residual breast tissue is substantially less likely to remain after a complete or total mastectomy with excision of the nipple–areola complex. The age at which the operation is performed influences the benefit derived, with the estimated maximal gain in life expectancy from surgery in patients in their thirties and little gain at age 60 or later (43).

One alternative to prophylactic mastectomy is careful clinical follow-up with frequent mammography, clinical examination, and breast self-examination. The potential contributions of magnetic resonance imaging (MRI) and positron emission tomography (PET) scanning to early carcinoma detection in high-risk women with documented hereditary breast carcinoma susceptibility have not been determined.

Chemoprevention of breast carcinoma has been effective in prospective trials of women at high risk, although no study to date has been devoted specifically to women with documented BRCA1 or BRCA2 mutations. Tamoxifen reduces the risk of developing breast cancer in women with several high-risk factors, including a history of one or more first-degree relatives with breast carcinoma (44). The risk reduction was 45% to 49%, depending on the number of affected relatives. The frequency of contralateral carcinoma also is reduced by the use of tamoxifen in adjuvant therapy for ipsilateral carcinoma and contributes to lowering the frequency of breast recurrence after conservation therapy (45). Analysis of competing causes of mortality suggests adjuvant tamoxifen treatment results in a significant decrease in mortality by reducing deaths from contralateral carcinoma and from cardiovascular disease, despite predisposing to endometrial carcinoma and thromboembolic events (44,46).

Genetic changes associated with transitions from normal epithelium to hyperplasia and ultimately carcinoma involve a series of events referred to as *initiation, transformation, and progression*. Few proliferative lesions actually advance through all of these steps to become invasive carcinomas, and it is likely that most never progress beyond the early stages of initiation that may be represented in some but not necessarily in all instances by hyperplasia.

One interesting prospect is suggested by studies of markers associated with pulmonary carcinoma (47). These investigators used immunohistochemistry to examine retrospectively the distribution of hnRNP and a ceramide related to Lewis-X antigens, two markers associated with carcinoma, in "moderately atypical sputum epithelial cells" preserved in archived cytology specimens. The samples were obtained in a screening program for persons at high risk of developing pulmonary carcinoma. Expression of the markers was found in atypical cells from 91% of patients who later developed carcinoma and in only 5 of 40 (12.5%) who did not develop carcinoma. A second study used the same markers to investigate previously treated patients with follow-up for evidence of new primary or recurrent carcinomas. Only 6% of subsequent lung carcinomas were anticipated by finding abnormal cells on routine cytologic examination in this population. By using quantitative immunohistochemistry, these researchers were able to detect marker overexpression in sputum samples from 92% of patients with second primary carcinomas (48).

The hypothesis underlying the aforementioned investigations of pulmonary carcinoma patients is equally applicable as a model for mammary carcinogenesis. This is based on the concept of field carcinogenesis (49), which holds that transformation occurs widely in epithelium exposed to a carcinogenic stimulus but that progression occurs unevenly. Molecular alterations associated with some stages of this process, especially those that precede phenotypic changes recognizable by cytologic or histologic examination, may occur during development of the mammary gland and are likely to be the earliest indicators of transformation in this as well as in other organs.

A provocative observation that relates genetic alterations to breast cancer risk is the finding of loss of heterozygosity (LOH) in morphologically normal lobular glands near breast carcinomas (50). Among 10 specimens with LOH at 3p22-25 in a breast carcinoma, six exhibited the same LOH in histologically normal lobules taken from tissue surrounding the carcinoma. Corresponding LOH in normal lobules was found less often for carcinomas that displayed LOH at 17p13.1 and 11p15.5. Several explanations have been suggested for these findings. One is the possibility that isolated carcinoma cells could be present in seemingly normal lobules as a result of pagetoid spread from the primary tumor. Alternatively, some stages in the process of transformation to carcinoma could occur in cells that retain a "normal" phenotype before the appearance of histologically detectable hyperplasia. The latter scenario includes the possibility that the hyperplastic phenotype is evanescent or entirely bypassed during carcinogenesis. The absence of hyperplasia at the site

of or in the vicinity of some mammary carcinomas is consistent with this hypothesis.

The clonality of histologically normal breast tissue was investigated by studying the pattern of X-chromosome inactivation in normal contiguous lobules and ducts (51). The analysis revealed patches of glands with a single X-chromosome inactivated, indicating the existence of discrete clonal regions within the breast. The existence of genetically different but histologically identical appearing patches of breast glandular parenchyma could provide an explanation for the heterogenous distribution of proliferative and neoplastic lesions in the breasts. This observation was confirmed by Diallo et al., who demonstrated monoclonal origin of terminal duct–lobular units, duct hyperplasia, intraductal papillomas, and intraductal carcinomas (52) and by Larson et al. (53).

Another approach to the study of clonality in the normal breast was described by Lakhani et al., who performed LOH analysis on colonies of epithelial and myoepithelial cells isolated *in vitro* from fresh breast specimens (54). LOH present in invasive carcinomas also was identified in adjacent normal tissue and under the conditions of the study was not attributable to pagetoid spread of carcinoma cells. LOH was detected in epithelial and in myoepithelial cells, providing evidence that the lobule is a clonal structure with both cell types derived from a common stem cell. Analysis of clones derived from normal tissue not in proximity to a carcinoma also revealed LOH, which indicates that genetic alterations that probably occur early in breast development can be heterogeneously distributed in the breast and not limited to a localized region. LOH also was found in epithelial/myoepithelial clones from samples of breast tissue obtained in reduction mammoplasties in the absence of carcinoma.

Clonal analysis also has been applied to the study of bilateral breast carcinomas. Discordant distribution of six immunohistochemical markers in paired samples of bilateral tumors from 51 women reported by Dawson et al. was indicative of independent origin of the carcinomas (55). Independent clonal origin of bilateral breast carcinomas also was demonstrated by Noguchi et al. (56). Shibata et al. detected different X-chromosome inactivation patterns of the androgen receptor gene between left and right breast tumors in three patients, indicating independent clonal origin of the neoplasms (57). Two patients had nonidentical p53 mutations in both tumors, and in nine cases, p53 mutations were identified in only one of the two neoplasms. The absence of concordant results with either procedure is further evidence in support of the strong probability that bilateral breast carcinomas are not only clonally independent but that they can arise from genetically distinct epithelial patches, possibly through differing genetic mechanisms.

## PROLIFERATIVE (FIBROCYSTIC) BREAST CHANGES

Biopsy-proven benign proliferative or fibrocystic changes, previously referred to as *fibrocystic disease,* have been identified as morphologic markers of risk for the development of breast carcinoma. The most extensive studies have been retrospective investigations in which the diagnosis of biopsy specimens was reclassified many years after surgery and correlated with follow-up. Few investigations have been prospective analyses that related the initial diagnostic classification to subsequent outcome. Most investigators have analyzed groups consisting of many hundreds or thousands of patients (58–62), and a few have dealt with highly selected, smaller series (63–65). Numerous observations and conclusions can be drawn from these reports. The reader should also see Chapter 9 for additional information about atypical hyperplasia.

- **The causes of proliferative changes in the human breast have received less attention than the precancerous risk associated with these lesions.**

Because of the association of proliferative changes with the development of carcinoma, it is reasonable to speculate that both conditions could have common predisposing factors. This speculation has been borne out by the finding that the risk of biopsy-proven benign breast disease is increased significantly by nulliparity, late age of first birth, and late menopause, factors also associated with increased risk of breast carcinoma (66–69). Dietary risks factors for breast cancer, such as high intake of meat fat (70) and caffeine (71), also have been associated with a greater risk of benign breast disease. Whereas most of the foregoing investigations did not specify a relationship with particular categories of benign breast disease, the analysis of meat fat revealed a strong association between frequent consumption and an elevated risk for severe atypia and *in situ* carcinoma (70). Boyle et al. reported that excess caffeine consumption was associated with atypical lobular hyperplasia and with sclerosing adenosis accompanied by duct hyperplasia (71). An inverse relationship between dietary fiber content and the risk of benign proliferative breast disease has been reported (72,73). A similar relationship was observed between dietary fiber intake and breast density (74). The mechanism by which dietary fiber influences mammary epithelial proliferation is unknown, but it might involve intestinal estrogen metabolism or substances associated with fiber-containing foods such as phytoestrogens.

No consistent association between proliferative changes in the breast and a family history of breast carcinoma has been found (66,75), although one study reported a slightly higher frequency of atypical hyperplasia in women with a positive family history than among those without this situation (76). Obesity or excess body mass (67,77) and the use of oral contraceptives (67,68,75) are factors associated with a decreased risk for benign breast disease.

Ionizing radiation is a well-documented cause of breast carcinoma after doses associated with exposure to an atomic bomb, multiple diagnostic radiographic tests, or radiation therapy for benign conditions (78–80). There is also a significant positive association between radiation exposure

from the atomic bomb and the prevalence of proliferative changes, particularly with atypical hyperplasia, in the breasts of survivors (81). The latter association was strongest in women exposed when they were 40 to 49 years old. The increased risk for breast carcinoma after exposure to atomic bomb radiation occurs largely in women exposed before the age of 40 years.

- **Surgical biopsy and needle core biopsy are currently the most reliable methods for establishing the presence of prognostically significant atypical hyperplasia in individual patients. Fine needle aspiration (FNA) cytology and mammography are useful adjunctive procedures.**

Stereotaxic needle core biopsy is being used with increasing frequency as an alternative to FNA to sample nonpalpable mammographically detected breast lesions. A broad spectrum of pathologic abnormalities is encountered in this material, including a substantial number of proliferative foci with varying degrees of atypia (82,83). The mammographic appearance of these lesions is usually not predictive of specific histologic abnormalities, but atypical duct hyperplasia (ADH) is not infrequently present. Surgical biopsy is indicated if the sampling obtained with a needle core biopsy results in a diagnosis of atypical hyperplasia because these abnormalities may be associated with intraductal carcinoma (83) (see Chapters 9 and 13).

Numerous published studies have assessed the criteria for the diagnosis of proliferative breast lesions in FNA cytology specimens. The major consideration in these investigations has been to develop reliable standards for distinguishing between atypical hyperplasia and intraductal carcinoma. Several methods for interpreting FNA specimens have been proposed, but investigators have had limited success when FNA diagnoses were compared with the findings in subsequent biopsy specimens (84–87). Bibbo et al. achieved a high level of concordance in specimens with severe atypia but were less effective in correctly recognizing mild to moderate atypia in FNA specimens (84). Stanley et al. found that only 40% of biopsies showed significant proliferative lesions after an FNA diagnosis that suggested the presence of such a process (88).

A combination of cytologic and architectural features investigated by Sneige and Staerkel proved useful for identifying some examples of orderly intraductal carcinoma in FNA samples (87). Nonetheless, these investigastors observed that "overlapping features" of ductal hyperplasia, ADH, and low-grade intraductal carcinoma "make separation of some of these lesions difficult." In this series, 7 of 11 (64%) samples of intraductal carcinoma were diagnosed correctly by FNA, whereas 2 of 9 (22%) biopsies interpreted cytologically as atypical hyperplasia had been classified as intraductal carcinoma. Similar results were obtained by Abendroth et al., who interpreted the FNA from 1 of 12 (8%) specimens with atypical hyperplasia as "suspicious" (89). Six cases were interpreted as having cytologic atypia, and five were reported to be "negative." Six of nine aspirates from patients with intraductal carcinoma were interpreted as suspicious or positive. In the series described by Abendroth et al., 11 of the 35 (31%) aspirates from patients with atypia or *in situ* carcinoma contained insufficient cellular material for diagnosis (89). This experience highlights a significant limitation of FNA as a procedure for the diagnosis of proliferative foci, which are often small, ill-defined lesions.

Cytologic features that suggest a diagnosis of hyperplasia include clusters and three-dimensional groups of cohesive cells, distinct cell borders, the presence of myoepithelial cells at the periphery of cell groups, the absence of coarse chromatin, and little or no nuclear pleomorphism (90). In one study, the only feature among 13 studied that was significantly more often present in aspirates from patients with proliferative breast disease when compared with nonproliferative lesions was a "swirling pattern of cells" (91). Irregular nuclear borders, nuclear hyperchromasia, dispersed noncohesive epithelial cells, irregular cell clusters, and overlapping nuclei were features that favored atypical hyperplasia or carcinoma in an FNA specimen. An inflammatory background, stromal fragments, increased nuclear:cytoplasmic ratio, nuclear enlargement, and nucleoli were nonspecific features found with relatively equal frequency in atypical hyperplasia and intraductal carcinoma.

One application of FNA has been in the study of asymptomatic women in families with a known history of breast carcinoma. Using aspirates from four quadrants, Skolnick et al. compared 77 women from 20 families with two first-degree affected relatives to 31 controls (92). Proliferative breast disease characterized as the cytologic diagnosis of "moderate to marked ductal hyperplasia or atypical hyperplasia" was found significantly more often (35%) in relatives of breast carcinoma patients than in controls (13%). Genetic analysis suggested that inherited susceptibility was responsible for the proliferative breast changes and for breast carcinoma in the families. Khan et al. did a similar study using FNA to assess the contralateral breasts of 32 women with sporadic breast carcinoma in one breast and 38 control subjects without breast carcinoma (93). Cytospin preparations from pooled four-quadrant aspirations revealed a significantly higher frequency of proliferative changes and atypical hyperplasia in samples from the contralateral breasts of patients with breast carcinoma. Overall, 40% of the specimens were deemed inadequate because of insufficient cellularity. Low cellularity was significantly more common in control samples and was associated with obesity and age greater than 50 years. An important limitation of these studies is that surgical biopsies were not performed to confirm the cytologic interpretations and to characterize the proliferative lesions histologically.

Mammographic patterns have been studied extensively as possible indicators of breast carcinoma risk. A classification of patterns introduced by Wolfe in the 1970s had four categories that proved to be associated with increasing risk (94). N1 described the predominantly fatty breast with the least risk. Intermediate risk was associated with P1 and P2 mammograms marked by linear densities indicative of a prominent ductal pattern. DY, the highest risk category, described nodular or plaque-like densities referred to in radiologic terms as "mammographic dysplasia." Quantitative classifications based on estimates of the proportion of the breast volume affected by parenchymal patterns such as DY were introduced to improve mammographic risk estimates (95,96).

Studies of the association between Wolfe's mammographic patterns and specific histopathologic findings in the breast did not result in consistent findings. Some investigators reported significant associations between proliferative epithelial changes, epithelial hyperplasia, and radiographic patterns (97,98). In one study, follow-up of women enrolled in a screening program revealed a 9.7-fold increased risk for subsequent carcinoma *in situ* or atypical hyperplasia in women with the greatest mammographic density compared with women with no mammographic density (97). They also found a 12.2-fold greater risk of hyperplasia without atypia in the group of women with the greatest density. Urbanski et al. reported a trend to more frequent atypical hyperplasia in women whose concurrent preoperative mammograms showed the greatest mammographic "dysplasia" (98). On the other hand, Moskowitz et al. (99) and Arthur et al. (100) found no association between mammographic pattern and histopathologic changes in concurrent biopsies.

Unfortunately, the foregoing mammography studies and others on this subject are not comparable because of substantial methodologic differences in mammographic classification and pathology review. It seems likely that a major component of dense mammographic parenchymal patterns is the fibrous stroma, an association noted in some studies (101,102). Proliferative epithelial lesions are accompanied by stromal proliferation to a greater extent in premenopausal than in postmenopausal women; however, premenopausal women with constitutionally dense mammary stroma and abundant glandular tissue lacking proliferative changes may not be distinguishable mammographically.

- **A minority of women with biopsies classified as nonproliferative or proliferative subsequently develop carcinoma in either breast.**

In published reports, the overall proportion of women with an antecedent breast biopsy who later developed breast carcinoma rarely exceeded 10% even with follow-up of two decades or longer. Bodian et al. detected subsequent breast carcinoma in 139 of 1,521 patients (9.1%) with proliferative changes and in 18 of 278 (6.5%) with nonproliferative biopsies within a follow-up period of 21 years (103). Overall, 8.7% of the patients developed breast carcinoma. In other reports involving at least 1,000 patients, the proportions of women who developed carcinoma were 2.2% (104), 2.9% (58), 4.1% (105), 4.6% (106), and 4.9% (63) (Table 10.1). The proportion of patients with subsequent carcinoma tended to increase with length of follow-up, being least in a group with follow-up of fewer than 5 years (107) and

**TABLE 10.1.** *Frequency of breast carcinoma following biopsy-proven atypical hyperplasia*

| Reference | Length of follow-up (yr mean or average) | Total no. patients | Total Ca patients no. (%) | Total no. AH patients (% AH of total patients) | No. of AH patients with Ca | Ca in AH patients | |
|---|---|---|---|---|---|---|---|
| | | | | | | % AH patients | % Total Ca patients |
| Kodlin et al. (104)[a] | — | 2,931 | 64 (2.2) | 4 (1.7) | 3 | 6.1 | 4.7 |
| Carter et al. (58) | 8.3 | 16,692 | 485 (2.9) | 1,305 (7.8) | 67 | 5.1 | 13.8 |
| Dupont and Page (105) | 17 | 3,303 | 135 (4.1) | 232 (7.0) | 30 | 12.9 | 22.2 |
| Krieger and Hiatt (63)[a] | 16 | 2,731 | 135 (4.9) | 52 (1.9) | 5 | 9.6 | 3.7 |
| Bodian et al. (103) | 21 | 1,799 | 157 (8.7) | 342[b] (19) | 33 | 9.6 | 21 |
| | | | | 272[c] | 25 | 9.1 | 15.9 |
| | | | | 70[d] | 8 | 11.4 | 5 |

AH, atypical hyperplasia; Ca, carcinoma.
[a] Atypical hyperplasia defined as Black–Chabon grade 4.
[b] Data below represent subsets of 342.
[c] Hyperplasia with mild atypia.
[d] Hyperplasia with moderate to severe atypia.

highest when follow-up was a decade or longer (63,105, 106). This observation is consistent with the rising risk for developing breast carcinoma with advancing age. Against this background, there is evidence that the relative risk (RR) associated with proliferative changes may be attenuated or may decrease with time and advancing age (108).

The frequency of breast carcinoma in women with previous biopsies that showed proliferative changes exceeds that of normal controls that did not undergo biopsy, but only a small proportion of patients with proliferative lesions develop carcinoma. Proliferative breast changes are one of several so-called attributable risk factors, a list that also includes family history of breast carcinoma, parity, age at menarche, age of first birth, and others. An American Cancer Society survey published in 1982 found that not more than 30% of women with breast carcinoma had any known attributable risk factor (109). Data from the first National Health and Nutrition Examination Survey reported in 1995 indicated that about 47% [95% confidence interval (CI): 17%–77%] of breast carcinoma in the study cohort was attributable to known risk factors (first birth after age 20 or nulliparity, family history of breast carcinoma, and high income) and by extrapolation for about 41% (95% CI: 2%–80%) of breast carcinoma cases in the United States (110). Breast carcinoma in women with an antecedent benign breast biopsy constitutes a small proportion of all breast carcinomas. Consequently, intervention to prevent breast carcinoma limited to women with "precancerous" proliferative changes may have a relatively small impact on the overall frequency of and mortality from breast carcinoma unless additional therapeutic indications that apply to many more persons can be identified to select women for chemoprevention therapy.

• **The risk of carcinoma subsequent to unilateral biopsy-proven proliferative changes affects both breasts.**

The bilaterality of risk was noted by Davis et al. in a review of 297 patients with "cystic disease" (111). These investigators also tabulated data from 11 studies that included at least 100 patients who had "cystic disease," showing that 0.7% to 4.9% of patients subsequently developed carcinoma, with 50% of the carcinomas in the contralateral breast.

Krieger and Hiatt found that only 56% of carcinomas diagnosed subsequent to a benign biopsy occurred in the previously biopsied breast that had shown benign proliferative changes (63). Laterality of subsequent carcinoma was not influenced significantly by the type of antecedent proliferative change or the age at biopsy. The mean interval to subsequent ipsilateral carcinomas (11.2 years) was shorter than for contralateral carcinomas (14 years). Page et al. reported that 8 of 18 (44%) carcinomas subsequent to ADH and 5 of 16 (31%) carcinomas following atypical lobular hyperplasia occurred in the contralateral breast (61). Involvement of the contralateral breast in similar proportions of patients also was described by Connolly et al. (112).

An exception to the foregoing reports of bilateral risk was described by Tavassoli and Norris, who found carcinoma in the ipsilateral breast of 10 of 14 (71%) women who had lesions they classified as duct hyperplasia or ADH (65). Although this unusual distribution of laterality could have been a chance event in a relatively small series of cases, it is more likely reflective of the authors' method for defining atypical hyperplasia with a size criterion that can result in classifying some intraductal carcinomas, lesions associated with the greatest increased ipsilateral risk, as atypical hyperplasia.

These data from various sources suggest that the risk for carcinoma is divided nearly equally between the two breasts after proliferative changes are detected in one breast. It appears that epithelial hyperplasia is a marker of a disturbance that may variably affect the entire mammary epithelium. The bilateral risk for subsequent carcinoma associated with proliferative lesions is in striking contrast to the strong tendency for subsequent invasive carcinoma to arise in the ipsilateral breast following intraductal carcinoma. This difference in laterality reflects fundamental biological changes affecting the mammary epithelium, associated with transitions from marker to precursor, and ultimately to obligate precursor lesions for invasive mammary carcinoma.

- **The chance of developing breast carcinoma is influenced by factors that may modify the level of risk associated with benign proliferative changes.**

The pathologic findings in a biopsy from an individual patient cannot be viewed out of the clinical context. Age at diagnosis proved to be an additive factor in a study by Carter et al., who found a sixfold increase in the rate of subsequent breast carcinoma among patients younger than 46 years who had undergone biopsy and who had atypical hyperplasia compared with normal women (58). The rate was increased 3.7-fold in women with atypical hyperplasia who were 46 to 55 years of age and 2.3-fold in women older than 55. London et al. also observed an inverse relationship of age and risk in which the relative risk increased 2.6-fold among premenopausal women who had biopsy-proven atypia compared with postmenopausal subjects (59). Page et al. reported that the risk associated with atypical lobular hyperplasia was inversely related to age, being greatest in women who underwent biopsy before the age of 45 (62). In the latter study, increased risk attributable to ADH was observed only in patients older than 45 at biopsy.

A history of breast carcinoma among first-degree female relatives is a particularly strong additive factor in women who have atypical hyperplasia. Page et al. (61) and Dupont et al. (113) found that the risk associated with atypical lobular and ADH was more than doubled in women with a positive family history compared with the risk without this factor. London et al. found that the increased risk associated with family history was strongest in patients with atypical hyperplasia (59). Relative risk was not increased by a positive family history in women with nonproliferative biopsies.

Ahmed et al. compared women with breast carcinoma and a prior benign breast biopsy with a cohort of breast carcinoma patients who had not undergone previous biopsy (114). Epidemiologic factors present significantly more often among women with a prior benign breast biopsy were a positive family history of breast carcinoma and postmenopausal hormone use. Age at the time of breast carcinoma diagnosis did not differ significantly between the two groups, and the groups did not differ significantly with respect to reproductive factors (age at menarche, age of first pregnancy, or number of pregnancies). Patients with a prior benign breast biopsy were more likely to have lobular carcinoma, smaller tumors, and fewer axillary lymph nodes with metastatic carcinoma, although the overall frequencies of nodal involvement were not significantly different. The frequency of estrogen receptor–positive tumors did not differ significantly between the two groups. Patients with prior benign breast disease had a significantly better 10-year disease-free survival than those without a history of benign breast disease. Prior benign biopsies were not reviewed in this study.

- **Among women who have had a benign breast biopsy, the risk for developing subsequent carcinoma is related to the histologic components of the antecedent biopsy.**

In 1978, Page et al. stated that "women with . . . sclerosing adenosis . . . were at no greater risk of subsequent carcinoma than women in the general population" (62). Subsequently, the same investigators reported that sclerosing adenosis was an additive factor, increasing the risk of women with a family history of breast carcinoma (115). When assessed independently, sclerosing adenosis has been associated with an increased risk in several studies (65,104,106,113,115,116). Some of these investigators reported a greater increase in risk for relatively small groups of women who had atypical hyperplasia and sclerosing adenosis (65,113,115). Bodian et al. reported a high relative risk associated with adenosis but no significant difference in risk between patients who had adenosis with or without coexistent atypical hyperplasia (103).

The relative risk associated with other proliferative lesions exclusive of atypical hyperplasia is less well documented. Increased risk has been associated with papillary apocrine metaplasia (61), with "pink cell" metaplasia (116) and with the presence of microcalcifications detected histologically (106,113).

A detailed analysis of the relationship of apocrine change to breast carcinoma risk was reported by Page et al. in 1996 (117). Lesions were subdivided on the basis of proliferative pattern into three categories: simple, complex, and highly complex. The relative risk for developing subsequent carcinoma compared with the expected frequency from the Third National Cancer Survey was increased slightly in women with simple (RR = 1.39) and complex lesions (RR = 1.30) and substantially increased by the presence of highly complex apocrine change (RR = 3.14). Further analysis revealed that atypical hyperplasia in nonapocrine tissue contributed to the risk associated with apocrine change. After exclusion of patients with coexisting atypical nonapocrine hyperplasia, the relative risks were 1.29, 0.90, and 2.0 for simple, complex, and high complex apocrine changes, respectively. Although none of these relative risks represented a statistically significant increase, the relative risk for highly complex lesions remained substantially higher than the other two categories and the 95% CI for patients with complex apocrine change and coexisting atypical hyperplasia (RR = 3.14; 95% CI: 1.3–7.6) and patients without coexisting atypical hyperplasia (RR = 2.0; 95% CI: 0.77–7.4) were nearly identical. The fact that patients in this study considered to have highly complex apocrine change exhibited the greatest relative risk for subsequent carcinoma may have resulted from the inclusion of patients with apocrine intraductal carcinoma in the highly complex apocrine category. These investigators acknowledged this with their observation "that patterns within the highly complex category of (papillary apocrine change) are close to the patterns noted in McDivitt et al. (118) as indicating carcinoma *in situ* of ductal pattern." A further explanation of the distinction between highly complex papillary apocrine change (PAC) and apocrine intraductal carcinoma was offered:

**TABLE 10.2.** *Relative risk for invasive carcinoma associated with benign lesions in a prior breast biopsy[a]*

No increased risk[b]
  Adenosis, other than sclerosing adenosis
  Duct ectasia
  Fibroadenoma lacking complex features
  Fibrosis
  Mastitis
  Hyperplasia without atypia
  Cysts, gross or microscopic
  Simple apocrine metaplasia without associated hyperplasia or adenosis
  Squamous metaplasia
Slightly increased risk (1.5–2.0)
  Complex fibroadenoma
  Moderate or florid hyperplasia without atypia
  Sclerosing adenosis
  Solitary papilloma without atypical hyperplasia
Moderately increased risk (4.0–5.0)
  Atypical ductal hyperplasia
  Atypical lobular hyperplasia

[a] Based on Fitzgibbons PL, Henson DE, Hutter RV. Benign breast changes and the risk for subsequent breast cancer: an update of the 1985 consensus statement. Cancer Committee of the College of American Pathologists. *Arch Pathol Lab Med* 1998;122:1053–1055, with permission.
[b] Relative risk determined by comparison with women who did not have a breast biopsy.

This is little problem in differential diagnosis, as is usually the case, the alteration of PAC is <2 mm in extent. When the lesion is >4–8mm in size or has >25% of nuclei with alternate patterns, some form of atypia or low-grade DCIS (duct carcinoma *in situ*) may be diagnosed. . . . We believe that these relatively concise rules foster interobserver agreement in this area, but there is no practical reason to separate simple PAC from complex PAC. Also, the occurrence of highly complex PAC is of practical importance only in avoiding overdiagnosing a borderline lesion, which it is not.

Upon reflection, the report does not provide a crisp distinction between highly complex PAC and apocrine intraductal carcinoma, and the authors themselves suggested that some of the lesions they included as "highly complex PAC" might be interpreted as intraductal carcinoma. On this basis,

highly complex PAC, as described by Page et al., should be distinguished from a simple and complex PAC, and it is likely that most of the increased relative risk in the highly complex PAC group was attributable to contamination by a subset of women who had apocrine intraductal carcinoma.

A report published in 1998 by the Cancer Committee of the College of American Pathologists defined the relative risk for breast carcinoma associated with proliferative breast lesions based on published data (119) (Table 10.2).

• **A higher relative risk is associated with atypical hyperplasia than with other proliferative lesions.**

The proportion of patients who develop carcinoma is highest in the group of women with atypical hyperplasia, intermediate in those with proliferative changes without atypia, and least when there are no proliferative changes (Tables 10.2 and 10.3).

Proliferative changes were identified in 152 (85%) of 1,799 biopsies studied by Bodian et al. (103). Moderate to severe atypia was present in 70 specimens, representing 3.8% of all cases and 4.6% of specimens with proliferative changes. Follow-up revealed that the relative risk of developing carcinoma compared with the general population represented by data from the Connecticut Tumor Registry was higher in women with any proliferative changes (RR = 2.2) than for those with nonproliferative biopsies (RR = 1.6). Within the group with proliferative changes, the relative risk ranged from 3.0 for moderate to severe atypia, to 2.3 for mild atypia, and 2.1 for hyperplasia without atypia. These differences in relative risk were not statistically significant, but the relative risk for each of the categories of hyperplasia was increased significantly compared with controls. The relative risks associated with proliferative changes in ducts and lobules were similar except for severe atypia, where the risk for duct lesions (RR = 3.9) was significantly greater than that for severe atypia in lobules (RR = 2.6). Because the combined number of cases with severe atypia in ducts or in lobules was 70, and five carcinomas occurred in this group, this distinction may not be clinically important, even if it is statistically significant.

**TABLE 10.3.** *Breast carcinoma following benign breast biopsy*

| Reference | Length of follow-up (average or mean) (yr) | No. patients | No. NP (% total patients) | No. Ca in NP patients (% total patients) | No. PDWA (% total patients) | No. Ca in PDWA patients (% PDWA) | No. AH (% total patients) | No. Ca in AH patients (% AH) | No. total Ca (% total patients) |
|---|---|---|---|---|---|---|---|---|---|
| Bodian et al. (103) | 21 | 1,799 | 362 (20) | 30 (8.2) | 1,095 (60.8) | 94 (8.6) | 272[a] (15.1) 70[b] (3.9) | 25 (9.1) 8 (11.4) | 157 (8.7) |
| Dupont and Page (105) | 17 | 3,303 | 1,378 (41.7) | 31 (2.2) | 1,693 (51.2) | 74 (4.3) | 232 (7) | 30 (12.9) | 135 (4.1) |
| Carter et al. (58) | 8 | 16,692 | 6,615 (39.6) | 147 (2.2) | 8,772 (52.5) | 271 (3.1) | 1,305 (7.8) | 67 (5.1) | 485 (2.9) |
| Moskowitz et al.4 (approximate) (107) | 1,408 | 832 (59) | 2 (0.02) | 503 (35.7) | 6 (1.1) | 76 (5.3) | 5 (6.6) | 13 (0.09) |

AH, atypical hyperplasia; Ca, carcinoma; NP, nonproliferative; PDWA, proliferative without atypia.
[a] All atypical hyperplasias.
[b] Moderate and severe atypical hyperplasias.

Page et al. found the relative risks to be 4.7 and 5.8, respectively, for women with ADH and atypical lobular hyperplasia compared with women who had nonproliferative biopsies (61). The relative risk for women with ADH and a family history of breast carcinoma was increased when further compared with women with nonproliferative biopsies who had a positive family history (61). London et al. found the relative risk for atypical hyperplasia to be 3.7, which is significantly greater than in women who had proliferative (RR = 1.6) and nonproliferative (RR = 1.0) biopsies without atypia (59). Premenopausal women with atypical hyperplasia had a higher relative risk (RR = 5.9) than postmenopausal patients (RR = 2.3).

Ma and Boyd undertook a metanalysis of studies that investigated the association between atypical hyperplasia and breast cancer risk (120). Fifteen reports between 1960 and 1992 fulfilled these investigators' requirements for inclusion in the study, resulting in a total sample size of 182,980 women. The overall OR compared with controls for the development of carcinoma in women with atypical hyperplasia was 3.67 (95% CI = 3.16–4.26).

- **Regardless of the definition of atypia, most carcinomas subsequent to a benign biopsy occur in women who did not have atypical hyperplasia.**

As shown in Table 10.1, the proportion of all subsequent carcinomas that occurred in women with prior biopsy-proven atypical hyperplasia ranged from 3.7% to 22.2%. More than 75%, and in some studies more than 90%, of subsequent carcinomas developed in women without antecedent atypical hyperplasia. This conclusion is also supported by several case-control studies (59,60,121,122). In these reports, subsequent carcinomas were preceded by biopsy-proven atypical hyperplasia in 14.7% (121) to 22.2% (59) of cases, and atypical hyperplasia was present in 2.2% (122) to 10.5% (59) of controls who did not develop carcinoma.

- **Atypical hyperplasia is diagnosed in a small proportion of benign breast biopsies. The frequency of atypia is influenced by the strictness of criteria defining the condition, rarely exceeding 10% of specimens studied.**

In the studies listed in Tables 10.1 and 10.3, the frequency of atypical hyperplasia varied from 1.7% to 7.8% of biopsies, except for the report by Bodian et al. in which 19% of biopsies were classified as atypical hyperplasia (103). Most of these, however, were classified as mild atypical hyperplasia, and the 70 specimens with moderate to severe atypia constituted only 5.3% of all biopsies in the series.

- **Despite attempts to refine and improve the specificity of definitions of atypical hyperplasia, there are substantial differences in the interpretation of these lesions.**

In 1916, Bloodgood introduced the term *borderline* for lesions about which "both the surgeon and pathologist are in doubt," and he stated that ". . . if women come *early* we shall find that the borderline group is large" (123). In this prophetic statement, Bloodgood anticipated current circumstances achieved after decades of effort to improve the early detection and diagnosis of breast carcinoma. The recent emergence of so-called borderline proliferative lesions as a major diagnostic and therapeutic problem is a result of several factors. These include the widespread use of mammography (which has made it possible to detect many of these abnormalities clinically), epidemiologic studies relating increased risk for developing breast carcinoma to proliferative breast changes, and growing interest in preventing breast carcinoma. Bloodgood tested the level of agreement among pathologists on the diagnosis of borderline lesions and reported the results of his trial as follows:

> I have submitted over sixty borderline cases to a number of pathologists, and have found that in not a single one has there been uniform agreement as to whether the lesion was benign or malignant. . . . This is no reflection on the diagnostic abilities of the pathologists; it is simply evidence that at the present time there are certain lesions of the breast about which we apparently do not agree from the microscopic appearance only (123).

Five years later, Bloodgood reported the following conclusion about the diagnosis of proliferative lesions:

> In breast lesions, when good pathologists disagree as to malignancy, the patient lives; when there is agreement, there is always a large percentage of deaths from cancer (124).

The problem of diagnosing borderline lesions persists, as illustrated in a report by Bodian et al. (125). To assess diagnostic reproducibility, 63 cases were chosen at random to be interspersed twice in a review of 1,799 biopsies in a manner that was inapparent to the reviewers. There were no disagreements on the diagnosis of intraductal or invasive carcinoma in five cases and of lobular neoplasia/lobular carcinoma *in situ* in 10 cases. Disagreements were encountered in 17 of the remaining 48 cases. Interpretations differed in 9 of the 48 cases (19%) with respect to the presence of hyperplasia, resulting in a low estimated concordance of 0.29. Among 39 cases in which hyperplasia was diagnosed on both reviews, the anatomic site of hyperplasia (ductal or lobular) differed in 11 cases. In a separate analysis by the same investigators, 219 of 240 cases (91%) originally diagnosed as hyperplasia without atypia by one pathologist were confirmed by a second pathologist, and 21 were reclassified as having mild or moderate atypia. These researchers concluded that there are ". . . sufficient problems with reproducibility of these criteria to suggest caution in making precise risk estimates for specific features of borderline conditions, particularly at the individual patient level" (125).

Others also documented disagreement on the diagnosis of proliferative or borderline lesions. Rosai invited five pathologists with recognized expertise in the diagnosis of breast lesions to review a set of 17 slides, each of which had a specific proliferative lesion circled for diagnosis (126). All participants reviewed the same slides and recorded one of three diagnoses for each circled lesion: hyperplasia, atypical hyperplasia, or *in situ* carcinoma. No case received a unanimous diagnosis from the five pathologists. At the extremes, one pathologist diagnosed *in situ* carcinoma in nine cases, whereas another pathologist interpreted all circled lesions as hyperplasia or atypical hyperplasia.

Clayton et al. described a study designed to examine the reproducibility of diagnoses in a setting similar to clinical practice because clinical information was provided at the time of review (127). After two pathologists prepared for the study by reviewing a standard set of diagnostic criteria, there was concurrence on the diagnosis of atypical hyperplasia in 8 (31%) of 26 cases that had been assigned this diagnosis by one reviewer. Agreement was reached in 76% of cases of intraductal carcinoma. The authors concluded that "atypical hyperplasias . . . are not sufficiently well defined to be clinically useful. More precise and reproducible criteria for these lesions are needed" (127).

One of the largest and most complex attempts to assess the reproducibility of histologic diagnosis of proliferative lesions and carcinomas was conducted in Italy (128). This project involved 16 pathologists practicing in university or community hospitals in 10 Italian cities. A single set of 82 slides was circulated to the participants "after an initial meeting in which general criteria were discussed." Each case was classified in one of five diagnostic categories using a slight modification of groupings previously outlined at a consensus meeting in the United States (129). Diagnostic categories adopted for the study were (a) non proliferative or proliferative without atypia; (b) ADH or lobular hyperplasia; (c) carcinoma *in situ*, ductal or lobular; and (d) invasive carcinoma. For analysis, comparisons were made with a standard that was defined as the diagnosis most frequently reported by the panel. The overall kappa value for agreement with the consensus diagnosis was 0.72. High levels of agreement were reached for invasive carcinoma (0.89) and benign lesions without atypia (0.77). Agreement was "relatively good" (0.69) for *in situ* carcinoma and "poor" for atypical hyperplasia (0.33).

A study similar to the one reported by Palli et al. was undertaken in the United States by 10 pathologists from academic and community hospitals (130). A set of 31 slides representing ductal, lobular, and papillary lesions was reviewed by each participant. Overall agreement on the diagnosis of carcinoma was recorded for 10 (32.3%) cases (kappa 0.347), on lesion type (ductal, lobular, papillary) in 17 (54.8%) cases (kappa 0.789), and for diagnosis in 8 (25.8%) cases (kappa 0.537). Results among eight pathologists who used standardized diagnostic criteria of Page did not differ substantially from the group as a whole.

Pathologists do not differ appreciably from their clinical colleagues in regard to problems of observer reproducibility. The decision-making process that leads a pathologist to classify specific microscopic findings as hyperplasia, atypical hyperplasia, or carcinoma *in situ* is similar to that of a radiologist interpreting an x-ray or a clinician presented with a patient's clinical findings and diagnostic tests. The diagnosis or therapeutic decision made in these circumstances is a judgment based on experience applied to a specific patient. In the routine diagnostic setting, specific lesions are interpreted in the context of the pathologic changes in all slides from the specimen or specimens. The diagnosis is sometimes influenced by the appearance of associated findings. Consequently, the levels of reproducibility and interobserver disagreement described in various research settings are not directly applicable to routine diagnostic pathology.

- **Pathologists can be "trained" to lower the level of their disagreement on the diagnosis of "borderline" lesions but a substantial level of uncertainty remains.**

Schnitt et al. demonstrated 58% complete agreement among six pathologists who reviewed a series of proliferative ductal lesions after being trained to use agreed-on specified diagnostic criteria (131). Participants prepared for the review by studying a common set of histologic slides and written definitions of proliferative lesions. After this intensive effort, five of the six pathologists classified 16 of 24 specimens as atypical hyperplasia or carcinoma *in situ*. Disagreement between the diagnosis of atypical hyperplasia and carcinoma *in situ* occurred in 33% of the cases.

Dupont et al. examined interobserver reproducibility among pathologists who had worked together in one department "for many years" (121). These investigators examined a common set of slides to standardize diagnostic criteria. The two review pathologists agreed on diagnoses in 63% of cases, achieving a kappa statistic of 0.39, described by these researchers as "suggesting a fair level of agreement beyond that which would be expected by chance alone" (121). Under these nearly ideal circumstances, the two pathologists did not agree on the interpretation of 37% of the specimens.

- **There is no consensus presently on criteria which should be adopted and how they should be applied for the distinctions between hyperplasia, atypical hyperplasia and carcinoma *in situ*.**

The lack of consensus is illustrated not only by the previously described problem of observer reproducibility but also in the definitions used by various investigators. Pathologists have agreed for decades with the concept that atypical proliferative lesions exhibit some but not all features of carcinoma *in situ*, but differences have arisen over specific criteria, particularly with respect to qualitative and quantitative aspects of the lesions (60–62,65,121,132–134). One definition characterizes ADH as having "the cytologic and architectural features of the non-necrotic forms of IDCa [intraductal carcinoma] and the changes may involve two or more ducts or ductules . . . [but] . . . the involved ducts/ductules measure less than 2 mm in aggregated diameter" (65). Others require ". . . at least 2 spaces completely involved . . ." by cells with appropriate cytologic features but do not include a measured dimension in their definition (61). Differences also exist in regard to definitions of structural growth patterns designated *micropapillary* and *cribriform* that are frequently seen in nonnecrotic variants of intraductal carcinoma.

In view of the foregoing problems in defining proliferative lesions and in diagnostic reproducibility, it has been suggested that the effort to distinguish between atypical hyperplasia and *in situ* carcinoma should be abandoned and the lesions amalgamated in a single diagnostic category that could be termed *mammary intraepithelial neoplasia* (MIN) (126). A precedent for this approach can be found in the uterine cervix, where the term *cervical intraepithelial neoplasia* (CIN) describes a spectrum of proliferative changes that include dysplasia and carcinoma *in situ*.

Important clinical differences exist between the cervix and mammary glands that limit applying the concept of intraepithelial neoplasia to lesions of the breast. The cervix is accessible to direct observation and nonexcisional methods of sampling that permit correlation of specific cytologic and histologic features of the lesions with clinical progression. In the breast, the absence of equivalent nonexcisional, nondestructive sampling techniques currently makes it impossible to observe and characterize the evolution of individual proliferative epithelial lesions. Furthermore, there appear to be clinical differences in the breast between lesions classified as proliferative and as *in situ* carcinoma, especially those arising in the ducts. The risk for subsequent invasive carcinoma is nearly equally distributed for the two breasts after biopsy-proven proliferative changes, whereas carcinoma following intraductal carcinoma tends to occur in the ipsilateral breast. The frequency of subsequent invasive carcinoma is considerably higher after intraductal carcinoma than after lesions usually diagnosed as hyperplasia. Presently, it would be prudent to retain the terms *hyperplasia, atypical hyperplasia*, and in situ *carcinoma* because these categories correspond in general terms with the concept that carcinogenesis is a multistage process. Rather than abandoning this concept, we should seek markers that will improve our ability to discriminate among these groups of proliferative change. For additional discussion of this issue, see Chapter 9.

- **The risk for subsequent breast carcinoma attributed to atypical hyperplasia may be exaggerated if this category includes a substantial number of patients with lesions that are regarded as *in situ* carcinoma in some classifications of proliferative lesions.**

In 1978, Page et al. reported finding no significant difference in the risk for subsequent breast carcinoma between biopsies classified as ADH and those described as "ordinary" ductal hyperplasia (62). To improve the discriminating power of their assessment of proliferative duct lesions, these investigators redefined the category of ADH by making ". . . a conscious effort . . . to exclude the complex and more solid examples of florid hyperplasia and recognize as ADH only those cases with features of DCIS" (108). Application of the revised criteria yielded a significantly increased risk associated with lesions that fulfilled the new definition of atypical hyperplasia. The process of refining morphologic definitions

to maximize risk differences also was exemplified by the study of papillary apocrine changes by Page et al. discussed earlier in this chapter (117).

Bodian et al. based their classification of proliferative lesions largely on the criteria of Page et al. but noted that the requirement to classify a lesion as atypical hyperplasia if features of intraductal carcinoma were restricted to a single duct could not be met because cases with single duct involvement had been treated consistently by mastectomy and thus were not available for inclusion in the study (103). They speculated that the primary difference between their results and those of Dupont and Page related to ". . . the threshold at which the pathologists recognized various levels of hyperplasia" and that there might be a lower threshold for diagnosing *in situ* carcinoma at their institution.

- **Morphologic criteria for the diagnosis of "atypia," implying increased breast cancer risk, and *in situ* carcinoma may be improved when it is possible to relate proliferative lesions to specific genetic or biochemical markers.**

As stated by London et al., "The specific characteristics of atypical hyperplasia that confer the highest risk remain unclear" (59). There is currently no laboratory test that serves as a "gold standard" or marker for *in situ* carcinoma of the breast or that distinguishes between hyperplasia and carcinoma *in situ* (135). Some interesting observations involving proliferative lesions have been reported, however, which suggest that significant differences ultimately will be uncovered.

Morphometric analysis of the nuclear cytology of intraductal carcinoma and proliferative duct lesions has revealed modest differences, and this technique may prove to be a useful quantitative method for assessing the risk associated with various types of hyperplasia (136,137). The pattern of nuclear distribution in fenestrated duct hyperplasia and in cribriform intraductal carcinoma was studied by Ozaki and Kondo, who calculated the angle of the longest nuclear diameter to a horizon in histologic sections (138). The nuclear pattern was more often multidirectional in intraductal carcinomas, reflecting "vertical nuclear arrangements toward acinar lumens," whereas hyperplastic lesions featured a more unidirectional nuclear distribution "forming a complex streaming pattern." These results tend to support current histologic criteria for distinguishing between these groups of lesions.

Norris et al. reported that "at best, 69% of well differentiated intraductal carcinomas, could be distinguished from atypical hyperplasia using a combination of DNA content and nuclear perimeter measurements," a level of distinction not deemed to be clinically useful by these investigators (139). A study of cell proliferation in hyperplasias and *in situ* carcinomas using *in vivo* labelling with bromodeoxyuridine (BrdU) found no significant difference between the proliferative fraction of hyperplasia without atypia and atypical hyperplasias (140). BrdU labelling was significantly increased in *in situ* and invasive carcinomas.

When examined by *flow cytometry,* DNA aneuploidy has been found more often in atypical hyperplasia (13%) than in hyperplasia without atypia (7%) (141). Others reported aneuploidy in 30% and 36% of proliferative lesions with atypia and in 30% and 72% of intraductal carcinomas, respectively (136,142). Similar frequencies of aneuploidy in intraductal and *in situ* lobular carcinoma have been detected in tissues studied by fluorescence *in situ* hybridization (143). In the latter study, none of the proliferative lesions exhibited a chromosome gain, and only one example of adenosis had evidence of chromosome 7 monosomy.

Investigations of the role of *oncogenes* in mammary carcinogenesis suggest that activation of *ras* oncogenes occurs at an early stage in the process (144,145). On the other hand, overexpression of the HER-2/*neu* oncogene (HER2) is rarely detected by immunohistochemistry in hyperplastic lesions (146–148). Nonetheless, studies using the MTSVI-7 cell line suggest that overexpression of HER2 can interfere with morphogenesis *in vitro* (149). Cells transfected with HER2 failed to form characteristic aggregates to an extent inversely proportional to expression of HER2, and this loss of organization was associated with reduced expression of $\alpha_2\beta_1$ integrin (150).

Weak immunohistochemical membrane staining for HER2 has been observed in normal breast epithelium, corresponding to the nonamplified level of a single gene copy (151–153). Two case-control studies investigated the relevance of HER2 immunoreactivity in a benign breast biopsy to the risk of subsequent carcinoma, Rohan et al. compared antecedent benign biopsies from 71 women who later developed carcinoma and benign biopsies from 291 women who did not develop carcinoma (154). Membrane staining for HER2 was detected in 3 of 71 (4.2%) benign biopsies from study patients and in 14 of 291 (4.7%) control biopsies. The odds ratio (OR) for subsequent carcinoma among women with HER2 detected by immunohistochemistry in a benign breast biopsy was 0.65 (95% CI = 0.27–1.53), indicating no increased risk.

A second case-control study by Stark et al. used immunohistochemistry and analyzed DNA extracted from archival tissues for HER2 amplification (155). None of the benign tissue samples from cases (women who later developed carcinoma) and from controls (no subsequent carcinoma) displayed membrane immunoreactivity for HER2 in ≥10% of cells. None of the 7 of 154 (4.5%) control specimens with HER2 amplification detected by the polymerase chain reaction (PCR) of DNA samples had membrane staining. Among the remaining 147 samples without HER2 amplification, 6 had immunostaining of fewer than 10% of cells, representing 3.9% of the entire control group. HER2 was amplified in 13 of 147 (9.5%) benign samples from study patients who later developed carcinoma, but none of these specimens exhibited membrane reactivity for HER2. Weak immunostaining (<10% of cells) was detected in four samples without amplified HER2 from study patients, representing 2.8% of the entire study group. In this study, HER2 amplification, but not immunohistochemical detection, in a benign breast biopsy was associated with an increased risk of breast carcinoma (OR = 2.2; 95% CI = 0.9–5.8). Among women who had HER2 amplification and proliferative benign changes, typical or atypical, the risk was substantially greater (OR = 7.2; 95% CI = 0.9–60.8). Immunoreactivity for HER2 was present in 30% of subsequent carcinomas. These data suggest that HER2 amplification in benign breast tissue may be a marker of risk for subsequent carcinoma and that this effect may interact with the type of benign alteration that is present.

Nuclear *p53 expression* was detected in 12% of 109 *in situ* ductal carcinomas but not in any of 89 samples of benign or hyperplastic tissue studied by Eriksson et al. (141). Other investigators also failed to detect p53 expression in normal proliferative epithelium in tissue sections (156–160) or in cytologic specimens (161). Mommers et al. found p53 nuclear reactivity in 10 of 124 (8%) examples of ductal hyperplasia, with no appreciable difference in the frequency of staining between mild, moderate, and florid lesions (162). One extensive study of biopsies revealed nuclear staining in 16% of 248 benign specimens (163). The highest frequency of reactivity was observed in fibroadenomas (30%), whereas only 8% of lesions characterized as fibrocystic disease were positive. The latter specimens were not subclassified with regard to the types of proliferative changes present. Follow-up revealed subsequent carcinoma in 12% of patients with a p53-positive biopsy and in 7% of p53-negative cases, a difference that was not statistically significant. In another study, the expression of p53 in breast carcinomas did not appear to be associated with antecedent benign breast disease or a family history of breast carcinoma (164).

Data linking p53 mutations and overexpression to increased breast carcinoma risk have come from several sources. A case-control study conducted by Rohan et al. used immunohistochemistry to detect p53 overexpression in benign biopsies from 71 study women who later developed breast carcinoma and 288 controls who did not develop carcinoma subsequently (154). Immunoreactivity for p53 was present in 10 (14%) of the study samples and in 19 (6.6%) of control samples. The presence of p53 immunoreactivity in an antecedent breast biopsy was associated with an increased risk for subsequent carcinoma (OR = 2.55; 95% CI = 1.01–6.40). The risk was higher when a greater proportion of cells was positive (<10% versus >10%) and when p53 reactivity coexisted with typical and atypical hyperplasia (OR = 4.62; 95% CI = 1.02–20.94). No consistent relationship was found between p53 expression in a benign biopsy and in a subsequent carcinoma. Both were negative in 66.7% of cases, and both were positive in 9.8%. A p53-negative benign specimen occurred in 19.6% of cases with a p53-positive carcinoma; the reverse relationship was observed in 3.9%.

Kamel et al. used FNA to obtain cytologic specimens for p53 immunostaining from women at high risk of developing carcinoma (165). The cohort included women with a family history of breast carcinoma, prior contralateral carcinoma, or a prior biopsy showing atypical hyperplasia or carcinoma *in situ*. Nuclear p53 reactivity was present in 29% of the patients and was highly correlated with the presence of atypical hyperplasia. Five of the seven women who were later found to have intraductal or invasive carcinoma during follow-up had p53-positive cells in their FNA specimens. Only one of the subsequent carcinomas had a p53 mutation when microdissected tumor samples were studied by PCR.

The foregoing studies indicate that p53 accumulation detected by immunohistochemistry in benign breast tissue is associated with an increased risk for subsequent carcinoma and that this effect interacts with the presence of hyperplasia to increase the risk. The p53 status of an antecedent benign breast biopsy is predictive of p53 expression in about 75% of subsequent carcinomas. Mutation of the p53 gene occurs with greater frequency in breast carcinomas from BRCA1 carriers than in tumors from noncarriers (166).

The *bcl*-2 gene encodes a protein that inhibits apoptosis and participates in the control of cell proliferation. When studied by immunohistochemistry, *bcl*-2 is found in virtually all normal ductal epithelial cells and ductal hyperplasias (158,159,162). One study reported no difference in the intensity of reactivity between normal and hyperplastic lesions (typical and atypical), but others reported reduced staining in 16% of hyperplastic foci, with differences in intensity not related to the degree of hyperplasia (mild, moderate, florid). Among intraductal carcinomas, *bcl*-2 reactivity was related to the degree of differentiation, being highest in low-grade foci (158) and noncomedo lesions (159) and substantially lower in comedo intraductal carcinoma (158,159). These observations suggest that loss of *bcl*-2 reactivity is not an early event in the evolution of proliferative lesions and the development of intraductal carcinoma. The role of other genes such as *Fas*, which is involved in promoting apoptosis (167) and survivin, an inhibitor of apoptosis (168), in proliferative breast lesions has received little attention.

Several genes that participate in the regulation of other aspects of the cell cycle also have been investigated in proliferative breast lesions. *Cyclin D1* is involved in controlling progression from G1 into the S-phase. Cells that overexpress cyclin D1 show reduced cyclin from G1 to G0. Amplification of cyclin D1 and overexpression of the protein were investigated by differential PCR of microdissected specimens and immunohistochemistry in benign proliferative lesions and carcinoma by Zhu et al. (169). Cyclin D1 gene amplification was present in 15% of normal tissues, 19% with epithelial hyperplasia without atypia, 27% with ADH and 35% with intraductal carcinoma. The corresponding frequencies of overexpression detected by immunohistochemistry were 13%, 13%, 57%, and 50%. These findings suggest that cyclin D1 expression can be altered in the absence of a histologically detectable abnormality and that the frequency of altered cyclin D1 expression as well as amplification tends to increase with the severity of the proliferative abnormality.

*In situ* hybridization detected increased cyclin D1 mRNA expression in the same proportion (18%) of proliferative le-

sions without and with atypia. A significantly higher frequency of overexpression was found in intraductal carcinomas; 76% in low-grade lesions and 87% in high-grade lesions (170). A study of cyclin D1 overexpression detected by immunohistochemistry reported an overall frequency of 6%, with no significant difference between mild, moderate, and florid hyperplasia (162). These data appear to indicate a more abrupt increase in cyclin D1 overexpression in the transition from hyperplasia to intraductal carcinoma than the foregoing study of Zhu et al. Overall, these investigations demonstrated that cyclin D1 amplification and overexpression are associated more strongly with intraductal carcinoma than with hyperplasia.

*Telomerase,* an enzyme responsible for maintaining the telomere segments at the ends of chromosomes, is present in extremely low levels in normal tissues. Telomerase activity is significantly increased in a variety of carcinomas, including intraductal and invasive duct carcinomas, but only very rarely in normal tissue (171,172). Telomerase activation is associated with increased cellular proliferation (173), but one study did not find a significant correlation with Ki67 immunoreactivity in breast carcinoma (171). The relevance of telomerase activation to proliferative breast lesions and breast cancer risk remains to be determined.

The *BRCA1 gene* has a tumor suppressor function mediated through the BRCA1 protein, a negative regulator of the cell cycle. Immunolocalization in nuclei is detected when a BRCA1-specific antibody is used. Almost all nuclei in normal tissue display immunoreactivity (174). Among sporadic carcinomas examined in one study, about 75% displayed nuclear immunoreactivity, and staining was absent from about 20% of tumors (174). Loss of BRCA1 reactivity was correlated significantly with high-grade carcinoma but not with other prognostic markers. The relationship of altered BRCA1 immunoexpression to BRCA1 mutation status as well as to the phenotype of proliferative lesions and breast carcinoma risk remains to be determined.

*Growth factors* are a group of substances produced locally in tissues that modulate cellular development and may contribute to carcinogenesis. *Epidermal growth factor* (EGF) is a protein involved in the proliferation of normal and neoplastic cells in the breast. The activity of EGF is induced by its interaction with a transmembrane receptor, the *epidermal growth factor receptor*, or EGF-R. Little information is available about expression of EGF-R in proliferative breast lesions. EGF-R is present in all benign tissue, although when measured biochemically, the level of expression appears to be lower than in EGF-R-positive breast carcinomas (175). Specimens classified as benign or fibrocystic have slightly higher EGF-R levels than samples of fat and fibrous tissue. Immunohistochemical studies also have detected fairly widespread EGF-R expression in benign or normal breast tissue samples (176,177). EGF-R positivity is detected in about 45% of breast carcinomas studied by various methods (178). A noteworthy difference in expression between carcinomas and noncarcinomatous tissues exists in relation to estrogen receptor (ER). EGF-R expression in carcinomas is inversely related to ER expression, being significantly more frequent in ER-negative tumors (175,176,179,180). On the other hand, EGF-R expression is directly related to ER in noncarcinomatous breast samples (175,178,179). The mechanisms for these differences in expression and their relationship to proliferative breast disease have not been explored adequately.

*Insulin-like growth factors* (IGFs) are potent mitogens known to influence the proliferation of normal and transformed cells. The action of IGFs is mediated through binding to an *insulin-like growth factor receptor* (IGF-R) localized to the cell membrane. The adult form, IGF-I, reportedly was found in the stroma associated with normal or noncarcinomatous proliferative breast tissue (181). Stromal cells associated with carcinoma cells, benign epithelial cells, and carcinoma cells did not express IGF-I. IGF-II, a form of IGF associated with immature fetal cells was localized to the stroma around carcinoma cells and has been detected in breast carcinomas (181,182). These observations provide an illustration of epithelial-stromal interaction that may be involved in paracrine regulation of cell growth in proliferative as well as carcinomatous breast lesions.

Nuclear immunoreactivity for *estrogen and progesterone receptors* (ERs and PRs) can be found in nonneoplastic breast tissue. Specific types of benign lesions do not differ significantly in the frequency of positivity (183). Khan et al. compared the immunohistochemical expression of ERs and PRs in benign breast tissue from women with and without documented breast carcinoma (184). There was a significant association between ER positivity in the benign epithelium (not further classified with respect to proliferative activity) and the presence of breast carcinoma. Within the various age groups analyzed, the strongest association with concurrent carcinoma was observed in patients with ER-positive, PR-negative benign epithelium.

Estrogen receptors play a critical role in modulating the effect of estrogen on breast epithelial development and growth. This is manifested clinically in part by the observed association between the use of hormone-replacement therapy (HRT) and the risk of benign breast disease, which had a relative risk of 1.70 (95% CI = 1.06–2.72) after 8 years of use in one study (185). Carcinomas that arise in women using HRT tend to be smaller, better differentiated, and less proliferative than tumors that arise in nonusers of HRT (186). These differences are attributable to the association of these prognostic factors with ER-positive but not with ER-negative tumors. Reduced proliferation was observed predominantly in tumors from patients receiving HRT at the time of diagnosis. This finding is consistent with the observation that patients with a breast carcinoma who have used HRT had reduced mortality, with the greatest reduction among those women under treatment at the time of diagnosis (187).

*pS2 protein,* an estrogen-inducible gene product, has been associated with ER-positive mammary carcinomas (188,189). Nuclear expression of pS2, detected by immunohistochemistry, has been found in about 65% of intraductal carcinomas, with no appreciable differences among various histologic subtypes (190). There was a stronger correlation of pS2 expression with immunoreactivity for PR than for ER in intraductal carcinomas. pS2 immunoreactivity also was encountered in a variety of benign proliferative lesions, with 50% exhibiting some staining. This staining was typically weak and limited to relatively few cells compared with the more extensive staining found in intraductal carcinomas. Scattered pS2-positive nuclei also were found in normal lobular epithelial cells. The relationships of pS2 protein expression in benign breast tissue and breast carcinoma risk has not been determined.

Changes in *cell polarity* are found histologically in proliferative breast lesions as well as in mammary carcinomas. Hyperplasia is characterized by an increased number of cells that fill part or all of duct or lobular gland lumens. Common abnormal patterns of cellular distribution in hyperplastic lesions include uneven positioning of cells with respect to the basement membrane, accumulation of cells in a multilayered fashion, polarization of cells around newly formed secondary lumens, and arrays of cells described as "swirling" or "streaming."

Recent studies of *proteins associated with cell adhesion and polarity* uncovered alterations in these substances that may prove to be markers for classifying proliferative changes and assessing risks for progression to carcinoma (191). Cell surface receptors for laminin are important nonintegrin proteins for adhesion to laminin, a component of the basement membrane (192). They participate in the process whereby epithelial cells are organized around the normal duct lumen. Focal loss of laminin has been observed in the basement membrane region of intraductal carcinomas (193). Myoepithelial cells appear to exert a tumor suppressor effect by contributing to basement membrane integrity (194) as well as through paracrine factors, which inhibit tumor invasion, metastasis, and possibly progression of precancerous epithelial alteration (195).

The apical and basolateral membrane regions of individual cells have distinctive biochemical and physiologic properties (196). The presence and distribution of these membrane domains are altered in proliferative lesions. Most hyperplastic cells accumulate in and tend to fill glandular lumens, away from the basement membrane. Apical membrane differentiation may be maintained around secondary lumens in hyperplastic epithelium at the surface of the hyperplastic proliferation. A substantial number of cells within the solid portions of proliferative foci, however, have no exposure to lumens or to the basement membrane.

*Fodrin* is a structural protein involved in the maintenance of cell polarity. It has been localized to basolateral cell membranes in normal terminal and intralobular ducts and in lesions such as sclerosing adenosis that are characterized by proliferation of glands with little increase in cell numbers within individual glands. In hyperplastic epithelium, which has increased cell numbers, fodrin is found around the entire cell membrane (197). Circumferential staining of the cell membrane has been observed in mammary and colonic carcinomas (197,198).

*Integrins* are a family of complex proteins composed of α and β subunits that are involved in binding to extracellular matrix and proteins in cell to cell adhesion. Their expression in various normal tissues and neoplasms is complex (199). Data presently available suggest that an understanding of the distribution of integrins may prove useful in distinguishing between proliferative lesions and carcinoma. Integrin expression in fibroadenomas is similar to levels in normal breast tissue, whereas expression is decreased in carcinomas of the breast (200–202). Zutter et al. observed that the level of integrin mRNA expression detected by *in situ* hybridization was correlated to the degree of differentiation, being lowest in poorly differentiated carcinomas and intermediate in well to moderately differentiated tumors (202). Other researchers also reported diminished expression of α4 and β6 subunits in carcinomas and in benign breast tissue from patients with carcinoma (203). The specimens examined did not include examples of "florid epithelial hyperplasia," but these investigators suggested that loss of α4β6 expression might be a marker of premalignant change (203). Down-regulation of integrin expression may be related in part to a loss of contact with basement membranes.

The ability of proliferative epithelial cells to produce *angiogenesis factor* and to induce *angiogenesis* in surrounding tissue has been demonstrated in hyperplastic mammary lesions as well as in established carcinomas (204,205). Bose et al. found that some types of intraductal carcinoma are characterized by a marked increase in the amount of periductal angiogenesis when compared to normal ducts (206). Heffelfinger et al. reported that periductal vascularity in normal tissue was greater in breasts with invasive carcinoma than in breasts lacking invasive carcinoma (207). Vascularity was greater around proliferative foci than in normal tissue, and the degree of vascularity increased in proportion to the severity of the lesion (hyperplasia, atypical hyperplasia, or *in situ* carcinoma). These observations suggest that proliferative lesions are capable of inducing angiogenesis and that angiogenesis is not exclusively associated with carcinoma. The extent to which the capacity to produce angiogenesis factor correlates with the morphologic classification of proliferative breast lesions and *in situ* carcinoma remains to be determined.

Evidence also exists that alterations in *stromal proteins* may accompany proliferative changes in the breast and carcinomatous transformation. This is illustrated by investigations of tenascin, a matrix glycoprotein. Some forms of tenascin act as antiadhesive molecules. Stromal cells produce predominantly two isoforms of tenascin of low (190 kDa) and high (330 kDa) molecular weight (208). Antiadhesive properties reside largely in the latter isoform, the predominant type found in the activated stroma in some fibroadenomas, cystosarcomas, and invasive carcinomas (208,209). Stroma associated with most benign lesions and atypical hyperplasias expresses mainly the 190-kDa form. Jones et al. reported finding an inverse relationship between integrin and tenasin expression in breast carcinomas (203). Differences in the distribution of fibronectins also have been observed when stroma from normal and hyperplastic breast was compared with stroma in carcinomas (210). Specific oncofetal isoforms associated with carcinomas were not found in benign specimens, an observation suggesting that the expression of these markers is associated with carcinomatous transformation.

Numerous studies examined the expression of different *cytokeratins* in proliferative breast lesions and in breast carcinomas. Normal luminal epithelial cells are reactive with antibodies directed against keratins 7, 8, 18, and 19 (211–213). These antibodies do not stain myoepithelial cells, which are immunoreactive with markers of keratins 5/14 (211,212). As might be expected, tubular carcinoma is immunoreactive with antibodies to keratins 18 and 19 but not to the 5/14 keratin complex, whereas both antibodies are reactive in sclerosing adenosis (211). Hyperplastic proliferative ductal lesions retain a myoepithelial component and are immunoreactive with both types of antibody, whereas staining in intraductal carcinomas is limited almost entirely to antibodies against keratins 8, 18, and 19 (211). Moinfar et al. studied the distribution of reactivity for 34BE12 (K903), an antibody against high-molecular-weight cytokeratins 1, 5, 10, and 14, in normal breast epithelium, proliferative lesions, and intraductal carcinoma (214). Reactivity for 34BE12 was stronger and present in a greater proportion of myoepithelial than epithelial cells in normal epithelium. A similar pattern of staining was observed in hyperplasias, whereas atypical hyperplasia and intraductal carcinoma were characterized by complete or nearly complete absence of epithelial 34BE12 reactivity.

The similarity of cytokeratin staining patterns in lesions classified as atypical duct hyperplasia and as intraductal carcinoma by Moinfar et al. may be largely the result of criteria for defining these groups of lesions rather than a manifestation of intrinsic biological characteristics. Lesions were classified as atypical intraductal proliferations if "they had the cytologic appearances of low-grade DCIS without recognizable architectural features of DCIS or both cytologic and architectural features suggestive of, but not sufficient for, a diagnosis of DCIS, with partial involvement of one or more ducts. . . . There were cases with atypical intraductal proliferations qualitatively identical to an intraductal carcinoma, quantitatively less than 2 mm in aggregate cross-sectional diameter and therefore insufficient to warrant a diagnosis of carcinoma *in situ*." By definition, the category of ADH differed from intraductal carcinoma not so much because of structural phenotypic differences in the appearance of proliferative foci, but largely as a result of quantitative criteria. In view of the clonal nature of carcinoma, quantitative criteria for distinguishing carcinoma from hyperplasia are not biologically meaningful, although lesion size may be relevant clinically to diagnosis and planning treatment. Consequently, results from studies such as those of Moinfar et al. (214) and Page et al. (117) may be misleading by suggesting that there is little difference between atypical hyperplasia and low-grade intraductal carcinoma and proposing that the two groups be merged. By including small intraductal carcinomas among atypical hyperplasias, these investigators contaminate the latter group and thereby obscure any biological differences that might exist. Applying biomarkers in this situation, as for example by Moinfar et al., inevitably shows little difference in patterns of reactivity between the "atypical hyperplasia" and intraductal carcinoma groups because the former category includes cases the authors themselves stated have qualitative features of carcinoma. This approach to the study of "precancerous" breast lesions is more likely to fulfill preconceived concepts about the phenotypic characterization of these abnormalities than to contribute to a clinically relevant understanding of their pathobiology.

- **As suggested in the introduction to this chapter, the molecular characterization of mammary epithelium may prove to be as important as, or more significant than, the histologic phenotype. Under these circumstances, much of the current controversy over the classification of proliferative lesions will have less relevance to clinical practice. This will be especially true if important molecular changes associated with transformation can be present in cells that do not have an abnormal histologic phenotype and if progression to carcinoma can occur in such cells with at most a transient phase corresponding to changes now referred to as hyperplasia.**

It is clear that many elements are involved in the conundrum that lies at the heart of the process of neoplastic transformation. Evidence to date summarized in this chapter suggests that it is highly unlikely that a single key marker will emerge as the gold standard for assessing the risk of carcinoma associated with proliferative lesions. Instead, the significant information will come from a panel of indicators assayed in tissues, blood, or both. The availability of increasingly effective chemoprevention agents as an alternative to surgery combined with data from future studies of cancer risk related to biomarkers probably will shift the focus of risk assessment away from histopathology. Ultimately, such developments are essential if chemoprevention is to be most widely effective because relatively few women undergo biopsies that yield "benign" tissue that can be used for microscopic risk assessment. The development of reliable biomarkers of risk is likely to be more successful if it is based on the clinical detection of breast carcinoma rather than through correlations with intermediate markers of risk such a histologic categories of proliferative lesions. This is because most current criteria for stratifying these histologic changes are not strictly morphologic and also include factors relevant to making therapeutic decisions such as lesion size.

## REFERENCES

1. Friedman LS, Ostermeyer EA, Szabo CI, et al. Confirmation of BRCA1 by analysis of germline mutations linked to breast and ovarian cancer in ten families. *Nat Genet* 1994;8:399–404.
2. King M-C. Linkage of early-onset familial breast cancer to chromosome 17q21. *Science* 1990;250:1684–1689.
3. Miki Y, Swensen J, Shattuck-Eidens D, et al. A strong candidate for the breast and ovarian cancer susceptibility gene BRCA1. *Science* 1994;266:66–71.
4. Wooster R, Bignell G, Lancaster J, et al. Identification of the breast cancer susceptibility gene BRCA2. *Nature* 1995;378:789–792.
5. Couch FJ, Weber BL. Mutations and polymorphisms in the familial early-onset breast cancer (BRCA1) gene: Breast Cancer Information Core. *Hum Mutat* 1996;8:8–18.
6. Tavtigian SV, Simard J, Rommens J, et al. The complete BRCA2 gene and mutations in chromosome 13q-linked kindreds. *Nat Genet* 1996;12:333–337.
7. Struewing JP, Brody LC, Erdos MR, et al. Detection of eight BRCA1 mutations in 10 breast/ovarian cancer families, including 1 family with male breast cancer. *Am J Hum Genet* 1995;57:1–7.
8. Struewing JP, Hartge P, Wacholder S, et al. The risk of cancer associated with specific mutations of BRCA1 and BRCA2 among Ashkenazi Jews. *N Engl J Med* 1997;336:1401–1408.
9. Ford D, Easton DF, Stratton M, et al. Genetic heterogeneity and penetrance analysis of the BRCA1 and BRCA2 genes in breast cancer families. The Breast Cancer Linkage Consortium. *Am J Hum Genet* 1998;62:676–689.
10. Thorlacius S, Struewing JP, Hartge P, et al. Population-based study of risk of breast cancer in carriers of BRCA2 mutation. *Lancet* 1998;352:1337–1339.
11. Easton DF, Bishop DT, Ford D, et al. Genetic linkage analysis in familial breast and ovarian cancer: results from 214 families. The Breast Cancer Linkage Consortium. *Am J Hum Genet* 1993;52:678–701.
12. Easton DF, Ford D, Bishop DT. Breast and ovarian cancer incidence in BRCA1-mutation carriers: Breast Cancer Linkage Consortium. *Am J Hum Genet* 1995;56:265–271.
13. Ford D, Easton DF, Bishop DT, et al. Risks of cancer in BRCA1-mutation carriers. Breast Cancer Linkage Consortium. *Lancet* 1994;343:692–695.
14. Rebbeck TR, Kantoff PW, Krithivas K, et al. Modification of BRCA1-associated breast cancer risk by the polymorphic androgen-receptor CAG repeat. *Am J Hum Genet* 1999;64:1371–1377.
15. Andrieu N, Smith T, Duffy S, et al. The effects of interaction between familial and reproductive factors on breast cancer risk: a combined analysis of seven case-control studies. *Br J Cancer* 1998;77:1525–1536.
16. Narod SA, Goldgar D, Cannon-Albright L, et al. Risk modifiers in carriers of BRCA1 mutations. *Int J Cancer* 1995;64:394–398.
17. Rebbeck TR, Blackwood MA, Walker AH, et al. Association of breast cancer incidence with NAT2 genotype and smoking in BRCA1 variant carriers. *Am J Hum Genet* 1998;61:A46.
18. Brunet JS, Ghadirian P, Rebbeck TR, et al. Effect of smoking on breast cancer in carriers of mutant BRCA1 or BRCA2 genes. *J Natl Cancer Inst* 1998;90:761–766.
19. Ursin G, Henderson BE, Haile RW, et al. Does oral contraceptive use increase the risk of breast cancer in women with BRCA1/BRCA2 mutations more than in other women? *Cancer Res* 1997;57:3678–3681.
20. Rebbeck TR. Inherited genetic predisposition in breast cancer: a population-based perspective. *Cancer* 1999;86:1673–1681.
21. Grade K, Hoffken K, Kath R, et al. BRCA1 mutations and phenotype. *J Cancer Res Clin Oncol* 1997;123:69–70.
22. Gayther SA, Mangion J, Russell P, et al. Variation of risks of breast and ovarian cancer associated with different germline mutations of the BRCA2 gene. *Nat Genet* 1997;15:103–105.
23. Couch FJ, De Shano ML, Blackwood MA, et al. BRCA1 mutations in women attending clinics that evaluate the risk of breast cancer. *N Engl J Med* 1997;336:1409–1415.
24. Noguchi S, Kasugai T, Miki Y, et al. Clinicopathologic analysis of BRCA1- or BRCA2-associated hereditary breast carcinoma in Japanese women. *Cancer* 1999;85:2200–2205.
25. Marcus JN, Watson P, Page DL, et al. BRCA2 hereditary breast cancer pathophenotype. *Breast Cancer Res Treat* 1997;44:275–277.
26. Marcus JN, Watson P, Page DL, et al. Hereditary breast cancer: patho-

biology, prognosis, and BRCA1 and BRCA2 gene linkage. *Cancer* 1996;77:697–709.

27. Verhoog LC, Brekelmans CT, Seynaeve C, et al. Survival and tumour characteristics of breast-cancer patients with germline mutations of BRCA1. *Lancet* 1998;351:316–321.

28. Johannsson OT, Idvall I, Anderson C, et al. Tumour biological features of BRCA1-induced breast and ovarian cancer. *Eur J Cancer* 1997;33:362–371.

29. Crook T, Crossland S, Crompton MR, et al. p53 mutations in BRCA1-associated familial breast cancer. *Lancet* 1997;350:638–639.

30. Li FP, Fraumeni JFJ, Mulvihill JJ, et al. A cancer family syndrome in twenty-four kindreds. *Cancer Res* 1988;48:5358–5362.

31. Birch JM, Hartley AL, Ticker KJ, et al. Prevalence and diversity of constitutional mutations in the p53 gene among 21 Li-Fraumeni families. *Cancer Res* 1994;54:1298–1304.

32. Li J, Yen C, Liaw D, et al. PTEN, a putative protein tyrosine phosphatase gene mutated in human brain, breast, and prostate cancer. *Science* 1997;275:1943–1947.

33. Jenne DE, Reimann H, Nezu J, et al. Peutz-Jeghers syndrome is caused by mutations in a novel serine threonine kinase. *Nat Genet* 1998;18:38–43.

34. Helzlsouer KJ, Selmin O, Huang HY, et al. Association between glutathione S-transferase M1, P1, and T1 genetic polymorphisms and development of breast cancer. *J Natl Cancer Inst* 1998;90:512–518.

35. Maugard CM, Charrier J, Bignon YJ. Allelic deletion at glutathione S-transferase M1 locus and its association with breast cancer susceptibility. *Chem Biol Interact* 1998;111–112:365–375.

36. Rebbeck TR, Kantoff PW, Krithivas K, et al. Modification of breast cancer risk in BRCA1 mutation carriers by the AIB1 gene. *Proc Am Assoc Cancer Res* 1999;40:194.

37. Seery LT, Knowlden JM, Gee JM, et al. BRCA1 expression levels predict distant metastasis of sporadic breast cancers. *Int J Cancer* 1999;84:258–262.

38. Lee JS, Wacholder S, Struewing JP, et al. Survival after breast cancer in Ashkenazi Jewish BRCA1 and BRCA2 mutation carriers. *J Natl Cancer Inst* 1999;91:259–263.

39. Verhoog LC, Brekelmans CT, Seynaeve C, et al. Survival in hereditary breast cancer associated with germline mutations of BRCA2. *J Clin Oncol* 1999;17:3396–3402.

40. Foulkes WD, Wong N, Brunet JS, et al. Germ-line BRCA1 mutation is an adverse prognostic factor in Ashkenazi Jewish women with breast cancer. *Clin Cancer Res* 1997;3:2465–2469.

41. Robson M, Levin D, Federici M, et al. Breast conservation therapy for invasive breast cancer in Ashkenazi women with BRCA gene founder mutations. *J Natl Cancer Inst* 1999;91:2112–2117.

42. Hughes KS, Papa MZ, Whitney T, et al. Prophylactic mastectomy and inherited predisposition to breast carcinoma. *Cancer* 1999; 86:1682–1696.

43. Schrag D, Kuntz KM, Garber JE, et al. Decision analysis—effects of prophylactic mastectomy and oophorectomy on life expectancy among women with BRCA1 or BRCA2 mutations. *N Engl J Med* 1997;336:1465–1471.

44. Fisher B, Costantino JP, Wickerham DL, et al. Tamoxifen for prevention of breast cancer: report of the National Surgical Adjuvant Breast and Bowel Project P-1 Study. *J Natl Cancer Inst* 1998;90:1371–1388.

45. Dalberg K, Johansson H, Johansson U, et al. A randomized trial of long term adjuvant tamoxifen plus postoperative radiation therapy versus radiation therapy alone for patients with early stage breast carcinoma treated with breast-conserving surgery: Stockholm Breast Cancer Study Group. *Cancer* 1998;82:2204–2211.

46. Ragaz J, Coldman A. Survival impact of adjuvant tamoxifen on competing causes of mortality in breast cancer survivors, with analysis of mortality from contralateral breast cancer, cardiovascular events, endometrial cancer, and thromboembolic episodes. *J Clin Oncol* 1998;16:2018–2024.

47. Tockman MS. Monoclonal antibody detection of premalignant lesions of the lung. In: Fortner JG, Sharp PA, eds. *Accomplishments in cancer research*. Philadelphia: Lippincott-Raven Publishers, 1995:169–177.

48. Tockman MS, Gupta PK, Pressman NJ, et al. Cytometric validation of immunocytochemical observations in developing lung cancer. *Diagn Cytopathol* 1993;9:615–622.

49. Slaughter DP, Southwick HW, Smejkal W. "Field cancerization" in oral stratified squamous epithelium. *Cancer* 1953;6:963–968.

50. Deng G, Lu Y, Zlotnikov G, et al. Loss of heterozygosity in normal tissue adjacent to breast carcinomas. *Science* 1996;274:2057–2059.

51. Tsai YC, Lu Y, Nichols PW, et al. Contiguous patches of normal human mammary epithelium derived from a single stem cell: implications for breast carcinogenesis. *Cancer Res* 1996;56:402–404.

52. Diallo R, Schafer K-L, Poremba C, et al. Monoclonality in normal epithelium, hyperplastic and neoplastic lesions of the breast. *Mod Pathol* 2000;13:20A.

53. Larson PS, de las Morenas A, Cupples LA, et al. Genetically abnormal clones in histologically normal breast tissue. *Am J Pathol* 1998;152:1591–1598.

54. Lakhani SR, Chaggar R, Davies S, et al. Genetic alterations in 'normal' luminal and myoepithelial cells of the breast. *J Pathol* 1999;189:496–503.

55. Dawson PJ, Maloney T, Gimotty P, et al. Bilateral breast cancer: one disease or two? *Breast Cancer Res Treat* 1991;19:233–244.

56. Noguchi S, Motomura K, Inaji H, et al. Differentiation of primary and secondary breast cancer with clonal analysis. *Surgery* 1994; 115:458–462.

57. Shibata A, Tsai YC, Press MF, et al. Clonal analysis of bilateral breast cancer. *Clin Cancer Res* 1996;2:743–748.

58. Carter CL, Corle DK, Micozzi MS, et al. A prospective study of the development of breast cancer in 16,692 women with benign breast disease. *Am J Epidemiol* 1988;128:467–477.

59. London SJ, Connolly JL, Schnitt SJ, et al. A prospective study of benign breast disease and the risk of breast cancer. *JAMA* 1992; 267:941–944.

60. McDivitt RW, Stevens JA, Lee NC, et al., and the Cancer and Steroid Hormone Study Group. Histologic types of benign breast disease and the risk for breast cancer. *Cancer* 1992;69:1408–1414.

61. Page DL, DuPont WD, Rogers LW, et al. Atypical hyperplastic lesions of the female breast. A long-term follow-up study. *Cancer* 1985;55:2698–2708.

62. Page DL, Van der Zwaag R, Rogers LW, et al. Relation between component parts of fibrocystic disease complex and breast cancer. *J Natl Cancer Inst* 1978;61:1055–1063.

63. Krieger N, Hiatt RA. Risk of breast cancer after benign breast diseases. Variation by histologic type, degree of atypia, age at biopsy, and length of follow-up. *Am J Epidemiol* 1992;135:619–631.

64. Ris H-B, Niederer U, Stirremann H, et al. Long-term follow-up of patients with biopsy-proven benign breast disease. *Ann Surg* 1988;207:404–408.

65. Tavassoli FA, Norris HJ. A comparison of the results of long-term follow-up for atypical intraductal hyperplasia and intraductal hyperplasia of the breast. *Cancer* 1990;65:518–529.

66. Nomura A, Comstock GW, Tonascia JA. Epidemiologic characteristics of benign breast disease. *Am J Epidemiol* 1977;105:505–512.

67. Parazzini F, La Vecchia C, Franceschi S, et al. Risk factors for pathologically confirmed benign breast disease. *Am J Epidemiol* 1984;120:115–122.

68. Sartwell PE, Arthes FG, Tonascia JA. Benign and malignant breast tumours. Epidemiological similarities. *Int J Epidemiol* 1978;7:217–221.

69. La Vecchia C, Parazzini F, Franceschi S, et al. Risk factors for benign breast disease and their relation with breast cancer risk. Pooled information from epidemiologic studies. *Tumori* 1985;71:167–178.

70. Hislop TG, Band PR, Deschamps M, et al. Diet and histologic types of benign breast disease defined by subsequent risk of breast cancer. *Am J Epidemiol* 1990;131:263–270.

71. Boyle CA, Berkowitz GS, LiVolsi VA, et al. Caffeine consumption and fibrocystic breast disease: a case-control epidemiologic study. *J Natl Cancer Inst* 1984;72:1015–1019.

72. Baghurst PA, Rohan TE. Dietary fiber and risk of benign proliferative epithelial disorders of the breast. *Int J Cancer* 1995;63:481–485.

73. Vobecky J, Simard A, Vobecky JS, et al. Nutritional profile of women with fibrocystic breast disease. *Int J Epidemiol* 1993;22:989–999.

74. Brisson J, Verreault R, Morrison AS, et al. Diet, mammographic features of breast tissue, and breast cancer risk. *Am J Epidemiol* 1989;130:14–24.

75. Kelsey JL, Lindfors KK, White C. A case-control study of the epidemiology of benign breast diseases with reference to oral contraceptive use. *Int J Epidemiol* 1974;3:333–340.

76. Page DL, Dupont WD. Proliferative breast disease: diagnosis and implications. *Science* 1991;253:915–916.

77. Cole P, Elwood JM, Kaplan SD. Incidence rates and risk factors of benign breast neoplasms. *Am J Epidemiol* 1978;108:112–120.

78. Mackenzie I. Breast cancer following multiple fluoroscopies. *Br J Cancer* 1965;19:1–8.

79. Mettler Jr FA, Hempelmann LH, Dutton AM, et al. Breast neoplasms in women treated with x rays for acute postpartum mastitis: a pilot study. *J Natl Cancer Inst* 1969;43:803–811.

80. Wanebo CK, Johnson KG, Sato K, et al. Breast cancer after exposure to the atomic bombings of Hiroshima and Nagasaki. *N Engl J Med* 1968;279:667–671.

81. Tokunaga M, Land CE, Aoki Y, et al. Proliferative and nonproliferative breast disease in atomic bomb survivors: results of a histopathologic review of autopsy breast tissue. *Cancer* 1993;72:1657–1665.

82. Parker SH, Burbank F, Jackman RJ, et al. Percutaneous large-core breast biopsy: a multi-institutional study. *Radiology* 1994;193:359–364.

83. Liberman L, Cohen MA, Abramson AF, et al. Atypical ductal hyperplasia diagnosed at stereotaxic core biopsy of breast lesions: an indication for surgical biopsy. *AJR Am J Roentgenol* 1995;164:1111–1113.

84. Bibbo M, Scheiber M, Cajulis R, et al. Stereotaxic fine needle aspiration cytology of clinically occult malignant and premalignant breast lesions. *Acta Cytol* 1988;32:193–201.

85. Dziura BR, Bonfiglio TA. Needle cytology of the breast: a quantitative and qualitative study of the cells of benign and malignant ductal neoplasia. *Acta Cytol* 1979;23:332–340.

86. Masood S, Frykberg ER, McLellan GL, et al. Cytologic differentiation between proliferative and nonproliferative breast disease in mammographically guided fine-needle aspirates. *Diagn Cytopathol* 1991;7:581–590.

87. Sneige N, Staerkel GA. Fine-needle aspiration cytology of ductal hyperplasia with and without atypia and ductal carcinoma in situ. *Hum Pathol* 1994;25:485–492.

88. Stanley MW, Henry-Stanley MJ, Zera R. Atypia in breast fine-needle aspiration smears correlates poorly with the presence of a prognostically significant proliferative lesion of ductal epithelium. *Hum Pathol* 1993;24:630–635.

89. Abendroth CS, Wang HH, Ducatman BS. Comparative features of carcinoma in situ and atypical ductal hyperplasia of the breast on fine-needle aspiration biopsy specimens. *Am J Clin Pathol* 1991;96:654–659.

90. Masood S. Cytomorphology of fibrocystic change, high-risk, and premalignant breast lesions. *Breast J* 1995;1:210–223.

91. Frost AR, Aksu A, Kurstin R, et al. Can nonproliferative breast disease and proliferative breast disease without atypia be distinguished by fine-needle aspiration cytology? *Cancer* 1997;81:22–28.

92. Skolnick MH, Cannon-Albright LA, Goldgar DE, et al. Inheritance of proliferative breast disease in breast cancer kindreds. *Science* 1990;250:1715–1720.

93. Khan SA, Masood S, Miller L, et al. Random fine needle aspiration of the breast of women at increased breast cancer risk and standard risk controls. *Breast J* 1998;4:420–425.

94. Wolfe JN. Risk for breast cancer development determined by mammographic parenchymal pattern. *Cancer* 1976;37:2486–2492.

95. Brisson J, Morrison AS, Kopans DB, et al. Height and weight, mammographic features of breast tissue and breast cancer risk. *Am J Epidemiol* 1984;119:371–381.

96. Wolfe JN, Saftlas AF, Salane M. Mammographic parenchymal patterns and quantitative evaluation of mammographic densities: a case-control study. *AJR Am J Roentgenol* 1987;148:1087–1092.

97. Boyd NF, Jensen HM, Cooke G, et al. Relationship between mammographic and histological risk factors for breast cancer. *J Natl Cancer Inst* 1992;84:1170–1179.

98. Urbanski S, Jensen HM, Cooke G, et al. The association of histological and radiological indicators of breast cancer risk. *Br J Cancer* 1988;58:474–479.

99. Moskowitz M, Gartside P, McLauglin C. Mammographic patterns as markers for high-risk benign breast disease and incident cancers. *Radiology* 1980;134:293–295.

100. Arthur JE, Ellis IO, Flowers C, et al. The relationship of "high-risk" mammographic patterns to histological risk factors for development of cancer in the human breast. *Br J Radiol* 1990;63:845–849.

101. Bright RA, Morrison AS, Brisson J, et al. Histologic and mammographic specificity of risk factors for benign breast disease. *Cancer* 1989;64:653–657.

102. Fisher ER, Paleker A, Kim WS, et al. The histopathology of mammographic patterns. *Am J Clin Pathol* 1978;69:421–426.

103. Bodian CA, Perzin KH, Lattes R, et al. Prognostic significance of benign proliferative breast disease. *Cancer* 1993;71:3896–3907.

104. Kodlin D, Winger EE, Morgenstern NL, et al. Chronic mastopathy and breast cancer: a follow-up study. *Cancer* 1977;39:2603–2607.

105. Dupont WD, Page DL. Breast cancer risk associated with proliferative disease, age at first birth, and family history of breast cancer. *Am J Epidemiol* 1987;1225:769–779.

106. Hutchinson WB, Thomas DB, Hamlin WB, et al. Risk of breast cancer in women with benign breast disease. *J Natl Cancer Inst* 1980;65:13–20.

107. Moskowitz M, Gartside P, Wirman JA, et al. Proliferative disorders of the breast as risk factors for breast cancer in a self-selected screened population: pathologic markers. *Radiology* 1980;134:289–291.

108. Dupont WD, Page DL. Relative risk of breast cancer varies with time since diagnosis of atypical hyperplasia. *Hum Pathol* 1989;20:723–725.

109. Seidman H, Seidman SD, Mushinski MH. A different perspective on breast cancer risk factors: some implications of the nonattributable risk. *Cancer* 1982;32:301–313.

110. Madigan MP, Ziegler RG, Benichou J, et al. Proportion of breast cancer cases in the United States explained by well-established risk factors. *J Natl Cancer Inst* 1995;87:1681–1685.

111. Davis HH, Simons M, Davis JB. Cystic disease of the breast: relationship to carcinoma. *Cancer* 1964;17:957–978.

112. Connolly J, Schnitt S, London S, et al. Both atypical lobular hyperplasia (ALH) and atypical ductal hyperplasia (ADH) predict for bilateral breast cancer risk. *Lab Invest* 1992;66:13A.

113. Dupont WD, Page DL. Risk factors for breast cancer in women with proliferative breast disease. *N Engl J Med* 1985;312:146–151.

114. Ahmed S, Tartter PI, Jothy S, et al. The prognostic significance of previous benign breast disease for women with carcinoma of the breast. *J Am Coll Surg* 1996;183:101–104.

115. Jensen RA, Page DL, Dupont WD, et al. Invasive breast cancer risk in women with sclerosing adenosis. *Cancer* 1989;64:1977–1983.

116. Roberts MM, Jones V, Elton RA, et al. Risk of breast cancer in women with history of benign disease of the breast. *BMJ* 1984;288:275–278.

117. Page DL, Dupont WD, Jensen RA. Papillary apocrine change of the breast: associations with atypical hyperplasia and risk of breast cancer. *Cancer Epidemiol Biomarkers Prev* 1996;5:29–32.

118. McDivitt RW, Stewart FW, Berg JW. *Tumors of the breast.* Washington DC: Armed Forces Institute of Pathology, 1968.

119. Fitzgibbons PL, Henson DE, Hutter RV. Benign breast changes and the risk for subsequent breast cancer: an update of the 1985 consensus statement. Cancer Committee of the College of American Pathologists. *Arch Pathol Lab Med* 1998;122:1053–1055.

120. Ma L, Boyd NF. Atypical hyperplasia and breast cancer risk: a critique. *Cancer Causes Control* 1992;3:517–525.

121. Dupont WD, Parl FF, Hartmann WH, et al. Breast cancer associated with proliferative breast disease and atypical hyperplasia. *Cancer* 1993;71:1258–1265.

122. Palli D, DelTurco MR, Simoncici R, et al. Benign breast disease and breast cancer: a case-control study in a cohort in Italy. *Int J Cancer* 1991;47:703–706.

123. Bloodgood JC. Cancer of the breast: figures which show that education can increase the number of cures. *JAMA* 1916;66:552–553.

124. Bloodgood JC. The pathology of chronic cystic mastitis of the female breast. *Arch Surg* 1921;111:445–542.

125. Bodian CA, Perzin KH, Lattes R, et al. Reproducibility and validity of pathologic classifications of benign breast disease and implications for clinical applications. *Cancer* 1993;71:3908–3913.

126. Rosai J. Borderline epithelial lesions of the breast. *Am J Surg Pathol* 1991;15:209–221.

127. Clayton F, Bodian CA, Banogon P, et al. Reproducibility of diagnosis in noninvasive breast disease. *Lab Invest* 1992;66:12A.

128. Palli D, Galli M, Bianchi S, et al. Reproducibility of histological diagnosis of breast lesions: results of a panel in Italy. *Eur J Cancer* 1996;32A:603–607.

129. [No authors listed.] Is "fibrocytic disease" of the breast precancerous? *Arch Pathol Lab Med* 1986;110:171–173.

130. Palazzo J, Hyslop T. Hyperplastic ductal and lobular lesions and carcinomas in situ of the breast: reproducibility of current diagnostic criteria among community- and academic-based pathologists. *Breast J* 1998;4:230–237.

131. Schnitt SJ, Connolly JL, Tavassoli FA, et al. Interobserver reproducibility in the diagnosis of ductal proliferative lesions using standardized criteria. *Am J Surg Pathol* 1992;16:1133–1143.

132. Black MM, Barclay THC, Cutler SJ, et al. Association of atypical characteristics of benign breast disease with subsequent risk of breast cancer. *Cancer* 1972;29:338–343.

133. Black MM, Chabon AB. *In situ* carcinoma of the breast. *Pathobiol Annu* 1969;4:185–210.

134. Page DL, Rogers LW. Combined histologic and cytologic criteria for the diagnosis of mammary atypical ductal hyperplasia. *Hum Pathol* 1992;23:1095–1097.

135. Rosen PP. "Borderline" breast lesions. *Am J Surg Pathol* 1991; 15:1100–1102.

136. Crissman JD, Visscher DW, Kubus J. Image cytophotometric DNA analysis of atypical hyperplasias and intraductal carcinomas of the breast. *Arch Pathol Lab Med* 1990;114:1249–1253.

137. King EB, Chew KL, Hom JD, et al. Characterization by image cytometry of duct epithelial proliferative disease of the breast. *Mod Pathol* 1991;4:291–296.

138. Ozaki D, Kondo Y. Comparative morphometric studies of benign and malignant intraductal proliferative lesions of the breast by computerized image analysis. *Hum Pathol* 1995;26:1109–1113.

139. Norris HJ, Bahr GF, Mikel UV. A comparative morphometric and cytophotometric study of intraductal hyperplasia and intraductal carcinoma of the breast. *Anal Quant Cytol Histol* 1988;10:1–9.

140. Christov K, Chew KL, Ljung B-M, et al. Cell proliferation in hyperplastic and in situ carcinoma lesions of the breast estimated by in vivo labeling with bromodeoxyuridine. *J Cell Biochem* 1994; 19(Suppl):165–172.

141. Eriksson ET, Schimmelpenning H, Aspenblad U, et al. Immunohistochemical expression of the mutant p53 protein and nuclear DNA content during the transition from benign to malignant breast disease. *Hum Pathol* 1994;25:1228–1233.

142. Carpenter R, Gibbs N, Matthews J, et al. Importance of cellular DNA content in pre-malignant breast disease and pre-invasive carcinoma of the female breast. *Br J Surg* 1987;74:905–906.

143. Visscher DW, Wallis TL, Crissman JD. Evaluation of chromosome aneuploidy in tissue sections of preinvasive breast carcinomas using interphase cytogenetics. *Cancer* 1996;77:315–320.

144. Kumar R, Sukumar S, Barbacid M. Activation of ras oncogenes preceding the onset of neoplasia. *Science* 1990;248:1101–1104.

145. Ohuchi N, Thor A, Page DL, et al. Expression of the 21,000 molecular weight ras protein in a spectrum of benign and malignant human mammary tissues. *Cancer Res* 1986;46:2511–2519.

146. Allred DC, Clark GM, Molina R, et al. Overexpression of HER-2/neu and its relationship with other prognostic factors change during the progression of in situ to invasive breast cancer. *Hum Pathol* 1992;23:974–979.

147. Lodato RF, Maguire Jr HC, Greene MI, et al. Immunohistochemical evaluation of c-erbB-2 oncogene expression in ductal carcinoma *in situ* and atypical ductal hyperplasia of the breast. *Mod Pathol* 1990;3:449–454.

148. De Potter CR, van Daele S, van de Vijver MJ, et al. The expression of the neu oncogene product in breast lesions and in normal fetal and adult human tissues. *Histopathology* 1989;15:351–362.

149. D'Souza B, Berdichevsky F, Kyprianou N, et al. Collagen induced morphogenesis and expression of the alpha 2-integrin subunit is inhibited by c-erbB2 transfected human mammary epithelial cells. *Oncogene* 1993;8:1797–1806.

150. Taylor-Papadimitriou J, D'Souza B, Berdichevsky F, et al. Human models for studying malignant progression in breast cancer. *Eur J Cancer Prev* 1993;2(Suppl):77–83.

151. Press MF, Cordon-Cardo C, Slamon DJ. Expression of the HER-2/neu proto-oncogene in normal human adult and fetal tissues. *Oncogene* 1990;5:953–962.

152. Natali PG, Nicotra MR, Bigotti A, et al. Expression of the p185 encoded by HER2 oncogene in normal and transformed human tissues. *Int J Cancer* 1990;45:457–461.

153. Ratcliffe N, Wells W, Wheeler K, et al. The combination of in situ hybridization and immunohistochemical analysis: an evaluation of Her2/neu expression in paraffin-embedded breast carcinomas and adjacent normal-appearing breast epithelium. *Mod Pathol* 1997; 10:1247–1252.

154. Rohan TE, Hartwick W, Miller AB, et al. Immunohistochemical detection of c-erbB-2 and p53 in benign breast disease and breast cancer risk. *J Natl Cancer Inst* 1998;90:1262–1269.

155. Stark A, Hulka BS, Joens S, et al. HER-2/*neu* amplification in benign breast disease and the risk of subsequent breast cancer. *J Clin Oncol* 2000;18:267–274.

156. Chitemerere M, Andersen TI, Holm R, et al. TP53 alterations in atypical ductal hyperplasia and ductal carcinoma *in situ* of the breast. *Breast Cancer Res Treat* 1996;41:103–109.

157. Done SJ, Arneson NC, Ozcelik H, et al. p53 mutations in mammary ductal carcinoma in situ but not in epithelial hyperplasias. *Cancer Res* 1998;58:785–789.

158. Siziopikou KP, Prioleau JE, Harris JR, et al. *bcl-2* expression in the spectrum of preinvasive breast lesions. *Cancer* 1996;77:499–506.

159. Zhang GJ, Kimijima I, Abe R, et al. Correlation between the expression of apoptosis-related bcl-2 and p53 oncoproteins and the carcinogenesis and progression of breast carcinomas. *Clin Cancer Res* 1997;3:2329–2335.

160. Bartek J, Bartkova J, Vojtesek B, et al. Patterns of expression of the p53 tumor suppressor in human breast tissues and tumors in situ and in vitro. *Int J Cancer* 1990;46:839–844.

161. Hall PA, Ray A, Lemoine NR, et al. p53 immunostaining as a marker of malignant disease in diagnostic cytopathology. *Lancet* 1991;338:513.

162. Mommers EC, van Diest PJ, Leonhart AM, et al. Expression of proliferation and apoptosis-related proteins in usual ductal hyperplasia of the breast. *Hum Pathol* 1998;29:1539–1545.

163. Younes M, Lebovitz RM, Boomer KE, et al. p53 accumulation in benign breast biopsy specimens. *Hum Pathol* 1955;26:155–158.

164. Seth A, Palli D, Mariano JM, et al. p53 gene mutations in women with breast cancer and a previous history of benign breast disease. *Eur J Cancer* 1994;30A:808–812.

165. Kamel S, Zeiger S, Zalles C, et al. p53 immunopositivity and gene mutation in a group of women at high risk for breast cancer. *Breast J* 1998;4:396–404.

166. Phillips KA, Nichol K, Ozcelik H, et al. Frequency of p53 mutations in breast carcinomas from Ashkenazi Jewish carriers of BRCA1 mutations. *J Natl Cancer Inst* 1999;91:469–473.

167. Mullauer L, Mosberger I, Grusch M, et al. Fas ligand is expressed in normal breast epithelial cells and is frequently up-regulated in breast cancer. *J Pathol* 2000;190:20–30.

168. Singh M, Jarboe EA, Shroyer KR. Survivin expression in benign, premalignant and malignant lesions of the breast. *Mod Pathol* 2000;13:47A.

169. Zhu XL, Hartwick W, Rohan T, et al. Cyclin D1 gene amplification and protein expression in benign breast disease and breast carcinoma. *Mod Pathol* 1998;11:1082–1088.

170. Weinstat-Saslow D, Merino MJ, Manrow RE, et al. Overexpression of cyclin D mRNA distinguishes invasive and in situ breast carcinomas from non-malignant lesions. *Nat Med* 1995;1:1257–1260.

171. Shpitz B, Zimlichman S, Zemer R, et al. Telomerase activity in ductal carcinoma in situ of the breast. *Breast Cancer Res Treat* 1999;58:65–69.

172. Hiyama E, Gollahon L, Kataoka T, et al. Telomerase activity in human breast tumors. *J Natl Cancer Inst* 1996;88:116–122.

173. Belair CD, Yeager TR, Lopez PM, et al. Telomerase activity: a biomarker of cell proliferation, not malignant transformation. *Proc Natl Acad Sci U S A* 1997;94:13677–13682.

174. Lee WY, Jin YT, Chang TW, et al. Immunolocalization of BRCA1 protein in normal breast tissue and sporadic invasive ductal carcinomas: a correlation with other biological parameters. *Histopathology* 1999;34:106–112.

175. Barker S, Panahy C, Puddefoot JR, et al. Epidermal growth factor receptor and oestrogen receptors in the non-malignant part of the cancerous breast. *Br J Cancer* 1989;60:673–677.

176. van Agthoven T, Timmermans M, Foekens JA, et al. Differential expression of estrogen, progesterone, and epidermal growth factor receptors in normal, benign, and malignant human breast tissues using dual staining immunohistochemistry. *Am J Pathol* 1994;144: 1238–1246.

177. Möller P, Mechtersheimer G, Kaufmann M, et al. Expression of epidermal growth factor receptor in benign and malignant primary tumours of the breast. *Virchows Arch [A]* 1989;414:157–164.

178. Klijn JGM, Berns PMJJ, Schmitz PIM, et al. The clinical significance of epidermal growth factor receptor (EGF-R) in human breast cancer: a review on 5232 patients. *Endocr Rev* 1992;13:3–17.

179. Bolufer P, Miralles F, Rodriguez A, et al. Epidermal growth factor receptor in human breast cancer: correlation with cytosolic and nuclear ER receptors and with biological and histological tumor characteristics. *Eur J Cancer* 1990;26:283–290.

180. Dittadi R, Donisi PM, Brazzale A, et al. Epidermal growth factor

receptor in breast cancer: comparison with nonmalignant breast tissue. *Br J Cancer* 1993;67:7–9.

181. Paik S. Expression of IGF-I and IGF-II mRNA in breast tissue. *Breast Cancer Res Treat* 1992;22:31–38.

182. Cullen KJ, Allison A, Martire I, et al. Insulin-like growth factor expression in breast cancer epithelium and stroma. *Breast Cancer Res Treat* 1992;22:21–29.

183. Giri DD, Dundas SAC, Nottingham JF, et al. Oestrogen receptors in benign epithelial lesions and intraduct carcinomas of the breast: an immunohistological study. *Histopathology* 1989;15:575–584.

184. Khan SA, Rogers MAM, Obando JA, et al. Estrogen receptor expression of benign breast epithelium and its association with breast cancer. *Cancer Res* 1994;54:993–997.

185. Rohann TE, Miller AB. Hormone replacement therapy and risk of benign proliferative epithelial disorders of the breast. *Eur J Cancer Prev* 1999;8:123–130.

186. Holli K, Isola J, Cuzick J. Low biologic aggressiveness in breast cancer in women using hormone replacement therapy. *J Clin Oncol* 1998;16:3115–3120.

187. Schairer C, Gail M, Byrne C, et al. Estrogen replacement therapy and breast cancer survival in a large screening study. *J Natl Cancer Inst* 1999;91:264–270.

188. Henry JA, Nicholson S, Hennessy C, et al. Expression of the estrogen regulated pNR-2 mRNA in human breast cancer: relation to estrogen receptor mRNA levels and response to tamoxifen therapy. *Br J Cancer* 1989;61:32–38.

189. Rio MC, Bellocq JP, Gairard B, et al. Specific expression of the pS2 gene in sub-classes of breast cancers in comparison with expression of the estrogen and progesterone receptors and the oncogene erbB2. *Proc Natl Acad Sci U S A* 1987;84:9243–9247.

190. Luqmani YA, Campbell T, Soomro S, et al. Immunohistochemical localisation of pS2 protein in ductal carcinoma in situ and benign lesions of the breast. *Br J Cancer* 1993;67:749–753.

191. Pignatelli M, Vessey CJ. Adhesion molecules: novel molecular tools in tumor pathology. *Hum Pathol* 1994;25:849–856.

192. Terranova VP, Rao CN, Kabelic T, et al. Laminin receptor on human breast cancer cells. *Proc Natl Acad Sci U S A* 1983;80:444–448.

193. Henning K, Berndt A, Katenkamp D, et al. Loss of laminin-5 in the epithelium-stroma interface: an immunohistochemical marker of malignancy in epithelial lesions of the breast. *Histopathology* 1999;34:305–309.

194. Slade MJ, Coope RC, Gomm JJ, et al. The human mammary gland basement membrane is integral to the polarity of luminal epithelial cells. *Exp Cell Res* 1999;247:267–278.

195. Sternlicht MD, Kedeshian P, Shao ZM, et al. The human myoepithelial cell is a natural tumor suppressor. *Clin Cancer Res* 1997;3:1949–1958.

196. Molitoris BA, Nelson WJ. Alterations in the establishment and maintenance of epithelial cell polarity as a basis for disease processes. *J Clin Invest* 1990;85:3–9.

197. Simpson JF, Page DL. Altered expression of a structural protein (fodrin) within epithelial proliferative disease of the breast. *Am J Pathol* 1992;141:285–298.

198. Younes M, Harris AS, Morrow JS. Fodrin as a differentiation marker: redistributions in colonic neoplasia. *Am J Pathol* 1989;135:1197–1212.

199. Albelda SM. Biology of disease: role of integrins and other cell adhesion molecules in tumor progression and metastasis. *Lab Invest* 1993;68:4–17.

200. Koukoulis GK, Virtanen I, Korhonen M, et al. Immunohistochemical localization of integrins in the normal, hyperplastic and neoplastic breast. *Am J Pathol* 1991;139:787–799.

201. Zutter MM, Mazoujian G, Santoro SA. Decreased expression of integrin adhesive protein receptors in adenocarcinoma of the breast. *Am J Pathol* 1990;137:863–870.

202. Zutter MM, Krigman HR, Santoro SA. Altered integrin expression in adenocarcinoma of the breast. Analysis by in situ hybridization. *Am J Pathol* 1993;142:1439–1448.

203. Jones JL, Critchley DR, Walker RA. Alteration of stromal protein and integrin expression in breast—a marker of premalignant change? *J Pathol* 1992;167:399–406.

204. Brem SS, Jensen HM, Gullino PM. Angiogenesis as a marker of preneoplastic lesions of the human breast. *Cancer* 1978;41:239–244.

205. Folkman J. Tumor angiogenesis factor. *Cancer Res* 1974;34:2109–2113.

206. Bose S, Lesser ML, Rosen PP. Immunophenotype of intraductal carcinoma. *Arch Pathol Lab Med* 1996;120:81–85.

207. Heffelfinger SC, Yassin R, Miller MA, et al. Vascularity of proliferative breast disease and carcinoma in situ correlates with histological features. *Clin Cancer Res* 1996;2:1873–1878.

208. Borsi L, Carnemolla B, Nicolò G, et al. Expression of different tenascin isoforms in normal, hyperplastic and neoplastic human breast tissues. *Int J Cancer* 1992;52:688–692.

209. Nicolò G, Salvi S, Oliveri G, et al. Expression of tenascin and of the ED-B containing oncofetal fibronectin isoform in human cancer. *Cell Diff Devel* 1990;32:401–408.

210. Kaczmarek J, Castellani P, Nicolo G, et al. Distribution of oncofetal fibronectin isoforms in normal, hyperplastic and neoplastic human breast tissues. *Int J Cancer* 1994;58:11–16.

211. Jarasch E-D, Nagle RB, Kaufmann M, et al. Differential diagnosis of benign epithelial proliferations and carcinomas of the breast using antibodies to cytokeratins. *Hum Pathol* 1988;19:276–289.

212. Gould VE, Koukoulis GK, Jansson DS, et al. Coexpression patterns of vimentin and glial filament protein with cytokeratins in the normal, hyperplastic, and neoplastic breast. *Am J Pathol* 1990;137:1143–1155.

213. Böcker W, Bier B, Ludwig A, et al. Benign proliferative lesions and in situ carcinoma of the breast: new immunohistological findings and their biological implications. *Eur J Cancer Prevent* 1993;2(Suppl):41–49.

214. Moinfar F, Man YG, Lininger RA, et al. Use of keratin 35BE12 as an adjunct in the diagnosis of mammary intraepithelial neoplasia-ductal type—benign and malignant intraductal proliferations. *Am J Surg Pathol* 1999;23:1048–1058.

# CHAPTER 11

# *In Situ* (Intraepithelial) Carcinoma

## An Overview

The epithelial origin of mammary carcinoma has been widely accepted for at least 75 years, but there still is considerable controversy about many aspects of the diagnosis, the "natural history" or clinical course, and the treatment of these lesions. This chapter provides an overview of the concept of *in situ* mammary carcinoma as a prelude to separate detailed discussions of the specific features of *in situ* lobular and intraductal carcinoma.

The terminology used to describe the preinvasive stages of breast carcinoma lesions has been varied and confusing. Broders (1) proposed the term *in situ* in 1932 to describe

> a condition in which malignant epithelial cells and their progeny are found in or near the positions occupied by their ancestors before the ancestors underwent malignant transformation. At least they have not migrated beyond the juncture of the epithelium and connective tissue or the so-called basement membrane. The diagnosis of carcinoma *in situ* as of carcinoma in general, is based chiefly on altered cellular characteristics in contradistinction to the cellular situation. If, in a specimen obtained for biopsy, carcinoma *in situ* is associated with infiltrating carcinoma, there is little chance of missing the diagnosis of carcinoma.

Although Broders' study dealt with neoplastic changes in the oral mucosa, it was applicable to other organs. In the breast, the term *in situ* was first associated with carcinoma originating in the lobules following the description of lobular carcinoma *in situ* in 1941 (2). Intraepithelial carcinoma of mammary ducts is referred to as intraductal carcinoma or ductal carcinoma *in situ*. Because of its intraepithelial location, *in situ* carcinoma is separated from the lymphatic and vascular circulation by the basement membrane complex, and in this respect, it also may be described as *noninvasive*.

Accurate assessment of the integrity of the basement membranes by light microscopy has limitations that will be mentioned here briefly and discussed later in more detail. Ultrastructural studies demonstrated protrusion of carcinoma cells through the basement membrane, even when this could not be appreciated in routine histologic sections (3,4). This phenomenon may be responsible for some extremely unusual cases where metastases apparently originated from lesions that appeared to be *in situ* when studied with the light microscope (5,6). It is impractical to use electron microscopy to prove that a carcinoma is truly noninvasive when it appears so by light microscopy. With very rare exceptions, the clinical course is consistent with the histologic impression. Immunohistochemical methods to assess the integrity of basement membranes may show areas of discontinuity, but usually these procedures have not been effective for proving that the epithelial process has actually invaded the surrounding stroma.

Another term proposed to describe *in situ* carcinoma is *preinvasive*. This adjective connotes more than the current state of the lesion at the time of diagnosis, because it refers to the capacity of intraepithelial carcinoma to evolve into or progress to an invasive state. This implication may be viewed as advantageous, because it suggests a dynamic condition and provides a better appreciation of the clinical course in some patients. Conversely, however, it now is apparent that such progression does not occur clinically in the lifetime of all patients and that satisfactory methods for assessing the likelihood of this sequence of events in individual patients have not been developed. On the other hand, analyses of groups of patients provided statistical data in the form of relative probabilities that offer general guidance for patient management.

It now is well established that mastectomy is curative in virtually all patients with *in situ* carcinoma of the breast. Removal of all of the affected breast tissue eradicates the disease, because at this clinical stage the sequence of invasion and metastasis has not begun. However, progression to invasion does not occur in all patients with biopsy-proven *in situ* lesions if they are not treated by mastectomy. There is evidence that some patients have multifocal lesions at the time of diagnosis or may develop such foci later, but there are individuals whose only focus of *in situ* carcinoma is removed in the diagnostic specimen. Among those with multifocal lesions, foci of *in situ* carcinoma may remain dormant for long periods, perhaps indefinitely. It is not inconceivable that they may regress and even disappear. There presently are no methods to accurately predict the propensity to develop new multifocal lesions, to identify all patients with multifocal *in situ* carcinoma preoperatively, to determine *in vivo* the morphologic characteristics of such multifocal lesions, or to determine with a high degree of certainty the likelihood of progression to invasion in individual patients. Dilemmas about the treatment of *in situ* carcinoma stem largely from a dearth of information about these issues.

Intraductal carcinoma occasionally may produce a mass, but until the advent of mammography, it was typically a microscopic lesion detected in a biopsy performed for a "lump." Lobular carcinoma *in situ* is, by its nature, a microscopic process that rarely has direct clinical manifestations, such as calcifications detected by mammography. As long as *in situ* carcinoma was a fortuitous finding, it remained an uncommon clinical problem engendering little controversy about therapy. The fact that an increasing number of patients have significant nonpalpable lesions detected preoperatively by mammography has focused greater attention on issues of treating *in situ* carcinoma, especially intraductal carcinoma. Among cases reviewed in a nationwide breast cancer screening program, 143 (67%) of 212 intraductal carcinomas were found in biopsies performed on the basis of mammographic indications alone and 2% were detected in biopsies initiated entirely because of clinical abnormalities (7).

It has been customary to distinguish two types of intraepithelial carcinoma in the breast on the basis of the anatomic distribution of the lesions in the duct-lobular system, as well as their growth patterns and their cytologic features. In most cases, generally accepted histologic criteria serve to distinguish *in situ* lobular from intraductal carcinoma. However, under some circumstances, the distinction is difficult. The two processes may coexist in the breast within a single duct-lobular unit (8), duct carcinoma may extend into the epithelium of lobules (9), and lobular carcinoma *in situ* has been observed within ductal epithelium (10). There also is evidence indicating that the site of origin of many carcinomas may be in the terminal duct epithelium, regardless of histologic type (11), but this concept has not led to a widely accepted modification of the scheme for classifying *in situ* breast carcinoma. Present evidence suggests that loss of E-cadherin immunoreactivity is a marker specifically associated with lobular carcinoma. The consistency of this finding and the presence of genetic alterations in the E-cadherin gene lends support to the concept that *in situ* lobular "neoplasia" is truly *in situ* carcinoma.

The fact that total mastectomy was curative for virtually all patients with *in situ* carcinoma of lobules or ducts led some to question whether it was appropriate to refer to these lesions as carcinoma. Some authors preferred to substitute the term *neoplasia* for intraepithelial or *in situ* carcinoma. It was felt that designating the disease as *intraepithelial neoplasia* or *lobular neoplasia* emphasized the high curability of the lesion and encouraged treatment other than radical surgery (12). Difficulty in distinguishing between hyperplasia and *in situ* carcinoma in borderline lesions also has been cited as a reason for using the term neoplasia.

The concerns raised by enthusiasts for the term *intraepithelial neoplasia* were addressed by Hutter (13) in an essay entitled, "Is Cured Early Cancer Truly Cancer?" He concluded,

> The real issue here is not whether the pathologic diagnosis of microscopic cancer is valid. . . . The real issue is how to manage patients with these lesions today; acknowledging that we do not yet have the diagnostic capability to separate those patients with lesions which will progress from those which will not.

As the foregoing discussion indicates, each of these terms has limitations. The presentation in this book will use the terms intraductal carcinoma and lobular carcinoma *in situ* to describe specific histologic lesions. Most information about intraepithelial carcinoma was acquired from retrospective studies prior to the last decade. The results described patients treated almost exclusively by mastectomy. Prospective data for women treated by breast conservation are now available. Despite notable differences in methodology in these studies, some general conclusions are warranted.

1. Total mastectomy is curative in virtually all patients with biopsy-proven intraepithelial breast carcinoma.
2. If intraepithelial carcinoma is treated by breast conservation, the organ is at risk to develop invasive carcinoma. The likelihood of developing subsequent ipsilateral carcinoma is greater for intraductal carcinoma than for lobular carcinoma *in situ*.
3. The average interval to the development of subsequent carcinoma is shorter for patients with intraductal carcinoma than for those with *in situ* lobular carcinoma.
4. In most cases, lobular carcinoma *in situ* can be managed by careful clinical follow-up. Antiestrogen therapy appears to be beneficial for these patients.
5. The majority of patients with intraductal carcinoma treated by breast conservation do not develop invasive carcinoma of either breast following excisional biopsy, even after follow-up for more than 20 years. The risk for subsequent ipsilateral invasive carcinoma in the conserved breast is reduced by administering postoperative radiotherapy and, in some cases, by antiestrogen treatment.
6. A patient with intraepithelial carcinoma in one breast is at risk of having carcinoma in the opposite breast. For women with *in situ* lobular carcinoma alone or in combination with intraductal carcinoma, the contralateral risk is greater than for those who have only intraductal carcinoma.

## REFERENCES

1. Broders AC. Carcinoma *in situ* contrasted with benign penetrating epithelium. *JAMA* 1932;99:1670–1674.
2. Foote FW Jr, Stewart FW. Lobular carcinoma *in situ*: a rare form of mammary cancer. *Am J Pathol* 1941;17:491–496.
3. Ozzello L. The behavior of basement membranes of intraductal carcinoma of the breast. *Am J Pathol* 1959;35:887–899.
4. Ozzello L. Ultrastructure of intraepithelial carcinomas of the breast. *Cancer* 1971;28:1508–1515.
5. Haupt HM, Rosen PP, Kinne DW. Breast carcinoma presenting with axillary lymph node metastases: an analysis of specific histopathologic features. *Am J Surg Pathol* 1985;9:165–176.
6. Rosen PP. Axillary lymph node metastases in patients with occult noninvasive breast carcinoma. *Cancer* 1980;46:1298–1306.
7. Beahrs O, Shapiro S, Smart C. Report of the working group to review the National Cancer Institute-American Cancer Society Breast Cancer Detection Demonstration Projects. *J Natl Cancer Inst* 1979;62:640–709.
8. Rosen PP. Coexistent lobular carcinoma *in situ* and intraductal carcinoma in a single lobular-duct unit. *Am J Surg Pathol* 1980;4:241–246.
9. Fechner RE. Ductal carcinoma involving the lobule of the breast. A source of confusion with lobular carcinoma *in situ*. *Cancer* 1971;28:274–281.
10. Fechner RE. Epithelial alterations in extralobular ducts of breasts with lobular carcinoma. *Arch Pathol* 1972;93:164–171.
11. Wellings SR, Jensen HM. On the origin and progression of ductal carcinoma in the human breast. *J Natl Cancer Inst* 1973;50:1111–1118.
12. Haagensen CD, Lane N, Lattes R, et al. Lobular neoplasia (so-called lobular carcinoma *in situ*) of the breast. *Cancer* 1978;42:737–769.
13. Hutter RVPH. Is cured early cancer truly cancer? *Cancer* 1981;47:1215–1220.

# CHAPTER 12

# Staging of Breast Carcinoma

Staging has several important applications in the study and treatment of breast diseases. It may be used to select therapeutic options for patients, and it forms the basis for assessing response to treatment as well as prognosis. Staging is essential for comparing the results of different forms of therapy or the results obtained by different groups of investigators who use similar treatments in clinical trials (1). This latter function is well illustrated by the National Cancer Data Base formed by the American Cancer Society and the American College of Surgeons (2). Data collected in a standardized fashion from institutions across the United States make it possible to identify general and regional trends in breast cancer treatment and outcome.

One of the earliest staging systems introduced by Steinthal (3) in 1905 stratified patients into three groups that are still used today for the broad categorization of patients: localized disease, regional spread, and advanced metastatic disease. Subsequent decades were marked by the development of more detailed staging systems based on clinical and pathologic features (4–6). Lack of comparability between these and other staging schemes resulted in the creation of the TNM system, which was adopted by the International Union Against Cancer (UICC) and the American Joint Committee for Cancer Staging and End Results Reporting (AJC). The TNM system formed the basis for the *Manual for Staging of Cancer* first published in 1978 by the AJC (7) and in later editions concurrently with the UICC (8). The most recent versions of TNM staging were published in 1997 (9,10).

TNM staging is based on characteristics of the primary tumor (T), extent of regional axillary nodal metastases (N), and extent of distant metastases (M). The designation TNM has been chosen for clinical classification, whereas pTNM refers to pathologic staging. However, this distinction is not always made in published reports (11). The current fifth edition of TNM classification has been expanded substantially beyond the fourth edition published in 1992 (12) by the addition of information about prognostic factors other than TNM (13). The following text is adapted from the American Joint Committee on Cancer (AJCC) *AJCC Cancer Staging Manual,* fifth edition (10). Staging described herein applies to carcinoma of the female and male breast.

## RULES FOR CLASSIFICATION

The TNM classification applies only to carcinoma that has been histologically confirmed. The anatomic subsite in the breast of the primary tumor should be recorded, but it is not an element in classification. The seven defined sites identified in the female breast are the nipple, the central subareolar region, the four quadrants (upper inner, upper outer, lower inner, and lower outer), and the axillary tail. A carcinoma positioned so that it involves more than one of these sites is described as an "overlapping lesion." The male breast is considered to be a single site not further subdivided. All other staging categories apply equally to carcinoma of the male breast.

When multiple simultaneous ipsilateral infiltrating macroscopically measurable carcinomas are present in one breast, "use the largest primary carcinoma to classify T . . . and record that this is a case of multiple simultaneous ipsilateral primary carcinomas. Such cases should be analyzed separately" (10). "These criteria do not apply to one macroscopic carcinoma associated with multiple separate microscopic foci" (10). When there are simultaneous *bilateral* breast cancers, "each carcinoma is staged as a separate primary carcinoma in a separate organ" (10).

*Clinical staging* may be used in some circumstances, but it is less accurate than pathologic staging. Clinical staging uses physical examination of the skin, mammary gland, and axillary lymph nodes, imaging studies, and pathologic examination of tissue from the breast or other tissue to establish the diagnosis of breast carcinoma. Operative findings, such as tumor size or chest wall invasion and the presence or absence of metastases in regional or distant sites, also contribute to clinical staging.

Dimpling of the skin, nipple retraction, or any other skin change except those described under T4b and T4d may occur in T1, T2, or T3 without changing the classification. Chest wall refers to ribs, intercostal muscles, and the serratus anterior muscle, but not to the pectoral muscle.

Clinical measurement of the size of the primary tumor should be based on the most accurate method in a given case (e.g., physical examination or mammography).

The major deficiencies of clinical staging are a tendency to overestimate the size of the primary tumor and inaccurate assessment of the axillary lymph nodes. The false-positive and false-negative rates for clinical axillary lymph node staging are 30% to 40% (14). Rosen et al. compared clinical and pathologic staging of the axillary lymph nodes in 203 patients treated by modified or radical mastectomy (15). The overall error rates were 33% and 38% for patients with T1 and T2 tumors, respectively. After surgery, 48% of patients classified clinically as T2N0 proved to be pathologically T2N1 (false-negative), and 41% of women staged clinically as T1N1 were pathologically staged as T1N0 (false-positive). Other noninvasive diagnostic procedures, such as lymphoscintigraphy (16–18), ultrasound (19,20), and magnetic resonance imaging have not proven to be reliable substitutes for the pathologic examination of lymph nodes from an axillary dissection. Procedures for sentinel lymph node mapping are able to identify one or more lymph nodes most likely to harbor metastatic carcinoma, but current methods cannot determine prior to excision whether metastases are present in the lymph nodes. Mammography is able to detect axillary lymph nodes in about 75% of women, but the number found radiographically is substantially less than in the pathologic examination of an axillary dissection and the procedure is not able to detect metastatic carcinoma consistently (21). There also is evidence that axillary dissection may be associated with an improved prognosis, especially in patients with early stage carcinoma (22), thus justifying the procedure for therapy as well as staging.

*Pathologic staging* uses "all data used for clinical staging, surgical exploration and resection as well as pathologic examination of the primary carcinoma, including not less than excision of the primary carcinoma with no macroscopic tumor in any margin of resection by pathologic examination. If there is tumor in the margin of resection by macroscopic examination, it is coded TX because the extent of the primary tumor cannot be assessed" (10). If there is only microscopic, but not macroscopic, tumor at the margin, the case can be assigned to a pT group. The pathologic determination of tumor size for the classification of T is a measurement of the invasive component. The size of the primary tumor should be measured before any tissue is removed for special studies.

For purposes of TNM staging, microinvasion is defined as "the extension of cancer cells beyond the basement membrane into the adjacent tissues with no focus no more than 0.1 cm in greatest dimension. When there are multiple foci of microinvasion, the size of only the largest focus is used to classify the microinvasion. (Do not use the sum of all the individual foci.) The presence of multiple foci of microinvasion should be noted" (10).

Paget's disease of the nipple without a clinically palpable mass or pathologically identified invasive carcinoma is clas-sified as Tis. When a mass is evident clinically or invasive carcinoma is present on microscopic pathologic examination, the carcinoma is staged according to the size of the tumor or invasive component.

## REGIONAL LYMPH NODES

The lymphatic drainage of the breast follows three major pathways: axillary, transpectoral, and internal mammary. Intramammary lymph nodes are coded as axillary lymph nodes (N) for staging purposes. Metastases in any other lymph node sites (including supraclavicular, cervical, and contralateral internal mammary) are considered distant metastases and coded as M1.

1. *Axillary* (ipsilateral) and *interpectoral* (Rotter's): lymph nodes and lymph nodes along the axillary vein and its tributaries, which may be (but are not required to be) divided into the following levels:
   *Level I* (low axilla): lymph nodes lateral to the lateral border of pectoralis minor muscle
   *Level II* (mid axilla): lymph nodes between the medial and lateral borders of the pectoralis minor muscle and the interpectoral (Rotter's) lymph nodes
   *Level III* (apical axilla): lymph nodes medial to the medial margin of the pectoralis minor muscle, including those designated as the subclavicular, infraclavicular, or apical
2. *Internal mammary* (ipsilateral): lymph nodes in the intercostal spaces along the edge of the sternum in the endothoracic fascia

For accurate pN staging, resection of at least the lower axillary lymph nodes (level I) is recommended to provide six or more lymph nodes for histologic examination. Nodules of metastatic carcinoma in fat without residual lymph node architecture are considered to be regional lymph node metastases. It should be noted that the AJCC requirement for axillary dissection as a basis for pN predated the availability of data from sentinel lymph node mapping and that this may not apply to patients who undergo this procedure.

## TNM CLINICAL CLASSIFICATION

Definitions for classifying the primary tumor are the same for clinical and pathologic classification. If the measurement is made by physical examination, only the major headings (T1, T2, or T3) are used. If mammographic or pathologic measurements are used, the carcinoma can be assigned to one of the T1 subsets.

### Primary Tumor (T)

TX  Primary tumor cannot be assessed
T0  No evidence of primary tumor
Tis  Carcinoma *in situ:* intraductal carcinoma, or lobular carcinoma *in situ,* or Paget's disease of the nipple with no tumor

Paget's disease associated with a tumor is classified according to the size of the tumor.

| | |
|---|---|
| T1 | Tumor 2 cm or less in greatest dimension |
| T1mic | Microinvasion 0.1 cm or less in greatest dimension |
| T1a | Tumor more than 0.1 but not more than 0.5 cm in greatest dimension |
| T1b | Tumor more than 0.5 cm but not more than 1 cm in greatest dimension |
| T1c | Tumor more than 1 cm but not more than 2 cm in greatest dimension |
| T2 | Tumor more than 2 cm but not more than 5 cm in greatest dimension |
| T3 | Tumor more than 5 cm in greatest dimension |
| T4 | Tumor of any size with direct extension to (a) chest wall or (b) skin, only as described as follows: |
| T4a | Extension to chest wall |
| T4b | Edema (including *peau d'orange*) or ulceration of the skin of the breast, or satellite skin nodules confined to the same breast |
| T4c | Both (T4a and T4b) |
| T4d | Inflammatory carcinoma |

Inflammatory carcinoma of the breast is a clinicopathologic entity characterized by diffuse, brawny induration of the skin with an erysipeloid edge. Radiologically, there may be a detectable mass and characteristic thickening of the skin over the breast. This clinical presentation is due to tumor embolization of dermal lymphatics.

Dimpling of the skin, nipple retraction, or any other skin change, except those described under T4b and T4d, may occur in T1, T2, or T3 without changing the classification.

### Regional Lymph Nodes (N)

| | |
|---|---|
| NX | Regional lymph nodes cannot be assessed (e.g., previously removed) |
| N0 | No regional lymph node metastasis |
| N1 | Metastasis to movable ipsilateral axillary node(s) |
| N2 | Metastasis to ipsilateral axillary node(s) fixed to one another or to other structures |
| N3 | Metastasis to ipsilateral internal mammary lymph node(s) |

### Pathologic Classification (pN)

| | |
|---|---|
| pNX | Regional lymph nodes cannot be assessed (e.g., previously removed or not removed for pathologic study) |
| pN0 | No regional lymph node metastasis |
| pN1 | Metastasis to movable ipsilateral axillary node(s) |
| pN1a | Only micrometastasis (none larger than 0.2 cm) |
| pN1b | Metastasis in lymph node(s), any larger than 0.2 cm |
| pN1bi | Metastasis in one to three lymph nodes, any more than 0.2 cm and all less than 2.0 cm in greatest dimension |
| pN1bii | Metastasis in four or more lymph nodes, any more than 0.2 cm and all less than 2.0 cm in greatest dimension |
| pN1biii | Extension of tumor beyond the capsule of a lymph node metastasis less than 2.0 cm in greatest dimension |
| pN1biv | Metastasis in a lymph node 2.0 cm or more in greatest dimension |
| pN2 | Metastasis in ipsilateral axillary lymph nodes that are fixed to one another or to other structures |
| pN3 | Metastasis in ipsilateral internal mammary lymph node(s) |

### Distant Metastasis (M)

| | |
|---|---|
| MX | Presence of distant metastasis cannot be assessed |
| M0 | No distant metastasis |
| M1 | Distant metastasis (includes metastasis to supraclavicular lymph node[s]) |

## HISTOPATHOLOGIC TYPES

Carcinoma, NOS (not otherwise specified)
Ductal
  Intraductal (*in situ*)
  Invasive with predominant intraductal component
  Invasive, NOS (not otherwise specified)
  Various special types
Lobular
  *In situ*
  Invasive with predominant *in situ* component
  Invasive
Paget's disease
  NOS (not otherwise specified)
  With intraductal carcinoma
  With invasive ductal carcinoma
Undifferentiated carcinoma

## HISTOPATHOLOGIC GRADE (G)

| | |
|---|---|
| GX | Grade cannot be assessed |
| G1 | Well differentiated |
| G2 | Moderately differentiated |
| G3 | Poorly differentiated |
| G4 | Undifferentiated |

## STAGE GROUPING

| Stage 0 | Tis | N0 | M0 |
|---|---|---|---|
| Stage I | T1* | N0 | M0 |
| Stage IIA | T0 | N1 | M0 |
| | T1* | N1 | M0 |
| | T2 | N0 | M0 |

| Stage IIB | T2 | N1 | M0 |
|---|---|---|---|
| | T3 | N0 | M0 |
| Stage IIIA | T0 | N2 | M0 |
| | T1* | N2 | M0 |
| | T2 | N2 | M0 |
| | T3 | N1 | M0 |
| | T3 | N2 | M0 |
| Stage IIIB | T4 | Any N | M0 |
| | Any T | N3 | M0 |
| Stage IV | Any T | Any N | M1 |

*T1 includes T1mic

# REFERENCES

1. Henson DE, Ries L, Freedman LS, et al. Relationship among outcome, stage of disease, and histologic grade for 22,616 cases of breast cancer. The basis for a prognostic index. *Cancer* 1991;68:2142–2149.
2. Osteen RT, Karnell LH. The National Cancer Data Base Report on Breast Cancer. *Cancer* 1994;73:1994–2000.
3. Steinthal CD. Zur Dauerheilung des Brustkrebses. *Beitr Z Klin Chir* 1905;47:226.
4. Haagensen CD, Stout AP. Carcinoma of the breast. II. Criteria of operability. *Ann Surg* 1943;118:1032–1051.
5. Lee BJ, Stubenbord JG. A clinical index of malignancy for carcinoma of the breast. *Surg Gynecol Obstet* 1928;47:812–814.
6. Portmann UV. Classification of mammary carcinomas to indicate preferable therapeutic procedures. *Radiology* 1937;29:391–402.
7. American Joint Committee for Cancer Staging and End-Results Reporting. In: *Manual for staging of cancer.* Chicago: AJC. 1978: 101–107.
8. Hutter RVP. At last—worldwide agreement on staging of cancer. *Arch Surg* 1987;122:1235–1239.
9. UICC International Union Against Cancer. Breast tumours. In: Sobin LH, Wittekind C, eds. *TNM classification of malignant tumours,* 5th ed. New York: Wiley-Liss, 1997:123–130.
10. American Joint Committee on Cancer. Breast. In: *AJCC cancer staging manual,* 5th ed. Philadelphia: Lippincott-Raven Publishers, 1997: 171–180.
11. Nachlas MM. Irrationality in the management of breast cancer. I. The staging system. *Cancer* 1991;68:681–690.
12. American Joint Committee on Cancer. The breast. In: Beahrs OH, Henson DE, Hutter RVP, et al., eds. *Manual for staging of cancer,* 4th ed. Philadelphia: JB Lippincott Co., 1992:149–154.
13. Hermanek P, Sobin LH, Fleming ID. What do we need beyond TNM? *Cancer* 1996;77:815–817.
14. Kinne DW. Staging and follow-up of breast cancer patients. *Cancer* 1991;67:1196–1198.
15. Rosen PP, Fracchia AA, Urban JA, et al. "Residual" mammary carcinoma following simulated partial mastectomy. *Cancer* 1975; 35:739–747.
16. McLean RG, Ege GN. Prognostic value of axillary lymphoscintography in breast carcinoma patients. *J Nucl Med* 1986;27:1116–1124.
17. Gasparini M, Andreoli C, Rodari A, et al. Lack of efficacy of lymphoscintigraphy in detecting axillary lymph node metastases from breast cancer. *Eur J Cancer Clin Oncol* 1987;23:475–480.
18. Tjandra JJ, Sacks NPM, Thompson CH, et al. The detection of axillary lymph node metastases from breast cancer by radiolabelled monoclonal antibodies: a prospective study. *Br J Cancer* 1989;59:296–302.
19. Bruneton JN, Caramella E, Hery M, et al. Axillary lymph node metastases in breast cancer: preoperative detection by US. *Radiology* 1986;158:325–326.
20. Tate JJT, Lewis V, Archer T, et al. Ultrasound detection of axillary lymph node metastases in breast cancer. *Eur J Surg Oncol* 1989; 15:139–141.
21. Dershaw DD, Panicek DM, Osborne MP. Significance of lymph nodes visualized by the mammographic axillary view. *Breast Dis* 1991; 4:271–280.
22. Cabanes PA, Salmon RJ, Vilcoq JR, et al., for the Breast Carcinoma Collaborative Group of the Institut Curie. Value of axillary dissection in addition to lumpectomy and radiotherapy in early breast cancer. *Lancet* 1992;339:1245–1248.

# CHAPTER 13

# Intraductal Carcinoma

## HISTORICAL BACKGROUND

Intraductal carcinoma was defined pathologically early in the twentieth century, largely by surgeons interested in the microscopic study of tumors they encountered clinically. Among the first studies are those of J.C. Warren, a surgeon practicing in Boston (1). Warren's investigation of "abnormal involution" or cystic disease led him to conclude that carcinoma might develop by transition from hyperplastic duct lesions:

> It is precisely under these conditions that we most frequently find the combination of abnormal involution and carcinoma. The transition stage is observed when the epithelium no longer confines itself to the cyst cavity, but breaks through the limiting membrane and infiltrates the adjacent structures (1).

Fundamental pathological and clinical studies of proliferative duct lesions of the breast were made during the early decades of the twentieth century by two other surgeons, Sir G. Lenthal Cheatle of Kings College Hospital, London, and Joseph Colt Bloodgood of Johns Hopkins University Hospital, Baltimore, Maryland. The extent to which Bloodgood and Cheatle influenced each other is difficult to ascertain from their published articles, which rarely contained references to work other than their own. Contemporaries separated by the Atlantic Ocean, they seem to have pursued independent routes in their efforts to distinguish more clearly between benign and malignant lesions of the breast.

Cheatle drew heavily from his own detailed studies of whole-organ sections of the breast to examine the relationships of various lesions to carcinoma as part of a systematic exploration of pathologic processes in the breast. Bloodgood's approach was case oriented, dealing largely with an analysis of patients under his personal care at Johns Hopkins University over several decades. Because of his concern with current diagnostic and therapeutic problems in the operating room, much of Bloodgood's attention was directed to biopsy specimens. He was therefore able to relate the morphology of many lesions to clinical follow-up, sometimes of the unresected breast.

Early descriptions of intraductal carcinoma outlined the major structural patterns of the disease that are recognized today. Micropapillary carcinoma was illustrated by Cheatle in 1920 (2) and by Bloodgood (3) in 1921, but this term was not used by either author. Bloodgood also drew attention to the problem of distinguishing between "borderline" hyperplastic lesions and intraductal carcinoma (4). Cheatle referred to the micropapillary proliferation as *laciform* and noted the "cartwheel" appearance of carcinoma in a nearby duct. Today, many would describe the "cartwheel" focus as *cribriform*. Muir (5) attributed the term *cribriform* to Schultz-Brauns' article on breast carcinoma contained in Henke and Lubarsch's 1933 *Handbook* (6).

The existence of comedo and cribriform patterns of intraductal carcinoma is readily apparent in Bloodgood's picture, which illustrated a tumor classified as *comedocarcinoma* (7). The accompanying description provides an interesting historical vignette:

> In 1893, forty-one years ago, I assisted Dr. Halstead in exploring a clinically benign tumor of the breast. The patient was sixty-seven years of age and had observed a small tumor for about eleven months. . . . The moment we cut into and pressed on it, there extruded from its surface many grayish-white, granular cylinders, which I called at that time comedos. From the gross appearance the tumor was diagnosed as malignant, and the radical operation was performed. The nodes were not involved . . . [and] the patient lived nineteen years after operation, dying at age eighty-six. (7)

Bloodgood recognized two types of comedoadenocarcinoma, which he referred to as "pure comedoadenocarcinoma and comedoadenocarcinoma with areas of fully developed cancer of the breast," the former being entirely intraductal and the latter partly invasive. He observed that large tumors with gross comedo features were more likely to be in the invasive category. Follow-up revealed that 30% of node-negative patients with invasive comedodenocarcinoma developed metastases and died of the disease.

Bloodgood's 1934 paper described a patient who had a remarkable clinical course (7). One year after treatment by excision alone in 1896, the patient developed recurrent carcinoma at the site of the prior surgery. A radical mastectomy then was performed. The lymph nodes were negative, and the patient lived more than 15 years without additional recurrence. Because of the apparent curability of the "pure comedo tumor," Bloodgood preferred the term *comedoadenoma*. Treatment by local excision was recommended "when the palpable tumor is small and can be excised completely by cutting through normal breast tissue and closing the wound without injury to the symmetry of the breast" (7).

This description ranks as one the earliest of breast-conservation surgery for intraductal carcinoma. Needle aspiration and cytologic examination were used by Bloodgood for the diagnosis of breast tumors, especially so that "older women could be spared the complete operation for cancer by an aspiration biopsy when pure comedo tumor involving a large part of, or the entire breast, is recognized" (7). He found, however, that aspiration cytology could not be relied on for making a distinction between intraductal and invasive carcinoma. In the case of a woman with a 1.5-cm lesion, "the tumor had been aspirated before it was explored, and from examination of the stained aspirated cells we could only decide that they suggested a malignant tumor. We did not recognize the comedo tumor" (7).

In 1938, Lewis and Geschickter described 40 patients treated for comedocarcinoma, reporting a 5-year cure rate of 85%, with most 5-year survivors having remained well for 10 years (8). Included were eight women whose initial treatment was local excision only. Six of the eight developed recurrent carcinoma within 1 to 4 years. Unfortunately, these investigators did not distinguish between lesions that were entirely intraductal and those with concomitant invasive carcinoma.

Until recently, there was little clinical interest in the histologic subtypes of intraductal carcinoma. This situation probably derived from the fact that almost all patients were treated by mastectomy and the observation that the lesions rarely consisted of a single growth pattern, for as Cheatle observed, "whole sections reveal that all these varieties may occur in the same mass of disease" (9).

Confusion over the precise use of the term *intraductal carcinoma* can have a significant effect on clinical studies of the disease. Failure to distinguish clearly between noninvasive and invasive ductal carcinomas was reflected in Haagensen's conclusion that intraductal carcinomas "all are infiltrating and fully malignant even though we do not happen to see actual infiltration." This approach led him "to classify as intraductal only those carcinomas in which at least 50% of the carcinoma grew intraductally." When defined in this fashion, it was not surprising that 24% of his patients with Columbia stage A intraductal carcinoma had axillary metastases when treated by radical mastectomy and that the 10-year survival in this group was 74% (10). The fact that the National Breast Cancer Survey reported a 5-year disease-free survival of 74% for intraductal carcinoma suggests that some cases in this report were classified by criteria similar to those of Haagensen (11).

To avoid these problems, names such as *intraductal noninfiltrating carcinoma* and *preinvasive intraductal carcinoma* have been advocated (12,13). Whether one uses these terms or not, it is necessary to limit the diagnosis of intraductal carcinoma to lesions with no invasion demonstrable in light microscopic histologic sections if the term is to be meaningful clinically.

## CLINICAL PRESENTATION

The reported *frequency of intraductal carcinoma* in different studies is influenced by clinical circumstances. A review of approximately 1,000 consecutive women treated at a cancer center in the United States in the late 1970s revealed that 5% had intraductal carcinoma (14). Data from nine population-based registries included in the National Cancer Institute's Surveillance, Epidemiology and End Results (SEER) program for 1975 indicated that 2.9% of patients had intraductal carcinoma (15). A review of SEER data published in 1996 demonstrated a striking increase in the incidence of intraductal carcinoma after 1983 (16). This change was observed in black and white populations and in all age groups. Among women 30 to 39 years of age, the average annual increase in the incidence rate changed from 0.3% between 1973 and 1983 to 12.0% between 1983 and 1992. Similar increases were found for women 40 to 49 years of age (from 0.4% to 17.4%) and for women 50 years and older (from 5.2% to 18.1%). The estimated total number of cases of intraductal carcinoma in 1992 was 200% higher than expected based on 1983 rates. In this series, the anatomic distribution of intraductal carcinoma in the breast was similar to that of invasive carcinomas, with 44% of lesions in the upper outer quadrant. Further analysis of the SEER data indicated that the estimated number of new cases of intraductal carcinoma in 1993 was 23,275 (17). Approximately 4,676 cases were in women 40 to 49 years of age, representing about 15% of breast carcinoma in this age group.

The National Cancer Database reported that 3.7% of 31,930 breast carcinomas registered were classified as intraductal (18). The percentage rose to 7.0% and 9.5%, respectively, in 1990 (65,255 cases) and 1993 (93,915 cases). During the same period, the reported frequency of lobular carcinoma *in situ* was quite stable, accounting for 1.3% to 1.6% of cases annually.

A population-based study of Danish women in the 1980s revealed that 4% of newly diagnosed carcinomas were intraductal (19). Review of the records of the Connecticut Tumor Registry revealed a yearly increase in the number of cases in intraductal carcinoma reported (20). In 1979, the 33 diagnoses of intraductal carcinoma represented 1.8% of breast carcinomas, and in 1988 the 200 cases constituted 7.4% of breast carcinomas. Data from the New Mexico Tumor Registry revealed stable incidence figures for intraductal carcinoma in Hispanic-White, non-Hispanic-White, and Native American women for more than a decade before 1984 (21). Thereafter, the incidence rate increased annually in each ethnic group. In 1994, the incidence rates per 100,000 were 13.8, 9.7 and approximately 7.0, respectively, for non-Hispanic-White, Hispanic-White, and Native American women. The lower incidence rates in the latter groups may reflect less access to mammography rather than intrinsic ethnic differences in the biology of intraductal carcinoma.

The increased age-adjusted incidence of *in situ* breast carcinoma in the United States coincides with a leveling off in the overall age-adjusted incidence of invasive carcinoma and of localized carcinoma, and a decline in the incidence of invasive carcinoma classified as *regional* (22). These changes in incidence by stage have been accompanied by a significant decline in age-adjusted breast cancer mortality (22). The beneficial effects of mammography as a diagnostic or screening modality and of improved systemic therapy are reflected in these trends.

Data on *epidemiologic risk factors* for intraductal carcinoma are limited (23,24). There appear to be some age-related differences in associations, but overall the risk factors for intraductal carcinoma and invasive carcinoma appear to be similar (23). The risk for both lesions increases with age, an association that is stronger for invasive carcinoma.

*Mammography* is the most sensitive diagnostic procedure now available for detecting intraductal carcinoma (25). On initial screening, 8% to 43% of mammographically detected carcinomas were intraductal (26–32). From 25% to 30% of nonpalpable carcinomas detected by mammography were intraductal lesions (29,33–35). In a series of nearly 20,000 patients, 30 of 70 carcinomas (43%) found in biopsies performed only for clustered calcifications detected by mammography were intraductal carcinomas (30). Mammographically detected calcifications were found in 72% to 98% of intraductal carcinomas (36–38). The proportion of intraductal carcinomas was not substantially higher in subsequent mammography screening, but some investigators described a greater frequency of small invasive tumors in later examinations (26,31).

The interval between screening examinations can influence the clinical characteristics of intraductal carcinoma detected by mammography (39). The size of intraductal carcinoma determined by mammographic measurement was significantly smaller in women examined annually (mean, 1.69 cm; range, 0.3–7.7 cm) than in those examined on a biennial (mean, 2.27 cm; range, 0.4–10 cm) or triennial (mean, 3.49 cm; range, 0.6–10 cm) schedule. Comedo-type intraductal carcinomas were significantly more frequent in the biennial (73.7%) than in the annual (46.8%) screening group. Tumor size and nuclear grade were inversely related; the mean sizes for low, intermediate, and high-grade lesions were determined to be 1.19 cm, 1.85 cm, and 2.82 cm, respectively. The frequency of microinvasion tended to increase with longer intervals between examinations, but the differences were not statistically significant.

Approximately 10% to 15% of intraductal carcinomas are discovered as incidental lesions in biopsies performed for other indications, usually a palpable abnormality (25,35,38). Radiologic findings that lead to the detection of a small pro-

portion of "incidental" intraductal carcinomas are densities and asymmetric soft tissue changes, sometimes with microcalcifications in the noncarcinomatous abnormality. Calcifications alone are more likely to be the mammographic indicator of intraductal carcinoma in women younger than 50 years, whereas coexistent soft tissue abnormalities are evident more often in women older than 50, a distinction that probably results from variation in overall breast density in these age groups rather than from intrinsic tumor differences (38).

*Calcifications* associated with intraductal carcinoma are generally described as linear "casts" or as granular on mammography (Fig. 13.1). Round or oval, well-circumscribed calcifications are less common in intraductal carcinoma. Predominantly linear, granular, or mixed types of calcifications occur with about equal frequency. Calcifications may be clustered, dispersed, or dispersed around clustered foci. Branching calcifications with linear patterns that outline the distribution of one or more ducts may consist of casts or granular particles. The type of calcifications is not related to age at diagnosis or to the size of the area involved mammographically (38). The level of suspicion for intraductal carcinoma is a function of the character and the number of calcifications. Most intraductal carcinomas have five or more calcifications (38).

Despite the well-documented relationship between mammographically detected calcifications and intraductal carcinoma, it must be emphasized that calcifications may not be present in every duct segment involved by intraductal carcinoma, and that a minority of intraductal carcinomas have few or no detectable calcifications when examined histologically. Goldstein et al. reported that calcifications were not found histologically in 17% of intraductal carcinomas examined in a study of pathologic features associated with breast recurrence after conservation therapy (38a). Features associated with absence of histologically identifiable calcifications were little or no necrosis, and low nuclear grade and low grade growth pattern. Absence of microcalcifications identified histologically was significantly associated with an increased risk of breast recurrence after conservation therapy.

Calcifications observed in mammograms are often referred to in diagnostic reports and published articles with terms such as "benign," "indeterminate," "suspicious," or "malignant." Unfortunately this terminology has been misunderstood, especially by those outside the medical community as adjectives that apply to the calcifications themselves. In fact, all calcifications in breast tissue are inanimate precipitates containing calcium and other salts combined with proteins which are concentrated in many secretions. Calcifications do not invade breast tissue or metastasize, as does the carcinoma that arises from the cellular component of intraductal carcinoma. On occasion, invasive carcinoma in the breast and metastatic breast carcinoma also harbor calcifications, but these are newly formed in the invasive or metastatic foci.

The mammographic distribution of calcifications and

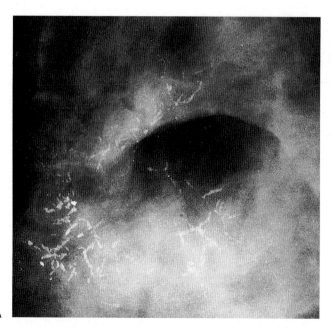
A

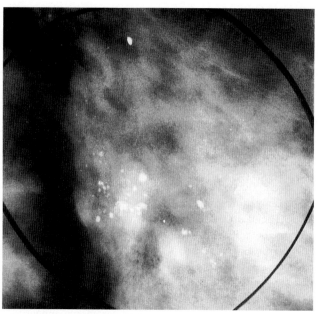
B

**FIG. 13.1.** *Intraductal carcinoma.* **A:** Mammogram showing branching linear calcifications found at biopsy to be an intraductal carcinoma, comedo type. **B:** Clustered irregular calcifications at the site of solid and cribriform intraductal carcinoma.

tissue density are guides to the extent of intraductal carcinoma or the dimensions of the involved area; however, these measurements tend to underestimate the size of the lesion compared with careful histologic sampling (40). When the extent of lesions was measured mammographically and pathologically, discrepancies were found more often between the interpretations for cases that were predominantly cribriform or micropapillary than for comedo intraductal carcinomas. A discrepancy of more than 20 mm was found in 44% of pure cribriform–micropapillary lesions, in 12% of pure comedocarcinomas, and in 50% of cases with both patterns (40). In patients who undergo mastectomy, extension of intraductal carcinoma to the nipple or subareolar region is more frequent with comedo than with cribriform–micropapillary intraductal carcinoma (40). The likelihood of detecting multifocal intraductal carcinoma radiologically and pathologically is related to the size of the lesion as determined by either procedure (36,41). Multifocality is appreciably more frequent in lesions larger than 2.0 to 2.5 cm than in smaller foci of intraductal carcinoma. Carlson et al. reported that the mean size of multifocal intraductal carcinoma (3.1 cm) was significantly greater than the size of nonmultifocal lesions (1.95 cm) (39).

The mammographic appearance of microcalcifications bears some relationship to the histologic type of the lesion; but, as noted by Stomper et al., "there is considerable overlap, and the predominant histologic subtype cannot be predicted on the basis of the microcalcification type with a high degree of accuracy" (42). Predominantly linear calcifications are found significantly more often in comedocarcinomas than in cribriform, papillary, or solid types, which typically contain granular calcifications (40,42). Nonetheless, 22% of linear calcifications were associated with noncomedocarcinomas, and 47% of granular calcifications occurred

in comedocarcinomas in one series (42). Computer programs developed for image analysis of calcifications have had some success in discriminating between comedo and noncomedo intraductal carcinomas (43). Abnormal mammograms without calcifications are more likely to call attention to intraductal carcinoma of the small cell type than the large cell type, regardless of the growth pattern (solid, cribriform, or mixed) of the lesion (44). Linear calcifications are a marker of necrosis, and granular calcifications are associated with intraductal carcinoma without necrosis (44). Intraductal carcinomas that express the HER2/*neu* oncogene are more likely to have calcifications detected by mammography than are HER2/*neu*-negative carcinomas (45).

*Unusual mammographic presentations* of intraductal carcinoma occur when the lesion has a configuration that suggests a benign tumor or invasive carcinoma. These patterns, which are reflective of associated soft tissue masses, are found in fewer than 10% of mammographically detected intraductal carcinomas (37,46–48). In one series, 8% of intraductal carcinomas were represented mammographically by stellate lesions without calcifications (48); in another report, 3.6% of intraductal carcinomas presented as stellate opacities (46). Three were pure intraductal carcinomas, and four proved to be intraductal carcinoma arising in benign radial sclerosing lesions or "radial scars." Microinvasion was found in only one case, despite the radiologic appearance suggesting invasive carcinoma in all instances. At the other end of the spectrum, intraductal carcinoma may be harbored by radiologically circumscribed lesions and appear to be benign (47). In addition to carcinoma arising in a fibroadenoma, these are usually examples of solid papillary intraductal carcinomas or nodular foci of comedocarcinoma. Microinvasion may be present (47).

*Magnetic resonance imaging* (MRI) may prove to be an effective method for detecting intraductal carcinomas that lack calcifications. Lesion detection is based on the finding of contrast enhancement in breast parenchyma after injection of a gadolinium contrast agent compared with the preinjection image (49–51). Orel et al. described three patterns of enhancement associated with intraductal carcinoma: ductal, regional, and a peripherally enhancing mass (52). The mean size of MRI-detected intraductal carcinomas was 10 mm. Correlation of immunohistochemical studies for vascularity and MRI characteristics of the lesions suggested that tumor angiogenesis contributed to MRI enhancement in one series (49).

Before the widespread use of mammography, *palpable tumors* were reportedly present in 50% to 65% of women who had intraductal carcinoma (53–55). A study comparing breast carcinomas diagnosed during 1973 through 1974 in Japan and the United States reported a higher frequency of intraductal carcinoma in Japanese patients and noted that the carcinomas tended to form bulky, palpable tumors in Japanese women (56). Pandya et al. compared the characteristics of intraductal carcinomas detected in preceding eras

(1969–1985) and after the "intensified use of screening" (1986–1990) at the Lahey Clinic (55). The proportion of mammographically detected cases increased from 19% to 80%, whereas palpable lesions decreased from 54% to 12%. The proportion of cases presenting with duct discharge and Paget's disease also decreased. Comedo intraductal carcinoma was found in 7% and 38% of palpable and mammographic lesions, respectively. These investigators observed that palpable intraductal carcinoma tended to be of lower grade than mammographically detected lesions and concluded that "mammographically detected ductal carcinoma *in situ* is not an inconsequential finding" (55).

Currently, intraductal carcinoma is not palpable in most patients who have this disease (57). Negative mammograms may be reported in up to 25% of cases, with a sensitivity ranging from 56% in women younger than 40 years to 67% in the 40- to 49-year age group and 76% in those 50 years or older (25). Nonpalpable lesions are detected because of mammographic findings, Paget's disease, nipple discharge, or as an incidental finding in a biopsy for a concurrent palpable benign tumor (33,57) (Fig. 13.2). About 25% of

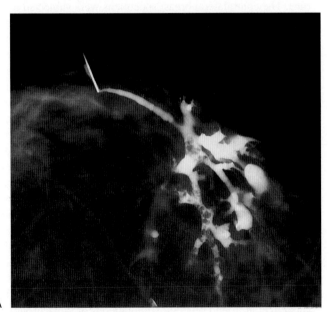

**FIG. 13.2.** *Intraductal carcinoma.* **A:** Ductogram from an 84-year-old woman with bloody nipple discharge. The cannulated lactiferous duct is seen in the *upper center.* Numerous defects in the white dye in ducts represent intraductal papillary lesions. **B:** Orderly papillary intraductal carcinoma in the lumen and micropapillary carcinoma at the periphery. **C:** Micropapillary intraductal carcinoma.

A

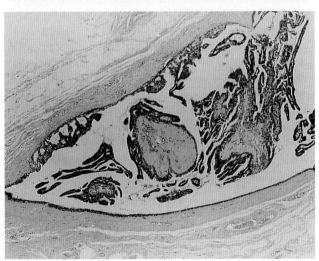

B

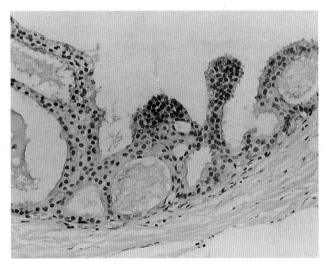

C

biopsies performed for "suspicious" calcifications reveal carcinoma, largely of the intraductal type (58,59). Duct hyperplasia and sclerosing adenosis account for most "significant" calcifications that do not prove to be carcinoma. Comedocarcinoma is the type most frequently detected by mammography alone, whereas micropapillary intraductal carcinoma is more often found as a result of a palpable lesion or other clinical sign (57).

The diagnosis of intraductal carcinoma requires histologic sections of excised breast tissue. Intraductal carcinoma can be recognized in *frozen sections,* but if any difficulty is encountered, the decision should be deferred immediately to permanent sections because there is a significant risk of trimming away the lesional area as more sections are made (60). Frozen section is not appropriate for the diagnosis of mammographically detected, nonpalpable lesions unless there are exceptional clinical circumstances. In one study of intraductal carcinomas, 50% of the lesions were diagnosed at the time of frozen section, 36% were reported to be benign, 8% were deferred, 5% were diagnosed as atypical hyperplasia, and one case was diagnosed as invasive (61). Approximately 3% of biopsies reported to be benign at frozen section prove to contain carcinoma when paraffin sections were examined (60). Because sampling of a biopsy is limited during surgery, approximately 20% of patients with a frozen-section diagnosis of intraductal carcinoma prove to have invasion after multiple paraffin sections of the same biopsy specimen have been examined (62).

Intraductal carcinoma occurs throughout the *age range* of breast carcinoma in women. The mean age at diagnosis of patients in multiple studies was between 50 and 59 years, quite similar to the mean age of women with invasive ductal carcinoma (25,57,63,64). There are no significant differences in the age distribution of structural subtypes of intraductal carcinoma (57). Young age at diagnosis, particularly before age 50, has been associated with an increased risk of recurrence in the breast after conservation therapy (38a,64a). Szelei-Stevens et al. (64a) reported that the impact of young age at diagnosis was seen largely in women treated by tylectomy without radiotherapy, and especially among patients with a family history of breast carcinoma. On the other hand, Harris et al. (64b) reported that a family history of breast carcinoma did not have a significant influence on local recurrence or survival among women treated by excision with radiotherapy, and that a family history was not significantly related to cosmesis or the risk of complications.

Limited data are available describing the frequency of *bilaterality* associated with intraductal carcinoma. Among 112 patients with intraductal carcinoma reported by Ashikari et al., 16 (14%) had concurrent contralateral carcinoma and 17 (15%) had undergone mastectomy previously for carcinoma (53). Westbrook and Gallager excluded an unstated number of patients with previous or concurrent contralateral invasive carcinoma from their study of intraductal carcinoma (54). Subsequent contralateral biopsies obtained from 14 of the 64 women included in the report revealed intraductal carcinoma

in five and invasion in three others, for an overall frequency of subsequent carcinoma in the opposite breast of 12.5%. The average length of follow-up was not stated. Brown et al. found that 10% of patients with intraductal carcinoma in one breast had contralateral invasive carcinoma, including three women treated previously for the contralateral lesion and one who subsequently developed contralateral carcinoma (12). No information about concurrent contralateral biopsies was provided. A population-based study of cases identified in the Connecticut Tumor Registry found that 22% of 217 patients with intraductal carcinoma in one breast had intraductal or invasive carcinoma in the opposite breast (20). Overall, 17% of the patients with intraductal carcinoma also had a nonmammary malignant neoplasm.

A systematic evaluation of the contralateral breast was reported by Urban, who biopsied the opposite breast in 70% of his cases (65). Among 16 women with intraductal carcinoma treated between 1966 and 1968, he found that three (19%) had undergone a prior contralateral mastectomy. No patients had simultaneous bilaterality. Ringberg et al. carried out bilateral mastectomy in patients with unilateral carcinoma (66). The contralateral breast specimens were subjected to a detailed pathologic analysis. Among 23 women with intraductal carcinoma in one breast, the distribution of contralateral disease was as follows: lobular carcinoma *in situ* (LCIS), two cases (9%); intraductal carcinoma, three cases (13%); invasive carcinoma, two cases (9%). Simultaneous contralateral mastectomy in 25 of 78 patients who had noncomedo intraductal carcinoma in one breast revealed contralateral intraductal carcinoma in 3 (12%) (67). The type of intraductal carcinoma and indications for performing the operation in these cases were not indicated. Schuh et al. reported that 7 of 52 (13%) patients with intraductal carcinoma had previously undergone a contralateral mastectomy for carcinoma (68). Simultaneous bilateral carcinoma was found in 3 of the remaining 45 (7%) women, including two contralateral invasive lesions and one with LCIS. Schwartz et al. reported that 3 of 47 (6%) patients with nonpalpable intraductal carcinoma treated by mastectomy had clinically detected intraductal carcinoma in the opposite breast (69). Silverstein et al. found bilateral simultaneous or metachronous carcinoma in 22 of 208 (11%) patients with pure or microinvasive intraductal carcinoma, including 5 (2.4%) with bilateral intraductal lesions (64). Ciatto et al. reported contralateral carcinoma in 44 of 350 (13%) women with intraductal carcinoma, including nine (3%) with synchronous bilateral intraductal, 9(3%) with synchronous invasive, two (6%) with metachronous invasive, and five (1.4%) with metachronous intraductal carcinoma (25). After excluding synchronous contralateral carcinoma, Ciatto et al. calculated the frequency of metachronous contralateral carcinoma based on breast-years at risk to be 8.5%, 5.6 times the expected risk of 1.5% for unilateral breast carcinoma in a normal population (25).

The occurrence of contralateral carcinoma in women with intraductal carcinoma was studied in a population-based cancer registry from the state of Washington by Habel et al. (70). These investigators identified 1,929 women with intraductal carcinoma diagnosed in one breast between 1974 and 1993. Contralateral invasive carcinoma developed at a rate twice that of the control population. When contralateral *in situ* carcinoma was found, it was intraductal in 78% of these patients. The detection rate for contralateral intraductal carcinoma was highest in the first year after diagnosis of the ipsilateral lesion, with a relative risk (RR) compared with controls of 21.4 [95% confidence interval (CI) 11.8–38.7]. Five years or longer after ipsilateral diagnosis, the RR was 3.1 [95% CI, 1.0–9.8]. The RR for detecting contralateral invasive carcinoma remained fairly constant during follow-up (RR = 1.9: 95% CI = 1.0–3.6 up to 1 year and 2.1: 95% CI = 1.4–3.3 after 4 years).

The frequency of subsequent invasive carcinoma in the contralateral breast of women with intraductal carcinoma was 4.3% in one series, considerably less than for patients with LCIS (71). A similar observation was recorded by Habel et al. (70), who found that the RR of contralateral invasive carcinoma was 1.8 (95% CI = 1.4–2.4) for women with ipsilateral intraductal carcinoma and 3.0 (95% CI = 1.7–5.1) for women with LCIS when compared with a control population.

Most deaths from breast carcinoma recorded in patients with intraductal carcinoma in one breast have been due to invasive carcinoma of the contralateral breast (25,33,53). Deaths from contralateral invasive carcinoma were reported in 3.6% (53), 1.9% (46), and 1.0% (25) of cases; in two of these studies, deaths caused by invasive recurrence in the ipsilateral breast occurred in 2 of 140, or 1.4% (25) and in 2 of 61, or 3.2% (46) of patients treated with breast conservation.

## GROSS PATHOLOGY

Nonpapillary intraductal carcinoma is usually not evident grossly. Comedocarcinoma involving multiple ducts occasionally produces a firm mass (Fig. 13.3). These lesions tend to be well-defined, tan tumors with white to pale yellow flecks composed of necrotic intraductal carcinoma (comedos) that extrude from the cut surface when the lesion is compressed. Abundant calcification in the lesion imparts a gritty sensation on cutting into the tumor. Although these findings are suggestive of comedocarcinoma, an identical gross appearance is found in some cases of stasis and mastitis.

Most classifications of intraductal carcinoma have been based on histopathologic features of the lesions, but some investigators have drawn attention to the distinction between grossly apparent and microscopic lesions. Gump et al. studied 70 consecutive patients treated in one institution for lesions classified as intraductal carcinoma on an initial biopsy (72). Fifty-four (77%) had lesions classified as "gross" because the patient presented with a palpable tumor, nipple discharge, or Paget's disease. Most of these patients (48 of 54, or 89%) had a mass. Microscopic intraductal carcinoma in

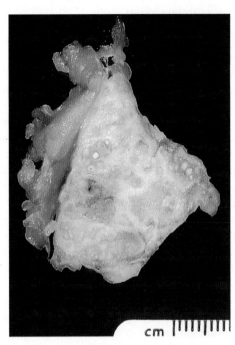

**FIG. 13.3.** *Intraductal carcinoma, comedo.* Gross biopsy specimen showing numerous round, pale yellow foci of comedonecrosis.

16 (23%) was nonpalpable and detected by mammographic calcifications or as an incidental finding. Invasive carcinoma was found in six (12%) surgical specimens subsequent to an initial biopsy that revealed gross intraductal carcinoma but not in the patients who had microscopic intraductal carcinoma. Axillary lymph node metastases were found in only one patient with a gross lesion and not in any patient with microscopic intraductal carcinoma.

A slightly more complex classification based on anatomic distribution was proposed by Andersen et al. (73), who identified three types of growth patterns, which can occur individually or in combinations. "Microfocal" lesions involved "one or a few lobules or ducts" measuring up to 5 mm. "Diffuse" intraductal carcinoma involved a region of 5 to 10 mm or an entire segment of the breast, and the "tumor-forming" type consisted of closely connected glandular structures that may occupy an area of 60 to 70 mm, resulting in a palpable mass. Microfocal and diffuse types of intraductal carcinoma were typically not palpable. A population-based review of cases revealed that 18 of 35 (51%) patients with intraductal carcinoma had microfocal lesions, 13 (37%) had the diffuse type, and 4 (11%) had tumor-forming intraductal carcinoma (19). No axillary lymph node metastases were found in any of the patients who had an axillary dissection.

The classifications proposed by Gump et al. and Andersen et al. drew a distinction between clinically apparent ("gross") and clinically inapparent ("microscopic") presentations of intraductal carcinoma. These groupings are applicable in current clinical practice because they are related to lesion size and therefore to local control in patients treated by breast-conservation therapy.

## MICROSCOPIC PATHOLOGY

The microanatomic site of origin of many intraductal carcinomas appears to be in the *terminal duct–lobular unit (TDLU)*. The most convincing evidence for this conclusion comes from the subgross microdissection studies of Wellings et al. (74). Expanded TDLUs sometimes resemble primary or secondary segmental ducts, but their lobular origin is suggested by an excessive number of duct structures within a low-power microscopic field. Exceptions can be found to the concept of the TDLU origin of intraductal carcinoma. For example, it does not readily describe intraductal carcinoma limited to major central lactiferous ducts, which sometimes is associated with Paget's disease or presents with nipple discharge. Occasionally, random sections disclose foci of intraductal carcinoma in sections of one or more segmental ducts with no apparent lobular connection, even when the lesion is traced with serial sections. The relative frequency of origin from the TDLU or from larger duct structures and the clinical significance of this distinction remain to be determined.

The historical origins of the terminology used to describe the conventional structural variants of intraductal carcinoma are discussed in Chapter 11. The microscopic classification of intraductal carcinoma became the subject of heightened interest after the widespread introduction of breast conservation therapy. Concern with factors associated with the success or failure of this therapy directed attention not only to variants described on the basis of growth pattern, but also to finer cytologic details.

The spectrum of histologic patterns of intraductal carcinoma in men does not differ appreciably from the appearance of the disease in women, but there is a higher proportion of papillary intraductal carcinoma and comedocarcinoma is less frequent in men.

In standard histologic sections, intraductal carcinoma is confined within the lumens of ducts and lobules involved in the process. When studied by immunohistochemistry for laminin or type IV collagen, basement membranes in intraductal carcinomas appear intact or focally discontinuous (75–77). The presence or absence of mitotic figures is not a definitive feature in the diagnosis of intraductal carcinoma because mitoses also may be found rarely in normal and hyperplastic epithelium; however, the finding of one or more mitoses per 10 high-power fields suggests intraductal carcinoma. Myoepithelial cells may be retained in intraductal carcinoma, and they are occasionally hyperplastic at the periphery of the duct (Fig. 13.4). Experimental evidence suggests that myoepithelial cells may have a paracrine tumor suppressor effect on intraductal carcinoma, acting to inhibit invasion (78). Carcinoma cells nearest to the basement membrane exhibit loss of basal polarity and cellular crowding. Rarely, remnants of nonneoplastic normal or hyperplastic duct epithelium persist in ducts involved by intraductal carcinoma.

The range of subtle differences in cell type found in intraductal carcinomas usually engenders little comment, but certain distinct variants have been identified and described by specific names. *Signet-ring cells*, usually associated with lobular carcinoma, also occur in intraductal carcinomas, most often in the papillary and cribriform types (Fig. 13.5). The presence of signet-ring cells with cytoplasmic mucin demonstrated with the mucicarmine, periodic-acid Schiff, or Alcian blue stains is convincing evidence for a diagnosis of intraductal carcinoma. These cells are present only rarely in hyperplastic duct lesions. Signet-ring cells have eccentric nuclei that are often indented along the nuclear border, which abuts on the cytoplasmic mucin vacuole. A minute droplet of secretion may be apparent in the vacuole. Nonspecific clear holes in the cytoplasm can be mistaken for signet-ring vacuoles. These cytoplasmic defects, sometimes the site of glycogen accumulation, are not reactive with stains for mucin, they usually do not indent the nucleus, and there is ordinarily no secretion evident in the lumen.

*Apocrine cytology* is encountered in all of the structural types of intraductal carcinoma (Fig. 13.6). Apocrine intraductal carcinoma cells have abundant cytoplasm that ranges from granular and eosinophilic to vacuolated or clear. There is variable nuclear pleomorphism, sometimes manifested by prominent nucleoli. A more complete discussion of apocrine carcinoma can be found in Chapter 21.

*Clear cell intraductal carcinoma* is a poorly defined variant that typically is encountered with solid and comedo patterns (Fig. 13.7). Some clear cell intraductal carcinomas are composed of cells with an arrangement described as "mosaic" because of the appearance created by sharply defined cell borders (Fig. 13.7). A subset of lesions classified under this heading are forms of apocrine carcinoma. The presence of a monomorphic clear cell population is highly suggestive of intraductal carcinoma. Occasionally, clear cell intraductal carcinomas are strongly mucicarmine positive. Other clear cell lesions are probably the *in situ* form of lipid-rich or glycogen-rich carcinomas, which are discussed in Chapters 29 and 30, respectively.

The cellular composition of intraductal carcinomas is typically *monomorphic*. This term has been applied especially to cribriform, solid, and micropapillary carcinomas as well as to LCIS. In this context, monomorphic means that there is overall homogeneity in the cytologic appearance of the lesion, although all cells are not identical in such features as the amount of cytoplasm or nuclear size. Variability in these parameters derives in part from differences in the plane in which they are sectioned. Cell and nuclear shape may be altered by the presence or absence of crowding in one or another part of the duct. The presence of a myoepithelial cell layer is not a consideration in judging whether a ductal proliferation is monomorphic as long as these cells are confined to the periphery of the duct.

Dimorphic variants of intraductal carcinoma consisting of two distinctly different populations of cells are unusual. Most dimorphic intraductal carcinomas are papillary carcinomas (see Chapter 16). A dimorphic papillary intraductal

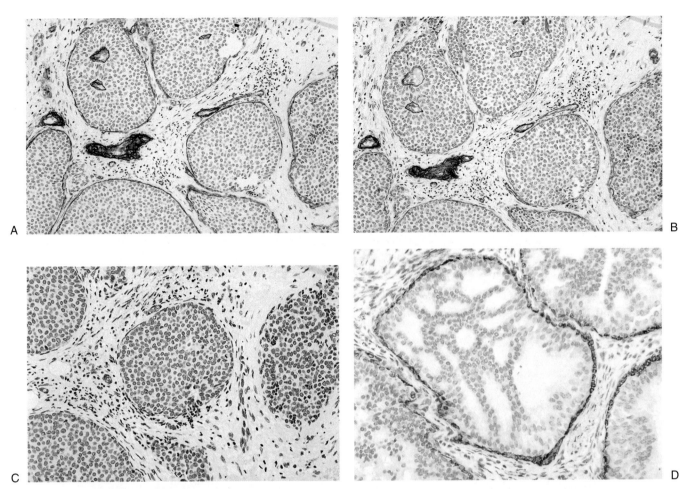

**FIG. 13.4.** *Intraductal carcinoma, basal lamina and myoepithelial cells.* Images **A–C** are from the same specimen. **A:** The basal lamina is highlighted by the immunostain for collagen type IV. Reactivity is also present around small blood vessels, including vessels in the upper two ducts. **B:** Laminin reactivity shown here has the same distribution as collagen type IV. **C:** There is no reactivity for smooth-muscle actin, indicating absence of myoepithelial cells. **D:** In this example of cribrifrom intraductal carcinoma, myoepithelial cells are highlighted by the smooth-muscle actin immunostain (avidin-biotin).

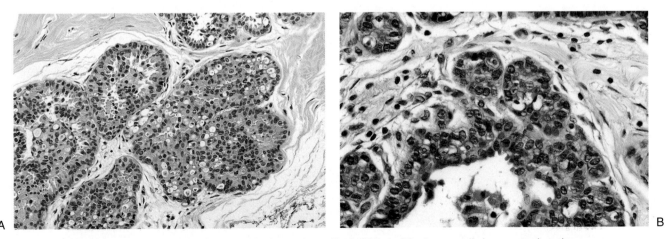

**FIG. 13.5.** *Intraductal carcinoma with signet-ring cells.* **A:** Many of the tumor cells have cytoplasmic vacuoles that contain condensed secretion. **B:** The secretion is strongly positive with the mucicarmine stain shown here.

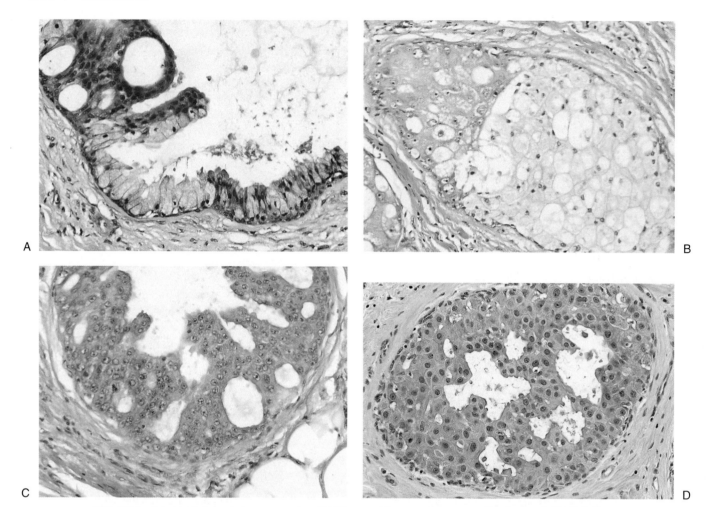

**FIG. 13.6.** *Intraductal carcinoma, apocrine.* **A:** Micropapillary carcinoma, partly clear cell. **B:** Cribriform carcinoma, partly clear cell. **C:** Cribriform carcinoma with high nuclear grade. **D:** Cribriform carcinoma with low and intermediate nuclear grade.

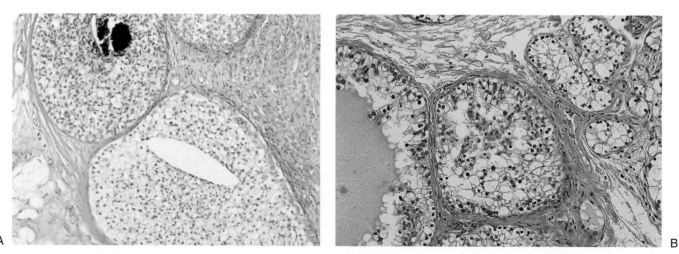

**FIG. 13.7.** *Intraductal carcinoma, clear cell.* **A:** Solid carcinoma with calcification. **B:** Solid carcinoma with intermediate nuclear grade. Note the mosaic-like appearance created by well-defined cell borders. *(continued)*

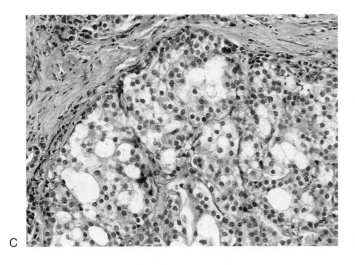

C

**FIG. 13.7.** *Continued.* **C:** Cribriform carcinoma.

carcinoma with a small invasive component of mucinous carcinoma is illustrated in Fig. 13.8. Other manifestations of dimorphic intraductal carcinoma are cited in the following discussion.

Intraductal carcinoma in a given patient can have more than a single microscopic structural, cytologic, or immuno-

cytochemical phenotype (57). Mixed histologic patterns are found in 30% to 40% of cases. Whereas some structural combinations, such as papillary– or micropapillary–cribriform and solid–comedo, occur relatively more often than others, there is considerable heterogeneity with respect to growth patterns (79). The probability of structural variability

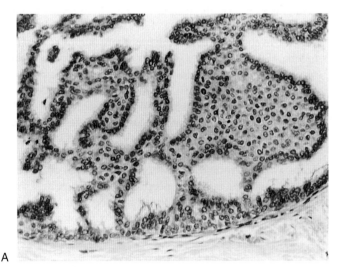

A

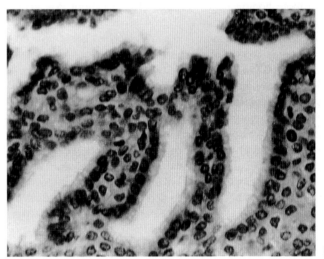

B

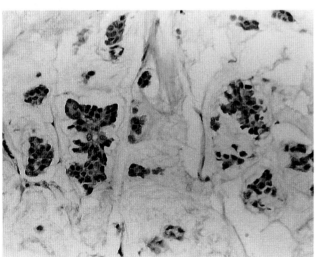

C

**FIG. 13.8.** *Intraductal carcinoma, dimorphic.* **A:** Papillary structure with two cell types. **B:** Cuboidal cells with basally oriented nuclei on the surface and intervening bands of polygonal cells. The two cell types have similar nuclear cytology. **C:** Invasive mucinous carcinoma that arose from this dimorphic intraductal carcinoma.

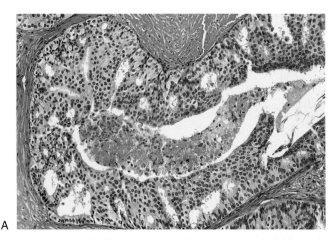
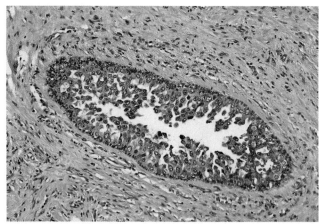

**FIG. 13.9.** *Intraductal carcinoma, discordant structure and nuclear grade.* **A:** Cribriform intraductal carcinoma with low nuclear grade and necrosis. **B:** Micropapillary intraductal carcinoma with high nuclear grade.

increases with the size of the lesion. The histologic diagnosis of intraductal carcinoma should list the structural types present in order of decreasing prominence, placing the dominant pattern first.

Cytologic features, especially at the nuclear level, tend to be more homogeneous than the growth pattern in a given case. Some combinations of growth patterns and cytologic appearances occur more frequently, such as classic comedocarcinoma composed of poorly differentiated pleomorphic cells or the low nuclear grade typically present in micropapillary carcinoma. Heterogeneity is illustrated by lesions with small, cytologically low-grade nuclei growing in a solid pattern or by high-grade nuclei found in some examples of micropapillary carcinoma (Fig. 13.9). The presence of two or more structural patterns that have different cytologic features is particularly unusual (Fig. 13.10). Classification schemes developed to take cognizance of the heterogeneous distribution of nuclear grade and necrosis across the spectrum of structural patterns are considered subsequent to a discussion of the current conventional structural classification.

*Micropapillary intraductal carcinoma* consists of ducts lined by a layer of neoplastic cells giving rise at intervals to papillary fronds or arcuate formations protruding into the lumen. When micropapillae are inconspicuous or absent, this type of intraductal carcinoma has been described as flat or "clinging" because the neoplastic epithelium seems to hug the basement membrane (Fig. 13.11) (80). The papillae are variable in appearance, ranging from short bumps or mounds to long, slender processes (Fig. 13.12). The papillae lack a fibrovascular core and are composed of cytologically homogenous carcinoma cells. Lesions in which the carcinomatous epithelium is supported by fibrovascular stroma should be classified as papillary carcinomas, even if the growth pattern is predominantly micropapillary (Fig. 13.13). Arcuate structures, commonly referred to as *Roman bridge arches*, occur when microlumens are formed by adjacent coalescent fronds or within a mound of neoplastic cells. These fenestrations resemble the lumens formed in cribriform intraductal carcinoma (Fig. 13.14). In conjunction with micropapillae, these arches are a feature of micropapillary intraductal carcinoma and do not warrant a diagnosis of cribriform

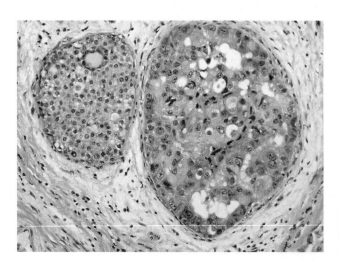

**FIG. 13.10.** *Intraductal carcinoma.* The smaller duct contains solid carcinoma with low nuclear grade, and the larger duct contains cribriform carcinoma with necrosis and high nuclear grade.

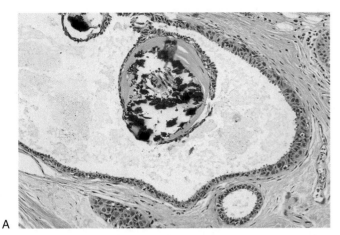

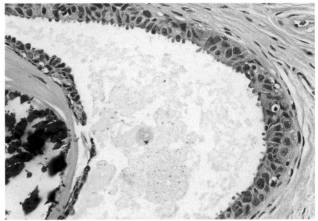

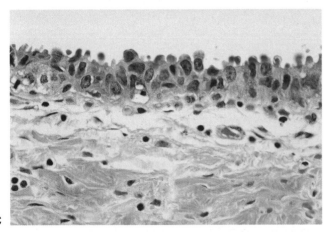

FIG. 13.11. *Intraductal carcinoma, flat ("clinging") micropapillary type.* **A:** The papillary structures in this cystically dilated duct contain fractured calcifications of the ossifying type typically associated with columnar cell lesions. **B:** Carcinoma cells with pleomorphic nuclei and a disorderly distribution line the duct and overlie the calcification. **C:** Magnified view of the flat ductal epithelium, which displays apical apocrine-type cytoplasmic "snouts."

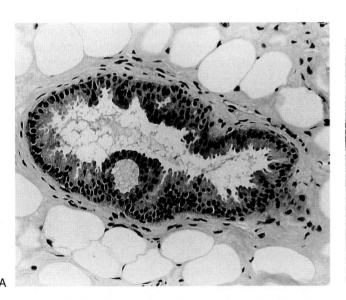

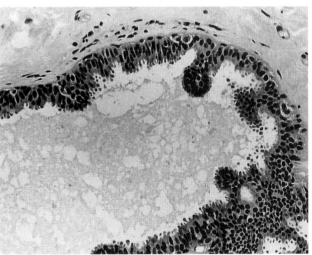

FIG. 13.12. *Intraductal carcinoma, micropapillary.* **A:** Mixed flat and low micropapillary carcinoma. Note the nuclear hyperchromasia. **B:** Crowded epithelium forming blunt micropapillary carcinoma. *(continued)*

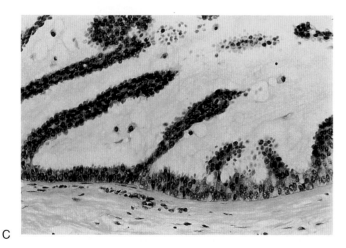

C

**FIG. 13.12.** *Continued.* **C:** Long micropapillary fronds.

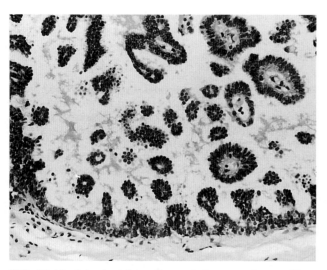

**FIG. 13.13.** *Intraductal papillary carcinoma, micropapillary.* Some epithelial fronds have fibrovascular centers.

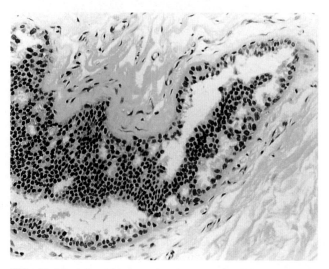

**FIG. 13.14.** *Intraductal carcinoma, micropapillary.* Intraductal growth developing a cribriform structure.

intraductal carcinoma, but in some situations the micropapillary and cribriform patterns merge (Fig. 13.15). Some samples of micropapillary intraductal carcinoma develop complex frond-forming structures without evolving into cribriform growth (Fig. 13.16).

The appearance of the micropapillary fronds varies somewhat with the plane of individual histologic sections. Whereas some micropapillae are cut perpendicular to their long axis, others are sectioned tangentially or transversely, resulting in irregular nests of seemingly detached cell clusters in the duct lumen (Fig. 13.16). Ducts with low-nuclear-grade micropapillary intraductal carcinoma are usually relatively free of cellular debris or inflammatory cells. Calcifications that are granular, crystalline, or laminated occur in a minority of cases, particularly when carcinoma arises in a background of columnar cell hyperplasia (Fig. 13.11).

In micropapillary intraductal carcinoma, the normal epithelial layer of the duct is replaced by a population of neoplastic cells. In any given case, the appearance of the carcinoma cells is relatively homogeneous, but cytologic heterogeneity can occur between individual cases. Most often, micropapillary intraductal carcinoma is composed of cytologically low-grade homogeneous cells with a high nuclear:cytoplasmic ratio and dense, hyperchromatic nuclei (Figs. 13.12, 13.14, and 13.15). The nuclei typically vary little in size, and chromatin density is consistent between cells at the base and tip of micropapillae. Nuclei may be slightly smaller and darker at the surface, but marked disparity in these characteristics is a feature of micropapillary hyperplasia (see Chapter 9). At the margin of the duct, between papillary and arcuate structures, the neoplastic cells typically are arranged in a layer that rarely exceeds three cells in depth. The nuclei of the cells in the epithelium between micropapillae usually are distributed unevenly in relation to the basement membrane (Figs. 13.12, 13.14, and 13.16). Persistent nonneoplastic epithelium between micropapillae is more often a feature of micropapillary hyperplasia rather than of micropapillary carcinoma. Mitoses are rarely present

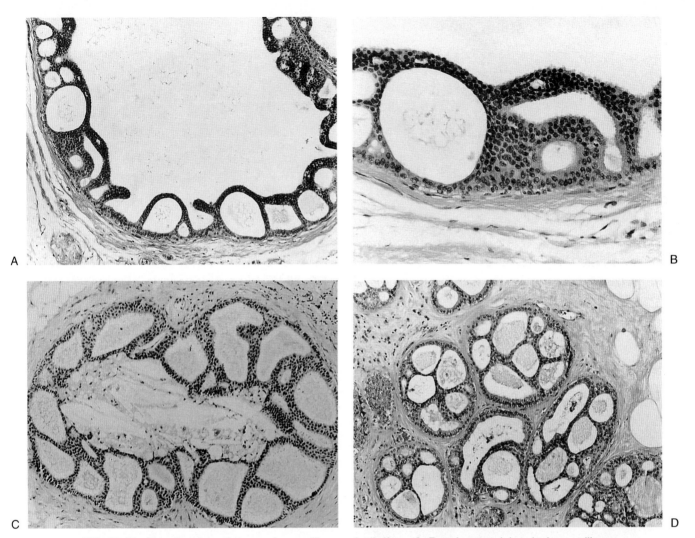

**FIG. 13.15.** *Intraductal carcinoma, micropapillary and cribriform.* **A:** Prominent peripheral micropapillary arches with secondary cribriform microlumens. (From Rosen PP. The pathology of breast carcinoma. In: Harris JR, Hellman S, Henderson IC, et al. eds. *Breast diseases.* Philadelphia: JB Lippincott, 1987:150, with permission.) **B:** Enlarged view of **A** showing low-grade nuclei. **C:** Large peripheral arcades that encroach on the lumen, which contains histiocytes. (From Rosen PP, Oberman HA. Tumors of the mammary gland. In: *Atlas of tumor pathology.* Washington, DC.: Armed Forces Institute of Pathology, 1993, with permission.) **D:** Intraductal carcinoma with a fully developed cribriform structure that can arise in the patient with micropapillary intraductal carcinoma.

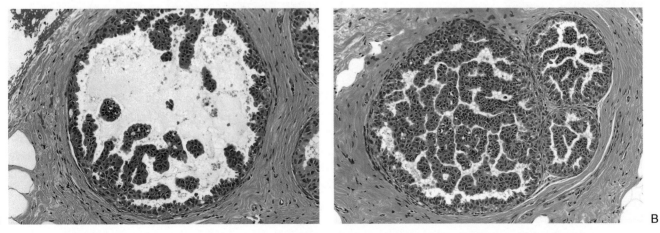

**FIG. 13.16.** *Intraductal carcinoma, micropapillary.* **A:** An example of relatively uncomplicated micropapillary intraductal carcinoma with apocrine cytology and intermediate nuclear grade. **B:** Florid micropapillary intraductal carcinoma with numerous epithelial fronds filling the duct lumen. Both images are from the same patient.

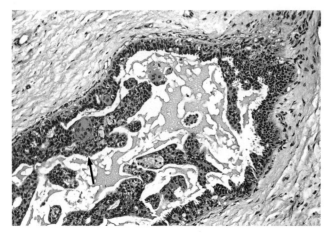

**FIG. 13.17.** *Micropapillary intraductal carcinoma with squamous metaplasia.* Squamous metaplasia is present in the micropapillary carcinomatous epithelium *(arrow).*

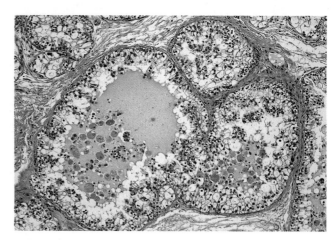

**FIG. 13.18.** *Intraductal carcinoma, micropapillary clear cell type.*

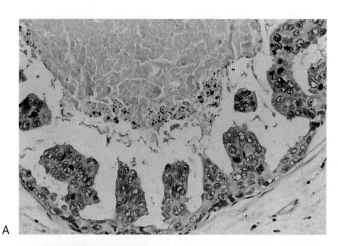

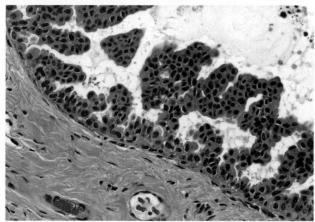

**FIG. 13.19.** *Intraductal carcinoma, micropapillary.* **A:** The cells have a poorly differentiated nuclear grade, and there is central necrosis in the duct. **B:** Apocrine cytology and intermediate nuclear grade. **C:** An unusual micropapillary intraductal carcinoma with intermediate nuclear grade and crystalloids.

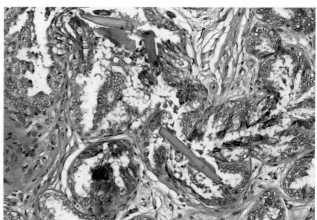

in cytologically low-grade micropapillary intraductal carcinoma. The carcinoma cells tend to be so crowded and overlapping that their individual borders and cytoplasm cannot be identified. Occasionally, the cells have slightly more abundant cytoplasm, with apocrine-type protrusions at the luminal border. In one variant of this cell type, the nuclei of the tumor cells are contained in cytoplasmic blebs that are extruded into the duct lumen. Low-grade micropapillary intraductal carcinoma can be found near some tubular carcinomas. These patients often have multifocal columnar cell hyperplasia with atypia and LCIS (see Chapter 9). Squamous metaplasia can be encountered in micropapillary intraductal carcinoma (Fig. 13.17). Clear cell micropapillary intraductal carcinoma is extremely uncommon (Fig. 13.18).

A minority of micropapillary carcinomas are composed of cells with intermediate or high-grade (poorly differentiated) cytologic characteristics (Figs. 13.9, 13.16, and 13.19). Cells forming this type of carcinoma differ from those in the conventional micropapillary lesions by being larger and having more abundant cytoplasm. Nuclei are also correspondingly larger, and nucleoli may be apparent. Mitoses can be found in this epithelium, and the cells often have a distinctly apocrine appearance. The cytologically high-grade form of micropapillary intraductal carcinoma is more likely to have calcifications than the low-grade variant, and necrotic cellular debris may be found in the duct lumen.

Two subtypes of micropapillary carcinoma have been given specific designations. *Cystic hypersecretory intraductal carcinoma* is discussed in Chapter 26. The term *flat micropapillary carcinoma* (clinging carcinoma) refers to intraductal carcinoma with the cytologic appearance of the micropapillary lesion that is lacking in fully developed epithelial fronds (Fig. 13.11). Lesions composed entirely of flat micropapillary intraductal carcinoma are uncommon, and more often one or more epithelial fronds or bridges are present (Fig. 13.11). In the absence of calcification or necrosis, flat micropapillary intraductal carcinoma can be easily overlooked microscopically. This type of intraductal carcinoma is encountered most often in a background of columnar cell hyperplasia (CCH), which occurs mainly in women 35 to 55 years of age. The lesions are typically multifocal or multicentric and can be bilateral. Calcifications with distinctive crystalline, ossifying and laminated appearances tend to occur in CCH, leading to mammographic detection. Patients with CCH may have tubular carcinoma, LCIS, and invasive lobular carcinoma as well as micropapillary intraductal carcinoma.

*Cribriform intraductal carcinoma* is a fenestrated epithelial proliferation in which microlumens are formed by neoplastic epithelium that bridges most or all of the duct lumen. Cribriform carcinoma can be found at all levels of the main duct system from major ducts to terminal intralobular ductules. Extension of intraductal carcinoma into lobular epithelium (so-called lobular cancerization) or into the main lactiferous ducts of the nipple is uncommon. Markedly dilated ducts with cribriform intraductal carcinoma can be mistaken for adenoid cystic carcinoma or a complex papilloma. Collagenous spherulosis, which usually is associated with hyperplastic duct lesions, in rare instances, can be involved by intraductal carcinoma (Fig. 13.20). The resultant structure resembles cribriform intraductal carcinoma because the spherules simulate microlumens. The presence of collagenous spherulosis can be confirmed with an actin immunostain, which will highlight myoepithelial cells at the perimeter of spherules or immunostains for basement membrane components. LCIS also can inhabit collagenous spherulosis. The distinction between intraductal and lobular carcinoma in collagenous spherulosis depends on the cytologic features of the lesion. Immunoreactivity for E-cadherin is weak and discontinuous in lobular carcinoma that involves collagenous spherulosis, whereas strong E-cadherin reactivity occurs in intraductal carcinoma in this setting. A mucin stain is useful for detecting intracytoplasmic mucin, which more often occurs in LCIS. The appearance of coexisting *in situ* carcinoma

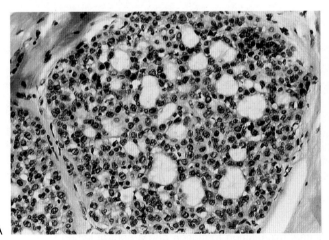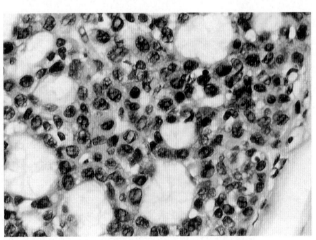

**FIG. 13.20.** *Intraductal carcinoma in collagenous spherulosis.* **A:** The spherules simulate a cribriform pattern. **B:** Stellate fibrils are visible in some spherules. Note the thin bands that define the perimeter of spherules. The carcinoma cells show moderate nuclear pleomorphism and intermediate nuclear grade. The carcinoma cells were immunoreactive for E-cadherin.

not in collagenous spherulosis also can be helpful (see Chapter 33).

The secondary microlumens in cribriform intraductal carcinoma tend to be round or oval, with smooth luminal edges bordered by cuboidal cells (Fig. 13.21). The distribution of microlumens is variable. In some instances, the spaces are spread across the entire duct or concentrated toward the center. The presence of microlumens entirely at the periphery of the duct is usually an indication of hyperplasia with atypia, but this appearance may be mimicked in cribriform intraductal carcinoma when the center of the duct is destroyed by necrosis (Fig. 13.22). It is a hallmark of cribriform intraductal carcinoma that the microlumens be surrounded by a homogeneous cell population that is uniformly distributed throughout the duct. The microlumens may contain secretion, small numbers of degenerated or necrotic cells, and punctate calcifications.

Bands of neoplastic cells between and around the microlumens in cribriform carcinoma are described as "rigid," a term that refers to the uniform, nonoverlapping, distribution of polygonal cells, in contrast to the streaming pattern of overlapping, frequently oval cells in duct hyperplasia (Fig. 13.23). Polarization of the cells in an orderly fashion around the microlumens contributes to the "rigid" appearance. The most orderly type of cribriform intraductal carcinoma is composed of cuboidal to low columnar monomorphic cells with low nuclear grade. Nucleoli are inconspicuous or absent, and mitoses are rarely encountered. The cells usually have sparse cytoplasm. An apocrine variant is composed of cells with low- to intermediate-grade nuclei and more abundant granular eosinophilic cytoplasm (Fig. 13.24). Secretion is found in some but not all cribriform microlumens, and, when present, it can form small calcifications. Cribriform intraductal carcinoma with necrosis, mitotic activity, and

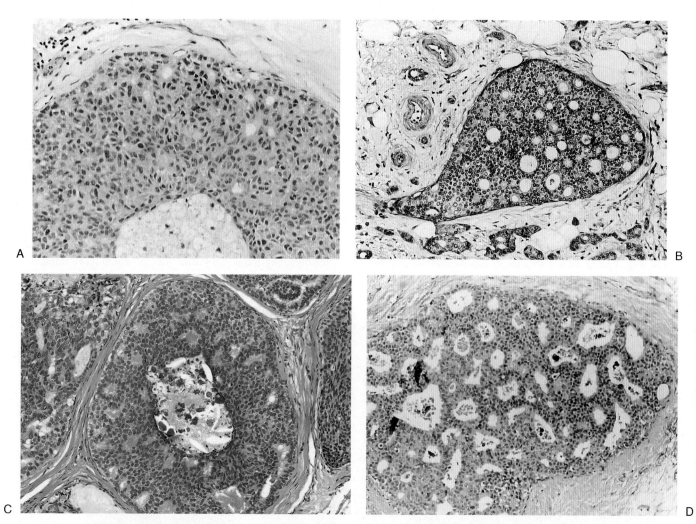

**FIG. 13.21.** *Intraductal carcinoma, cribriform.* **A:** Minimal microlumen formation and a central lumen (*lower border*) that contains histiocytes. Nuclei are low grade. **B:** Round microlumens throughout the duct. Invasive carcinoma is present in the surrounding stroma. **C:** Central and peripheral microlumens with central necrosis and calcifications. **D:** Microlumens with irregular contours containing cellular debris and calcifications.

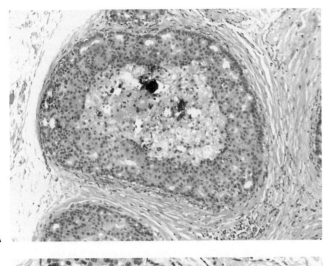

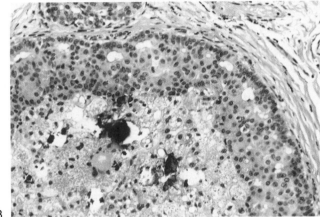

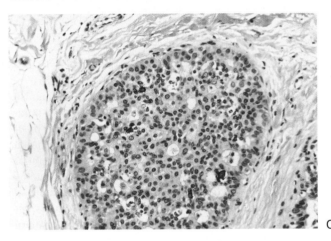

**FIG. 13.22.** *Intraductal carcinoma, cribriform.* **A:** Peripheral microlumens, some of which are slit-shaped, and a prominent central lumen with degenerating cells and calcification. **B:** Magnified view showing degenerating tumor cells in the lumen. **C:** Another duct from the same specimen with a conventional cribriform structure.

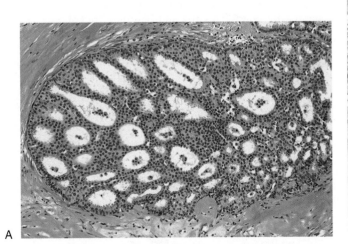

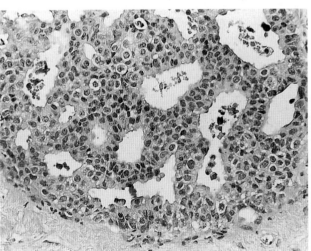

**FIG. 13.23.** *Intraductal carcinoma, cribriform.* **A:** Round and oval microlumens with smooth contours. **B:** Microlumens with irregular shapes and scalloped contours.

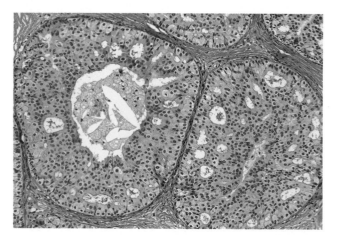

**FIG. 13.24.** *Intraductal carcinoma, cribriform.* Apocrine features with low to intermediate nuclear grade.

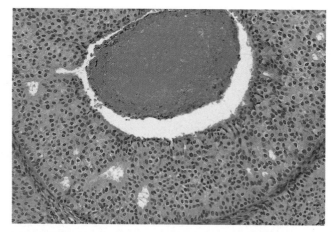

**FIG. 13.26.** *Intraductal carcinoma, predominantly solid with microlumens.* Central necrosis is present in this duct with low nuclear grade.

poorly differentiated nuclear grade is rare, and these lesions tend to have less well-defined microlumens (Fig. 13.25).

In some circumstances, it may be difficult to distinguish between cribriform and other structural subtypes of intraductal carcinoma, and in these instances the choice is sometimes arbitrary. Fibrovascular stroma and myoepithelial cells are not present in the epithelium of cribriform intraductal carcinoma, but myoepithelial cells may persist at the periphery of the involved duct (Fig. 13.4). Solid intraductal papillary carcinoma, in which fibrovascular stroma is detectable, occasionally has a prominent fenestrated pattern that mimics intraductal cribriform carcinoma. The stromal component of solid, papillary carcinoma may be quite inconspicuous and easily overlooked. Another ambiguous situation arises when there is prominent secondary lumen formation in micropapillary carcinoma (Fig. 13.15). This process can encompass a substantial part of the overall duct lumen. Generally, the growth pattern of micropapillary car-

cinoma is oriented to the circumference of the duct, whereas in cribriform intraductal carcinoma, there is a more even distribution of microlumens across the duct without peripheral orientation. Difficulty in classification also arises when the intraductal proliferation is almost entirely solid with rare microlumens (Fig. 13.26).

The differential diagnosis of cribriform intraductal carcinoma includes adenoid cystic carcinoma, invasive cribriform carcinoma, and collagenous spherulosis.

*Comedo intraductal carcinoma* is described classically as a solid growth of large carcinoma cells with poorly differentiated nuclei, central necrosis with calcification, and, in some but not all cases, a high mitotic rate (Fig. 13.27). The myoepithelial cell layer is variably affected and sometimes completely eliminated by the carcinomatous proliferation. In some instances, the myoepithelial cells are hyperplastic with hyperchromatic nuclei, producing a distinct ring between the neoplastic epithelial cells and basement membrane. This

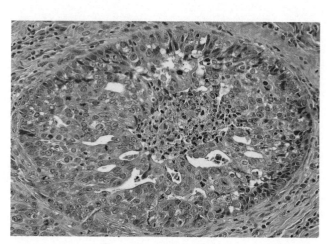

**FIG. 13.25.** *Intraductal carcinoma, cribriform.* This duct has central necrosis, high nuclear grade, and mitotic activity.

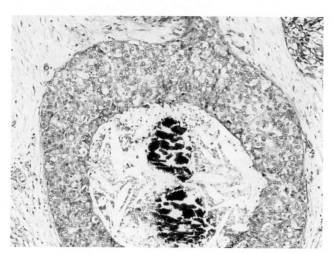

**FIG. 13.27.** *Intraductal carcinoma, comedo.* Central necrosis and calcification are evident.

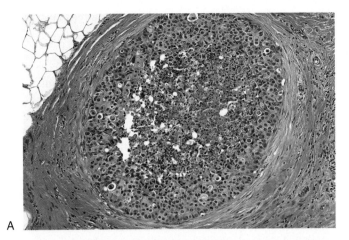

A

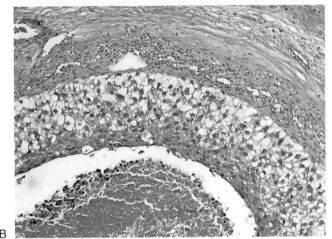

B

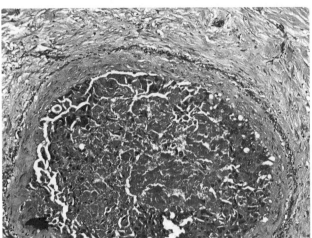

C

**FIG. 13.28.** *Intraductal carcinoma, comedo, with periductal fibrosis.* **A:** Solid intraductal carcinoma with central necrosis and concentric periductal fibrosis. **B:** Unusually prominent periductal neovascularity forms a distinct zone between comedo intraductal carcinoma and peripheral concentric fibrosis. **C:** A remarkably thick, reduplicated basement membrane forms a broad collar around this duct between intraductal carcinoma and a zone of neovascularization.

configuration often is accompanied by accentuation of the basement membrane itself as well as a circumferential periductal collar of desmoplastic stroma. Elastosis occurs around some ducts with this periductal reaction. Rarely, pronounced neovascularity is represented by a partial or complete ring of capillaries external to the basement membrane (77) (Fig. 13.28). A variable inflammatory infiltrate is present in the periductal stroma. In some instances, this consists of lymphocytes and histiocytes in amounts ranging from sparse to abundant. A more conspicuous inflammatory reaction may be elicited in foci where the duct wall is partially disrupted, and it appears that necrotic contents of the duct have been discharged or microinvasion is suspected (Fig. 13.29). Calcification can be displaced from the duct into the stroma at such sites. This appears to be the mechanism responsible for the presence of calcifications in the stroma associated with intraductal carcinoma when no invasion is evident. Accentuation and duplication of basement membrane components in the form of a thick eosinophilic band also may be evident in such foci (Fig. 13.30).

It is important to distinguish between comedonecrosis and the accumulation of secretion accompanied by an inflammatory reaction that occurs in duct stasis. Both conditions are prone to the formation of irregular microcalcifications that are indistinguishable on mammography. Cellular necrosis is rarely seen in duct stasis, and when present the degenerated cells are usually histiocytes. The duct contents in comedocarcinoma consist of necrotic carcinoma cells

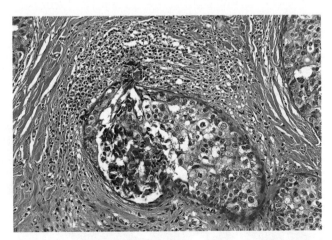

**FIG. 13.29.** *Intraductal carcinoma, comedo type.* Periductal lymphocytic reaction is concentrated at a site of possible microinvasion at the upper border of this duct.

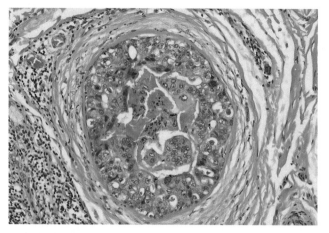

**FIG. 13.30.** *Intraductal carcinoma, comedo type.* Note concentric periductal fibrosis, lymphocytic reaction *(left)* and the eosinophilic band formed by the thickened basement membrane at the perimeter of the duct.

represented by ghost cells and karyorrhectic debris, typically with little or no intraductal inflammation. There is a sharp demarcation between viable carcinoma cells at the periphery and the necrotic core (Figs. 13.28 and 13.30). A space may be formed between the surviving cells and cellular debris, presumably as a result of shrinkage of the latter during tissue processing. Dying cells at the inner edge of the viable zone

have pyknotic nuclei and frayed cytoplasmic borders. The outlines of necrotic carcinoma cells (ghost cells) may be visible in the center of the duct.

*Dystrophic calcification* develops in the necrotic core. The calcification tends to be finely granular and mixed with cellular debris in some instances, whereas in others it forms more solid irregular fragments (Fig. 13.27). Calcifications in comedocarcinoma almost always consist of calcium salts, mainly calcium phosphate, rather than crystalline calcium oxalate, which is typically found in benign apocrine lesions. Calcium oxalate calcifications have been described in apocrine intraductal carcinoma (81,82). In routine hematoxylin and eosin–stained sections, calcifications are magenta to purple, whether in the comedo or other varieties of intraductal carcinoma. Large calcifications may be fractured in the course of histologic processing, and fragments can be physically pushed by the microtome blade from the duct into the surrounding stroma. Neoplastic epithelium may be coincidentally displaced as well. This artefact usually can be readily recognized because the path of the displaced calcification through the tissue is indicated by one or more linear scratches.

*Crystalloids* are eosinophilic, noncalcific protein deposits that occur in various types of intraductal carcinoma (Figs. 13.19 and 13.31). They appear to be formed by crystallization of proteins in necrotic debris formed in some intraductal carcinomas (see Chapter 46).

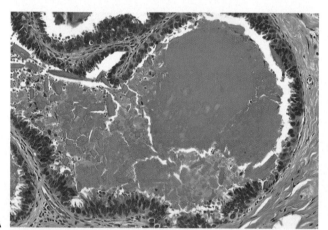

A

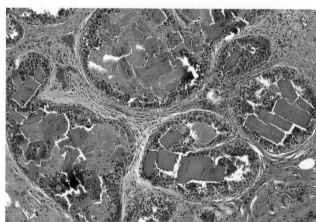

B

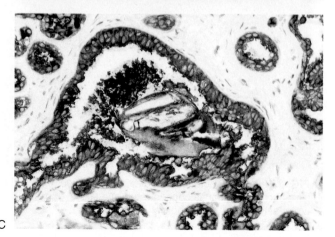

C

**FIG. 13.31.** *Intraductal carcinoma with crystalloids.* **A:** Small crystalloids are being formed in the necrotic debris in this duct. **B:** Numerous crystalloids are present in another part of the specimen shown in **A**. **C:** The needle-shaped crystalloids appear transparent in this preparation in which the epithelium and intraductal cellular debris are immunoreactive for epithelial membrane antigen (avidin-biotin). **C** is from the specimen shown in Fig. 13.19.

Morphometric analysis has demonstrated a correlation between duct diameter and the presence of necrosis in solid intraductal carcinoma (83). In one study, the mean diameter of ducts with necrosis was 470 μm compared with a mean diameter of 192 μm for solid nonnecrotic ductal carcinoma (83). A radius of 180 μm proved to be important for distinguishing between ducts with and without necrosis. Necrosis occurred in 94% of ducts greater than 180 μm in radius and in 34% of smaller ducts. The viable rim of carcinomatous epithelium surrounding the necrotic core averaged 105 μm and exceeded 180 μm in fewer than 10% of cases. These observations suggest that central necrosis occurs because cells at the center of ducts with an excessive radius are deprived of one or more essential metabolites, such as oxygen, as a result of limited diffusion in the nonvascularized intraductal neoplastic epithelium. It has been theorized that the presence of an hypoxic compartment in intraductal carcinomas with comedo necrosis renders this type of intraductal carcinoma relatively radioresistant and contributes to the high risk of local recurrence after breast conservation and radiotherapy for carcinomas with this feature (84).

*Apoptosis*, genetically programmed cell death, also appears to contribute to necrosis in comedo and other types of intraductal carcinoma. Evidence of apoptosis in intraductal carcinoma is derived from morphologic observations supported by terminal deoxynucleotidyl transferase-mediated dUPT-biotin end labeling staining (TUNEL) to demonstrate nuclear fragmentation. Morphologic criteria of apoptosis include nuclear shrinkage, condensation of chromatin, nuclear fragmentation, the formation of apoptotic bodies, and the absence of inflammation. Bodis et al. reported that TUNEL-positive staining was present in foci of necrosis with the features of apoptotic cell death in 19 examples of intraductal carcinoma (85). No TUNEL staining was found in low-grade intraductal carcinoma without necrosis. Nuclear immunoreactivity for p53 did not correlate significantly with apoptosis or necrosis.

Harn et al. studied the distribution of apoptosis in intraductal, invasive, and metastatic ductal carcinomas (86). The apoptosis-labelling index determined by the TUNEL method was significantly higher in intraductal carcinoma than in invasive or metastatic carcinoma. There was also a significant positive correlation between the apoptotic index and p53 expression in intraductal and invasive carcinoma, leading these researchers to speculate that p53 played a role in the regulation of apoptosis and the development of necrosis in intraductal carcinoma.

Further evidence that altered control of apoptosis may contribute to necrosis in intraductal carcinoma comes from studies of bcl-*2 expression*. The *bcl*-2 gene located on chromosome 18 plays an important role in regulating growth by inhibiting apoptosis. *Bcl*-2 expression is inversely related to differentiation as well as to the expression of the estrogen receptor (ER), p53, and HER2/*neu* proteins in intraductal carcinoma (87). Intraductal carcinomas with biological features most often associated with necrosis are characterized by down-regulation of apoptosis inhibiting *bcl*-2 (Fig. 13.32).

Sneige et al. correlated the frequency of central necrosis in intraductal carcinoma with nuclear grade (88). Central necrosis was much more frequent in lesions with poorly differentiated nuclear grade (80%) than in those with intermediate (35%) or low (22%) nuclear grade.

*Marked periductal fibrosis* on occasion can be associated with extensive obliteration of intraductal carcinoma, a process referred to as "healing" by Muir and Aitkenhead (89) (Fig. 13.33). The residual ductal structures typically consist of round to oval scars composed of circumferential layers of collagen and elastic tissue. The core representing the center of the duct may contain a few residual carcinoma cells, fragments of calcification, or histiocytes. End-stage scars of periductal mastitis may not be distinguishable from those of obliterated comedocarcinoma. After a study of 425 breasts, Davies concluded that " . . . ductal hyperelastosis, obliteration and fibrous plaques are not limited to breasts that are the seat of carcinoma. Indeed the prevalence of these three lesions in major ducts that are unaffected by microscopic changes do not differ significantly in 'normal' and carcinomatous breasts" (90). At the other extreme, perhaps also representing the result of host response to the tumor or its products, one can encounter a severe inflammatory reaction that may lead to a mistaken diagnosis of mastitis because intraductal carcinoma is masked by the inflammation.

*Solid intraductal carcinoma* is formed by neoplastic cells that fill most or all of the duct space (Fig. 13.34). Microlumens and papillary structures are absent, but calcifications may be present. Necrosis is not a conspicuous feature of solid intraductal carcinoma, but small foci may be present in affected ducts (Fig. 13.35). Patients with comedocarcinoma often have coexistent foci of solid intraductal carcinoma. In contrast to solid intraductal hyperplasia, the polygonal cells are typically of a single type with low to moderate nuclear grade. The cytoplasm has a spectrum of cytologic appearances, including clear, granular, amphophilic and eosinophilic, and apocrine.

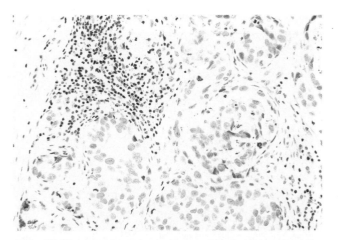

**FIG. 13.32.** *Intraductal carcinoma*, bcl-*2 expression*. Immunoreactivity for *bcl*-2 is present in lymphocytes which appear brown, but not in the nuclei of high-grade intraductal carcinoma cells (avidin-biotin).

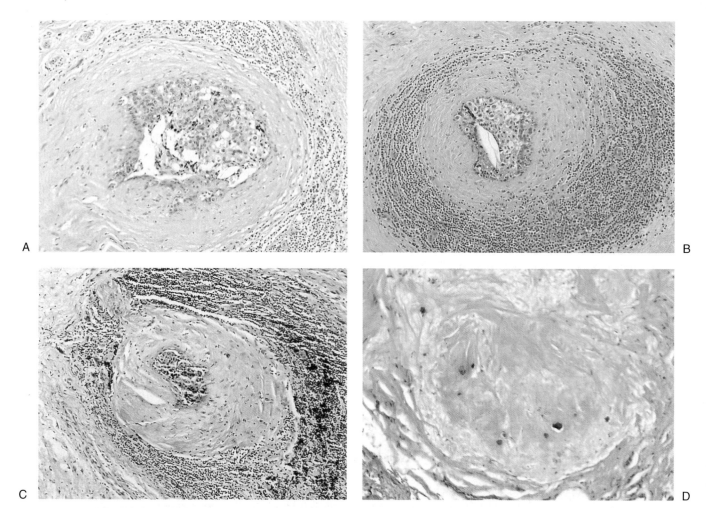

**FIG. 13.33.** *Intraductal carcinoma, "healing."* **A:** Prominent periductal fibrosis and chronic inflammation. **B,C:** Severe periductal fibrosis with intense lymphocytic reaction. The epithelial element is greatly reduced. **D:** Scar composed of collagen and elastin fibers with calcifications at the site of "healed" intraductal carcinoma. All images are from a single specimen.

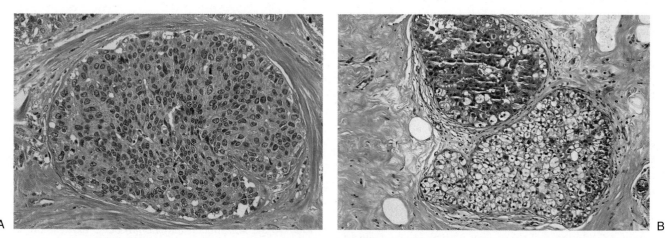

**FIG. 13.34.** *Intraductal carcinoma, solid.* **A:** The duct is filled by a compact growth of carcinoma cells with pleomorphic nuclei of intermediate to high nuclear grade. **B:** Solid apocrine intraductal carcinoma with clear cell change.

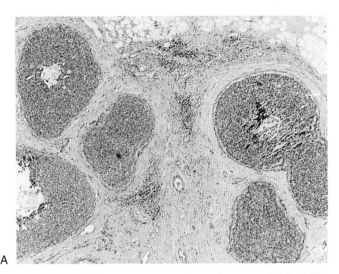 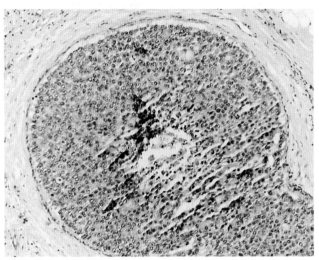

**FIG. 13.35.** *Intraductal carcinoma, solid.* **A,B:** Traces of central degeneration and calcification are evident.

Myoepithelial cells are variably present at the periphery of ducts with solid intraductal carcinoma.

*Papillary intraductal carcinoma* is distinguished by the presence of a fibrovascular stromal architecture supporting one or more of the foregoing structural patterns. *Endocrine in-*

*traductal carcinoma*, described by Cross et al. (91), and some examples of *spindle cell intraductal carcinoma* are variants of papillary carcinoma (see Chapter 16); however, spindle cell growth can be encountered in nonpapillary intraductal carcinoma (Fig. 13.36). *Small cell intraductal carcinoma* occurs in

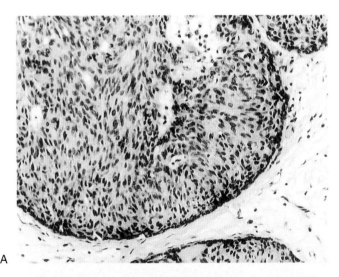

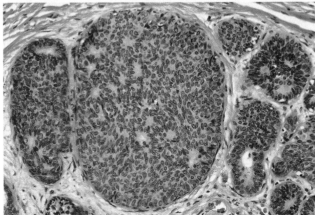

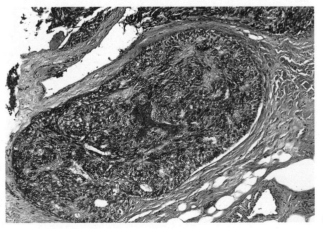

**FIG. 13.36.** *Intraductal carcinoma, spindle cell.* **A:** The carcinoma cells have spindle-shaped nuclei with traces of palisading. **B:** Rosette-like microlumens are present. **C:** Spindle cell carcinoma with a central fibrovascular stromal core. This focus was part of a complex papillary carcinoma with an extensive spindle cell component.

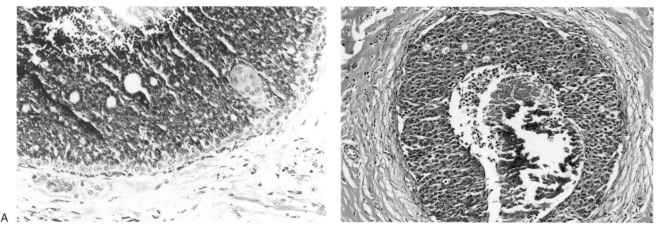

A

B

**FIG. 13.37.** *Intraductal carcinoma, small cell.* **A:** Focal squamous differentiation and central necrosis are shown. **B:** Central necrosis with calcification.

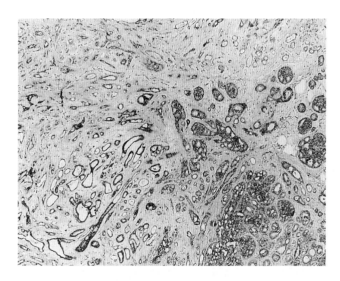

**FIG. 13.38.** *Intraductal carcinoma in sclerosing adenosis.* Cribriform carcinoma is present on the *right*. Sclerosing adenosis is present throughout the photograph.

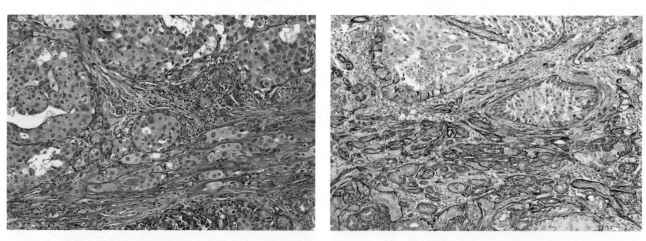

A

B

**FIG. 13.39.** *Intraductal carcinoma in sclerosing adenosis.* **A:** Apocrine intraductal carcinoma occupies the structure of sclerosing adenosis. Elongated groups of carcinoma cells near the *upper border* resemble invasive carcinoma cells. **B:** The immunostain for smooth-muscle myosin heavy chain on a section parallel to **A** reveals myoepithelial cells surrounding all groups of carcinoma cells (avidin-biotin).

association with invasive small cell (oat cell) carcinoma (see Chapter 23) or as an isolated lesion (Fig. 13.37).

*Intraductal carcinoma arising in sclerosing adenosis* assumes the structural configuration of the underlying adenosis and may be mistaken for invasive carcinoma (92–95) (Fig. 13.38). Most of these patients are premenopausal. Because sclerosing adenosis is fundamentally a lesion formed by altered lobules, this presentation can be viewed as a form of intralobular extension of the ductal lesion. The condition usually occurs focally rather than diffusely and is diagnosed when the proliferative epithelium has the structural and cytologic appearance of intraductal carcinoma. The growth patterns are usually solid and cribriform (Figs. 13.38 and 13.39). An organoid appearance may result from the alveolar expansion of lobular structures in the adenosis. Microcalcifications may be present in the underlying adenosis or as part of the intraductal carcinoma. Intraductal carcinoma can be limited to the sclerosing adenosis, or there may be foci in the surrounding breast (93). The underlying architecture of sclerosing adenosis can be appreciated with stains for basement membranes such as periodic acid-Schiff, reticulin, or laminin and immunostains for actin to identify myoepithelial cells (93,95). The antibody for smooth-muscle myosin-heavy chain is especially useful in this circumstance because it is more specific for myoepithelial cells and avoids most of the obscuring effect produced by actin reactivity in myofibroblasts encountered with other anti-actin antibodies (Fig. 13.39). Rarely, invasive carcinoma can have an adenosis-like pattern that is difficult to distinguish from intraductal carcinoma in adenosis. In this situation, immunostains for basement membrane components collagen type IV and laminin are useful if the basement membrane is absent (See the discussion of Microinvasion in this chapter). Invasive carcinoma arising in sclerosing adenosis is difficult to detect unless the invasive component has clearly grown beyond the area of adenosis and has an architectural pattern that differs from the adenosis (Figs. 13.40 and 13.41). A double immunostain for cytokeratin and actin can be helpful for identifying microinvasion when intraductal carcinoma inhabits sclerosing adenosis (Fig. 13.42).

Nerves may be incorporated in sclerosing adenosis when no carcinoma is present (96). The presence of this unusual

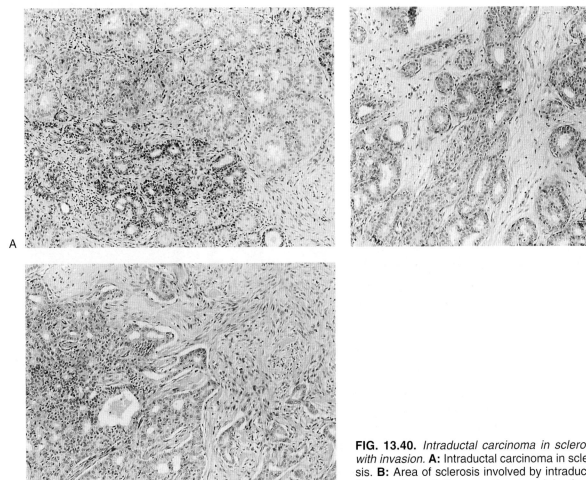

**FIG. 13.40.** *Intraductal carcinoma in sclerosing adenosis with invasion.* **A:** Intraductal carcinoma in sclerosing adenosis. **B:** Area of sclerosis involved by intraductal carcinoma. **C:** Invasive cribriform carcinoma originating in sclerosing adenosis.

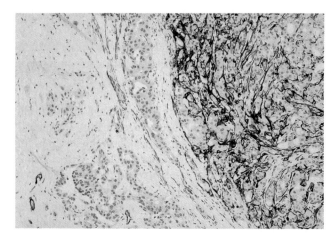

**FIG. 13.41.** *Invasive carcinoma arising in sclerosing adenosis.* Intraductal carcinoma in sclerosing adenosis is shown on the *right* in this section prepared with the immunostain for smooth-muscle myosin heavy chain. Invasive carcinoma in the stroma to the left of the sclerosing adenosis is not encased in actin-positive myoepithelial cells.

finding when there is intraductal carcinoma in the adenosis is not indicative of invasion. Neural entrapment also has been observed in areas of sclerosing papillary intraductal carcinoma not associated with sclerosing adenosis (97).

Intraductal carcinoma has been found to arise near and in *radial sclerosing lesions*, so-called radial scars (Figs. 13.43 and 13.44). The presence of an underlying radial sclerosing lesion is indicated by the overall configuration and the presence of benign proliferative foci such as duct hyperplasia, cysts, sclerosing adenosis, and apocrine metaplasia. Intraductal carcinoma with a stellate growth pattern can manifest as a radial sclerosing lesion (Fig. 13.45).

*Concurrent intraductal and* in situ *lobular carcinoma* are present when there are separate foci of carcinoma with these histologic features in the breast. This situation is illustrated by instances in which the lobular lesion with the classic small cell phenotype of lobular carcinoma is limited to lobular–terminal duct units that are separate from ducts with the classic features of comedo, papillary, or cribriform intraductal carcinoma (Fig. 13.46).

In some instances, the distinction is less clear, especially when the proliferation in the ducts and lobules is composed of uniform cells, with cytologically well to moderately differentiated nuclei (Fig. 13.47). The difficulty presented by these lesions is whether they should be classified as entirely intraductal carcinoma with "lobular cancerization" or as LCIS with duct extension. The presence of a homogeneous population of small cells with low-grade nuclei and signet-ring cells in ducts and lobules supports classification as florid LCIS (see Chapter 33). Some of the affected ducts may be markedly distended, exhibiting central necrosis and calcification. Loss of cohesion among the neoplastic cells is a feature associated with LCIS. The most extreme examples of this version of *in situ* lobular carcinoma occur when the expanded ducts are sufficiently numerous to produce a palpable lesion or calcifications are present on mammography. Absence of E-cadherin in most of these lesions supports classifying them as a florid form of LCIS (see Chapter 33).

The presence of a cribriform pattern suggests intraductal carcinoma with lobular extension. Cells with apocrine differentiation are more consistent with ductal carcinoma. Some cases defy classification and a diagnosis may require resolution by the E-cadherin immunostain. Further studies of E-cadherin expression may help in the classification of these lesions (Fig. 13.48).

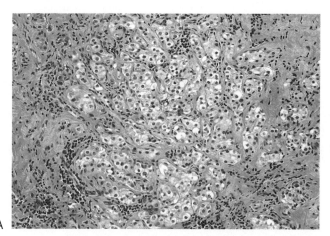

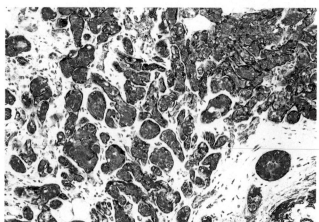

A                                    B

**FIG. 13.42.** *Intraductal carcinoma in sclerosing adenosis.* **A:** This pattern of apocrine intraductal carcinoma in sclerosing adenosis might be mistaken for invasive carcinoma. **B:** The combined cytokeratin *(red)* and actin *(brown)* immunostain demonstrates actin-positive myoepithelial cells around all of the cytokeratin-positive epithelial cells (anti-CK, alkaline phosphatase; anti–smooth muscle actin, avidin-biotin).

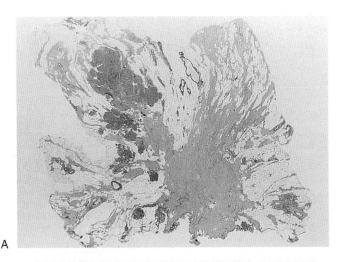

A

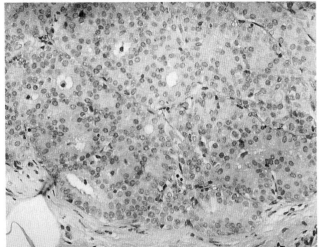

B

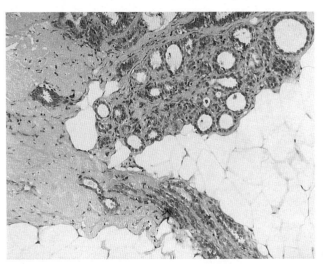

C

**FIG. 13.43.** *Intraductal carcinoma near a radial sclerosing lesion.* **A:** A whole-mount histologic section showing dark areas of intraductal carcinoma in the *upper left* and a lighter staining stellate radial sclerosing lesion that did not contain carcinoma. **B:** Cribriform intraductal carcinoma from the *upper left* region of **A**. **C:** Sclerosing adenosis and elastosis, which formed the rest of the radial sclerosing lesion.

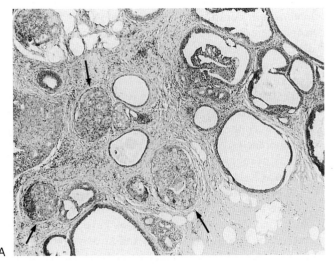

A

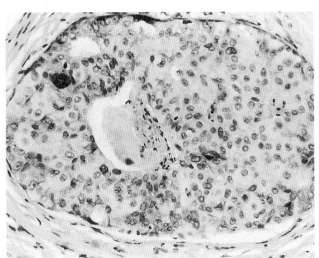

B

**FIG. 13.44.** *Intraductal carcinoma in a radial sclerosing lesion.* **A:** Intraductal carcinoma (*arrows*) surrounded by duct hyperplasia and cysts in a radial sclerosing lesion. **B:** Intraductal carcinoma shown in **A**.

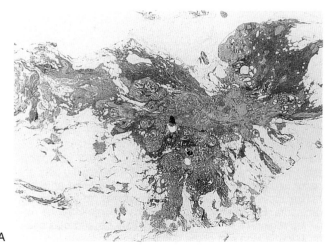

A

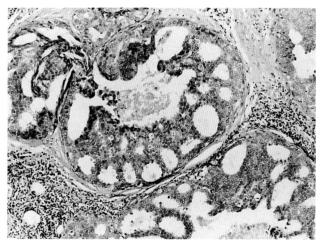

B

**FIG. 13.45.** *Intraductal carcinoma, radial configuration.* **A:** Stellate lesion with a scleroelastotic center. **B:** Cribriform intraductal carcinoma shown here is present throughout the tumor.

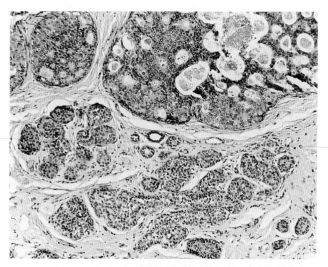

**FIG. 13.46.** *Concurrent cribriform intraductal and* in situ *lobular carcinoma.* (From Rosen PP. Coexistent lobular carcinoma *in situ* and intraductal carcinoma in a single lobular-duct unit. *Am J Surg Pathol* 1980;4:241–246, with permission.)

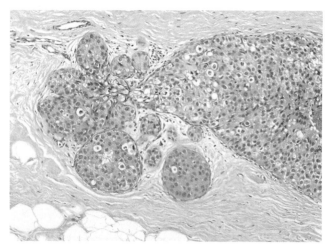

**FIG. 13.47.** *Lobular extension of intraductal carcinoma.* Solid intraductal carcinoma extending into lobular glands. The relatively abundant eosinophilic cytoplasm and low nuclear grade favor classification as ductal carcinoma.

Little attention has been paid to these poorly defined lesions. Because the treatments for LCIS and intraductal carcinoma are in many cases different, there is considerable clinical pressure to distinguish between *in situ* ductal carcinoma and LCIS and to minimize diagnostic uncertainty. This circumstance undoubtedly causes pathologists to arbitrarily classify some of these lesions as ductal carcinoma or lobular carcinoma. It is best to make this distinction whenever possible. A diagnosis of combined intraductal and LCIS is preferable to arbitrarily assigning one or the other diagnosis. Immunoreactiviy for E-cadherin warrants classification as intraductal carcinoma, and lack thereof indicates lobular carcinoma *in situ*.

*Coexistent intraductal and LCIS in a single duct–lobular unit* constitutes one of the most unusual microscopic patterns of noninvasive breast carcinoma (98). This diagnosis depends on finding carcinoma with two distinctly different cytologic and structural patterns in a single duct. In these combined lesions, LCIS with the conventional small cell cytology is typically present within lobular glands as well as in a pagetoid distribution in the ductal epithelium (Figs. 13.49 and 13.50). E-cadherin immunoreactivity is weak, discontinuous, or absent in regions occupied by *in situ* lobular carcinoma in such combined lesions. The ductal lumen contains a papillary, solid, or cribriform proliferation composed of more pleomorphic cells than typically are found in an intraductal carcinoma. Coexistent *in situ* lesions have been found in association with invasive ductal and invasive lobular carcinoma. This pattern of *in situ* carcinoma should be distinguished from lobular extension of intraductal carcinoma, so-called lobular cancerization. In the latter condition, the nonneoplastic lobular epithelium is replaced by carcinoma cells with the same cytologic appearance as the intraductal carcinoma.

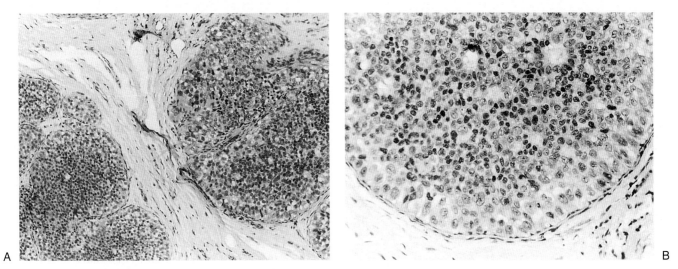

**FIG. 13.48.** *Intraductal carcinoma with lobular features.* **A:** Carcinoma in a duct *(right)* and distended lobular glands *(left)*. **B:** Small and large cell populations are present. Microlumens have been formed in an area composed of small cells in a duct. This lesion was immunoreactive for E-cadherin.

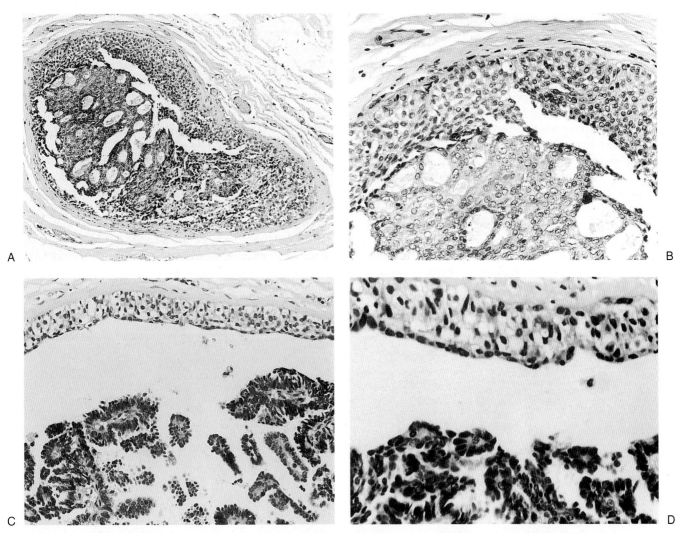

**FIG. 13.49.** *Coexistent intraductal and* in situ *lobular carcinoma in a single duct-lobular unit.* **A,B:** Cribriform intraductal carcinoma surrounded by *in situ* lobular carcinoma. **C,D:** Papillary intraductal carcinoma with *in situ* lobular carcinoma at the periphery of the duct. (From Rosen PP. Coexistent lobular carcinoma *in situ* and intraductal carcinoma in a single lobular-duct unit. *Am J Surg Pathol* 1980;4:241–246, with permission.)

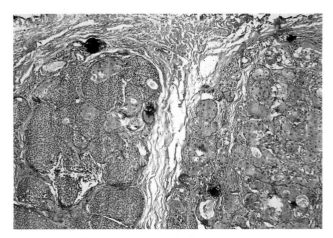

**FIG. 13.50.** *Coexistent intraductal and* in situ *lobular carcinoma in a single duct-lobular unit.* Intraductal carcinoma, apocrine type, is present in adenosis on the *right.* Lobular carcinoma *in situ* fills expanded lobular glands on the *left.* Apocrine intraductal carcinoma is surrounded by lobular carcinoma *in situ* in the *upper left* area. Calcifications are present in the ductal and lobular *in situ* carcinoma.

## GRADING

Grading of intraductal carcinoma has been investigated to determine whether it would be useful for predicting the risk for breast recurrence after conservation therapy. When there is an invasive element associated with intraductal carcinoma, both components tend to have similar nuclear grades (99). Grading schemes consisting of two categories (high grade and all others) and three categories (high, intermediate, and low) have been devised for intraductal carcinoma. The determination of grade is based mainly on nuclear cytology (100). Nuclear grade tends to be relatively constant in a given patient, even when there is substantial variation in architectural pattern (99). The presence or absence of necrosis and the architecture of the intraductal carcinoma also may be considered.

*Comedocarcinoma* is high grade by definition. Poorly differentiated nuclei, sometimes accompanied by necrosis, are also infrequently encountered in papillary, micropapillary, and cribriform intraductal carcinomas (99) (Figs. 13.19, 13.25, and 13.51). Intraductal carcinoma is in the intermediate grade category when it has a cribriform, solid, or papillary pattern with necrosis but lacks the nuclear anaplasia of comedocarcinoma or if one of these growth patterns is composed of atypical cells in the absence of necrosis (Figs. 13.9, 13.11, 13.21, and 13.26). Any pattern of intraductal carcinoma composed of uniform cells without atypia or necrosis is classified as low grade (Figs. 13.2, 13.4, 13.7, 13.15, 13.21, 13.43, and 13.52). A case usually is classified on the basis of the highest grade present (101). Rarely, high- and low-grade components coexist in a patient or even in one duct (Figs. 13.10 and 13.53).

Silverstein et al. proposed a classification of intraductal carcinoma based on nuclear grade (high or nonhigh) and the presence or absence of necrosis as part of a prognostic index (102). Three prognostic categories resulting from consideration of these variables were as follows: group 1, nonhigh nuclear grade without necrosis; group 2, nonhigh nuclear grade with necrosis; and group 3, high nuclear grade with or without necrosis. The Van Nuys Prognostic Index (VNPI) includes margin status and tumor size as well as these histologic groups (103). Follow-up revealed a significant correlation between the VNPI and the risk of recurrence in the breast after conservation therapy.

Grading has been a component of other classification schemes for assessing the effectiveness of breast-conservation therapy in the treatment of intraductal carcinoma. Including those cited already, at least six classifications have been proposed (104). These have been based on some or all of the following features: architecture, nuclear grade, presence or absence of necrosis, lesion size, and cell polarity. Most classifications emphasize nuclear grade, necrosis, and architecture. Generally, three grades have been proposed: high, intermediate, and low grade. There is a significant cor-

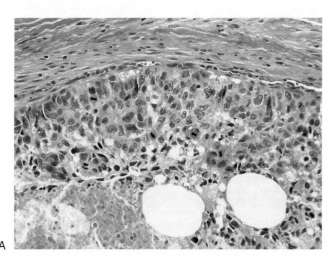

A

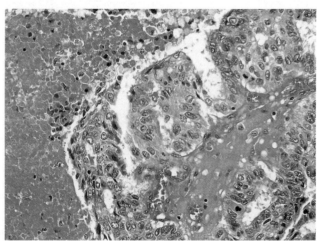

B

**FIG. 13.51.** *Intraductal carcinoma, high grade.* **A:** Comedocarcinoma. **B:** Papillary carcinoma with necrosis.

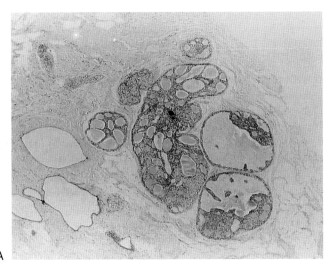 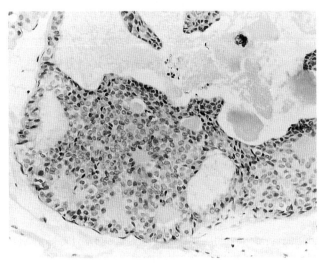

A                                      B

**FIG. 13.52.** *Intraductal carcinoma, low grade.* **A:** Papillary and cribriform architecture. **B:** Low nuclear grade.

relation between the grade of intraductal carcinoma and a corresponding invasive component, if present, regardless of grading system (104). The grading categories also have significant associations with biological characteristics of intraductal carcinoma, especially lesions typically classified as high and low grade. As discussed elsewhere in this chapter, high-grade lesions exhibit the following features: absence of estrogen and progesterone receptor expression, aneuploidy, high proliferative rate, periductal angiogenesis, membrane reactivity for HER2/*neu*, nuclear reactivity for p53, and abnormal *bcl*-2 expression. Conversely, low-grade intraductal carcinomas usually have been characterized by the following: presence of estrogen and progesterone receptors, absence of aneuploidy, low proliferative rate, little periductal angiogenesis, absence of HER2/*neu* and p53 expression, and normal *bcl*-2. Intermediate-grade intraductal carcinomas tend to have mixed patterns of biological marker expression.

No single grading system for intraductal carcinoma has been demonstrated to be notably superior, and none has gained widespread acceptance. A consensus conference convened in 1997 did not endorse any single system of classification but recommended that a pathology report for intraductal carcinoma provide information about the descriptive characteristics considered to be essential in most grading schemes (101). The three essential elements noted were nuclear grade, necrosis, and architectural pattern(s).

In the 1997 consensus report, nuclear grade was stratified in three categories (Table 13.1). Pleomorphic nuclei of similar size were not consistent with low nuclear grade. The pathology report should reflect the highest nuclear grade but may indicate the relative proportions of grade when there is heterogeneity. *Necrosis* was defined as the "presence of ghost cells and karyorrhectic debris" (Table 13.2). Five architectural patterns were identified: comedo, cribriform,

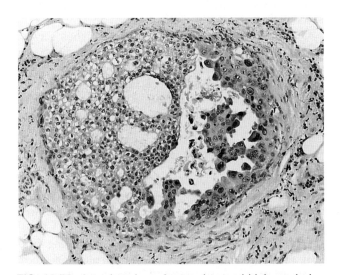

**FIG. 13.53.** *Intraductal carcinoma, low and high grade in a single duct.*

**TABLE 13.1.** *Consensus committee recommendation for nuclear grading of intraductal carcinoma*

Low nuclear grade (NG1)
  Monomorphic (monotonous) appearance
  Size of duct epithelial nuclei or 1.5–2.0 normal red blood
    cells
  Chromatin diffuse, finely dispersed
  "Occasional nucleoli and mitoses"
  Cells usually polarized
High nuclear grade (NG3)
  "Markedly pleomorphic"
  Size usually more than 2.5 duct epithelial nuclei
  Chromatin vesicular with irregular distribution
  "Prominent, often multiple nucleoli"
  "Mitoses may be conspicuous"
Intermediate nuclear grade (NG2)
  "Nuclei that are neither NG1 nor NG3"

Based on The Consensus Conference Committee. Consensus Conference on the classification of ductal carcinoma *in situ*. *Cancer* 1997;80:1798–1802, with permission.

**TABLE 13.2.** *Consensus committee recommendation for reporting necrosis in intraductal carcinoma*

Comedonecrosis
 "Central zone necrosis within a duct, usually exhibiting a linear pattern within ducts if sectioned longitudinally"
Punctate
 "Nonzonal type necrosis (foci of necrosis that do not exhibit a linear pattern if longitudinally sectioned)"

Based on The Consensus Conference Committee. Concensus Conference on the classification of ductal carcinoma *in situ. Cancer* 1997;80:1798–1802, with permission.

papillary, micropapillary, solid. It was specified that comedo referred "to solid intraepithelial growth within the basement membrane with central (zonal) necrosis. Such lesions are often but not invariably of high nuclear grade."

Other elements recommended by the 1997 consensus report for inclusion in the diagnosis were cell polarization around intraductal microlumens, lesion "size (extent, distribution)," and margin status. No particular method for assessing size or margins was suggested.

Interobserver variability is an important consideration in applying a grading system in clinical practice. This issue has been addressed in a limited number of studies, and the results suggest that architectural descriptions (e.g., cribriform, micropapillary, comedo) are less reproducible than nuclear grade and necrosis (88,104–106a). This probably reflects the heterogeneity of architectural patterns that may be encountered in a single case, whereas nuclear grade tends to be relatively more consistent. The description of necrosis also can be a source of disagreement if quantification of necrosis is an element in classification as the comedo type (105). The usual quantitative descriptors of necrosis are: present, focally present, or absent.

Sneige et al. studied interobserver reproducibility among six pathologists who assessed nuclear grade in 125 examples of intraductal carcinoma (88). Complete agreement on nuclear grade was reported in 43 (35%) cases, and five of six pathologists agreed in 45 (36%) cases. The generalized kappa for distinctions between grades 1 and 2 and between 2 and 3 were 0.29 and 0.48, respectively (SE = 0.02). These levels of agreement were regarded as fair and moderate by the authors. Pair-wise correlations between individual pathologists and the consensus grade included a range of kappa values from 0.44 to 0.76, with five of six having values greater than 0.60, representing "substantial" agreement. Douglas-Jones et al. circulated 60 "unselected" examples of intraductal carcinoma among 19 "practicing histopathologists" and found the following degrees of agreement: cytological grade (three categories) 71%, weighted kappa (κw) 0.36; and intraductal necrosis (absent, present, extensive) 76%, κw 0.57 (106a).

Some researchers have suggested that apocrine and micropapillary intraductal carcinomas be listed as separate cat-

egories and not included in a three-tiered grading scheme (106). This proposal appears to derive from perceived difficulty in assigning these lesions to one of the three conventional grades because of inconsistent expression of individual criteria for grading. In practice, however, intraductal carcinomas with apocrine or micropapillary features express the same range of diverse histologic variation as nonapocrine and nonmicropapillary intraductal carcinomas, and separate characterization is not recommended. In regard to apocrine lesions, nuclear grade is based on comparison with nuclei in ordinary benign apocrine metaplasia. Assessment of features listed in Table 13.1 is based on this standard. The distribution of architectural patterns and necrosis is not different in apocrine and nonapocrine intraductal carcinomas. Micropapillary intraductal carcinoma is subject to variations in nuclear grade and to necrosis illustrated in this chapter, which do not differ from other architectural types of intraductal carcinoma.

## ANGIOGENESIS

Studies of the microvascular pattern of capillaries in breast tissue from patients with intraductal carcinoma have demonstrated increased periductal vascularity associated with some but not all intraductal carcinomas. The most reliable information has been obtained from histologic sections immunostained with vascular markers such as factor VIII, CD31, or CD34. Increased microvessel size has been observed at sites of intraductal carcinoma compared with normal breast tissue (107). Neovascularization has been described around intraductal carcinoma associated with invasive lesions (108). Periductal neovascularity found around 21 of 55 (38%) pure intraductal carcinomas studied by Guidi et al. was not related to histologic subtype, the presence of necrosis, proliferative index, or HER2/*neu* expression (109). These investigators observed that stromal vascularity was increased in comedo carcinoma with marked stromal desmoplasia, but the increased vascularity was not specifically periductal in distribution.

Other investigators also studied the association between the architectural pattern of intraductal carcinoma and periductal neovascularity. Heffelfinger et al. recorded the distribution of capillaries in contact with the basement membrane of ducts in various conditions, including proliferative disease and intraductal carcinoma (110). The mean score for vascularity was increased significantly between normal and proliferative ducts (0.187 versus 0.836) and between both of these categories and intraductal carcinomas as a group (1.525). Variations in mean scores were seen in subtypes of intraductal carcinoma, ranging from 0.962 for micropapillary to 2.216 for comedocarcinoma, but the differences were not statistically significant.

Bose et al. analyzed periductal angiogenesis using factor VIII and CD34 immunostains in comedo and noncomedo types of intraductal carcinoma (77). Small capillaries were usually present in the connective tissue, but they were found only rarely in the region of the basement membrane around normal ducts. New vessel formation associated with intraductal carcinoma was limited to the region of the basement membrane in ducts with intraductal carcinoma (Fig. 13.54). Evidence of angiogenesis was found in 80% of intraductal carcinomas consisting of a ring of neovascularity completely or partially encircling the affected duct. A complete ring was found more often in comedocarcinomas, whereas noncomedo lesions tended to have a partial ring or no periductal neovascularity (Figs. 13.28 and 13.54). Using a different method of quantitation, Guidi and Schnitt confirmed that maximal periductal neovascularity was associated with comedocarcinoma, the expression of HER2/neu, and with a high proliferative index (111).

Engels et al. compared intraductal carcinomas with increased stromal vascularity between affected ducts, which they termed "pattern I," and lesions in which neovascularity formed a dense rim around the basement membrane ("pattern II") (112). Patterns I and II were present alone in 11% and 16%, respectively, of 75 cases. Increased vascularity with either pattern alone or in combination was associated with high-grade forms of intraductal carcinoma.

The observed pattern of angiogenesis may be related in part to the fate of the myoepithelial (ME) cell layer in ducts that develop intraductal carcinoma. ME cells are more likely to persist in low-grade intraductal carcinoma, and they are usually markedly attenuated or absent in high-grade comedo intraductal carcinoma. Barsky et al. suggested that ME cells may exert a tumor-suppressor influence on the development or progression of intraductal carcinoma (113,114). Several lines of evidence appear to support this hypothesis. *In vitro* and *in situ* tissue studies have demonstrated that myoepithelial cells express high amounts of proteinase inhibitors including maspin, protease nexin II, and α-1-antitrypsin and that these inhibitory proteins are concentrated in the surrounding stroma (115,116). The effect of these inhibitors of matrix metalloproteinases is to decrease tumor invasiveness and to reduce angiogenesis (115). Another paracrine effect of myoepithelial cells appears to be an antiproliferative effect that has been detected in *in vitro* studies (117).

Angiogenesis associated with intraductal carcinoma also may be modulated by the ability of the neoplastic cells to express angiogenic proteins such as the vascular endothelial growth factor (VEGF). High-grade intraductal carcinoma and a significantly higher microvessel count have been associated with stronger VEGF mRNA expression detected by *in situ* hybridization (118).

## HORMONE RECEPTORS

Because intraductal carcinoma is often a lesion of microscopic dimension, little information was available about

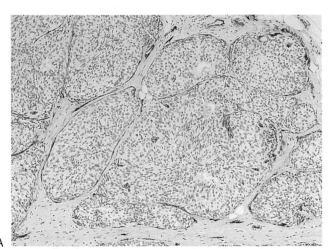

A

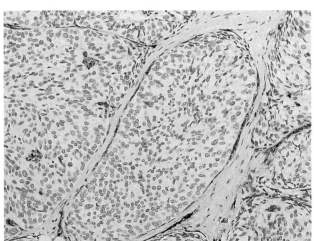

B

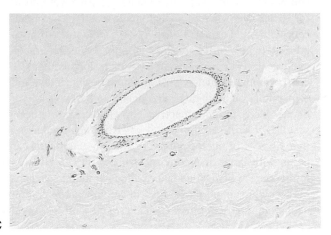

C

**FIG. 13.54.** *Intraductal carcinoma, angiogenesis.* **A,B:** Intraductal carcinoma solid type with low nuclear grade is partially encircled by capillaries in these immunostained sections. **C:** Capillaries are present in the stroma, but they are not concentrated around this normal duct (anti-CD34, avidin-biotin).

hormone receptor expression until immunohistochemical methods became available. Biochemical analysis using homogenized tissue samples contained a substantial proportion of nonneoplastic tissue, and as a consequence, most specimens of intraductal carcinoma were reportedly receptor negative. In one study, the median level of ER in intraductal carcinoma was 5 fmol/mg of cytosol protein, significantly less than the median of 11 fmol/mg for infiltrating duct carcinoma (119). Hawkins et al. found a similar difference between intraductal and invasive carcinomas studied biochemically (120). After adjusting for variation in cellularity, these authors concluded that invasive carcinomas had significantly higher concentrations of ER than intraductal carcinomas.

Barnes and Masood in 1990 described an immunohistochemical study of ER in intraductal carcinoma (121). Nuclear reactivity, usually heterogeneously distributed when present, was found in 75% of pure intraductal carcinomas, in 73% of intraductal carcinomas associated with invasive duct carcinoma, and in 100% of 36 examples of atypical duct hyperplasia. Nuclear ER reactivity was less frequent in comedo intraductal carcinoma than in other variants (Fig. 13.55). The same pattern of ER expression usually was found in the intraductal and the infiltrating portions of carcinomas with both components. ER positivity was more frequent in tumors from women older than 55 years than in younger patients.

A more detailed analysis of ER immunohistochemistry was provided by Bur et al. in 1992 (122), who classified 80% of intraductal carcinomas as ER positive, with a significantly higher frequency of receptor positivity in noncomedo (91%) than in comedo (57%) lesions. The frequencies of ER positivity among variants of noncomedo intraductal carcinoma did not differ significantly (cribriform, 89%; solid, 94%; micropapillary–papillary, 100%). Cellular features associated with the absence of ER were large cell size, nuclear pleomorphism, and necrosis. These investigators also confirmed

the observation of Barnes and Masood that ER immunoreactivity was almost always the same in the intraductal and invasive portions of a lesion. A comparison of women younger and older than 50 years did not reveal a significant difference in the frequency of ER positivity in intraductal carcinoma, but the intensity of reactivity tended to be greater in the older group.

Holland et al. studied the response of intraductal carcinoma to estrogens in human breast tissue *in vivo* using nude mouse xenografts (123). Samples of ER-negative comedo intraductal carcinoma had a high proliferative rate before transplantation, and this was maintained but did not increase when xenografts were exposed to estrogen. On the other hand, noncomedo, ER-positive intraductal carcinoma exhibited increased proliferation after exposure to estrogens, although the proliferative levels did not reach those of the comedocarcinoma. These results suggest that ER-negative intraductal carcinoma is estrogen independent and that antiestrogen therapy may not be beneficial to patients with these lesions.

## ONCOGENES

### HER2/*neu*

Immunohistochemical studies demonstrated membrane immunoreactivity for the HER2/*neu* (HER-2) oncogene in 42% to 61% of intraductal carcinomas (124–128) (Fig. 13.56). HER2/*neu* gene amplification was reported in 40% to 48% of intraductal carcinoma specimens isolated by microdissection and studied by the differential polymerase chain reaction (PCR) (129,130). Ho et al. found significantly higher frequencies of HER2/*neu* amplification in comedo than in noncomedo intraductal carcinomas (69% versus 18%) and in lesions with high rather than low nuclear grade (63% versus 14%) (130). Expression of HER2/*neu* occurs in 85% to 100% of comedocarcinomas and is associated with the pleomorphic nuclear cytology in these lesions (124,128,131).

Most investigators have not detected HER2/*neu* in small cell micropapillary and cribriform intraductal carcinomas (124,128,132). Using actual measurements of nuclear size, Bartkova et al. observed that 94% of intraductal carcinomas composed of cells with large nuclei (20 μm) were positive for HER2/*neu*, whereas no membrane reactivity was seen in cells with small nuclei (10 μm) (124). Immunoreactivity was present in 71% of intraductal carcinomas with intermediate nuclear size (15 μm) and in 91% of lesions composed of cells with mixed nuclear size. In this series, a small number of papillary and clinging intraductal carcinomas with large nuclei were immunoreactive for HER2/*neu*. Other researchers confirmed the finding of HER2/*neu* immunoreactivity in 85% of micropapillary or clinging intraductal carcinoma with large or pleomorphic nuclei (133). HER2/*neu* immunoreactivity is found more often in intraductal carcinomas with aneuploid nuclei than in carcinomas with diploid nuclei, an association that correlates well with the reported

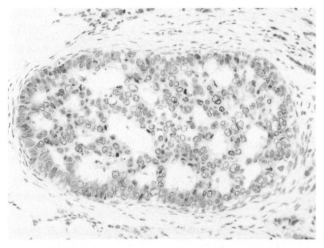

**FIG. 13.55.** *Intraductal carcinoma, estrogen receptor.* Nuclear immunoreactivity for estrogen receptor in cribriform intraductal carcinoma (antiestrophilin, avidin-biotin).

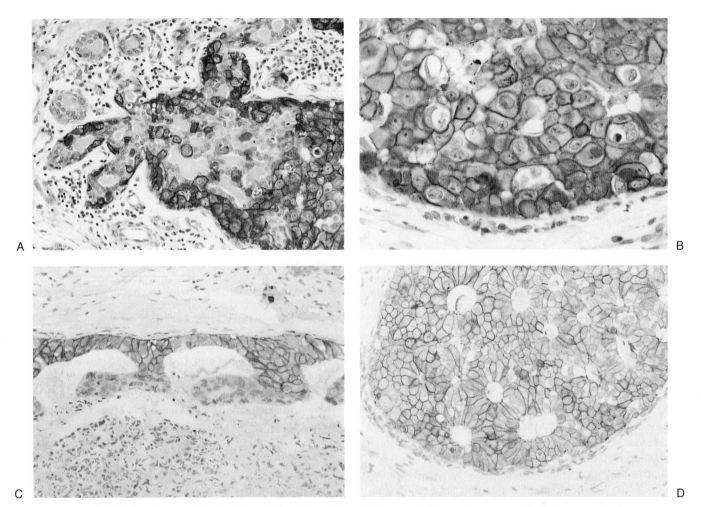

**FIG. 13.56.** *Intraductal carcinoma, HER 2/*neu. **A:** HER 2/*neu* membrane immunoreactivity is present in the intraductal carcinoma extending into a lobule but not in nonneoplastic epithelial cells. **B:** HER 2/*neu*-positive, poorly differentiated, solid, intraductal carcinoma. **C:** HER 2/*neu* positive micropapillary intraductal carcinoma with poorly differentiated nuclear grade and necrosis. **D:** Cribriform intraductal carcinoma with intermediate nuclear grade (avidin-biotin).

relationship of HER2/*neu* to nuclear size (127,131). There is also a strong association between positive HER2/*neu* reactivity and a high proliferative rate represented by the thymidine and MIB1 labeling indices (131,134). HER2/*neu* expression was significantly associated with large cell intraductal carcinomas and with the extent of the lesion (135). HER2/*neu* occurred in 10% of intraductal carcinomas smaller than 10 mm and in 61% of lesions larger than 20 mm (135). Immunohistochemical detection of HER2/*neu* was inversely related to the detection of immunostaining for neuron-specific enolase in intraductal carcinoma (136).

The extracellular domain of HER2/*neu* can be detected in the serum of patients with invasive breast carcinoma, and this finding has been associated with overexpression in the carcinoma detected by immunohistochemistry (137). Serum analysis for HER2/*neu* may prove to be a useful method for identifying patients with microinvasive duct carcinoma. Esteva-Lorenzo et al. described a patient with elevated serum extracellular domain of HER2/*neu* at the time a breast biopsy

demonstrated comedo–intraductal carcinoma that was immunoreactive for HER2/*neu* (138). Reexcision, which was performed because carcinoma involved the initial excision margin, revealed a microinvasive focus. Thereafter, the serum level of HER2/*neu* decreased to normal. No elevation of serum extracellular domain HER2/*neu* was detected by these researchers in specimens from eight other patients with intraductal carcinoma, including three with intraductal carcinoma immunoreactive for HER2/*neu* or in 27 patients with benign biopsies. In women with clinically invasive carcinoma, serial HER2/*neu* serum levels during the course of chemotherapy did not correlate well with the clinical status of the patients (139).

### p53

Investigators using a monoclonal antibody to wild and mutant forms of the p53 protein reported nuclear reactivity in 10% (140), 18.5% (141), 19.2% (132), 25.2% (142), and

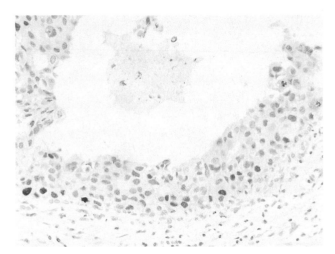

**FIG. 13.57.** *Intraductal carcinoma, p53.* Nuclear immunoreactivity is evident in this lesion with intermediate nuclear grade and central necrosis (polyclonal anti-p53, avidin-biotin).

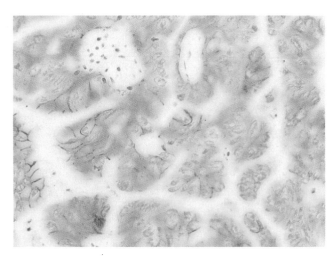

**FIG. 13.58.** *Intraductal carcinoma, epidermal growth factor receptor (EGF-R).* Membrane immunoreactivity for EGF-R forms slender beaded lines between cells in a papillary intraductal carcinoma. Background cytoplasmic staining is also evident (anti–EGF-R, avidin-biotin).

37% (143) of intraductal carcinomas examined (Fig. 13.57). In some studies, expression of p53 was significantly associated with large or pleomorphic cell type, intraductal necrosis, and comedo intraductal carcinoma (132,134,140–142), but others did not find a significant correlation between grade or histologic subtype and p53 expression (143) or p53 mutations (130). Nuclear p53 was found only rarely in small cell intraductal carcinomas (142). No p53 reactivity was found in 17 cystic papillary carcinomas studied by O'Malley et al. (140). When present, p53 mutations have been identical in most instances where intraductal and invasive carcinoma samples from a single tumor have been examined (144). In one study, no p53 mutations were identified in microdissected hyperplastic lesions from patients who had p53 mutations in coexisting intraductal and invasive duct carcinoma (144).

Carcinomas expressing p53 tend to be ER and progesterone receptor (PR) negative when studied by immunohistochemistry (134,142), and they show evidence of a higher than median proliferative rate manifested by a relatively high MIB1 labeling index (134). Molecular analysis using direct sequencing of PCR products revealed mutant p53 protein accumulation in comedo intraductal carcinoma (140). There was no significant trend for coexpression of p53 and HER2/*neu* in any subset of carcinomas, despite the independent association of p53 and HER2/*neu* with large cell or comedo intraductal carcinoma in some studies (126,130,142,145).

## OTHER MARKERS

A variety of other markers have been studied in intraductal carcinoma. The *nm23 gene product* is associated with a low metastatic potential in some cell culture systems and in invasive human breast carcinomas (146). Cytoplasmic immunoreactivity for nm23 is found in normal breast epithelium and in most noninvasive carcinomas (147). Strong staining was found in LCIS. Comedocarcinomas without associated invasion exhibited more intense nm23 reactivity than comedocarcinomas with invasion, a difference not observed when noncomedo intraductal and invasive carcinoma were compared (147). These observations suggest that reduced nm23 expression in comedo intraductal carcinomas may be a marker for the acquisition of invasive characteristics. The relationship of growth factors and their receptors to the morphology and prognosis of intraductal carcinoma has not been determined (Fig. 13.58).

*E-cadherin* is a cell–cell adhesion molecule expressed by epithelial cells. Loss of expression resulting from mutations in the E-cadherin gene has been associated with invasive lobular carcinoma and LCIS (148). E-cadherin expression may be reduced in intraductal carcinoma, but it is rarely absent. Vos et al. studied 150 examples of intraductal carcinoma and detected E-cadherin in all cases, with reduced expression in 11% (148). In one study, there was significantly less expression in high-grade than in low-grade lesions (149). Bankfalvi et al. also reported reduced E-cadherin reactivity in high-grade intraductal carcinoma and confirmed the absence of E-cadherin expression in lobular carcinomas (150). The reduced cell–cell adhesion in high-grade intraductal carcinomas may contribute to the relatively high frequency of microinvasion observed in these lesions.

## PLOIDY AND PROLIFERATIVE RATE

When studied by flow cytometry, the frequency of aneuploidy in intraductal carcinoma has ranged from 21% to 71% (151–156). Aneuploidy has been found in 55% to more than 90% of comedocarcinomas (151,152,154,155) and in 65% of intraductal carcinomas with high or poorly differentiated nuclear grade (153). Image analysis of Feulgen-stained tissue sections revealed aneuploidy in 77.5% of intraductal carcinomas, predominantly in lesions with poorly differentiated (100%) and intermediate (80%) nuclear grade (157).

Thymidine labelling and flow cytometry studies demonstrated a significantly higher proliferative rate in comedocarcinoma than in cribriform–micropapillary intraductal carcinoma (126,158). All papillary intraductal carcinomas examined in one series were diploid (155). Cribriform intraductal carcinomas tend to be diploid with a low S-phase fraction (154,156). Sataloff et al. reported that micropapillary carcinoma was typically diploid with a low S-phase fraction (156). Using nonfluorescent *in situ* hybridization with centromeric probe specific for chromosome 8, Juarez et al. detected increased signals in intraductal carcinoma indicative of aneuploidy compared with benign ductal cells (159). The frequency of increased signals ranged from 18% to 95%. Chromosome 8 aneuploidy was most pronounced in high-grade intraductal carcinoma.

Numeric alterations in individual chromosomes have been studied by fluorescence *in situ* hybridization (FISH) using specific probes. Using this method in paraffin sections of archival tissue samples, Visscher et al. detected chromosomal aneuploidy in 7 to 10 specimens of intraductal carcinoma (160). Aneuploidy was more frequent in specimens from patients with concurrent invasive carcinoma. Patterns of aneuploidy consisted of gains only, losses only, or gains and losses involving different chromosomes. Aneuploidy was most frequent for chromosomes 16 and 17.

*Proliferative activity* in intraductal carcinoma is now usually analyzed by immunohistochemistry with the Ki67 and MIB1 antibodies (Fig. 13.59). Albonico et al. reported the highest proliferative index (PI) in lesions of the comedo type, with 52.7% of cases exhibiting nuclear staining in more than 13% of nuclei (132). Other types of intraductal carcinoma had much lower PIs: solid, 14.4%; papillary, 13.4%; cribriform, 4.5%; and micropapillary, 0%.

The *bcl*-2 gene plays a role in the control of cell growth by inhibiting apoptosis (Fig. 13.32). The expression of *bcl*-2 in intraductal carcinoma is inversely related to grade. Loss of *bcl*-2 expression is most pronounced in high-grade intraductal carcinoma and is directly related to p53 expression (87). High-grade intraductal carcinomas exhibit a higher rate of apoptosis (*apoptotic index*) than do low-grade lesions (161).

## CYTOGENETICS AND MOLECULAR GENETICS

Before the development of microdissection techniques, few genetic studies of intraductal carcinoma were reported

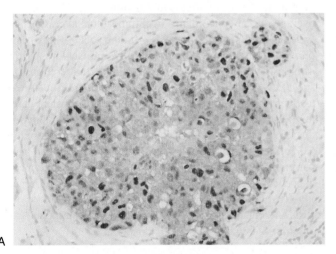

A

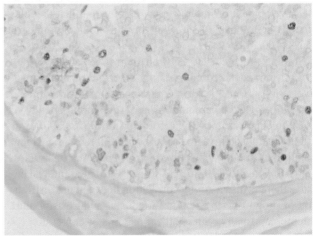

B

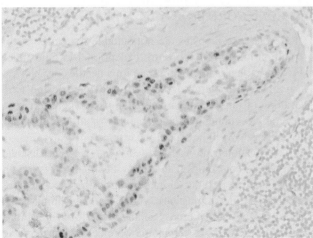

C

**FIG. 13.59.** *Intraductal carcinoma, proliferating cell nuclear antigen (PCNA).* **A:** Nuclear immunoreactivity for PCNA is present in almost all cells in this solid intraductal carcinoma. **B:** Most cells are not reactive for PCNA in this solid intraductal lesion. **C:** PCNA in micropapillary carcinoma. Nuclear reactivity is localized to the basal region (anti-PCNA, avidin-biotin).

because of the technical difficulties inherent in isolating the epithelium of these microscopic lesions. One study involved classic genetic analysis of cells obtained from tumor-forming intraductal carcinomas (162). Abnormal metaphases were found in all cases, and marker chromosome abnormalities were found most often on chromosome 1.

The DNA extracted from ducts containing intraductal carcinoma isolated by microdissection provided the material for the molecular analysis of genetic alterations. Using this method, Radford et al. reported loss of heterozygosity (LOH) on 17p in 29% of intraductal carcinomas compared with normal control DNA (163). No significant difference in the frequency of LOH was observed among subtypes of intraductal carcinoma (comedo versus noncomedo) or in regard to nuclear grade. Another study revealed LOH on chromosome 17p13.1 in 5 of 15 informative cases studied (164). Three samples with LOH were obtained from comedo intraductal carcinoma, coincident with a micropapillary component in one, and two others had micropapillary intraductal carcinoma. LOH on 11p15 has been reported in a high proportion of microdissected samples of intraductal carcinoma (165). Chuaqui et al. reported finding LOH on 11q13 in 6 of 22 (27.3%) intraductal carcinomas (166). All the lesions with LOH were high grade. LOH also was found in 1 of 11 (9%) lesions classified as atypical duct hyperplasia. The accumulated data suggest that LOH occurs often and early in the development of intraductal carcinoma and that the sites of LOH are probable loci of one or more tumor suppressor genes (167,168).

Stratton et al. detected LOH on 16q in 28% and on 17p in 29% of intraductal carcinomas not associated with an invasive lesion (169). Intraductal carcinoma found in conjunction with invasive carcinomas had a greater frequency of LOH on chromosomes 16q (55%) and 17p (52%). Analysis of intraductal and invasive carcinoma from the same patient usually but not always showed similar patterns of LOH in both components (170–173). This is of particular interest because there is also a strong correlation between the distribution of prognostic markers in intraductal and invasive duct carcinoma, usually with identical patterns of expression for hormone receptors, HER2/*neu*, p53, epidermal growth factor (EGF) receptor, and cyclin D1. Studies by Barsky et al. suggested that intraductal carcinoma often has acquired many of the biological characteristics of invasive carcinoma, and they hypothesized that the most significant difference between *in situ* and invasive carcinoma lies in the inhibitory influences of myoepithelial cells (174). Studies performed by these investigators indicated that one or more proteins secreted by myoepithelial cells inhibit invasion and angiogenesis.

A study of alterations in chromosome 1 revealed that the cells in individual ducts from a single specimen of intraductal carcinoma may have different genetic patterns (171). Similar observations were reported by Marsh and Varley, who analyzed LOH at 9p in multiple microdissected ducts from individual patients (175). LOH was found in 12 of 13 cases studied. Loss of at least one marker was detected in all

subtypes (comedo, solid, cribriform, and micropapillary), but the most extensive loss was present in comedo and cribriform lesions. In a few instances, heterogeneity was observed among different ducts from the same patient. The pattern of LOH in intraductal carcinoma was present in the corresponding invasive carcinoma in some but not in all tumors. Aubele et al. applied comparative genomic hybridization to microdissected examples of extensive intraductal carcinoma with small foci of invasive carcinoma (176). The procedure detected "multiple genetic changes affecting 6–19 different chromosomal regions per tumor (mean 13.6 ± 5.4)" in intraductal carcinoma. "Chromosomal alterations identified in more than one-third of the invasive lesions were mainly identical" to those in the corresponding intraductal carcinoma, except for gains of DNA on 3p and 12q, which were found more frequently in invasive carcinomas. Lymph node metastases in three cases showed 6 to 12 chromosomal changes (mean, 9.7 ± 3.2), representing a lower frequency than in the primary tumor.

A remarkable molecular genetic study of intraductal carcinoma reported by Waldman et al. used comparative genomic hybridization (CGH) to detect chromosomal alterations in primary lesions and in subsequent recurrences (177). Paired samples from 18 patients were studied, with all recurrences being entirely intraductal and detected 16 months to 9.3 years after initial treatment. In 17 cases, the average rate of concordance in chromosomal alterations between paired samples was 81% (range, 65%–100%), and pairs of lesions were morphologically similar. One pair of samples had no agreement, having 2 and 20 alterations, respectively. These findings indicate that situations classified as *recurrence* in 17 cases were instances of persistent carcinoma and that the 18th patient most likely had two independent foci of intraductal carcinoma. The mean number of CGH changes was lower in the initial lesions (8.8) than in recurrent intraductal carcinoma (10.7). The degree of concordance was not significantly related to the time to recurrence.

Allelic imbalance was detected in the region of the BRCA1 gene in nearly 75% of 34 samples of intraductal carcinoma studied by Munn et al. (178).

## NEEDLE CORE BIOPSY

Needle core biopsies are not suitable for frozen section examination unless there are exceptional circumstances. Frozen section is not appropriate for a needle core biopsy of a nonpalpable mammographically detected lesion (179). Grading of intraductal carcinoma in needle core biopsies is generally accurate, but the probability of structural variability increases with the size of the lesion.

Calcifications and necrotic debris may become dislodged in a needle core biopsy, and rarely this material is the only component of intraductal carcinoma in the specimen (Fig. 13.60). In this circumstance, serial sections should be prepared. An excisional biopsy should be performed even if no epithelial elements of carcinoma were detected in serial sec-

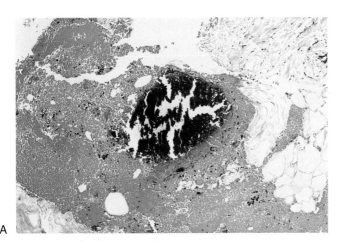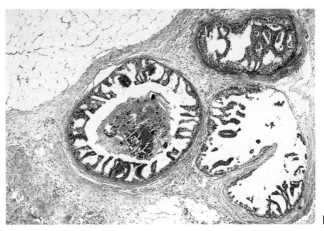

A                                                                                                       B

**FIG. 13.60.** *Intraductal carcinoma, needle core biopsy.* **A:** A fragmented calcification surrounded by necrotic debris and sparse isolated atypical cells in blood was the significant finding in a needle core biopsy. **B:** Subsequent surgical excision revealed this micropapillary intraductal carcinoma with calcifications.

tions that showed displaced calcification of a type that might occur in intraductal carcinoma. A dislodged fragment of intraductal carcinoma that becomes embedded in fat or stroma as part of a needle core biopsy sample may have an appearance that can be mistaken for invasive carcinoma (Fig. 13.61).

"Healed" intraductal carcinoma and end-stage periductal mastitis both can result in indistinguishable scarred ductal structures with calcifications (Fig. 13.62). When this type of structure is found in a needle core biopsy specimen, multiple serial sections should be prepared to search for scant foci of carcinoma that may be present. The extremely limited epithelial abnormalities found in some of these cases may result in a diagnosis of atypical ductal hyperplasia. A surgical excision is indicated for the latter diagnosis and in some situations may be appropriate when ductal scars are present without epithelial atypia if the mammographic findings raise concern about carcinoma. It is not unusual to find duct stasis and periductal mastitis in the vicinity of "healing" intraductal carcinoma.

The distinction between invasive carcinoma and sclerosing adenosis or radial sclerosing lesions can be challenging in needle core biopsies. This difficulty is compounded when intraductal carcinoma arises in sclerosing lesions (Fig. 13.63). It is important to consider this potential diagnostic pitfall and to use immunohistochemical stains for actin or smooth muscle myosin heavy chain to define the distribution of myoepithelial cells in the specimen. Incomplete samples of radial sclerosing lesions obtained in a needle core biopsy are difficult to assess for intraductal or invasive carcinoma, and they may be reported as atypical hyperplasia.

A needle core biopsy cannot be relied on to accurately measure the size of an intraductal carcinoma lesion, even if the procedure is performed for calcifications alone and calcifications are no longer present in a follow-up mammogram. The needle biopsy rarely provides a single intact sample of

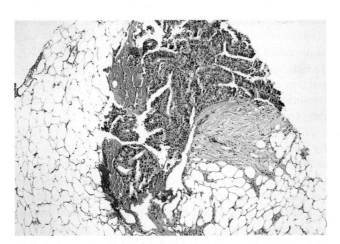

**FIG. 13.61.** *Intraductal carcinoma, needle core biopsy with displaced epithelium.* A fragment of papillary carcinoma is lodged in fat. This is not invasive carcinoma.

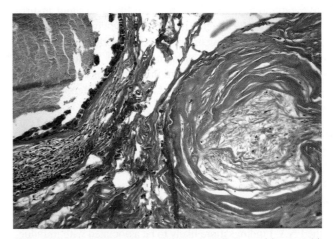

**FIG. 13.62.** *Intraductal carcinoma, needle core biopsy with scar.* Concentric layers of collagen probably represent the scar formed at the site of "healed" intraductal carcinoma. A dilated duct with a thin layer of intraductal carcinoma is shown on the *left*.

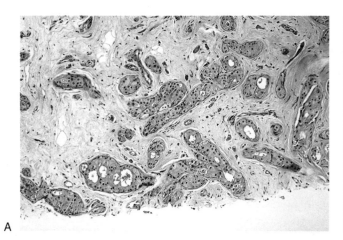
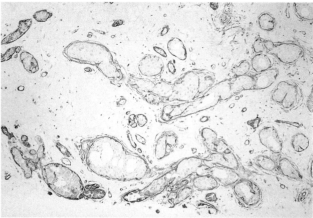

**FIG. 13.63.** *Intraductal carcinoma, apocrine type in sclerosing adenosis, needle core biopsy.* **A:** Apocrine intraductal carcinoma occupying sclerosing adenosis resembles invasive carcinoma. **B:** A section parallel to **A** prepared with the immunostain for smooth muscle actin demonstrating myoepithelial cells around all glandular structures.

the lesion, and it is not feasible to reassemble the intraductal carcinoma foci from multiple samples to obtain a single measurement. At best, needle core biopsy samples can be used to get a rough estimate of the extent of intraductal carcinoma.

The diagnosis of intraductal carcinoma in a needle core biopsy does not exclude the possibility of invasive carcinoma in the affected breast. The reported frequency of invasive carcinoma detected in excisional biopsies performed after a needle core biopsy diagnosis of intraductal carcinoma was 15% to 20% (180–182). The diagnosis of intraductal carcinoma was reported to be more reliable with a directional vacuum-assisted biopsy procedure than with an automated needle biopsy system (182).

## CYTOLOGIC DIAGNOSIS

Fine needle aspiration (FNA) specimens from intraductal carcinomas tend to be less cellular than aspirates from invasive carcinomas, and they are more likely to yield insufficient material for diagnosis (183). These circumstances are especially likely to occur when FNA is performed on a nonpalpable lesion detected by mammography. Failure to obtain diagnostic material by FNA in this setting is one indication for excisional biopsy because of the high frequency of intraductal carcinoma.

In most cases, when the FNA specimen is diagnostic of carcinoma, the distinction between intraductal and infiltrating duct carcinoma cannot be made with confidence (183,184). Correlation with the mammogram is useful, but intrinsic limitations of these samples make it impossible to exclude the presence of invasive carcinoma outside the site of the FNA procedure or even to exclude microinvasion in the region of the FNA. Findings more likely to be associated with intraductal than with invasive carcinoma are admixed cytologically benign cells and histiocytes. Invasive carcinoma is more likely to be present if carcinoma cells, singly or in groups, are intimately mingled with adipose tissue fibrous stroma or fat cells.

Venegas et al. identified criteria that they felt were helpful for detecting intraductal carcinoma in a FNA sample (185). These features were cohesive groups of atypical cells or hyperplastic ductal cells associated with malignant cells or a necrotic background and tissue fragments of cohesive cells with a cribriform arrangement. One or more of these findings were present in 81% of FNA specimens diagnosed as suspicious or positive for intraductal carcinoma. These criteria also proved useful for identifying intraductal carcinoma in invasive duct carcinomas because one or more of these features was present in 73% of lesions with extensive intraductal carcinoma and in 35% of those with a minor intraductal component.

Subclassification of intraductal carcinoma, distinguishing between comedo and noncomedo variants, may be suggested by FNA cytology (184,186,187). The aspirate from comedo intraductal carcinoma typically consists of pleomorphic, loosely cohesive cells with poorly differentiated nuclei and prominent nucleoli, sometimes accompanied by mitotic figures. Necrotic debris that may contain calcifications is usually present. Specimens from noncomedo intraductal carcinoma tend to contain more cohesive three-dimensional cell clusters with a papillary or cribriform configuration as well as dispersed cells distributed singly or in small groups (Fig. 13.64). Nuclei are intermediate to low grade cytologically, and they usually lack prominent nucleoli. Necrosis and an inflammatory background are found much less often in aspirates from noncomedo intraductal carcinomas.

Although the foregoing cytologic features may be reliable for distinguishing between classic examples of lesions, such as comedo intraductal carcinoma and orderly cribriform intraductal carcinoma, in some circumstances, the findings are not specific. This can occur when the intraductal lesion has comedo and noncomedo components. If the comedo portion of the lesion is not represented in the FNA sample, its presence will not be appreciated and the lesion will be classified as noncomedo carcinoma. In this respect, FNA is not only unreliable for distinguishing intraductal from invasive carci-

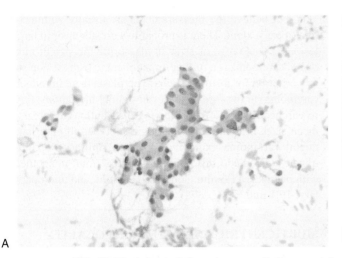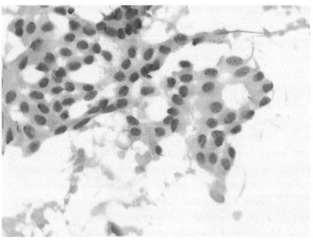

A                                               B

**FIG. 13.64.** *Intraductal carcinoma, cribriform, cytology.* **A:** Irregular, flat sheet of cells with a microlumen in a fine needle aspiration smear. **B:** Three adjacent microlumens are apparent in the epithelium with low-grade nuclear cytology.

noma, but it also can be inaccurate in subclassification of the lesion.

## SIZE AND QUANTITY OF INTRADUCTAL CARCINOMA

There is no widely accepted method for routinely measuring the actual size of intraductal carcinoma (101). Even when a patient has a palpable lesion found to harbor intraductal carcinoma, it is not unusual to find that the intraductal lesion extends microscopically beyond the gross lesion. Many intraductal carcinomas currently detected by mammography do not form a clinically or pathologically palpable lesion. Fisher et al. reported that approximately 80% of the 573 cases included in the National Surgical Adjuvant Breast Project (NS-ABP) protocol B-17 were not palpable (188). The extent (size) of intraductal carcinoma can be estimated by mammography, largely on the basis of the distribution of calcifications. Coombs et al. reported that mammography underestimated size in 23% of cases compared with pathologic size determination (189). In the same study, lesions pathologically larger than 15 mm were more likely to be multifocal or multicentric than those 15 mm or less, and these investigators reported no significant correlation between nuclear grade, necrosis, histologic subtype, proliferative index, ploidy, and size (189).

It is sometimes possible to determine the size of a lesion microscopically if it is limited to a single group of contiguous ducts *(unifocal)*, especially when the area is confined to the histologic section from a single paraffin block. Reporting the size of the small lesions in this category is confounded by the fact that some investigators exclude abnormalities smaller than 2.0 mm from the diagnosis of intraductal carcinoma regardless of histologic appearance (79,190).

A significant proportion of intraductal carcinomas are multifocal and are not confined to a single coherent palpable lesion or to a microscopic focus that will fit in the confines of a single paraffin block. It is noteworthy that the dimensions of an intraductal carcinoma limited to one standard paraffin block ordinarily would not exceed 2.0 to 2.5 cm (or 1 inch). Lagios et al. studied mastectomy specimens from patients with intraductal carcinoma by a serial subgross method and reported that the frequency of multicentricity and occult invasion was substantially greater for lesions larger than 2.5 cm (191). It is on the basis of these studies that 2.5 cm came to be viewed as an important size criterion in the selection of patients for breast-conserving therapy. More recently, Lagios expressed skepticism about the quantitation of ductal carcinoma in situ (DCIS), observing that "quantitation of DCIS will remain a problem since the association of the extent of DCIS, and the extent of microcalcifications, the only preoperative measure available at present, is quite variable" (192). The prognostic significance attributed to size is discussed in a subsequent section of this chapter devoted to Treatment and Prognosis.

Because of the problems inherent in determining the extent of intraductal carcinoma by direct measurement of the lesion, indirect methods of quantitation have been used. One of these methods has been to count the number of ducts involved by intraductal carcinoma as seen in the histologic sections. Equating the number of duct cross sections with the measurement of tumor size is at best an approximation of the actual dimensions of the lesional area. Without preparing serial sections and a three-dimensional reconstruction, it is impossible to correlate the number of duct cross sections in a two-dimensional histologic slide with the actual number of independent ducts containing carcinoma because a single duct may pass through the plane of section more than once. In one instance, a given number of duct cross sections may be concentrated in a relatively small area, whereas in another, an equal or lesser number of sections of ducts may be distributed in a larger area.

Another approach has been the suggestion to report the number of slides and the proportion of slides containing intraductal carcinoma (193). Kestin et al. reported a significant association between the number of slides showing intraductal carcinoma and the frequency of local failure in the breast after breast-conserving surgery and radiotherapy (194). Recurrences were significantly more frequent if intraductal carcinoma involved six or more slides than if it was seen on five or fewer sections. In this study, margin status (close/positive versus negative) was not significantly related to local or systemic failure.

Tornos et al. correlated the number of slides with intraductal carcinoma in a lumpectomy and the likelihood of there being residual carcinoma in the breast by examining mastectomy or reexcision specimens (195). They found residual intraductal carcinoma in the second specimen in 78% of cases when there was intraductal carcinoma in at least 50% of the initial excision slides and in 48% when fewer than 50% of the slides showed intraductal carcinoma. Margin width (<2 mm versus ≥2 mm) was not significantly related to finding residual carcinoma. These researchers recommended that reexcision be performed if at least 50% of the slides in an initial biopsy were involved by intraductal carcinoma. The distinction between finding residual carcinoma in 78% versus 48% of cases is not great enough to make the 50% of slides rule a reliable criterion.

Presently, there is no consensus on a method for determining the extent of intraductal carcinoma on the basis of the proportion of slides showing the lesion. This approach is highly dependent on the completeness of sampling and biopsy size, both of which determine the denominator. This issue would be partially addressed if the denominator were biopsy weight in grams, with a numerator representing the number of slides showing intraductal carcinoma. This calculation would be most useful in situations where all tissue has been processed for histologic examination. Until a standardized method has been validated and widely adopted, the proportion of slides with intraductal carcinoma will remain a crude measure of the extent of intraductal carcinoma.

Many patients have more then one operation performed (e.g., excision followed by reexcision) with intraductal carcinoma in more than one specimen. It is not practical to reassemble the intraductal foci from two or more specimens to obtain a single measurement.

For the foregoing reasons, a 1997 consensus report on the classification of intraductal carcinoma left the issue of size largely unanswered and was unable to address this question (101). A classification system for intraductal carcinoma that includes lesion size is currently impractical. Nonetheless, data purportedly describing the "size" of intraductal carcinoma are reported. The mean size of 227 lesions in one series was 2.1 cm, ranging from 1.5 cm in cribriform to 2.5 cm in comedo intraductal carcinoma (196). In a study of cases referred for consultation, Lennington et al. recorded size from the "outside surgical pathology report" for "extensive lesions"; but for "smaller, less extensive lesions, size was measured directly from the glass slides" (79). Lesions 2 mm or smaller in diameter were excluded by definition because they were classified as atypical hyperplasia. These researchers stated that they " . . . recognize the lack of preci-

sion, but believe the measurements are usually within 3–5 mm of true extent. There is probably a greater error in larger lesions." This range of error in measuring the size of intraductal carcinoma is a further impediment to using lesion size as a criterion for distinguishing hyperplasia from intraductal carcinoma. In the face of these substantial limitations, these researchers reported the following distribution of "precise" mean sizes in relation to histologic subtype: all pure intraductal carcinoma exclusive of micropapillary, 8.5 mm; mixed noncomedo histologic types, 13.1 mm; noncomedo with necrosis, 11.6 mm; comedo, 16.2 mm; and micropapillary, 19.1 mm (79).

## MULTICENTRICITY AND MULTIFOCALITY

There is no uniformly accepted definition of multicentricity in intraductal carcinoma. The concept of multicentricity was advanced by Cheatle and Cutler and by Charteris as a result of observations made on whole-organ sections of mastectomy specimens (9,197,198). Carcinoma was considered multicentric when there were foci that were separate from the clinically detected tumor. Lagios et al. defined multicentricity as " . . . the presence of separate independent foci of carcinoma within the breast—separate from the lesion which is clinically or mammographically evident, that is, the reference tumor" (199). In practical terms, multicentricity refers to foci of carcinoma in distinctly different regions of the breast, usually in two or more quadrants.

Multicentricity should be distinguished from intraepithelial extension within ducts and lobules of a single carcinomatous focus typically limited to one region or quadrant. The later condition is commonly referred to as multifocality. One commonly used criterion for establishing the presence of multifocality depends on the number of histologic sections that show intraductal carcinoma. For example, Fisher et al. stated that "ductal carcinoma in situ in only one section of two or more obtained from different blocks was considered to be unifocal. Its presence in sections from two or more different blocks was considered multifocal" (188). On the basis of this definition, 329 of 541 (60.8%) evaluable specimens of intraductal carcinoma were classified as multifocal in data from the NSABP B-17 (188). Silverstein et al. considered intraductal carcinoma to be multifocal when " . . . separate foci of DCIS [duct carcinoma in situ] more than 2 cm from primary site . . . " were found in a mastectomy specimen (196). On the basis of this criterion, multifocality was present in 41 of 98 (41%) of breasts examined after mastectomy. Multicentricity, defined as carcinoma outside the index quadrant, was present in 15% of these breasts. Multifocality and multicentricity were not significantly related to the histologic category of intraductal carcinoma when stratified as comedo and noncomedo type (196). Hardman et al. found multicentric carcinoma in 27% of mastectomy specimens from patients with carcinoma of the comedo type (200). Multicentricity was reported in 33% (12) and 37% (201) of mastectomies performed for diverse types of intraductal carcinoma.

In an effort to circumvent these technical issues, some investigators set anatomic limits on the distribution of carcinoma to somewhat arbitrarily distinguish between unicentric and multicentric disease. For example, carcinoma has been deemed to be multicentric if it was detected in more than one quadrant or if it is 5 cm from the index lesion (69,201–203). Silverstein et al. classified intraductal carcinoma as multicentric if two foci were separated by more than 2.0 cm (204).

Schwartz et al. studied the frequency of multicentricity in the breasts of patients with intraductal carcinoma who underwent mastectomy (69,205). Multicentricity was defined as " . . . the presence [of] invasive ductal or lobular carcinoma, microinvasive ductal carcinoma, or DCIS in an area or quadrant outside the biopsy site. . . . If the lesion was centrally located . . . the cancer was considered multicentric only if additional foci of carcinoma were found outside a perimeter of 5 cm from the edge of the nipple and areola" (69). Multicentricity was found in 18 of 50 (36%) (69) and in four of 11 (36%) (205) breasts. Multicentricity was present more often in lesions detected because of nipple discharge (71%) or Paget's disease (50%) than in those found by mammography (38%) (69). When classified on the basis of the predominant growth pattern, micropapillary intraductal carcinoma was more often multicentric (86%) than papillary (33%) or comedo (42%) carcinomas. No multicentricity was encountered in five cribriform and seven solid intraductal carcinomas. Bellamy et al. also found multicentricity to be present significantly more often in patients with micropapillary intraductal carcinoma than in those with other patterns of intraductal carcinoma (63).

Faverly et al. applied a method for the stereoscopic examination of breast tissue to 60 mastectomy specimens from patients with intraductal carcinoma (206). This procedure allowed the investigators to observe the three-dimensional distribution of intraductal carcinoma. Overall, intraductal carcinomas measured 2 to 140 mm, with a median size of 65 mm. Of these lesions, 47% involved more than one quadrant. *Multicentric carcinoma,* defined as discontinuity of 4 cm or more between carcinomatous foci, was found in only one case. *Multifocal carcinoma,* defined as discontinuous foci less than 4 mm apart, was more common in well-differentiated (70%) and moderately differentiated (56%) forms of intraductal carcinoma than in poorly differentiated lesions (10%). Conversely, continuous growth was found in 30% of well-differentiated and in 90% of poorly differentiated tumors. The gaps between foci in multifocal intraductal carcinomas were less than 10 mm in 83% of the cases.

If the sample provided for histologic diagnosis is an excisional biopsy limited to the region of the index lesion, the material is not suitable for determining whether the patient has multicentric carcinoma. According to some definitions, more than a quadrantectomy is necessary to detect multicentricity. In practice, the distinction between multifocality and multicentricity is difficult to make with certainty in slides prepared by conventional methods of sampling breast specimens for diagnostic purposes. Investigative techniques such as serial sectioning, stereoscopic dissection, and subgross microscopic–radiologic correlative studies are more reliable methods for identifying true multicentricity, but they are too costly and time consuming to be practical procedures for routine diagnostic work. Given the limited resources available in most pathology laboratories, it is unrealistic to expect diagnostic reports on breast biopsies to routinely distinguish multicentricity from multifocality.

## MICROINVASION

Ultrastructural studies have detected foci of discontinuity in the basement membranes of ducts with intraductal carcinoma (207,208), and similar observations have been reported in tissues studied by immunohistochemistry (209). Breaks in the basement membrane were more common when intraductal carcinoma was of the comedo type or had a high nuclear grade. Carcinoma cells have been observed by electron microscopy protruding through gaps in the basal lamina when invasion was not apparent by light microscopy (210). At sites where the basement membrane is intact, the periductal stromal cells are fibroblasts, whereas myofibroblastic proliferation mingles with the fibroblasts where there is basement membrane disruption (210). On the basis of electron microscopy, Tulusan et al. concluded that true microinvasion involves penetration of basal lamina and the basement membrane (211). This was found to occur in two ways: protrusion of intraductal carcinoma through gaps in the basement membrane or the passage of single cancer cells through similar defects. The latter mechanism may be more common in invasive lobular carcinoma. These ultrastructural observations are of biological and theoretical interest, but it remains to be determined whether protruding cells still attached to their intraductal counterparts are capable of metastatic spread. In addition, the limited sampling possible with the electron microscope makes this an impractical method for detecting invasion.

Basement membrane integrity at sites of microinvasion has been investigated by immunohistochemistry (Fig. 13.65). Barksy et al. detected fragmentation and disruption of basement membranes in areas of microinvasion by using antibodies to laminin and collagen type IV (75) (Fig. 13.66). Type IV collagen is degraded by type IV collagenase, a metalloproteinase, which specifically cleaves type IV collagen. The active enzyme is absent from normal and proliferative ducts, variably present in comedocarcinoma and prominent in invasive carcinoma (212). These and other observations suggest that the ability of carcinoma cells to form latent type IV collagenase and convert it to the active form is an important attribute associated with the invasive phenotype. As noted earlier in this chapter, myoepithelial cells also appear to play a significant role in inhibiting invasion by intraductal carcinoma (116). One important function of myoepithelial cells is the elaboration of protease inhibitors, which appear to counteract the invasion-promoting effects of metalloproteinases produced by intraductal carcinoma cells.

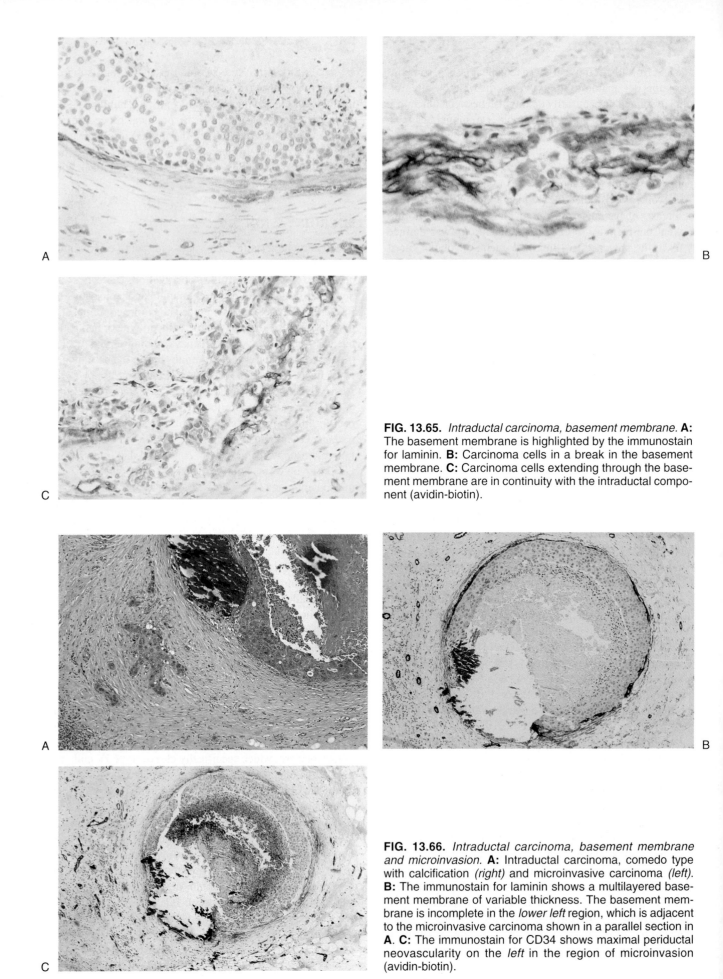

**FIG. 13.65.** *Intraductal carcinoma, basement membrane.* **A:** The basement membrane is highlighted by the immunostain for laminin. **B:** Carcinoma cells in a break in the basement membrane. **C:** Carcinoma cells extending through the basement membrane are in continuity with the intraductal component (avidin-biotin).

**FIG. 13.66.** *Intraductal carcinoma, basement membrane and microinvasion.* **A:** Intraductal carcinoma, comedo type with calcification *(right)* and microinvasive carcinoma *(left).* **B:** The immunostain for laminin shows a multilayered basement membrane of variable thickness. The basement membrane is incomplete in the *lower left* region, which is adjacent to the microinvasive carcinoma shown in a parallel section in **A**. **C:** The immunostain for CD34 shows maximal periductal neovascularity on the *left* in the region of microinvasion (avidin-biotin).

The type IV collagen molecule consists of a number of distinctive α-chain subunits. The cross-linked α-chains form a macromolecular network that is a major structural component of the basement membrane. Studies using A(IV) chain-specific antibodies and *in situ* hybridization showed that the expression of selected α-chains is dependent on the presence of myoepithelial cells (213). Discontinuous or absent expression of type IV collagen α-chain subunits has been observed in invasive carcinomas (213,214).

The laminin molecule is also composed of cross-linked subunits designated alpha, beta, and gamma chains. Immunohistochemical studies using chain-specific antibodies revealed discontinuous or absent expression of most subunits in invasive carcinomas and no expression of the $\beta_2$ chain (214).

The importance of determining whether invasion is present outweighs the information that might be obtained from a variety of studies that can be performed on a specimen known or suspected to contain intraductal carcinoma. Frozen section is not recommended in most instances, and a sample should not be taken for ancillary assays, such as flow cytometry or molecular studies, because the tissue removed is no longer available for histologic examination.

*Microinvasion* should be distinguished from *minimally invasive carcinoma*, a term that refers to invasive lesions less than 1.0 cm in diameter (215–217). *Microinvasive carcinoma* is a subcategory of minimally invasive carcinoma. *Microinvasion* is defined in the current staging system for breast carcinoma as *T1mic,* an invasive focus 0.1 cm or less in greatest dimension (see Chapter 12).

A controversial aspect of the histologic diagnosis of microinvasion relates to the interpretation of ducts that have poorly defined walls and there is an indistinct basement membrane zone. In such regions, the neoplastic epithelium may appear to protrude from the duct, seeming to come in direct contact with the stroma, although it remains connected with the intraductal neoplasm (218) (Figs. 13.29 and 13.67). This finding often elicits diagnostic uncertainty reflected in such caveats as "suspect microinvasion" or "microinvasion cannot be ruled out." Retrospective studies have given no indication that these ambiguous findings are associated with an appreciable risk of systemic metastases, but they may account for some instances in which micrometastases have been detected in sentinel lymph nodes from patients with intraductal carcinoma (see Chapter 46).

To qualify for the term *microinvasion,* the cells deemed to be invasive must be distributed in a fashion that does not represent tangential sectioning of a duct or a lobular gland with intraductal carcinoma (Figs. 13.67 and 13.68). Tangentially sectioned *in situ* carcinoma that simulates microinvasion usually occurs as compact groups of tumor cells that have a smooth border surrounded by a circumferential layer of myoepithelial cells and stroma. These "organoid" foci are dis-

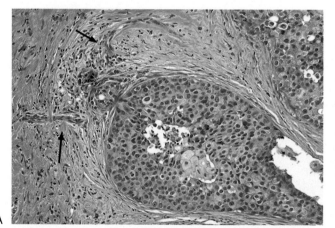

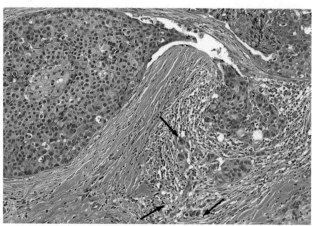

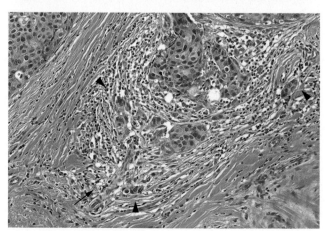

**FIG. 13.67.** *Intraductal carcinoma, microinvasion.* **A:** Carcinoma protrudes from a duct with solid intraductal carcinoma. Note the stromal reaction including two small blood vessels directed toward the protruding carcinoma *(arrows).* In this plane of section, the finding is ambiguous and not diagnostic of invasion because this could be a tangential section of a small secondary duct exiting the large duct. Immunostains for basement membrane components, myoepithelial cells, and cytokeratin are helpful in analyzing such foci. **B,C:** This focus from the same case as **A** provides stronger evidence for microinvasion because there appears to be greater disruption of the protruding epithelium including isolated cell clusters in the stroma *(arrowheads).* Note the small blood vessel directed a the site of probable invasion *(arrow).*

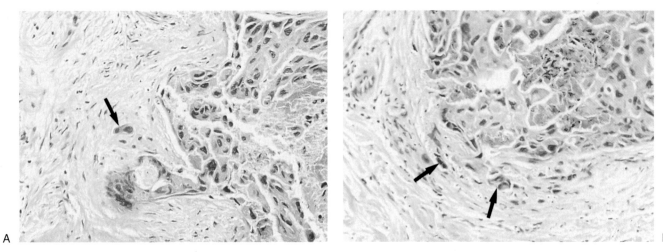

A

B

**FIG. 13.68.** *Intraductal carcinoma, microinvasion.* **A:** Two isolated carcinoma cells *(arrow)* in the periductal stroma adjacent to a tangentially sectioned duct containing intraductal carcinoma. **B:** Disruption of the basement membrane is evident and there are carcinoma cells in the periductal stroma *(arrows)*.

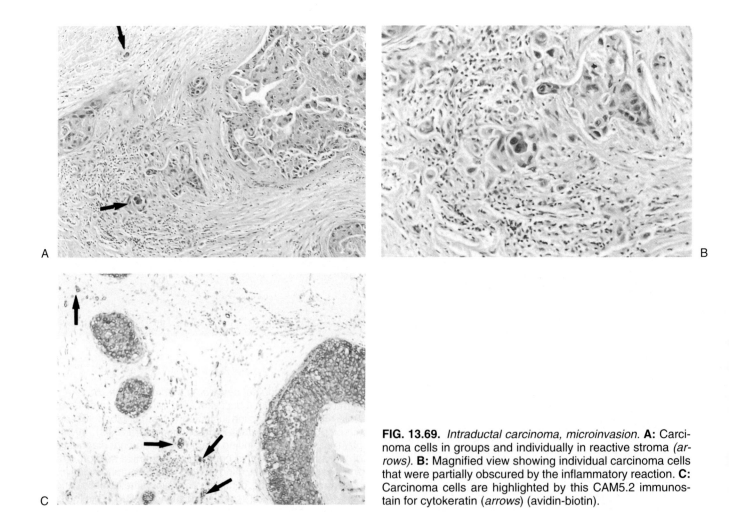

A

B

C

**FIG. 13.69.** *Intraductal carcinoma, microinvasion.* **A:** Carcinoma cells in groups and individually in reactive stroma *(arrows)*. **B:** Magnified view showing individual carcinoma cells that were partially obscured by the inflammatory reaction. **C:** Carcinoma cells are highlighted by this CAM5.2 immunostain for cytokeratin *(arrows)* (avidin-biotin).

tributed in the specialized periductal or intralobular stroma. In many instances, immunostains are helpful in resolving the problem by demonstrating the presence or absence of basement membrane components or myoepithelial cells at these sites. The conventional immunostain for smooth-muscle actin highlights myofibroblasts as well as myoepithelial cells. The resultant appearance can interfere with the assessment of foci suspected to harbor microinvasion. Immunostains for calponin or smooth-muscle myosin heavy chain are preferable in this setting because they have greater specificity for myoepithelial cells (219), although immunoreactivity with the smooth-muscle actin antibody is typically more intense. Unfortunately, myoepithelial cells are not present in many intraductal carcinomas, and therefore their absence in these cases is not a reliable indication of invasion.

At sites of microinvasive ductal carcinoma, tumor cells are distributed singly or as small groups that have irregular shapes reminiscent of conventional invasive carcinoma with no particular orientation (Figs. 13.66, 13.68, and 13.69). Microinvasion can be identified more readily in nonspecialized interlobular stroma. Sometimes the intralobular or periductal stroma appears less dense at sites of microinvasion than in other areas around these structures, and microinvasive foci appear to attract lymphocytic reaction. Detecting carcinoma cells in the stroma can be difficult when there is a marked periductal inflammatory and stromal cell reaction. Microinvasion may be suspected at sites where there is a pronounced lymphocytic accumulation near ducts with intraductal carcinoma (Fig. 13.70). A granulomatous reaction may be elicited at foci of microinvasion (220). The tumor cells can resemble histiocytes, and immunostains for cytokeratin might be required to confirm the presence of microinvasion. Double immunolabeling for cytokeratin and actin is an elegant method for visualizing foci of microinvasion (Fig. 13.42) (221).

Microinvasion more often is associated with high-grade and comedo intraductal carcinoma, but it may occur in other types of intraductal carcinoma (57). Thorough histologic sectioning is recommended for all cases of high-grade intraductal carcinoma, especially comedocarcinoma, and for other types of intraductal carcinoma that form a cohesive lesion

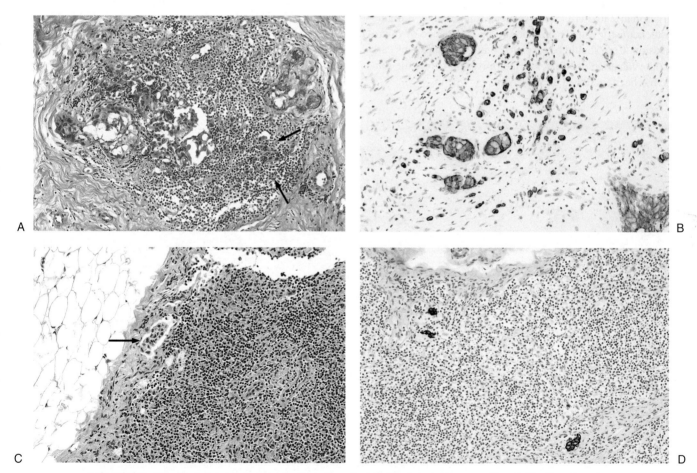

**FIG. 13.70.** *Intraductal carcinoma, microinvasion.* **A:** Intraductal carcinoma with calcifications in a terminal duct–lobular structure. Isolated invasive carcinoma cells are obscured by a lymphocytic reaction *(arrows).* **B:** The CAM5.2 cytokeratin immunostain highlights invasive carcinoma cells (avidin-biotin). **C:** A cluster of metastatic carcinoma cells *(arrow)* in a peripheral sinusoid of the sentinel lymph node. **D:** Isolated CAM5.2 cytokeratin immunoreactive cells in the sentinel lymph node (avidin-biotin). The patient was staged as T1micN1.

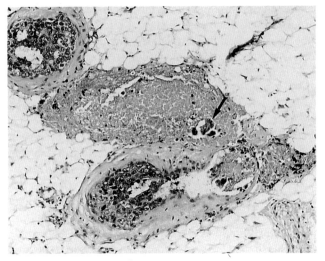

**FIG. 13.71.** *Intraductal carcinoma, displaced epithelium.* Fragment of carcinoma in a fibrin clot next to intraductal carcinoma *(arrow).* The site of duct disruption is evident on the *right.* The patient had a fine-needle aspiration biopsy before surgical excision.

larger than 2 to 3 cm. Serial sections supported by immuno-histochemistry usually provide the best evidence of microinvasion. Care should be taken to obtain immunostains early in the evaluation of suspected microinvasion before the sample has been sectioned excessively.

Carcinomatous epithelium displaced by needling procedures should not be interpreted as intrinsic invasive carcinoma (Fig. 13.71). The presence of carcinoma cells in vascular or lymphatic channels after a needle biopsy of intraductal carcinoma, however, can be associated with carcinoma cells in axillary lymph nodes, even when intrinsic invasion is not detected (Fig. 13.72).

The histologic diagnosis of microinvasion is confounded in some cases by the capacity of invasive carcinoma to assume a growth pattern that simulates intraductal carcinoma (Fig. 13.73). This occurrence is appreciated most easily in metastatic deposits at sites outside the breast, such as the axillary lymph nodes, and less frequently in visceral metastases. The phenomenon was described by Cowen in 1980 (222) and in a later paper, Cowen and Bates reported finding metastatic carcinoma with an intraductal carcinoma-like appearance in lymph nodes from 35 of 391 (9%) patients with axillary metastases (223). In two of these cases, no intraductal component was found in the primary tumor, but in the others the "pseudointraductal" carcinoma in metastases resembled intraductal carcinoma in the primary lesion. Barsky et al. reported finding intraductal carcinoma-like metastases in axillary lymph nodes from 21% of 200 cases (224). These foci were termed *revertant* intraductal carcinoma to reflect the hypothesis that this phenomenon is a manifestation of a condition in which metastatic potential is inhibited or reversed by local factors. These investigators observed complete concordance between primary and revertant intra-

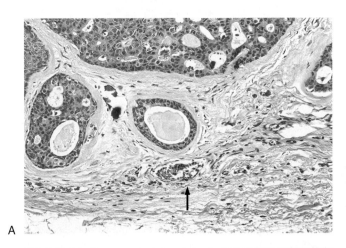

A

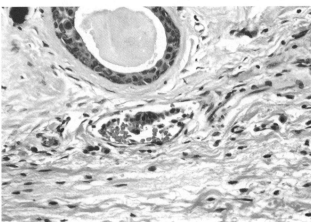

B

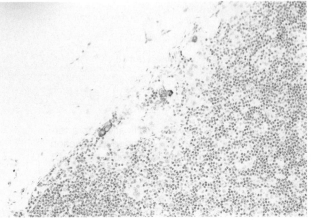

C

**FIG. 13.72.** *Intraductal carcinoma with vascular tumor emboli.* **A,B:** After a needle core biopsy revealed intraductal carcinoma, this patient underwent excisional biopsy. The specimen contained cribriform intraductal carcinoma, shown here with carcinoma cells in an adjacent vascular channel *(arrow).* **C:** Isolated cytokeratin (AE1/AE3)-positive cells were present in subcapsular sinuses of the sentinel lymph node.

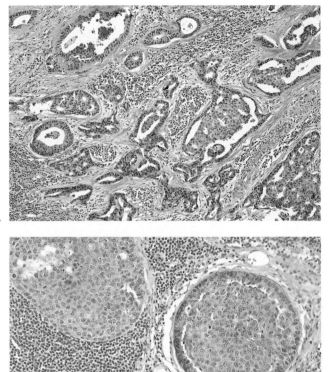

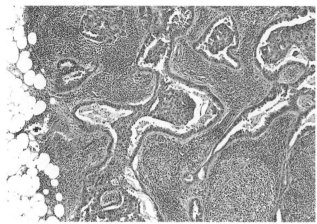

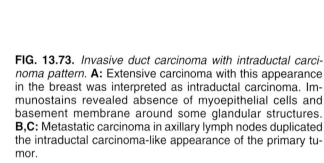

**FIG. 13.73.** *Invasive duct carcinoma with intraductal carcinoma pattern.* **A:** Extensive carcinoma with this appearance in the breast was interpreted as intraductal carcinoma. Immunostains revealed absence of myoepithelial cells and basement membrane around some glandular structures. **B,C:** Metastatic carcinoma in axillary lymph nodes duplicated the intraductal carcinoma-like appearance of the primary tumor.

ductal carcinoma with respect to architectural pattern, nuclear size determined by digital image analysis, as well as the expression of the prognostic markers p53, HER2/*neu*, and Ki67. Revertant intraductal carcinoma featured circumferential basement membranes demonstrated by immunoreactivity for laminin and collagen type IV but lacked myoepithelial cells.

The capacity of invasive carcinoma to assume an appearance that resembles its *in situ* counterpart is a significant confounding factor, especially in the diagnosis of microinvasive carcinoma. Cowen and Bates concluded that, "since invasive breast carcinoma may mimic intraductal growth some cases of breast cancer diagnosed histologically as intraductal carcinoma may in reality be invasive" (223). This phenomenon may be responsible for some of the rare patients found to have axillary nodal metastases, especially as a result of sentinel lymph node mapping, when the breast appears to be the site of intraductal carcinoma with no demonstrable invasion.

The difficulties raised by the structural similarities of *in situ* and invasive duct carcinoma are complicated by the results of studies that demonstrated the presence of basement membrane components around groups of invasive carcinoma cells (Fig. 13.74). Arihiro et al. found immunoreactivity for laminin at sites of invasive carcinoma in 54% of 71 carcinomas (225). The presence of laminin was associated with a greater degree of tubule formation. These findings correlate with data obtained by Nadji et al., who reported that the ex-

pression of a 67-kDa laminin-binding protein, 67LR, was significantly related to low histologic and nuclear grade (226). Henning et al. found a complete absence of immunoreactivity for laminin-5 in 45% of 44 invasive carcinomas studied (227).

The foregoing investigations were not directed specifically at assessing basal lamina at sites where microinvasion was a concern. This issue was addressed by Damiani et al., who compared invasive carcinomas to lesions "suggestive of invasive carcinoma" (228). Intraductal carcinomas were characterized by a "well-formed basal lamina and/or an evident myoepithelial layer. These features were lacking in the invasive areas." The study was conducted using antibodies for laminin, collagen type IV, α-smooth-muscle actin, and calponin. These authors achieved a definitive diagnosis in 9 of 11 cases initially regarded as "suggestive of invasive carcinoma." Five were classified as invasive and four as intraductal carcinoma "according to the absence or presence of a continuous myoepithelial layer and/or basal lamina." The studies were not diagnostic in two cases (18%) in which immunostains were difficult to interpret or the lesions were not present in all sections. These researchers found that the calponin stain was more specific for myoepithelial cells than the antibody for smooth-muscle actin and that it was less sensitive with less intense staining. They also noted that the staining for basement membrane components was "discontinuous or lacking" at the site of invasion.

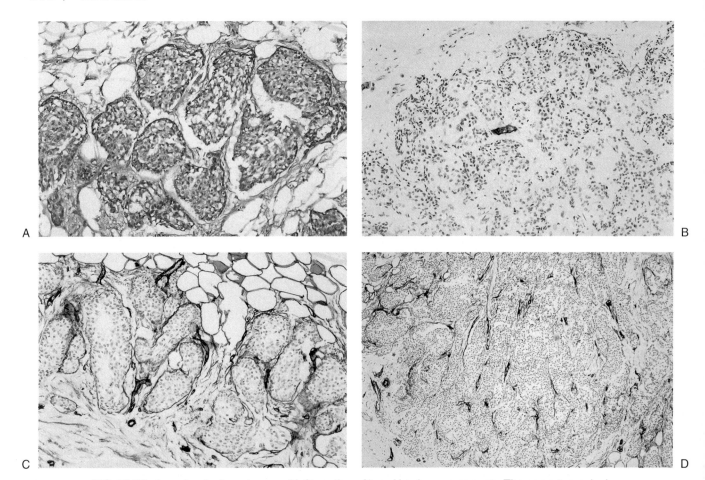

**FIG. 13.74.** *Invasive duct carcinoma with formation of basal lamina components.* The same tumor is depicted in all images. **A:** The carcinoma with an alveolar structure invades fat. There are compressed cells that resemble myoepithelial cells at the perimeter of some of the rounded tumor cell clusters. **B:** The immunostain for actin reveals reactivity in a small central blood vessel but not in the carcinoma, indicating absence of myoepithelial cells. **C:** Alveolar nests of carcinoma cells are encircled here by a thin band of laminin reactivity. **D:** The alveolar groups of carcinoma cells are only partially encompassed by reactivity for collagen type IV. Some of the collagen type IV reactivity is associated with small blood vessels in the tumor. (All immunostains avidin-biotin).

In light of the foregoing discussion, it is evident that there are instances in which the presence or absence of microinvasion can be difficult to determine with certainty, even with the immunohistochemical reagents currently available. Some guidelines can be suggested based on the author's experience in examining numerous specimens in which microinvasion was a concern.

1. The presence of myoepithelial cells is the most convincing evidence of intraductal carcinoma, especially if demonstrated with an actin immunostain. It is helpful to use more than one immunostain because reactivity is not equally intense with all reagents.
2. Absence of demonstrable actin reactivity usually means that myoepithelial cells are not present, although they can be severely attenuated and difficult to recognize. Loss of the myoepithelial cell layer occurs in a substantial proportion of intraductal carcinomas. By itself, the absence of myoepithelial cells is not indicative of invasive carcinoma, and the interpretation of this finding depends on the complete histologic appearance of the lesion.
3. Immunostains for basement membrane components, laminin, and collagen type IV are also helpful. Absence of reactivity for both components indicates a strong likelihood of invasive carcinoma, especially if coupled with absence of myoepithelial cells.
4. Reactivity for one or both basal lamina components in the absence of myoepithelial cells presents the most difficult diagnostic situation that requires assessment of the entire lesion, including multple levels if possible. The presence of laminin and collagen-type IV favors a diagnosis of *in situ* carcinoma; however, consideration must be given to the possibility that basal lamina may be formed at sites of invasion. With present routine diagnostic techniques, the distinction between basal lamina formed at sites of invasion and basement membranes in *in situ* carcinoma cannot be resolved with confidence in all cases.

It is preferable to use the term *microinvasion* for invasive lesions smaller than 1 mm in largest diameter. This definition was adopted by the Tumor, Node, Metastasis (TNM) staging system, with the rubric T1mic to provide a descriptive identity for these unusually small invasive lesions that are otherwise not separately categorized. When multiple foci of such microinvasion are present, there is no agreed on method for estimating their aggregate diameter, and these cases still qualify as intraductal carcinoma with microinvasion. Foci of invasion 1 mm or larger are diagnosed as invasive duct carcinoma and are reported on the basis of measured size.

Before acceptance of the category T1mic, there was no consensus as to the amount or extent of invasive carcinoma described by the term *microinvasion*. A variety of definitions were proposed involving arbitrary criteria, estimated measurements, or a combination of both elements. Shuh et al. stated that "the sections were examined for evidence of stromal invasion, and if this was present the patient was designated as having DCIS with microinvasion" (68). The amount of invasion needed to qualify for this type of microinvasion was not specified. Fifty-two patients with pure intraductal carcinoma and 30 with microinvasive carcinoma according to the definition of Shuh et al. were compared. Patients with microinvasion more often had a mass (63% versus 33%) than those with pure intraductal carcinoma. The frequency of detection by mammography did not differ greatly between patients with pure and microinvasive intraductal carcinoma (33% versus 23%). Patients with microinvasion were more likely to have multicentric carcinoma. Axillary nodal metastases were found in 1 of 52 (2%) patients with pure intraductal carcinoma and in 6 of 30 (20%) of patients with microinvasion.

Wong et al. defined microinvasion as "only a microscopic focus of malignant cells invading beyond the basement membrane as determined by light microscopy" and found no lymph node metastases in 33 patients who underwent an axillary dissection (229).

Solin et al. limited microinvasion to a "maximal extent of invasion of <2 mm or invasive carcinoma comprising <10% of the tumor" (230). Axillary lymph node metastases were found in 2 of 39 (5%) patients with microinvasion. Most (67%) had comedocarcinoma, but microinvasion also was found in patients with cribriform, papillary, micropapillary, and solid types of intraductal carcinoma. After a median follow-up of 55 months, one (7%) patient had developed a distant recurrence. and there were 9 (24%) instances of local recurrence in the breast after conservation therapy. Rosner et al. referred to " . . . limited microscopic stromal invasion below the basement membrane in one or several ducts, but not invading more than 10% of the surface of the histologic sections examined" (231). This definition was based on previously established criteria that characterized microinvasion as occurring in " . . . predominantly intraductal tumors showing either focal infiltration outside the basement membrane or stromal invasion that accounted for less than an estimated surface area of 10% in the sections examined" (35). These researchers found 36 such patients (8.8%) in a series of 408 women with node-negative invasive breast carcinoma. Fifty-six percent of the lesions were detected by mammography. All patients remained recurrence-free after a mean follow-up of 57 months.

Silverstein et al. used the term microinvasion if "one or two microscopic foci of possible invasion no more than 1 mm in maximum diameter were found or if the pathologists were uncertain as to whether or not a cancerous lobule was tangentially sectioned or infiltrating" (64). Microinvasion as so defined was detected in 28 of 208 (13%) cases. Most microinvasive lesions were comedocarcinoma (21 of 28, 75%), representing 20% of intraductal comedocarcinomas. Microinvasion also was encountered in 3 of 23 (13%) micropapillary, 2 of 15 (13%) papillary, 1 of 22 (5%) solid, and 1 of 43 (2%) cribriform intraductal carcinomas. One of the 28 (4%) patients with microinvasive carcinoma had axillary lymph node metastases.

Lagios et al. reported a higher frequency of "occult invasion" associated with intraductal carcinomas larger than 25 mm, with most of the risk in lesions 50 mm or larger (199). Silver and Tavassoli defined microinvasion as " single focus of invasive carcinoma ≤2 mm or up to 3 foci of invasion, each ≤1 mm in greatest dimension" in a study of 38 patients (232). Comedo intraductal carcinoma was present in 31 (82%), and 7 (18%) had papillary or other types of intraductal carcinoma. All patients were treated by mastectomy with axillary dissection, and no lymph node metastases were found. After a mean follow-up of 7.5 years, no patient had developed recurrent breast carcinoma.

Little information is presently available about patients with microinvasion defined as T1mic. Jimenez and Visscher described 75 patients with microinvasion defined as one focus smaller than 5 mm or multiple foci with an aggregate diameter smaller than 10 mm (233). Two or more histologically separate foci of invasion were present in 59% of the cases. Microinvasion consisting of isolated cell clusters smaller than 1 mm was present in 25 cases (33%). Axillary lymph node dissection performed in 69 cases revealed metastatic carcinoma in 5 (7%). Two of these patients had invasive foci measuring smaller than 1 mm (T1mic), and in a third case, the invasive lesion measured 1.1 mm.

Walker et al. compared the clinical and pathologic features of intraductal carcinoma detected by mammography to patients who had symptoms, usually a mass or nipple discharge (234). Microinvasion (T1mic) was found in 5 of 92 (5%) cases mammographically detected and in 10 of 74 (13.5%) symptomatic cases. All but one of the 15 intraductal carcinoma lesions with microinvasion were larger than 2 cm. Most intraductal carcinomas with microinvasion had a comedo growth pattern or necrosis and high nuclear grade.

de Mascarel analyzed 77 patients with microinvasive carcinoma defined as "infiltration of the periductal stroma by a few tumor cells singly," a description that probably corresponds to T1mic (235). Axillary nodal metastases were found in 1.6% and the disease-free survival at 10 years was 96%. By comparison, 191 patients with invasive carcinoma that involved 5% or less of the tumor area had a higher frequency of axillary nodal metastases and a 10-year disease-free survival of 88%.

By using a double-immunostaining procedure for actin and cytokeratin, Prasad et al. were able to confirm microinvasion (T1mic) in 21 of 109 cases originally diagnosed as microinvasion or in which microinvasion was suspected (236). Eighteen lesions were ductal, and three were lobular. The carcinoma had high nuclear grade and necrosis in 16 of the 18 (89%) ductal lesion, including 13 (72%) described as *comedo type.* Axillary dissection performed in 15 patients revealed metastatic carcinoma in two cases, each with one lymph node involved. One of the 18 patients had recurrent carcinoma in the same breast after conservation surgery and radiotherapy, and another developed a chest wall recurrence of invasive duct carcinoma after a mastectomy. No systemic metastases were found after a median follow-up of 28 months.

Sentinel lymph node mapping has been used to assess axillary nodal status in patients with microinvasion ductal carcinoma. Zavotsky et al. found metastatic carcinoma in the sentinel lymph node(s) from 2 of 14 (14.3%) patients (237). Completion axillary dissection revealed no other nodal metastases. Dauway et al. described nine patients with microinvasive intraductal carcinoma (T1mic) (238). Three (33%) of these patients had micrometastases detected in a sentinel lymph node by cytokeratin immunohistochemistry and no other metastases in a complete axillary dissection. These investigators also reported that 5 of 86 (6%) patients with lesions classified as intraductal carcinoma had metastases in a sentinel lymph node. Four of the nodal metastases were detected only by cytokeratin immunohistochemistry. Four of the five patients had comedointraductal carcinoma, and the fifth had a 9.5-cm low-grade micropapillary and cribriform lesion. Completion axillary dissection in four cases yielded no additional metastases.

## MARGINS OF EXCISION

Microscopic examination of histologic sections is necessary to determine whether intraductal carcinoma is present at the margin of a surgical biopsy specimen. The general issue of margin assessment is discussed extensively in Chapter 46.

A transected duct containing intraductal carcinoma that is present at a margin identified by ink applied to the gross specimen or some other standardized marking procedure is reported as a "positive" margin (239). Intraductal carcinoma involving lobular glands (cancerization of lobules) is considered to be a risk factor for local recurrence and should be reported as a positive margin if present at the border of the specimen (240). In cases with a positive margin, the report should indicate the extent of involvement with terms such as *focal* (limited to one or two microscopic fields) or more than focal. When the margin is not directly involved, the closest approach of intraductal carcinoma to the margin should be

stated, preferably with a measurement in millimeters. The term *close* has been variably defined, but the most frequent usage is for carcinoma within 1 mm of the margin.

In addition to sampling the surface of an excisional biopsy specimen, margin status has been assessed by obtaining samples of the surface of the postexcision biopsy cavity. These specimens, termed *margin* or *shave biopsies,* are difficult to orient, and any intraductal carcinoma found microscopically in this tissue is considered indicative of a positive margin (101).

## TREATMENT AND PROGNOSIS

### Mastectomy

Until the last quarter of the twentieth century, the standard treatment for intraductal carcinoma was mastectomy. Before the introduction of modified mastectomy procedures, this operation was a classic radical mastectomy. Even after the widespread adoption of the modified radical mastectomy, an *en bloc* axillary dissection was routinely performed, yielding axillary lymph node metastases in only isolated instances (12,13,53,54). These operations ensured at least a 99% cure rate (13,53,54,241). Systemic recurrences that occurred in 1% or fewer of patients after such treatment resulted from contralateral carcinomas or foci of invasion that were undetected or overlooked (53,54,242,243). The operation was deemed justified because of these extremely unusual recurrences and the presence of unsuspected frankly invasive foci discovered in the mastectomy specimens from about 5% of breasts that had only intraductal carcinoma in the biopsy specimen (62,244).

Mastectomy remains a treatment option for patients with intraductal carcinoma and may be indicated for fewer than 25% of patients under several circumstances outlined by a Consensus Conference on the Treatment of In Situ Ductal Carcinoma (DCIS) (179). The situations in which mastectomy was recommended were:

1. "Large areas of DCIS of a size that the lesion cannot be removed by an oncologically acceptable excision . . . while still conserving a cosmetically acceptable breast."
2. "Patients with multiple areas of DCIS in the same breast that cannot be encompassed through a single incision."
3. "Patients who cannot undergo radiation therapy because of other medical problems, such as collagen vascular diseases, or prior therapeutic radiation to the chest for another illness, and for whom treatment by excision alone is not appropriate."

Local recurrence on the chest wall is an unusual complication in the treatment of intraductal carcinoma by total mastectomy. A metanalysis of published studies reported that the frequency of local recurrence following mastectomy alone was 1.4% (95% CI =0.7–2.1) (245). The recurrent lesion may consist of intraductal carcinoma (246), or it may manifest as invasion (247). Some of these recurrences occur in residual breast parenchyma, which may harbor persistent intraductal carcinoma (248). Most published descriptions of local recurrence after mastectomy for intraductal carcinoma do not comment on the presence or absence of breast parenchyma associated with the recurrence. It is essential that persistent breast tissue be looked for and mentioned in the report that describes the specimen from the site of any local recurrence, regardless of whether the primary lesion was *in situ* or invasive.

Recurrent carcinoma in residual breast tissue constitutes persistence of the original primary tumor or a new primary carcinoma and has a more favorable prognosis than the more frequent true local recurrence in a mastectomy scar, which is usually a manifestation of systemic metastases. Recurrent carcinoma in persistent breast tissue is adequately treated in most cases by local excision supplemented by radiotherapy or systemic chemotherapy or both, depending on the size of the lesion and whether invasion is present (53,249). In one report, the 5- and 10-year survival of patients with an invasive local recurrence after mastectomy for intraductal carcinoma was 83% and 63%, respectively (247). This result suggests that the chest wall recurrences were a manifestation of persistent carcinoma rather than evidence of systemic metastases in a substantial number of these patients.

Recurrence in the preserved nipple is a rare complication of subcutaneous mastectomy for intraductal carcinoma. In one instance, recurrence as invasive carcinoma occurred 17 years after a subcutaneous mastectomy that was accompanied by irradiation of the nipple (250). Additional examples of recurrence in the preserved nipple after subcutaneous mastectomy were described by Price et al. (251). Another unusual type of recurrence consisted of two separate foci of invasive carcinoma at subcutaneous drainage sites 8 years after a patient underwent a modified mastectomy for intraductal carcinoma (248). No mammary parenchyma was seen at the sites of recurrence. It was suggested that intraductal carcinoma cells dislodged at operation persisted at the drain sites and gave rise to recurrent carcinoma.

Recurrent intraductal carcinoma has been detected as a result of the mammographic appearance of calcifications in residual breast tissue after total mastectomy and saline implant reconstruction (246). Helvie et al. reported six patients who developed recurrent invasive carcinoma at the mastectomy site after TRAM flap reconstruction (252). All were described as having had extensive intraductal carcinoma, and four patients had undergone a skin-sparing mastectomy. Five of the recurrent lesions were palpable. Two of four patients who underwent axillary dissection had nodal metastases. The report did not mention whether breast glandular tissue was associated with the recurrent carcinoma lesions.

## Breast-conserving Surgery and Radiotherapy

Despite the widespread reliance on mastectomy, alternative therapies involving excisional surgery and radiotherapy were employed as early as the 1930s. After reviewing the record of his cases of intraductal comedocarcinoma, Bloodgood commented that "the striking feature is that none of the cases of pure comedo-adenocarcinoma was associated with metastasis to the axillary nodes, and not a single patient died of cancer" (7). He also noted that "if the tumor is too large to exclude the presence of malignant areas by frozen section, a radical mastectomy should be done" (7). Bloodgood described four patients with "pure" or noninvasive comedocarcinoma who were "completely excised with postoperative irradiation" and remained well up to 3 years later. These observations led him to conclude that "when the tumor is small and a frozen section shows a pure comedo neoplasm, it is sufficient to excise only the tumor" (7).

Occasional patients treated by local excision were mentioned in reviews of intraductal carcinoma published in the 1960s and 1970s. Farrow reported on 25 patients treated by local excision alone (241). Histologic features of the intraductal carcinomas were not specified. Further carcinoma developed in the same breast 1 to 8 years after excision in 5 of the 25 women. The subsequent lesions were "within or nearby the previous local excisional site." Gillis et al. cited one patient with an unspecified type of intraductal carcinoma who seemingly remained well during follow-up after excisional surgery (13). In 1971, Ashikari et al. mentioned two patients, one of whom refused surgery and a second with a medical contraindication who were treated by local excision and did not develop recurrent carcinoma (53). Four of 64 patients with intraductal carcinoma described by Westbrook and Gallager received only radiation therapy after biopsy because of patient preference or comorbid conditions (54).

The changing trend in the treatment of intraductal carcinoma in the United States was reported by Winchester et al. in 1997, who analyzed data for over 39,000 women diagnosed between 1985 and 1993 (18). The use of breast-conservation therapy increased from 31% to 54%, and overall 33.4% of patients did not undergo mastectomy during the 8-year interval. Radiotherapy was used in 38% of patients treated by breast-conserving surgery in 1985 and in 54% in 1993. Axillary dissection was performed in 49% of cases with or without mastectomy, but the frequency of this procedure decreased from 52% in 1985 to 40% in 1993.

The relationship between histologic characteristics of intraductal carcinoma treated by local excision and outcome was first investigated during the 1960s and 1970s. Kraus and Neubecker identified four patients with papillary carcinomas that were initially diagnosed as benign and treated by local excision (253). In two of these women, infiltrating carcinoma was found in the same breast 10 and 12 years, respectively, after the initial excision, and both patients had axillary lymph node metastases. The other two patients were disease free with follow-up of 6 and 13 years. McDivitt et al. evaluated 267 patients with papillary carcinoma and found 15 who had previously undergone a biopsy of the same breast (254). On review, 10 of these previous biopsies were found to contain low-grade papillary intraductal carcinoma.

Two of nine patients treated by local excision developed breast recurrences in a series described by Millis and Thynne (255). A patient with comedo intraductal carcinoma had a mastectomy for local recurrence 6 months after excision and remained well for 15 years. A second woman with micropapillary carcinoma had a breast recurrence seven years after excision and a second recurrence 1 year thereafter treated by mastectomy. Two patients with micropapillary and one each with comedo, cribriform, and intracystic intraductal carcinoma remained well for 5 to 15 years after excision alone.

Long-term follow-up of intraductal carcinoma treated by local excision was documented in several retrospective reports. The patients were identified in reviews of breast biopsies initially deemed to be benign but found to contain foci of intraductal carcinoma on review. One of the earliest series consisted of eight patients with intraductal carcinoma detected by Kiaer in a review of patients with "fibroadenomatosis" (proliferative breast changes) (256). "Follow-up revealed that 6 of these 8 patients had died of mammary carcinoma which had become clinically manifest $1\frac{1}{2}$ to 16 years after the first operation" (256). A second series consisted of 10 patients who in retrospect had low-grade papillary or micropapillary intraductal carcinoma identified in 8,609 biopsies from 1940 to 1950 (257). During follow-up averaging 21.6 years, seven patients were found to have subsequent carcinoma in the same breast after an average interval of 9.7 years. Six of the seven subsequent carcinomas were invasive. Four of these women developed metastatic carcinoma, which was fatal in two cases. In a later report, the series was expanded to 15 patients, eight of whom developed subsequent carcinoma (258). Harvey and Fechner reviewed 879 breast biopsies from 1962 to 1966 reported to be benign (259). They identified six patients with previously undiagnosed papillary intraductal carcinoma, all of whom remained well, with four followed for less than 5 years and two for less than 2 years. Page et al. found 28 women with intraductal carcinoma treated by excision only in a review of 11,760 biopsies from 1950 to 1968 (260). The intraductal carcinomas were described as cribriform and micropapillary. Invasive carcinoma developed in the ipsilateral breasts of 7 of 25 women who had follow-up of at least 3 years. All subsequent carcinomas were at or near the site of the original intraductal lesion. The observed frequency of subsequent invasive carcinoma was 11 times the expected rate. A later report with follow-up averaging nearly 30 years found that 9 (32%) of the 28 women subsequently developed ipsilateral invasive carcinoma (261). This frequency was 9.1 times expected (95% CI = 4.73–17.5).

Eusebi et al. found 28 examples of previously undiagnosed intraductal carcinoma in a review of 4,397 biopsies performed from 1965 to 1971 (262). Twenty-one of the lesions were forms of micropapillary carcinoma, four cribriform, one papillary–cribriform, and two comedocarcinoma. Two patients had ipsilateral recurrences. One of these women who originally had comedocarcinoma developed an invasive recurrence 5 years after biopsy. The other patient was found to have recurrent micropapillary carcinoma 8.8 years after biopsy. In this series, the observed frequency of subsequent carcinoma was 4.3 times (90% CI = 1.1–11.1) the expected risk, somewhat higher for nonmicropapillary (5.4) than for micropapillary (3.9) intraductal carcinoma.

Before the emergence of clinical trials, little information was available prospectively about the treatment of intraductal carcinoma by breast-conserving therapy. In 1982, Lagios et al. reported that 3 of 15 patients (15%) treated for intraductal carcinoma by local excision developed recurrences in the ipsilateral breast during follow-up averaging 44 months (191). An expanded series consisting of 79 patients with average follow-up of 48 months was reported in 1989 (263). Eight patients had developed recurrent carcinoma, four entirely intraductal and four invasive. Seven of eight recurrences in the breast were in patients with comedocarcinoma or cribriform carcinoma with comedonecrosis. The eighth recurrence was associated with "intraductal carcinoma with anaplasia." No recurrences occurred in women with micropapillary intraductal carcinoma. There were no systemic recurrences. Included in the series were 20 women with lesions 2.5 cm or smaller who had been followed for an average of 124 months. Four (20%) had ipsilateral recurrences, two of which were invasive. Further information about this series was reported in 1994 (264). At that time, the local failure rate in the conserved breast was 14.7% after a mean follow-up of 106 months. Half the recurrences were described as "minimally invasive carcinomas," and the others were intraductal. When correlated with histologic features of the initial lesion, the recurrence rate for intraductal carcinoma of high nuclear grade with comedonecrosis was 30.5%, and for those with intermediate nuclear grade, it was 10%. There were no breast recurrences in patients with low-grade intraductal carcinoma.

After follow-up averaging 39 months, Fisher et al. found a local recurrence rate of 23% in 22 patients treated by excisional biopsy alone (265). These patients had been entered into a clinical trial for invasive carcinoma in which one of the randomized treatments was excision alone, and the diagnosis was corrected to intraductal carcinoma during a subsequent pathology review. The same report described recurrences in 2 of the 29 women (7%) with retrospectively diagnosed intraductal carcinoma who had been randomized to receive radiation therapy. Ciatto et al. reported that infiltrating carcinoma developed in the ipsilateral breast in 7 of 55 women (12.7%) treated by local excision or quadrantectomy (46). The intraductal carcinoma had been detected through routine examinations or mammographic screening in Florence, Italy, from 1968 to 1988. The length of follow-up was not stated.

Several population-based prospective analyses of excisional surgery alone have been reported. The largest series, from Denmark, consisted of 112 women with a median follow-up of 53 months (266). Recurrent invasive carcinoma occurred in 5 women (4.4%), and 19 (17%) had recurrent intraductal carcinoma. The initial lesions ranged from 1 to 80 mm, with a median size of 10 mm. Features favoring recurrence were large nuclear size, lesion size greater than 10 mm, and the presence of comedonecrosis regardless of the histologic subtype (solid, micropapillary, or cribriform). Papillary lesions, of which there were few, had a high recurrence rate whether or not comedonecrosis was present. Heterogeneity of growth pattern was found in all but 3 of the 112 lesions. Margin status, evaluable in about one-third of the cases, did not appear to be a good predictor of recurrence. Recurrences occurred in 33% of cases with negative margins. Review of 132 patients with intraductal carcinoma diagnosed in Malmo, Sweden, revealed that 3 of 21 women (14%) treated by breast conserving surgery developed ipsilateral invasive carcinoma after a median follow-up of 7 years (267).

Two additional studies described the follow-up of women with intraductal carcinoma detected in regional mammography screening programs and treated by excisional surgery alone. Arnesson et al. identified 38 women with lesions detected with a single-view mammography technique who were treated only by "sector resection" with negative margins (268). After a median follow-up of 60 months, five (13%) patients had recurrent carcinoma consisting of two invasive and three intraductal lesions. The primary lesions associated with recurrence measured 3 to 15 mm. Cribriform intraductal carcinoma preceded the two invasive lesions, whereas comedocarcinoma was followed by recurrent intraductal carcinoma. Carpenter et al. reported on 28 women with lesions detected through screening mammography and clinical examination (269). Treatment consisted of quadrantectomy or segmental resection. No data were given about margin status. After a median follow-up of 38 months, five recurrences detected mammographically as microcalcifications in the region of prior excision consisted of one invasive and four intraductal lesions. No significant association was found to exist between the development of recurrent carcinoma and the size of the primary lesions, the size of the excisional biopsy specimen, or the presence of multifocality.

Schwartz et al. selected patients with mammographically detected nonpalpable or incidentally discovered intraductal carcinoma for treatment by excision alone (270). Patients were eligible for inclusion if the mammographic diameter of the area of calcifications did not exceed 25 mm. Comedocarcinoma was present to some extent in 51% of the lesions and was the predominant type in 29%. At least two subtypes of intraductal carcinoma were present in 41% of the cases. The excisions were not consistently studied for margin status. After a median follow-up of 47 months, 11 recurrences were detected in the ipsilateral breasts of 70 women (15.3%), consisting of three invasive and eight intraductal lesions. All recurrent intraductal carcinomas were detected mammographically because of the appearance of calcification. Comedocarcinoma was present in 10 of 11 lesions followed by recurrence (one was papillary), and all recurrent intraductal carcinoma was of the comedo type. No correlation

was found between the number of duct cross sections with intraductal carcinoma in the primary lesion and recurrence.

Another series of clinically selected patients treated by excision alone was reported by Hetelekidis et al. (271). The group consisted of 59 women, almost all of whom had mammographically detected lesions. Local recurrence in the breast was detected in 10 women (17%) 5 to 132 months after excision with a median interval of 37 months and a 5-year recurrence rate of 10%. Four recurrent lesions were invasive, and six were intraductal. Eight recurrences were at the site of prior excision. Factors associated with local recurrence were high nuclear grade, lesions occupying more than five low magnification ($4\times$) microscopic fields, and tumor 1 mm or less from the margin. Lesion size was the only statistically significant indicator of recurrence. The local recurrence rate was 18% for lesions with poor nuclear grade and less than 10% when nuclear grade was intermediate or well differentiated ($p$ = nonsignificant). Intraductal carcinoma involving fewer than 5 low-power fields had a 3% recurrence rate compared with more extensive lesions with a 17% recurrence rate ($p$ = 0.02). The local recurrence rates for negative and close margins were 8% and 25%, respectively.

### Risk Factors for Breast Recurrences after Conservation Therapy

Data presented in many of the foregoing reports suggest that pathologic features of intraductal carcinoma might contribute to the success or failure of treatment by excisional surgery alone. It appears that low-grade, noncomedocarcinoma is more amenable to this approach. A case-control study by Badve et al. examined the value of five histologic classification schemes for predicting local recurrence in the breast after excisional surgery alone (272). The exercise involved reviewing slides of excisional biopsies from 43 patients who developed recurrences and from 81 controls matched for age at diagnosis who did not develop a recurrence. The median time to recurrence was 39 months, and for recurrence-free controls, median follow-up was 68 months. None of the classification systems was clearly superior for predicting local recurrence. The characteristics of intraductal carcinoma most strongly associated with recurrence were the presence of necrosis and poorly differentiated nuclear grade.

Radiation therapy has been used in conjunction with excisional surgery in an effort to improve local control after breast-conserving therapy of intraductal carcinoma. Data are available from a number of prospective investigations of patients treated by excisional surgery with radiation therapy and from a randomized trial comparing the results of excision alone to excision with radiotherapy. Initial reports published in the 1980s described selected patients and noted a recurrence rate in the conserved breast of 10% or less after a median follow-up of approximately 5 years (273–275). Bornstein et al. reported an actuarial 8-year breast recurrence rate of 27% in a series of 38 selected patients (276). Five of the eight recurrences were invasive, and one of these women developed metastatic carcinoma. Solin et al. identified 259 women treated in nine institutions in the United States and Europe and found a 10-year actuarial breast failure rate of 16% (277). Of the 28 recurrences, 50% were invasive. and four patients developed metastatic carcinoma. In a later report, the 15-year actuarial rate for local failure in the series was 19% after a median follow-up of 10.3 years (278). The overall survival rate for the patient group was 87%, and the breast carcinoma-specific survival rate was 96%. Fifty-three percent of local recurrences in the breast were invasive. No clinical or pathologic parameter was found to be predictive of local failure in this study. Distant metastases occurred in 3% of patients. Contralateral carcinoma was diagnosed in 6% of patients; most of the lesions were invasive.

Several studies in addition to those previously cited have identified necrosis in intraductal carcinoma or comedo-type intraductal carcinoma as having an especially high risk for breast recurrence after breast conservation with radiotherapy. In one report, the average diameter of lesions treated by breast conservation was 1.5 cm (279). The recurrence rate in the breast was higher for patients with comedo (11%) than for those with noncomedo (2%) carcinoma. One patient who initially had comedocarcinoma died of metastatic disease after an invasive breast recurrence. Solin et al. found that the presence of necrosis was a significant risk factor when it occurred in intraductal carcinoma with poorly differentiated nuclear grade (280). Kuske et al. reported significantly poorer local control in patients with comedo (75%) than in those with noncomedo (98%) carcinoma but did not offer a definition of comedo intraductal carcinoma (281).

Goonewardene et al. studied the significance of necrosis as a risk factor for local recurrence in 166 women who had been treated for intraductal carcinoma by excision alone (282). After an average follow-up of 6.5 years, recurrences were detected in 40 (24%) patients, and 12 recurrences were invasive. Substantial necrosis was present in the original intraductal carcinoma in 70% of the cases with recurrence and in 83% with invasive recurrence. Necrosis was present in only 25% of intraductal carcinomas not followed by recurrence.

The VNPI was developed to stratify patients with intraductal carcinoma to distinguish between women who are most likely to be treated successfully by breast conservation and those who might be candidates for mastectomy because of a relatively high risk of breast recurrence (283,284). The VNPI is a numeric score of 3 to 9 based on the assessment of three variables: size of intraductal carcinoma, distance between intraductal carcinoma and margin, and a pathologic classification based on necrosis and nuclear grade. Each variable is divided into three categories, which are ranked (scored) from most to least favorable as 1 to 3 (Table 13.3). The VNPI is derived from the sum of scores for individual variables.

Follow-up of patients with intraductal carcinoma grouped into three VNPI categories (scores 3, 4; scores 5, 6, 7; and

**TABLE 13.3.** *Scoring system for the Van Nuys Prognostic Index*

| Variable | Score | | |
|---|---|---|---|
| | 1 | 2 | 3 |
| Size (mm) | ≤ 15 | 16–40 | ≥ 41 |
| Margin (mm) | ≥ 10 | 1–9 | < 1 |
| Pathology | Not HG; necrosis absent | Not HG; necrosis present | HG; necrosis present or absent |

HG, high nuclear grade.
Based on Silverstein MJ, Weisman JR, Gierson ED, et al. Radiation therapy for intraductal carcinoma: is it an equal alternative? *Arch Surg* 1991;126:424–426, with permission.

scores 8, 9) showed significant differences in recurrence-free survival, with the most favorable outcome associated with the lowest scores. Patients were stratified within the VNPI groups according to whether they received radiotherapy in addition to excision. Radiated patients in the VNPI 3, 4 group did not differ significantly from those who were not radiated, but radiation did appear to be beneficial in the intermediate VNPI group. Recurrences were "unacceptably" frequent in the VNPI 8, 9 group, even when radiotherapy was administered (283). On the basis of these observations, it was suggested that women with intraductal carcinoma classified as VNPI 3, 4 could be treated by excision alone, that excision with radiotherapy be used for the VNPI 5–7 group, and that mastectomy should be recommended if the VNPI is 8 or 9.

The VNPI should be validated in a prospective randomized trial before acceptance as a basis for clinical practice. This is especially important because of significant concerns about the database from which it was derived. A major issue is the lack of a consistent treatment program illustrated by the following quotation (284):

> Until 1988 all patients with DCIS who elected breast conservation were advised to add breast irradiation to their treatment. Most patients accepted this recommendation; a few refused and were treated with careful clinical follow-up without irradiation. Beginning in 1989, the physicians within The Breast Center were no longer convinced of the overall value of radiation therapy for DCIS and all breast conservation patients with uninvolved biopsy margins (clear by 1 mm or more) were offered the option of careful clinical follow-up without radiation therapy. Many patients accepted this option; some refused and were treated with breast irradiation. Outside patients with DCIS referred to our radiation oncologists for radiation therapy continued to be treated with radiation therapy in accord with the wishes of their referring physicians.

Other uncontrolled variables included differing radiation schedules and inconsistent boost treatment (284).

Lesion size is one of the three variables included in the VNPI. As discussed elsewhere in this chapter, there is no reliable or generally accepted method for measuring the size or extent of intraductal carcinoma, especially with a precision that would consistently discriminate size as required for the VNPI scoring system. In lesions limited to a single tissue block, it may be possible to distinguish between foci smaller and larger than 15 mm, but the distinction between 15 to 40 mm and larger than 40 mm is likely to be quite unreliable. Determining size when intraductal carcinoma is distributed in more than one tissue block from a single biopsy or if it is in more than one biopsy specimen is very imprecise. The methods for determining lesion extent by counting 4× fields of involvement or the number of slides with intraductal carcinoma do not provide measurements suitable for the VNPI. There are likely to be many patients for whom a VNPI cannot be determined or for whom the calculated VNPI is of questionable accuracy, as reported by Kestin et al., who were unable to determine tumor size in 58% of the cases they analyzed (194). Warnberg et al. reported no statistically significant differences in relapse-free survival between patients with intraductal carcinoma stratified into the three Van Nuys prognostic groups (285).

An updated report from the Van Nuys Center published in 1998 did not classify patients according to the VNPI (286). The series of 707 of nonrandomized patients included 208 women treated by lumpectomy and radiotherapy and 240 treated by excision alone. Breast recurrences were detected in 36 women in each group, representing 17% and 15%, respectively, and approximately half of the recurrences were invasive in each group. Distant metastases were diagnosed in six patients, five of whom had been treated originally by lumpectomy and radiotherapy. Five of the patients (0.7%) in the entire series died of breast carcinoma, with four in the radiated group. The median follow-up for the 35 patients who had invasive recurrent carcinoma was 127 months (58 months from initial diagnosis to invasive recurrence and 69 additional months after recurrence). The distant recurrence rate in the subset of 35 patients with invasive recurrence in the breast was 27.1%, and the mortality rate from breast carcinoma was 14.4% at 8 years.

A large-scale prospective randomized trial to compare lumpectomy alone with lumpectomy and radiation was undertaken by the NSABP as Protocol 17 (287). After a mean follow-up of 90 months, breast recurrences were significantly more frequent in women treated by lumpectomy alone (26.8%) than in those who had radiation after lumpectomy (12.1%). The proportion of invasive recurrences was lower in the radiated (36%) than in the nonradiated (51%) group. Six patients developed distant metastases, three each in the radiated and nonradiated groups. Features associated with increased risk for local recurrence after either form of treatment were the presence of moderate to marked comedonecrosis, regardless of histologic subtype, margins that were positive or indeterminate, multifocality, and a moderate to marked lymphocytic infiltrate (288). The size of the lesion (<10 or ≥ 10 mm) did not prove to be a statistically significant predictor for breast recurrence. Necrosis proved to be the only statistically significant independent risk factor for recurrence in both treatment groups in multivariate analysis (288).

Few studies have analyzed data based exclusively on mammographically detected intraductal carcinoma treated by breast conservation with radiotherapy (289,290). The 10-year breast recurrence rates ranged from 4% to 7% in patients with negative final excision margins to as high as 30% for women with positive or close margins. Time to recurrence appeared to be shorter for patients with positive margins (median, 3.6 years) than for those with negative (median, 4.3 years) or indeterminate (median, 5.2 years) margins (289). In patients with mammographically detected intraductal carcinoma, pathologic features such as nuclear grade, necrosis, and architecture (comedo versus noncomedo) were not significantly related to the risk for local recurrence. The lack of association with pathologic characteristics indicates the importance of stratifying patients by detection modality in the analysis of risk factors for local breast recurrence after conservation therapy.

Age at diagnosis (<45 versus ≥45 years) was a significant predictor of local recurrence after breast-conserving surgery with radiation in patients with mammographically detected intraductal carcinoma (194). In this study, the 10-year actuarial rate of local failure in the breast was 23.4% for women less than 45 years of age when treated and 7.1% among those 45 years or older. These investigators were unable to apply the VNPI to their analyses because tumor size could not be measured in 58% of the cases. Pathological study of the intraductal carcinomas revealed several factors that might have predisposed the younger women to local recurrence (291). These factors included smaller diagnostic biopsy specimens and more frequent lesions with high nuclear grade and necrosis.

Hillner et al. applied decision analysis to hypothetical cohorts of 55-year-old white women with nonpalpable intraductal carcinoma to compare the impact on outcome of mastectomy, breast-conservation surgery with radiation, and breast-conservation surgery alone (292). Recurrence rates were based on published data. The actuarial 20-year breast cancer-free survival rates were 74.5% for mastectomy, 63.3% for breast conservation with radiotherapy, and 46.8% for breast-conserving surgery alone.

A metanalysis of published reports compared recurrence rates for patients with intraductal carcinoma after treatment with one of three modalities (245). The summary recurrence rates were 1.4% (95% CI = 0.7–2.1), 8.9% (95% CI = 6.8–11.0), and 22.5% (95% CI = 16.9–28.2), respectively, for mastectomy, lumpectomy with radiotherapy and lumpectomy alone. The proportions of invasive recurrence in each group were 76%, 50%, and 43%, respectively. The nearly threefold higher rate of recurrence after lumpectomy without radiotherapy compared with women who underwent radiation is especially striking in view of the likelihood that excision alone was most often recommended for patients with low-grade, relatively small lesions with negative margins. These researchers observed that "patients with risk factors of presence of necrosis, high-grade cytologic features or comedo subtype were found to derive the greatest improvement in local control" from the addition of radiotherapy to conservation surgery.

## Treatment Recommendations

The treatment recommendation is made on the basis of clinical and pathologic findings in consultation with the patient. Important considerations include the manner of clinical presentation (e.g., palpable, incidental, or mammographic), extent by mammography, size measured grossly or microscopically, margin status of the lumpectomy, and histologic features of the intraductal carcinoma such as nuclear grade, growth pattern (e.g., cribriform, comedo, solid, papillary), and the presence or absence of necrosis. The issue is complicated by the many different combinations of these and other features that can occur in a given case.

On the basis of numerous studies cited herein, it appears likely that margin status and the biological characteristics of intraductal carcinoma represented histologically most directly by nuclear grade and the presence or absence of necrosis are the most important predictors of local recurrence in the breast after breast-conservation surgery with or without radiotherapy. Tumor size, which is particularly difficult to assess accurately, correlates well with the extent of the lesion and thus influences margin status. For example, Cheng et al. reported positive lumpectomy margins in 15%, 28%, and 69% of patients with intraductal carcinoma lesions measured as smaller than 1.0 cm, 1.0 to 2.4 cm, and 2.5 cm or larger, respectively (293). Biological characteristics, at least partially reflected in the histologic appearance of intraductal carcinoma, have a complex influence on the success of treatment by affecting the rate of growth, (and to some extent the time to detection of clinical recurrences) and radiosensitivity of residual intraductal carcinoma after lumpectomy. Consequently, it is possible for patients with comparable amounts of incompletely excised residual high-grade (comedo) and low-grade (cribriform) intraductal carcinoma who receive the same treatment to have similar absolute risks for breast recurrence, but they may differ in time to clinical detection of recurrence, especially of invasive lesions, and in responsiveness to radiotherapy or antiestrogens. Follow-up for more than 10 years of large, uniformly treated patient groups with diverse types of intraductal carcinoma will be needed to assess reliably the interplay of these factors.

Age at diagnosis appears to be an independent risk factor which increases the risk for breast recurrence in young women, especially those under 45 years of age and treated by conservation therapy with or without radiotherapy.

Mammography is an essential component of the clinical follow-up of women treated by breast-conserving surgery with or without radiotherapy (179). In one series of 162 women, 33 (20%) developed recurrent ipsilateral carcinoma 6 to 168 months (median, 26 months) after primary therapy (294). Review of mammograms from 20 patients with recurrent carcinoma revealed that 17 (85%) of these recurrences were detected solely on the basis of calcifications, which had a pattern similar to that of calcifications seen before the ini-

tial excision in 82% of cases. Intraductal carcinoma alone was present in 65% of recurrences, whereas 35% also had invasive carcinoma.

Some patients may choose mastectomy even if they are candidates for breast conservation. Mastectomy is preferable for the patient with such widespread intraductal carcinoma that negative margins cannot be achieved with a cosmetically acceptable surgical procedure. Many, but not all, of these patients have dispersed calcifications on mammography. Lumpectomy with or without radiation will suffice for most women with intraductal carcinoma limited to a single focus on the basis of pathologic and clinical findings, if the margins of excision are negative, if the lesion is not comedo type with necrosis and high nuclear grade, and it is small (variously defined as <1.0 cm or <2.5 cm). Radiation after lumpectomy is recommended regardless of extent if the intraductal carcinoma has comedocarcinoma features or the margins are indeterminate or are involved.

The assessment of margins is only a guide to and not a precise measurement of the completeness of excision for intraductal carcinoma. This was demonstrated by Silverstein et al., who compared the findings in reexcision specimens from patients who had positive margins and patients who had negative margins in their initial excisional biopsy (295). Although the chance of finding residual intraductal carcinoma was significantly greater if the original margins were positive, 43% of those with negative margins initially had carcinoma in the reexcision. There was also a higher risk (76%) for residual intraductal carcinoma if the primary focus was 2.5 cm or larger, but residual carcinoma was present in 57% of reexcisions for lesions smaller than 2.5 cm. Goldstein et al. analyzed the quantitative relationship between the amount of intraductal carcinoma in a lumpectomy and in the subsequent reexcision (296). The study was based on 98 patients who had a reexcision performed after a lumpectomy for intraductal carcinoma. Residual intraductal carcinoma was present in 52 (53%) reexcision specimens. Features that were significantly related to finding intraductal carcinoma in the reexcision were multifocal involvement of margins by intraductal carcinoma or by intraductal carcinoma extending into terminal duct–lobular units and extensive intraductal carcinoma represented by the number of slides with the lesion. When intraductal carcinoma was limited to one or two slides in the initial excision, no intraductal carcinoma was detected in 62% of reexcisions, whereas intraductal carcinoma was present in 100% of excisions after initial biopsies with intraductal carcinoma in more than six slides.

It must be reemphasized that methods for the quantitation of intraductal carcinoma are imprecise. No method for measuring the size of intraductal carcinoma has gained wide acceptance. Lagios observed that "quantitation, or better, estimating the extent of DCIS, should be a collaborative exercise between mammographer and pathologist, but is more a fictional practice than a reliable fact" (192). For this and other reasons summarized by Schnitt et al. (297), classifications for assessing the prognosis of intraductal carcinoma, such as the VNPI, which depend on and offer precise size categories, may be viewed, at best, as general guidelines rather than as a strict criteria for making therapeutic decisions.

Axillary dissection is not indicated in most patients with intraductal carcinoma (298). Some low axillary lymph nodes may be taken with the axillary tail of the breast in the course of a mastectomy. If the lesion is extensive intraductal carcinoma, especially comedo type with marked duct distortion, low axillary dissection or sentinel lymph node mapping may be performed because of concern for undetected invasion. Micrometastases were detected in axillary sentinel lymph nodes from 4 of 87 (4.6%) patients with intraductal carcinoma studied by Haigh and Giuliano (299) and in 11 of 150 (7.3%) patients reported by Cox et al. (300). As noted by Haigh and Giuliano, "if metastases are detected, microinvasion can be assumed" (299).

Treatment of most patients with microinvasive duct carcinoma previously described in the literature has been mastectomy, as discussed earlier in this chapter. The outcome overall was relatively favorable after mastectomy, but the studies were not directly comparable because of differing criteria for defining microinvasion. Patients treated by breast conservation were described in several reports, with results indicating that this was equally effective as mastectomy. Wong et al. described 41 patients with microinvasion ("a microfocus of malignant cells invading beyond the basement membrane"), including 15 treated by breast conservation (229). Nine had excision with radiotherapy. All patients were recurrence free after a median follow-up of 37 months.

Microinvasion was defined as "DCIS with limited microscopic stromal invasion below the basement membrane in one or several ducts but not invading more than 10% of the surface of the histologic sections examined" by Rosner et al. (231). Thirty-five of 36 patients fulfilling this definition underwent an axillary dissection, yielding metastatic carcinoma in one case. Thirty-three patients were treated by mastectomy and three by excision alone. Residual microinvasive duct carcinoma was found in five (15%) patients, and six (18%) had "frank invasive" carcinoma. All patients remained recurrence free after a mean follow-up of 57 months.

Breast-conserving therapy consisting of excision and radiation therapy was used for 39 patients with microinvasive duct carcinoma described as "predominantly intraductal carcinoma with microscopic or early invasion" and more specifically defined as "either maximal extent of invasion of <2 mm or invasive carcinoma comprising <10% of the tumor" (231). Two patients had axillary lymph node metastases. Recurrence was detected in the conserved breast in nine patients, including one woman with coincidental systemic recurrence, after a median follow-up of 55 months.

These and other published reports indicate that the presence of microinvasion, as variously defined in the past or as currently described in the TNM staging system (T1mic), probably has little independent impact on the effectiveness of conservation for local control in the breast. The characteristics of the intraductal carcinoma that are associated with microinvasion, such as high grade, the presence of necrosis, and greater lesion extent are crucial determinants for treatment. The significance of multiple microinvasive foci is yet to be determined. The presence or suspicion of microinvasion will lead to axillary lymph node staging, often by sentinel lymph node mapping, in many patients before consideration of systemic therapy (300).

## REFERENCES

1. Warren JC. Abnormal involution of the mammary gland with its treatment by operation. *Am J Med Sci* 1907;134:521–535.
2. Cheatle GL. Cysts, and primary cancer in cysts of the breast. *Br J Surg* 1920–1921;8:149–166.
3. Bloodgood JC. The pathology of chronic cystic mastitis of the female breast. *Arch Surg* 1921;3:445–542.
4. Bloodgood JC. Border-line breast tumors. *Ann Surg* 1931; 93:235–249.
5. Muir R. The evolution of carcinoma of the mamma. *J Pathol Bacteriol* 1941;52:155–172.
6. Schultz-Brauns O. Die geschwulste der Brustbrüse. In: Henke F, Lubarsch O, eds. *Handbuch der speziellen Pathologischen anatomie und Histologie*, VII. Berlin: Verlag von Julius Springer, 1933.
7. Bloodgood JC. Comedo carcinoma or comedo-adenoma of the female breast. *Am J Cancer* 1934;22:842–853.
8. Lewis D, Geschickter CF. Comedocarcinoma of the breast. *Arch Surg* 1938;36:225–244.
9. Cheatle GL, Cutler M. *Tumors of the breast.* Philadelphia: JB Lippincott, 1931.
10. Haagenson CD. Special pathological forms of breast carcinoma. *Diseases of the breast*, 2nd ed. Philadelphia: WB Saunders, 1971:586–590.
11. Rosner D, Bedwani RN, Vana J, et al. Noninvasive breast carcinoma. Results of a national survey by the American College of Surgeons. *Ann Surg* 1980;92:139–147.
12. Brown PW, Silverman J, Owens E, et al. Intraductal "noninfiltrating" carcinoma of the breast. *Arch Surg* 1976;111:1063–1067.
13. Gillis DA, Dockerty MB, Clagett OT. Preinvasive intraductal carcinoma of the breast. *Surg Obstet Gynecol* 1960;110:555–562.
14. Rosen PP. The pathological classification of human mammary carcinoma: past, present and future. *Ann Clin Lab Sci* 1979;9:144–156.
15. Smart CR, Myers MH, Gloecker LA. Implications from SEER data on breast cancer management. *Cancer* 1978;41:787–789.
16. Ernster VL, Barclay J, Kerlikowske K, et al. Incidence of and treatment for ductal carcinoma in situ of the breast. *JAMA* 1996;275:913–918.
17. Ernster VL, Barclay J. Increases in ductal carcinoma in situ (DCIS) of the breast in relation to mammography: a dilemma. *J Natl Cancer Inst Monogr* 1997;22:151–156.
18. Winchester DJ, Menck HR, Winchester DP. National treatment trends for ductal carcinoma in situ of the breast. *Arch Surg* 1997; 132:660–665.
19. Blichert-Toft M, Graversen HP, Andersen J, et al. *In situ* breast carcinomas: a population-based study on frequency, growth pattern, and clinical aspects. *World J Surg* 1988;12:845–851.
20. Ward BA, McKhann CF, Ravikumar TS. Ten-year follow-up of breast carcinoma in situ in Connecticut. *Arch Surg* 1992;127: 1392–1395.
21. Adams-Cameron M, Gilliland FD, Hunt WC, et al. Trends in incidence and treatment for ductal carcinoma *in situ* in Hispanic, American Indian, and non-Hispanic white women in New Mexico, 1973–1994. *Cancer* 1999;85:1084–1090.
22. Chu KC, Tarone RE, Kessler LG, et al. Recent trends in U.S. breast cancer incidence, survival, and mortality rates. *J Natl Cancer Inst* 1996;88:1571–1579.
23. Kerlikowske K, Barclay J, Grady D, et al. Comparison of risk factors for ductal carcinoma in situ and invasive breast cancer. *J Natl Cancer Inst* 1997;89:76–82.
24. Weiss HA, Brinton LA, Brogan D, et al. Epidemiology of in situ and invasive breast cancer in women aged under 45. *Br J Cancer* 1996;73:1298–1305.
25. Ciatto S, Bonardi R, Cataliotti L, et al. Intraductal breast carcinoma. Review of a multicenter series of 350 cases. *Tumori* 1990; 76:552–554.
26. Andersson I. Breast cancer screening in Malmo. *Recent Results Cancer Res* 1984;90:114–116.

27. Andersson I, Andren L, Hildell J, et al. Breast cancer screening with mammography: a population-based randomized trial with mammography as the only screening mode. *Radiology* 1979;132:273–276.

28. Hendricks JHCL. *Population screening for breast cancer by means of mammography in Nijmegen, 1975–1982.* [M.D. Thesis]. Nijmegen University, 1982.

29. Lewis JD, Milbrath JR, Shaffer KA, et al. Implications of suspicious findings in breast cancer screening. *Arch Surg* 1975;110:903–907.

30. Sigfusson BF, Anderson I, Aspergren K, et al. Clustered breast calcifications. *Acta Radiol* 1983;24:273–281.

31. Tabar L, Akerlund E, Gad A. Five-year experience with single-view mammography randomized controlled screening in Sweden. *Recent Results Cancer Res* 1984;90:105–113.

32. Verbeek ALM, Hendriks JHCL, Holland R, et al. Reduction of breast cancer mortality through mass screening with modern mammography: first results of the Nijmegen Project, 1975–1981. *Lancet* 1984;1:1222–1224.

33. Ciatto S, Cataliotti L, Distante V. Nonpalpable lesions detected with mammography: review of 512 consecutive cases. *Radiology* 1987;165:99–102.

34. Meyer JS. Cell kinetics of histologic variants of in situ breast carcinoma. *Breast Cancer Res Treat* 1986;7:171–180.

35. Patchefsky AS, Shaber GS, Schwartz GF, et al. The pathology of breast cancer detected by mass population screening. *Cancer* 1977;40:1659–1670.

36. Dershaw DD, Abramson A, Kinne DW. Ductal carcinoma *in situ*: mammographic findings and clinical implications. *Radiology* 1989;170:411–415.

37. Ikeda DM, Andersson I. Atypical mammographic presentation of ductal carcinoma in situ. *Radiology* 1989;172:661–666.

38. Stomper PC, Connolly JL, Meyer JE, et al. Clinically occult ductal carcinoma in situ detected with mammography: analysis of 100 cases with radiologic-pathologic correlation. *Radiology* 1989;172:235–241.

38a. Goldstein NS, Kestin L, Vicini F. Intraductal carcinoma of the breast. Pathologic features associated with local recurrence in patients treated breast-conserving therapy. *Am J Surg Pathol* 2000;24:1058–1067.

39. Carlson KL, Helvie MA, Roubidoux MA, et al. Relationship between mammographic screening intervals and size and histology of ductal carcinoma in situ. *AJR Am J Roentgenol* 1999;172:313–317.

40. Holland R, Hendriks JHCL, Verbeek ALM, et al. Extent, distribution, and mammographic/histological correlations of breast ductal carcinoma *in situ. Lancet* 1990;335:519–522.

41. Lagios MD. Multicentricity of breast carcinoma demonstrated by routine correlated subgross and radiographic examination. *Cancer* 1977;40:1726–1734.

42. Stomper PC, Connolly JL. Ductal carcinoma *in situ* of the breast: correlation between mammographic calcification and tumor subtype. *AJR Am J Roentgenol* 1992;159:483–485.

43. Parker J, Dance DR, Davies DH, et al. Classification of ductal carcinoma in situ by image analysis of calcifications from digital mammograms. *Br J Radiol* 1995;68:150–159.

44. Evans A, Pinder S, Wilson R, et al. Ductal carcinoma *in situ* of the breast: correlation between mammographic and pathologic findings. *AJR Am J Roentgenol* 1994;162:1307–1311.

45. Evans AJ, Pinder SE, Ellis IO, et al. Correlations between the mammographic features of ductal carcinoma *in situ* (DCIS) and c-erb-s oncogene expression. *Clin Radiol* 1994;49:559–562.

46. Ciatto S, Grazzini G, Iossa A, et al. *In situ* ductal carcinoma of the breast—analysis of clinical presentation and outcome in 156 consecutive cases. *Eur J Surg Oncol* 1990;16:220–224.

47. Mitnick JS, Roses DF, Harris MN, et al. Circumscribed intraductal carcinoma of the breast. *Radiology* 1989;170:423–425.

48. Reiff DB, Cooke J, Griffin M, et al. Ductal carcinoma in situ presenting as a stellate lesion on mammography. *Clin Radiol* 1994;49:396–399.

49. Gilles R, Zafrani B, Guinebretiere J-M, et al. Ductal carcinoma in situ: MR imaging-histopathologic correlation. *Radiology* 1995;196:415–419.

50. Orel S, Schnall M, Livolsi V, et al. Suspicious breast lesions: MR imaging with radiologic-pathologic correlation. *Radiology* 1994;190:485–493.

51. Heywang-Köbrunner S. Contrast-enhanced magnetic resonance imaging of the breast. *Invest Radiol* 1994;29:94–104.

52. Orel SG, Mendonca MH, Reynolds C, et al. MR imaging of ductal carcinoma *in situ. Radiology* 1997;202:413–420.

53. Ashikari R, Hajdu SI, Robbins GF. Intraductal carcinoma of the breast (1960–1969). *Cancer* 1971;28:1182–1187.

54. Westbrook KC, Gallager HS. Intraductal carcinoma of the breast. A comparative study. *Am J Surg* 1975;130:667–670.

55. Pandya S, Mackarem G, Lee AKC, et al. Ductal carcinoma in situ: the impact of screening on clinical presentation and pathologic features. *Breast J* 1998;4:146–151.

56. Rosen PP, Ashikari R, Thaler H, et al. A comparative study of some pathologic features of mammary carcinoma in Tokyo, Japan and New York, USA. *Cancer* 1977;39:429–434.

57. Patchefsky AS, Schwartz GF, Finkelstein SD, et al. Heterogeneity of intraductal carcinoma of the breast. *Cancer* 1989;63:731–741.

58. Rosen P, Snyder RE, Urban JA, et al. Correlation of suspicious mammograms and x-rays of breast biopsies during surgery. Results in 60 cases. *Cancer* 1973;31:656–660.

59. Snyder R, Rosen P. Radiography of breast specimens. *Cancer* 1971;28:1608–1611.

60. Rosen PP. Frozen section diagnosis of breast lesions: recent experience with 556 consecutive biopsies. *Ann Surg* 1978;187:17–19.

61. Cheng L, Al-Kaisi NK, Liu AY, et al. The results of intraoperative consultations in 181 ductal carcinomas *in situ* of the breast. *Cancer* 1997;80:75–79.

62. Rosen PP, Senie R, Schottenfeld D, et al. Noninvasive breast carcinoma: frequency of unsuspected invasion and implication for treatment. *Ann Surg* 1979;189:98–103.

63. Bellamy COC, McDonald C, Salter DM, et al. Noninvasive ductal carcinoma of the breast: the relevance of histologic categorization. *Hum Pathol* 1993;24:16–23.

64. Silverstein MJ, Waisman JR, Gamagami P, et al. Intraductal carcinoma of the breast (208 cases): clinical factors influencing treatment choice. *Cancer* 1990;66:102–108.

64a. Szelei-Stevens KA, Kuske RR, Yantsos VA, et al. The influence of young age and positive family history of breast cancer on the prognosis of ductal carcinoma in situ treated by excision with or without radiation therapy or by mastectomy. *Int J Radiat Oncol Biol Phys* 2000;48:943–949.

64b. Harris EER, Schultz DJ, Peters CA, et al. Relationship of family history and outcome after breast conservation therapy in women with ductal carcinoma in situ of the breast. *Int J Radiat Oncol Biol Phys* 2000;48:933–942.

65. Urban JA. Biopsy of the "normal" breast in treating breast cancer. *Surg Clin North Am* 1969;49:291–301.

66. Ringberg A, Palmer B, Linell F. The contralateral breast at reconstructive surgery after breast cancer operation—a histological study. *Breast Cancer Res Treat* 1982;2:151–161.

67. Griffin A, Frazee RC. Treatment of intraductal breast cancer—noncomedo type. *Am Surg* 1993;59:106–109.

68. Schuh ME, Nemoto T, Penetrante RB, et al. Intraductal carcinoma. Analysis of presentation, pathologic findings, and outcome of disease. *Arch Surg* 1986;121:1303–1307.

69. Schwartz GF, Patchefsky AS, Finklestein SD, et al. Nonpalpable in situ ductal carcinoma of the breast: predictors of multicentricity and microinvasion and implications for treatment. *Arch Surg* 1989;124:29–32.

70. Habel LA, Moe RE, Daling JR, et al. Risk of contralateral breast cancer among women with carcinoma *in situ* of the breast. *Ann Surg* 1997;225:69–75.

71. Webber BL, Heise H, Neifeld JP, et al. Risk of subsequent contralateral breast carcinoma in a population of patients with *in-situ* breast carcinoma. *Cancer* 1981;47:2928–2932.

72. Gump FE, Jicha DL, Ozello L. Ductal carcinoma *in situ* (DCIS): a revised concept. *Surgery* 1987;102:790–795.

73. Andersen JA, Nielsen M, Blichert-Toft M. The growth pattern of *in situ* carcinoma in the female breast. *Acta Oncol* 1988;27:739–743.

74. Wellings SR, Jensen HM, Marcum RG. An atlas of subgross pathology of the human breast with special reference to possible precancerous lesions. *J Natl Cancer Inst* 1975;55:231–273.

75. Barsky SH, Siegal GP, Jannotta F, et al. Loss of basement membrane components by invasive tumors but not by their benign counterparts. *Lab Invest* 1983;49:140–147.

76. Henning K, Berndt A, Katenkamp D, et al. Loss of laminin-5 in the epithelium-stroma interface: an immunohistochemical marker of malignancy in epithelial lesions of the breast. *Histopathology* 1999;34:305–309.

77. Bose S, Lesser ML, Norton L, et al. Immunophenotype of intraductal carcinoma. *Arch Pathol Lab Med* 1996;100:81–85.

78. Sternlicht MD, Kedeshian P, Shao ZM, et al. The human myoepithelial cell is a natural tumor suppressor. *Clin Cancer Res* 1997;3:1949–1958.

79. Lennington WJ, Jensen RA, Dalton LW, et al. Ductal carcinoma in situ of the breast. Heterogeneity of individual lesions. *Cancer* 1994;73:118–124.

80. Azzopardi JG. *Problems in breast pathology.* Philadelphia: WB Saunders, 1979:192–203.

81. Martin HM, Bateman AC, Theaker JM. Calcium oxalate (Weddellite) crystals within ductal carcinoma in situ. *J Clin Pathol* 1999;52:932.

82. Singh N, Theaker JM. Calcium oxalate crystals (Weddellite) within the secretions of ductal carcinoma *in situ*—a rare phenomenon. *J Clin Pathol* 1999;52:145–146.

83. Mayr NA, Staples JJ, Robinson RA, et al. Morphometric studies in intraductal breast carcinoma using computerized image analysis. *Cancer* 1991;67:2805–2812.

84. Lindley R, Bulman A, Parsons P, et al. Histologic features predictive of an increased risk of early local recurrence after treatment of breast cancer by local tumor excision and radical radiotherapy. *Surgery* 1989;105:13–20.

85. Bodis S, Siziopikou KP, Schnitt SJ, et al. Extensive apoptosis in ductal carcinoma *in situ* of the breast. *Cancer* 1996;77:1831–1835.

86. Harn HJ, Shen KL, Yueh KC, et al. Apoptosis occurs more frequently in intraductal carcinoma than in infiltrating duct carcinoma of human breast cancer and correlates with altered p53 expression: detected by terminal-deoxynucleotidyl-transferase-mediated dUTP-FITC nick end labelling (TUNEL). *Histopathology* 1997;31:534–539.

87. Quinn CM, Ostrowski JL, Harkins L, et al. Loss of *bcl-2* expression in ductal carcinoma in situ of the breast relates to poor histological differentiation and to expression of p53 and *c-erb*B-2 proteins. *Histopathology* 1998;33:531–536.

88. Sneige N, Lagios MD, Schwarting R, et al. Interobserver reproducibility of the Lagios nuclear grading system for ductal carcinoma in situ. *Hum Pathol* 1999;30:257–262.

89. Muir R, Aitkenhead AC. The healing of intraduct carcinoma of the mamma. *J Pathol Bacteriol* 1934;38:117–127.

90. Davies JD. Hyperelastosis, obliteration and fibrous plaques in major ducts of the human breast. *J Pathol* 1973;110:13–26.

91. Cross AS, Azzopardi JG, Krausz T, et al. A morphologic and immunocytochemical study of a distinctive variant of ductal carcinoma *in situ* of the breast. *Histopathology* 1985;9:21–37.

92. Chan JKC, Ng WF. Sclerosing adenosis cancerized by intraductal carcinoma. *Pathology* 1987;19:425–428.

93. Eusebi V, Collina G, Bussolati G. Carinoma *in situ* in sclerosing adenosis of the breast: an immunocytochemical study. *Semin Diagn Pathol* 1989;6:146–152.

94. Oberman HA, Markey BA. Non-invasive carcinoma of the breast presenting in adenosis. *Mod Pathol* 1991;4:31–35.

95. Ichihara S, Aoyama H. Intraductal carcinoma of the breast arising in sclerosing adenosis. Case report. *Pathol Int* 1994;44:722–726.

96. Taylor HB, Norris HJ. Epithelial invasion of nerves in benign diseases of the breast. *Cancer* 1967;20:2245–2249.

97. Tsang WYW, Chan JKC. Neural invasion in intraductal carcinoma of the breast. *Hum Pathol* 1992;23:202–204.

98. Rosen PP. Coexistent lobular carcinoma *in situ* and intraductal carcinoma in a single lobular-duct unit. *Am J Surg Pathol* 1980;4:241–246.

99. Goldstein NS, Murphy TM. Intraductal carcinoma associated with invasive carcinoma of the breast: a comparison of the two lesions with implications for intraductal carcinoma classification systems. *Am J Clin Pathol* 1996;106:312–318.

100. Shoker BS, Sloane JP. DCIS grading schemes and clinical implications. *Histopathology* 1999;35:393–400.

101. The Consensus Conference Committee. Consensus Conference on the classification of ductal carcinoma *in situ.* *Cancer* 1997;80:1798–1802.

102. Silverstein MJ, Poller DN, Waisman JR, et al. Prognostic classification of breast ductal carcinoma-in-situ. *Lancet* 1995;345:1154–1157.

103. Silverstein MJ, Lagios MD, Craig PH, et al. A prognostic index for ductal carcinoma *in situ* of the breast. *Cancer* 1996;77:2267–2274.

104. Douglas-Jones AG, Gupta SK, Attanoos RL, et al. A critical appraisal of six modern classifications of ductal carcinoma *in situ* of the breast (DCIS): correlation with grade of associated invasive carcinoma. *Histopathology* 1996;29:397–409.

105. Sloane JP, Amendoeira I, Apostolikas N, et al. Consistency achieved by 23 European pathologists in categorizing ductal carcinoma in situ of the breast using five classifications. European Commission Working Group on Breast Screening Pathology. *Hum Pathol* 1998;29:1056–1062.

106. Scott MA, Lagios MD, Axelsson K, et al. Ductal carcinoma in situ of the breast: reproducibility of histological subtype analysis. *Hum Pathol* 1997;28:967–973.

106a. Douglas-Jones AG, Morgan JM, Appleton MAC, et al. Consistency in the observation of features used to classify duct carcinoma in situ (DCIS) of the breast. *J Clin Pathol* 2000;53:596–602.

107. Ottinetti A, Sapino A. Morphometric evaluation of microvessels surrounding hyperplastic and neoplastic mammary lesions. *Breast Cancer Res Treat* 1988;11:241–248.

108. Weidner N, Semple JP, Welch WR, et al. Tumor angiogenesis and metastasis—correlation in invasive breast cancer. *N Engl J Med* 1991;324:1–8.

109. Guidi AJ, Fischer L, Harris JR, et al. Microvessel density and distribution in ductal carcinoma in situ of the breast. *J Natl Cancer Inst* 1994;86:614–619.

110. Heffelfinger SC, Yassin R, Miller MA, et al. Vascularity of proliferative breast disease and carcinoma *in situ* correlates with histological features. *Clin Cancer Res* 1996;2:1873–1878.

111. Guidi AJ, Schnitt SJ. Angiogenesis in preinvasive lesions of the breast. *Breast J* 1996;2:364–369.

112. Engels K, Fox SB, Whitehouse RM, et al. Distinct angiogenic patterns are associated with high-grade *in situ* ductal carcinomas of the breast. *J Pathol* 1997;181:207–212.

113. Sternlicht MD, Barksy SH. The myoepithelial defense: a host defense against cancer. *Med Hypotheses* 1997;48:37–46.

114. Barsky SH, Nguyen M, Grossman DA, et al. Myoepithelial cells limit DCIS metastasis by blocking invasion and angiogenesis. *Mod Pathol* 1997;10:16A.

115. Basset P, Okada A, Chenard MP, et al. Matrix metalloproteinases as stromal effectors of human carcinoma progression: therapeutic implications. *Matrix Biol* 1997;15:535–541.

116. Sternlicht MD, Safarians S, Rivera SP, et al. Characterizations of the extracellular matrix and proteinase inhibitor content of human myoepithelial tumors. *Lab Invest* 1996;74:781–796.

117. Shao ZM, Nguyen M, Alpaugh ML, et al. The human myoepithelial cell exerts antiproliferative effects on breast carcinoma cells characterized by p21WAF1/CIP1 induction, G2/M arrest, and apoptosis. *Exp Cell Res* 1998;241:394–403.

118. Guidi AJ, Schnitt SJ, Fischer L, et al. Vascular permeability factor (vascular endothelial growth factor) expression and angiogenesis in patients with ductal carcinoma *in situ* of the breast. *Cancer* 1997;80:1945–1953.

119. Lesser ML, Rosen PP, Senie RT, et al. Estrogen and progesterone receptors in breast carcinoma: correlations with epidemiology and pathology. *Cancer* 1981;48:299–309.

120. Hawkins RA, Tesdale AL, Ferguson WA, et al. Oestrogen receptor activity in intraduct and invasive breast carcinomas. *Breast Cancer Res Treat* 1987;9:129–133.

121. Barnes R, Masood S. Potential value of hormone receptor assay in carcinoma *in situ* of breast. *Am J Clin Pathol* 1990;94:533–537.

122. Bur ME, Zimarowski MJ, Schnitt SJ, et al. Estrogen receptor immunohistochemistry in carcinoma *in situ* of the breast. *Cancer* 1992;69:1174–1181.

123. Holland PA, Knox WF, Potten CS, et al. Assessment of hormone dependence of comedo ductal carcinoma in situ of the breast. *J Natl Cancer Inst* 1997;89:1059–1065.

124. Bartkova J, Barnes DM, Millis RR, et al. Immunohistochemical demonstration of c-erbB-2 protein in mammary ductal carcinoma *in situ.* *Hum Pathol* 1990;21:1164–1167.

125. Gusterson BA, Machin LG, Gullick WJ, et al. Immunohistochemical distribution of c-erbB-2 in infiltrating and *in situ* breast cancer. *Int J Cancer* 1988;42:842–845.

126. Poller DN, Silverstein MJ, Galea M, et al. Ductal carcinoma in situ of the breast: a proposal for a new simplified histological classification association between cellular proliferation and c-erbB-2 protein expression. *Mod Pathol* 1994;7:257–262.

127. Schimmelpenning H, Eriksson ET, Pallis L, et al. Immunohistochemical c-erbB-2 proto-oncogene expression and nuclear DNA content in human mammary carcinoma *in situ.* *Am J Clin Pathol* 1992;97(Suppl 1):S48–S52.

128. van de Vijver MJ, Peterse JL, Mooi WJ, et al. Neu-protein overex-

pression in breast cancer: association with comedo-type ductal carcinoma in situ and limited prognostic value in stage II breast cancer. *N Engl J Med* 1988;319:1239–1245.

129. Liu E, Thor A, He M, et al. The HER2 (c-erbB-2) oncogene is frequently amplified in in situ carcinomas of the breast. *Oncogene* 1992;7:1027–1032.

130. Ho GH, Calvano JE, Bisogna M, et al. HER2/*neu* amplification but not p53 mutation is associated with comedo and high grade ductal carcinoma in situ. *Cancer* 2000;89:2153–2160.

131. Barnes DM, Meyer JS, Gonzalez JG, et al. Relationship between c-erbB-2 immunoreactivity and thymidine labelling index in breast carcinoma in situ. *Breast Cancer Res Treat* 1991;18:11–17.

132. Albonico G, Querzoli P, Ferretti S, et al. Biological heterogeneity of breast carcinoma in situ. *Ann NY Acad Sci* 1996;784:458–461.

133. De Potter CR, Foschini MP, Schelfhout A-M, et al. Immunohistochemical study of *neu* protein overexpression in clinging in situ duct carcinoma of the breast. *Virchows Arch* 1993;422:375–380.

134. Rudas M, Neumayer R, Gnant MFX, et al. p53 protein expression, cell proliferation and steroid hormone receptors in ductal and lobular *in situ* carcinomas of the breast. *Eur J Cancer* 1997;33:39–44.

135. De Potter CR, Schelfhout A-M, Verbeeck P, et al. *Neu* overexpression correlates with extent of disease in large cell ductal carcinoma in situ of the breast. *Hum Pathol* 1995;26:601–606.

136. Lilleng R, Hagmar BM, Nesland JM. C-erbB-2 protein and neuroendocrine expression in intraductal carcinomas of the breast. *Mod Pathol* 1992;5:41–47.

137. Isola JJ, Holli K, Oksa H, et al. Elevated erbB-2 oncoprotein levels in preoperative and follow-up serum samples define an aggressive disease course in patients with breast cancer. *Cancer* 1994;73:652–658.

138. Esteva-Lorenzo FJ, Paik S, Harris LN. Serum erbB-2 in ductal carcinoma in situ of the breast—a marker of microinvasion. *Acta Oncol* 1997;36:651–652.

139. Volas GH, Leitzel K, Teramoto Y, et al. Serial serum c-erbB-2 levels in patients with breast carcinoma. *Cancer* 1996;78:267–272.

140. O'Malley FP, Vnencak-Jones CL, Dupont WD, et al. p53 mutations are confined to the comedo type ductal carcinoma *in situ* of the breast. Immunohistochemical and sequencing data. *Lab Invest* 1994; 71:67–72.

141. Rajan PB, Scott DJ, Perry RH, et al. p53 protein expression in ductal carcinoma in situ (DCIS) of the breast. *Breast Cancer Res Treat* 1997;42:283–290.

142. Poller DN, Bell RJA, Elston CW, et al. p53 protein expression in mammary ductal carcinoma *in situ:* relationship to immunohistochemical expression of estrogen receptor and c-erbB-2 protein. *Hum Pathol* 1993;24:463–468.

143. Leal CB, Schmitt FC, Bento MJ, et al. Ductal carcinoma in situ of the breast. Histologic categorization and its relationship to ploidy and immunohistochemical expression of hormone receptors, p53 and c-erbB-2 protein. *Cancer* 1995;75:2123–2131.

144. Done SJ, Arneson NCR, Ozcelik H, et al. p53 mutations in mammary ductal carcinoma *in situ* but not in epithelial hyperplasia. *Cancer Res* 1998;58:785–789.

145. Walker RA, Dearing SJ, Lane DP, et al. Expression of p53 protein in infiltrating and in-situ breast carcinomas. *J Pathol* 1991; 165:203–211.

146. Barnes R, Masood S, Barker E, et al. Low nm23 protein expression in infiltrating ductal breast carcinomas correlates with reduced patient survival. *Am J Pathol* 1991;139:245–250.

147. Simpson JF, O'Malley F, Dupont WD, et al. Heterogeneous expression of nm23 gene product in noninvasive breast carcinoma. *Cancer* 1994;73:2352–2358.

148. Vos CB, Cleton-Jansen AM, Berx G, et al. E-cadherin inactivation in lobular carcinoma in situ of the breast: an early event in tumorigenesis. *Br J Cancer* 1997;76:1131–1133.

149. Gupta SK, Douglas-Jones AG, Jasani B, et al. E-cadherin (E-cad) expression in duct carcinoma in situ (DCIS) of the breast. *Virchows Arch* 1997;430:23–28.

150. Bankfalvi A, Terpe HJ, Breukelmann D, et al. Immunophenotypic and prognostic analysis of E-cadherin and beta-catenin expression during breast carcinogenesis and tumour progression: a comparative study with CD44. *Histopathology* 1999;34:25–34.

151. Aasmundstad TA, Haugen OA. DNA ploidy in intraductal breast carcinomas. *Eur J Cancer* 1990;26:956–959.

152. Crissman JD, Visscher DW, Kubus J. Image cytophotometric DNA analysis of atypical hyperplasias and intraductal carcinomas of the breast. *Arch Pathol Lab Med* 1990;114:1239–1253.

153. Killeen JL, Namiki H. DNA analysis of ductal carcinoma in situ of the breast. A comparison with histologic features. *Cancer* 1991;68:2602–2607.

154. Locker AP, Horrocks C, Gilmour AS, et al. Flow cytometric and histological analysis of ductal carcinoma *in situ* of the breast. *Br J Surg* 1990;77:564–567.

155. Pallis L, Skoog L, Falkmer U, et al. The DNA profile of breast cancer in situ. *Eur J Surg Oncol* 1992;18:108–111.

156. Sataloff DM, Russin Vl, Sohn M, et al. DNA flow cytometric analysis in ductal carcinoma in situ of the breast. *Breast Dis* 1993;6:195–205.

157. Leal CB, Schmitt FC, Bento MJ, et al. Ductal carcinoma in situ of the breast: histologic categorization and its relationship to ploidy and immunohistochemical expression of hormone receptors, p53 and c-erbB-2 protein. *Cancer* 1995;75:2123–2131.

158. Meyer JE, Kopans DB, Stomper PC, et al. Occult breast abnormalities: percutaneous preoperative needle localization. *Radiology* 1984;150:335–337.

159. Juarez D, Jenkins S, Zervoudis M, et al. Aneuploidy of breast intraductal carcinomas detected on tissue sections by non-fluorescent in situ hybridization. *Mod Pathol* 1997;10:21A.

160. Visscher DW, Wallis TL, Crissman JD. Evaluation of chromosome aneuploidy in tissue sections of preinvasive breast carcinomas using interphase cytogenetics. *Cancer* 1996;77:315–320.

161. Gandhi A, Holland PA, Knox WF, et al. Evidence of significant apoptosis in poorly differentiated ductal carcinoma in situ of the breast. *Br J Cancer* 1998;78:788–794.

162. Nielsen KV, Andersen JA, Blichert-Toft M. Chromosome changes of in situ carcinomas in the female breast. *Eur J Surg Oncol* 1987;13:225–229.

163. Radford DM, Fair K, Thompson AM, et al. Allelic loss on chromosome 17 in ductal carcinoma in situ of the breast. *Cancer Res* 1993;53:2947–2950.

164. Alburquerque A, Kennedy S, Bryant B, et al. LOH on chromosome 17p and 17q in the histologic spectrum of DCIS. *Mod Pathol* 1997;10:15A.

165. Lichy JH, Zavar M, Tsai MM, et al. Loss of heterozygosity on chromosome 11p15 during histological progression in microdissected ductal carcinoma of the breast. *Am J Pathol* 1998;153:271–278.

166. Chuaqui RF, Zhuang Z, Emmert-Buck MR, et al. Analysis of loss of heterozygosity on chromosome 11q13 in atypical ductal hyperplasia and *in situ* carcinoma of the breast. *Am J Pathol* 1997;150:297–303.

167. Chen T, Sahin A, Aldaz CM. Deletion map of chromosome 16q in ductal carcinoma in situ of the breast: refining a putative tumor suppressor gene region. *Cancer Res* 1996;56:5605–5609.

168. Fujii H, Szumel R, Marsh C, et al. Genetic progression, histological grade, and allelic loss in ductal carcinoma in situ of the breast. *Cancer Res* 1996;56:5260–5265.

169. Stratton MR, Collins N, Lakhani SR, et al. Loss of heterozygosity in ductal carcinoma in situ of the breast. *J Pathol* 1995;175:195–201.

170. Radford DM, Phillips NJ, Fair KL, et al. Allelic loss and the progression of breast cancer. *Cancer Res* 1995;55:5180–5183.

171. Munn KE, Walker RA, Varley JM. Frequent alterations of chromosome 1 in ductal carcinoma in situ of the breast. *Oncogene* 1995;10:1653–1657.

172. Zhuang Z, Merino MJ, Chuaqui R, et al. Identical allelic loss on chromosome 11q13 in microdissected *in situ* and invasive human breast cancer. *Cancer Res* 1995;55:467–471.

173. James LA, Mitchell ELD, Menasce L, et al. Comparative genomic hybridisation of ductal carcinoma *in situ* of the breast: identification of regions of DNA amplification and deletion in common with invasive breast carcinoma. *Oncogene* 1997;14:1059–1065.

174. Barsky SH, Shao ZM, Bose S. Should DCIS be renamed carcinoma of the ductal system? *Breast J* 1999;5:70–72.

175. Marsh KL, Varley JM. Loss of heterozygosity at chromosome 9p in ductal carcinoma *in situ* and invasive carcinoma of the breast. *Br J Cancer* 1998;77:1439–1447.

176. Aubele M, Mattis A, Zitzelsberger H, at al. Extensive ductal carcinoma *in situ* with small foci of invasive ductal carcinoma: evidence of genetic resemblance by CGH. *Int J Cancer* 2000;85:82–86.

177. Waldman FM, DeVries S, Chew KL, et al. Chromosomal alterations in ductal carcinomas in situ and their *in situ* recurrences. *J Natl Cancer Inst* 2000;92:313–320.

178. Munn KE, Walker RA, Menasce L, et al. Allelic imbalance in the re-

gion of the BRCA1 gene in ductal carcinoma *in situ* of the breast. *Br J Cancer* 1996;73:636–639.

179. Schwartz GF, Solin LJ, Olivotto IA, et al. The Consensus Conference on the treatment of in situ ductal carcinoma of the breast, April 22–25, 1999. *Hum Pathol* 2000;31:131–139.

180. Jackman RJ, Nowels KW, Shepard MJ, et al. Stereotaxic large-core needle biopsy of 450 nonpalpable breast lesions with surgical correlation in lesions with cancer or atypical hyperplasia. *Radiology* 1994;193:91–95.

181. Liberman L, Dershaw DD, Rosen PP, et al. Stereotaxic core biopsy of breast carcinoma: accuracy at predicting invasion. *Radiology* 1995;194:379–381.

182. Burbank F. Stereotactic breast biopsy of atypical ductal hyperplasia and ductal carcinoma *in situ* lesions: improved accuracy with directional, vacuum-assisted biopsy. *Radiology* 1997;202:843–847.

183. Wang HH, Ducatman BS, Eick D. Comparative features of ductal carcinoma in situ and infiltrating ductal carcinoma of the breast on fine-needle aspiration biopsy. *Am J Clin Pathol* 1989;92:736–740.

184. Sneige N, Singletary SE. Fine-needle aspiration of the breast: diagnostic problems and approaches to surgical management. *Pathol Annu* 1994(Pt1);29:281–301.

185. Venegas R, Rutgers JL, Cameron BL, et al. Fine needle aspiration cytology of breast ductal carcinoma *in situ*. *Acta Cytol* 1994;38:136–139.

186. Malamud YR, Ducatman BS, Wang HH. Comparative features of comedo and noncomedo ductal carcinoma in situ of the breast on fine-needle aspiration biopsy. *Diagn Cytopathol* 1992;8:571–576.

187. McKee GT, Tildsley G, Hammond S. Cytologic diagnosis and grading of ductal carcinoma in situ. *Cancer* 1999;87:203–209.

188. Fisher ER, Costantino J, Fisher B, et al., for the National Surgical Adjuvant Breast and Bowel Project Collaborating Investigators. Pathologic findings from the National Surgical Adjuvant Breast Project (NSABP) Protocol B-17. Intraductal carcinoma (ductal carcinoma *in situ*). *Cancer* 1995;75:1310–1319.

189. Coombs JH, Hubbard E, Hudson K, et al. Ductal carcinoma in situ of the breast: correlation of pathologic and mammographic features with extent of disease. *Am Surg* 1997;63:1079–1083.

190. Tavassoli FA, Norris HJ. A comparison of the results of long-term follow-up for atypical intraductal hyperplasia of the breast. *Cancer* 1990;65:518–529.

191. Lagios MD, Westdahl PR, Margolin FR, et al. Duct carcinoma *in situ*: relationship of extent of noninvasive disease to the frequency of occult invasion, multicentricity, lymph node metastases, and short-term treatment failures. *Cancer* 1982;50:1309–1314.

192. Lagios MD. Ductal carcinoma *in situ*: biological and therapeutic implications of classification. *Breast J* 1996;2:32–34.

193. Schnitt SJ, Connolly JL. Classification of ductal carcinoma in situ: striving for clinical relevance in the era of breast conserving therapy. *Hum Pathol* 1997;28:877–880.

194. Kestin L, Goldstein NS, Lacerna MD, et al. Factors associated with local recurrence of mammographically detected ductal carcinoma in situ in patients given breast-conserving therapy. *Cancer* 2000;88:596–607.

195. Tornos C, O'Hea B. Ductal carcinoma in situ (DCIS) of the breast: pathologic features predictive of residual disease (RD) after initial excisional biopsy. *Mod Pathol* 2000;13:48A.

196. Silverstein MJ, Cohlan BF, Gierson ED, et al. Duct carcinoma *in situ*: 227 cases without microinvasion. *Eur J Cancer* 1992;28:630–634.

197. Charteris AA. On the changes in the mammary gland preceding carcinoma. *J Pathol* 1930;33:101–117.

198. Cheatle GL. Benign and malignant changes in duct epithelium of the breast. *Br J Surg* 1920/21;8:285–306.

199. Lagios MD, Westdahl PR, Rose MR. The concept and implications of multicentricity in breast carcinoma. *Pathol Annu* 1981;16:1123–1130.

200. Hardman PDJ, Worth A, Lee U. The risk of occult invasive breast cancer after excisional biopsy showing *in-situ* ductal carcinoma of comedo pattern. *Can J Surg* 1989;32:56–60.

201. Ashikari R, Huvos AG, Snyder RE. Prospective study of non-infiltrating carcinoma of the breast. *Cancer* 1977;39:435–439.

202. Gallager HS, Martin JE. Early phases in the development of breast cancer. *Cancer* 1969;24:1170–1178.

203. Morgenstern L, Kaufman PA, Friedman ND. The case against tylectomy for carcinoma of the breast. The factor of multicentricity. *Am J Surg* 1975;130:251–258.

204. Silverstein MJ, Rosser RJ, Gierson ED, et al. Axillary lymph node dis-

section for intraductal carcinoma: is it indicated? *Cancer* 1987;59:1819–1824.

205. Schwartz GF, Patchefsky AS, Feig SA, et al. Multicentricity of non-palpable breast cancer. *Cancer* 1980;45:2913–2916.

206. Faverly DRG, Burgers L, Bult P, et al. Three dimensional imaging of mammary ductal carcinoma in situ: clinical implications. *Sem Diagn Pathol* 1994;11:193–198.

207. Ozzello J, Sentipak P. Epithelial-stromal junction of intraductal carcinoma of the breast. *Cancer* 1970;26:1186–1198.

208. Ozzello L. Ultrastructure of intra-epithelial carcinomas of the breast. *Cancer* 1971;28:1508–1515.

209. Rajan PB, Perry RH. A quantitative study of patterns of basement membrane in ductal carcinoma *in situ* (DCIS) of the breast. *Breast J* 1995;1:315–321.

210. Tamimi SO, Ahmed A. Stromal changes in early invasive and non-invasive breast carcinoma: an ultrastructural study. *J Pathol* 1986;150:43–49.

211. Tulusan AH, Grünsteidel W, Ramming I, et al. A contribution to the natural history of breast cancer. III. Changes in the basement membranes in breast cancers with stromal microinvasion. *Arch Gynecol* 1982;231:209–218.

212. Barsky SH, Togo S, Garbisa S, et al. Type IV collagenase immunoreactivity in invasive breast carcinoma. *Lancet* 1983;1:296–297.

213. Nakano S, Iyama K, Ogawa M, et al. Differential tissular expression and localization of type IV collagen alpha-1(IV), alpha-5(IV), and alpha-6(IV) chains and their mRNA in normal breast and in benign and malignant breast tumors. *Lab Invest* 1999;79:281–292.

214. Hewitt RE, Powe DG, Morrell K, et al. Laminin and collagen IV subunit distribution in normal and neoplastic tissues of colorectum and breast. *Br J Cancer* 1997;75:221–229.

215. Frazier TG, Copeland EM, Gallager HS, et al. Prognosis and treatment in minimal breast cancer. *Am J Surg* 1977;133:697–701.

216. Gallager HS, Martin JE. An orientation to the concept of minimal breast cancer. *Cancer* 1971;28:1505–1507.

217. Hutter RVP. The pathologist's role in minimal breast cancer. *Cancer* 1971;28:1527–1536.

218. Ozzello L. The behaviour of basement membranes in intraductal carcinoma of the breast. *Am J Pathol* 1959;35:887–899.

219. Yaziji H, Sneige N, Gown AM. Comparative sensitivities and specificities of myoepithelial markers in the detection of stromal invasion in breast cancer. *Mod Pathol* 2000;13:50A.

220. Coyne J, Haboubi NY. Micro-invasive breast carcinoma with granulomatous stromal response. *Histopathology* 1992;20:184–185.

221. Prasad ML, Hyjek E, Giri DD, et al. Double immunolabeling with cytokeratin and smooth-muscle actin in confirming early invasive carcinoma of breast. *Am J Surg Pathol* 1999;23:176–181.

222. Cowen PN. Recognition of intraduct mammary carcinoma. *J Clin Pathol* 1980;33:797.

223. Cowen PN, Bates C. The significance of intraduct appearances in breast cancer. *Clin Oncol* 1984;10:67–72.

224. Barsky SH, Doberneck SA, Sternlicht MD, et al. 'Revertant' DCIS in human axillary breast carcinoma metastases. *J Pathol* 1997;183:188–194.

225. Arihiro K, Inai K, Kurihara K, et al. Distribution of laminin, type IV collagen and fibronectin in the invasive component of breast carcinoma. *Acta Pathol Japonica* 1993;43:758–764.

226. Nadji M, Nassiri M, Fresno M, et al. Laminin receptor in lymph node negative breast carcinoma. *Cancer* 1999;85:432–436.

227. Henning K, Berndt A, Katenkamp D, et al. Loss of laminin-5 in the epithelium-stroma interface: an immunohistochemical marker of malignancy in epithelial lesions of the breast. *Histopathology* 1999;34:305–309.

228. Damiani S, Ludvikova M, Tomasic G, et al. Myoepithelial cells and basal lamina in poorly differentiated *in situ* duct carcinoma of the breast. *Virchows Arch* 1999;434:227–234.

229. Wong JH, Kopald KH, Morton DL. The impact of microinvasion on axillary node metastases and survival in patients with intraductal breast cancer. *Arch Surg* 1990;125:1298–1302.

230. Solin LJ, Fowble BL, Yeh I-T, et al. Microinvasive ductal carcinoma of the breast treated with breast-conserving surgery and definitive irradiation. *Int J Radiat Oncol Biol Phys* 1992;23:961–968.

231. Rosner D, Lane WW, Penetrante R. Duct carcinoma *in situ* with microinvasion: a curable entity using surgery along without need for adjuvant therapy. *Cancer* 1991;67:1498–1503.

232. Silver SA, Tavassoli FA. Mammary ductal carcinoma *in situ* with microinvasion. *Cancer* 1998;82:2382–2390.

233. Jimenez RE, Visscher DW. Clinicopathologic analysis of microscopically invasive breast carcinoma. *Hum Pathol* 1998;29:1412–1419.

234. Walker RA, Dearing SJ, Brown LA. Comparison of pathological and biological features of symptomatic and mammographically detected ductal carcinoma in situ of the breast. *Hum Pathol* 1999;30:943–948.

235. de Mascarel I, MacGrogan G, Soubeyran I, et al. Breast ductal carcinoma *in situ* with microinvasion (DCIS-MI): a definition supported by a long-term study of 1401 serially sectioned ductal carcinomas: 268 DCIS-MI versus 829 DCIS and versus 304 infiltrating ductal carcinomas with a predominant DCIS component (IDC<DCIS). *Mod Pathol* 2000;13:19A.

236. Prasad ML, Osborne MP, Giri DD, et al. Microinvasive carcinoma (T1mic) of the breast. Clinicopathologic profile of 21 cases. *Am J Surg Pathol* 2000;24:422–428.

237. Zavotsky J, Hansen N, Brennan MB, et al. Lymph node metastasis from ductal carcinoma in situ with microinvasion. *Cancer* 1999;85:2439–2443.

238. Dauway EL, Giuliano R, Pendas S, et al. Lymphatic mapping: a technique providing accurate staging for breast cancer. *Breast Cancer* 1999;6:145–154.

239. Pathology Working Group Breast Cancer Task Force. Standardized management of breast cancer specimens. *Am J Clin Pathol* 1973;60:789–798.

240. Goldstein NS, Lacerna M, Vicini F. Cancerization of lobules and atypical ductal hyperplasia adjacent to ductal carcinoma *in situ* of the breast. *Am J Clin Pathol* 1998;110:357–367.

241. Farrow JH. Current concepts in the detection and treatment of the earliest of the early breast cancers. *Cancer* 1970;25:458–479.

242. Kinne DW, Petrek JA, Osborne MP, et al. Breast carcinoma *in situ*. *Arch Surg* 1989;124:33–36.

243. Sunshine JA, Moseley HS, Fletcher WS, et al. Breast carcinoma *in situ*: a retrospective review of 112 cases with minimum 10 year follow-up. *Am J Surg* 1985;150:44–51.

244. Carter D, Smith AL. Carcinoma *in situ* of the breast. *Cancer* 1977;40:1189–1193.

245. Boyages J, Delaney G, Taylor R. Predictors of local recurrence after treatment of ductal carcinoma *in situ*: a meta-analysis. *Cancer* 1999;85:616–628.

246. Clark L, Ritter E, Glazebrook K, et al. Recurrent ductal carcinoma *in situ* after total mastectomy. *J Surg Oncol* 1999;71:182–185.

247. Montgomery RC, Fowble BL, Goldstein LJ, et al. Local recurrence after mastectomy for ductal carcinoma *in situ*. *Breast J* 1998;4:430–436.

248. Finkelstein SD, Sayegh R, Thompson WR. Late recurrence of ductal carcinoma in situ at the cutaneous end of surgical drainage following total mastectomy. *Am Surg* 1993;59:410–414.

249. Fisher DE, Schnitt SJ, Christian R, et al. Chest wall recurrence of ductal carcinoma *in situ* of the breast after mastectomy. *Cancer* 1993;71:3025–3028.

250. Srivastava A, Webster DJT. Isolated nipple recurrence seventeen years after subcutaneous mastectomy for breast cancer—a case report. *Eur J Surg Oncol* 1987;13:459–461.

251. Price P, Sinnett HD, Gusterson B, et al. Duct carcinoma in situ: predictors of local recurrence and progression in patients treated by surgery alone. *Br J Cancer* 1990;61:869–872.

252. Helvie MA, Wilson TE, Roubidoux MA, et al. Mammographic appearance of recurrent breast carcinoma in six patients with TRAM flap breast reconstructions. *Radiology* 1998;209:711–715.

253. Kraus FT, Neubecker RD. The differential diagnosis of papillary tumors of the breast. *Cancer* 1962;15:444–455.

254. McDivitt RW, Holleb AI, Foote Jr FW. Prior breast disease in patients treated for papillary carcinoma. *Arch Pathol* 1968;85:117–124.

255. Millis RR, Thynne GSJ. *In situ* intraduct carcinoma of the breast: a long term follow-up study. *Br J Surg* 1975;62:957–962.

256. Kiaer W. *Relation of fibroadenomatosis ("chronic mastitis") to cancer of the breast*. Copenhagen: Ejnar Munksgaard, 1954:69.

257. Betsill Jr WL, Rosen PP, Lieberman PH, et al. Intraductal carcinoma: long-term follow-up after treatment by biopsy alone. *JAMA* 1978;239:1863–1867.

258. Rosen PP, Braun Jr DW, Kinne DW. The clinical significance of preinvasive breast carcinoma. *Cancer* 1980;46:919–925.

259. Harvey DG, Fechner RE. Atypical lobular and papillary lesions of the breast: a follow-up study of 30 cases. *South Med J* 1978;71:361–364.

260. Page DL, Dupont WD, Rogers LW, et al. Intraductal carcinoma of the breast: follow-up after biopsy only. *Cancer* 1982;49:751–758.

261. Page DL, Dupont WD, Rogers LW, et al. Continued local recurrence of carcinoma 15–25 years after a diagnosis of low grade ductal carcinoma in situ of the breast treated only by biopsy. *Cancer* 1995;76:1197–1200.

262. Eusebi V, Foschini MP, Cook MG, et al. Long-term follow-up of in situ carcinoma of the breast with special emphasis on clinging carcinoma. *Diagn Pathol* 1989;6:165–173.

263. Lagios MD, Margolin FR, Westdahl PR, et al. Mammographically detected duct carcinoma in situ. Frequency of local recurrence following tylectomy and prognostic effect of nuclear grade on local recurrence. *Cancer* 1989;63:618–624.

264. Lagios MD. Evaluation of surrogate endpoint biomarkers for ductal carcinoma *in situ*. *J Cell Biochem* 1994;19(Suppl):186–188.

265. Fisher ER, Sass R, Fisher B, et al. Pathologic findings from the National Surgical Adjuvant Breast Project. (protocol 6). I. Intraductal carcinoma (DCIS). *Cancer* 1986;57:197–208.

266. Ottesen GL, Graversen HP, Blichert-Toft M, et al., on behalf of the Danish Breast Cancer Cooperative Group. Ductal carcinoma in situ of the female breast: short-term results of a prospective nationwide study. *Am J Surg Pathol* 1992;16:1183–1196.

267. Ringberg A, Andersson I, Aspegren K, et al. Breast carcinoma in situ in 167 women—incidence, mode of presentation, therapy and follow-up. *Eur J Surg Oncol* 1991;17:466–476.

268. Arnesson L-G, Smeds S, Fagerberg G, et al. Follow-up of two treatment modalities for ductal cancer in situ of the breast. *Br J Surg* 1989;76:672–675.

269. Carpenter R, Boulter PS, Cooke T, et al. Management of screen detected ductal carcinoma in situ of the female breast. *Br J Surg* 1989;76:564–567.

270. Schwartz GF, Finkel GC, Garcia JC, et al. Subclinical ductal carcinoma in situ of the breast. *Cancer* 1992;70:2468–2474.

271. Hetelekidis S, Collins L, Silver B, et al. Predictors of local recurrence following excision alone for ductal carcinoma *in situ*. *Cancer* 1999;85:427–431.

272. Badve S, A'Hern RP, Ward AM, et al. Prediction of local recurrence of ductal carcinoma *in situ* of the breast using five histological classifications: a comparative study with long follow-up. *Hum Pathol* 1998;29:915–923.

273. Montague ED. Conservative surgery and radiation therapy in the treatment of operable breast cancer. *Cancer* 1984;53:700–704.

274. Recht A, Danoff BS, Solin LJ, et al. Intraductal carcinoma of the breast: results of treatment with excisional biopsy and irradiation. *J Clin Oncol* 1985;3:1339–1343.

275. Zafrani B, Fourquet A, Vilcoq JR, et al. Conservative management of intraductal breast carcinoma with tumorectomy and radiation therapy. *Cancer* 1986;57:1299–1301.

276. Bornstein BA, Recht A, Connolly JL, et al. Results of treating ductal carcinoma in situ of the breast with conservative surgery and radiation therapy. *Cancer* 1991;67:7–13.

277. Solin LJ, Recht A, Fourquet A, et al. Ten-year results of breast-conserving surgery and definitive irradiation for intraductal carcinoma (ductal carcinoma *in situ*) of the breast. *Cancer* 1991;68:2337–2344.

278. Solin LJ, Kurtz J, Fourquet A, et al. Fifteen-year results of breast-conserving surgery and definitive breast irradiation for the treatment of ductal carcinoma *in situ* of the breast. *J Clin Oncol* 1996;14:754–763.

279. Silverstein MJ, Waisman JR, Gierson ED, et al. Radiation therapy for intraductal carcinoma. Is it an equal alternative? *Arch Surg* 1991;126:424–428.

280. Solin LJ, Yeh I-T, Kurtz J, et al. Ductal carcinoma *in situ* (intraductal carcinoma) of the breast treated with breast-conserving surgery and definitive irradiation: correlation of pathologic parameters with outcome of treatment. *Cancer* 1993;71:2532–2542.

281. Kuske RR, Bean JM, Garcia DM, et al. Breast conservation therapy for intraductal carcinoma of the breast. *Int J Radiat Oncol Biol Phys* 1993;26:391–396.

282. Goonewardene S, Palazzo J, Cornfield D, et al. Prognostic significance of necrosis in evaluating risk for recurrence of ductal carcinoma *in situ* of the breast and progression to invasive carcinoma: survey of 166 conservatively treated patients. *Am J Clin Pathol* 1999;112:531–532.

283. Silverstein MJ. Incidence and treatment of ductal carcinoma in situ of the breast. *Eur J Cancer* 1997;33:10–11.

284. Silverstein MJ. Ductal carcinoma in situ of the breast: the Van Nuys experience by treatment. *Breast J* 1997;3:232–237.

285. Warnberg F, Nordgren H, Bergh J, et al. Ductal carcinoma in situ of the breast from a population-defined cohort: an evaluation of new histopathological classification systems. *Eur J Cancer* 1999;35:714–720.

286. Silverstein MJ, Lagios MD, Martino S, et al. Outcome after invasive local recurrence in patients with ductal carcinoma *in situ* of the breast. *J Clin Oncol* 1998;16:1367–1373.

287. Fisher B, Dignam J, Wolmark N, et al. Lumpectomy and radiation therapy for the treatment of intraductal breast cancer: findings from National Surgical Adjuvant Breast and Bowel Project B-17. *J Clin Oncol* 1998;16:441–452.

288. Fisher ER, Dignam J, Tan-Chiu E, et al. Pathologic findings from the National Surgical Adjuvant Breast Project (NSABP) eight-year update of Protocol B-17: intraductal carcinoma. *Cancer* 1999; 86:429–438.

289. Solin LJ, McCormick B, Recht A, et al. Mammographically detected, clinically occult ductal carcinoma in situ treated with breast-conserving surgery and definitive breast irradiation. *Cancer J Sci Am* 1996;2:158–165.

290. Fowble B. The results of conservative surgery and radiation for mammographically detected ductal carcinoma in situ. *Breast J* 1997; 3:238–241.

291. Thomas M, Goldstein NS, Vicini FA, et al. The association of age at diagnosis with pathologic features in patients with duct carcinoma *in situ* of the breast. *Mod Pathol* 2000;13:47A.

292. Hillner BE, Desch CE, Carlson RW, et al. Trade-offs between survival and breast preservation for three initial treatments of ductal carcinoma-in-situ of the breast. *J Clin Oncol* 1996;14:70–77.

293. Cheng L, Al-Kaisi NK, Gordon NH, et al. Relationship between the size and margin status of ductal carcinoma in situ of the breast and residual disease. *J Natl Cancer Inst* 1997;89:1356–1360.

294. Liberman L, Van Zee KJ, Dershaw DD, et al. Mammographic features of local recurrence in women who have undergone breast-conserving therapy for ductal carcinoma in site. *AJR Am J Roentgenol* 1997;168:489–493.

295. Silverstein MJ, Gierson ED, Colburn WJ, et al. Can intraductal breast carcinoma be excised completely by local excision? *Cancer* 1994;73:2985–2989.

296. Goldstein NS, Kestin L, Vicini F. Pathologic features of initial biopsy specimens associated with residual intraductal carcinoma on reexcision in patients with ductal carcinoma *in situ* of the breast referred for breast-conserving therapy. *Am J Surg Pathol* 1999;23:1340–1348.

297. Schnitt SJ, Harris JR, Smith BL. Developing a prognostic index for ductal carcinoma *in situ* of the breast: are we there yet? *Cancer* 1996;77:2189–2192.

298. Wood WC. Should axillary dissection be performed in patients with DCIS? *Ann Surg Oncol* 1995;2:193–194.

299. Haigh PI, Giuliano AE. The Cox et al. article reviewed. *Oncology* 1998;12:1293–1294.

300. Cox CE, Haddad F, Bass S, et al. Lymphatic mapping in the treatment of breast cancer. *Oncology* 1998;12:1283–1292.

# CHAPTER 14

# Invasive Duct Carcinoma

## Assessment of Prognosis, Morphologic Prognostic Markers, and Tumor Growth Rate

Invasive duct carcinoma is the largest group of malignant mammary tumors constituting 65% to 80% of mammary carcinomas (1,2). Included under this heading are lesions characterized variously as duct carcinoma with productive fibrosis, scirrhous carcinoma, and carcinoma simplex. A generic term sometimes used is invasive duct carcinoma, not otherwise specified (NOS). This is a useful designation, because it recognizes the distinction between these tumors and the many other specific forms of duct carcinoma, such as tubular, medullary, metaplastic, colloid, and adenoid cystic carcinoma.

Invasive duct carcinoma includes tumors that express, in part, one or more characteristics of the specific types of breast carcinoma, but do not constitute pure examples of the individual tumors. Examples of this phenomenon are invasive duct carcinomas that have limited microscopic foci of tubular, medullary, papillary, or mucinous differentiation. The relatively favorable prognosis associated with some specific histologic types has been found to apply only to those tumors composed entirely or in very large part of the designated pattern. Where these features are less extensively represented, the tumors are appropriately relegated to the broader group of invasive duct carcinoma, NOS. Tumors combining invasive duct carcinoma with associated Paget's disease are included in this category.

Approximately one-third of the lesions characterized as invasive duct carcinoma in one detailed review of 1,000 carcinomas expressed one or more combined features (3). Slightly more than half of the combined tumors were invasive duct carcinomas with a tubular carcinoma component. Combinations with invasive lobular carcinoma were detected in 6% of the tumors. Thus far, prognostic differences have not been identified for most of the combined histologic patterns, and, as a consequence, they frequently have been grouped together as invasive duct carcinoma. The present section considers invasive duct carcinoma in the context of this broad definition, and reference will be made to specific combined histologic patterns where relevant.

The growth pattern of a coexisting intraductal component usually is reflected in the structure of the invasive carcinoma. There is a significant association between the grade of intraductal and invasive duct carcinoma in tumors that have both components (4). This observation suggests that important prognostic features of the tumor are established in the preinvasive stage and that the clinical course sometimes may be predetermined by the *in situ* component before invasion occurs. Studies of genetic alterations in the intraductal and invasive components of individual tumors have shown similar patterns of loss of heterozygosity (LOH) in both parts, a finding that further supports this hypothesis.

Tubular carcinoma invariably arises from an orderly micropapillary or cribriform intraductal carcinoma that features cytologically low-grade nuclei. The intraductal component of medullary carcinoma typically is solid with poorly differentiated nuclei. Invasive poorly differentiated duct carcinoma, NOS, tends to develop from solid or comedo intraductal carcinoma. Comedonecrosis may occur in invasive areas of a tumor with solid or comedo intraductal carcinoma duplicating the intraductal pattern. It can be difficult to distinguish between intraductal and invasive components in some primary tumors. Foci that resemble comedo intraductal carcinoma can be encountered in metastatic lesions derived from such tumors (5).

Moderately differentiated invasive duct carcinoma, NOS, most often originates from cribriform or papillary intraductal components. Invasive cribriform carcinoma is a subtype of invasive duct carcinoma with a prominent cribriform structure. These tumors arise from cribriform intraductal carcinoma. The presence of invasive components that mimic cribriform intraductal carcinoma can complicate the measurement of the invasive tumor area, and foci with an *in situ* cribriform pattern can occur in metastatic lesions. Invasive lesions that are entirely cribriform and those with a mixture of cribriform and tubular components are relatively low grade and have a very good prognosis. If less well-differentiated elements are present in the tumor, the prognosis is not as favorable. Invasive cribriform carcinoma sometimes is mistaken for adenoid cystic carcinoma (6).

## THE COMPLEXITY OF ASSESSING PROGNOSIS

Innumerable studies have attempted to assess the prognosis of breast cancer patients on the basis of clinical and pathologic parameters. Because nearly three-fourths of the patients have invasive duct carcinoma, the characteristics of these tumors have a considerable influence on laboratory, clinical, or pathologic studies of breast carcinoma.

Breast carcinoma is a heterogeneous disease clinically and pathologically. As noted by Sistrunk and MacCarty (7) almost 80 years ago, "It is impossible to foretell the duration of life of all patients with carcinoma of the breast, because the degree of malignancy varies widely, and persons react differently to the disease." More recently, Heimann and Hellman (8) commented on this subject as follows:

> The varied outcomes of similarly staged patients is most consistent with breast cancer not being a homogeneous disease, but rather a spectrum of disease states that have varying capacities for growth and metastasis. . . . Required of tumors is the development of critical phenotypic attributes: growth, invasion, metastagenicity, and angiogenesis. . . . Recognizing tumor heterogeneity emphasizes the need to determine an individual tumor's place in the evolutionary spectrum. This may be accomplished using clinical features such as size, nuclear grade and patient age, as well as by examining angiogenesis, metastatic capacity, and proliferation. Identification of the extent of tumor progression with regard to these major tumor phenotypes should allow individual therapy to be fashioned for each patient.

In a subsequent report, Heimann and Hellman (9) analyzed data from approximately 1,500 patients treated by mastectomy without systemic therapy, with a median follow-up of 145 months among survivors. Follow-up revealed that the risk for recurrence ("metastagenicity" or M) and time to recurrence ("virulence" or V) were dependent on tumor size and nodal status. The calculated percent of risk for recurrence expended in different periods of follow-up revealed an inverse relationship between virulence and the distribution of risk over time (Table 14.1). Among node-positive patients, most of the risk of recurrence was expended in the first 10 years of follow-up, with only 5% to 10% remaining thereafter. In the node-negative group, 30% of the risk for recurrence remained after 10 years. A cured group with a negligible remaining risk for recurrence was identified in each stage group, although the proportion of "cured" patients diminished with greater tumor size and increased nodal involvement.

A similar type of analysis was reported by Blamey et al. (10), who examined tumor grade as well as size and nodal status. The study included 4,500 patients, among whom 1,756 died of breast carcinoma. Presentation of survival curves in logarithmic form revealed two components. The first part of the curve was a relatively rapid decline with a duration determined by tumor grade (grade I, 28 years; grade II, 12 years; grade III, 7 years). Thereafter, an inflection point was reached in each curve to a slow decline that was parallel for all grades. The authors observed that 90% of recurrences occurred within 9, 7, and 5 years for patients with grade I, II, and III tumors, respectively. The rate of death due to breast carcinoma also was influenced by grade, with 90% occurring in 40, 13, and 8 years among patients with grade I, II, and III tumors, respectively. In this study, histologic grade proved to be an additional determinant of metastagenicity and virulence among patient groups stratified by tumor size and nodal status.

**TABLE 14.1.** *Percent risk of distant disease recurrence expended at 2, 5, 10, and 15 years from diagnosis[a]*

| Size of tumor | No. of lymph nodes | No. of patients | No. of patients recurred | Total risk M | Percent risk expended | | | |
|---|---|---|---|---|---|---|---|---|
| | | | | | 2 years | 5 years | 10 years | 15 years |
| All | 0 | 796 | 177 | 0.30 | 20 | 50 | 70 | 85 |
| | 1–3 | 434 | 232 | 0.62 | 45 | 75 | 95 | 99 |
| | >4 | 360 | 276 | 0.86 | 45 | 75 | 90 | 99 |
| ≤2 cm | 0 | 367 | 56 | 0.20 | 15 | 40 | 65 | 80 |
| | 1–3 | 115 | 36 | 0.36 | 20 | 65 | 100 | 100 |
| | ≥4 | 60 | 43 | 0.81 | 30 | 70 | QNS | QNS |
| >2 cm | 0 | 428 | 121 | 0.38 | 10 | 50 | 75 | 87 |
| | 1–3 | 317 | 195 | 0.70 | 50 | 75 | 90 | 98 |
| | ≥4 | 300 | 233 | 0.89 | 45 | 75 | 90 | 98 |

[a]Calculated from Kaplan-Meier curves.
M, metastagenicity; QNS, quantity not sufficient (<40 patients).
From Heimann R, Hellman S. Clinical progression of breast cancer malignant behavior: what to expect and when to expect it. *J Clin Oncol* 2000;18:591–599, with permission.

## Genetic Factors

A genetic basis for differences in rates of cancer progression is suggested by analysis of LOH in primary and locally recurrent lesions. Regitnig et al. (11) studied primary and recurrent specimens from 26 patients and reported that all LOH identified in the primary tumor also was present in the local recurrence, but that there was a significant increase in "total LOH" in recurrent tumors. Early recurrence was associated with LOH at specific loci (TP53 and D5S107). Lymph node metastases were associated with LOH at these sites and at D35.

Data relating race to prognosis have compared black and white patients. In one study, black women were significantly younger at diagnosis (mean, 55 years) than white women (mean, 60 years) (12). Black patients were more likely to have larger tumors and tumors with necrosis after adjustment for differences in income, medical insurance, and method of tumor detection. Analysis of a national database composed of more than 115,000 breast carcinoma patients by Edwards et al. (13) revealed that, compared to whites, black women had a reduced likelihood of cure and that black women who were not cured had a shorter survival after diagnosis.

The impact on prognosis of specific germline mutations, such as BRCA1 and BRCA2, has not been fully investigated. BRCA-associated breast carcinomas are significantly more likely than non–BRCA-associated carcinomas to have poorly differentiated histologic grade, lack estrogen receptors, be HER2/neu negative, and manifest high Ki67 labeling indicative of a high proliferative rate (14–29). Robson et al. (19) found no significant differences in the expression of epidermal growth factor receptor (EGFR), cathepsin D, bcl-2, p27, p53, or cyclin D, and there was not a significant difference in relapse-free or overall survival between BRCA-associated and non–BRCA-associated tumors despite the relatively unfavorable tumor characteristics of the former group.

Robson et al. (19) also reported that the presence of a germline BRCA mutation did not significantly increase the risk of local breast recurrence after breast conservation with lumpectomy and radiotherapy when compared to stage-matched controls. Patients with BRCA germline mutations had a substantial 5-year risk for contralateral breast carcinoma (12.2%) and ovarian carcinoma (8.1%). These additional carcinoma events resulted in significantly reduced event-free survival when compared with the controls (53.2% vs. 73.3%).

Armes et al. (20) compared the histologic features of BRCA1- and BRCA2-associated breast carcinomas in a population-based study. The cases were drawn from a cohort of Australian women found to have breast carcinoma before age 40. It is noteworthy that 70% of BRCA1 carriers and 40% of BRCA2 carriers did not have a family history of breast carcinoma in a first- or second-degree relative. When compared to tumors from BRCA2 carriers and age-matched controls, carcinomas in BRCA1 carriers were more often high grade with a higher mean mitotic rate. They also were more likely to be classified as medullary or atypical medullary carcinomas. Carriers of BRCA2 mutations had an increased frequency of pleomorphic lobular carcinoma, but in other respects their tumors did not differ significantly from controls in histologic appearance. No follow-up data were provided.

BRCA1-associated invasive breast carcinomas are reported to have a significantly lower frequency of associated intraductal carcinoma than sporadic or nonhereditary carcinomas (18,21). This observation is consistent with the low frequency of pure intraductal carcinoma observed in studies of BRCA1-associated tumors (22). BRCA2 tumors did not have a significantly different frequency of intraductal carcinoma when compared with sporadic control tumors (18).

## Bilaterality

The impact of bilateral breast carcinoma on prognosis has received considerable attention. Among women treated by mastectomy, prognosis is similar after unilateral and bilateral disease, compared on the basis of the higher stage tumor in bilateral cases (23,24). Several studies that analyzed outcome in women with simultaneous bilateral breast carcinoma treated by breast conservation therapy reported no differences in overall survival when compared to women treated by bilateral mastectomy or in comparison to women treated by unilateral breast conservation (25–27). When compared to patients with unilateral carcinoma, tumors in patients with bilateral carcinoma had a greater frequency of multicentricity in one or both breasts (19% vs. 3%) (28).

Some reports noted that patients with simultaneous bilateral breast carcinoma were older than women with unilateral tumors at the time of diagnosis (29) or that patients with metachronous bilaterality tended to be younger (30,31). Patients with bilateral carcinoma report a positive family history more often than women with unilateral tumors (25,32). Lee et al. (27) reported a positive family history of breast carcinoma in 28% of women with unilateral tumors and 40% in bilateral breast carcinoma patients, a statistically significant difference. The possibility of genetic susceptibility in some cases was suggested by the finding of a 70% incidence of other malignant tumors in women with a first-degree relative affected by breast carcinoma. Testing for BRCA mutations was not reported in this series of patients.

## Method of Tumor Detection and Screening

The method of tumor detection influences prognosis and disease-free survival. Among patients diagnosed before widespread mammography screening, tumor detection by clinical breast examination was associated with a significant reduction in recurrence compared with detection by self-palpation (33). Screening examinations using mammography with or without physical examination have been shown to reduce mortality due to breast carcinoma in the screened population. When compared with unscreened controls, a 1985 report of data from a study conducted by the Health Insurance Plan of New York (HIP) revealed a 30% lower death rate due to breast carcinoma among women enrolled in a program of annual breast palpation and mammography (34). An updated report in 1997 revealed that the screened group had about a 25% lower breast cancer mortality among women aged 40 to 64 years at entry into the study than did the control group after 18 years (35). Reduction in mortality in women 40 to 49 years old at entry was in part due to treatment of carcinomas detected after screening when these women were 50 to 54 years old. When compared to controls, the reduction in mortality for carcinomas diagnosed when women were in the 40- to 49-year age group was 14% 18 years after entry into the study.

Tabár et al. (36) demonstrated a reduction in mortality of nearly 30% in Sweden with mammography screening at 2- and 3-year intervals. A later analysis of the Swedish two-county study revealed a 13% difference in breast cancer mortality between women invited and not invited to be screened in the 40- to 49-year age group (37). In the 50- to 74-year age group, the difference in mortality was 35% favoring the invited group. The relatively small impact of screening on mortality in the younger age group was attributed to failure to detect high-grade tumors sufficiently early with the screening intervals then being used in the study; consequently, more frequent screening was proposed for women younger than 50 years (38).

In the nationwide Breast Cancer Diagnosis Demonstration Project in the United States, there was a greater than 50% reduction in "case fatality for all stages . . . for cases that were screen-detected than for cases that were not screen detected" (39). The favorable effect of screening on prognosis also has been documented with 20-year follow-up (40).

When compared to breast carcinomas presenting clinically, carcinomas detected by screening with mammography tend to be smaller, to be lower grade, and to have fewer nodal metastases (41–43). This difference is most pronounced in the first or prevalent screening examination (44). Tumors detected in the first round of mammography screening have flow cytometry features associated with slow growth, such as a low S-phase (45,46). However, the relationship between nodal status and tumor size is similar among patients with carcinomas detected by screening and clinically; the frequency of nodal metastases does not differ significantly according to the method of detection within any category of tumor size (47). No differences in the expression of HER2/neu and EGFR were reported in one study of screen and clinically detected carcinomas (42). In a series of 65 patients treated by mastectomy for nonpalpable, screen-detected invasive carcinomas, 26% had multicentric invasive carcinoma and 35% had residual invasive carcinoma at the biopsy site (48).

Interval carcinomas detected between screening examinations have been reported by some to have less favorable prognostic features than screen-detected tumors, such as high S-phase, aneuploidy, larger size, lower estrogen receptor content (45,49,50), fewer tubular carcinomas, and more invasive lobular, medullary, and comedocarcinomas (51). Although these observations have suggested that interval carcinomas would have a less favorable clinical course than screen-detected tumors (52), follow-up studies have not consistently revealed a less favorable outcome among women with interval carcinomas (53,54).

Vitak et al. (50) analyzed patients with prevalent, incident, and interval-detected carcinomas using data from the Östergötland county screening program in Sweden. The end points for assessing benefit derived from screening were the time to, or frequency of, systemic recurrence. The probability of systemic recurrence was significantly greater for women with interval-detected tumors and for women who did not participate in screening than in the screened group. The recurrence rate was significantly higher for interval tumors detected within 1 year of the last screen than for those detected later. These observations support the notion that interval carcinomas as a group tend to be clinically more aggressive than screen-detected tumors. However, when screen-detected and interval cases with similar characteristics (size, grade, etc.) were compared in multivariate analysis, the method of detection (screening vs. interval) was not significantly related to metastatic potential.

The possibility that a noninvasive diagnostic procedure might also detect prognostically significantly biologic features of breast carcinoma has been explored with positron emission tomography (PET) using 2-deoxy-2-fluoro[$^{18}$F]-D-glucose (FDG) to obtain information about glucose metabolism. Cancer cells exhibit a higher rate of glycolysis than normal cells, and they overexpress the immunohistochemically detected glucose transport molecule GLUT1, which may be responsible for glucose accumulation (55). PET has successfully identified breast carcinomas in several studies (56,57), and it has been effective as a method for distinguishing between benign and malignant tumors (58,59), with a sensitivity of 68% to 94% and specificity of 84% to 97% (59). Response of breast carcinoma to preoperative chemotherapy has been evaluated by PET (60). Oshida et al. (61) studied the differential absorption rate (DAR) of FDG in breast carcinomas by PET and related the calculated DAR to prognosis in 70 patients after a mean follow-up 41 months. The mean DAR was 2.61 ± standard deviation (SD) 1.61 (range 0.65 to 9.39). When patients were stratified into two groups with DAR ≥3.0 or DAR <3.0, patients with high DAR had a significantly worse overall and relapse-free survival. DAR proved to be a significant independent indicator of relapse-free survival in multivariate analysis. DAR also was significantly related to microvessel density (MVD) in the primary tumors of patients with and without axillary lymph node metastases.

## Time to Recurrence

The interval to recurrence (disease-free or recurrence-free interval) and length of survival are basic measurements of prognosis. In general, these factors are closely related; hence, factors associated with a high frequency of recurrence correlate with reduced survival. Treatment that delays but does not reduce the overall frequency of recurrence may increase the duration of survival without reducing overall mortality due to the disease. These concepts are supported by a report from Edwards et al. (62), who analyzed nearly 2,000 patients to assess the relationships between time from treatment to relapse, time from treatment to death, and time from relapse to death. In this series, the likelihood of cure was similar for time to relapse and time to death, but time to relapse was not significantly correlated with time from relapse to death. Touboul et al. (63) analyzed 528 patients treated by breast conservation with radiotherapy. In this clinical setting, the risk of distant metastases was related to the incidence of local recurrence. After local recurrence, the disease-free interval from start of treatment to local recurrence influenced survival so that a shorter interval to local recurrence was associated with shorter overall survival. Factors predicting local failure and systemic metastases differed somewhat. Local recurrence was significantly associated with diagnosis at age less than 40 years, premenopausal status, two tumor foci rather than one, and an extensive intraductal component. The probability of systemic recurrence was significantly related to the number of lymph nodes with metastases, high histologic grade, and presence of a local recurrence.

Survival after recurrence is influenced by characteristics of the primary tumor and of the recurrence. The range of reported median survival after recurrence is 11 to 37 months (64). Factors associated with shorter postrecurrence survival include short recurrence-free interval, visceral metastases, estrogen receptor-negative tumor, larger primary tumor size, presence of axillary nodal metastases at diagnosis, and premenopausal menstrual status at the time of initial treatment (64–66). Patients with stage I disease at the time of diagnosis are more likely to have an initial recurrence that is local-regional, whereas stage II patients are more likely to have a systemic recurrence initially (67). If local-regional recurrences are excluded, stage I and II patients have similar patterns of recurrence at systemic sites (67). Systemic adjuvant therapy tends to increase the disease-free interval, and there is evidence that patients given adjuvant therapy relapse in fewer sites (68).

## Local Radiotherapy

Radiotherapy administered to the chest wall after mastectomy or to the breast after lumpectomy reduces the risk of local recurrence at these sites. Whether this beneficial effect on local recurrence is translated into improved overall survival in patients who receive radiation to the chest wall after mastectomy remains controversial, and the benefit, if any, may not be sufficient to offset potential complications such as cardiovascular disease (69–71). Data from one study suggest that the survival benefit of reduced local recurrence after

mastectomy for node-negative patients at 10 years may be 2% and 6% for women with axillary nodal metastases (72). To assess the cardiovascular effects of chest wall radiation, Hojris et al. (73) analyzed data from a trial in which patients were randomized to systemic treatment with or without local-regional radiotherapy after mastectomy. After a median follow-up of 10 years, mortality due to breast carcinoma was lower in the radiated group (44.2%) than in the nonradiated group (52.5%), whereas the two groups experienced very similar rates of death due to ischemic heart disease. The hazard rate for mortality due to ischemic heart disease in the radiated versus nonradiated group did not increase with time after treatment.

The laterality of the carcinoma and subsequent radiotherapy proved to be a significant risk factor for mortality due to myocardial infarction in a study of cancer registry data for United States patients treated from 1973 to 1992 (74). The analysis did not distinguish between surgical treatment by lumpectomy or mastectomy. The relative risk for a fatal myocardial infarction (controlling for age) was 1.17 (95% confidence interval [CI] 1.01 to 13.6) among women with left versus right breast carcinoma. The relative risk was increased for women treated before age 60 (1.98; 95% CI-sign 1.31 to 2.97), but not in women older than 60 years. The age-related effect was observed in patients with regional disease at diagnosis, but no difference related to age was found for women with local disease. These data suggest that chest wall radiation after left breast carcinoma increases the risk of cardiovascular disease in women younger than 60 years at the time of treatment.

## Local Recurrence in Conserved Breast or Chest Wall

In patients treated by breast-conserving surgery and radiation therapy, the time to breast recurrence is significantly related to the risk of systemic metastases and survival at 5 years (75). Patients with breast recurrences 2 to 4 years after diagnosis have a significantly greater risk of developing systemic metastases and poorer survival than those who manifest breast recurrence more than 4 years after initial treatment (75,76). The rates of local breast recurrence and distant metastases after breast conservation appear to differ. In one series, the yearly frequency of local breast recurrence was about 1% per year up to 10 years, whereas the probability of systemic metastases was 5% at 2 years and decreased thereafter (76). Tumor size and axillary lymph node metastases were predictors of systemic metastases, but they were not related to local recurrence in patients treated by breast conservation.

Whether recurrence in the breast or chest wall is a marker for tumors more likely to disseminate or a source of metastases remains to be determined. The two scenarios are not mutually exclusive, and one or both may apply in individual cases. One study relevant to this issue was described by Schnitt et al. (77), who reported that breast recurrences were detected in 14 (16%) of 87 patients with node-negative invasive breast carcinoma treated by lumpectomy without radiotherapy. The median follow-up period was 56 months. Tumor size ranged from 2 to 25 mm (median, 9 mm), and 76% of the tumors were detected by mammography alone. All patients underwent reexcision of the initial biopsy site, with residual tumor detected in only two reexcisions; all had negative margins of excision. In addition to the 14 patients with local recurrence, 4 (11%) other women had systemic metastases with no prior local recurrences. Breast recurrence was observed in one of these four women after systemic metastases were detected. A comparison group treated with conservation surgery and radiotherapy had no breast recurrences, and the 3-year metastatic rate was 7%. Neither group of patients received systemic adjuvant therapy. These data suggest that local breast recurrence after conservation therapy and systemic metastases are not necessarily linked temporally and may be independent events. Recurrence in the breast often occurs without clinical evidence of concurrent systemic metastases, and patients may develop systemic metastases when local recurrence is not evident. The "natural history" in these circumstances may be influenced by breast irradiation and adjuvant systemic therapy.

### Early Detection of Recurrence

Most recurrences are documented because patients present with symptoms or they are evident on physical examination (78,79). The detection of asymptomatic metastases by screening patients with x-ray or laboratory tests during follow-up after primary therapy has resulted in a reduction in the lead time to diagnosis of recurrence in some (79,80), but not all, studies (81–83). In one study, patients with asymptomatic recurrences detected by screening at scheduled times had a longer postrecurrence survival than patients with symptomatic lesions detected during intervals between scheduled examinations (83). This may reflect more favorable prognostic features associated with occult recurrences (79). Routine screening of patients treated by mastectomy using scans, radiography, and laboratory tests to detect asymptomatic, clinically unapparent recurrences has not been shown to improve the overall survival of patients with breast carcinoma (79–83). After reviewing the usefulness of routine imaging studies in the follow-up of patients with mammary and colonic carcinoma, Kagan and Steckel (84) concluded "that earlier detection of a local recurrence or metastatic disease through periodic tests in the asymptomatic patient with breast or colon cancer rarely alters the treatment or the outcome." This conclusion must be reevaluated as more effective systemic therapy becomes available.

### Time Dependence of Prognostic Variables

There is evidence indicating that the prognostic importance of a given pathologic variable does not apply uniformly throughout the course of follow-up, but the time dependency of prognostic variables has not been thoroughly analyzed (85–87). Some variables are associated with short-term outcome, whereas others appear to exert an effect later. This is illustrated by the observation that the main influence of tumor necrosis on prognosis is manifested early in follow-up (88). In another study, nuclear grade, nodal status, and peritumoral lymphocytic infiltration were related to prognosis in time-dependent patterns (89).

Analysis by Nab et al. (90) of the long-term follow-up of 462 consecutively treated patients revealed that the risk of recurrence decreased progressively from 10% in the first 2 years after diagnosis to 1% beyond 10 years. After 10 years, 72% of T1N0 patients were recurrence-free, and only one of the remaining 79 disease-free women developed a recurrence thereafter. During the first 5 years of follow-up, nodal status and tumor size each had approximately equal significance as prognostic markers. In the 5- to 10-year interval, only tumor size remained prognostically significant.

Combined data from several adjuvant therapy trials under the aegis of the Eastern Cooperative Oncology Group (ECOG) have been analyzed to determine the annual hazard for recurrence in this clinical setting (91). The peak hazard rate for recurrence occurred 1 to 2 years after diagnosis and the initiation of therapy. A consistent decline in the hazard rate was observed in years 2 to 5, with a more slowly declining rate thereafter through year 12. Most patients followed this overall pattern; subsets of patients at greater risk for recurrence, such as women with three or more nodal metastases, had a higher hazard for recurrence at all intervals of follow-up than those at lower risk. For years 5 to 12 after diagnosis, the mean hazard for recurrence was 4.3% per year.

### Methods of Analysis: Univariate and Multivariate

Analysis of prognostic variables can be performed by univariate and multivariate methods. The former approach examines each prognostic factor separately, being influenced by other factors only to the extent that the analysis is restricted by stratification for other variables (e.g., stage, menstrual status). Multivariate analysis compares the relative prognostic importance of the individual variables included in an analysis. A factor that has prognostic significance in univariate analysis may prove not to be significant when compared to other variables in multivariate analysis.

There have been attempts to assess combinations of variables as a means for developing a prognostic profile or prognostic index (92–94). For example, a prognostic model based on S-phase fraction (SPF), progesterone receptor status, and tumor size distinguished between node-negative patients with an increased risk for distant relapse and those with an age-adjusted survival similar to a control population (95). The Nottingham Prognostic Index (NPI) uses tumor size, lymph node status, and histologic grade to stratify patients into significantly different prognostic groups (96,97). Various methods of grading and axillary lymph node staging have been used to determine components of the index (97).

This concept deserves more attention in clinical practice because of the growing interest in a greater variety of clinical, pathologic, and biologic prognostic factors. Because the influence of all prognostic factors in a given case may not be unidirectional (favorable or unfavorable), it is likely that multiple combinations of these variables may be associated with equivalent outcomes (94).

### Impact of Therapy on Prognosis

It is important to consider the impact of primary treatment on the evaluation of prognostic factors. Until the 1960s, radical mastectomy was the most widely used form of primary treatment. A large body of data was accumulated with respect to the importance of stage at diagnosis, type of tumor, and other clinical and morphologic parameters in relation to this form of treatment. The past two decades have witnessed major changes in treatment, with a shift from total mastectomy to partial mastectomy, quadrantectomy, or lumpectomy combined with primary radiation therapy and axillary dissection, or more recently, sentinel lymph node mapping. The evaluation of prognostic factors has been complicated further by the introduction of adjuvant chemotherapy for women with nodal metastases and for most patients with uninvolved lymph nodes. At present, reports documenting the follow-up of patients treated with various modalities suggest that pathologic prognostic variables determined to be significant in populations treated by mastectomy are equally relevant to survival and systemic recurrence for patients treated by breast-conserving surgery and radiotherapy (98,99). The extent to which the prognostic importance of conventional pathologic parameters influences response to adjuvant chemotherapy is uncertain. Pinder et al. (100) reported that response to chemotherapy was more favorable in patients with high-grade carcinoma if they had lymph node metastases, but this effect was not evident in node-negative cases.

### Changing Incidence and Mortality

Data from the National Cancer Institute's Surveillance, Epidemiology and End Results (SEER) program have been used to estimate the incidence rate of breast cancer and mortality due to the disease in the United States (101). Between 1973 and 1992, the overall incidence rose from 82.5 per 100,000 women to 110.6, rising steadily from 1973 to 1987 and stabilizing in the period from 1988 to 1992. From 1973 to 1992, the death rate varied between approximately 26 and 27 per 100,000 women, with a decline to 26.2 in the period from 1989 to 1992. Data from Sweden also documented an increasing incidence of and declining mortality due to breast carcinoma in Malmö when compared to the rest of Sweden (102). The reduction of mortality in Malmö was 43% compared to 12% throughout Sweden. The increase in and subsequent stabilization of incidence and the decline in the death rate have been attributed to the combined effects of screening by mammography and clinical examination and improved methods of treatment. A decline in mortality due to breast cancer among women born after 1920 has been documented in several countries (103).

## MORPHOLOGIC PROGNOSTIC MARKERS

For the most part, there are no clinical features that distinguish invasive duct carcinoma from other types of invasive carcinoma and some benign tumors. An exception is palpable breast carcinoma associated with Paget's disease of the nipple. The underlying invasive carcinoma in these cases is almost always of the duct type, NOS. However, Paget's disease may derive from intraductal carcinoma without invasion limited to the lactiferous ducts. Coincidentally, there may be a palpable lesion formed by another separate carcinoma, possibly of a different histologic type, such as a tubular carcinoma. Invasive duct carcinoma occurs throughout the age range of breast carcinoma, but is most common in patients in their mid to late 50s.

### Gross Pathology

Invasive duct carcinoma invariably forms a solid tumor. The consistency and appearance of the cut surface vary considerably depending on the composition of the lesion. Cystic change is extremely uncommon in this group of lesions, but it may be a manifestation of necrosis, usually accompanied by hemorrhage in the degenerated area. Noncystic areas of necrosis may be soft and chalky white or hemorrhagic (Fig. 14.1). Carcinomas with a relatively abundant scirrhous or fibrotic stroma can be extremely firm to hard, with a gray-to-white surface. When there is prominent elastosis of the stroma, a yellow tinge may be observed. Chalky white streaks in the tumor tissue usually are indicative of necrosis (Fig. 14.2), calcification, or elastosis. Carcinomas with less abundant stroma that are composed largely of neoplastic cells and inflammatory cells tend to be softer and tan. The cut surfaces of such cellular neoplasms are likely to bulge slightly when bisected (Fig. 14.3).

#### Tumor Size

The measured gross size of a mammary carcinoma is one of the most significant prognostic variables. Numerous studies have shown that survival decreases with increasing tumor size and that there is a coincidental rise in the frequency of axillary nodal metastases (89,104–106). This phenomenon applies not only to the overall spectrum of primary tumor size, but also within subsets such as those defined by TNM staging. For example, among T1 breast carcinomas, (2 cm or less in diameter), there is a significant relationship between size, the frequency of nodal metastases, and prognosis when the tumors are stratified in 5-mm groups (107,108). Roger et al. (109) reported the following significant ($p < 0.0001$) distribution of the frequency of axillary nodal involvement in relation to tumor size in a series of 534 patients: T1a (0 to 0.5

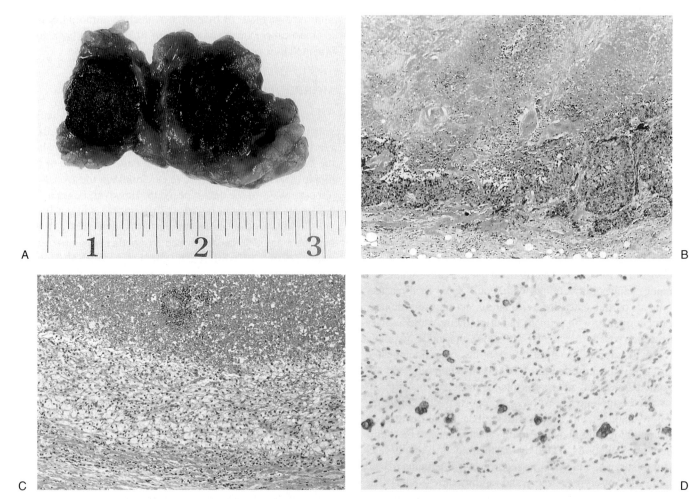

**FIG. 14.1.** *Invasive duct carcinoma.* **A:** The dark, well-defined area is necrotic invasive carcinoma with hemorrhage. **B:** A thin border of intact, poorly differentiated duct carcinoma is present at the edge of the tumor around extensive tumor necrosis. **C:** Another invasive duct carcinoma with almost complete infarction. **D:** Isolated carcinoma cells at the border are highlighted by the CK7 cytokeratin immunostain (avidin-biotin).

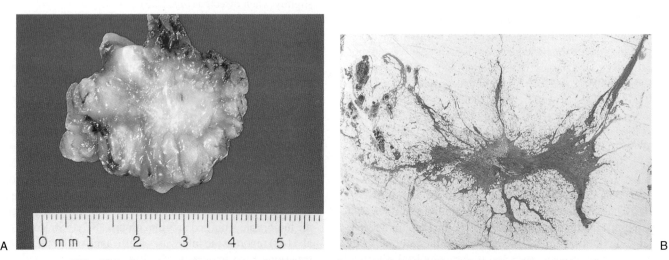

**FIG. 14.2.** *Invasive duct carcinoma.* **A:** This tumor has a stellate border and chalky white streaks of necrosis. **B:** Whole-mount histologic section of a stellate invasive duct carcinoma.

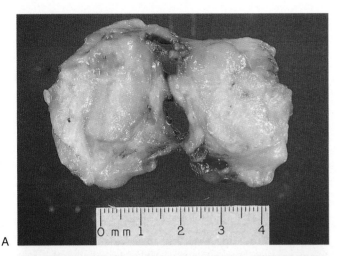

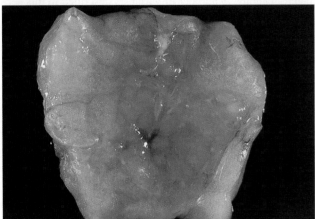

**FIG. 14.3.** *Invasive duct carcinoma.* **A:** Tumor has a circumscribed border and bulges above the surrounding tissue. **B:** This fleshy invasive duct carcinoma was poorly differentiated and had a lymphocytic infiltrate, which may have contributed to the tan color.

cm) (3%); T1b (0.6 to 1.0 cm) (10%); 1.1 to 1.5 cm (21%); and 1.6 to 2.0 cm (35%) (109). Others have reported finding axillary lymph node metastases in 31% of 336 patients treated for invasive carcinoma 1 cm or less in diameter (110).

A recent detailed analysis of tumor size and nodal status in women with T1 breast carcinoma was reported by Abner et al. (111), who studied 118 patients treated by breast-conserving surgery and radiation therapy. Macroscopic gross tumor size and microscopically measured invasive tumor diameter were equal in 22% of cases. The macroscopic size was smaller than microscopic size in 31% and larger in 47% of cases. Overall, 21% of patients had axillary lymph node metastases. The risk of lymph node metastases was not significantly different between patients with tumors less than 1 cm (T1a to T1b) and patients with tumors 1.1 to 2.0 cm (T1c), regardless of whether tumor size was based on macroscopic or microscopic measurements. The 10-year actuarial rate of recurrence-free survival was 91% of N0 patients with tumors measured macroscopically as less than 1.0 cm compared to 77% for patients with macroscopic tumors 1.1 to 2.0

cm. The rates for tumors measured microscopically were 96% and 72%, respectively. These data indicate somewhat greater prognostic discrimination when T1 tumor size is measured microscopically to define the diameter of the invasive component.

### Size and Nodal Status

Among node-negative patients considered to be at high risk for recurrence (any size tumor estrogen receptor-negative or estrogen receptor-positive tumor larger than 2 cm), the addition of systemic chemotherapy resulted in a 34% reduction in the risk of death due to breast carcinoma after 10 years and a 10.1% absolute benefit in overall survival (112).

Long-term follow-up is necessary to fully assess the prognosis of patients who had invasive carcinoma with a favorable stage, such as T1N0M0. The 20-year overall survival in a Finish Cancer Registry study was 54% (95% CI = 48% to 60%), and the survival rate corrected for nonbreast carcinoma deaths was 81% (95% CI = 75% to 87%) (113). In patients with T1a to T1b tumors, the corrected 20-year survival rate was 92% (95% CI = 86% to 96%). In the T1c group, the corrected 20-year survival was 75% (95% CI = 64% to 86%). During the first 5 years of follow-up, the risk of death due to breast carcinoma was 0.70% per year of follow-up, rising to 0.80%, 1.51%, and 1.19% per year in each of the subsequent 5-year intervals. During the same period, the risk of death due to nonmammary carcinoma was 0.23%, 0.45%, 0.88%, and 0.71% per year in each 5-year period.

The interaction of the number of involved lymph nodes and tumor size is important prognostically in stage II patients. Quiet et al. (114) found that disease-free survival after mastectomy was 81% in patients with one lymph node metastasis and a tumor 2 cm or smaller as compared with 59% if the tumor was larger than 2 cm.

### Measuring Tumor Size

Because most carcinomas have asymmetric shapes, measurement of size generally is reported in terms of the greatest diameter. It is important that the tumor be submitted intact to the pathologist, so that the configuration of the lesion can be assessed by palpation. This makes it possible to bisect the specimen in a plane that exposes the longest diameter. The measurement should be made before any samples are taken for frozen section or any other procedure. When a frozen section is prepared, the grossly measured diameter can be reported with the intraoperative histologic diagnosis and entered as part of the frozen section record.

The gross measurement of the size of a carcinoma is only an approximation of the actual amount of invasive tumor present. Benign tissue with hyperplastic or reactive changes may contribute to the palpable lesion. In some tumors, a considerable part of the mass is composed of invasive carcinoma, whereas in other lesions of comparable gross size, varying proportions of the bulk may be intraductal carcinoma with a lesser invasive component or nonneoplastic elements such as connective tissue or inflammatory cells (115,116). Measurement of the invasive component exclusive of peripheral extensions of intraductal carcinoma is recommended when it is practical to make this distinction on the basis of histologic sections. In some cases, there is microscopic extension of the invasive component beyond the grossly measurable tumor. These contiguous peripheral invasive elements should be included in the measurement of tumor size, especially in lesions 2.0 cm or less in diameter, which can be represented by a complete cross section on a histologic slide. If invasive carcinoma is dispersed across the entire tumor diameter in histologic sections, the largest dimension from point to point across the entire invasive diameter is the measured tumor size even if there are interspersed zones of intraductal carcinoma or benign tissue. A comment can be made to indicate the proportion of the cross-sectional area that is occupied by invasive carcinoma.

### Tumor Configuration or Shape

The majority of invasive duct carcinomas can be described on the basis of gross tumor configuration as stellate (spiculated, infiltrative, radial, serrated), circumscribed (rounded, pushing, encapsulated, smooth), or having a mixed contour (Figs. 14.2–14.5). Approximately one-third of the tumors have grossly circumscribed margins. A minority of tumors have indistinct borders and cannot be described in these terms. In general, the gross appearance of the tumor duplicates the configuration visualized by mammography.

However, carcinomas that appear to have circumscribed margins grossly or mammographically may exhibit an invasive growth pattern when studied microscopically.

Some investigators observed a more favorable prognosis associated with circumscribed carcinomas determined by gross inspection of the tumor or by mammography (117,118). Infiltrative tumors tend to be larger when detected, and they are more likely to have axillary lymph node metastases than those with circumscribed margins (117–119). Tumors with a stellate configuration in which there is focal necrosis were found to have an especially poor prognosis (119).

### Microscopic Histopathologic Prognostic Factors

The histologic appearance of invasive duct carcinoma is heterogeneous. A number of variables described in this section should be included in the microscopic diagnosis of invasive duct carcinomas in order to characterize the histologic and prognostic features of a particular tumor. Additional discussion about reporting prognostic features of breast carcinoma can be found in the discussion of specific tumor types and in Chapter 46.

### Grading

Grading of carcinomas is an estimate of differentiation. Unless otherwise indicated, grading is limited to the invasive portion of the tumor. *Nuclear grading* is the cytologic evaluation of tumor nuclei in comparison with the nuclei of normal mammary epithelial cells. Because nuclear grading does

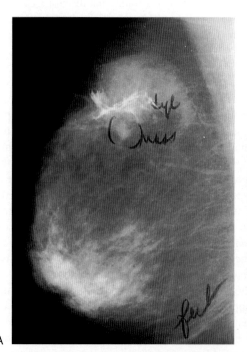
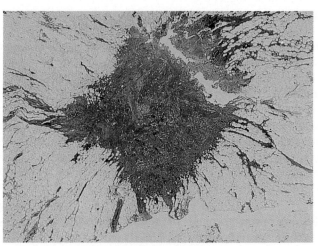

**FIG. 14.4.** *Invasive duct carcinoma.* **A:** Small, nonpalpable stellate tumor *(circled)* in the upper central area on the mammogram. Dye injected for localization is present above the lesion. **B:** Whole-mount histologic section of the stellate invasive duct carcinoma.

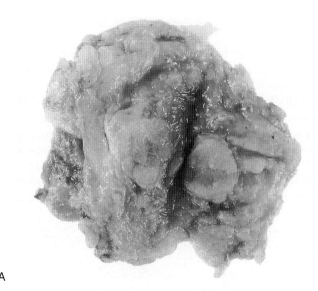

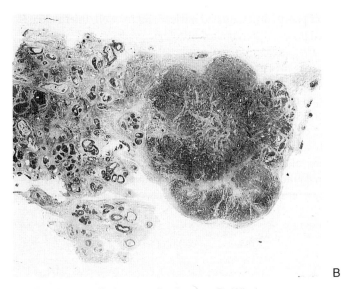

A B

**FIG. 14.5.** *Invasive duct carcinoma.* **A:** Gross specimen showing a well-circumscribed tumor. **B:** Whole-mount histologic section of a multinodular invasive duct carcinoma with a circumscribed lobulated border.

not involve assessment of the growth pattern of the tumor, this procedure is applicable not only to invasive duct carcinoma, but also to other subtypes of mammary carcinoma. The most widely used system for nuclear grading, introduced by Black et al. (120,121), usually is reported in terms

of three categories: well differentiated, intermediate, and poorly differentiated (Fig. 14.6). The sequence of numerical designations used by Black et al. for nuclear grading was the reverse of the sequence used in histologic grading. Current grading systems use grades 1, 2, and 3 for well, intermediate,

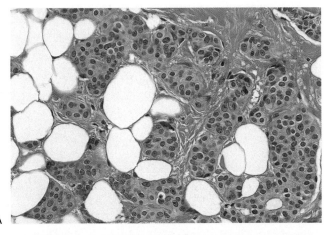

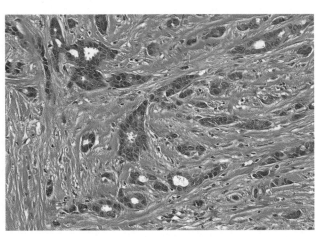

A B

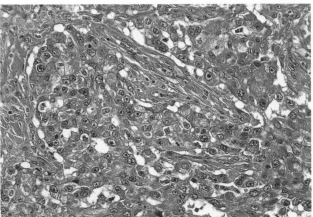

C

**FIG. 14.6.** *Invasive duct carcinoma, nuclear grade.* **A:** Low nuclear grade with small nuclei lacking nucleoli. **B:** Intermediate nuclear grade. **C:** High-grade pleomorphic nuclei with prominent nucleoli.

and poorly differentiated nuclear and for well, intermediate, and poorly differentiated histologic grades.

*Histologic grading* describes the microscopic growth pattern of invasive ductal carcinomas as well as cytologic features of differentiation. The most widely used histologic grading systems are based on criteria established by Bloom and Richardson (122,123). The parameters measured are (a) the extent of tubule formation; (b) nuclear hyperchromasia, pleomorphism, and size; and (c) mitotic rate. Each of the three elements is assigned a score on a scale of 1 to 3, and the final grade is determined from the sums of the scores. Histologic grade traditionally is expressed in three categories:

scores 3 to 5, well differentiated (grade I); scores 6 to 7, intermediate (grade II); and scores 8 to 9, poorly differentiated (grade III) (Fig. 14.7). The relative importance of the components in histologic grading has not been determined; therefore, their values are given equal weight.

*Mitotic rate* was reported by Parham et al. (124) to be the most important feature of the Bloom-Richardson grading system. They found that a grading system or prognostic index grade based on mitotic rate and the presence or absence of necrosis was a better predictor of outcome than the Bloom-Richardson grading method. Other authors also emphasized the importance of mitotic activity as an indicator of

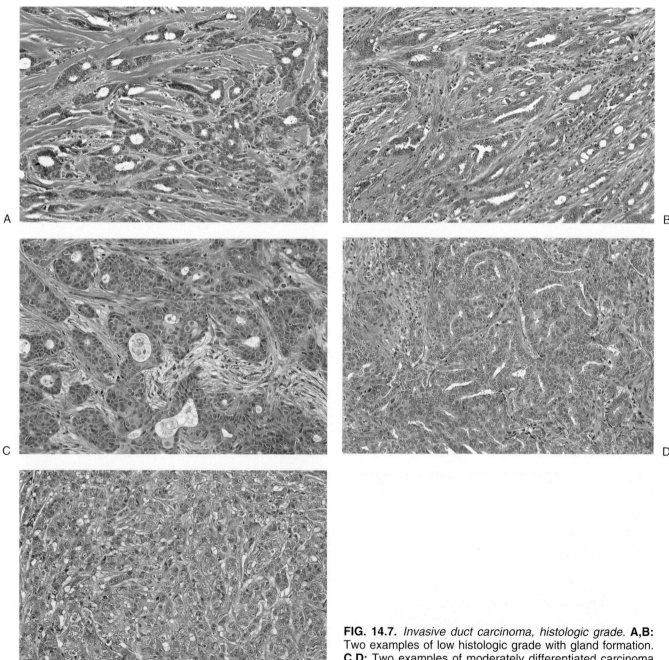

**FIG. 14.7.** *Invasive duct carcinoma, histologic grade.* **A,B:** Two examples of low histologic grade with gland formation. **C,D:** Two examples of moderately differentiated carcinoma with complex glandular growth patterns. **E:** Poorly differentiated carcinoma with a solid, nonglandular architecture.

prognosis. Jannink et al. (125) compared four methods for assessing mitotic activity and concluded that the traditional mitotic activity index (MAI) was preferable because it was "easy to apply and less time consuming." In their report, MAI was measured in a 0.5 × 0.5-cm area "in the most cellular region at the periphery of the tumor . . . (selected to) avoid areas of necrosis, inflammation, calcification and large vessels." Counting was done at 400× magnification and counting was limited to invasive tumor in 10 consecutive fields. When determined by a standardized protocol, MAI has proven to be a reliable and reproducible method that added significantly to the prognostic value of lymph node status and tumor size (126). Baak et al. (127) evaluated the prognostic importance of MAI in a prospective study of Dutch premenopausal women entered into a systemic adjuvant therapy trial. When node-negative patients were compared after stratification by MAI <10 versus MAI ≥10, MAI was the strongest prognostic factor.

The importance of using a standardized counting method and especially a fixed *field size* has been emphasized by several observers. Kuopio and Collan (128) demonstrated substantial variation of grading in the Bloom-Richardson system depending on field size and mitotic rate. Variation in field size had the greatest effect on the scoring of mitotic counts (classified as scores 1, 2, or 3 in the Bloom-Richardson system) when the mitotic count per mm$^2$ was between 7 and 20. The larger the field diameter or area measured in mm$^2$, the greater the probability of obtaining a score of 3 at a given mitotic rate. As a method of overcoming this difficulty, a table has been created listing mitotic rates per 10 high-power fields for different microscopes (129,130), and conversion factors have been developed for converting counts per 10 high-power fields to counts per mm$^2$ (131).

The range of *field areas* (mm$^2$) for 26 combinations of microscope types and eyepieces was tabulated by Ellis and Whitehead (132). Field areas ranged from 0.071 to 0.385 mm$^2$ with an objective of 40× in each instance. An important variable in these calculations is the field number or index, a factor that varies among microscopes and can be obtained from the manufacturer.

A table for converting mitotic count and field diameter data to mitotic scores in the modified Bloom-Richardson grading system was devised by Kuopio and Collan (128).

Another factor influencing mitotic counting is the choice of fields to count. The most widely used approach is to select a cellular invasive region at the periphery of the tumor where mitotic activity is likely to be highest (129). An alternative method has been to count mitoses in 10 randomly selected 40× high-power fields, starting from a field previously determined to have "the highest density of mitotic figures" (125).

Definitions of *mitotic figures* have not been standardized. The original Bloom-Richardson grading system considered hyperchromatic nuclei to be mitotic, but subsequent modifications of the Bloom-Richardson grading system introduced more specific criteria for identifying mitoses. The Notting-

ham histologic grade excludes hyperchromatic nuclei when this is the only mitosis-related feature (100). van Diest et al. (126) offered detailed specifications for mitotic figures (Table 14.2). It should be noted that the counting of metaphase figures as two separate mitoses, as cited in Table 14.2, in order to achieve comparability with image analysis is not customarily used in routine light microscopy where a metaphase figure would be counted as a single mitosis.

Baehner and Weidner (133) reported improved specificity in mitosis counting by using the mitosis-specific antibody antiphosphohistone-H3 (PHH3). The antibody tags some prophase nuclei as well as cells in mitosis. The antibody enhanced recognition of mitotic figures, and after prophase nuclei labeled with PHH3 were excluded, the resultant counts were highly correlated with traditional mitotic counts and with Ki67 labeling.

Several variants of Bloom-Richardson grading have been described. The system of Schauer and Weiss (134) subdivided Bloom-Richardson grade II into two subcategories, resulting in a total of four grades. The modification of Le Doussal et al. (135) created five grades based on nuclear pleomorphism and mitotic index, omitting the degree of structural differentiation. Modification of Bloom-Richardson grading with more rigorous criteria for most parameters resulted in the development of the Nottingham histologic grade (Table 14.3) (129,136).

### Grading and Prognosis

Presently, most methods for grading use the previously cited three-tiered systems for describing tumor structure in terms of tubule formation, nuclear grade, and mitotic count, with the latter usually expressed as the number of mitoses per 10 high-magnification fields (40×). Each element is scored on a scale from 1 to 3 according to criteria of the specific grading system, and the final grade is determined by the

---

**TABLE 14.2.** *Specifications for mitotic figures*

Nuclear membrane
  "absent, so cells must have passed the prophase"

Nuclear structure
  "clear, hairy extensions of nuclear material (condensed chromosomes) must be present, either clotted (beginning metaphase), in a plane (metaphase/anaphase), or in separate clots (telophase). Regular extensions with an empty central zone favor a nonmitosis."

Mitotic figure
  "two parallel, clearly separate chromosome clots are to be counted as if they are separate mitoses, however, obvious it is that only one mitotic figure is concerned. This is in view of future automated mitotic figure recognition with image analysis."

From van Diest PJ, Baak JPA, Matze-Cok P, et al. Reproducibility of mitosis counting in 2,469 breast cancer specimens: results from the Multicenter Morphometric Mammary Carcinoma Project. *Hum Pathol* 1992;23:603–607, with permission.

**TABLE 14.3.** *Modified Bloom-Richardson histologic grading*

Tubule formation
　　Score 1: >75% of tumor has tubules
　　Score 2: 10% to 75% of tumor has tubules
　　Score 3: <10% tubule formation

Nuclear size
　　Score 1: tumor nuclei similar to normal duct cell nuclei (2–3 × RBC)
　　Score 2: intermediate-size nuclei
　　Score 3: very large nuclei, usually vesicular with prominent nucleoli

Mitotic count
(per 10 hpf with 40× objective and field area of 0.196 mm$^2$)
　　Score 1: 0–7 mitoses
　　Score 2: 8–14 mitoses
　　Score 3: ≥15 mitoses

hpf, high-power field; RBC, red blood cell.
From Robbins P, Pinder S, deKlerk N, et al. Histological grading of breast carcinomas: a study of interobserver agreement. *Hum Pathol* 1995;26:873–879, with permission.

sum of the scores. The Bloom-Richardson and Nottingham histologic grades have very similar predictive values and are probably the most frequently used methods.

Pinder et al. (100) analyzed histologic grade as a prognostic factor and as an indicator of response to chemotherapy in an International Breast Cancer Study Group trial involving 465 patients. There was a strong correlation between grading assigned with the Bloom-Richardson and Nottingham systems, although a greater proportion of tumors were classified as grade 1 with Nottingham grading, and Bloom-Richardson grading identified a greater proportion of tumors as grade 3. The authors reported that "no apparent differences in overall and disease-free survival were observed between the two systems."

The histologic and nuclear grades of a given tumor coincide in many, but not all, invasive duct carcinomas (137). There is a significant correlation between nuclear grade and SPF, and it has been suggested that nuclear grade can be used to predict whether a carcinoma has a high SPF (138). Numerous studies demonstrated that patients with high-grade or poorly differentiated invasive duct carcinoma treated by mastectomy had a significantly higher frequency of axillary lymph node metastases and of four or more positive lymph nodes, that they developed more systemic recurrences, and that more of these patients died of metastatic disease than did women with low-grade tumors (89,107,120–123,139–142). Nuclear and histologic grade have been shown to be useful predictors of prognosis for patients stratified by stage of disease, especially among those without axillary lymph node metastases (107,135,141). The absence of tubule formation is a particularly unfavorable histologic feature when combined with poorly differentiated nuclear cytology.

The impact of grade on prognosis in stage II patients is uncertain. Some authors reported a significant correlation, noting a more favorable outcome associated with low-grade lesions (140,141). However, these analyses did not take into

consideration stratification on the basis of tumor size and the number of affected lymph nodes. In a carefully defined series of T1N1M0 patients, neither histologic nor nuclear grade was significantly correlated with outcome (108). On the other hand, a case-control analysis of patients who survived 25 years after radical mastectomy for invasive carcinoma revealed a significantly higher proportion of histologically grade 1 tumors (43%) among long-term survivors when compared with controls matched on the basis of tumor size, number of lymph nodes with metastases, and age at diagnosis (143). Histologic grade was reportedly a prognostically significant factor in the response of stage II patients to adjuvant chemotherapy (144), especially patients who received prolonged rather than perioperative treatment (97). Higher failure rates were observed in patients with higher-grade tumors. This negative effect of grade was independent of nodal status, tumor size, hormone receptors, and several other prognostic factors. Histologic grade also was a significant indicator of response among patients who received endocrine treatment for systemic recurrence (145,146). Histologic type of tumor (duct, lobular, or other) was not significantly related to response to treatment.

Histologic grade is significantly related not only to the frequency of recurrence and death due to invasive ductal carcinoma, but also to the disease-free interval and overall length of survival after mastectomy regardless of clinical stage (89). High-grade carcinomas result in early treatment failures, whereas later recurrences are observed more often among low-grade tumors. For this reason, an unequal distribution of patients by grade could significantly influence the results of a randomized trial if this factor is not considered in stratification. The effect would be most marked early in the study.

The relationship of histologic tumor grade to local recurrence after breast-conserving therapy with lumpectomy and radiotherapy is uncertain. Increasing tumor grade has been associated with several factors that are related to an increased risk for breast recurrence after conservation therapy, including greater tumor size, diagnosis at a relatively young age, and absence of estrogen receptor expression. Some investigators found a significant relationship between grade and local recurrence (147–149), but others concluded that grade was not significant (150–152). In patients with relatively favorable stage I carcinomas treated by lumpectomy with radiotherapy, it has been observed that tumor grade was a significant factor for time to recurrence, as recurrences occurred sooner and with greater frequency after a median follow-up of 58 months in patients with high-grade carcinomas (153).

### Reproducibility of Grading

The subjective nature of histologic grading has been evaluated in studies of interobserver agreement on the assessment of the components that determine grade and grading itself (132,154,155). In one report, the kappa value for tubule formation was 0.64, indicating a substantial level of interobserver agreement on this variable, with lower levels of agreement for mitotic count (kappa = 0.52) and nuclear pleomorphism (kappa = 0.40) (132). Others reported a range of observer agreement for overall modified Bloom-Richardson grading, with kappa values of 0.73 (136), 0.70 (154), and 0.43 (155), respectively. Technical factors, such as the method of fixation, may have a significant influence on the level of observer agreement, which was higher for tissues fixed with B5 than with buffered formaldehyde in one study (136).

Tsuda et al. (156) investigated the relationship between histologic grade and genetic alterations manifested by LOH in invasive node-negative carcinomas. Alterations were most extensive in grade 3 tumors, and the number of genetic changes proved to be a significant prognostic indicator. After adjustment for grade in a multivariate analysis, alterations in 18q and int were independent prognostic markers.

The clinical importance of histologic grading was aptly summarized by Schumacher et al. (157), who concluded that "tumor grade is able to separate a small subgroup of patients with very good prognosis and a small subgroup of patients with very poor prognosis. The majority remains in an intermediate group. Here other prognostic factors are necessary to split the patients into groups with different prognoses."

### Necrosis

The independent prognostic significance of tumor necrosis has been studied extensively (Fig. 14.8) (85,119,124, 158,159). Controversy exists about the definition and classification of necrosis, with respect to the amount of necrosis that is considered to be significant as well as the relative distribution of necrosis within intraductal and invasive components of the tumor. There is evidence indicating that the prognostic significance of tumor necrosis is time dependent. For example, Gilchrist et al. (88) found that tumor necrosis defined as the "presence of confluent necrosis of any dimension in a section of invasive cancer that could be distinguished at

intermediate magnification" was a significant predictor of time to recurrence and overall survival with 10-year follow-up. However, the effect was manifested only during the first 2 years of follow-up. For patients who remained disease free beyond 10 years, having had necrosis in the primary tumor no longer was a significant prognostic factor.

Extensive necrosis rarely destroys most of the tumor, but this process may be so extreme as to leave few or no apparently viable elements (Fig. 14.1). This situation has been encountered in ordinary invasive duct carcinoma as well as in special tumor types such as papillary carcinoma (see Chapter 16). Visscher et al. (160) studied 28 "centrally necrotizing carcinomas." The tumors typically were circumscribed, unicentric lesions with a mean size of 2.8 cm (±1.3%). Histologic examination revealed central necrosis surrounded by a peripheral zone of poorly differentiated high-grade carcinoma bordered by a "sparse lymphocytic infiltrate and focal ductal carcinoma *in situ.*" Mean patient age was 59.8 ± 11.9 years, and 43% had axillary nodal metastases (mean positive, 1.2 ± 1.9). Among tumors with available tissue, all 10 were aneuploid, and 10 of 11 did not express estrogen receptors. After a median follow-up of nearly 40 months, 16 (67%) of 24 evaluable patients died of breast carcinoma, with a median survival of 19.5 months. These data add further support to the perception that extensive necrosis is a prognostically unfavorable feature in invasive mammary carcinoma, possibly reflecting a growth rate so rapid that it exceeds angiogenesis to a substantial degree.

### Apoptosis

Apoptosis is an important mechanism of cell death. Apoptotic cells are characterized in routine histologic sections by condensation of chromatin and cytoplasm, as well as intracellular and extracellular chromatin fragments as small as 2 μm. An apoptotic index (AI) can be measured by counting the number of apoptotic cells using the same method as for a mitotic index (161). In one study of 288 carcinomas, the AI was significantly related to tumor grade, SPF, mitotic index, and the expression of hormone receptors and p53 (161). High mean AI was associated with poorly differentiated grade, high SPF and mitotic rate, absence of hormone receptor expression, and presence of p53 (162). Increased apoptosis has been associated with comedo intraductal carcinoma and concomitant invasive carcinoma (162). Shen et al. (163) reported that the mean frequency of apoptotic cells determined by the terminal deoxynucleotidyl transferase-mediated dUTP-biotin end labeling (TUNEL) method was greater in intraductal than in invasive carcinomas, whereas intraductal carcinoma had a relatively low proliferative rate, a finding suggesting that apoptosis might contribute to maintaining a steady state in intraductal carcinoma. Conversely, the invasive carcinomas featured a higher proliferative rate manifested by Ki67 immunoreactivity and a lower apoptotic rate. When examined in multivariate analysis, apoptosis was not an independent prognostic factor.

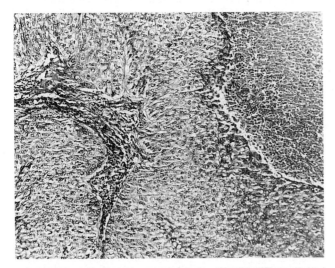

**FIG. 14.8.** *Invasive duct carcinoma.* Poorly differentiated carcinoma with necrosis on the *right.*

### BCL-2

Bcl-2, part of the *bcl*-2 gene family located at chromosome 18q21, was first identified during studies of the t(14:18) chromosome translocation that occurs in B-cell lymphomas. Individual genes in this family have an inhibiting or promoting effect on cell death. One group of genes, including *bcl*-2, *Bcl*-x, and *MCL1*, suppresses programmed cell death (apoptosis), whereas others, such as *Bax* and *Bak*, promote cell death. These antagonistic functions play an important role in mammary epithelial differentiation and possibly in mammary neoplasia (164). The mechanism by which *bcl*-2 contributes to tumorigenesis appears to be through suppression of apoptosis, thereby conferring a survival advantage on *bcl*-2–expressing cells. The prolonged life span of cells with enhanced *bcl*-2 expression may contribute to the greater cellularity of proliferative lesions and increase the risk for these cells to acquire oncogenic genetic changes. p53, which induces apoptosis as well as $G_1$ arrest, down-regulates *bcl*-2 and coincidentally up-regulates *Bax* to promote apoptosis (165,166).

Immunohistochemical studies of bcl-2 in tissue reveal cytoplasmic localization. In normal breast tissue, expression is highest in the hormonally regulated lobular epithelium, being maximal at the midpoint of the menstrual cycle (167). Expression of bcl-2 was reportedly detected in all examples of atypical duct hyperplasia and lobular carcinoma *in situ* studied by Siziopikou et al. (168). In intraductal carcinoma, bcl-2 expression was found to correlate with the grade of the lesion and to be inversely related to the expression of Bax (169). Low-grade intraductal carcinomas featured predominate bcl-2 staining relative to Bax, intermediate grade lesions tended to coexpress both proteins, and high-grade intraductal carcinomas expressed Bax more prominently. Expression of bcl-2 has been detected in 58% (170), 64% (171), 68% (172), 75% (173), and 79% (174,175) of carcinomas studied (Fig. 14.9). By comparison, Alsabeh at al. (174) found expression in only 5.6% and 8.3% of gastric and pulmonary carcinomas, respectively, and staining of these nonmammary tumors was usually not as intense as in breast carcinomas (174). Bcl-2 expression is significantly associated with the presence of estrogen and progesterone receptors (170,172–178). Some investigators reported an inverse relationship between bcl-2 expression and the immunohistochemical detection of EGFR, HER2, and p53 (171, 175–180), whereas others reported no significant association with p53 (173,174,181,182) or with transforming growth factor-α (176).

The relationship of bcl-2 to proliferative activity in breast carcinoma is not clear. Alsabeh et al. (174) reported that bcl-2 expression was significantly more frequent in breast carcinomas with low MIB1 expression (174). Joensuu et al. (183) observed bcl-2 expression significantly more often in tumors with a low mitotic count, low S-phase, and a diploid deoxyribonucleic acid (DNA) content, and Silverstrini et al. (181) found that bcl-2 staining was inversely related to the thymidine index, another marker of proliferative activity.

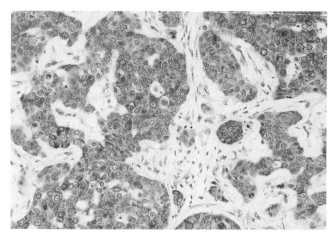

**FIG. 14.9.** *Invasive duct carcinoma*, bcl-*2*. Cytoplasmic immunolocalization in a moderately differentiated carcinoma (avidin-biotin).

Gee et al. (176) found no association between bcl-2 and Ki67 proliferative status. Most investigators found bcl-2 immunoreactivity to be more frequent in low-grade carcinomas (170,172,174,178,179,183,184). Stage at diagnosis and axillary lymph node status were not significantly related to bcl-2 immunoreactivity (172–174,183,184).

The relationship of bcl-2 expression to prognosis and response to therapy in breast carcinoma remains uncertain. The subject was reviewed in 1998 by Zhang et al. (185), who concluded the following: (a) bcl-2 expression is associated with a better response to hormone therapy; and (b) the expression of bcl-2 is a favorable prognostic factor regardless of nodal status. Because bcl-2 blocks apoptosis, lower levels of apoptosis induced by bcl-2 expression would be expected to result in the accumulation of malignant cells in a carcinoma and thereby have an unfavorable effect on outcome. However, Berardo et al. (186) found no association between bcl-2 expression and apoptosis in patients with node-positive carcinoma. High bcl-2 expression was associated with a significantly improved disease-free and overall survival, and in multivariate analysis, bcl-2 expression was associated with a more favorable disease-free survival. Analysis of apoptosis revealed that a greater apoptotic rate was associated with unfavorable features, such as an increased number of positive lymph nodes, p53 expression, estrogen and progesterone receptor negativity, aneuploidy, and higher proliferative rate. Despite these characteristics in tumors with a higher apoptotic rate, these cases did not have a significantly worse prognosis. Gee et al. (176) found that patients with estrogen receptor and bcl-2–positive tumors were particular responsive to endocrine therapies that included antiestrogen. van Slooten et al. (184) found no association between bcl-2 expression and response to perioperative chemotherapy (5-fluorouracil, doxorubicin, and cyclophosphamide) in node-negative patients. Bonetti et al. (187) reported a higher response rate to chemotherapy among tumors classified as bcl-2 positive, with immunostaining in 40% or more of tumor cells.

### Telomerase

Telomerase is a polymerase that adds telomeric DNA to the ends of chromosomes (188). This process prevents the shortening of these chromosome ends during replication. In normal cells, the replicating DNA loses terminal segments (telomeres). With repeated cell divisions, shortened telomere length reaches a critical point that signals cessation of division followed by cell senescence. Increased telomerase activity is associated with telomere repair and may serve as an immortalization marker by inhibiting normal progression to senescence and death.

Telomerase activity has been detected in 79% (189), 82% (190), and 85% (191) of breast carcinoma studies. In one report, there was no association with lymph node status, tumor size, and hormone receptor status (189), but others did not confirm these associations (190). Telomerase has been detected in fibroadenomas (192) and not in normal tissue samples. High telomerase activity was associated with overexpression of cyclin D1 and/or cyclin E by Landberg et al. (191) and with p53 overexpression (193). Tumors with high telomerase activity had a relatively unfavorable prognosis in node-negative but not in node-positive patients studied by Roos et al. (193). However, Carey et al. (190) reported that telomerase activity was not predictive of survival regardless of nodal status.

### Lymphoplasmacytic Infiltrate

The prognostic significance of stromal lymphoplasmacytic infiltration within and around invasive duct carcinomas has been the subject of considerable interest and some controversy (Fig. 14.10). The reaction consists mainly of mature lymphocytes with a variable admixture of plasma cells and macrophages. Rarely, plasma cells or eosinophils predominate. Tumors with plasma cell predominance usually are medullary carcinomas or carcinomas with medullary features. The marked lymphoplasmacytic reaction observed in medullary carcinoma also occurs in a minority of non-medullary invasive duct carcinomas (4,58). A subset of these tumors with some, but not all, of the features of medullary carcinoma, referred to as infiltrating duct carcinoma with medullary features, may have a slightly more favorable prognosis than infiltrating duct carcinomas generally, but the difference is not statistically significant (194). Most nonmedullary duct carcinomas with a prominent lymphocytic reaction tend to be poorly differentiated and have a circumscribed rather than infiltrative contour. Medullary carcinomas and invasive duct carcinomas with a marked lymphocytic reaction almost always are estrogen and progesterone receptor negative.

Whereas the favorable prognosis of medullary carcinoma has been ascribed to the lymphoplasmacytic reaction that characterized these tumors, it is less clear that the same conclusion can be drawn about nonmedullary invasive duct carcinomas. Some investigators found carcinomas with a "host response" to have a relatively favorable prognosis (89,121,195,196), but others found no significant difference or reported a less favorable outcome associated with the presence of a prominent lymphoplasmacytic infiltrate (107,143,159). Subset analysis in one study suggested that the influence of a lymphoplasmacytic reaction on prognosis was related to nodal status, tumor grade, and overexpression of the HER2/neu oncogene (197).

Studies of the lymphocyte subgroups infiltrating mammary carcinomas indicate that they are largely T lymphocytes (198–200) consisting mainly of T4 (CD4$^+$ helper) and T8 (CD8$^+$ cytotoxic suppressor) cells (199,200). Macrophages may be relatively more abundant than T lymphocytes in poorly differentiated carcinomas and in carcinomas that are HER2/neu positive (197). However, using direct immunofluorescence of frozen sections, Bilik et al. (198) found that the T4:T8 ratio exceeded 1.0 in only 34% of tumors, indicating that T8 cells were more numerous in the majority of carcinomas. Whitford et al. (201) also reported a predominance of T8 cells when lymphocytes were isolated from breast carcinomas and analyzed by flow cytometry. Ordinarily, few B cells are found in benign or in carcinomatous

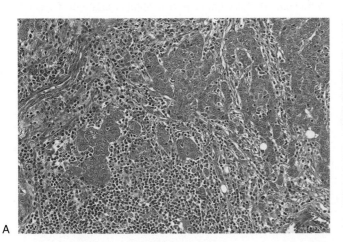
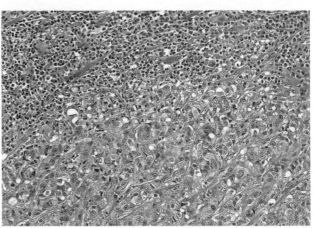

**FIG. 14.10.** *Invasive duct carcinoma.* **A:** Lymphoplasmacytic infiltrate fills the stroma of invasive poorly differentiated duct carcinoma. **B:** Invasive duct carcinoma with stromal eosinophils.

breast tissue, but the proportion of B cells tends to be relatively increased in carcinomas (202). By applying a variety of procedures, including *in situ* hybridization in a small series of cases, Parkes et al. (203) demonstrated that the presence of plasma cells that expressed high levels of immunoglobulin kappa-chain mRNA was associated with a poor prognosis.

The intensity of mast cell infiltration in the substance or at the periphery of an invasive breast carcinoma is not significantly related to prognosis (204).

### Lymphatic Tumor Emboli

The presence of *lymphatic tumor emboli* in the breast is an unfavorable prognostic finding. For this purpose, lymphatics are defined as vascular channels lined by endothelium without supporting smooth muscle or elastica (Fig. 14.11). Most lymphatics do not contain red blood cells, but undoubtedly some blood capillaries are included in this definition. Artifactual spaces are sometimes formed around nests of tumor cells within an invasive carcinoma as a result of tissue shrinkage during processing so-called *shrinkage artifact* (Fig. 14.12). Because it is very difficult to distinguish these artifacts from true lymphatic spaces, assessment for lymphatic invasion is more reliably accomplished in breast parenchyma adjacent to, or well beyond, the invasive tumor

margin (205,206). Efforts to identify intratumoral lymphatic spaces by using immunoperoxidase reagents associated with endothelial cells (factor VIII, CD34 or CD31, and blood group antigens) have met with limited success (207–209). Strong staining of tumor cells in artifactual spaces can be associated with diffusion of reactivity into the surrounding stroma, and the resultant staining may be most intense at the margin of the space (208,210). CD34 and CD31 are immunoreactive with myofibroblasts and will outline the artifactual nonvascular spaces in pseudoangiomatous stromal hyperplasia. Factor VIII antigen has not been consistently demonstrable in all endothelium-lined capillary or lymphatic channels. False-negative immunohistochemical results usually can be recognized in extratumoral breast tissue, but the fact that they occur means these reagents are not reliable for detecting lymphatic emboli within a tumor (207). The prognostic significance of intratumoral lymphatic emboli has not been determined.

Extratumoral lymphatic tumor emboli in the breast are found associated with approximately 15% of invasive duct carcinomas. Lymphatic tumor emboli were found in the breast surrounding invasive duct carcinomas in 5% to 10% of patients who have pathologically negative lymph nodes. Several studies showed that lymphatic emboli were prognostically unfavorable in node-negative patients treated by mastectomy (107,159,206,211–215) and by breast conserva-

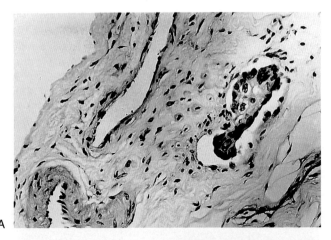

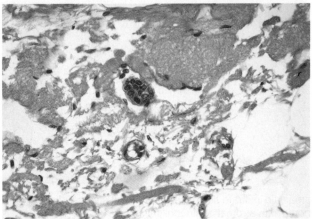

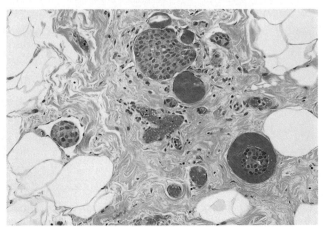

**FIG. 14.11.** *Invasive duct carcinoma, lymphatic invasion.* **A:** Intralymphatic carcinoma shown next to a small artery and vein. The space around the clump of tumor cells is lined by endothelium. **B:** Carcinoma in a lymphatic channel. **C:** Carcinoma in a lymphatic channel *(left)* and in a dilated capillary *(right).*

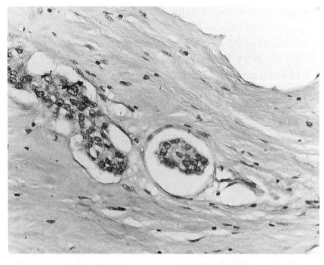

A

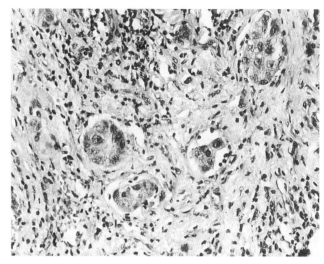

B

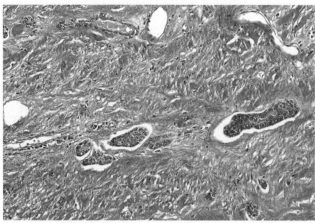

C

**FIG. 14.12.** *Invasive duct carcinoma, shrinkage artifact.* **A:** Shrinkage artifact resembling lymphatic invasion. The groups of carcinoma cells are partly attached to the stroma, and there is no endothelium. **B:** Groups of carcinoma cells resembling lymphatic tumor emboli in an invasive carcinoma. Such foci are interpreted as shrinkage artifact. **C:** Invasive carcinoma in stroma with shrinkage artifact. The shape of the carcinoma corresponds closely to the space in which it lies.

tion therapy (216). The deleterious effect was most pronounced in women with T1N0M0 disease. In a 10-year follow-up study of 378 patients treated for T1N0M0 carcinoma, 33% of 30 women with lymphatic emboli died of disease. Death due to breast carcinoma was observed in 10% of the 348 women who did not have lymphatic emboli (107). Another study comparing similar subsets of T1N0M0 patients found recurrences in 32% of those with lymphatic emboli and in 10% of controls (159). In stage I patients with tumors larger than 2 cm (T2N0M0), those with lymphatic emboli also experienced a higher recurrence rate (206,208,215). Recurrences that developed in node-negative patients who had peritumoral lymphatic emboli tended to occur more than 5 years after diagnosis, and they were almost always systemic. Lymphatic tumor emboli did not predispose to local recurrence in patients treated by mastectomy, but they were associated with an increased risk for recurrence in the breast after breast conservation therapy (216). Liljegren et al. (217) reported that the relative risk for recurrence in the breast after conservation therapy was 1.9 (95% CI = 1.1 to 3.5) comparing women with and without peritumoral lymphatic tumor emboli.

The unfavorable effect of lymphatic emboli in lymph node-negative patients probably is not due to occult metas-

tases in their axillary lymph nodes. Serial sections of lymph nodes detected metastases in nine of 28 patients originally classified as T1N0M0 with lymphatic tumor emboli in the breast. The recurrence rate was not higher among those with occult metastases than in the subset with truly negative lymph nodes (218).

The significance of lymphatic tumor emboli for prognosis in patients already proven to have lymph node metastases is uncertain. Among T1N1M0 patients treated by mastectomy prior to the era of adjuvant chemotherapy, lymphatic tumor emboli did not significantly influence disease-free survival at 10-year follow-up (108). One group of investigators found that lymphatic invasion did not have an independent effect on disease-free survival at 10 years in patients who received adjuvant chemotherapy (219). Others reported significantly lower overall and disease-free survival in stage II patients with "peritumoral vessel invasion" in an adjuvant therapy trial (220). Analysis of 863 consecutive node-positive patients who received adjuvant therapy at the University of Naples revealed that the presence of lymphatic tumor emboli was a significant, prognostically unfavorable factor in this setting (215). This effect was independent of the number of lymph nodes with metastases, tumor size, or tumor grade.

### Blood Vessel Invasion

Blood vessel invasion is defined as penetration by tumor cells into the lumen of an artery or vein (Fig. 14.13). These vascular structures can be identified by the presence of a smooth muscle wall supported by elastic fibers. It usually is necessary to use special histochemical procedures (e.g., orcein or Verhoeff-van Gieson stains) that selectively stain elastic tissue in order to detect this component of the vascular wall. Elastic fibers often are deposited around ducts that contain intraductal carcinoma within an invasive tumor, and the resulting appearance in an elastic tissue stain may be difficult to distinguish from vascular invasion. An immunostain for actin is useful for defining the smooth muscle structure of blood vessels. Because larger vascular components in the breast usually consist of a paired artery and vein, vascular invasion can be diagnosed with confidence when tumor is detected within one or both of a pair of vessels, as demonstrated by the elastic tissue and actin stains.

The reported frequency of blood vessel invasion varies from about 5% to nearly 50% (107,108,159,221–223). These widely divergent observations reflect major differences in these studies with respect to the number of patients evaluated, clinical and pathologic characteristics of the study population, and the methods by which blood vessel invasion was identified. Some investigators reported that blood vessel invasion denoted a poorer prognosis in node-positive patients with two or more positive lymph nodes (223). Others concluded that this finding was prognostically significant only in the absence of axillary lymph node metastasis (221).

Thorough assessment of blood vessel invasion was provided by 10-year follow-up data for 524 women treated consecutively for invasive carcinomas 2 cm or less in diameter (T1) by modified or standard radical mastectomy (107,108).

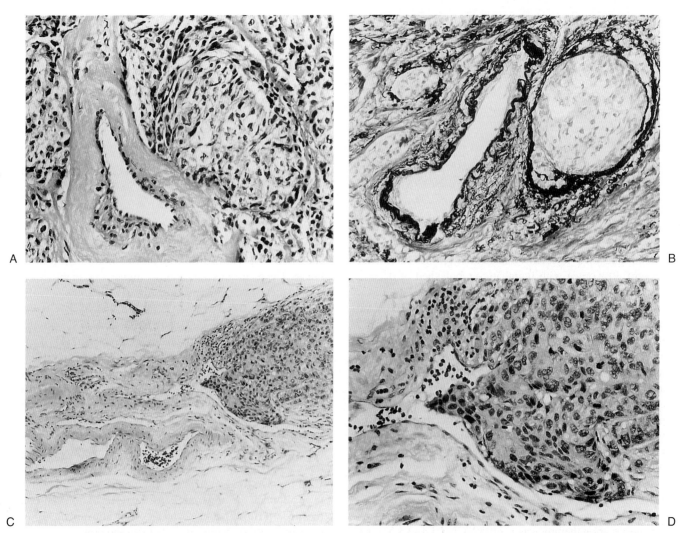

**FIG. 14.13.** *Invasive duct carcinoma, blood vessel invasion.* **A:** Oval mass of carcinoma in a vein on the *right* is next to a thick-walled artery. **B:** Adjacent section stained to highlight elastic tissue in the same focus demonstrating the presence of carcinoma in the vein and an elastic lamina in the artery (van Gieson elastic stain). **C:** On the *right*, carcinoma is present in the lumen of a vein cut longitudinally. **D:** Magnified view of carcinoma in the vein.

It was possible to evaluate 502 tumors for blood vessel invasion using one section per case stained to demonstrate elastic tissue. Blood vessel invasion was identified in 47 (13%) of 362 T1N0M0 cases. Recurrence of breast carcinoma was more frequent when blood vessel invasion was present (12/47 [26%]) than in its absence (50/315 [16%]), and death due to disease also occurred more often among women with blood vessel invasion (present: 9/47 [19%]; absent: 38/315 [12%]). However, these differences in recurrence and death rates were not statistically significant. Visceral metastases occurred in 67% of patients with blood vessel invasion and in 35% when it was not present. Bone recurrences were more frequent in the absence of demonstrable blood vessel invasion. Others also observed a similar trend toward a higher recurrence rate associated with blood vessel invasion in T1N0M0 patients (159).

Blood vessel invasion was found in 23 (16%) of 117 stage II T1 tumors (T1N1M0) (108). Deaths due to metastatic breast carcinoma occurred with significantly greater frequency among women with blood vessel invasion ($p < 0.03$), whether they had a single positive lymph node or two or more affected nodes.

The distinction between lymphatic tumor emboli and blood vessel invasion is not always clear-cut. Small capillaries lack a distinct smooth muscle wall or elastica, and red blood cells may be present in the lumens of lymphatic spaces. Markers of endothelial cells, such as factor VIII, have limited value because staining is absent in some true blood vessels (210). For these reasons, some investigators have referred to all carcinoma in endothelial-lined channels as *vascular invasion,* making no distinction between lymphatic and blood vessel invasion. Using this definition, Pinder et al. (224) identified vascular invasion in 22.8% of 1,704 consecutive invasive T1 and T2 breast carcinomas. Another 17.4% of the tumors were described as having probable vascular invasion because of the presence of tumor "in a space with the appearances of a vessel but without a clear endothelial layer." The presence of vascular invasion was significantly associated with larger tumors, poorly differentiated carcinoma, presence of axillary lymph node metastases, and invasive ductal carcinoma. Multivariate analysis revealed that tumor size, nodal status, histologic grade, histologic tumor type, and vascular invasion were significantly associated with survival. Vascular invasion was a significant predictor of local recurrence in patients treated by mastectomy or by wide local excision. Among lymph node–negative patients, vascular invasion was not a significant independent prognostic factor in multivariate analysis. In an overall analysis of all patients regardless of stage, those with probable vascular invasion had a significantly higher frequency of local recurrence and a lower survival rate.

Vascular invasion has been associated with increased expression of E-cadherin in the intravascular carcinoma in the breast and other sites when compared to the extravascular invasive component (225). This difference between parenchymal and intravascular invasive carcinoma suggests that the biologic properties of the cells may change after entry into the circulatory system. Up-regulation of E-cadherin expression in intravascular carcinoma could reflect the absence of inhibitory factors that might be present in the stroma, a stimulatory effect of the intravascular milieu, or the association of E-cadherin expression with other factors involved in vascular invasion. If confirmed in additional studies, enhanced expression of E-cadherin might prove to be a useful marker for identifying vascular invasion.

### Angiogenesis

The angiogenesis associated with breast carcinomas has attracted interest as a prognostic indicator. The capacity of neoplastic (226) and preneoplastic (227,228) tissues to induce vascular proliferation is well documented. Conversion from *in situ* carcinoma, a stage not dependent on neovascularization, to an enlarging invasive carcinoma is associated with conversion to the angiogenic phenotype. Early expansion of the invasive lesion in the prevascular stage is guided by a balance between the growth rate and apoptosis, a phenomenon observed in experimental studies at sites of primary tumors and micrometastases (229).

Acquisition of the angiogenic phenotype is attributed to the overexpression of angiogenic factors, such as vascular endothelial growth factor (VEGF), also termed vascular permeability factor (VPF) and basic fibroblast growth factor (bFGF). When studied *in vitro,* VEGF and bFGF have a synergistic effect on angiogenesis (230).

Several sources of angiogenic factors have been identified. *In vitro* studies showed that mammary stromal fibroblasts produce VEGF and that expression of this protein is up-regulated by exposure of the cells to hypoxic conditions (231). Angiogenic proteins can be present in the stroma and are produced by inflammatory cells such as macrophages. A significant correlation between stromal cell cathepsin D reactivity and stromal vascular (232) density has been observed, suggesting that up-regulation of matrix proteinases might facilitate invasion and angiogenesis (232).

VEGF has been detected in the cytoplasm of human breast carcinoma cells by immunohistochemistry (233). Anan et al. (234) demonstrated that VEGF mRNA expression determined by the reverse transcriptase-polymerase chain reaction and Southern blotting on samples obtained by fine needle aspiration correlated significantly with neovascularization in invasive ductal carcinomas stained with anti-CD31 antibody (234). There was a high degree of correlation between VEGF mRNA in the fine needle aspiration and excision specimens ($r = 0.874$). Expression of VEGF protein and mRNA was higher in invasive ductal than in invasive lobular carcinomas studied by Lee et al. (235), although MVD did not differ significantly between the tumor types. Expression of VEGF protein and mRNA correlated significantly with MVD in invasive ductal and not in invasive lobular carcinomas, an observation suggesting that other angiogenic factors might play a greater role in invasive lobular carcinoma. The concentration of VEGF in human breast carcinomas measured by immunoassay has been found to correlate with tumoral MVD determined by immunohistochemistry in the same lesions (233). Concentrations of VEGF were not significantly related to measured levels of bFGF. The angiogenic phenotype also is promoted by down-regulation of inhibitors of angiogenesis, such as thrombospondin (236,237) and angiostatin (238). The tumor suppressor gene p53 may play a role in controlling the expression of thrombospondin (237).

Tumor growth is enhanced not only by increased perfusion associated with neovascularization, but also by the paracrine mitogenic effects of growth factors, such as insulin-like growth factor-1 and platelet-derived growth factor produced by endothelial cells (239). Expression of receptors for VPF (VEGF) has been detected in endothelial cells in small blood vessels adjacent to some types of breast carcinoma in which tumor cells were found to express VPF mRNA (240). Inhibition of tumor growth has been achieved experimentally with antibodies to VEGF (241) and to bFGF (242). The angiogenic phenotype usually is expressed by a subset of cells in a carcinoma. Acquisition of this phenotype may be an important hallmark in the evolution of a carcinoma (Fig. 14.14).

Pathologic studies of angiogenesis in breast carcinoma have examined the relevance of tumor vascularity to known prognostic markers and to prognosis. To perform such studies, histologic sections of paraffin-embedded tissue are stained with immunohistochemical markers for endothelial cells such as factor VIII (antihuman von Willebrand factor [anti-VWF]), CD34, and CD31 (243). Comparative studies using these markers of vascular differentiation have not yielded consistent results for determining the optimal method by which angiogenesis should be measured in breast carcinoma. Data from one study indicated that CD31 was the most sensitive reagent and that it gave the highest vessel counts (243). However, others reported that "anti-CD34 and anti-VWF showed better staining performance than anti-CD31, although the staining results with different antibodies were comparable" (244).

Using manual methods, vessel counts are recorded in foci of greatest vascular density, so-called *hotspots*, by counting the number of immunostained structures in a predetermined number of fields at a fixed magnification (Fig. 14.15) (245,246). A significant problem in the method of assessment based on detecting hotspots is the heterogeneity of vascularity with breast carcinomas. Martin et al. (247) studied vascular heterogeneity in breast carcinomas by performing angiograms and comparing the radiographic results with MVD counts in histologic sections of the same tumors. The specimen angiograms revealed two basic patterns of vascularity: (i) an anastomosing pattern exhibiting numerous interconnecting branches, and (ii) a radiating pattern with relatively few anastomoses. Vascular density in the specimen x-ray images was found to correlate with the histologic assessment of vascularity using CD34 immunostaining. However, vessel counts on three sections from each tumor varied by more than 20% in 30% of the cases. Analysis of MVD in three tumor zones (central, intermediate, and peripheral) carried out on 147 invasive duct carcinomas revealed significantly greater vascularity at the periphery (248). The average microvessel counts per 200× field were 34.4, 39.4, and 51.5 in the central, intermediate, and peripheral zones, respectively. A study of angiogenesis in multiple blocks from individual carcinomas revealed an average coefficient of variation (CV) of 11.1% for vessel counts in hotspots in different sections from a single paraffin block and a CV of 24.4% when hotspots in sections from different blocks from the same tumor were compared (249). The authors concluded that "one must carefully scan all the available tumor material in each case for the best spot." Counts based on limited samples, such as needle core biopsies or one section of a tumor, may be highly misleading.

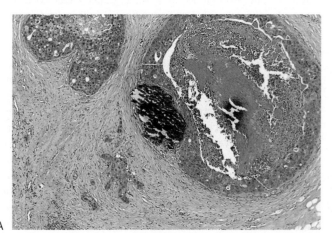 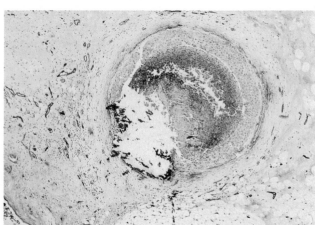

A    B

FIG. 14.14. *Angiogenesis, microinvasive duct carcinoma.* **A:** Intraductal carcinoma, comedo type with calcification. Microinvasive duct carcinoma is present *(lower left)*. **B:** Parallel section of the intraductal carcinoma in **A** with the CD34 immunostain shows greater vascularity in the region of the microinvasive carcinoma *(lower left)* than in the remaining perimeter of the duct (avidin-biotin).

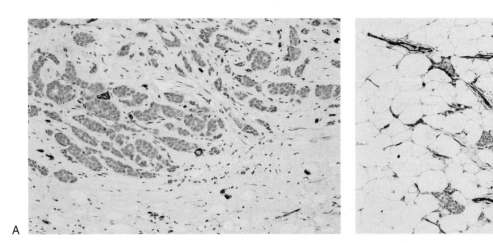

**FIG. 14.15.** *Angiogenesis, invasive duct carcinoma.* **A:** Sparse angiogenesis present at the border of this invasive duct carcinoma. **B:** Conspicuous angiogenesis at the border of an invasive duct carcinoma (both anti-CD34, avidin-biotin).

Numerical microvessel counts have been analyzed by comparing cases above and below the mean number in a given study, or by comparing cases with fewer than or more than a mean of microvessels per standardized field (200× or 400×) (244,246,250–254). Recommended methods for reporting vessel counts include Chalkley counting and MVD determined in one hotspot, as the mean of three hotspots or as the highest count in one of three hotspots. In one study, analysis of microvessel count as a continuous numerical value revealed that more than 80 microvessels provided "the optimal cut-off value for stratifying patients into relatively good and poor prognosis groups." Subjective grading of MVD on a scale from 1 to 4 also has been used (246). Image analysis has been used to determine the endothelial area or the surface area that is immunoreactive for a vascular marker (250,255,256). One study compared two methods of manual counting to image analysis of endothelial area (250). One manual procedure involved counting vessels on the monitor of an image analysis instrument. The other manual method used counts of vessels in photomicrographs.

High MVD has been shown in some studies to be associated with a poor grade of histologic differentiation in invasive duct carcinomas (232,243,245,257–260) and with a greater probability of axillary nodal metastases (243, 246,257,261,262). Some authors found high microvessel counts to be associated with greater tumor size (243,257, 260,263), HER2/*neu* expression (261), estrogen receptor-negative status (232,244,253), cathepsin D expression by the carcinoma (232,255), and age at diagnosis less than 50 years (264). Others reported no significant relationship between vessel counts and primary tumor grade (244,251–253, 255,264,265), size (232,244,245,251–253, 255,258,261, 265,266), lymph node status (232,253,255, 264,265), expression of p53 (243,251,252,255,259,260) or HER2/*neu* (243,244,251,255,259,260), or estrogen receptor status (251,252,260,261).

Angiogenesis has been reported to be an independent prognostic indicator by some investigators. High microves-

sel counts have been associated with a poor prognosis in node-negative (245,250,253,254,257,263,266) and in node-positive (250,253,257,266) breast carcinoma. Angiogenesis determined by Chalkley counts proved to be a prognostically significant factor in an adjuvant therapy trial of tamoxifen administrated to node-positive patients (262). However, others failed to detect a significant relationship to prognosis (244,251,252,256,258,267) or to recurrence in the breast after wide excision and breast conservation (268).

Substantial methodologic variability may be an important factor in the failure of published studies to detect a consistent relationship between angiogenesis and prognostic factors or prognosis. These technical differences include the use of different markers to highlight vessels (CD31, CD34, factor VIII), different methods for counting (manual, image analysis), different quantitation methods (average microvessel count per square millimeter vs. highest microvessel count per square millimeter), and variability in microvessel distribution in different parts of a tumor. Hansen et al. (269) examined observer variability using four different methods of vessel counting in tissue sections stained with anti-CD34. The counting methods were Chalkley counting, MVD estimated in one hotspot, mean MVD in three hotspots, and highest MVD in one of three hotspots. The CV values for intraobserver variability were approximately 20% for each method (14% to 23%). A lower coefficient of interobserver variation was achieved with the Chalkley method (8% to 9%) than with the microvessel methods (30%). Presently, the immunohistochemical assessment of angiogenesis in tissue sections requires further standardization before it is accepted as a independent prognostic variable.

Efforts to assess tumor vascularity using magnetic resonance imaging (MRI) with gadolinium enhancement have not yielded consistent results. Buadu et al. (270) reported that the pattern and rate of contrast uptake observed in MRI studies of the breast were directly correlated with the distribution of angiogenesis in the tumors. Two studies reported an association between MRI enhancement and MVD

(271,272). However, there was considerable variability in the measurements and it was concluded that "MRI cannot be used to predict MVD in vivo" (271) and that "gadolinium enhancement of breast lesions is not an accurate predictor of vessel density" (271). It was reported more recently that a modified dynamic MRI technique with high resolution revealed an association between early signal enhancement with rapid washout of contrast and high tumor vascularity (273).

A different application of contrast-enhanced MRI to the study of breast carcinoma vascularity was described by Siewert et al. (274). In this study of 18 breast carcinomas, contrast-enhanced MRI was used to enumerate the number of major vessels associated with the tumor by three-dimensional analysis. The mean number of vessels ($3 \pm 2.1$; range, 1 to 10) was found to be significantly related to tumor size, with larger tumors having more vessels. Microscopic vessel counts were not reported.

VEGF and other angiogenesis-related proteins in invasive carcinomas have been evaluated as independent prognostic markers. Linderholm et al. (275) determined cytosolic levels of VEGF in tumors from 525 consecutive node-negative patients. VEGF level was inversely related to estrogen receptor and directly correlated with tumor size and grade. Patients with VEGF levels higher than the median had a significantly poorer prognosis after a median follow-up of 46 months, and higher VEGF levels when analyzed as a continuous variable also were prognostically less favorable. Among patients with estrogen receptor-positive tumors, survival was significantly reduced among those with VEGF expression higher than the median level. A similar association of VEGF and prognosis was reported by Eppenberger et al. (276), who studied 305 patients with a median follow-up of 37 months. Other angiogenesis factors (angiogenin and bFGF), the plasminogen activator inhibitor-1, and the tumor proteolysis factor urokinase-type plasminogen activator (uPA) also were studied. By multivariate Cox regression analysis, VEGF and uPA were significantly associated with relapse-free survival in node-negative patients. The most favorable relapse-free survival was observed in women with tumors classified as VEGF($-$)/uPA($-$), with intermediate and relatively poor relapse-free survival in the groups classified as VEGF($+$)/uPA($-$) and VEGF($+$)/uPA($+$), respectively.

The angiogenic capacity of neoplasms is a potential basis for cancer treatment through the use of chemotherapeutic and antiangiogenic agents. Current data indicate that response to conventional forms of chemotherapy is not correlated significantly with tumor angiogenesis. Consequently, tumors with marked angiogenesis do not appear to be more sensitive in the adjuvant setting than tumors with low levels of neovascularization (260,277). Paulsen et al. (278) reported that MVD was not associated with responsiveness to doxorubicin therapy in patients with locally advanced carcinoma. Experimental evidence suggests that antiangiogenic therapy may potentiate chemotherapy as well as inhibit neovascularization of the tumor bed (279). In an experimental animal model, microtubule inhibitors such as paclitaxel (Taxol) and 2-methoxy-estradiol are able to inhibit neovascularization induced by VEGF and bFGF (280). Growth of tumor cells and neovascularity were decreased by the administration of 2-methoxy-estradiol in this system. Antiangiogenic agents presently under investigation, such as angiostatin, exert their effect by inhibiting endothelial cell proliferation. This is a relatively slow process that requires prolonged administration. Initial observations did not detect drug resistance in animal studies (281).

### Perineural Invasion

Carcinomas arising in various organs exhibit a capacity and, in some instances, a proclivity to invade around and into nerves—so-called *perineural invasion* (Fig. 14.16). This phenomenon is not frequently observed among invasive mammary carcinomas, perhaps in part because nerves of notable size are not numerous in mammary tissues. Perineural invasion can be found in approximately 10% of invasive carcinomas. It tends to occur in high-grade tumors, frequently associated with lymphatic tumor emboli, but it has not been proven to have independent prognostic significance.

### Stromal Characteristics

Tumors vary considerably with respect to the quantity and qualitative characteristics of their stroma. Extremes are represented by medullary carcinoma that contains virtually no fibrous stroma and scirrhous carcinoma characterized by marked collagenization. It is not clear that the character of stroma in an invasive duct carcinoma is an independent prognostic variable, because there are clear associations between this and other prognostically significant structural features of breast carcinomas. For example, tumors that contain minimal stromal reaction tend to have the following characteristics: circumscription, poorly differentiated nuclear and histologic grade, and prominent lymphoplasmacytic reaction. They also tend to be estrogen receptor negative. On the other hand, densely fibrotic or scirrhous carcinomas are more likely to be stellate, to be moderately differentiated, and to have little lymphoplasmacytic reaction. A greater proportion of these lesions are estrogen receptor positive. The pattern of growth of an invasive carcinoma can be determined by the architecture of the stroma, especially when there is pseudoangiomatous stromal hyperplasia (Fig. 14.17).

Attempts to assess the character or composition of stroma in invasive duct carcinomas have focused on the amount of elastic tissue present. Stromal elastic fibers can be detected by the same stains used to demonstrate the elastic components in blood vessels (orcein or Verhoeff-van Gieson stains) and by immunohistochemistry using antibodies to components of elastin (282). Although elastic tissue is minimally present in normal mammary stroma, increased amounts can be deposited around ducts with benign proliferative breast

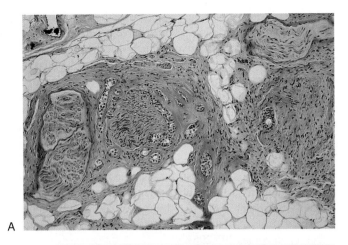

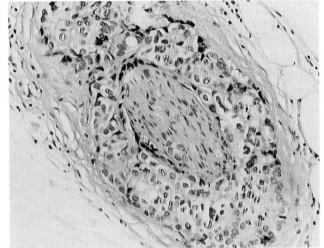

**FIG. 14.16.** *Invasive duct carcinoma, perineural invasion.* **A:** Carcinoma cells present in the fibrofatty stroma and in a thin band around the nerve. **B:** Carcinoma forming a thick collar around a nerve. **C:** Carcinoma present around and within the nerve.

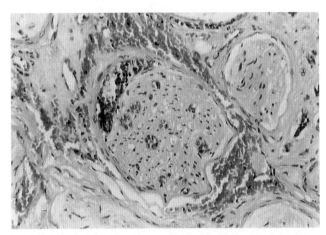

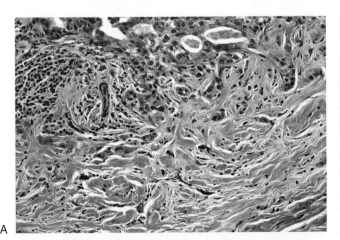

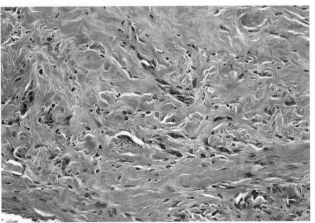

**FIG. 14.17.** *Invasive duct carcinoma in pseudoangiomatous stromal hyperplasia.* **A:** Moderately differentiated carcinoma on the *left* invades stroma that has pseudoangiomatous features. **B:** Part of the tumor where invasive duct carcinoma in pseudoangiomatous stroma resembles invasive lobular carcinoma.

changes (283,284). A similar phenomenon occurs around intraductal carcinoma, particularly when it is present in the invasive portion of the tumor, and to varying degrees in the stroma of invasive carcinoma (Fig. 14.18).

The cellular source of elastin is uncertain. *In vitro* cultured breast carcinoma cells secrete relatively little elastin when compared with fibroblasts (285,286). At the ultrastructural level, elastin fibrils have been found associated with myofibroblasts (287). Elastosis can develop in benign proliferative lesions, so it is not a specific product of carcinoma cells. It is likely that epithelial cells secrete a factor or factors that induce the production of elastin by stromal cells, thereby contributing to the development of elastosis. The observation that elastotic fibers associated with breast carcinoma bind lectins more strongly than the elastica of blood vessels indicates that they are newly formed and immature (288). Plasma protease inhibitors, including $\alpha_1$-antitrypsin, $\alpha_1$-antichymotrypsin, and C1 esterase inhibitor, have been detected in elastic tissue associated with carcinoma (288). These substances contribute to the accumulation of immature elastic fibers by inhibiting elastinolytic enzymes.

In the absence of a widely accepted method for describing elastosis, various grading schemes have been adopted in an effort to convey quantitative estimates of the extent of this process. The frequency of the most extreme or marked degrees of elastosis described in recent reports varied from 17% to 23%, whereas 12% to 55% of tumors in the same studies were characterized by little or no elastosis (289,290).

Abundant elastosis is significantly associated with estrogen receptor positivity (289–291). The importance of elastosis as an independent prognostic variable remains controversial. Although marked elastosis has been described by some investigators as a favorable prognostic feature (292,293), others found that elastosis did not correlate with prognosis (288,289,294), or that abundant elastosis had a negative effect on outcome (295,296).

Myofibroblastic proliferation occurs to a variable extent in invasive duct carcinomas. This stromal component is demonstrated with an actin immunostain (Fig. 14.19). Reactivity in myofibroblasts can be a confounding factor when assessing a lesion for possible microinvasion. Immunostains for calponin or smooth muscle myosin heavy chain exhibit

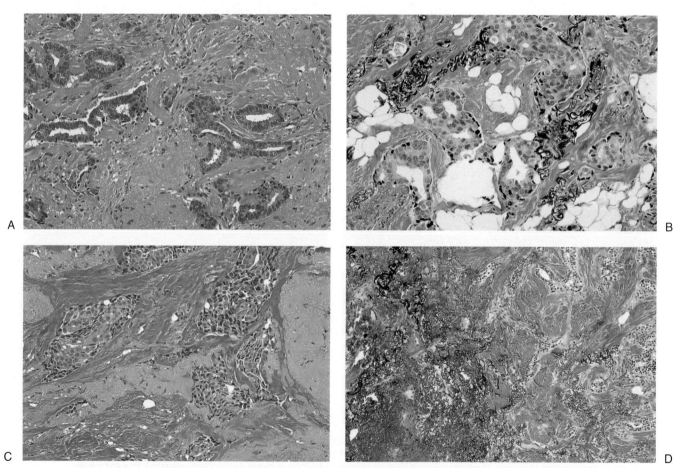

**FIG. 14.18.** *Invasive duct carcinoma, elastosis.* **A:** Fibrillar elastosis blends with collagen fibers in this well-differentiated invasive duct carcinoma. **B:** Coarse elastic fibers stained black are demonstrated in the collagen among the invasive carcinoma glands (elastin van Gieson stain). **C:** Amorphous elastosis deposited in a band-like distribution in collagenous stroma. **D:** Amorphous elastosis is shown highlighted with elastin van Gieson stain. **A** and **B** are from the same case; **C** and **D** are from another case.

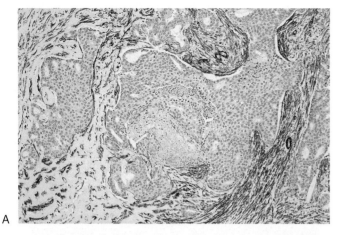

A

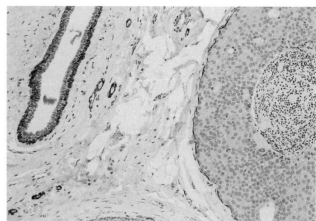

B

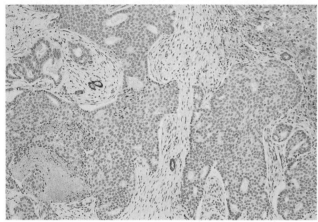

C

**FIG. 14.19.** *Invasive duct carcinoma, myofibroblastic reaction.* All images are from the same tumor. **A:** Immunostain for smooth muscle actin reveals myofibroblastic proliferation in the stroma of an invasive duct carcinoma. **B:** Immunostain for smooth muscle myosin heavy chain is reactive in capillaries, myoepithelial cells in a normal duct *(left),* and intraductal carcinoma *(right).* **C:** No myoepithelial cells are present in the invasive duct carcinoma, and myofibroblasts are not immunoreactive with the smooth muscle myosin heavy-chain antibody (all avidin-biotin).

reactivity in myoepithelial cells, and they are weakly positive or nonreactive in myofibroblasts.

### Extent of Intraductal Carcinoma and Atypia

Attention has been directed to the pattern and distribution of intraductal carcinoma as a prognostic variable in patients with invasive duct carcinoma. Tumors vary in the relative proportions of intraductal and invasive components, from lesions with only microscopic invasion that is not grossly measurable (Fig. 14.20) to lesions composed entirely of invasive carcinoma. Silverberg and Chitale (116) observed a trend to decreased nodal metastases and a more favorable prognosis when the intraductal component in the tumor was relatively more abundant. This is not unexpected, because the size of the invasive component tends to decrease as the proportion of intraductal carcinoma increases. In another report, little or no intraductal carcinoma was detected in sections from 72% of 974 tumors, and 11% were described as composed of at least 66% intraductal carcinoma (3). These authors noted that lesions with a prominent intratumoral intraductal component also tended to have intraductal carcinoma outside the main tumor and to have multicentric foci of carcinoma in other quadrants of the breast.

Although the distribution of intraductal carcinoma in and around the primary tumor appears to correlate with the risk

for recurrence in the breast after lumpectomy and radiation therapy (297), this feature has no bearing on the risk for systemic recurrence in women treated by mastectomy (298,299). Recurrence occurs more often in the breast after lumpectomy and radiation therapy in women who have comedo intraductal carcinoma or when there is extensive intraductal carcinoma defined as intraductal carcinoma within and around an invasive tumor that comprises at least 25% of the neoplasm. The increased risk for local recurrence attributable to an extensive intraductal component probably is a manifestation of a greater probability of there being carcinoma at the margin of excision and remaining in the breast. In patients with negative margins, the presence of extensive intraductal carcinoma does not increase the risk for local recurrence in the breast after breast conservation therapy (300,301).

Carcinomas with an extensive intraductal component frequently have microcalcifications, which help in determining the extent of the lesion on mammography. Lesions with calcifications that extend beyond 3 cm were significantly more likely to have an extensive intraductal component than those with calcifications of lesser extent (90% vs. 54%) (302). In most cases, the mammographic pattern was indicative of a segmental distribution resulting from continuous intraductal spread. This conclusion was supported by a study of the X-chromosome–linked phosphoglycerokinase gene, which

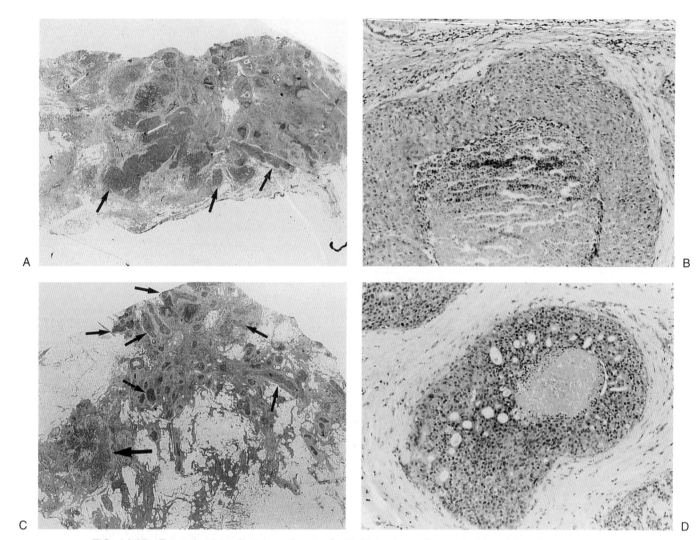

**FIG. 14.20.** *Extensive intraductal carcinoma.* **A:** Multiple ducts *(arrows)* with solid and comedo intraductal carcinoma radiating from invasive duct carcinoma. **B:** Intraductal carcinoma comedo type in **A**. **C:** Intraductal carcinoma *(small arrows)* occupies the large stellate area above an oval focus of invasive duct carcinoma on the *lower left (large arrow)*. **D:** Intraductal carcinoma, cribriform type with necrosis in **C**.

found a monoclonal pattern of gene expression when multiple areas of intraductal carcinoma from three cases were analyzed (303).

The pattern of ductal involvement around invasive duct carcinomas has been studied by three-dimensional reconstruction using computer graphics (304). Intraductal carcinoma usually was found extending in a continuous fashion from the invasive tumor into the duct-lobular system. The direction of involvement was more prominently central than peripheral. Although extension tended to be limited to one ductal system, spread to adjacent duct segments did occur through anastomosing ductal branches.

Jing et al. (305) studied the biologic characteristics of invasive carcinomas with extensive intraductal carcinoma. The intraductal component generally had the same pattern of expression for c-*erb*B-2 (HER2/*neu*) and p53 as the invasive tumor. Overexpression of c-*erb*B-2 was more frequent in

cases with extensive intraductal carcinoma, and these tumors had significantly more frequent lymphatic tumor emboli or venous invasion and the subareolar margin was more frequently involved.

The presence of atypical hyperplasia in the breast around an invasive carcinoma was not associated with an increased risk for tumor recurrence in the breast after conservative surgery with radiation, and it did not correlate significantly with 5- and 10-year survival rates (306).

### Other Histologic Variables

An array of other histologic variables has been assessed as potential prognostic indicators. Among these are the amount and type of mucin produced by the tumor cells, mucopolysaccharide content of tumor stroma, glycogen content of tumor cells, presence of calcifications in the tumor, and influence of associated benign or atypical proliferative changes in the breast (306). For the most part, none of these has been found to correlate strongly with overall prognosis or the risk of recurrence in the breast after breast conservation surgery with radiation.

## TUMOR GROWTH RATE

### Clinical Assessment of Tumor Growth Rate

Estimates of the growth rate of mammary carcinoma have been made clinically from serial mammography studies. Tabár et al. (37) reported that the mean preclinical state, the "sojourn time," was 2.46 years in women 40 to 49 years of age entered into a breast cancer screening trial. Mean sojourn time was longer in women 50 to 59 years (3.75 years) and among those 60 to 69 years (4.23 years) of age at diagnosis. Analysis of data from this study led the authors to conclude that the rate of tumor progression, manifested by "dedifferentiation" to less well-differentiated grade, larger size, and greater frequency of nodal metastases, was more rapid in women 40 to 49 years of age than in older women. The estimated annual progression rates from size smaller than 2 cm to size 2 cm or greater were 31%, 22%, and 20% for women 40 to 49, 50 to 59, and 60 to 69 years old, respectively, at entry into the screening program. Annual progression rates from lymph node negative to lymph node positive were 26%, 19%, and 16%, respectively, for the same age groups. Annual progression rates from grades 1 or 2 to grade 3 were 47%, 12%, and 15%, respectively, for these age groups.

Interval carcinomas are defined as tumors diagnosed clinically between screening intervals after a negative screening examination. Vitak et al. (50) reported that, in comparison to screen-detected carcinomas, interval carcinomas occurred more often in women 40 to 49 and 50 to 59 years of age on entry into the screening program than in women 60 years or older. Statistically significant unfavorable characteristics of interval carcinomas when compared with screen-detected tumors were larger size, greater frequency of nodal metastases, fewer stage I tumors, greater frequencies of estrogen receptor-negative or aneuploid carcinomas, and a higher proportion of tumors with high SPF.

Estimates of growth rate have been determined by examining serial mammograms from women who develop carcinoma detected mammographically after a prior "negative" radiographic examination. The radiograph that preceded the diagnostic image is considered to be a "false-negative" if, on review, an abnormality deemed not significant in initial review is found at the site where carcinoma was later detected. Peer et al. (307) used data from serial mammograms to estimate tumor growth rate for incident and interval carcinomas when the prior screening examination was negative. Growth rate expressed as estimated tumor doubling time was significantly greater for women less than 50 years old on entry into screening (geometric mean in days: 80; 95% CI = 44 to 147) than in those 50 to 70 years (geometric mean, 157; 95% CI = 121 to 204) or in women older than 70 years (geometric mean, 188; 95% CI = 120 to 295). A substantial proportion of carcinomas detected mammographically when no lesion was detectable retrospectively on the antecedent mammogram were *in situ* carcinomas. Other studies reported a similar correlation between younger age and shorter doubling time based on screening studies (308,309) or other data (310). Overall tumor doubling times reported in these studies, not stratified for age, were 220 days (308), 174 days (309), and 115 days (310). Daly et al. (311) analyzed 25 patients with breast carcinoma detected in a screening program after what proved, in retrospect, to be a false-negative mammography study. The average mammographic size of false-negative lesions was 6 mm, whereas the average size on mammography of the incident tumors found on subsequent screening examinations was 13.8 mm. The average histologic size of invasive carcinomas detected after false-negative mammography was 16.7 mm (range 7, to 30 mm).

### Determination of S-Phase Fraction and Ploidy by Flow Cytometry

In 1979, Atkin and Kay (312) described the relationship of modal DNA values to prognosis in 1,465 diverse malignant tumors, including some breast carcinomas. The study was based on microspectrophotometric DNA measurements made of Feulgen-stained imprints of fresh tumors. Most tumors exhibited a bimodal distribution of DNA values. Generally, patients whose tumors were in the near-diploid range had a better survival than those with an aneuploid DNA distribution. These results confirmed an earlier report by Atkin (313), who had described comparable results specifically for breast cancers.

Subsequently, Auer et al. (314,315) used fine needle aspiration biopsies of breast carcinomas to prepare Feulgen-stained smears and reported that the resultant DNA histograms correlated with survival time. In another study that also used needle aspiration smear material, Auer et al. (316) compared the DNA histograms of 18 primary breast carcinomas and metastases in the same patient. With one exception, little difference in DNA patterns was found between the two specimens from a given patient. When related to estrogen receptor content, tumors with a near-diploid DNA content tended to be receptor positive, whereas those with aneuploid DNA were likely to be receptor negative (317).

DNA ploidy distributions in breast carcinomas measured by flow cytometry have generally confirmed results obtained with the Feulgen-stained cytology procedure. The majority of carcinomas in most series have a bimodal distribution of DNA values, with more than 50% of cells in the hyperdiploid range (318–320). When measured by flow cytometry, tumors with a near-diploid DNA distribution tend to be estrogen and progesterone receptor positive, whereas receptor negativity has been associated with aneuploidy (318,321,322).

Pathologic studies have shown a close correlation between cytologic grading of tumor nuclei and DNA ploidy analyzed by flow cytometry (323,324). Low-grade tumors typically exhibit near-diploid DNA, whereas aneuploidy is most pronounced in tumors with high-grade nuclei. Subtypes of carcinoma that are histologically low grade, such as tubular, mucinous, and papillary carcinoma, usually are diploid, whereas medullary carcinoma, which is a cytologically high-grade neoplasm, generally is aneuploid (325). There appears to be a weak relationship between ploidy and stage at diagnosis, with a tendency to aneuploidy among cases with larger tumors and axillary nodal metastases, but in most reports the association was not statistically significant.

Estimates of the growth rate of breast cancer cells based on statistical models and clinical data have been supplemented and replaced by laboratory studies in the past decade. The proliferative proportion of cells in DNA synthesis determined by the thymidine labeling index (TLI) has been shown to correlate significantly with prognosis (326–329). High TLI has been associated with a higher frequency of recurrence, earlier recurrence, and shorter survival after recurrence (329–331). The unfavorable effect of high TLI was independent of stage at diagnosis (331–333), but it may not be a better guide to prognosis than histologic grade (329).

Flow cytometry provides a simple method of determining the proliferative fraction (SPF), which is reported to be equivalent to the TLI (334). In 1983, Hedley et al. (335) described a method of preparing paraffin-embedded tissues for flow cytometric DNA analysis. DNA histograms of cells from fixed material correlate well with suspensions of unfixed cells from the same tumor. This method is now widely used in retrospective studies of archival material, as well as for the analysis of specimens in clinical practice. For a variety of technical reasons, it is not possible to determine the SPF in subsets of breast carcinomas that may constitute as many as 45% of tumors studied. These problems arise largely in aneuploid tumors when the S-phase portion of the DNA histogram is obscured and cannot be resolved into distinct peaks. Difficulties are encountered more often with material extracted from paraffin blocks.

It has been observed that proliferative activity reflected in the SPF is correlated with ploidy to the extent that diploid carcinomas tend to have a lower SPF than aneuploid lesions (336,337). Tumors with a high SPF tend to be estrogen receptor negative (337–339). SPF has been found to correlate with the histologic differentiation of duct carcinomas and with nuclear differentiation (322,337,338). Some investigators reported that ploidy and/or SPF did not correlate with nodal status at the time of initial treatment (340), but others found a high SPF in node-positive compared with node-negative patients (341). Dressler et al. (341) found that the mean SPF of diploid node-positive tumors was significantly higher than the mean SPF of diploid node-negative tumors. A reduction in the SPF was found in 25% of nodal metastases from estrogen receptor-positive tumors. This phenomenon was not apparent when estrogen receptor-negative tumors were compared with their concurrent nodal metastases (342).

The relationship of the TLI to DNA ploidy and SPF was reviewed extensively by Meyer et al. (327), who concluded that "high S-phase fraction and aneuploidy may prove to have prognostic significance like thymidine labeling index." Numerous studies relating cell cycle kinetics and ploidy determined by flow cytometry to breast carcinoma prognosis have been published. Investigators have used paraffin-embedded tissue (335,343), stored frozen tissue (341), and fresh tumor samples (344). Procedures have been developed to perform flow cytometry on the small samples obtained by needle aspiration (345,346). Because of tumor heterogeneity, analyses based on needle aspiration samples are subject to considerable variability, which may be minimized if multiple samples are obtained at one time (347–349). Tumor heterogeneity limits the reliability of multiple sequential aspirates taken during the course of therapy to monitor changes in proliferative activity (349,350). Intratumoral variations in ploidy were found in 24% of 518 breast carcinomas studied by Kallioniemi (351). Fourteen percent had multiple aneuploid populations, and in 10% the DNA index was diploid in one sample and aneuploid in a second specimen from the same tumor. The DNA index of tumor samples from axillary lymph node metastases duplicates the ploidy of the primary tumor sample in more than 90% of cases (342,352).

Many reviews of the prognostic significance of ploidy and SPF have been published (353–356). Because of the close correlation between tumor grade, SPF, and ploidy, the significance of any one of these features as an independent prognostic factor is difficult to ascertain. Whereas patients with tumors that have a diploid DNA index tend to have a more favorable prognosis (357–360), "the magnitude of this advantage compared to tumors showing aneuploidy is small" (355). Bergers et al. (361) analyzed DNA ploidy data from breast carcinomas in a prospective study of 1,301 cases and concluded that "DNA ploidy seems to be of little clinical importance in breast cancer patients compared to other prognostic parameters." An association between high SPF and increased risk for recurrence has been documented in most studies (362–366), but others have failed to detect this relationship (359,367). Hietanen et al. (368) reported that metastatic breast carcinoma with a high SPF was significantly more responsive to chemotherapy than tumor with a low SPF.

## Immunohistochemical Assessment of Proliferation

*Bromodeoxyuridine (BrdU)*, a thymidine analogue, is incorporated into DNA during the S-phase of the cell cycle. Uptake of BrdU after *in vivo* administration to patients (369–371) or *in vitro* incubation of fresh biopsies with BrdU (372,373) can be measured in tissue sections by an immunohistochemical procedure that uses an anti-BrdU antibody (374–376) or by multiparameter flow cytometry (370). The results are comparable to those obtained by thymidine labeling (374,377). The procedures for *in vivo* and *in vitro* labeling do not require radioactive reagents, and they can be completed in considerably less time than is necessitated by autoradiography of $^3$H-thymidine–labeled tissues. BrdU incorporation requires fresh, unfixed tissue and cannot be used for retrospective studies of paraffin-embedded tumors.

*In vivo* BrdU administration yielded median labeling indices of 4.2% (370) and 10.3% (369) in two studies based on multiparameter flow cytometry and manual counting of immunohistochemical sections, respectively. Rew et al. (370) found no correlation between BrdU labeling index, lymph node status, tumor size, and tumor grade. Thor et al. (373) reported that the BrdU labeling index in 460 invasive duct carcinomas (median, 4%; mean, 6%; range, 0% to 40%) was significantly higher than in 26 invasive lobular carcinomas (median, 3.0%; mean, 3.5%; range, 0% to 12%) when BrdU was considered a continuous variable. BrdU labeling also was significantly associated with tumor grade, being lower in low-grade tumors, tumor size, nodal status, mitotic index, and MIB1 labeling (373). Weidner et al. (371) also found that *in vivo* BrdU labeling was significantly correlated with histologic grade and with the mitotic count. The *in vivo* BrdU labeling indices of primary carcinomas and concurrent axillary lymph node metastases are very similar.

A number of immunocytochemical assays have been developed that use antibodies to cell proliferation-related proteins. These reagents provide a static measure of proliferation at a point in time rather than the proliferative rate.

*Ki67* is a mouse monoclonal antibody to nuclear components of a cell line derived from Hodgkin's lymphoma (378). The antibody reacts with a nuclear antigen that is expressed in proliferating cells throughout the cell cycle but is absent from quiescent cells (379). It has been shown that there is a close correlation in breast carcinomas between the Ki67 growth fraction and SPF determined by flow cytometry (380–382), the TLI (383), the BrdU index (384), labeling with MIB1 (385), and mitotic counts (380,386).

Because Ki67 labeling occurs throughout the cell cycle, the percentage of positive cells is consistently higher and generally about twice the proportion in S-phase (TLI or BrdU positive). However, Ki67 positivity may not accurately reflect proliferative activity under some circumstances. Ki67 expression may be so low as to be undetectable at the outset of DNA replication, particularly in cells with a long $G_1$ phase (387). Cells with proliferation impaired or arrested by suboptimal growth conditions or drug treatment (e.g., tamoxifen) may retain immunohistochemically demonstrable Ki67 antigen. The difference between growth fraction determined by BrdU labeling and Ki67 positivity is accentuated when conditions are altered in a fashion that inhibits proliferation. A statistically significant positive correlation between Ki67 positivity and the number of nucleolar organizer regions in mammary carcinoma nuclei has been reported (388,389).

The mean value of Ki67-positive cells (3% to 4%) in benign breast lesions is substantially lower than the mean value (16% to 17%) in mammary carcinomas (383,390). The Ki67 growth fraction is significantly related to grade in most tumors, being highest in poorly differentiated carcinomas

and invasive duct carcinomas with comedo features (380, 390,391). Invasive lobular and mucinous carcinomas have a low-to-moderate growth fraction, whereas medullary carcinomas have more than 50% Ki67-positive cells. Estrogen and progesterone receptor-negative tumors tend to have a high Ki67-positive fraction (390,392). Ki67 reactivity does not correlate well with the stage of the primary carcinoma as reflected in tumor size and lymph node status in most studies, suggesting it may be an independent prognostic marker (393,394). Several studies reported a significant inverse association between Ki67 staining and disease-free and overall survival (386,392,395,396). A comparison of screen-detected and interval carcinomas revealed that interval carcinomas had higher Ki67 labeling and higher mitotic rates than tumors detected by screening (397).

*MIB1* is an antibody raised against recombinant parts of the Ki67 antigen that can be used on microwave-processed paraffin-embedded tissue (398). A significant correlation between Ki67 expression and MIB1 immunoreactivity was described in three studies (385,399,400), but Keshgegian and Cnaan (401) reported finding no significant correlation (401). Pinder et al. (402) reported that high MIB1 labeling was associated with poorly differentiated carcinomas, larger tumor size, earlier recurrence, and poorer survival. Thor et al. (373) reported that MIB1 labeling in invasive ductal carcinomas was significantly higher (mean, 32.2%; median, 28.6%; range, 0% to 99%) than in invasive lobular carcinomas (median, 20.8%; mean, 17.8%; range, 2% to 52%). High MIB1 labeling also was associated with diagnosis before age 50 years, estrogen and progesterone receptor negativity, high tumor grade, larger tumor size, and axillary lymph node metastases. In this study, MIB1 labeling was "more closely associated with outcome than mitotic index or BrdU" labeling, especially in patients with T1N0M0 tumors. A strong correlation between MIB1 labeling and disease-free survival also was reported by Arber et al. (403). Umemura et al. (404) found that high MIB1 labeling and high mitotic indices were independent prognostic factors for node-negative patients. On the other hand, Domagala et al. (405) reported that the MIB1 labeling index was prognostically significant in node-positive but not in node-negative patients.

*Proliferating cell nuclear antigen (PCNA)/cyclin* is a nonhistone nuclear protein that serves as a cofactor to DNA polymerase. It is expressed during the late $G_1$- and S-phases of the cell cycle. A number of monoclonal antibodies have been developed to antigenically distinct forms of PCNA. Some of these reagents, applicable to paraffin sections, are commercially available. Staining is localized to nuclei. PCNA positivity is significantly correlated with SPF determined by flow cytometry, and it is higher in aneuploid than in diploid carcinomas (406). PCNA staining has been significantly related to tumor size, histologic grade, and mitotic rate (407). Other investigators confirmed the association with mitotic rate but found no significant association with tumor size or axillary nodal status (408). In one study, high PCNA scores were associated with a less favorable prognosis than low scores (408), but another report concluded that PCNA expression was not a significant indicator of prognosis (409).

*Mitosin* is a nuclear phosphoprotein formed during the late G-, S-, $G_2$-, and M-phases of the cell cycle, but not in $G_0$. Immunohistochemical expression of mitosin was studied by Clark et al. (410) in 386 node-negative tumors. High mitosin expression was associated with an elevated SPF, negative estrogen and progesterone receptor, and unfavorable prognosis.

## NUCLEAR MORPHOMETRY

Nuclear morphometry provides a method for obtaining quantitative measurements of the size and shape of tumor cell nuclei. Among the parameters commonly recorded in these studies are nuclear diameter, nuclear area, and nuclear perimeter. Careful counts of mitotic activity also have been obtained in some of these studies. Measurements can be made using properly prepared histologic sections (411) and on aspiration cytology smears (412–414). Prognostic correlations have been made with the nuclear morphometry of the primary tumor (411–414) as well as with morphometric features of tumor cell nuclei in axillary nodal metastases (415). The morphometric feature that most often had a statistically significant association with prognosis has been nuclear area (411–413,415,416). Nuclear diameter, a parameter included in the calculation of area, has been significantly related to prognosis (412,414), as has the frequency of mitoses (411). Inverse relationships were observed between mean nuclear area, mean nuclear diameter, mitotic index, and prognosis. Concurrent assessment of nuclear and histologic grading proved prognostically significant in some of these studies (411,415). It remains to be determined as to how the observations of morphometry can be used to improve the assessment of prognosis beyond that more readily obtained by nuclear and histologic grading.

## REFERENCES

1. Rosen PP. The pathological classification of human mammary carcinoma: past, present and future. *Ann Clin Lab Sci* 1979;9:144–156.
2. Tulinius H, Bjarnason O, Sigvaldason H, et al. Tumours in Iceland. 10. Malignant tumours of the female breast. A histological classification, laterality, survival and epidemiological considerations. *APMIS* 1988;96:229–238.
3. Fisher ER, Gregorio RM, Fisher B, et al. The pathology of invasive breast cancer. A syllabus derived from findings of the National Surgical Adjuvant Breast Project (Protocol No. 4). *Cancer* 1975;36:1–85.
4. Gupta SK, Douglas-Jones AG, Fenn N, et al. The clinical behavior of breast carcinoma is probably determined at the preinvasive stage (ductal carcinoma in situ). Cancer 1997;80:1740–1745.
5. Cowen PN, Bates C. The significance of intraduct appearances in breast cancer. *Clin Oncol* 1984;10:67–72.
6. Wells CA, Ferguson DJP. Ultrastructural and immunocytochemical study of a case of invasive cribriform breast carcinoma. *J Clin Pathol* 1988;41:17–20.
7. Sistrunk WE, MacCarty WC. Life expectancy following radical amputation for carcinoma of the breast: a clinical and pathologic study of 218 cases. *Ann Surg* 1922;75:61–69.
8. Heimann R, Hellman S. Aging, progression, and phenotype in breast cancer. *J Clin Oncol* 1998;16:2686–2692.
9. Heimann R, Hellman S. Clinical progression of breast cancer malignant behavior: what to expect and when to expect it. *J Clin Oncol* 2000;18:591–599.
10. Blamey RW, Elston CW, Ellis IO. When is a patient cured of breast cancer? *Mod Pathol* 2000;13:18A.
11. Regitnig P, Heckermann H, Moser R, et al. Molecular genetic comparison of primary and recurrent breast carcinoma? Significant increase of loss of heterozygosity (LOH) in the recurrence and specific LOH associated with early recurrence. *Mod Pathol* 2000;13:45A.
12. Elmore JG, Moceri VM, Carter D, et al. Breast carcinoma tumor characteristics in black and white women. *Cancer* 1998;83:2509–2515.
13. Edwards MJ, Gamel JW, Vaughan WP, et al. Infiltrating ductal carcinoma of the breast: the survival impact of race. *J Clin Oncol* 1998;16:2693–2699.
14. Robson M, Rajan P, Rosen PP, et al. BRCA-associated breast cancer: absence of a characteristic immunophenotype. *Cancer Res* 1998;58:1839–1842.
15. Beckman MW, Picard F, An HX, et al. Clinical impact of detection of loss of heterozygosity of BRCA1 and BRCA2 markers in sporadic breast cancer. *Br J Cancer* 1996;73:1220–1226.
16. Karp SE, Tonin PN, Begin LR, et al. Influence of BRCA1 mutations on nuclear grade and estrogen receptor status of breast carcinoma in Ashkenazi Jewish women. *Cancer* 1997;80:435–441.
17. Eisinger F, Stoppa-Lyonnet D, Longy M, et al. Germ line mutation at BRCA1 affects the histoprognostic grade in hereditary breast cancer. *Cancer Res* 1996;56:471–474.
18. Breast Cancer Linkage Consortium. Pathology of familial breast cancer: differences between breast cancers in carriers of BRCA1 and BRCA2 mutations and sporadic cases. *Lancet* 1997;349:1505–1510.
19. Robson M, Levin D, Federici M, et al. Breast conservation therapy for invasive breast cancer in Ashkenazi women with BRCA gene founder mutations. *J Natl Cancer Inst* 1999;91:2112–2117.
20. Armes JE, Egan AJ, Southey MC, et al. The histologic phenotypes of breast carcinoma occurring before age 40 years in women with and without BRCA1 or BRCA2 germline mutations: a population-based study. *Cancer* 1998;83:2335–2345.
21. Jacquemier J, Guinebretiere J-M. Intraductal component and BRCA-1–associated breast cancer. *Lancet* 1996;348:1098.
22. Sun C, Lenoir G, Lynch H, et al. In-situ breast cancer and BRCA1. *Lancet* 1996;348:408.
23. Slack NH, Bross ID, Nemoto T, et al. Experiences with bilateral primary carcinoma of the breast. *Surg Gynecol Obstet* 1973;136:433–440.
24. Schell SR, Montague ED, Spanos WJ, et al. Bilateral breast cancer in patients with initial stage I and II disease. *Cancer* 1982;50:1191–1194.
25. de la Rochefordiere A, Asselain B, Scholl S, et al. Simultaneous bilateral breast carcinomas: a retrospective review of 149 cases. *Int J Radiat Oncol Biol Phys* 1994;30:35–41.
26. Gollamudi SV, Gelman RS, Peiro G, et al. Breast-conserving therapy for stage I-II synchronous bilateral breast carcinoma. *Cancer* 1997;79:1362–1369.
27. Lee MM, Heimann R, Powers P, et al. Efficacy of breast conservation therapy in early stage bilateral breast cancer. *Breast J* 1999;5:36–41.
28. Brown H, Vlastos G, Newman L, et al. Histopathologic features of bilateral and unilateral breast carcinoma: a comparative study. *Mod Pathol* 2000;13:18A.
29. Tulusan AH, Ronay G, Egger H, et al. A contribution to the natural history of breast cancer. V. Bilateral primary breast cancer: incidence, risks and diagnosis of simultaneous primary cancer in the opposite breast. *Arch Gynecol* 1985;237:85–91.
30. Healey EA, Cook EF, Orav EJ, et al. Contralateral breast cancer: clinical characteristics and impact on prognosis. *J Clin Oncol* 1993;11:1545–1552.
31. Schwartz AG, Ragheb NE, Swanson GM, et al. Racial and age differences in multiple primary cancers after breast cancer: a population-based analysis. *Breast Cancer Res Treat* 1989;14:245–254.
32. Chaudary MA, Millis RR, Bulbrook RD, et al. Family history and bilateral primary breast cancer. *Breast Cancer Res Treat* 1985;5:201–205.
33. Senie RT, Lesser M, Kinne DW, et al. Method of tumor detection influences disease-free survival of women with breast carcinoma. *Cancer* 1994;73:1666–1672.
34. Shapiro S, Venet W, Strax P, et al. Selection, follow-up, and analysis

in the Health Insurance Plan study: a randomized trial with breast cancer screening. *Natl Cancer Inst Monogr* 1985;67:65–74.

35. Shapiro S. Periodic screening for breast cancer: the HIP Randomized Controlled Trial. Health Insurance Plan. *J Natl Cancer Inst Monogr* 1997;(22):27–30.

36. Tabar L, Fagerberg CJ, Gad A, et al. Reduction in morality from breast cancer after mass screening with mammography. *Lancet* 1985;1: 829–832.

37. Tabár L, Chen HH, Fagerberg G, et al. Recent results from the Swedish Two-County Trial: the effects of age, histologic type, and mode of detection on the efficacy of breast cancer screening. *J Natl Cancer Inst Monogr* 1997;(22):43–47.

38. Tabár L, Duffy SW, Vitak B, et al. The natural history of breast carcinoma: what have we learned from screening? *Cancer* 1999;86: 449–462.

39. Morrison AS, Brisson J, Khalid N. Breast cancer incidence and mortality in the breast cancer detection demonstration project. *J Natl Cancer Inst* 1988;80:1540–1547.

40. Lopez MJ, Smart CR. Twenty-year follow-up of minimal breast cancer from the Breast Cancer Detection Demonstration Project. *Surg Oncol Clin N Am* 1997;6:393–401.

41. Anderson TJ, Lamb J, Donnan P, et al. Comparative pathology of breast cancer in a randomised trial of screening. *Br J Cancer* 1991;64:108–113.

42. Cowan WK, Angus B, Henry J, et al. Immunohistochemical and other features of breast carcinomas presenting clinically compared with those detected by cancer screening. *Br J Cancer* 1991;64:780–784.

43. Gibbs NM. Comparative study of the histopathology of breast cancer in a screened and unscreened population investigated by mammography. *Histopathology* 1985;9:1307–1318.

44. Anderson TJ, Alexander F, Chetty U, et al. Comparative pathology of prevalent and incident cancers detected by breast screening. *Lancet* 1986;1:519–523.

45. Arnerlöv C, Emdin SO, Lundgren B, et al. Breast carcinoma growth rate described by mammographic doubling time and S-phase fraction. Correlations to clinical and histopathologic factors in a screened population. *Cancer* 1992;70:1928–1934.

46. Kallioniemi O-P, Kärkkäinen A, Auvinen O, et al. DNA flow cytometric analysis indicates that many breast cancers detected in the first round of mammographic screening have a low malignant potential. *Int J Cancer* 1988;42:697–702.

47. Tabar L, Duffy SW, Krusemo UB. Detection method, tumour size and node metastases in breast cancers diagnosed during a trial of breast cancer screening. *Eur J Cancer Clin Oncol* 1987;23:959–962.

48. Tinnemans JGM, Wobbes T, van der Sluis R, et al. Multicentricity in nonpalpable breast carcinoma and its implications for treatment. *Am J Surg* 1986;151:334–338.

49. von Rosen A, Frisell J, Nilsson R, et al. Histopathologic and cytochemical characteristics of interval breast carcinomas from the Stockholm Mammography Screening Project. *Acta Oncol* 1992;31: 399–402.

50. Vitak B, Stal O, Manson JC, et al. Interval cancers and cancers in non-attenders in the Ostergotland Mammographic Screening Programme. Duration between screening and diagnosis, S-phase fraction and distant recurrence. *Eur J Cancer* 1997;33:1453–1460.

51. Ikeda DM, Andersson I, Wattsgård C, et al. Interval carcinomas in the Malmo Mammographic Screening Trial: radiographic appearance and prognostic considerations. *AJR Am J Roentgenol* 1992;159:287–294.

52. DeGroote R, Rush BF, Milazzo J, et al. Interval breast cancer: a more aggressive subset of breast neoplasias. *Surgery* 1983;94:543–547.

53. Shapiro S, Venet W, Strax P, et al. Ten to fourteen year effect of screening on breast cancer mortality. *J Natl Cancer Inst* 1982;69:349–355.

54. Holmberg LH, Adami HO, Tabar L, et al. Survival in breast cancer diagnosed between mammographic screening examinations. *Lancet* 1986;1:27–30.

55. Brown RS, Wahl RL. Overexpression of Glut-1 glucose transporter in human breast cancer. *Cancer* 1993;72:2979–2985.

56. Wahl RL, Cody RL, Hutchins GD, et al. Primary and metastatic breast carcinoma: initial clinical evaluation with PET with the radiolabeled glucose analogue 2-[F-18]-fluoro-2-deoxy-D-glucose. *Radiology* 1991;179:765–770.

57. Bruce DM, Evans NT, Heys SD, et al. Positron emission tomography: 2–deoxy-2-[18F]-fluoro-D-glucose uptake in locally advanced breast cancers. *Eur J Surg Oncol* 1995;21:280–283.

58. Adler LP, Crowe JP, Al-Kaisi NK, et al. Evaluation of breast masses and axillary lymph nodes with [F-18] 2-deoxy-2-fluoro-D-glucose PET. *Radiology* 1993;187:743–750.

59. Avril N, Dose J, Janicke F, et al. Metabolic characterization of breast tumors with positron emission tomography using F-18 fluorodeoxyglucose. *J Clin Oncol* 1996;14:1848–1857.

60. Bassa P, Kim EE, Inoue T, et al. Evaluation of preoperative chemotherapy using PET with fluorine-18-fluorodeoxyglucose in breast cancer. *J Nucl Med* 1996;37:931–938.

61. Oshida M, Uno K, Suzuki M, et al. Predicting the prognoses of breast carcinoma patients with positron emission tomography using 2-deoxy-2-fluoro[18F]-D-glucose. *Cancer* 1998;82:2227–2234.

62. Edwards MJ, Bonadonna G, Valagussa P, et al. End points in the analysis of breast cancer survival: relapse versus death from tumor. *Surgery* 1998;124:197–202.

63. Touboul E, Buffat L, Belkacémi Y, et al. Local recurrences and distant metastases after breast-conserving surgery and radiation therapy for early breast cancer. *Int J Radiat Oncol Biol Phys* 1999;43:25–38.

64. Vogel CL, Azevedo S, Hilsenbeck S, et al. Survival after first recurrence of breast cancer. The Miami experience. *Cancer* 1992;709: 129–135.

65. Aaltomaa S, Lipponen P, Eskelinen M, et al. Prediction of outcome after first recurrence of breast cancer. *Eur J Surg* 1992;158:13–18.

66. Clark GM, Sledge GW Jr, Osborne CK, et al. Survival from first recurrence: relative importance of prognostic factors in 1,015 breast cancer patients. *J Clin Oncol* 1987;5:55–61.

67. Kamby C, Rose C, Ejlertsen B, et al. Stage and pattern of metastases in patients with breast cancer. *Eur J Cancer Clin Oncol* 1987;23: 1925–1934.

68. Kamby C, Ejlertsen B, Andersen J, et al. The pattern of metastases in human breast cancer. Influence of systemic adjuvant therapy and impact on survival. *Acta Oncol* 1988;27:715–719.

69. Cuzick J, Stewart H, Rutqvist L, et al. Cause-specific mortality in long-term survivors of breast cancer who participated in trials of radiotherapy. *J Clin Oncol* 1994;12:447–453.

70. Fowble B. Postmastectomy radiation. A modest benefit prevails for high risk patients. *Cancer* 1997;79:1061–1066.

71. Rutqvist LE, Cedermark B, Fornander T, et al. The relationship between hormone receptor content and the effect of adjuvant tamoxifen in operable breast cancer. *J Clin Oncol* 1989;7:1474–1484.

72. Arriagada R, Rutqvist LE, Mattsson A, et al. Adequate locoregional treatment for early breast cancer may prevent secondary dissemination. *J Clin Oncol* 1995;13:2869–2878.

73. Hojris I, Overgaard M, Christensen JJ, et al. Morbidity and mortality of ischaemic heart disease in high-risk breast-cancer patients after adjuvant postmastectomy systemic treatment with or without radiotherapy: analysis of DBCG 82b and 82c randomised trials. Radiotherapy Committee of the Danish Breast Cancer Cooperative Group. *Lancet* 1999;354:1425–1430.

74. Paszat LF, Mackillop WJ, Groome PA, et al. Mortality from myocardial infarction after adjuvant radiotherapy for breast cancer in the surveillance, epidemiology, and end-results cancer registries. *J Clin Oncol* 1998;16:2625–2631.

75. Haffty BG, Reiss M, Beinfield M, et al. Ipsilateral breast tumor recurrence as a predictor of distant disease: implications for systemic therapy at the time of local relapse. *J Clin Oncol* 1996;14:52–57.

76. Veronesi U, Marubini E, Del Vecchio M, et al. Local recurrences and distant metastases after conservative breast cancer treatments: partly independent events. *J Natl Cancer Inst* 1995;87:19–24.

77. Schnitt SJ, Hayman J, Gelman R, et al. A prospective study of conservative surgery alone in the treatment of selected patients with stage I breast cancer. *Cancer* 1996;77:1094–1100.

78. Mansi JL, Earl HM, Powles TJ, et al. Tests for detecting recurrent disease in the follow-up of patients with breast cancer. *Breast Cancer Res Treat* 1988;11:249–254.

79. Tomin R, Donegan WL. Screening for recurrent breast cancer—its effectiveness and prognostic value. *J Clin Oncol* 1987;5:62–67.

80. Andreoli C, Buranelli F, Campa T, et al. Chest x-ray survey in breast cancer follow-up—a contrary view. *Tumori* 1987;73:463–465.

81. Rutgers EJT, van Slooten EA, Kluck HM. Follow-up after treatment of primary breast cancer. *Br J Surg* 1989;76:187–190.

82. Stierer M, Rosen HR. Influence of early diagnosis on prognosis of recurrent breast cancer. *Cancer* 1989;64:1128–1131.

83. Wagman LD, Sanders RD, Terz JJ, et al. The value of symptom directed evaluation in the surveillance for recurrence of carcinoma of the breast. *Surg Gynecol Obstet* 1991;172:191–196.

84. Kagan AR, Steckel RJ. Routine imaging studies for the posttreatment surveillance of breast and colorectal carcinoma. *J Clin Oncol* 1991;9:837–842.

85. Freedman LS, Edwards DN, McConnell EM, et al. Histological grade and other prognostic factors in relation to survival of patients with breast cancer. *Br J Cancer* 1979;40:44–45.

86. Lipponen P, Aaltomaa S, Eskelinen M, et al. The changing importance of prognostic factors in breast cancer during long-term follow-up. *Int J Cancer* 1992;51:698–702.

87. Stenkvist B, Bengtsson E, Dahlqvist B, et al. Predicting breast cancer recurrence. *Cancer* 1982;50:2884–2893.

88. Gilchrist KW, Gray R, Fowble B, et al. Tumor necrosis is a prognostic predictor for early recurrence and death in lymph node-positive breast cancer: a 10-year follow-up study of 728 Eastern Cooperative Oncology Group patients. *J Clin Oncol* 1993;11:1929–1935.

89. Yoshimoto M, Sakamoto G, Ohashi Y. Time dependency of the influence of prognostic factors on relapse in breast cancer. *Cancer* 1993;72:2993–3001.

90. Nab HW, Kluck HM, Rutgers EJT, et al. Long-term prognosis of breast cancer: an analysis of 462 patients in a general hospital in southeast Netherlands. *Eur J Surg Oncol* 1995;21:42–46.

91. Saphner T, Tormey DC, Gray R. Annual hazard rates of recurrence for breast cancer after primary therapy. *J Clin Onocl* 1996;14:2738–2746.

92. Haybittle JL, Blamey RW, Elston CW, et al. A prognostic index in primary breast cancer. *Br J Cancer* 1982;45:361–366.

93. McGuire WL, Clark GM, Fisher ER, et al. Predicting recurrence and survival in breast cancer. *Breast Cancer Res Treat* 1987;9:27–38.

94. Shek LL, Godolphin W. Model for breast cancer survival: relative prognostic roles of axillary nodal status, TNM stage, estrogen receptor concentration, and tumor necrosis. *Cancer Res* 1988;48:5565–5569.

95. Sigurdsson H, Baldetorp B, Borg Å, et al. Indicators of prognosis in node-negative breast cancer. *N Engl J Med* 1990;322:1045–1053.

96. Galea MH, Blamey RW, Elston CE, et al. The Nottingham Prognostic Index in primary breast cancer. *Breast Cancer Res Treat* 1992;22:207–209.

97. Balslev I, Axelsson CK, Zedeler K, et al. The Nottingham Prognostic Index applied to 9,149 patients from the studies of the Danish Breast Cancer Cooperative Group (DBCG). *Breast Cancer Res Treat* 1994;32:281–290.

98. Tubiana-Hulin M, Le Doussal V, Hacene K, et al. Sequential identification of factors predicting distant relapse in breast cancer patients treated by conservative surgery. *Cancer* 1993;72:1261–1271.

99. Winchester DJ, Menck HR, Winchester DP. The National Cancer Data Base report on the results of a large nonrandomized comparison of breast preservation and modified radical mastectomy. *Cancer* 1997;80:162–167.

100. Pinder SE, Murray S, Ellis IO, et al. The importance of the histologic grade of invasive breast carcinoma and response to chemotherapy. *Cancer* 1998;83:1529–1539.

101. *MMWR Morbid Mortal Wkly Rep* 1996 Oct 4:45:833–851.

102. Garne JP, Aspegren K, Balldin G, et al. Increasing incidence of and declining mortality from breast carcinoma. Trends in Malmö, Sweden, 1961–1992. *Cancer* 1997;79:69–74.

103. Hermon C, Beral V. Breast cancer mortality rates are levelling off or beginning to decline in many western countries: analysis of time trends, age-cohort and age-period models of breast cancer mortality in 20 countries. *Br J Cancer* 1996;73:955–960.

104. Adair F, Berg J, Joubert L, et al. Long term follow-up of breast cancer patients. The 30 year report. *Cancer* 1974;33:1145–1150.

105. Say CC, Donegan WL. Invasive carcinoma of the breast: prognostic significance of tumor size and involved axillary lymph nodes. *Cancer* 1974;34:468–471.

106. Smart CR, Myers MH, Gloecker LA. Implications for SEER data on breast cancer management. *Cancer* 1978;41:787–789.

107. Rosen PP, Saigo PE, Braun DW Jr, et al. Predictors of recurrence in Stage I ($T_1N_0M_0$) breast carcinoma. *Ann Surg* 1981;193:15–25.

108. Rosen PP, Saigo PE, Braun DW Jr, et al. Prognosis in Stage II ($T_1N_1M_0$) breast cancer. *Ann Surg* 1981;194:576–584.

109. Roger V, Beito G, Jolly PC. Factors affecting the incidence of lymph node metastases in small cancers of the breast. *Am J Surg* 1989;157:501–502.

110. Fentiman IS, Hyland D, Chaudary MA, et al. Prognosis of patients with breast cancers up to 1 cm in diameter. *Eur J Cancer* 1996;32A:417–420.

111. Abner AL, Collins L, Peiro G, et al. Correlation of tumor size and axillary lymph node involvement with prognosis in patients with T1 breast carcinoma. *Cancer* 1998;83:2502–2508.

112. Mansour EG, Gray R, Shatila AH, et al. Survival advantage of adjuvant chemotherapy in high-risk node-negative breast cancer: ten-year analysis—an intergroup study. *J Clin Oncol* 1998;16:3486–3492.

113. Joensuu H, Pylkkanen L, Toikkanen S. Late mortality from pT1N0M0 breast carcinoma. *Cancer* 1999;85:2183–2189.

114. Quiet CA, Ferguson DJ, Weichselbaum RR, et al. Natural history of node-positive breast cancer: the curability of small cancers with a limited number of positive nodes. *J Clin Oncol* 1996;14:3105–3111.

115. Seidman JD, Schnaper LA, Aisner SC. Relationship of the size of the invasive component of the primary breast carcinoma to axillary lymph node metastasis. *Cancer* 1995;75:65–71.

116. Silverberg SG, Chitale AR. Assessment of significance of proportions of intraductal and infiltrating tumor growth in ductal carcinoma of the breast. *Cancer* 1978;32:830–837.

117. Gold RH, Main G, Zippin C, et al. Infiltration of mammary carcinoma as an indicator of axillary metastases. A preliminary report. *Cancer* 1972;29:35–40.

118. Lane N, Goksel H, Salerno RA, et al. Clinicopathologic analyses of the surgical curability of breast cancers. A minimum ten year study. *Ann Surg* 1961;153:483–498.

119. Carter D, Pipkin RD, Shepard RH, et al. Relationship of necrosis and tumor border to lymph node metastases and 10 year survival in carcinoma of the breast. *Am J Surg Pathol* 1978;2:39–46.

120. Black MM, Speer FD. Nuclear structure in cancer tissues. *Surg Gynecol Obstet* 1957;105:97–105.

121. Cutler SJ, Black MM, Mork T, et al. Further observations on prognostic factors in cancer of the female breast. *Cancer* 1969;24:653–667.

122. Bloom HJG. Prognosis in carcinoma of the breast. *Br J Cancer* 1950;4:259–288.

123. Bloom HJG, Richardson WW. Histological grading and prognosis in breast cancer. A study of 1049 cases, of which 359 have been followed 15 years. *Br J Cancer* 1957;11:359–377.

124. Parham DM, Hagen N, Brown RA. Simplified method of grading primary carcinomas of the breast. *J Clin Pathol* 1992;45:517–520.

125. Jannick I, van Diest PJ, Baak JPA. Comparison of the prognostic value of four methods to assess mitotic activity in 186 invasive breast cancer patients: classical and random mitotic activity assessments with correction for volume percentage of epithelium. *Hum Pathol* 1995;26:1086–1092.

126. van Diest PJ, Baak JPA, Matze-Cok P, et al. Reproducibility of mitosis counting in 2,469 breast cancer specimens: results from the Multicenter Morphometric Mammary Carcinoma Project. *Hum Pathol* 1992;23:603–607.

127. Baak JPA, van Diest PJ, Peterse HL, other MMMCP collaborators. Selection of lymph node negative unfavourable premenopausal breast cancer patients for adjuvant systemic therapy can be done best by the mitotic activity index (MAI). *Mod Pathol* 2000;13:17A.

128. Kuopio T, Collan Y. Still more about counting mitoses. *Hum Pathol* 1996;27:1110–1111.

129. Elston CW, Ellis IO. Pathological prognostic factors in breast cancer. I. The value of histological grade in breast cancer: experience from a large study with long-term follow-up. *Histopathology* 1991;19:403–410.

130. National Co-ordinating Committee for Breast Screening Pathology. *Pathology reporting in breast cancer screening,* 2nd ed. Sheffield: NHSBSP Publications, 1995.

131. Rippey JJ. More about counting mitoses. *Hum Pathol* 1996;27:1109–1110.

132. Ellis PS, Whitehead R. Mitosis counting—a need for reappraisal. *Hum Pathol* 1981;12:3–4.

133. Baehner R, Weidner N. Enhanced mitotic figure counting in breast carcinomas using a mitosis-specific antibody: anti-phosphohistone-H3 (PHH3). *Mod Pathol* 2000;13:17A.

134. Schauer A, Weiss A. Bedeuting des Tumorgrading und der Blutgefäßeinbrüche für die Verlaufsbeurteilung des mammacarcinoms bei Stadium-I-Patientinnen. *Verh Dtsch Ges Pathol* 1981;65:382–394.

135. Le Doussal V, Tubiana-Hulin M, Friedman S, et al. Prognostic value of histologic grade nuclear components of Scarff-Bloom-Richardson (SBR). An improved score modification based on a multivariate analysis of 1262 invasive ductal breast carcinomas. *Cancer* 1989;643:1914–1921.

136. Robbins P, Pinder S, de Klerk N, et al. Histological grading of breast carcinomas: a study of interobserver agreement. *Hum Pathol* 1995;26:873–879.

137. Goldstein NS, Murphy T. Intraductal carcinoma associated with invasive carcinoma of the breast. A comparison of the two lesions with implications for intraductal carcinoma classification systems. *Am J Clin Pathol* 1996;106:312–318.

138. Dabbs DJ. Ductal carcinoma of breast: nuclear grade as a predictor of S-phase fraction. *Hum Pathol* 1993;24:652–656.

139. Andersen JA, Fischermann K, Hou-Jensen K, et al. Selection of high risk groups among prognostically favorable patients with breast cancer. An analysis of the value of prospective grading of tumor anaplasia in 1048 patients. *Ann Surg* 1981;194:1–3.

140. Henson DE. The histological grading of neoplasms. *Arch Pathol Lab Med* 1988;112:1091–1096.

141. Hopton DS, Thorogood J, Clayden AD, et al. Histological grading of breast cancer: significance of grade on recurrence and mortality. *Eur J Surg Oncol* 1989;15:25–31.

142. Thoresen S. Histological grading and clinical stage at presentation in breast carcinoma. *Br J Cancer* 1982;46:457–458.

143. Dawson PJ, Ferguson DJ, Karrison T. The pathologic findings of breast cancer in patients surviving 25 years after radical mastectomy. *Cancer* 1982;50:2131–2138.

144. Davis BW, Gelber RD, Goldhirsch A, et al. Prognostic significance of tumor grade in clinical trials of adjuvant therapy for breast cancer with axillary nodal metastases. *Cancer* 1986;58:2662–2670.

145. Masters JRW, Millis RR, Rubens RD. Response to endocrine therapy and breast cancer differentiation. *Breast Cancer Res Treat* 1986;7:31–34.

146. Williams MR, Blamey RW, Todd JH, et al. Histological grade in predicting response to endocrine treatment. *Breast Cancer Res Treat* 1986;8:165–166.

147. Clarke DH, Le MG, Sarrazin D, et al. Analysis of local-regional relapses in patients with early breast cancer treated by excision and radiotherapy: experience of the Institut Gustave-Roussy. *Int J Radiat Oncol Biol Phys* 1985;11:137–145.

148. Stadler B, Staffen A, Strasser K, et al. Prognostic factors for local recurrence in patients with limited surgery and irradiation of breast cancer. *Strahlenther Onkol* 1990;166:453–456.

149. Locker A, Ellis IO, Morgan DA, et al. Factors influencing local recurrence after excision and radiotherapy for primary breast cancer. *Br J Surg* 1989;76:890–894.

150. Nixon AJ, Schnitt SJ, Gelman R, et al. Relationship of tumor grade to other pathologic features and to treatment outcome of patients with early stage breast carcinoma treated with breast-conserving therapy. *Cancer* 1996;78:426–431.

151. Mate TP, Carter D, Fischer DB, et al. A clinical and histopathologic analysis of the results of conservation surgery and radiation therapy in stage I and II breast carcinoma. *Cancer* 1986;58:1995–2002.

152. Fourquet A, Campana F, Zafrani B, et al. Prognostic factors of breast recurrence in the conservative management of early breast cancer: a 25-year follow-up. *Int J Radiat Oncol Biol Phys* 1989;17:719–725.

153. Schnitt SJ, Hayman J, Gelman R, et al. A prospective study of conservative surgery alone in the treatment of selected patients with stage I breast cancer. *Cancer* 1996;77:1094–1100.

154. Dalton LW, Page DL, Dupont WD. Histologic grading of breast carcinoma. A reproducibility study. *Cancer* 1994;73:2765–2770.

155. Harvey JM, deKlerk NH, Sterrett GF. Histological grading in breast cancer: interobserver agreement, and relation to other prognostic factors including ploidy. *Pathology* 1992;24:63–68.

156. Tsuda H, Sakamaki C, Tsugane S, et al. Prognostic significance of accumulation of gene and chromosome alterations and histological grade in node-negative breast carcinoma. *Jpn J Clin Oncol* 1998;28:5–11.

157. Schumacher M, Schmoor C, Sauerbrei W, et al. The prognostic effect of histological tumor grade in node-negative breast cancer patients. *Breast Cancer Res Treat* 1993;25:235–245.

158. Fisher ER, Palikar AS, Gregorio RM, et al. Pathologic findings from the National Surgical Adjuvant Breast Project (protocol No. 4). IV. Significance of tumor necrosis. *Hum Pathol* 1978;9:523–530.

159. Roses DF, Bell DA, Flotte TJ, et al. Pathologic predictors of recurrence in Stage 1 (T1N0M0) breast cancer. *Am J Clin Pathol* 1982;78:817–820.

160. Visscher DW, Wallis T, Jimenez RE. Centrally necrotizing carcinoma: a distinct histologic subtype of breast cancer with an aggressive clinical behavior. *Mod Pathol* 2000;13:49A.

161. Lipponen P, Aaltomaa S, Kosma VM, et al. Apoptosis in breast cancer as related to histopathological characteristics and prognosis. *Eur J Cancer* 1994;30A:2068–2073.

162. Nishimura R, Nagao K, Miyayama H, et al. Apoptosis in breast cancer and its relationship to clinicopathological characteristics and prognosis. *J Surg Oncol* 1999;71:226–234.

163. Shen KL, Harn HJ, Ho LI, et al. The extent of proliferative and apoptotic activity in intraductal and invasive ductal breast carcinomas detected by Ki-67 labeling and terminal deoxynucleotidyl transferase-mediated digoxigenin-11-dUTP nick end labeling. *Cancer* 1998;82: 2373–2381.

164. Bargou RC, Daniel PT, Mapara MY, et al. Expression of the bcl-2 gene family in normal and malignant breast tissue: low bax-(alpha) expression in tumor cells correlates with resistance towards apoptosis. *Int J Cancer* 1995;60:854–859.

165. Miyashita T, Krajewski S, Krajewska M, et al. Tumor suppressor p53 is a regulator of bcl-2 and bax gene expression in vitro and in vivo. *Oncogene* 1994;9:1799–1805.

166. Haldar S, Negrini M, Monne M, et al. Down-regulation of bcl-2 by p53 in breast cancer cells. *Cancer Res* 1994;54:2095–2097.

167. Sabourin JC, Martin A, Baruch J, et al. bcl-2 expression in normal breast tissue during the menstrual cycle. *Int J Cancer* 1994;59:1–6.

168. Siziopikou KP, Prioleau JE, Harris JR, et al. bcl-2 expression in the spectrum of preinvasive breast lesions. *Cancer* 1996;77:499–506.

169. Kapucuoglu N, Losi L, Eusebi V. Immunohistochemical localization of Bcl-2 and Bax proteins in in situ and invasive duct breast carcinomas. *Virchows Arch* 1997;430:17–22.

170. Bhargava V, Kell DL, van de Rijn M, et al. Bcl-2 immunoreactivity in breast carcinoma correlates with hormone receptor positivity. *Am J Pathol* 1994;145:535–540.

171. Silvestrini R, Veneroni S, Daidone MG, et al. The bcl-2 protein: a prognostic indicator strongly related to p53 protein in lymph node-negative breast cancer patients. *J Natl Cancer Inst* 1994;86:499–504.

172. Visscher DW, Sarkar F, Tabaczka P, et al. Clinicopathologic analysis of bcl-2 immunostaining in breast carcinoma. *Mod Pathol* 1996;9:642–646.

173. Hellemans P, van Dam PA, Weyler J, et al. Prognostic value of bcl-2 expression in invasive breast cancer. *Br J Cancer* 1995;72:354–360.

174. Alsabeh R, Wilson CS, Ahn CW, et al. Expression of bcl-2 in breast cancer: a possible diagnostic application. *Mod Pathol* 1995;9:439–444.

175. Leek RD, Kaklamanis L, Pezzella F, et al. bcl-2 in normal human breast and carcinoma, association with oestrogen receptor-positive, epidermal growth factor receptor-negative tumours and in situ cancer. *Br J Cancer* 1994;69:135–139.

176. Gee JMW, Robertson JFR, Ellis IO, et al. Immunocytochemical localization of bcl-2 protein in human breast cancers and its relationship to a series of prognostic markers and response to endocrine therapy. *Int J Cancer* 1994;59:619–628.

177. Dueñas-González A, Abad-Hernández M, Cruz-Hernandez JJ, et al. Analysis of bcl-2 in sporadic breast carcinoma. *Cancer* 1997;80: 2100–2108.

178. Krajewski S, Thor AD, Edgerton SM, et al. Analysis of bax and bcl-2 expression in p53-immunopositive breast cancers. *Clin Cancer Res* 1997;3:199–208.

179. Barbareschi M, Caffo O, Veronese S, et al. Bcl-2 and p53 expression in node-negative breast carcinoma; a study with long-term follow-up. *Hum Pathol* 1996;27:1149–1155.

180. Geuna M, Palestro G, Malandrone LB, et al. Relationships between proliferative activity and oncogene expression in human breast cancer. *Ann N Y Acad Sci* 1996;784:555–563.

181. Silvestrini R, Benini E, Veneroni S, et al. p53 and bcl-2 expression correlates with clinical outcome in a series of node-positive breast cancer patients. *J Clin Oncol* 1996;14:1604–1610.

182. Nakopoulou L, Michalopoulou A, Giannopoulou I, et al. bcl-2 protein expression is associated with a prognostically favourable phenotype in breast cancer irrespective of p53 immunostaining. *Histopathology* 1999;34:310–319.

183. Joensuu H, Pylkkänen L, Toikkanen S. Bcl-2 immunoreactivity and long-term survival in breast cancer. *Am J Pathol* 1994;145: 1191–1198.

184. van Slooten H-J, Clahsen PC, van Dierendonck JH, et al. Expression of BCL-2 in node-negative breast cancer is associated with various prognostic factors, but does not predict response to one course of perioperative chemotherapy. *Br J Cancer* 1996;74:78–85.

185. Zhang GJ, Kimijima I, Tsuchiya A, et al. The role of bcl-2 expression in breast carcinomas [Review]. *Oncol Rep* 1998;5:1211–1216.

186. Berardo MD, Elledge RM, de Moor C, et al. bcl-2 and apoptosis in lymph node positive breast carcinoma. *Cancer* 1998;82:1296–1302.

187. Bonetti A, Zaninelli M, Leone R, et al. bcl-2 but not p53 expression is associated with resistance to chemotherapy in advanced breast cancer. *Clin Cancer Res* 1998;4:2331–2336.

188. Greider CW, Blackburn EH. Telomeres, telomerase and cancer. *Sci Am* 1996;274:92–97.

189. Nawaz S, Hashizumi TL, Markham NE, et al. Telomerase expression in human breast cancer with and without lymph node metastases. *Am J Clin Pathol* 1997;107:542–547.

190. Carey LA, Kim NW, Goodman S, et al. Telomerase activity and prognosis in primary breast cancers. *J Clin Oncol* 1999;17:3075–3081.

191. Landberg G, Nielsen NH, Nilsson P, et al. Telomerase activity is associated with cell cycle deregulation in human breast cancer. *Cancer Res* 1997;57:549–554.

192. Poremba C, Shroyer KR, Frost M, et al. Telomerase is a highly sensitive and specific molecular marker in fine-needle aspirates of breast lesions. *J Clin Oncol* 1999;17:2020–2026.

193. Roos G, Nilsson P, Cajander S, et al. Telomerase activity in relation to p53 status and clinico-pathological parameters in breast cancer. *Int J Cancer* 1998;79:343–348.

194. Ridolfi R, Rosen P, Port A, et al. Medullary carcinoma of the breast. A clinicopathologic study with 10 year follow-up. *Cancer* 1977;40:1365–1385.

195. Alderson MR, Hamlin I, Staunton MD. The relative significance of prognostic factors in breast carcinoma. *Br J Cancer* 1971;25:646–656.

196. Berg JW. Morphological evidence for immune response to cancer—an historical review. *Cancer* 1971;28:1453–1456.

197. Pupa SM, Bufalino R, Invernizzi AM, et al. Macrophage infiltrate and prognosis in c-erbB-2–overexpressing breast carcinomas. *J Clin Oncol* 1996;14:85–94.

198. Bilik R, Mor C, Haraz B, et al. Characterization of T-lymphocyte subpopulations infiltrating breast cancer. *Cancer Immunol Immunother* 1989;28:143–147.

199. Horny H-P, Horst H-A. Lymphoreticular infiltrates in invasive ductal breast cancer. A histological and immunohistological study. *Virchows Arch [A]* 1986;409:275–286.

200. Whiteside TL, Miescher S, Hurlimann J, et al. Clonal analysis and in situ characterization of lymphocytes infiltrating human breast carcinomas. *Cancer Immunol Immunother* 1986;23:169–173.

201. Whitford P, Mallon EA, George WD, et al. Flow cytometric analysis of tumour infiltrating lymphocytes in breast cancer. *Br J Cancer* 1990;62:971–975.

202. Zuk JA, Walker RA. Immunohistochemical analysis of HLA antigens and mononuclear infiltrates of benign and malignant breast. *J Pathol* 1987;152:275–285.

203. Parkes H, Collis T, Baildam A, et al. In situ hybridization and S1 mapping show that the presence of infitrating plasma cells is associated with poor prognosis in breast cancer. *Br J Cancer* 1988;58:715–722.

204. Fisher ER, Sass R, Watkins G, et al. Tissue mast cells in breast cancer. *Breast Cancer Res Treat* 1985;5:285–291.

205. Gilchrist KW, Gould VE, Hirschl S, et al. Interobserver variation in the identification of breast carcinoma in intramammary lymphatics. *Hum Pathol* 1982;13:170–172.

206. Rosen PP. Tumor emboli in intramammary lymphatics in breast carcinoma: pathologic criteria for diagnosis and clinical significance. *Pathol Annu* 1983;18[Pt 2]:215–232.

207. Hanau CA, Machera H, Miettinen M. Immunohistochemical evaluation of vascular invasion in carcinomas with five different markers. *Appl Immunohistochem* 1993;1:46–50.

208. Lee AKC, DeLellis RA, Wolfe HJ. Intramammary lymphatic invasion in breast carcinomas. Evaluation using ABH isoantigens as endothelial markers. *Am J Surg Pathol* 1986;10:589–594.

209. Saigo PE, Rosen PP. The application of immunohistochemical stains to identify endothelial-lined channels in mammary carcinoma. *Cancer* 1987;59:51–54.

210. Ordonez NG, Brooks T, Thompson S, et al. Use of *Ulex europaeus* agglutinin I in the identification of lymphatic and blood vessel invasion in previously stained microscopic slides. *Am J Surg Pathol* 1987;11:543–550.

211. Bettelheim R, Penman HG, Thornton-Jones H, et al. Prognostic significance of peritumoral vascular invasion in breast cancer. *Br J Cancer* 1984;50:771–777.

212. Fracchia AA, Rosen PP, Ashikari R. Primary carcinoma of the breast without axillary lymph node metastases. *Surg Gynecol Obstet* 1980;151:375–378.

213. Merlin C, Gloor F, Hardmeier T, et al. Hat die intrammarare lymphangiosis carcinomatosa bein nodel-negativen mammakarziom eine prognostische bedeutung? *Schweiz Med Wochenschr* 1980;110:605–606.

214. Nime F, Rosen PP, Thaler H, et al. Prognostic significance of tumor emboli in intramammary lymphatics in patients with mammary carcinoma. *Am J Surg Pathol* 1977;1:25–30.

215. Lauria R, Perrone F, Carlomagno C, et al. The prognostic value of lymphatic and blood vessel invasion in operable breast cancer. *Cancer* 1995;76:1772–1778.

216. Clemente CG, Boracchi P, Andreola S, et al. Peritumoral lymphatic invasion in patients with node-negative mammary duct carcinoma. *Cancer* 1992;69:1396–1403.

217. Liljegren G, Holmberg L, Bergh J, et al. 10-Year results after sector resection with or without postoperative radiotherapy for stage I breast cancer: a randomized trial. *J Clin Oncol* 1999;17:2326–2333.

218. Rosen PP, Saigo PE, Braun DW Jr, et al. Occult axillary lymph node metastases from breast cancers with intramammary lymphatic tumor emboli. *Am J Surg Pathol* 1982;6:639–641.

219. Fisher ER, Sass R, Fisher B. Pathologic findings from the National Surgical Adjuvant Project for breast cancers (Protocol No. 4). X. Discriminants of tenth year treatment failure. *Cancer* 1984;53:712–723.

220. Davis BW, Gelber R, Goldhirsch A, et al. Prognostic significance of peri-tumoral vessel invasion in clinical trials of adjuvant therapy for breast cancer with axillary lymph node metastases. *Hum Pathol* 1985;16:1212–1218.

221. Bell JR, Friedell GH, Goldenberg IS. Prognostic significance of pathologic findings in human breast carcinoma. *Surg Gynecol Obstet* 1969;129:258–262.

222. Sampat MB, Sirsat MV, Gangadharan P. Prognostic significance of blood vessel invasion in carcinoma of the breast in women. *J Surg Oncol* 1977;9:623–632.

223. Weigand RA, Isenberg WM, Russo J, et al., and the Breast Cancer Prognostic Study Associates. Blood vessel invasion and axillary lymph node involvement as prognostic indicators for human breast cancer. *Cancer* 1982;50:962–969.

224. Pinder SE, Ellis IO, Galea M, et al. Pathological prognostic factors in breast cancer. III. Vascular invasion: relationship with recurrence and survival in a large study with long-term follow-up. *Histopathology* 1994;24:41–47.

225. Cowley GP, Smith MEF. Modulation of E-cadherin expression and morphological phenotype in the intravascular component of adenocarcinomas. *Int J Cancer* 1995;60:325–329.

226. Folkman J. What is the evidence that tumors are angiogenesis dependent? *J Natl Cancer Inst* 1990;82:4–6.

227. Folkman J, Watson K, Ingber D, et al. Induction of angiogenesis during the transition from hyperplasia to neoplasia. *Nature* 1989;339:58–61.

228. Jensen HM, Chen I, DeVault MR, et al. Angiogenesis induced by "normal" human breast tissue: a probable marker for precancer. *Science* 1982;218:293–295.

229. Holmgren L, O'Reilly MS, Folkman J. Dormancy of micrometastases: balanced proliferation and apoptosis in the presence of angiogenesis suppression. *Nat Med* 1995;1:149–153.

230. Pepper MS, Ferrara N, Orci L, et al. Potent synergism between vascular endothelial growth factor and basic fibroblast growth factor in the induction of angiogenesis in vitro. *Biochem Biophys Res Commun* 1992;189:824–831.

231. Hlatky L, Tsionou C, Hahnfeldt P, et al. Mammary fibroblasts may influence breast tumor angiogenesis via hypoxia-induced vascular endothelial growth factor up-regulation and protein expression. *Cancer Res* 1994;54:6083–6086.

232. Gonzalez-Vela MC, Garijo MF, Fernandez F, et al. Cathepsin D in host stromal cells is associated with more highly vascular and aggressive invasive breast carcinoma. *Histopathology* 1999;34:35–42.

233. Toi M, Kondo S, Suzuki H, et al. Quantitative analysis of vascular endothelial growth factor in primary breast cancer. *Cancer* 1996;77:1101–1106.

234. Anan K, Morisaki T, Katano M, et al. Preoperative assessment of tumor angiogenesis by vascular endothelial growth factor mRNA expression in homogenate samples of breast carcinoma: fine-needle aspirates vs. resection samples. *J Surg Oncol* 1997;66:257–263.

235. Lee AH, Dublin EA, Bobrow LG, et al. Invasive lobular and invasive ductal carcinoma of the breast show distinct patterns of vascular en-

dothelial growth factor expression and angiogenesis. *J Pathol* 1998;185:394–401.

236. Rastinejad F, Polverini P, Bouck NP. Regulation of the activity of a new inhibitor of angiogenesis by a cancer suppressor gene. *Cell* 1989;56:345–355.

237. Dameron KM, Volpert OV, Tainsky MA, et al. Control of angiogenesis in fibroblasts by p53 regulation of thrombospondin-1. *Science* 1994;265:1582–1584.

238. O'Reilly MS, Holmgren L, Shing Y, et al. Angiostatin: a novel angiogenesis inhibitor that mediates the suppression of metastases by a Lewis lung carcinoma. *Cell* 1994;79:315–328.

239. Rak JW, St Croix BD, Kerbel RS. Consequences of angiogenesis for tumor progression, metastasis and cancer therapy. *Anticancer Drugs* 1995;6:3–18.

240. Brown LF, Berse B, Jackman RW, et al. Expression of vascular permeability factor (vascular endothelial growth factor) and its receptors in breast cancer. *Hum Pathol* 1995;26:86–91.

241. Kim KJ, Li B, Winer J, et al. Inhibition of vascular endothelial growth factor-induced angiogenesis suppresses tumour growth in vivo. *Nature* 1993;362:841–844.

242. Hori A, Sasada R, Matsutani E, et al. Suppression of solid tumor growth by immunoneutralizing monoclonal antibody against human basic fibroblast growth factor. *Cancer Res* 1991;51:6180–6184.

243. Horak ER, Leek R, Klenk N, et al. Angiogenesis, assessed by platelet/endothelial cell adhesion molecule antibodies, as indicator of node metastases and survival in breast cancer. *Lancet* 1992;340:1120–1124.

244. Siitonen SM, Haapasalo HK, Rantala IS, et al. Comparison of different immunohistochemical methods in the assessment of angiogenesis: lack of prognostic value in a group of 77 selected node-negative breast carcinomas. *Mod Pathol* 1995;8:745–752.

245. Gasparini G, Gullick WJ, Bevilacqua P, et al. Human breast cancer: prognostic significance of the c-erbB-2 oncoprotein compared with epidermal growth factor receptor, DNA ploidy, and conventional pathologic features. *J Clin Oncol* 1992;10:686–695.

246. Weidner N, Gasparini G. Determination of epidermal growth factor receptor provides additional prognostic information to measuring tumor angiogenesis in breast carcinoma patients. *Breast Cancer Res Treat* 1994;29:97–107.

247. Martin L, Holcombe C, Green B, et al. Is a histological section representative of whole tumour vascularity in breast cancer? *Br J Cancer* 1997;76:40–43.

248. Jitsuiki Y, Hasebe T, Tsuda H, et al. Optimizing microvessel counts according to tumor zone in invasive ductal carcinoma of the breast. *Mod Pathol* 1999;12:492–498.

249. de Jong JS, van Diest PJ, Baak JPA. Methods in laboratory investigation. Heterogeneity and reproducibility of microvessel counts in breast cancer. *Lab Invest* 1995;73:922–926.

250. Simpson JF, Ahn C, Battifora H, et al. Endothelial area as a prognostic indicator for invasive breast carcinoma. *Cancer* 1996;77:2077–2085.

251. Costello P, McCann A, Carney DN, et al. Prognostic significance of microvessel density in lymph node negative breast carcinoma. *Hum Pathol* 1995;26:1181–1184.

252. Axelsson K, Ljung B-ME, Moore DH II, et al. Tumor angiogenesis as a prognostic assay for invasive ductal breast carcinoma. *J Natl Cancer Inst* 1995;87:997–1008.

253. Ogawa Y, Chung Y-S, Nakata B, et al. Microvessel quantitation in invasive breast cancer by staining for factor VIII-related antigen. *Br J Cancer* 1995;71:1297–1301.

254. Obermair A, Kurz C, Czelwenka K, et al. Microvessel density and vessel invasion in lymph-node negative breast cancer: effect on recurrence-free survival. *Int J Cancer* 1995;62:126–131.

255. Charpin C, Devictor B, Bergeret D, et al. CD31 quantitative immunocytochemical assays in breast carcinomas. Correlation with current prognostic factors. *Am J Clin Pathol* 1995;103:443–448.

256. Goulding H, Nik Abdul Rashid NF, Robertson JF, et al. Assessment of angiogenesis in breast carcinoma: an important factor in prognosis? *Hum Pathol* 1995;26:1196–1200.

257. Harris AL, Horak E. Growth factors and angiogenesis in breast cancer. Recent results. *Cancer Res* 1993;127:35–41.

258. van Hoef MEHM, Knox WF, Dhesi SS, et al. Assessment of tumour vascularity as a prognostic factor in lymph node negative invasive breast cancer. *Eur J Cancer* 1993;29A:1141–1145.

259. Bevilacqua P, Barbareschi M, Verderio P, et al. Prognostic value of intratumoral microvessel density, a measure of tumor angiogenesis, in node-negative breast carcinoma—results of a multiparametric study. *Breast Cancer Res Treat* 1995;36:205–217.

260. Gasparini G. Clinical significance of the determination of angiogenesis in human breast cancer: update of the biological background and overview of the Vicenza studies. *Eur J Cancer* 1996;32A:2485–2493.

261. Toi M, Inada K, Suzuki H, et al. Tumor angiogenesis in breast cancer: its importance as a prognostic indicator and the association with vascular endothelial growth factor expression. *Breast Cancer Res Treat* 1995;36:193–204.

262. Gasparini G, Fox SB, Verderio P, et al. Determination of angiogenesis adds information to estrogen receptor status in predicting the efficacy of adjuvant tamoxifen in node-positive breast cancer patients. *Clin Cancer Res* 1996;2:1191–1198.

263. Heimann R, Ferguson D, Powers C, et al. Angiogenesis as a predictor of long-term survival for patients with node-negative breast cancer. *J Natl Cancer Inst* 1996;88:1764–1769.

264. Miliaras D, Kamas A, Kalekou H. Angiogenesis in invasive breast carcinoma: is it associated with parameters of prognostic significance? *Histopathology* 1995;26:165–169.

265. Kato T, Kimura T, Miyakawa R, et al. Clinicopathologic study of angiogenesis in Japanese patients with breast cancer. *World J Surg* 1997;21:49–56.

266. Toi M, Kashitani J, Tominaga T. Tumor angiogenesis is an independent prognostic indicator in primary breast carcinoma. *Int J Cancer* 1993;55:371–374.

267. Sightler HE, Borowsky AD, Dupont WD, et al. Evaluation of tumor angiogenesis as a prognostic marker in breast cancer. *Lab Invest* 1994;70:22A.

268. Cohen P, Guidi A, Harris J, et al. Microvessel density and local recurrence in patients with early stage breast cancer treated by wide excision above (WEA). *Lab Invest* 1994;70:14A.

269. Hansen S, Grabau DA, Rose C, et al. Angiogenesis in breast cancer: a comparative study of the observer variability of methods for determining microvessel density. *Lab Invest* 1998;78:1563–1573.

270. Buadu LD, Murakami J, Murayama S, et al. Breast lesions: correlation of contrast medium enhancement patterns on MR images with histopathologic findings and tumor angiogenesis. *Radiology* 1996;200:639–649.

271. Stomper PC, Winston JS, Herman S, et al. Angiogenesis and dynamic MR imaging gadolinium enhancement of malignant and benign breast lesions. *Breast Cancer Res Treat* 1997;45:39–46.

272. Buckley DL, Drew PJ, Mussurakis S, et al. Microvessel density of invasive breast cancer assessed by dynamic Gd-DTPA enhanced MRI. *J Magn Reson Imaging* 1997;7:461–464.

273. Esserman L, Hylton N, George T, et al. Contrast-enhanced magnetic resonance imaging to assess tumor histopathology and angiogenesis in breast carcinoma. *Breast J* 1999;5:13–21.

274. Siewert C, Oellinger H, Sherif HK, et al. Is there a correlation in breast carcinomas between tumor size and number of tumor vessels detected by gadolinium-enhanced magnetic resonance mammography? *MAGMA* 1997;5:29–31.

275. Linderholm B, Tavelin B, Grankvist K, et al. Vascular endothelial growth factor is of high prognostic value in node-negative breast carcinoma. *J Clin Oncol* 1998;16:3121–3128.

276. Eppenberger U, Kueng W, Schlaeppi JM, et al. Markers of tumor angiogenesis and proteolysis independently define high- and low-risk subsets of node-negative breast cancer patients. *J Clin Oncol* 1998;16:3129–3136.

277. Penault-Llorca F, Sun ZZ, Viens P, et al. Tumor angiogenesis is not a predictive marker of responsiveness to conventional adjuvant chemotherapy. *Mod Pathol* 1997;10:23A.

278. Paulsen T, Aas T, Borressen A-L. Angiogenesis does not predict clinical response to doxorubicin monotherapy in patients with locally advanced breast cancer [Letter]. *Int J Cancer (Pred Oncol)* 1997;74:138–140.

279. Teicher BA, Holden SA, Ara G, et al. Potentiation of cytotoxic cancer therapies by TNP-470 alone and with other anti-angiogenic agents. *Int J Cancer* 1994;57:920–925.

280. Klauber N, Parangi S, Flynn E, et al. Inhibition of angiogenesis and breast cancer in mice by the microtubule inhibitors 2-methoxyestradiol and taxol. *Cancer Res* 1997;57:81–86.

281. Brem H, Goto F, Budson A, et al. Minimal drug resistance after prolonged antiangiogenic therapy with AGM-1470. *Surg Forum* 1994;45:674–677.

282. Uchiyama S, Fukuda Y. Abnormal elastic fibers in elastosis of breast carcinoma. Ultrastructural and immunohistochemical studies. *Acta Pathol Jpn* 1989;39:245–253.

283. Davies JD. Hyperelastosis, obliteration and fibrous plaques in major ducts of the human breast. *J Pathol* 1973;110:13–26.

284. Reyes MG, Bazile DB, Tosch T, et al. Periductal elastic tissue of breast cancer. *Arch Pathol Lab Med* 1982;106:610–614.

285. Douglas JG, Shivas AA. The origins of elastosis in breast carcinoma. *J R Coll Surg Edinb* 1974;19:89–93.

286. Kao RT, Hall J, Stern R. Collagen and elastin synthesis in human stroma and breast carcinoma cell lines: modulation by extracellular matrix. *Connect Tissue Res* 1986;14:245–255.

287. Mera SL, Davies JD. Elastosis in breast carcinoma: I. Immunohistochemical characterization of elastic fibres. *J Pathol* 1987;151:103–110.

288. Davies JD, Mera SL. Elastosis in breast carcinoma: II. Association of protease inhibitors with immature elastic fibres. *J Pathol* 1987;151:317–324.

289. Humeniuk V, Forrest APM, Hawkins RA, et al. Elastosis and primary breast cancer. *Cancer* 1983;52:1448–1452.

290. Rasmussen BB, Pedersen BV, Thorpe SM, et al. Elastosis in relation to prognosis in primary breast carcinoma. *Cancer Res* 1985;45:1428–1430.

291. Masters JRW, Sangster K, Hawkins RA, et al. Elastosis and estrogen receptors in human breast cancer. *Br J Cancer* 1976;33:342–343.

292. Shivas AA, Douglas JG. The prognostic significance of elastosis in breast carcinoma. *J R Coll Surg Edinb* 1972;17:315–320.

293. Tamura S, Enjoji M. Elastosis in neoplastic and non-neoplastic tissues from patients with mammary carcinoma. *Acta Pathol Jpn* 1988;38:1537–1546.

294. Robertson AJ, Brown RA, Cree IA, et al. Prognostic value of measurement of elastosis in breast carcinoma. *J Clin Pathol* 1981;34:738–743.

295. Anastassiades OT, Bouropoulou V, Kontogeorgos G, et al. Duct elastosis in infiltrating carcinoma of the breast. *Pathol Res Pract* 1979;165:411–421.

296. Glaubitz LC, Bowen JH, Cox ED, et al. Elastosis in human breast cancer. Correlation with sex steroid receptors and comparison with clinical outcome. *Arch Pathol Lab Med* 1984;108:27–30.

297. Schnitt SJ, Connolly JL, Harris JR, et al. Pathologic predictors of early local recurrences in Stage I and II breast cancer treated by primary radiation therapy. *Cancer* 1984;53:1049–1057.

298. Rosen PP, Kinne DW, Lesser ML, et al. Are prognostic factors for local control of breast cancer treated by primary radiotherapy significant for patients treated by mastectomy? *Cancer* 1986;57:1415–1420.

299. Joura EA, Lösch A, Kainz CH, et al. Infiltrating ductal carcinoma of the breast: extensive intraductal component has no impact on lymph node involvement and survival. *Anticancer Res* 1995;15:2285–2286.

300. Hurd TC, Sneige N, Allen PK, et al. Impact of extensive intraductal component on recurrence and survival in patients with stage I and II breast cancer treated with breast conservation therapy. *Ann Surg Oncol* 1997;4:119–124.

301. Schnitt SJ, Abner A, Gelman R, et al. The relationship between microscopic margins of resection and the risk of local recurrence in patients with breast cancer treated with breast-conserving surgery and radiation therapy. *Cancer* 1994;74:1746–1751.

302. Stomper PC, Connolly JL. Mammographic features predicting an extensive intraductal component in early-stage infiltrating ductal carcinoma. *AJR Am J Roentgenol* 1992;158:269–272.

303. Noguchi S, Aihara T, Koyama H, et al. Discrimination between multicentric and multifocal carcinomas of the breast through clonal analysis. *Cancer* 1994;74:872–877.

304. Ohtake T, Abe R, Kimijima I, et al. Intraductal extension of primary invasive breast carcinoma treated by breast-conservation surgery. Computer graphic three-dimensional reconstruction of the mammary duct-lobular systems. *Cancer* 1995;76:32–45.

305. Jing X, Kakudo K, Murakami M, et al. Intraductal spread of invasive breast carcinoma has a positive correlation with c-erb B-2 overexpression and vascular invasion. *Cancer* 1999;86:439–448.

306. Fowble B, Hanlon AL, Patchefsky A, et al. The presence of proliferative breast disease with atypia does not significantly influence outcome in early-stage invasive breast cancer treated with conservative surgery and radiation. *Int J Radiat Oncol Biol Phys* 1998;42:105–115.

307. Peer PG, van Dijck JA, Hendriks JH, et al. Age-dependent growth rate of primary breast cancer. *Cancer* 1993;71:3547–3551.

308. von Fournier D, Weber E, Hoeffken W, et al. Growth rate of 147 mammary carcinomas. *Cancer* 1980;45:2198–2207.

309. Kuroishi T, Tominaga S, Morimoto T, et al. Tumor growth rate and prognosis of breast cancer mainly detected by mass screening. *Jpn J Cancer Res* 1990;81:454–462.

310. Tabbane F, Bahi J, Rahal K, et al. Inflammatory symptoms in breast cancer. Correlations with growth rate, clinicopathologic variables, and evolution. *Cancer* 1989;64:2081–2089.

311. Daly CA, Apthorp L, Field S. Second round cancers: how many were visible on the first round of the UK National Breast Screening Programme, three years earlier? *Clin Radiol* 1998;53:25–28.

312. Atkin NB, Kay R. Prognostic significance of modal DNA value and other factors in malignant tumors based on 1465 cases. *Br J Cancer* 1979;40:210–221.

313. Atkin NB. Modal deoxyribonucleic acid value and survival in carcinomas of the breast. *Br Med J* 1972;1:271–272.

314. Auer GU, Caspersson TO, Wallgren AS. DNA content and survival in mammary carcinomas. *Anal Quant Cytol Histol* 1980;2:162–165.

315. Auer GU, Eriksson E, Azavedo E, et al. Prognostic significance of nuclear DNA content in mammary adenocarcinomas in humans. *Cancer Res* 1984;44:394–396.

316. Auer GU, Falenius AG, Erhardt KY, et al. Progression of mammary adenocarcinomas as reflected by nuclear DNA content. *Cytometry* 1984;5:420–425.

317. Auer GU, Caspersson TO, Gustaffson SA, et al. Relationship between nuclear DNA distribution and estrogen receptors in human mammary carcinomas. *Anal Quant Cytol Histol* 1980;2:280–284.

318. Bichel P, Paulsen HS, Andersen J. Estrogen receptor content and ploidy of human mammary carcinomas. *Cancer* 1982;50:1771–1774.

319. Chessevent A, Daver A, Bertrand G, et al. Comparative flow DNA analysis of different cell suspensions in the breast carcinomas. *Cytometry* 1984;5:263–267.

320. Sven-Borje E, Langstrom E, Baldetorp B, et al. Flow cytometric DNA analysis in primary breast carcinomas and clinicopathologic correlations. *Cytometry* 1984;5:408–419.

321. Cornelisse CJ, de Koning HR, Moolenaar AJ, et al. Image and flow cytometric analysis of DNA content in breast cancer. Relation to estrogen receptor content and lymph node involvement. *Anal Quant Cytol Histol* 1984;6:9–18.

322. Raber MN, Barlogie B, Latreille J, et al. Ploidy, proliferative activity and estrogen receptor content in human breast cancer. *Cytometry* 1982;3:36–41.

323. Fisher B, Gunduz N, Constantino J, et al. DNA flow cytometric analysis of primary operable breast cancer. Relation of ploidy and S-phase fraction to outcome of patients in NSABP B-04. *Cancer* 1991;68:1465–1475.

324. Frierson HF Jr. Grade and flow cytometric analysis of ploidy for infiltrating ductal carcinomas. *Hum Pathol* 1993;24:24–29.

325. Cook DL, Weaver DL. Comparison of DNA content, S-phase fraction, and survival between medullary and ductal carcinoma of the breast. *Am J Clin Pathol* 1995;104:17–22.

326. Meyer JS, Friedman E, McCrate M, et al. Prediction of early course of breast carcinomas by thymidine labeling. *Cancer* 1983;51:1879–1886.

327. Meyer JS, McDivitt RW, Stone KR, et al. Practical breast carcinoma cell kinetics: review and update. *Breast Cancer Res Treat* 1984;4:79–88.

328. Tubiana M, Pejovic MH, Chavaudra N, et al. The long-term prognostic significance of the thymidine labeling index in breast cancer. *Int J Cancer* 1984;33:441–445.

329. Tubiana M, Pejovic MH, Koscielny S, et al. Growth rate, kinetics of tumor cell proliferation and long-term outcome in human breast cancer. *Int J Cancer* 1989;44:17–22.

330. Meyer JS, Prey MV, Babcock DS, et al. Breast carcinoma cell kinetics, morphology, stage and host characteristics. A thymidine labelling study. *Lab Invest* 1986;54:41–51.

331. Paradiso A, Mangia A, Barletta A, et al. Heterogeneity of intratumour proliferative activity in primary breast cancer: biological and clinical aspects. *Eur J Cancer* 1995;31A:911–916.

332. Klintenberg C, Stal O, Nordenskjold B, et al. Proliferative index, cytosol estrogen receptor and axillary nodal status as prognostic predictors in human mammary carcinoma. *Breast Cancer Res Treat* 1986;7[Suppl]:99–106.

333. Silvestrini R, Daidone MG, Valagussa P, et al. ³H-Thymidine-label-

ing index as a prognostic indicator in node-positive breast cancer. *J Clin Oncol* 1990;8:1321–1326.

334. Fossa SD, Thorud E, Vaage S, et al. DNA cytometry of primary breast cancer. A comparison of microspectrophotometry and flow cytometry and different preparation methods for flow cytometric measurements. *Acta Pathol Microbiol Immunol Scand (A)* 1983;91:235–243.

335. Hedley DW, Friedlander ML, Taylor IW, et al. Method for analysis of cellular DNA content of paraffin-embedded pathological material using flow cytometry. *J Histochem Cytochem* 1983;31:1333–1335.

336. Meyer JS, Hixon B. Advanced stage and early relapse of breast carcinomas associated with high thymidine labeling indices. *Cancer Res* 1979;39:4042–4047.

337. Moran RE, Black M, Alpert L, et al. Correlation of cell-cycle kinetics, hormone receptors, histopathology and nodal status in human breast cancer. *Cancer* 1984;54:1586–1590.

338. Olszewski W, Darzynkiewicz Z, Rosen PP, et al. Flow cytometry of breast carcinoma. II. Relation of tumor cell cycle distribution to histology and estrogen receptor. *Cancer* 1981;48:985–988.

339. Olszewski W, Darzynkiewicz A, Rosen PP, et al. Flow cytometry of breast carcinoma: I. Relation of DNA ploidy level to histology and estrogen receptor. *Cancer* 1981;48:980–984.

340. McDivitt RW, Stone KR, Craig B, et al. A proposed classification of breast cancer based on kinetic information derived from a comparison of risk factors in 168 primary operable breast cancers. *Cancer* 1986;57:269–276.

341. Dressler LG, Seamer LC, Owens MA, et al. DNA flow cytometry and prognostic factors in 1331 frozen breast cancer specimens. *Cancer* 1988;61:420–427.

342. Olszewski W, Darzynkiewicz Z, Rosen PP, et al. Flow cytometry of breast carcinoma. III. Possible altered kinetics in axillary node metastases. *Anal Quant Cytol Histol* 1982;4:275–278.

343. Kallioniemi O-P, Blanco G, Alavaikko M, et al. Tumour DNA ploidy as an independent prognostic factor in breast cancer. *Br J Cancer* 1987;56:637–642.

344. Meyer JS, Coplin MD. Thymidine labeling index, flow cytometric S-phase measurement, and DNA index in human tumors. *Am J Clin Pathol* 1988;89:586–595.

345. Eliasen CA, Opitz LM, Vamvakas EC, et al. Flow cytometric analysis of DNA ploidy and S-phase fraction in breast cancer using cells obtained by ex vivo fine-needle aspiration: an optimal method for sample collection. *Mod Pathol* 1991;4:196–200.

346. Remvikos Y, Magdelenat H, Zajdela A. DNA flow cytometry applied to fine needle sampling of human breast cancer. *Cancer* 1988;61:1629–1634.

347. Fuhr JE, Frye A, Kattine AA, et al. Flow cytometric determination of breast tumor heterogeneity. *Cancer* 1991;67:1401–1405.

348. Meyer JS, Wittliff JL. Regional heterogeneity in breast carcinoma: thymidine labelling index, steroid hormone receptors, DNA ploidy. *Int J Cancer* 1991;47:213–220.

349. Mullen P, Miller WR. Variations associated with the DNA analysis of multiple fine needle aspirates obtained from breast cancer patients. *Br J Cancer* 1989;59:688–691.

350. Spyratos F, Briffod M, Tubiana-Hulin M, et al. Sequential cytopunctures during preoperative chemotherapy for primary breast carcinoma. II. DNA flow cytometry changes during chemotherapy, tumor regression, and short-term follow-up. *Cancer* 1992;69:470–475.

351. Kallioniemi O-P. Comparison of fresh and paraffin-embedded tissue as starting material for DNA flow cytometry and evaluation of intratumor heterogeneity. *Cytometry* 1988;9:164–169.

352. Feichter GE, Kaufmann M, Müller A, et al. DNA index and cell cycle analysis of primary breast cancer and synchronous axillary lymph node metastases. *Breast Cancer Res Treat* 1989;13:17–22.

353. Frierson Jr HF. Ploidy analysis and S-phase fraction determination by flow cytometry of invasive adenocarcinomas of the breast. *Am J Surg Pathol* 1991;15:358–367.

354. Batsakis JG, Sneige N, El-Naggar AK. Flow cytometric (DNA content and S-phase fraction) analysis of breast cancer. *Cancer* 1993;71:2151–2153.

355. Hedley DW, Clark GM, Cornelisse CJ, et al. Consensus review of the clinical utility of DNA cytometry in carcinoma of the breast. *Cytometry* 1993;14:482–485.

356. O'Reilly SM, Richards MA. Is DNA flow cytometry a useful investigation in breast cancer? *Eur J Cancer* 1992;28:504–507.

357. Ellis CN, Frey ES, Burnette JJ, et al. The content of tumor DNA as an indicator of prognosis in patients with T1N0M0 and T2N0M0 carcinoma of the breast. *Surgery* 1989;106:133–138.

358. Keyhani-Rofagha S, O'Toole RV, Farrar WB, et al. Is DNA ploidy an independent prognostic indicator in infiltrative node-negative breast adenocarcinoma? *Cancer* 1990;65:1577–1582.

359. Witzig TE, Ingle JN, Cha SS, et al. DNA ploidy and the percentage of cells in S-phase as a prognostic factors for women with lymph node negative breast cancer. *Cancer* 1994;74:1752–1761.

360. Toikkanen S, Joensuu J, Klemi P. Nuclear DNA content as a prognostic factor in T1-2N0 breast cancer. *Am J Clin Pathol* 1990;93:471–479.

361. Bergers E, Baak JPA, van Diest PJ, et al. Prognostic value of DNA ploidy using flow cytometry in 1301 breast cancer patients: results of the prospective multicenter morphometric mammary carcinoma project. *Mod Pathol* 1997;10:762–768.

362. Bosari S, Lee AKC, Tahan SR, et al. DNA flow cytometric analysis and prognosis of axillary lymph nodes-negative breast carcinoma. *Cancer* 1992;70:1943–1950.

363. Camplejohn RS, Ash CM, Gillett CE, et al. The prognostic significance of DNA flow cytometry in breast cancer: results from 881 patients treated in a single centre. *Br J Cancer* 1995;71:140–145.

364. Clark GM, Mathieu M-C, Owens MA, et al. Prognostic significance of S-phase fraction in good-risk, node-negative breast cancer patients. *J Clin Oncol* 1992;10:428–432.

365. Haffty BG, Toth M, Flynn S, et al. Prognostic value of DNA flow cytometry in the locally recurrent, conservatively treated breast cancer patient. *J Clin Oncol* 1992;10:1839–1847.

366. Stål O, Dufmats M, Hatschek T, et al. S-phase fraction is a prognostic factor in stage I breast carcinoma. *J Clin Oncol* 1993;11:1717–1722.

367. Stanton PD, Cooke TG, Oakes SJ, et al. Lack of prognostic significance of DNA ploidy and S phase fraction in breast cancer. *Br J Cancer* 1992;66:925–929.

368. Hietanen P, Blomqvist C, Wasenius V-M, et al. Do DNA ploidy and S-phase fraction in primary tumour predict the response to chemotherapy in metastatic breast cancer? *Br J Cancer* 1995;71:1029–1032.

369. Goodson WH III, Ljung B-M, Moore DH II, et al. Tumor labeling indices of primary breast cancers and their regional lymph node metastases. *Cancer* 1993;71:3914–3919.

370. Rew DA, Campbell ID, Taylor I, et al. Proliferation indices of invasive breast carcinomas after in vivo 5-bromo-2′-deoxyuridine labelling: a flow cytometric study of 75 tumours. *Br J Surg* 1992;79:335–339.

371. Weidner N, Moore DH II, Ljung B-M, et al. Correlation of bromodeoxyuridine (BRDU) labeling of breast carcinoma cells with mitotic figure content and tumor grade. *Am J Surg Pathol* 1993;17:987–994.

372. Meyer JS, Nauert J, Koehm S, et al. Cell kinetics of human tumors by in vitro bromodeoxyuridine labeling. *J Histochem Cytochem* 1989;37:1449–1454.

373. Thor AD, Liu S, Moore DH, et al. Comparison of mitotic index, in vitro bromodeoxyuridine labeling, and MIB-1 assays to quantitate proliferation in breast cancer. *J Clin Oncol* 1999;17:470–477.

374. Gratzner HG. Monoclonal antibody to 5-bromo- and 5-iododeoxyuridine: a new reagent for detection of DNA replication. *Science* 1982;218:474–475.

375. Lloveras B, Edgerton S, Thor AD. Evaluation of in vitro bromodeoxyuridine labeling of breast carcinomas with the use of a commercial kit. *Am J Clin Pathol* 1991;95:41–47.

376. Sasaki K, Ogino T, Takahashi M. Immunological determination of labelling index on human tumor tissue sections using monoclonal anti-BrdU antibody. *Stain Technol* 1986;61:155–161.

377. Meyer JS, Koehm SL, Hughes JM, et al. Bromodeoxyuridine labeling for S-phase measurement in breast carcinoma. *Cancer* 1993;71:3531–3540.

378. Gerdes J, Schwab U, Lemke H, et al. Production of a mouse monoclonal antibody reactive with a human nuclear antigen associated with cell proliferation. *Int J Cancer* 1983;31:13–20.

379. Gerdes J, Lemke H, Baisch H, et al. Cell cycle analysis of cell proliferation-associated human nuclear antigen defined by the monoclonal antibody Ki-67. *J Immunol* 1984;133:1710–1715.

380. Isola JJ, Helin HJ, Helle MJ, et al. Evaluation of cell proliferation in breast carcinoma. Comparison of Ki-67 immunohistochemical study, DNA flow cytometric analysis, and mitotic count. *Cancer* 1990;65:1180–1184.

381. Sahin AA, Ro JY, El-Naggar AK, et al. Tumor proliferative fraction in solid malignant neoplasms. A comparative study of Ki-67 immunostaining and flow cytometric determinations. *Am J Clin Pathol* 1991;96:512–519.

382. Vielh P, Chevillard S, Mosseri V, et al. Ki67 index and S-phase fraction in human breast carcinomas. Comparison and correlations with prognostic factors. *Am J Clin Pathol* 1990;94:681–686.

383. Kamel OW, Franklin WA, Ringus JC, et al. Thymidine labeling index and Ki-67 growth fraction in lesions of the breast. *Am J Pathol* 1989;134:107–113.

384. Sasaki K, Matsumura K, Tsuji T, et al. Relationship between labeling indices of Ki-67 and BrdU in human malignant tumors. *Cancer* 1988;62:989–993.

385. Barbareschi M, Girlando S, Mauri FM, et al. Quantitative growth fraction evaluation with MIB1 and Ki67 antibodies in breast carcinomas. *Am J Clin Pathol* 1994;102:171–175.

386. Sahin AA, Ro J, Ro JY, et al. Ki-67 immunostaining in node-negative stage I/II breast carcinoma. Significant correlation with prognosis. *Cancer* 1991;68:549–557.

387. van Dierendonck JH, Keijzer R, van de Velde CJH, et al. Nuclear distribution of the Ki-67 antigen during the cell cycle: comparison with growth fraction in human breast cancer cells. *Cancer Res* 1989;49:2999–3006.

388. Dervan PA, Magee HM, Buckley C, et al. Proliferating cell nuclear antigen counts in formalin-fixed paraffin-embedded tissue correlate with Ki-67 in fresh tissue. *Am J Clin Pathol* 1992;97[Suppl 1]:S21–S28.

389. Raymond WA, Leong AS-Y. Nuclear organizer regions relate to growth fractions in human breast carcinoma. *Hum Pathol* 1989;20:741–746.

390. Gerdes J, Lelle RJ, Pickartz H, et al. Growth fractions in breast cancers determined in situ with monoclonal antibody Ki-67. *J Clin Pathol* 1986;39:977–980.

391. Kuenen-Boumeester V, Van Der Kwast TH, Van Laarhoven HAJ, et al. Ki-67 staining in histologic subtypes of breast carcinoma and fine needle aspiration smears. *J Clin Pathol* 1991;44:208–210.

392. Veronese SM, Gambacorta M. Detection of Ki-67 proliferation rate in breast cancer. Correlation with clinical and pathologic features. *Am J Clin Pathol* 1991;95:30–34.

393. Bouzubar N, Walker KJ, Griffiths K, et al. Ki67 immunostaining in primary breast cancer: pathological and clinical associations. *Br J Cancer* 1989;59:943–947.

394. Lelle RJ, Heidenreich W, Stauch G, et al. The correlation of growth fractions with histologic grading and lymph node status in human mammary carcinoma. *Cancer* 1987;59:83–88.

395. Weikel W, Beck T, Mitze M, et al. Immunohistochemical evaluation of growth fractions in human breast cancers using monoclonal antibody Ki-67. *Breast Cancer Res Treat* 1991;18:149–154.

396. Pierga J-Y, Leroyer A, Viehl P, et al. Long term prognostic value of growth fraction determination by Ki-67 immunostaining in primary operable breast cancer. *Breast Cancer Res Treat* 1996;37:57–64.

397. Porter PL, El-Bastawissi AY, Mandelson MT, et al. Breast tumor characteristics as predictors of mammographic detection: comparison of interval- and screen-detected cancers. *J Natl Cancer Inst* 1999;91:2020–2028.

398. Cattoretti G, Becker MH, Key G, et al. Monoclonal antibodies against recombinant parts of the Ki-67 antigen (MIB 1 and MIB 3) detect proliferating cells in microwave-processed formalin-fixed paraffin sections. *J Pathol* 1992;168:357–363.

399. McCormick D, Chong H, Hobbs C, et al. Detection of the Ki-67 antigen in fixed and wax-embedded sections with the monoclonal antibody MIB1. *Histopathology* 1993;22:355–360.

400. Remmele W, Mühlfait V, Keul HG. Estimation of the proliferative activity of human breast cancer tissue by means of the Ki-67 and MIB-1 antibodies—comparative studies on frozen and paraffin sections. *Virchows Arch* 1995;426:435–439.

401. Keshgegian AA, Cnaan A. Proliferation markers in breast carcinoma. Mitotic figure count, S-phase fraction, proliferating cell nuclear antigen, Ki-67 and MIB1. *Am J Clin Pathol* 1995;104:42–49.

402. Pinder SE, Wencyk P, Sibbering DM, et al. Assessment of the new proliferation marker MIB1 in breast carcinoma using image analysis: associations with other prognostic factors and survival. *Br J Cancer* 1995;71:146–149.

403. Arber JM, Riggs MW, Arber DA. Correlation among MIB-1, paraffin section proliferation index, and recurrence in low stage breast carcinoma. *Appl Immunohistochem* 1997;5:117–124.

404. Umemura S, Komaki K, Noguchi S, et al. Prognostic factors for node-negative breast cancers: results of a study program by the Japanese Breast Cancer Society. *Breast Cancer* 1998;5:243–249.

405. Domagala W, Markiewski M, Harezga B, et al. Prognostic significance of tumor cell proliferation rate as determined by the MIB-1 antibody in breast carcinoma: its relationship with vimentin and p53 protein. *Clin Cancer Res* 1996;2:147–154.

406. Visscher DW, Wykes S, Kubus J, et al. Comparison of PCNA/cyclin immunohistochemistry with flow cytometric S-phase fraction in breast cancer. *Breast Cancer Res Treat* 1992;22:111–118.

407. Frierson HF Jr. Immunohistochemical analysis of proliferating cell nuclear antigen (PCNA) in infiltrating ductal carcinomas: comparison with clinical and pathologic variable. *Mod Pathol* 1993;6:290–294.

408. Tahan SR, Neuberg DS, Dieffenbach A, et al. Prediction of early relapse and shortened survival in patients with breast cancer by proliferating cell nuclear antigen score. *Cancer* 1993;71:3552–3559.

409. Haerslev T, Jacobsen GK, Zedeler K. Correlation of growth fraction by Ki-67 and proliferating cell nuclear antigen (PCNA) immunohistochemistry with histopathological parameters and prognosis in primary breast carcinomas. *Breast Cancer Res Treat* 1996;37:101–113.

410. Clark GM, Allred DC, Hilsenbeck SG, et al. Mitosin (a new proliferation marker) correlates with clinical outcome in node-negative breast cancer. *Cancer Res* 1997;57:5505–5508.

411. Baak JPA, VanDop H, Kurver PHJ, et al. The value of morphometry to classic prognosticators in breast cancer. *Cancer* 1985;56:374–382.

412. Kuenen-Boumeester V, Hop WCJ, Blonk DE, et al. Prognostic scoring using cytomorphometry and lymph node status of patients with breast carcinoma. *Eur J Cancer Clin Oncol* 1984;20:337–345.

413. Stenkvist B, Bengtsson E, Eriksson O, et al. Correlation between cytometric features and mitotic frequency in human breast carcinoma. *Cytometry* 1981;1:287–291.

414. Zajdela A, DeLaRiva LS, Ghossein NA. The relation of prognosis to the nuclear diameter of breast cancer cells obtained by cytologic aspiration. *Acta Cytol* 1979;23:75–80.

415. Maehle B, Thoresen S, Skjaerve R, et al. Mean nuclear area and histological grade of axillary node tumor in breast cancer. Relation to prognosis. *Br J Cancer* 1982;46:95–100.

416. van der Linden HC, Baak JPA, Lindeman J, et al. Morphometry and breast cancer. II. Characterization of breast cancer cells with high malignant potential in patients with spread to lymph nodes: preliminary results. *J Clin Pathol* 1986;39:603–609.

# CHAPTER 15

# Tubular Carcinoma

Tubular carcinoma has been appreciated as a distinctive type of mammary carcinoma for more than a century (1). It has been described in the World Health Organization (WHO) monograph on the histologic classification of breast tumors as "a highly differentiated invasive carcinoma whose cells are regular and arranged in well-defined tubules typically one layer thick and surrounded by an abundant fibrous stroma" (2). The term "tubular" refers to the microscopic feature that defines the lesion, namely, the formation of neoplastic tubules that closely resemble breast ductules (3,4). The WHO monograph states that "tubular carcinoma should not be confused with invasive ductal carcinomas with gland-like structures whose cells are less well-differentiated" (2).

Tubular elements can be found focally in many infiltrating duct carcinomas, but few tumors are composed entirely of these structures, representing "pure" tubular carcinomas. Carcinomas with a tubular element forming part of the tumor have been termed duct carcinomas with tubular features or "mixed tubular" carcinomas. Currently, the preferred term is "duct carcinoma with tubular features." The minimum proportion of tubular growth necessary for inclusion in this category varies among published reports; consequently, "mixed tubular" carcinoma is a poorly defined diagnostic term.

Pure tubular carcinoma constitutes less than 2% of all breast carcinomas (5–9). Because they tend to be small, tubular carcinomas are relatively more frequent in reports of T1 breast carcinomas. In one series, 5% of 382 T1N0M0 breast carcinomas were classified as tubular (10). When further stratified by size, 9% of lesions 1.0 cm or smaller were tubular, which is a substantially higher proportion than the 2% of tubular carcinomas among tumors that measured 1.1 to 2.0 cm. Tubular carcinoma was uncommon among women with T1N1M0 disease (1.5% of 142 patients), because axillary metastases infrequently arise from these tumors (11).

Tubular carcinomas are encountered with increasing frequency as a result of the growing use of mammography. Although often quite small and nonpalpable, tubular carcinomas have structural features that render the lesions detectable by mammography. As a result, 8% of invasive carcinomas 1.0 cm or less in diameter detected in the Breast Cancer Detection Demonstration Projects were of the tubular variety (12). In one screening program in the United States, 7% of 138 carcinomas were tubular. All of the tubular carcinomas were detected by mammography, but only 30% also were evident clinically (13). Swedish investigators reported finding 25 pure tubular carcinomas among 116 carcinomas (21.5%) detected by mammography (14).

Mammographic findings may be suggestive of tubular carcinoma. In one study, the average radiographic size of tubular carcinomas was 0.8 cm in patients with nonpalpable lesions and 1.2 cm when the lesions were palpable (15). Most tubular carcinomas are spiculated and lack calcifications (Fig. 15.1) (16). Rounded lesions, densities with indistinct borders or calcifications in the absence of a mass, rarely prove to be tubular carcinoma. Difficulty in distinguishing tubular carcinoma from radial scar has been reported, because both lesions have similar growth patterns and tubular carcinoma may arise in a radial scar (17,18). Ultrasonography is helpful for detecting tubular carcinoma, especially small lesions that are not apparent on mammography (19).

## CLINICAL PRESENTATION

Unusual examples of tubular carcinoma of the male breast have been reported (20–22). These lesions constitute not more than 1% of male breast carcinomas (23,24).

Among women, the age at diagnosis ranges from 24 to 92 years (8,9,20,21,25). The age distribution is not exceptional. Occasionally, a palpable lesion reportedly has been present for a substantial period before biopsy or a relatively long duration can be established by retrospective review of mammograms. The median duration prior to histologic diagnosis is about 2 months (20,21,25). Superficial tumors may be fixed to the skin, producing retraction signs in about 15% of cases. Tubular carcinoma usually occurs in peripheral portions of the breast; as a consequence, nipple discharge is rarely a symptom (8). However, tubular carcinoma can arise from the major lactiferous ducts in the nipple or slightly lower in the subareolar region. In this setting, tubular carcinoma may be difficult to distinguish from florid papillomatosis of the

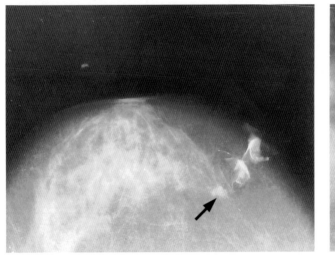
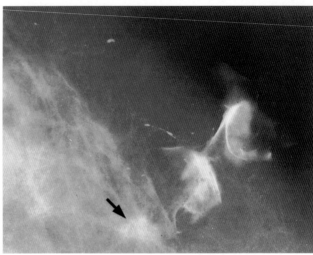

**FIG. 15.1.** *Tubular carcinoma.* **A:** Mammogram showing a nonpalpable tumor near the right border of the breast parenchyma (*arrow*). **B:** Magnified view of the stellate carcinoma near the lower border of the image (*arrow*) and two wisps of dye injected for surgical localization.

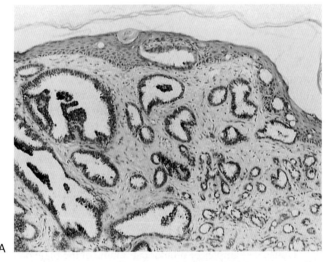
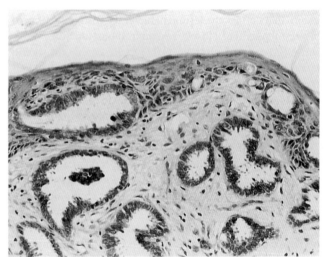
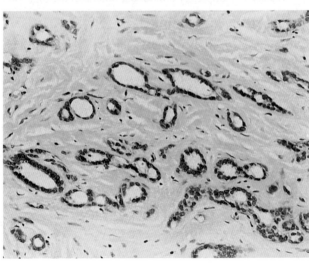

**FIG. 15.2.** *Tubular carcinoma in the nipple.* **A:** Invasive glands of tubular carcinoma in the nipple extending to the epidermis. **B:** Paget's disease composed of tubular carcinoma glands. **C:** Typical tubular carcinoma glands of the type seen in the lower right-hand corner of **A**.

nipple. The finding of Paget's disease supports the diagnosis of tubular carcinoma in this setting (Fig. 15.2), but Paget's disease usually is absent in patients with tubular carcinoma.

Tubular carcinoma was associated with a 40% frequency of positive family history of breast carcinoma among first-degree relatives in one study (26). This may reflect selective factors related to the specific population studied, which included many women who had mammography performed because they had a positive family history. Others have not found a disproportionately high frequency of positive family history among relatives of women treated for tubular carcinoma.

When studied by immunohistochemistry or biochemically, more than 90% of tubular carcinomas have been positive for estrogen receptor (27–30). Nuclear reactivity for progesterone receptor has been detected in 69% to 75% of tubular carcinomas (30,31). The tumors also rarely express MIB1, a marker of proliferative activity, and fewer than 5% are positive for HER2/*neu* or p53 (31).

## GROSS PATHOLOGY

Most tubular carcinomas are 2 cm or less in diameter, but they have been described as large as 4 cm (5,7,8,20,21,25); in one study, the largest tumor was 12 cm (32). In some instances, tumors reported to be larger than 5 cm may be examples of coalescent multifocal lesions. Two studies reported that 80% (21) and 87% (20) of tubular carcinomas were 1 cm or smaller. In the latter study, the median size of 90 "pure" tubular carcinomas was 0.8 cm. Fifty-two percent of duct carcinomas with tubular features were 1 cm or less. The median size of mixed duct and tubular lesions was 1.1 cm.

Tubular carcinoma is grossly an ill-defined firm or hard tumor. When bisected, the lesion often is stellate, and the cut surface is likely to retract, becoming depressed in relation to the surrounding noncarcinomatous tissue. Most tumors are described as gray to white. Lesions that appear tan or pale yellow tend to have extensive elastosis microscopically. The gross appearance may suggest tubular carcinoma, but without microscopic examination it is impossible to rule out a benign lesion such as sclerosing papillomatosis with a radial scar pattern or a less well-differentiated invasive carcinoma.

## MICROSCOPIC PATHOLOGY

Microscopically, tubular carcinoma is composed of small glands or tubules. The distribution of these neoplastic structures is largely haphazard, although the overall configuration tends to be stellate and has ill-defined borders. The glands of a tubular carcinoma are composed of a single layer of neoplastic epithelial cells, and they can have virtually any shape (Fig. 15.3). In very well-differentiated small tumors less than 1 cm, the lesion may be composed of round or oval glands of relatively uniform caliber that resemble microglandular adenosis (Fig. 15.4) (33). However, microglandular adenosis typically has a diffuse infiltrative growth pattern, rather than the localized growth found in tubular carcinoma. It is helpful to seek areas of intraductal carcinoma to establish a diagnosis of tubular carcinoma in this situation. A very uncommon variant of tubular carcinoma features mucin secretion (Fig. 15.5).

Most often, the glands of tubular carcinoma have irregular shapes and angular contours, leading one to consider the distinction between tubular carcinoma and sclerosing adenosis. The proliferative pattern of sclerosing adenosis is lobulocentric. At low magnification, it is almost always possible to perceive individual altered lobules even when the proliferation is so florid as to form a mass composed of coalescent lobules. Tubular carcinoma does not have a lobulocentric configuration, although it can be multicentric (discussed later).

At higher magnification, individual foci of sclerosing

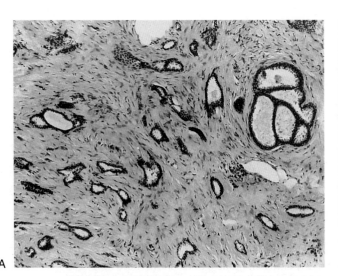
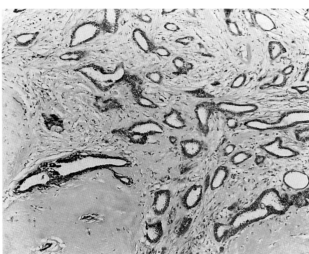

A                                                                                          B

**FIG. 15.3.** *Tubular carcinoma.* Various glandular patterns. **A:** Oval and angular glands in moderately cellular stroma. Note one duct with intraductal carcinoma on the *right*. **B:** Angular, oval, and tubular glands. *(continued)*

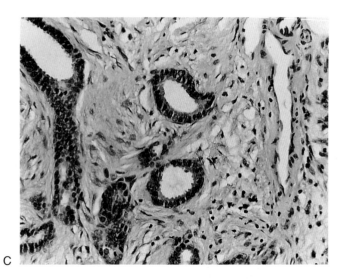

C

**FIG. 15.3.** *Continued.* **C:** Round, angular, and tubular glands lined by regular cuboidal cells that have low-grade nuclei.

adenosis are composed of compact whorled, elongated, and largely compressed glands with interlacing spindly myoepithelial cells. Varying numbers of round, oval, or angular glands with open lumens usually are dispersed in these foci. Proliferation of myoepithelial cells is a regular concomitant of sclerosing adenosis, but these cells are absent in tubular carcinoma. Whereas myoepithelial cells usually are readily evident in routine sections stained with hematoxylin and eosin, it is helpful to use immunohistochemical reagents when dealing with a particularly difficult problem. Myoepithelial cells are not present in tubular carcinomas. An actin immunostain is more reliable than S-100 or 34BE12 (K903) stains to demonstrate the absence of myoepithelial cells in this situation (34). Proliferation of myofibroblasts may make it difficult to demonstrate the absence of myoepithelial cells in a tubular carcinoma. The immunostains for smooth muscle myosin heavy chain and calponin are helpful in this cir-

cumstance, because they are relatively specific for myoepithelial cells and exhibit little or no reactivity with myofibroblasts (Fig. 15.6) (35).

Histochemical studies have documented the presence of basement membranes around the glands in sclerosing adenosis and incomplete or absent basement membrane constituents in tubular carcinoma (Fig. 15.7). Laminin, type IV collagen, and basement membrane proteoglycan were not detected in one series of nine tubular carcinomas (36), and other investigators also failed to find laminin (37) and type IV collagen (34) around the neoplastic glands of tubular carcinoma.

Maspin, a protease inhibitor in the serpin family, is highly expressed in myoepithelial cells. Immunoreactivity for maspin is present as a distinct ring around glandular structures in sclerosing adenosis and benign radial sclerosing lesions, a pattern not seen in tubular carcinoma (37a). Rarely,

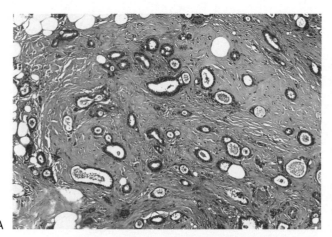

A

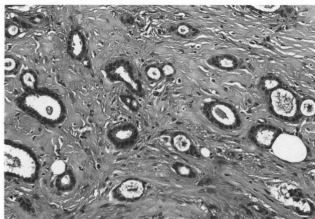

B

**FIG. 15.4.** *Tubular carcinoma.* **A,B:** Round or oval, orderly carcinomatous glands shown here resemble glands found in microglandular adenosis. Note evidence of stromal elastosis, which is not a feature of microglandular adenosis, and myofibroblastic proliferation in the stroma.

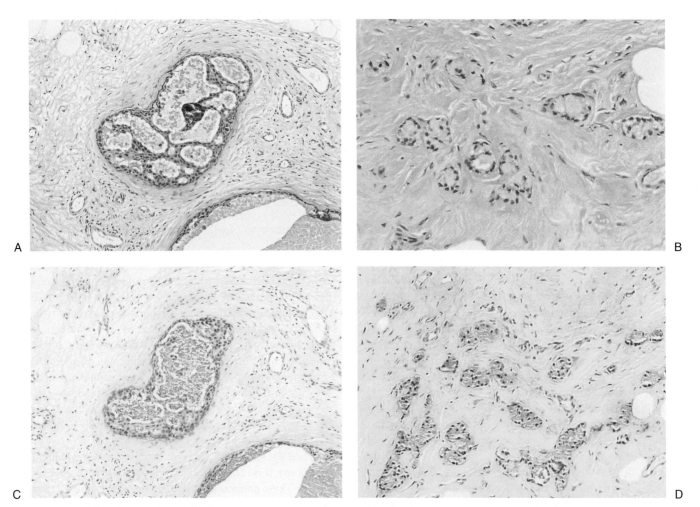

**FIG. 15.5.** *Tubular carcinoma, mucin forming.* **A:** Intraductal carcinoma associated with the tubular carcinoma. **B:** Invasive glands have clear cytoplasm and resemble microglandular adenosis. **C,D:** Mucin in the intraductal and infiltrating carcinoma stains pink with the mucicarmine stain.

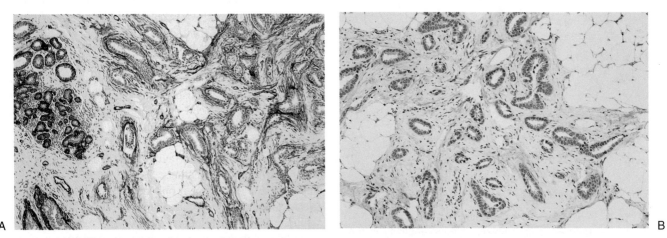

**FIG. 15.6.** *Tubular carcinoma.* **A:** Immunostain for smooth muscle actin shows reactivity in myoepithelial cells around lobular glands in adenosis *(left)* and in myofibroblasts in the carcinoma *(right)*. **B:** No reactivity is seen when the same tumor is stained for smooth muscle myosin heavy chain. *(continued)*

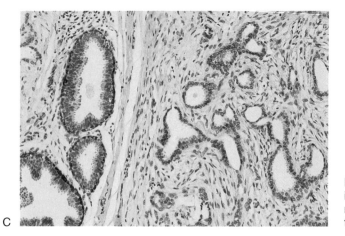

C

**FIG. 15.6.** *Continued.* **C:** Another specimen in which myoepithelial cells around ducts are stained for smooth muscle myosin heavy chain *(left)* and reactivity is absent from the tubular carcinoma *(right)* (all avidin-biotin).

the glandular elements in tubular carcinoma display cytoplasmic maspin immunoreactivity (37a).

The cells in tubular carcinoma glands usually are homogeneous in a given lesion. They may be cuboidal or columnar, with round or oval hyperchromatic nuclei that tend to be basally oriented (Fig. 15.8). Nucleoli are inconspicuous or inapparent. Mitoses are rarely seen. "Apocrine"-type cytoplasmic tufts or "snouts" usually are present at the luminal cell border (38). The cytoplasm usually is amphophilic or infrequently clear. Distinctly eosinophilic apocrine cytoplasmic staining rarely occurs in a pure tubular carcinoma.

The diagnosis of tubular carcinoma is made when virtually all of the tumor exhibits the tubular growth pattern. When tubular components are found in a carcinoma that does not fulfill this quantitative criterion, the lesion has been described as a duct carcinoma with tubular features. The latter tumors form a heterogeneous group with respect to the proportion of the tubular component and the degree of differentiation of the nontubular element (Fig. 15.9).

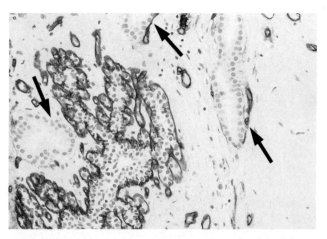

**FIG. 15.7.** *Tubular carcinoma.* Section stained with an anti-type IV collagen antibody reveals immunoreactivity in the basement membranes of lobular glands on the *left* and very faint reactivity around carcinomatous glands *(arrows)* (avidin-biotin).

In nontubular well-differentiated duct carcinoma, the pattern of glandular growth is largely tubular, but in part the epithelial proliferation tends to be more florid than in typical tubular carcinoma. As a consequence, the epithelial lining of the glands may be more than one cell thick. Some glands develop micropapillae, transluminal bridging, or microgland structures (Figs. 15.10 and 15.11). An occasional mitotic figure may be encountered, and there is a slight tendency to cytologic pleomorphism. The intraductal component is more likely to be cribriform than micropapillary in well-differentiated nontubular duct carcinoma.

When the tumor has areas of invasive lobular and tubular carcinoma, it is referred to as *tubulolobular carcinoma* (Fig. 15.12). These patients are more likely to have axillary lymph node metastases than women with pure tubular carcinoma, and they have a prognosis between that of pure tubular and invasive lobular carcinoma (39). Almost all tubulolobular carcinomas are immunoreactive for estrogen and progesterone receptors (40).

The precise position of tubulolobular carcinoma in the classification of breast carcinomas is uncertain. When studied by comparative genomic hybridization, a "high degree of genetic homology" was observed between lobular carcinoma *in situ* and well differentiated intraductal carcinoma, an observation which led the investigators to speculate that the two lesions might be "different phenotypic forms of a common genotype" (40a). Such a phenomenon is supported not only by the existence of the hybrid tubulolobular carcinoma phenotype, but also by the frequent coexistence of low-grade columnar cell ductal proliferations with lobular carcinoma *in situ* and tubular carcinoma (40b).

Tubulolobular carcinoma has been regarded as a variant of tubular carcinoma by some authors and as a form of invasive lobular carcinoma by others. As greater experience with tubulolobular carcinoma is obtained, it is likely to emerge as a separate subtype of mammary carcinoma, distinct from tubular and invasive lobular carcinoma. Presently, patients with tubulolobular carcinoma should be viewed as having a good prognosis, but not in the exceptionally favorable category of pure tubular carcinoma.

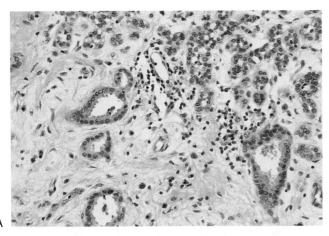

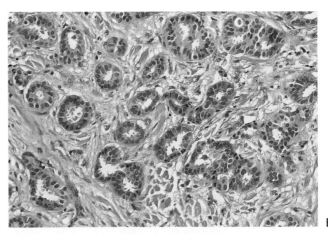

**FIG. 15.8.** *Tubular carcinoma.* **A:** Four round and angular carcinoma glands are shown near sclerosing adenosis *(upper right).* The carcinoma cells form a single cell layer with luminal apical "snouts." **B:** This tubular carcinoma exhibits cellular crowding with a few secondary microlumens and prominent apical "tufts."

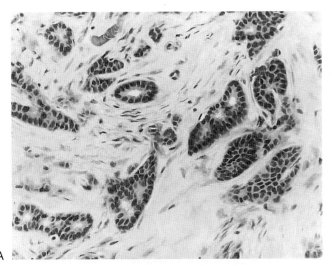

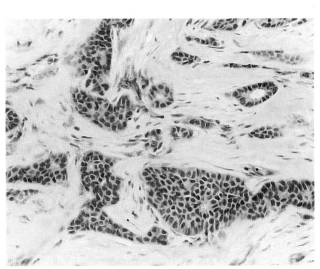

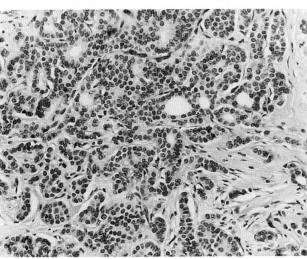

**FIG. 15.9.** *Duct carcinoma with tubular features.* Two histologic patterns. **A,B:** Areas in a tumor with some tubular glands and foci with trabecular growth. This tumor qualified as a well-differentiated duct carcinoma. **C:** Another tumor with a more complex glandular pattern. This carcinoma should be classified as a moderately differentiated duct carcinoma.

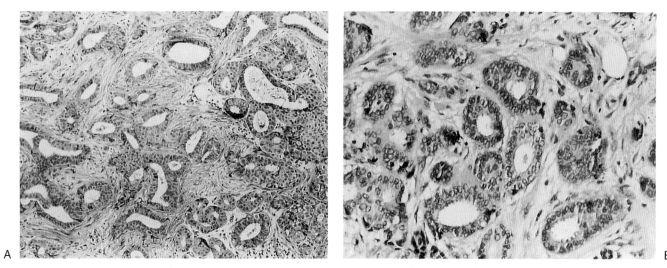

**FIG. 15.10.** *Well-differentiated invasive duct carcinoma.* **A:** Carcinoma with tubular-type glands, some of which have transluminal epithelial bridges and multilayered epithelium. **B:** Multilayered epithelium is present in some glands.

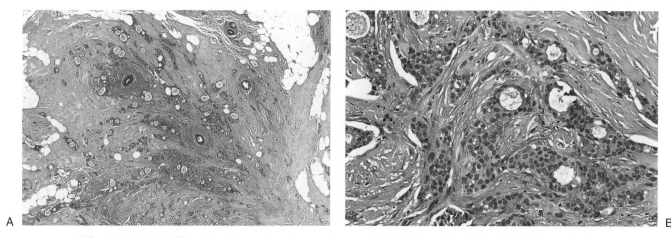

**FIG. 15.11.** *Well-differentiated invasive duct carcinoma.* **A,B:** Carcinoma with a radial sclerosing configuration. Basophilia of the stroma is due to elastosis.

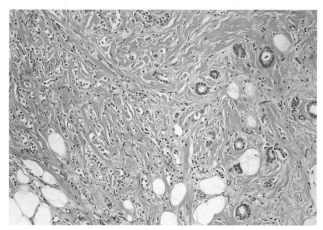

**FIG. 15.12.** *Tubulolobular carcinoma.* Invasive carcinoma with linear growth pattern and signet-ring cells of lobular carcinoma *(left)* and the round glands of tubular carcinoma *(right).*

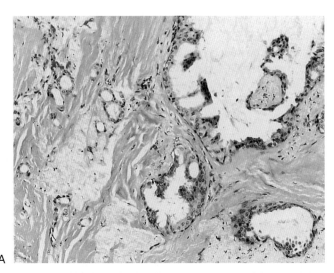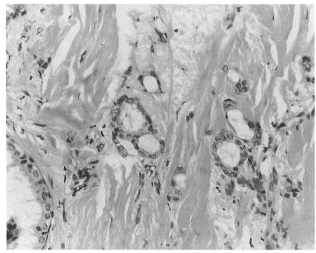

A  B

**FIG. 15.13.** *Tubular carcinoma.* **A:** Micropapillary intraductal carcinoma in the *upper right* and invasive glands of tubular carcinoma on the *left*. The pale stromal material is elastosis. **B:** Tubular carcinoma glands and elastosis.

Stroma between the glands in tubular carcinoma often appears different from stroma in the surrounding breast due to the presence of altered collagenous tissue that also may contain myofibroblasts, abundant elastic tissue, and myxoid matrix material (Figs. 15.4, 15.11, and 15.13) (41,42). Elastosis has been regarded as a hallmark of tubular carcinoma (41,42), but it is not present in all cases. It can be a prominent feature of nontubular carcinomas and some benign lesions, particularly those with the "radial scar" pattern.

Calcifications are reportedly found microscopically in at least 50% of tubular carcinomas. They may be distributed in the neoplastic glands, in the stroma, or in the intraductal carcinoma component. Intraductal carcinoma has been described in 60% to 84% of tubular carcinomas (7,20,21,43). With careful and thorough histologic examination it is possible to find intraductal carcinoma in the majority of tubular

carcinomas. It typically has papillary or cribriform patterns or a mixture of the two (20) (Figs. 15.13–15.16). Micropapillary intraductal carcinoma is especially common and sometimes the growth pattern of the intraductal carcinoma is so orderly that it is mistaken for hyperplasia. In some instances, tubular carcinoma appears to arise from or in association with a benign proliferative lesion with a radial scar configuration (44,45).

Tubular and tubulolobular carcinoma frequently arise in breast tissue that is the site of a multifocal, distinctive proliferation in terminal duct-lobular units and ducts previously designated informally as "pretubular" hyperplasia and now referred to as columnar cell change. A spectrum of proliferation occurs in columnar cell change, ranging from simple hyperplasia (columnar cell hyperplasia [CCH]) through CCH with atypia to intraductal carcinoma. Cystic dilation

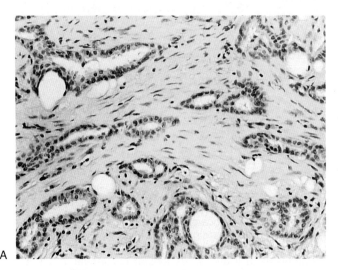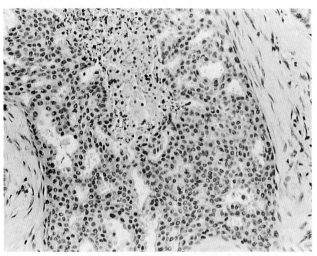

A  B

**FIG. 15.14.** *Tubular carcinoma.* **A:** Invasive component. **B:** Cribriform intraductal carcinoma in the tumor.

often accompanies these epithelial alterations, especially in terminal duct-lobular units where the condition seems to arise. Goldstein and O'Malley (46) referred to carcinoma in this setting as "cancerization of small ectatic ducts of the breast by ductal carcinoma *in situ* cells with apocrine snouts." Features common to all phases of CCH are nuclear hyperchromasia, a high nuclear-to-cytoplasmic ratio, and apocrine snouts at the luminal borders of ducts and ductules. The lesions are prone to develop calcifications. The most subtle expression of this condition is formed by cuboidal or low columnar cells with the foregoing cytologic features distributed in a single layer. Progressive hyperplasia is marked by crowding of cells that become increasingly compressed, columnar, and come to have nuclei distributed in a haphazard pattern with respect to the basement membrane. The presence of blunt micropapillae or cribriform growth composed of the same proliferative cells with "streaming" or condensation of cells toward the lumen is indicative of atypical CCH.

When encountered, "flat" micropapillary carcinoma is found in a background of CCH. The lesion is characterized by a nearly flat growth of neoplastic cells lacking polarity with respect to the basement membrane. The tumor cells have intermediate to poorly differentiated nuclear grade, and mitoses usually are evident. Conventional micropapillary intraductal carcinoma forming micropapillae of variable

height, arcades, and cribriform microlumens occur more frequently in CCH associated with tubular carcinoma than does "flat" micropapillary intraductal carcinoma.

Columnar cell lesions are associated with lobular carcinoma *in situ* as well as tubular carcinoma (Fig. 15.15). Because CCH is prone to develop calcifications, often at multiple sites, it is a relatively common finding in needle core biopsy samples from women with nonpalpable mammographically detected calcifications. Excisional biopsy should be performed after a needle core biopsy diagnosis of CCH with atypia or if the follow-up mammogram shows residual calcifications. Partially sampled surgical biopsies that harbor CCH should be entirely submitted for histologic examination. Additional discussion and illustrations of CCH can be found in Chapter 9.

Coexistent lobular carcinoma *in situ* has been described in 0.7% to 40% of patients with tubular carcinoma (7,20, 21,25). In retrospect, a subset of these lesions would be classified now as tubulolobular carcinoma (39). When present, lobular carcinoma *in situ* usually is found in the vicinity of the invasive tubular lesion. but it also has been identified separately in the same breast or in the contralateral breast. Foci of atypical lobular hyperplasia also are not unusual in association with, or in the absence of, fully developed *in situ* lobular carcinoma. Lobular proliferative lesions are encountered so commonly in association with tubular and tubu-

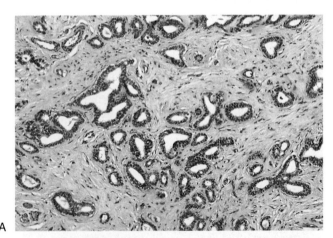

A

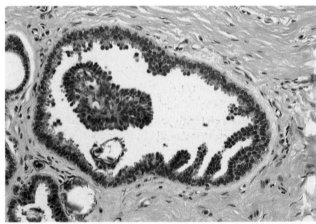

B

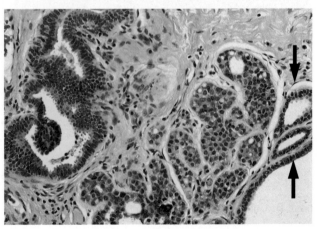

C

**FIG. 15.15.** *Tubular carcinoma.* All images are from a single case. **A:** Tubular carcinoma. **B:** Micropapillary intraductal carcinoma with calcifications *(lower left).* **C:** Columnar cell hyperplasia in a duct *(left),* lobular carcinoma *in situ* with signet ring cells *(right center),* and two tubular carcinoma glands *(arrows).*

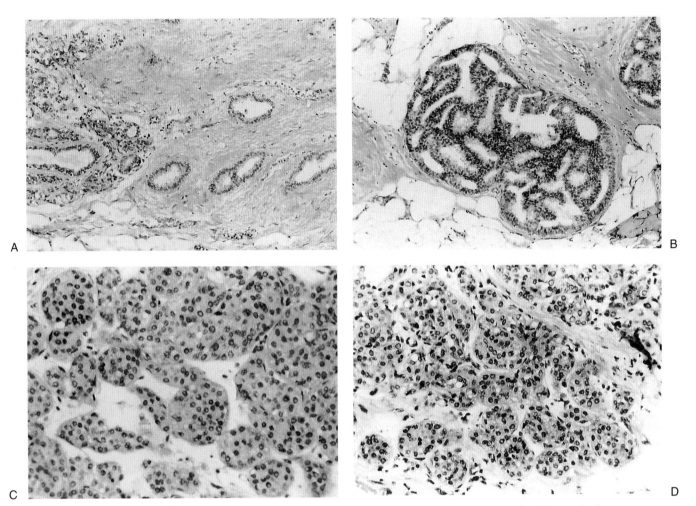

**FIG. 15.16.** *Tubular carcinoma.* **A:** Invasive tubular carcinoma. **B:** Papillary intraductal carcinoma in the same tumor. **C:** Lobular carcinoma *in situ* near the tubular carcinoma. **D:** Atypical lobular hyperplasia.

lolobular carcinoma that their presence may be regarded as secondary evidence supporting a diagnosis of tubular carcinoma (Fig. 15.16).

Tubular carcinoma does not elicit a notable lymphocytic reaction. Perineural invasion is uncommon (Fig. 15.17).

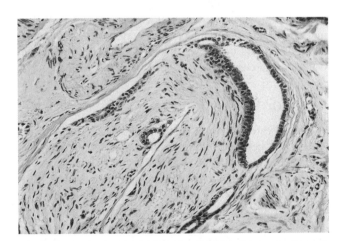

**FIG. 15.17.** *Tubular carcinoma.* Perineural invasion is evident around the perimeter of the nerve and one carcinomatous gland is present in the nerve.

Blood vessel invasion and lymphatic tumor emboli are virtually never seen, except after needling procedures (Fig. 15.18).

Tubular carcinoma usually is considered a unicentric lesion. Most patients present with a single mass detected by palpation or by mammography. When studied pathologically, 10% to 20% of patients are found to have multifocal tubular carcinoma lesions growing as separate foci in one or more quadrants (19,39). Multifocality is encountered in nearly 30% of patients with tubulolobular carcinoma (39). These are not intramammary metastases, because associated lymphatic tumor emboli are not found and intraductal carcinoma often is present in the individual carcinomatous areas. Associated multiple foci of CCH may be the source of multifocal tubular carcinoma.

The frequency and prognostic significance of this multifocal variant have not been carefully evaluated. Several studies have described multifocal carcinoma in patients with tubular carcinoma. The data in these reports are difficult to evaluate, because some authors incorrectly tabulated the intraductal portion of the tubular carcinoma as if it were a separate carcinoma. However, 10% to 56% of tubular carcinoma patients reportedly had independent foci of carcinoma

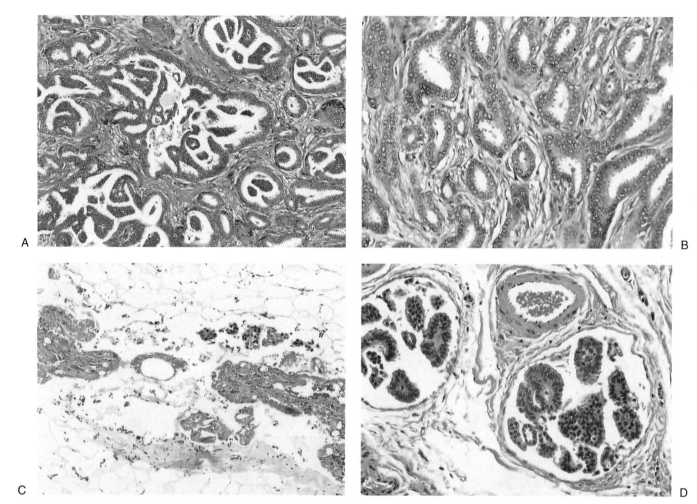

**FIG. 15.18.** *Tubular carcinoma, needling effect.* **A:** The intraductal component is papillary. **B:** Tubular carcinoma. **C:** Displaced epithelium in the needle track with hemorrhage. **D:** Clusters of carcinoma cells in dilated vascular channels, probably derived from the papillary intraductal component.

elsewhere in the same breast (7,20,25,26,43) consisting of various types of *in situ* and invasive carcinoma. Twenty (16.7%) of 120 patients treated by mastectomy had tubular carcinoma remaining at the biopsy site, six (5%) had a second separate infiltrating carcinoma, four (3.3%) had multifocal intraductal carcinoma, and three (2.5%) had lobular carcinoma *in situ* (20). Mitnick et al. (19) found invasive lobular carcinoma in 7% of patients with tubular carcinoma.

The reported frequency of contralateral carcinoma varies from 0% to 38% (8,20,21,25,26,29). Despite the relatively common coexistence of tubular and *in situ* lobular carcinoma, most contralateral tumors have been described as infiltrating duct carcinomas. Bilateral tubular carcinoma is uncommon (8,25,43).

## ELECTRON MICROSCOPY

Electron microscopy typically demonstrates uniform cells that form a single layer but may be slightly stratified within the neoplastic gland. Myoepithelial cells are scarce or not seen (47,48). Observations regarding the basal lamina have

not been consistent, but it is generally described as absent, incompletely formed, or discontinuous (47,48). Microvilli are seen at the luminal cell surface. The tumor cells are joined by numerous desmosomes and well-formed terminal bars. The cytoplasm contains mitochondria, rough endoplasmic reticulum, tonofilaments that may have a perinuclear distribution, and occasional cytoplasmic secretory lumina. Collagen and elastic fibers are present in the stroma.

## CYTOLOGY

Tubular carcinomas are characterized cytologically by the presence of cells exhibiting mild-to-moderate atypia, often in angular groups or singly (49,50). A lumen may be seen in the cell cluster. Tubular clusters and fragments with a cribriform structure may be present. The latter probably arise from associated intraductal carcinoma. The chromatin pattern of the carcinoma cells is bland in most cases, but fine chromatin clumps and small nucleoli sometimes are encountered. Bipolar stromal nuclei are commonly present. Calcifications may be present. Scattered actin-positive bipolar cells in the aspirate from tubular carcinoma are likely to be myofibroblasts from the stroma, whereas the specimen from a fibroadenoma contains a mixture of dispersed bipolar myofibroblasts and myoepithelial cells attached to epithelial cell clusters.

The cytologic differences between tubular carcinoma and complex sclerosing lesions were studied by Lamb and Mc-Googan (51), who compared 31 tubular carcinomas with 22 radial sclerosing lesions. Eight (36%) sclerosing lesions and 20 (65%) of the tubular carcinomas were 10 mm or less in diameter. Fourteen (45%) tubular carcinomas and 50% of the radial sclerosing lesions were palpable. The original diagnostic interpretations of these specimens revealed substantial difficulty in distinguishing the two lesions. Twenty-five (81%) of the tubular carcinomas were interpreted as malignant or suspicious, two (6%) as benign, and four (13%) as acellular. Nine (41%) specimens from radial sclerosing lesions were interpreted as suspicious or carcinomas, 10 (46%) as benign, and 3 (13%) as acellular. Mitnick et al. (19) reported greater accuracy in diagnosing tubular carcinoma by needle core biopsy than by fine needle aspiration.

Tubulolobular carcinoma will be suggested by an aspirate that demonstrates signet-ring cells and the features of tubular carcinoma (40).

## PROGNOSIS AND TREATMENT

Tubular carcinoma has a very favorable prognosis when the diagnosis is restricted to tumors that consist almost entirely of tubular elements (5–8,20,21,25,30). In a series of patients with T1N0 breast carcinomas treated by modified or radical mastectomy and followed for a median of 18 years, there were no recurrences among patients with tubular carcinoma (11).

The average frequency of axillary lymph node metastases resulting from tubular carcinoma is about 10% (5,8,10, 20,21,25,29,39,43,52,53), ranging from 0% (8,28) to 29% (16). In one series, three tumors with nodal metastases were smaller than 1 cm, including one 0.4-mm lesion (39). Brad-

ford et al. (53) reported that 13.3% of patients with tubular carcinoma 1 cm or larger had axillary nodal metastases. Axillary lymph node metastases are encountered in about 30% of patients with tubulolobular carcinoma who undergo an axillary dissection (Fig. 15.19) (39). Affected lymph nodes usually are in the low axilla (level I), and only exceptionally are more than three lymph nodes involved (20). Metastases in lymph nodes tend to reproduce the tubular growth pattern of the primary tumor. Metastatic deposits may be in the lymph node capsule or parenchyma (Fig. 15.20). It is not unusual for these well-differentiated metastases to be misinterpreted as benign glandular inclusions. Metastatic tubular carcinoma glands lack myoepithelial cells (Fig. 15.21). Rarely, metastases are less well differentiated or resemble infiltrating lobular carcinoma. The presence of multifocal carcinoma at the primary site appears to predispose patients with tubular and tubulolobular carcinoma to developing axillary lymph node metastases, perhaps because of the greater tumor volume associated with multifocality. Axillary lymph node metastases were found in 21% (5) and 29% (25) of patients with duct carcinomas with tubular features (mixed tubular carcinomas). In the latter study, 21% of patients with a stage II mixed tubular tumor had metastatic carcinoma in more than three lymph nodes.

For decades, patients with pure tubular carcinomas were treated by modified or radical mastectomy. Fewer than 10% of patients in the larger series were treated by simple mastectomy or excisional surgery with or without primary radiotherapy. In a review of several follow-up studies (7,8,20, 21,25,39,43) describing more than 400 women with pure tubular carcinoma, 3.0% had recurrences due to the tubular carcinoma. Six of the women had recurrent carcinoma in the same breast following simple excision after an interval of 2 to 22 years. One of these six women also had axillary nodal metastases when the breast recurrence was detected, but none were reported to have developed systemic metastases after a mastectomy was performed to treat the mammary recurrence.

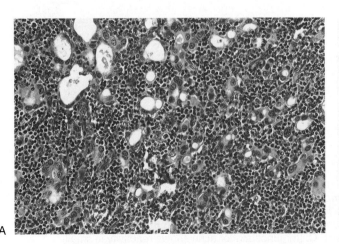
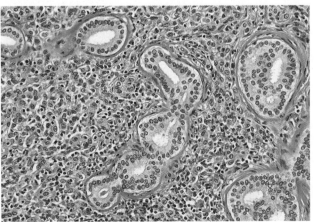

**FIG. 15.19.** *Metastatic tubulolobular carcinoma in a lymph node.* **A:** This nodal metastasis has a mixture of tubular carcinoma glands and signet-ring lobular carcinoma cells. **B:** Tubular carcinoma glands *(right)* are separate from lobular carcinoma *(left)* in this lymph node metastasis.

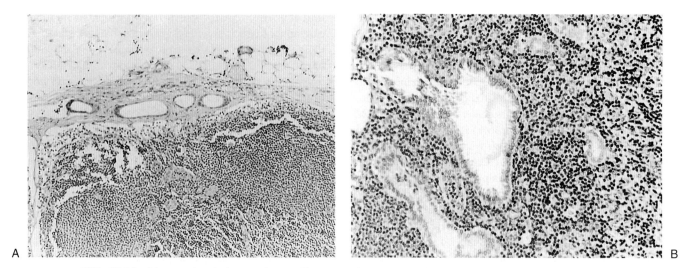

**FIG. 15.20.** *Metastatic tubular carcinoma.* Patterns of metastases in axillary lymph nodes that sometimes are mistaken for benign glandular inclusions. **A:** Metastatic carcinoma in the lymph node capsule. **B:** Metastatic carcinoma in cortical lymphoid tissue. The thin clear zone around the glands that resembles a basement membrane was not immunoreactive for laminin or type IV collagen.

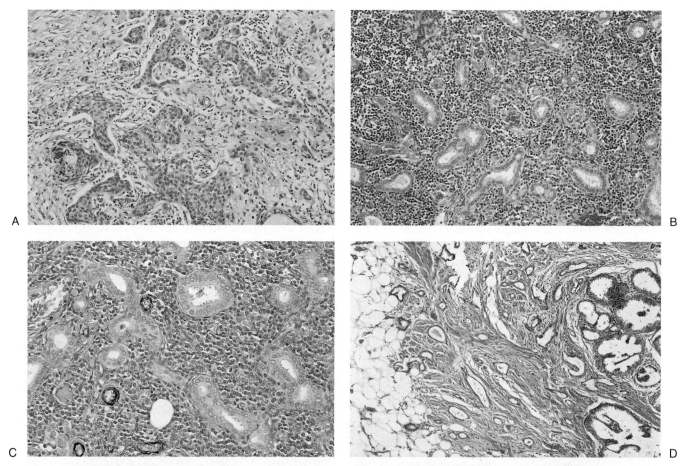

**FIG. 15.21.** *Metastatic tubular carcinoma in lymph node.* All images are from the same case. **A:** Lumpectomy was performed for the moderately differentiated invasive duct carcinoma shown here. **B:** Sentinel lymph node mapping revealed metastatic carcinoma of the tubular type in the sentinel lymph node. All other lymph nodes were free of metastases. **C:** Immunostain for actin shows reactivity in small blood vessels in the lymph node but not around the carcinoma glands (antismooth muscle actin, avidin-biotin). **D:** Extensive further sampling of the lumpectomy disclosed a separate, previously inapparent tubular carcinoma that was responsible for the lymph node metastasis.

Recurrence after primary treatment by mastectomy was reported in several other cases. Three of these patients had axillary lymph node metastases in the mastectomy specimen. One of the three developed a local recurrence, and the other two died of systemic metastases. One of two other patients with negative axillary lymph nodes developed systemic metastases and the other had "persistent carcinoma." A sixth patient with negative lymph nodes and a seventh with unreported nodal status had local recurrences. Death due to metastatic mammary carcinoma in several patients with bilateral carcinoma has been attributable to a less well-differentiated contralateral carcinoma when one breast had a tubular carcinoma (20,25). Recurrences have been reported in up to 32% of patients with mixed tubular carcinoma, and 6% to 28% of these patients reportedly died of metastatic mammary carcinoma (7,8,25).

Most patients with unifocal pure tubular carcinoma are now considered to be excellent candidates for breast conservation therapy. If a unifocal pure tubular carcinoma is excised with an adequate margin and there is no extensive intraductal carcinoma in the surrounding breast, postoperative radiotherapy has been omitted in selected cases. In one series, there were no breast recurrences among 21 patients with tubular carcinoma treated by lumpectomy and radiotherapy (54). Bradford et al. (53) reported no breast or systemic recurrences in 38 women treated by excision, including 17 women who did not have breast irradiation.

Patients with multifocal tubular carcinoma, coexistent extensive intraductal carcinoma, or evidence of other invasive lesions in the breast should have radiotherapy after excision, or they may require mastectomy. Low axillary dissection or sentinel lymph node mapping should be performed in patients with a tubular carcinoma larger than 1 cm, when there are multifocal invasive lesions, or if there are other indications suggesting axillary nodal metastases. In view of the extremely favorable prognosis of tubular carcinoma, there is no evidence that systemic adjuvant therapy would prove beneficial except for women with tumors larger than 3 cm, if there are axillary metastases or if there is also a less well-differentiated carcinoma in the ipsilateral or contralateral breast.

Patients with invasive duct carcinoma with tubular features should receive treatment appropriate for an infiltrating duct carcinoma of the grade of the nontubular component as determined by tumor size and stage. This is likely to include postoperative radiotherapy and systemic adjuvant therapy if the tumor is larger than 1 cm.

## REFERENCES

1. Cornil V, Ranvier L. *Manuel d'histologie pathologique*. Paris: Germer Bailliere, 1869:1167–1170.
2. World Health Organization. *Histological typing of breast tumours*, 2nd ed. International Histological Classification of Tumours No. 2. Geneva: World Health Organization, 1981:19.
3. Foote FW Jr. Surgical pathology of cancer of the breast. In: Parson WH, ed. *Cancer of the breast*. Springfield: Charles C Thomas, 1959:37–38.
4. McDivitt RW, Stewart FW, Berg JW. Tumors of the breast. In: *Atlas of tumor pathology. Series 2, Fascicle No. 2*. Washington, DC: Armed Forces Institute of Pathology, 1968:89–90.
5. Carstens PHB. Tubular carcinoma of the breast. A study of frequency. *Am J Clin Pathol* 1978;70:204–210.
6. Carstens PHB, Greenberg RA, Francis D, et al. Tubular carcinoma of the breast. A long term follow-up. *Histopathology* 1985;9:271–280.
7. Cooper HS, Patchefsky AS, Krall RA. Tubular carcinoma of the breast. *Cancer* 1978;42:2334–2342.
8. Peters GN, Wolff M, Haagensen CD. Tubular carcinoma of the breast. Clinical pathologic correlations based on 100 cases. *Ann Surg* 1981;193:138–149.
9. Rosen PP. The pathological classification of human mammary carcinoma: past, present and future. *Ann Clin Lab Sci* 1979;9:144–156.
10. Rosen PP, Saigo PE, Braun DW Jr, et al. Predictors of recurrence in Stage I (T1N0M0) breast carcinoma. *Ann Surg* 1981;193:15–25.
11. Rosen PP, Groshen S, Saigo PE, et al. A long-term follow-up study of survival in Stage I ($T_1N_0M_0$) and Stage II ($T_1N_1M_0$) breast carcinoma. *J Clin Oncol* 1989;7:355–366.
12. Beahrs O, Shapiro S, Smart C. Report of the working group to review the National Cancer Institute-American Cancer Society Breast Cancer Detection Demonstration Projects. *J Natl Cancer Inst* 1979;62:640–709.
13. Feig SA, Shaber GS, Patchefsky A, et al. Analysis of clinically occult and mammographically occult breast tumors. *AJR Am J Roentgenol* 1977;128:403–408.
14. Andersson I. Radiographic screening for breast carcinoma. II. Prognostic considerations on the basis of short-term follow-up. *Acta Radiol Diagn* 1982;22:227–233.
15. Leibman AJ, Lewis M, Kruse B. Tubular carcinoma of the breast: mammographic appearance. *AJR Am J Roentgenol* 1993;160:263–265.
16. Elson BC, Helvie MA, Frank TS, et al. Tubular carcinoma of the breast: mode of presentation, mammographic appearance, and frequency of nodal metastases. *AJR Am J Roentgenol* 1993;161:1173–1176.
17. Vega A, Garijo F. Radial scar and tubular carcinoma. Mammographic and sonographic findings. *Acta Radiol* 1993;34:43–47.
18. Frouge C, Tristant H, Guinebretière J-M, et al. Mammographic lesions suggestive of radial scars: microscopic findings in 40 cases. *Radiology* 1995;195:623–625.
19. Mitnick JS, Gianutsos R, Pollack AH, et al. Tubular carcinoma of the breast: sensitivity of diagnostic techniques and correlation with histopathology. *AJR Am J Roentgenol* 1999;172:319–323.
20. McDivitt RW, Boyce W, Gersell D. Tubular carcinoma of the breast. Clinical and pathological observations concerning 135 cases. *Am J Surg Pathol* 1982;6:401–410.
21. Oberman HA, Fidler WJ Jr. Tubular carcinoma of the breast. *Am J Surg Pathol* 1979;13:387–395.
22. Taxy JB. Tubular carcinoma of the male breast. Report of a case. *Cancer* 1975;36:462–465.
23. Heller KS, Rosen PP, Schottenfeld D, et al. Male breast cancer. A clinicopathologic study of 97 cases. *Ann Surg* 1978;188:60–65.
24. Norris HJ, Taylor HB. Carcinoma of the male breast. *Cancer* 1969;23:1428–1435.
25. Deos PH, Norris HJ. Well-differentiated (tubular) carcinoma of the breast. *Am J Clin Pathol* 1982;78:1–7.
26. Lagios MD, Rose MR, Margolin FR. Tubular carcinoma of the breast. Association with multicentricity, bilaterality and family history of mammary carcinoma. *Am J Clin Pathol* 1980;73:25–30.
27. Masood S, Barwick KW. Estrogen receptor expression of the less common breast carcinomas. *Am J Clin Pathol* 1990;93:437.
28. Berger AC, Miller SM, Harris MN, et al. Axillary dissection for tubular carcinoma of the breast. *Breast J* 1996;2:204–208.
29. Winchester DJ, Sahin AA, Tucker SL, et al. Tubular carcinoma of the breast. Predicting axillary nodal metastases and recurrence. *Ann Surg* 1996;223:342–347.
30. Diab SG, Clark GM, Osborne CK, et al. Tumor characteristics and clinical outcome of tubular and mucinous breast carcinomas. *J Clin Oncol* 1999;17:1442–1448.
31. Fasano M, Vamvakas E, Delgado Y, et al. Tubular carcinoma of the breast: immunohistochemical and DNA flow cytometric profile. *Breast J* 1999;5:252–255.
32. Andersen JA, Carter D, Linell F. A symposium on sclerosing duct lesions of the breast. *Pathol Annu* 1986;21[Pt 2]:145–180.
33. Rosen PP. Microglandular adenosis. A benign lesion simulating invasive mammary carcinoma. *Am J Surg Pathol* 1983;7:137–144.
34. Joshi MG, Lee AKC, Pedersen CA, et al. The role of immunocyto-

chemical markers in the differential diagnosis of proliferative and neoplastic lesions of the breast. *Mod Pathol* 1996;9:57–62.

35. Dabbs DJ, Gown AM. Distribution of calponin and smooth muscle myosin heavy chain in fine-needle aspiration biopsies of the breast. *Diagn Cytopathol* 1999;20:203–207.

36. Ekblom P, Miettinen M, Forsman L, et al. Basement membrane and apocrine epithelial antigens in differential diagnosis between tubular carcinoma and sclerosing adenosis of the breast. *J Clin Pathol* 1984;37:357–363.

37. Flotte TJ, Bell DA, Greco MA. Tubular carcinoma and sclerosing adenosis. The use of basal lamina as a differential feature. *Am J Surg Pathol* 1980;4:75–77.

37a. Lele SM, Graves K, Gatalica Z. Immunohistochemical detection of maspin is a useful adjunct in distinguishing radial sclerosing lesion from tubular carcinoma of the breast. *Appl Immunohistochem Molecul Morphol* 2000;8:32–36.

38. Eusebi V, Betts CM, Bussolati G. Tubular carcinoma: a variant of secretory breast carcinoma. *Histopathology* 1979;3:407–419.

39. Green I, McCormick B, Cranor M, et al. A comparative study of pure tubular and tubulolobular carcinoma of the breast. *Am J Surg Pathol* 1997;21:653–657.

40. Boppana S, Erroll M, Reiches E, et al. Cytologic characteristics of tubulolobular carcinoma of the breast. *Acta Cytol* 1996;40:465–471.

40a. Buerger H, Simon R, Schäfer KL, et al. Genetic relations of lobular carcinoma in situ, ductal carcinoma in situ, and associated invasive carcinoma of the breast. *J Clin Pathol* 2000;5:118–121.

40b. Rosen PP. Columnar cell hyperplasia is associated with lobular carcinoma in situ and tubular carcinoma. *Am J Surg Pathol* 1999;23:1561.

41. Eggor H, Dressler W. A contribution to the natural history of breast cancer. 1. Duct obliteration with periductal elastosis in the centre of breast cancers. *Arch Gynecol* 1982;231:191–198.

42. Tremblay G. Elastosis in tubular carcinoma of the breast. *Arch Pathol* 1974;98:302–307.

43. Carstens PHB, Huvos AG, Foote FW Jr, et al. Tubular carcinoma of the breast. A clinicopathologic study of 35 cases. *Am J Clin Pathol* 1972;58:231–238.

44. Linell F, Ljungberg O. Breast carcinoma, progression of tubular carcinoma and a new classification. *Acta Pathol Microbiol Scand (A)* 1980;88:59–60.

45. Linell F, Ljungberg O, Andersson I. Breast carcinoma. Aspects of early stages, progression and related problems. *Acta Pathol Microbiol Scand (A) Suppl* 1980;272:1–233.

46. Goldstein NS, O'Malley BA. Cancerization of small ectatic ducts of the breast by ductal carcinoma in situ cells with apocrine snouts. A lesion associated with tubular carcinoma. *Am J Clin Pathol* 1997;107:561–566.

47. Erlandson RA, Carstens PHB. Ultrastructure of tubular carcinoma of the breast. *Cancer* 1972;29:987–995.

48. Harris M, Ahmed A. The ultrastructure of tubular carcinoma of the breast. *J Pathol* 1977;123:79–83.

49. Dawson AE, Logan-Young W, Mulford DK. Aspiration cytology of tubular carcinoma. Diagnostic features with mammographic correlation. *Am J Clin Pathol* 1994;101:488–492.

50. Fischler DF, Sneige N, Ordonez NG, et al. Tubular carcinoma of the breast: cytologic features in fine-needle aspirations and application of monoclonal anti-alpha-smooth muscle actin in diagnosis. *Diagn Cytopathol* 1994;12:120–125.

51. Lamb J, McGoogan E. Fine needle aspiration cytology of breast in invasive carcinoma of tubular type and in radial scar/complex sclerosing lesions. *Cytopathology* 1994;2:17–26.

52. Rosen PP, Saigo PE, Braun DW Jr, et al. Prognosis in Stage II ($T_1N_1M_0$) breast cancer. *Ann Surg* 1981;194:576–584.

53. Bradford WZ, Christensen WN, Fraser H, et al. Treatment of pure tubular carcinoma of the breast. *Breast J* 1998;4:437–440.

54. Haffty BG, Perrotta PL, Ward B, et al. Conservatively treated breast cancer: outcome by histologic subtype. *Breast J* 1997;3:7–14.

# CHAPTER 16

# Papillary Carcinoma

About 1% to 2% of breast carcinomas in women can be classified as papillary (1–3). A slightly greater percentage of male breast carcinomas are papillary. A distinction should be made between invasive and noninvasive papillary carcinoma. As noted by Foote and Stewart (4), intracystic carcinoma is a variant of papillary carcinoma, "more distinctly a gross than a microscopic entity," that may have an invasive component. The many and varied definitions of papillary carcinoma have included intraductal carcinoma with papillary features in multiple ducts, solitary papillary tumors, cystic papillary carcinomas, and invasive carcinomas with a papillary growth pattern (2,5).

The relationship between benign and malignant papillary tumors of the breast has long been a controversial subject. As early as 1922, Bloodgood (6) classified papilloma as a benign condition best managed by local excision. However, other authors who concluded that papillomas frequently gave rise to carcinoma advocated simple mastectomy to treat breast papilloma (7–9). In 1946, Foote and Stewart (4) commented that surrounding some lesions "in which the presence of noninfiltrating papillary carcinoma is quite obvious, there will be additional outlying or adjacent foci in which the degree of structural change is distinctly less advanced and this leads one to believe that pre-existing papillomatosis had been present and had undergone malignant transformation."

A differing point of view was expressed by Stout (10) in 1952, when he made the following comment at the Second National Cancer Conference:

> Intraductal papillomas are altogether benign and the papillary carcinomas altogether malignant. I have never been able to detect cancer cells intermingled with the cells of a benign papilloma. Therefore in the breast I cannot say I have ever observed what may be interpreted as a carcinoma arising in a benign papilloma. Are benign papillomas precancerous lesions? It is almost impossible to get convincing evidence pro and con on this question for once a papilloma has been removed there is no further chance for that particular one to become malignant.

However, Stout acknowledged that *in situ* carcinoma could reside in a papilloma when he stated (11):

> Recognizable nodules of papillary carcinoma almost never show traces of benign intraductal proliferations, so that in doubtful cases if there are microscopic cells which one might be tempted to consider cancerous within an otherwise benign papillary tumor . . . either these are not cancer cells, or if one chooses to regard them as such, the condition is comparable to cancer *in situ*. Because we have no proof that this condition has ever led to the development of true clinical cancer, we have classified tumors showing epithelial proliferations of this sort with the rest of the benign intraductal papillary tumors.

One must presume that Stout used the term "clinical cancer" to mean invasive carcinoma. Because papillary lesions with *in situ* carcinoma did not produce metastases, he evidently chose to classify them as papillomas, but it is clear from the foregoing quotation that he appreciated the fact that areas with carcinomatous features could be found within benign papillary proliferative foci (12). He recognized the difficulties inherent in proving that carcinoma may have arisen from a previously excised papillary lesion (13):

> Most attempts to determine the incidence of cancer development from intraductal papillomas by follow-up studies are fruitless because when discovered the papilloma is removed. All that can then be demonstrated is that . . . the rate of breast cancer development in either breast following it is no higher than the expected breast cancer development rate for a comparable age group and time period.

Stout and Stewart took part in a study of benign intraductal papillomas from 125 patients treated at the New York Hospital (14). Carcinoma subsequently was detected in the ipsilateral breast of seven patients, typically in close proximity to the lesion previously described as a papilloma. They agreed that five lesions originally diagnosed as papillomas had actually been carcinomas. A sixth tumor was confirmed to be a papilloma, and the seventh prior lesion was not reviewed.

Overall, less than 5% of patients have reportedly developed breast carcinoma following excision of a papilloma, and nearly half of the subsequent cancers were detected in the opposite breast. In some cases, the close proximity of mammary carcinoma and a papilloma is such that they must be regarded as parts of a single lesion. Mingling of the two processes is evidence of carcinoma arising in a papilloma. Usually, the carcinomatous component in these lesions is *in situ* (intraductal). Papillary tumors that have progressed to invasion infrequently contain areas of papilloma. A solitary papilloma that has been excised and not found to contain carcinoma or severe atypical hyperplasia is not a precancerous lesion. The risk of detecting carcinoma subsequently in the same breast is low. A greater risk has been associated with the prior excision of multiple papillomas and with papillomas that contain *in situ* carcinoma.

## CLINICAL PRESENTATION

Women with cystic and solid papillary carcinoma of the breast are reportedly older than patients with other types of carcinoma (1–3,15). The mean age in several studies ranges from 63 to 67 years. In one series, the mean age of women with noncystic papillary carcinoma was 57 years. Papillary carcinoma was found in two (1.2%) of 169 women who were at least 75 years old when breast carcinoma was diagnosed (16). In the same series, there were three other women with papillary intraductal carcinoma in multiple ducts.

There is no clear evidence of a specific racial distribution of papillary carcinoma. This type of tumor was not found to be more frequent among Japanese women when compared with a series of predominantly white American patients (17). One group of authors commented on a relatively high proportion of nonwhite women in a series of patients with papillary carcinoma (2).

Nearly 50% of papillary carcinomas arise in the central part of the breast. As a consequence, nipple discharge has been described in 22% to 34% of patients (1,3). Bleeding from the nipple occurs in a higher percentage of patients with papillary carcinoma than in those with a papilloma. Galactography may be used to examine patients who have nipple discharge to determine if papillary lesions are multicentric (18). Filling defects in ducts outlined in a galactogram may be due to papillomas or papillary carcinoma. Paget's disease is rarely found in association with papillary carcinoma, but it may be present if the lesion arises from major lactiferous ducts within the nipple or there are additional foci of intraductal carcinoma in the nipple. Most papillary carcinomas have a slow growth rate. Patients have reported the presence of discharge or a mass for prolonged periods of time. A duration of symptoms for a year or more before biopsy is not unusual (1,3,15,19).

The average size clinically is 2 to 3 cm. Large cystic tumors may fill the entire breast (20), sometimes becoming fixed to, or invading, the skin. Axillary lymph node enlargement is unusual clinically, except in patients with massive tumors that tend to develop areas of hemorrhagic necrosis. Papillary carcinomas usually are estrogen and progesterone receptor-rich and they tend to have a low growth rate when measured by thymidine labeling (21,22). Cathepsin D may be demonstrable in the tumor cells and in stromal histiocytes

by immunohistochemistry (Fig. 16.1). Flow cytometry has not been helpful in distinguishing between benign and malignant papillary tumors. All benign lesions were diploid in one study. Only one of 15 borderline lesions and five of 19 carcinomas were aneuploid (23).

Solitary papillary carcinomas often appear as rounded, lobulated, circumscribed lesions on mammography (24,25), but ill-defined lesions also may be encountered (26). The differential diagnosis includes fibroadenoma, benign cystic lesions, and medullary or mucinous carcinoma. An invasive component may be suspected when part of the contour lacks circumscription (24,26). Extension of papillary carcinoma into adjacent ducts cannot be assessed reliably by mammography. Examination by ultrasound can suggest a papillary tumor when a solid area manifested by posterior enhancement is imaged in an otherwise hypoechoic cystic lesion (24,25,27,28). Calcifications are not abundant in most papillary carcinomas; when present, they tend to be punctate and associated with intraductal papillary carcinoma (28). Coarse, irregular calcifications may develop in areas of sclerosis or resolved hemorrhage in papillomas or in papillary carcinomas.

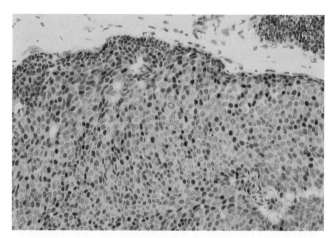

A

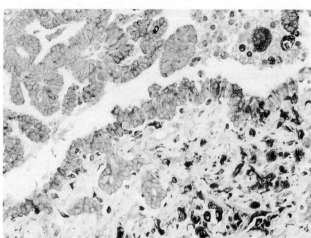

B

**FIG. 16.1.** *Papillary carcinoma.* **A:** Nuclear immunoreactivity for estrogen receptor in solid papillary carcinoma, (avidin-biotin). **B:** Cytoplasmic immunoreactivity for cathepsin D in papillary carcinoma cells and in stromal histiocytes *(lower right)* (avidin-biotin).

Biochemical analysis of the fluid from cystic papillary lesions may be helpful in the differential diagnosis between cystic papilloma and papillary carcinoma. Matsuo et al. (29) described finding an elevated carcinoembryonic antigen (CEA) content in aspirated fluid from a 10-cm cystic breast tumor. CEA was demonstrated immunohistochemically in the carcinoma cells in the resected specimen. Another study compared CEA and *erb*B-2 protein levels in fluid from six cystic papillomas, six papillary carcinomas, and 42 gross cystic disease lesions (30). Five (83%) of the six carcinomas had elevated levels of both proteins compared to two (33%) of the papillomas and two (5%) of the gross cysts.

## GROSS PATHOLOGY

The gross appearance of these tumors varies considerably, depending on the relative proportions of cystic and solid components (Fig. 16.2). Papillary carcinomas usually are well circumscribed grossly, and they may even appear encapsulated (Fig. 16.3). The tumor tissue is soft to moderately firm, depending on the extent of fibrosis. Bleeding into the tumor can impart a dark brown or hemorrhagic appearance,

but usually these lesions are described as tan or gray. Needle aspiration or needle core biopsy can produce more hemorrhage than occurs in a nonpapillary mammary carcinoma after these procedures due to the friable character of many papillary lesions, especially those without fibrosis or a healed prior hemorrhage.

Large cystic papillary carcinomas containing dark brown, partly clotted blood and detached degenerated papillary fragments of tumor should be examined carefully in order to separate the tumor tissue for microscopic study. The membrane that constitutes the cyst wall is formed of fibrous tissue, reactive inflammatory infiltrates, and varying amounts of proliferating epithelium. Residual papillary tumor usually can be found on the luminal surface or in the cyst wall. It is important that such areas be sampled extensively because they may contain foci of invasion (Fig. 16.4).

## MICROSCOPIC PATHOLOGY

The term "papillary" should be used to describe carcinomas in which the underlying microscopic pattern is predominantly frond-forming (Fig. 16.5). Although most of these

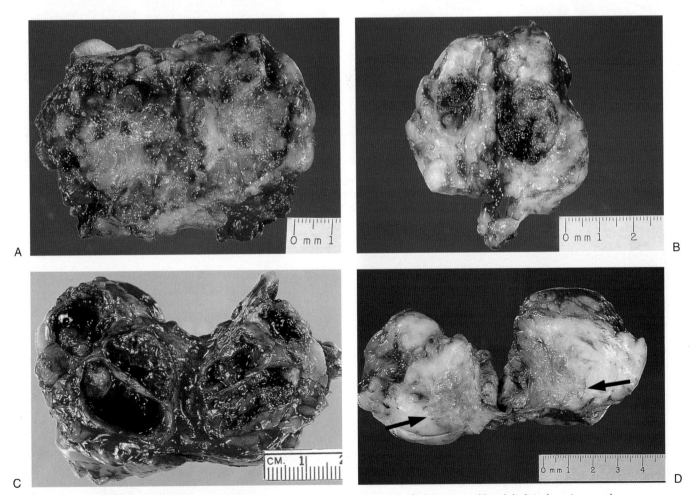

**FIG. 16.2.** *Papillary carcinoma.* Various gross appearances. **A:** Solid tumor with a lobulated contour and central fibrosis. **B:** Solid intracystic tumor. **C:** Multiloculated cystic tumor with intracystic papillary nodules. **D:** Cystic papillary carcinoma with a large invasive component represented by the tan areas (*arrows*) around the cyst.

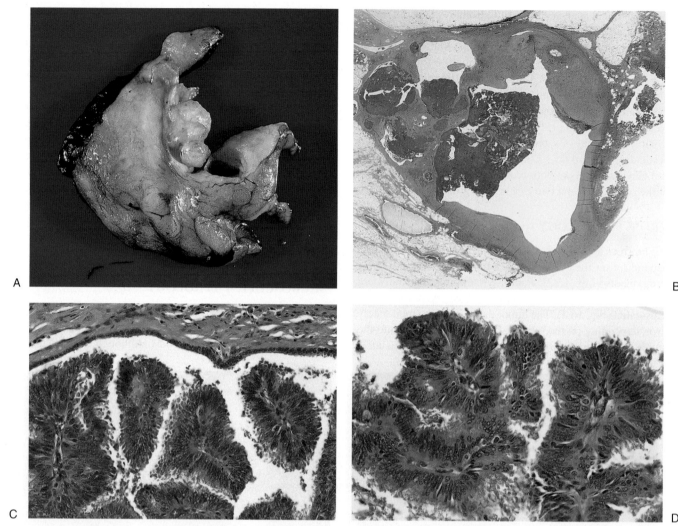

**FIG. 16.3.** *Papillary carcinoma, cystic.* **A:** The tumor forms a tan nodule that protrudes into the cyst. **B:** Whole-mount histologic section of a similar specimen showing a nodular papillary tumor protruding into the cyst lumen and the thick fibrous cyst wall. **C,D:** Histologic appearance of the orderly papillary carcinoma shown in **B**.

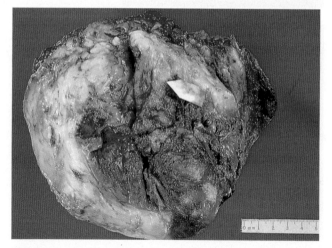

**FIG. 16.4.** *Cystic papillary carcinoma.* Opened cystic tumor that contains blood clot, tan mural nodules of papillary carcinoma below the *arrow,* and a focus of invasive carcinoma indicated by the *arrow.*

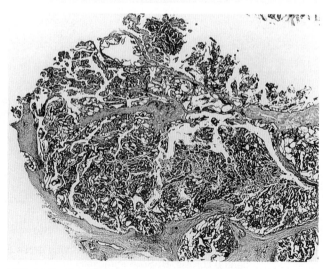

**FIG. 16.5.** *Papillary carcinoma.* Whole-mount histologic section. The epithelial pattern is largely cribriform.

tumors are large enough to form a palpable mass, the diagnosis also is applicable to microscopic lesions that have a papillary structure (Fig. 16.6). Many papillary carcinomas have cystic areas, but cyst formation is not necessary for the diagnosis of papillary carcinoma. Foote and Stewart (4) observed that "in some areas the cell proliferation becomes so dense that basic papillary properties are overgrown." Such a tumor is classified as *solid papillary carcinoma* (Fig. 16.7). The underlying papillary nature of these lesions is defined by a branching network of fibrovascular stroma, although individual papillary fronds are not separated by spaces.

Carcinoma usually extends into ducts at the periphery of a papillary carcinoma. When the interpretation of an orderly papillary tumor is difficult, careful examination of the surrounding ducts can be extremely helpful. The presence of foci of papillary, cribriform, or comedocarcinoma usually is evidence that *in situ* carcinoma also is present in the papillary tumor.

The distinction between a papilloma and papillary carcinoma is determined by the cytology and microscopic structure of the lesion. In 1962, Kraus and Neubecker (31) set forth often quoted criteria for distinguishing benign from malignant papillary tumors. The histologic characteristics cited be Kraus and Neubecker are summarized in Table 16.1. The application of these criteria is complicated by numerous exceptions and structural variations. In subsequent years, it has become apparent that myoepithelial cells can be detected in some papillary carcinomas.

The fundamental principle in evaluating papillary tumors is to determine whether the epithelium between adjacent fibrovascular cores has features diagnostic of intraductal carcinoma. In this sense, the space between the fibrovascular cores can be likened to a duct lumen bounded by these stromal elements. When present, intraductal carcinoma has papillary, micropapillary or filiform, cribriform, reticular, and solid appearances (Fig. 16.8). Supporting fibrovascular

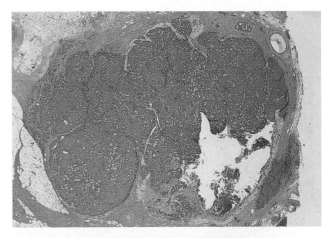

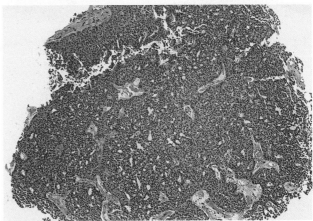

**FIG. 16.7.** *Solid papillary carcinoma.* **A:** Whole-mount histologic section showing the multinodular circumscribed tumor. A defect in the tumor is the site of a needle core biopsy. **B:** Needle core biopsy specimen obtained from **A** containing branching fibrovascular stroma.

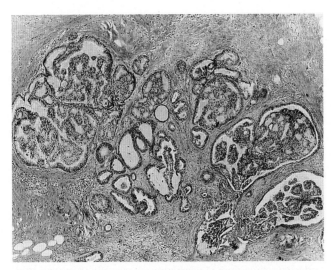

**FIG. 16.6.** *Papillary carcinoma.* Nonpalpable focus with a radial scar configuration. The lesion was detected by mammography.

**TABLE 16.1.** *Criteria of Kraus and Neubecker for diagnosis of papillary breast lesions[a]*

| Histologic feature | Papilloma | Papillary carcinoma |
|---|---|---|
| 1. Cell types | Epithelial/myoepithelial | Epithelial |
| 2. Chromasia | Normochromatic nuclei | Hyperchromatic nuclei |
| 3. Apocrine metaplasia | Present | Absent |
| 4. Glandular pattern | Complex | Cribriform |
| 5. Stroma | Prominent; fibrosis with epithelial entrapment | Delicate or absent; stroma invaded in invasive lesions |
| 6. Adjacent ducts | Hyperplasia | Intraductal carcinoma |
| 7. Sclerosing adenosis | Sometimes present in breast | Usually absent |

[a] See text for detailed discussion and interpretation of these criteria. From Kraus FT, Neubecker RD. The differential diagnosis of papillary tumors of the breast. *Cancer* 1962;15: 444–455, with permission.

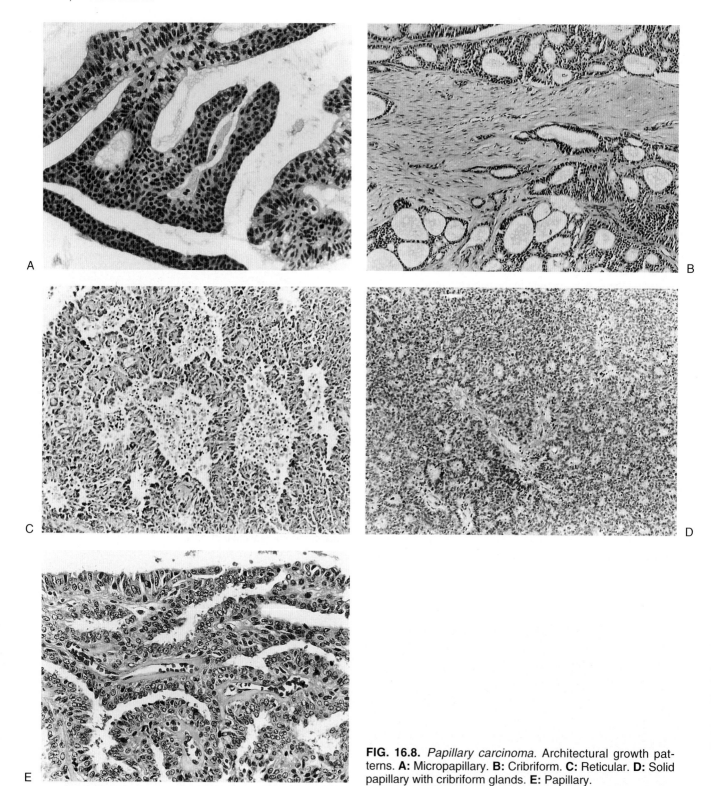

**FIG. 16.8.** *Papillary carcinoma.* Architectural growth patterns. **A:** Micropapillary. **B:** Cribriform. **C:** Reticular. **D:** Solid papillary with cribriform glands. **E:** Papillary.

stroma is present in virtually all papillary carcinomas, but it tends to be less conspicuous in carcinomas than in benign papillary lesions because of the more pronounced epithelial component in carcinomas. A minority of papillary carcinomas have areas where there are relatively broad fibrous stalks of extensive sclerosis; consequently, the character of

the stroma within the lesion is not by itself a reliable diagnostic feature (Fig. 16.9).

The epithelial cells in papillary carcinomas grow in a less orderly fashion than in papillomas as a result of uneven stratification and loss of polarity with respect to stromal elements within the lesion (Fig. 16.10). Nuclei are characteristically

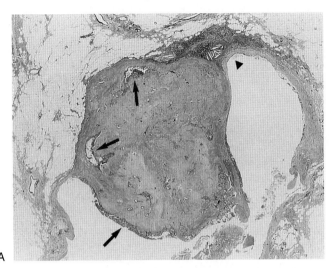
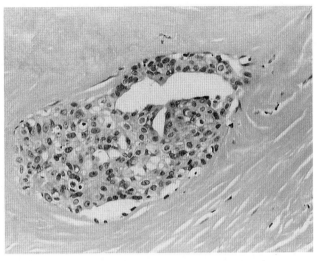

FIG. 16.9. *Papillary carcinoma with sclerosis.* **A:** Whole-mount histologic section of a cystic papillary carcinoma that has been reduced to a fibrotic nodule with a few neoplastic glands and a thin layer of residual carcinoma on the surface *(arrows)*. Chronic inflammation and fat necrosis are evident at the upper border of the tumor *(arrowhead)*. **B:** Carcinomatous gland within the fibrotic tumor.

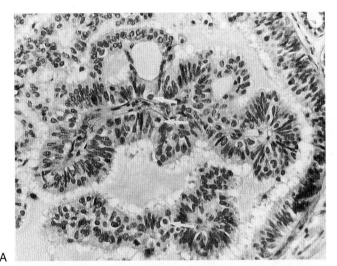
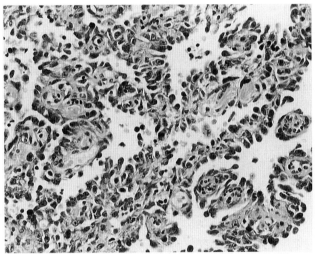
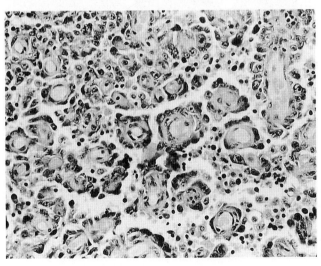

FIG. 16.10. *Papillary carcinoma.* **A:** Orderly papillary carcinoma composed of tall columnar cells that form papillary fronds. Myoepithelial cells are present *(arrows)*. **B:** Disorderly arrangement of neoplastic epithelial cells with hyperchromatic nuclei on papillary fronds. **C:** Pleomorphic carcinomatous cells on papillary fronds with degenerating cells in the intervening spaces. *(continued)*

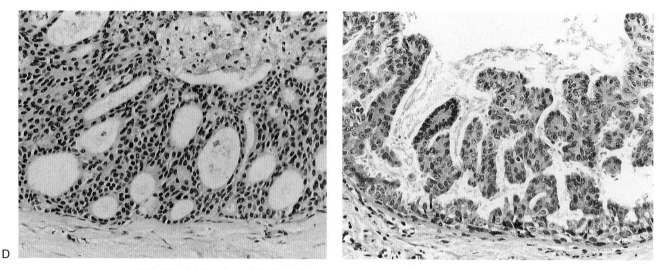

**FIG. 16.10.** *Continued.* **D:** Cribriform carcinoma. **E:** Micropapillary carcinoma.

hyperchromatic regardless of cytologic grade, and there usually is a high nuclear-to-cytoplasmic ratio. Mitotic figures are variably present in papillary carcinomas and are more numerous in lesions that exhibit the most severe cytologic atypia. Mitotic activity is very uncommon in papillomas. The presence of more than one mitosis per ten high-magnification (40×) fields is an atypical feature.

The tumor cells sometimes have secretory "snouts" at the luminal surface. The cytoplasm typically is amphophilic, but eosinophilic cells are found in a substantial number of lesions. Papotti et al. (32) found apocrine cells that were immunoreactive for gross cystic disease fluid protein 15 (GCDFP-15) in 75% of papillomas and in 50% of papillary carcinomas. Apocrine areas in a papillary carcinoma exhibit cytologic atypia consistent with the rest of the tumor and,

therefore, differ from the bland foci of apocrine metaplasia commonly encountered in papillomas (Fig. 16.11).

Myoepithelial cells, which are distributed relatively uniformly and proportionately with the epithelium in benign papillary lesions, may be overgrown in papillary carcinomas. However, the finding of myoepithelial cells in some parts of a papillary lesion is not inconsistent with a diagnosis of carcinoma (32–34). Myoepithelial cells are prominent mainly in residual areas of a papilloma that has given rise to a papillary carcinoma, and they tend to be less conspicuous or absent in the carcinomatous areas (Fig. 16.12).

Lefkowitz et al. (15) drew attention to the presence in papillary carcinomas of cuboidal cells with abundant clear or faintly eosinophilic cytoplasm (Fig. 16.13). These cells were located mainly near the basement membrane, singly, in small

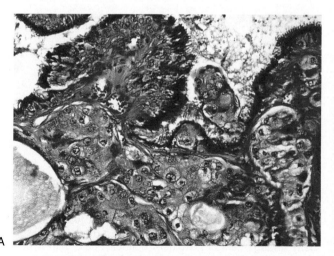
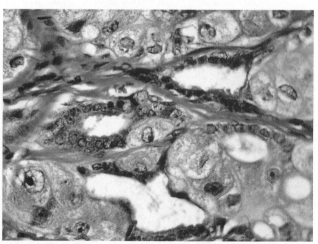

**FIG. 16.11.** *Papillary carcinoma.* **A:** Residual epithelium of a papilloma is present on the surface of these fronds, which are occupied by apocrine carcinoma *(below).* **B:** Apocrine carcinoma has almost completely replaced the benign epithelium of this papillary tumor, leaving a few glandular lumens surrounded by benign epithelium.

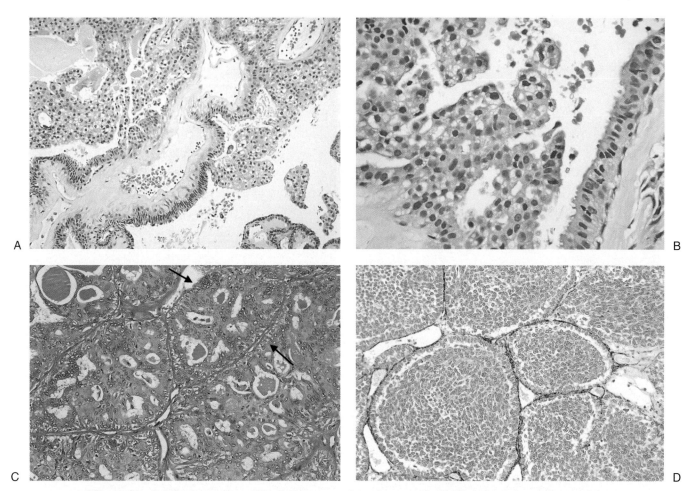

**FIG. 16.12.** *Papillary carcinoma.* **A:** Solid areas of carcinoma are distributed on the surfaces of the fronds of an underlying papilloma. **B:** Myoepithelial cells are seen in epithelium of the papilloma on the *right* and they are absent in the papillary carcinoma on the *left.* **C:** Papillary carcinoma with cribriform structure and myoepithelial cells *(arrows).* **D:** Solid papillary carcinoma with spindle cell growth in which attenuated myoepithelial cells are highlighted by an immunostain for smooth muscle actin (avidin-biotin).

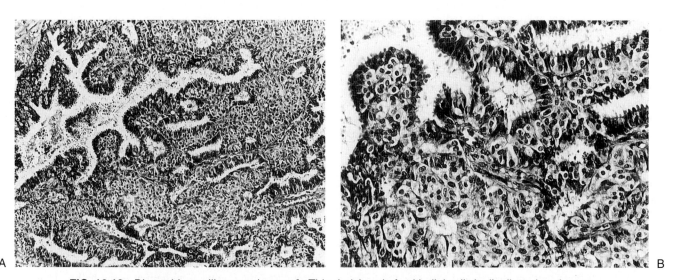

**FIG. 16.13.** *Dimorphic papillary carcinoma.* **A:** Thin dark band of epithelial cells is distributed on the surface of anastomosing broad papillary fronds that are filled with cells that have pale cytoplasm. **B:** Columnar epithelial cells on the surface and polygonal cells in the stroma of papillary fronds.

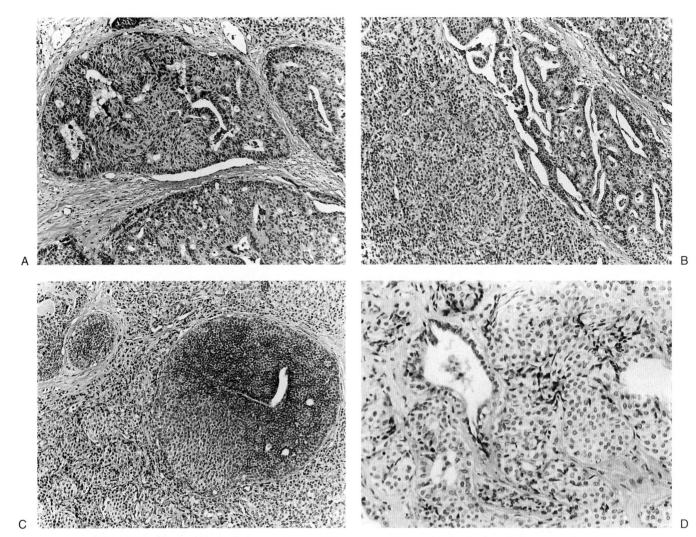

**FIG. 16.14.** *Dimorphic papillary carcinoma.* All images are from a single lesion. **A:** Intraductal component composed of glandular spaces lined by columnar epithelium with intervening small round and spindle cells. **B:** Separate areas consisting of cribriform carcinoma formed by columnar cells and solid carcinoma consisting of small cells. **C:** Intraductal and invasive small cell carcinoma. Columnar epithelium outlines the cleft in the large duct. **D:** Small cell carcinoma and a gland lined by remnants of cuboidal papillary epithelium. The regions shown in **C** and **D** resemble lobular carcinoma in the papillary carcinoma. Material was not available for E-cadherin immunostaining.

clusters, or in broad sheets, a distribution that suggested myoepithelial origin. Occasionally, the polygonal cells with pale cytoplasm were numerous, creating solid and cribriform regions beneath the superficial columnar epithelium (Fig. 16.14). The polygonal cells contrasted strikingly with the conventional columnar epithelial cells in a fashion that resembled pagetoid spread. Despite the difference in cytoplasmic features between the clear cells and the columnar carcinomatous cells, the nuclei of the two cell types were similar. Both cell types were immunoreactive for CAM5.2, which stained myoepithelial cells weakly or not at all, but there was no reactivity for S-100 protein or smooth muscle actin in the polygonal cells. On this basis, Lefkowitz et al. concluded that both cell types were epithelial, and they referred to the two cell populations as "dimorphic" carcinoma. Polygonal dimorphic carcinoma cells should not be mistaken for resid-

ual myoepithelial cells in a papillary lesion, which are immunoreactive for actin, myosin, and calponin, or for pagetoid lobular carcinoma *in situ*. E-cadherin reactivity is absent from lobular carcinoma *in situ* and present in myoepithelial cells.

Neoplasms with a characteristic papillary and cystic structure are readily recognized as papillary carcinoma, but the existence of a solid variant of papillary carcinoma is not widely appreciated (35). These tumors are formed by aggregated ducts completely filled by a solid neoplastic proliferation. They usually are well circumscribed and often are multinodular. The presence of a delicate network of fibrovascular stroma distributed in an arborizing pattern throughout the compact epithelium is the hallmark of solid papillary carcinoma (Figs. 16.7 and 16.15). Collagenization and sclerosis of stroma around and among the ducts is pre-

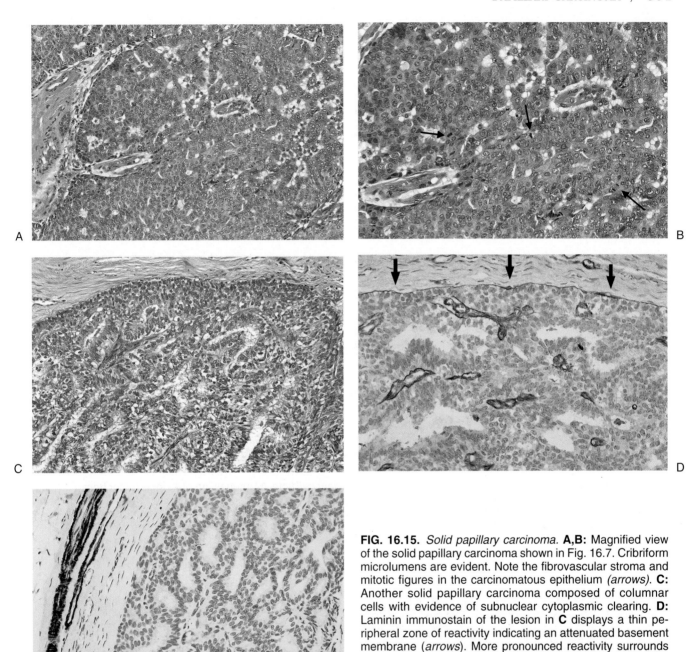

**FIG. 16.15.** *Solid papillary carcinoma.* **A,B:** Magnified view of the solid papillary carcinoma shown in Fig. 16.7. Cribriform microlumens are evident. Note the fibrovascular stroma and mitotic figures in the carcinomatous epithelium *(arrows).* **C:** Another solid papillary carcinoma composed of columnar cells with evidence of subnuclear cytoplasmic clearing. **D:** Laminin immunostain of the lesion in **C** displays a thin peripheral zone of reactivity indicating an attenuated basement membrane *(arrows).* More pronounced reactivity surrounds the internal fibrovascular stroma. **E:** Absence of myoepithelial cells in the carcinoma is evident in this immunostain for smooth muscle actin. A small blood vessel on the *left* is immunoreactive (avidin-biotin).

sent to a variable degree, in some cases producing a pattern with features of radial sclerosing lesion. Some solid papillary carcinomas have areas with an organoid growth pattern, in which solid masses of cells are outlined by a peripheral zone of palisaded cells. Occasionally, solid areas are broken up into ribbons or trabeculae of neoplastic cells by prominent fibrovascular stroma. Uncommon variants of solid papillary carcinoma include glycogen-rich clear cell tumors (Fig. 16.16), spindle cell tumors (Fig. 16.17), and carcinomas with mucoepidermoid features (Fig. 16.18). Cribriform foci and comedonecrosis are infrequent. Intraductal carci-

noma found in ducts at the periphery of a solid papillary carcinoma usually reflects the cytology and structure of the papillary neoplasm.

Papillary carcinoma that has arisen in a papilloma usually retains areas of papilloma that appear benign or atypical, as well as having foci of more cellular proliferation diagnostic of carcinoma (Figs. 16.11, 16.12, and 16.19). Small areas of papilloma in such lesions are of little consequence, and they should not impede recognition of the carcinomatous element. Foote and Stewart (4) noted that "in some instances in which the presence of noninfiltrating papillary carcinoma is

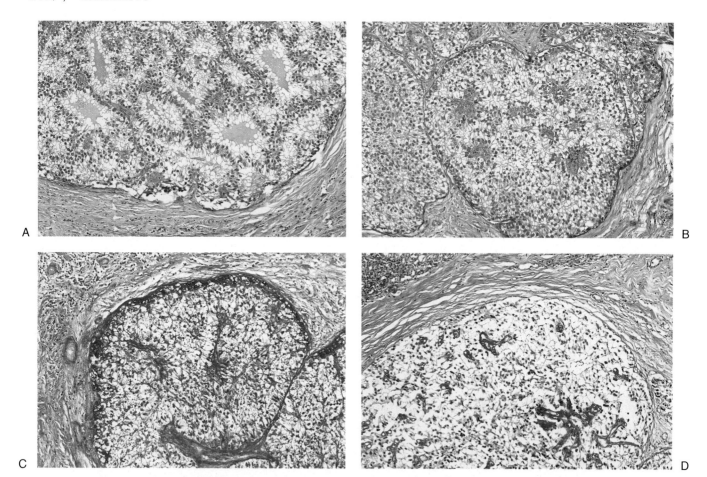

**FIG. 16.16.** *Solid papillary carcinoma, glycogen-rich clear cell type.* All images are of a single tumor from a 29-year-old woman. **A:** Columnar cells with clear cytoplasm are arranged on fibrovascular stroma, outlining glands that contain secretion. **B:** Another region in the tumor with solid, non–gland-forming growth. **C:** The tumor cells contain periodic acid-Schiff (PAS)-positive material, which has a purple color. **D:** PAS staining has been abolished in the carcinoma by diastase, and remains only in fibrovascular stroma.

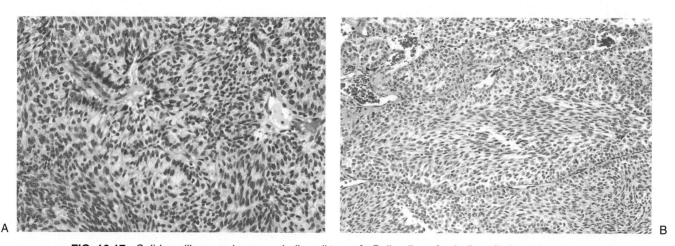

**FIG. 16.17.** *Solid papillary carcinoma, spindle cell type.* **A:** Palisading of spindle cells is evident around fibrovascular cores. **B:** Pronounced spindle cell growth.

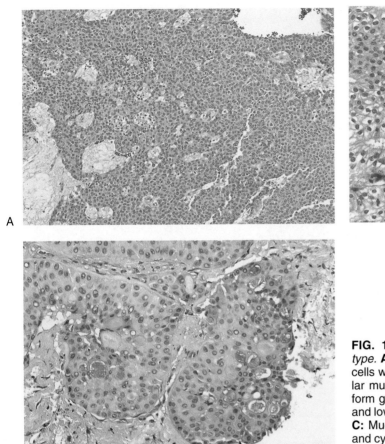

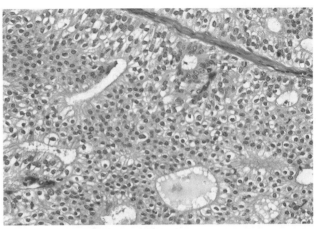

A

B

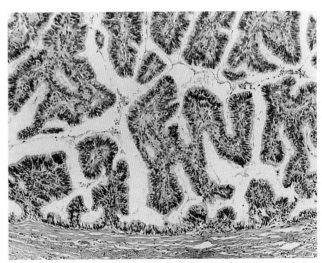

C

**FIG. 16.18.** *Solid papillary carcinoma, mucoepidermoid type.* **A:** Tumor consists of solid masses of polygonal tumor cells with inconspicuous fibrovascular structures. Extracellular mucin is shown in the *lower left* corner. **B:** Tumor cells form glands and have distinct cell borders. Nuclei are small and low grade. Cytoplasmic vacuolization is variably present. **C:** Mucicarmine stain demonstrates mucin in gland lumens and cytoplasm of tumor cells in an area with squamoid differentiation.

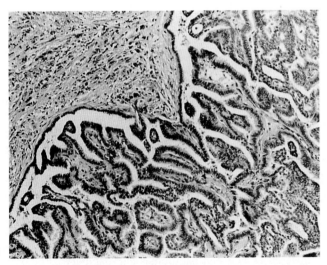

A

B

**FIG. 16.19.** *Papillary carcinoma arising in a papilloma.* **A:** Remnant of the underlying papilloma. (From Rosen PP, Oberman HA. Tumors of the mammary gland. In: *Atlas of tumor pathology.* Washington, DC: Armed Forces Institute of Pathology, 1993, with permission.) **B:** Papilloma with epithelial atypia. *(continued)*

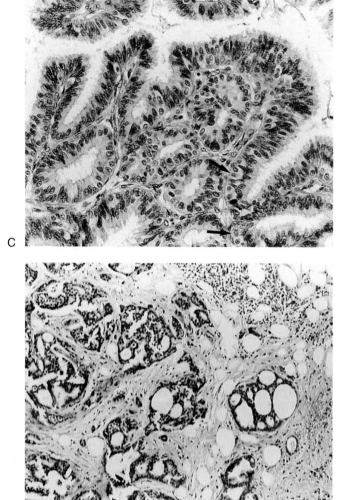

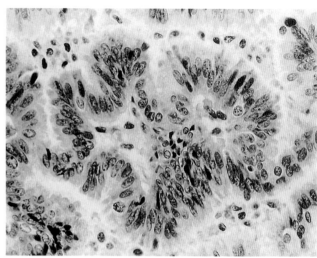

**FIG. 16.19.** *Continued.* **C:** Atypical epithelial hyperplasia on the surface of papillary fronds with underlying secondary gland formation indicative of carcinoma in the lesion. Myoepithelial cells are focally prominent (*arrows*). **D:** Orderly papillary carcinoma. **E:** Invasive cribriform carcinoma that arose from this papillary tumor.

quite obvious, there will be additional outlying or adjacent foci in which the degree of structural change is distinctly less advanced and this leads one to believe that pre-existing papillomatosis had been present and had undergone malignant transformation."

In some instances, the diagnosis of papillary carcinoma can be "a 'shadow land' even for the most experienced pathologist" (36), a situation that Foote and Stewart (4) referred to as "a zone of altered cell growth where the diagnosis of carcinoma versus atypical papillomatosis is a question of occult distinction and must be accepted or rejected on grounds of faith in the pathologist or lack of it." "Borderline" papillary lesions that fit this description often have modest or substantial areas of benign papillary proliferation, as well as more cellular and atypical components. To make a diagnosis of carcinoma in the latter setting, it is necessary to find one or more low-power microscopic fields where the growth pattern and cytologic appearance constitute one of the established patterns of duct carcinoma. Some authors illustrated focal intraductal carcinoma in papillomas but classified

these lesions as "papillomas with atypical ductal hyperplasia" (37,38). In one of these studies, the relative risk for "subsequent carcinoma" in women with such papillomas was more than four times the risk of women with papillomas that lacked atypical hyperplasia/intraductal carcinoma (38). Underdiagnosis of such lesions is likely to result in inadequate treatment, which is reflected in the outcome of patients in these reports.

Microcalcifications found in most papillary carcinomas usually are distributed in the glandular portions of the lesion, but they also may be found in the papillary stroma.

Three-dimensional reconstruction of the microscopic structure of papillary lesions has revealed some interesting differences between papillomas and papillary carcinomas (39,40). In papillomas and papillomatosis, the luminal spaces between the proliferating epithelial cells form a complex but diffusely anastomosing continuous network of channels. On the other hand, in intraductal carcinomas the luminal spaces tend to be separate and they do not form a continuous network. These elegant and painstaking studies

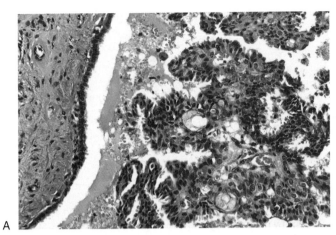 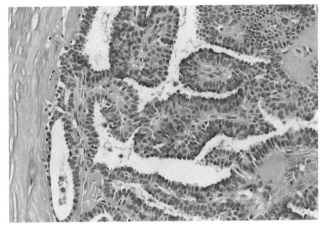

**FIG. 16.20.** *Papillary carcinoma with mucin secretion.* **A:** Blue mucin vacuoles are present in the epithelium. **B:** Mucin is stained blue with the Alcian blue–periodic acid-Schiff reaction.

have resulted in a more complete appreciation of the structural differences between hyperplastic and carcinomatous papillary lesions.

## HISTOCHEMISTRY AND MOLECULAR STUDIES

Immunohistochemical procedures have yielded inconsistent results in the evaluation of difficult papillary lesions. It was reported that areas of papilloma were negative for CEA but that cytoplasmic CEA was present in carcinomatous portions of the same papillary tumors (32,34). The authors concluded that "CEA-positive myoepithelial cell-free carcinomatous areas can be anatomically associated with and even present inside the benign-looking papillary lesions." The observations were seen "as evidence of a malignant transformation of intraductal papillomas, or less likely, of their 'cancerization' by ductal carcinoma." As noted previously, fluid aspirated from cystic papillary carcinomas is more likely to

contain increased amounts of CEA than fluid from cystic papillomas (30).

Saddik et al. (41) found that a significantly ($p < 0.0001$) greater proportion of cells expressed cyclin D1 in papillary carcinomas than in papillomas. The percentage of cyclin D1-positive cells was $89\% \pm 18\%$ (range, 53% to 98%) in papillary carcinomas and $8\% \pm 7\%$ (range, 0 to 19%) in papillomas. A significant difference ($p = 0.01$) also was observed for Ki67 immunoreactivity, but the values for papillary carcinoma ($13\% \pm 6\%$; range, 9% to 23%) and for papillomas ($8\% \pm 2\%$; range, 6% to 12%) showed some overlap, making this a less reliable diagnostic criterion.

There is a broad range of mucin secretion demonstrable with the mucicarmine, Alcian blue, and periodic acid-Schiff stains (Fig. 16.20). Few papillary carcinomas have no detectable mucin. In the majority, mucin secretion is not prominent, but a small number of papillary carcinomas have signet-ring cells (Fig. 16.21), or abundant and diffuse

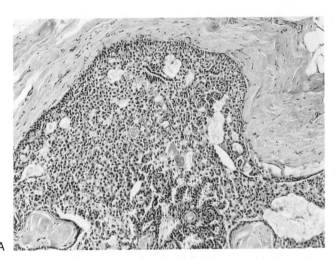 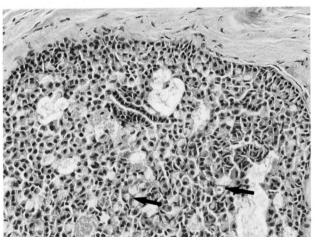

**FIG. 16.21.** *Papillary carcinoma with signet-ring cells.* **A:** Cells with clear cytoplasm were strongly reactive with the mucicarmine stain and focally positive with the Grimelius stain. **B:** Signet-ring cells (*arrows*).

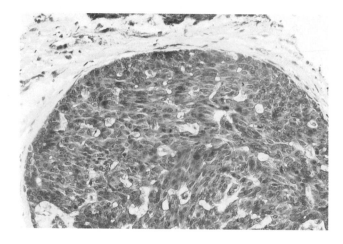

**FIG. 16.22.** *Solid papillary carcinoma with mucin.* Spindle cells show diffuse magenta staining with mucicarmine stain.

intracellular mucin secretion (Fig. 16.22). The accumulation of abundant extracellular mucin creates a pattern that resembles invasive mucinous carcinoma but does not represent invasion when confined within the tumor (Fig. 16.23).

The cells in a minority of papillary carcinomas contain Grimelius- and chromogranin-positive cytoplasmic granules that have not been demonstrated by histochemical methods in papillomas. These tumors, which typically have a solid papillary growth pattern, are immunoreactive for neuron-specific enolase and synaptophysin and have mucin-positive cells (Fig. 16.24) (42). They usually are estrogen receptor positive (Fig. 16.25).

Molecular analysis of deoxyribonucleic acid (DNA) isolated from papillomas and papillary carcinomas demonstrated significant differences. Loss of heterozygosity (LOH) on chromosome 16q was found in eight (67%) of 12 cystic papillary carcinomas and in seven (64%) of 11 low-grade invasive duct carcinomas, but in none of the 11

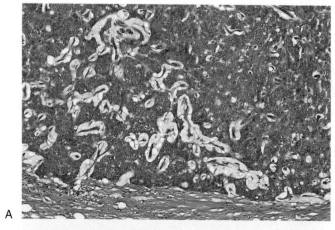

A

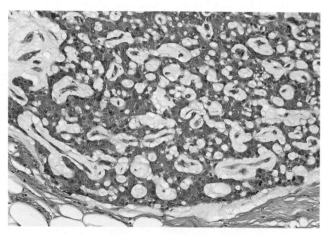

B

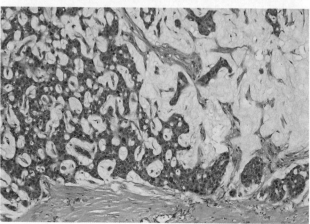

C

**FIG. 16.23.** *Solid papillary carcinoma with extracellular mucin.* These images from a single tumor illustrate progressive accumulation of extracellular mucin. **A:** Extracellular mucin is concentrated around fibrovascular structures rather than in gland lumens. **B:** Further expansion of the mucin is evident including at the interface of the tumor and stroma *(below)*. Vascular structures remain in virtually every mucin collection. **C:** Coalescent areas of mucin on the *right* contain the basic papillary vascular pattern. Note the retained sharply defined border *below*.

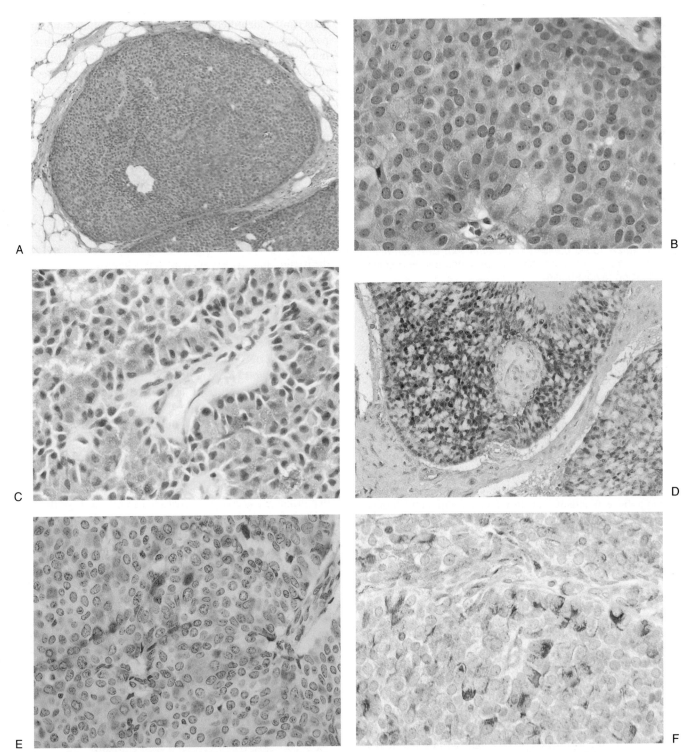

**FIG. 16.24.** *Solid papillary carcinoma with endocrine differentiation.* **A:** Fibrovascular cores containing capillaries are scattered through this solid papillary carcinoma. **B:** Tumor cells have amphophilic finely granular cytoplasm and focal intracytoplasmic vacuoles. **C:** Positive reaction for mucin is present in the cytoplasm of most carcinoma cells (mucicarmine stain). **D:** Immunoreactivity for neuron-specific enolase (NSE) (anti-NSE, avidin-biotin). **E:** Weak immunoreactivity for synaptophysin (avidin-biotin). **F:** Grimelius-positive black granules are present in many tumor cells (Grimelius stain).

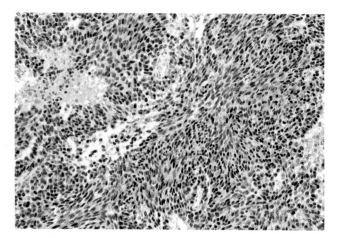

**FIG. 16.25.** *Solid papillary carcinoma with estrogen receptors.* Nuclear immunoreactivity is demonstrated in a spindle cell lesion (avidin-biotin).

papillomas studied (43). Other investigators who studied several loci of 16p13 reported finding LOH in eight (57%) of 14 papillary carcinomas and in six (60%) of 10 papillomas with florid hyperplasia (44).

## ELECTRON MICROSCOPY

Electron microscopy generally confirms the light microscopic characteristics of papillary carcinoma and is not regarded as particularly helpful in evaluating difficult cases (45,46). Myoepithelial cells are more numerous in benign papillary lesions than in papillary carcinomas. Papillomas tend to have abundant, well-formed microvilli at the luminal surfaces of epithelial cells, whereas in some papillary carcinomas, the microvilli are less abundant, stunted, and poorly formed (45). Intracytoplasmic lumens have been described in the cells of papillary carcinoma (46).

## INVASIVE PAPILLARY CARCINOMA

The microscopic diagnosis of minimally invasive papillary carcinoma can be difficult. Many papillary carcinomas are bounded by zones of fibrosis, recent or resolved hemorrhage, and chronic inflammation. Similar alterations also may occur within the lesion. Papillary or glandular clusters of epithelial cells routinely found within these areas present a challenging problem (Fig. 16.26). If one recalls that similar patterns of epithelial dispersal can occur in sclerotic portions of benign papillary lesions, it is possible in most cases to determine that these do not constitute foci of invasion. Groups of neoplastic cells distributed parallel to layers of reactive stroma at the border of a papillary carcinoma usually represent entrapped *in situ* epithelium rather than invasive carcinoma. An actin immunostain sometimes is helpful in this situation, although proliferating myofibroblasts can complicate the interpretation. Myofibroblastic staining is less of a problem if an antibody to smooth muscle myosin heavy chain or calponin is used. Isolated invasive carcinoma

cells can be identified with a cytokeratin immunostain, and persisting basement membranes can be detected with immunostains for collagen IV or laminin. In general, the most reliable histologic evidence of frank invasion is extension of tumor beyond the zone of reactive changes into the mammary parenchyma and fat (Figs. 16.27–16.29).

Papillary lesions that have been subjected to fine needle aspiration or needle core biopsy prior to excision exhibit alterations that complicate the issue of determining whether there is invasion. Hemorrhage is commonly found in and around the tumor grossly. The best microscopic clues to such manipulation of the tumor are the presence of fresh hemorrhage and acute inflammation associated with "unnatural" fragmentation of the lesion. Tumor cells can be found singly or in clusters deposited in areas of hemorrhage and along the course of the needle (Fig. 16.30). As long as it is known that the lesion was recently "needled," these detached cells are best regarded as the result of trauma rather than as evidence of invasion. Sometimes papillary clusters of epithelial cells, which may contain fibrovascular stroma, are seen in capillary or lymphatic channels after needle aspiration or core biopsy (Fig. 16.31). This uncommon finding should be described in the pathology report and may be regarded as a manifestation of invasive carcinoma in some instances (47) (see Chapter 46).

One unusual pattern of true invasion associated with solid papillary carcinomas may simulate epithelial displacement resulting from needling procedures. This type of invasion is characterized by the presence of one or more irregularly shaped cohesive sheets of carcinoma cells in surrounding fat or stroma unassociated with the reactive stromal changes that ordinarily accompany invasive carcinoma (Fig. 16.32). These invasive carcinomatous foci abut sharply on normal fat cells, or less often, on collagenous stroma in a fashion that suggests, on superficial inspection, that they were "pushed" or artifactually displaced to this location. In this situation,

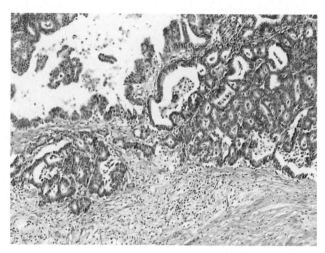

**FIG. 16.26.** *Papillary carcinoma, possibly microinvasive.* Epithelial nest in the fibrous wall around a papillary carcinoma. Irregular epithelial islands with this cribriform pattern are suggestive of invasion but could be part of the intracystic lesion trapped in the cyst wall.

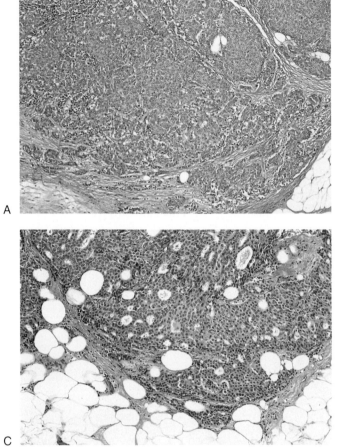

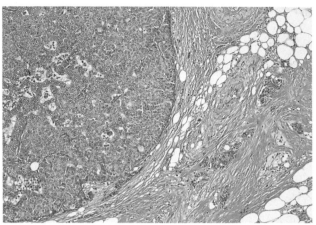

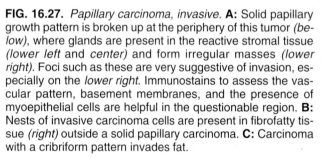

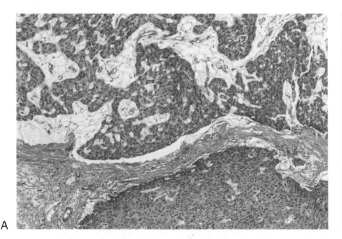

**FIG. 16.27.** *Papillary carcinoma, invasive.* **A:** Solid papillary growth pattern is broken up at the periphery of this tumor *(below)*, where glands are present in the reactive stromal tissue *(lower left* and *center)* and form irregular masses *(lower right)*. Foci such as these are very suggestive of invasion, especially on the *lower right*. Immunostains to assess the vascular pattern, basement membranes, and the presence of myoepithelial cells are helpful in the questionable region. **B:** Nests of invasive carcinoma cells are present in fibrofatty tissue *(right)* outside a solid papillary carcinoma. **C:** Carcinoma with a cribriform pattern invades fat.

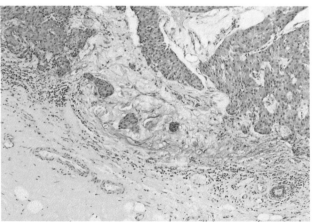

**FIG. 16.28.** *Papillary carcinoma, invasive mucinous.* **A:** Extracellular mucin in a solid papillary carcinoma confined to the tumor *(above)* does not constitute invasive carcinoma (see Fig. 16.23). **B:** Small clusters of carcinoma cells and mucin in the peritumoral stroma represent invasive mucinous carcinoma (mucicarmine stain).

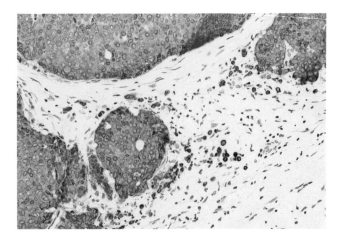

**FIG. 16.29.** *Papillary carcinoma, microinvasive.* Isolated microinvasive carcinoma cells are highlighted in the peritumoral stroma by a cytokeratin immunostain (CAM5.2, avidin-biotin).

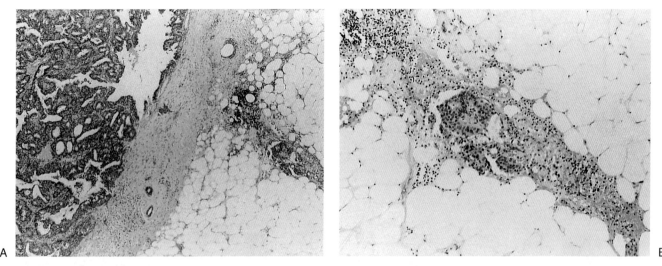

A

B

**FIG. 16.30.** *Papillary carcinoma, needle biopsy.* **A:** *In situ* papillary carcinoma surrounded by a thick capsule. The track of a needle aspiration biopsy is evident on the *right*. At this plane of section, the site of penetration into the tumor is not seen. **B:** Carcinomatous papillary epithelium displaced in the needle track.

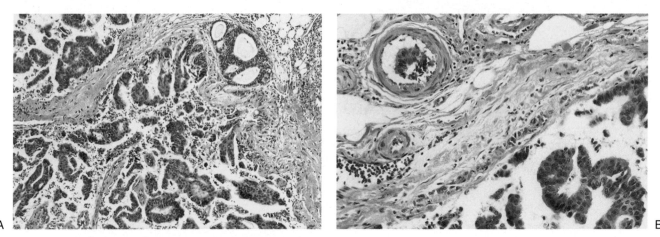

A

B

**FIG. 16.31.** *Papillary carcinoma, needle biopsy.* **A:** Tumor disruption and hemorrhage. **B:** Disrupted papillary neoplasm *(below)* and a fragment of papillary epithelium in a blood vessel *(above).*

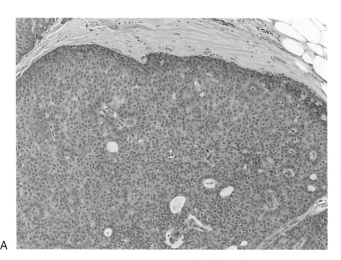
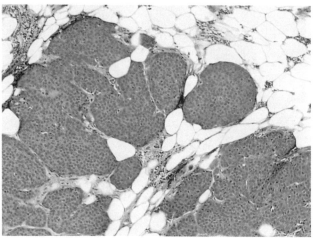

A

B

**FIG. 16.32.** *Solid papillary carcinoma with invasion.* **A:** Solid papillary carcinoma. This portion of the tumor is intraductal. **B:** Invasive carcinoma in fat without reactive stroma. Note the absence of tissue disruption, hemorrhage, or fat necrosis, which characterize a needle track.

features that favor true invasion include the absence at this site of evidence of needling such as hemorrhage, fat necrosis, a needle track, or tissue disruption. Perhaps the most telling observation is the intimate mingling of carcinoma and normal tissue that occurs in these foci, especially in fat where individual adipose cells may be found in the sheet of carcinoma cells. Carcinoma cells may be "molded" around fat cells within or at the border of such foci (Fig. 16.33).

The growth patterns found in areas of frankly invasive papillary carcinoma usually constitute variations on the architecture of *in situ* carcinoma in the underlying papillary tumor (Fig. 16.34). Cytologically, the invasive component of a papillary carcinoma also resembles the *in situ* portion of the lesion. Apocrine features may be seen in invasive papillary carcinoma. Cribriform, comedo, tubular, and mucinous foci also

may be present. The invasive element may grow partly or entirely as mucinous carcinoma, an occurrence usually associated with solid papillary carcinoma. Mucinous differentiation in solid papillary carcinoma is manifested not only by intracellular and intraluminal mucin, but also by the accumulation of extracellular mucin in limited amounts between the neoplastic epithelium and adjacent stroma (Fig. 16.23). This phenomenon can occur within the tumor, adjacent to fibrovascular stalks, and at the border of the tumor. The resultant small pools of mucin are not interpreted as invasive mucinous carcinoma unless they contain detached neoplastic cells. Larger accumulations may surround or disrupt portions of the epithelium, and the resultant appearance is interpreted as invasive carcinoma when the mucin accompanied by carcinoma cells extends into the surrounding stroma (Fig. 16.28).

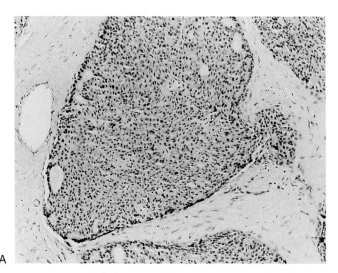
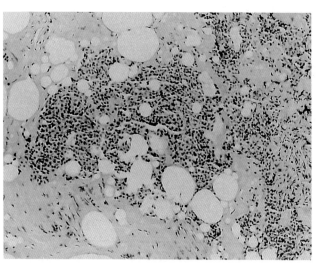

A

B

**FIG. 16.33.** *Solid papillary carcinoma with invasion.* **A:** Solid portion of the tumor with a knob of epithelium protruding into the stroma. This does not constitute invasion. **B:** Irregular groups of invasive carcinoma cells that mingle with fat and fibrous stroma at the periphery of the tumor. No preoperative or intraoperative needling procedure was performed in this case.

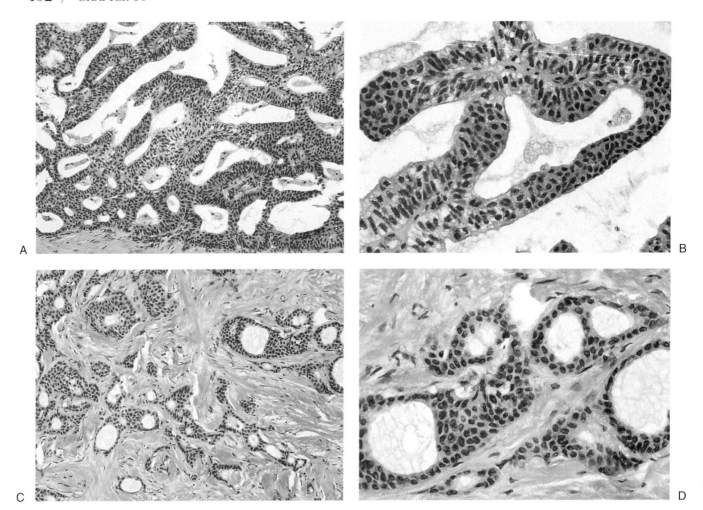

**FIG. 16.34.** *Invasive papillary carcinoma.* **A:** Papillary carcinoma. **B:** Carcinoma cells have dark cytologically low-grade nuclei and eosinophilic cytoplasm. **C:** Invasive cribriform carcinoma that arose in the papillary carcinoma. **D:** Cytologic features of the invasive component resemble the papillary *in situ* carcinoma.

Clusters of invasive papillary carcinoma cells may have shrinkage artifacts and appear to lie in spaces, creating the appearance of lymphatic tumor emboli. When one applies strict criteria for the diagnosis of lymphatic invasion, most such foci prove to be artifactual (48).

## CYTOLOGY

In view of the difficulty sometimes encountered in making a distinction between papilloma and papillary carcinoma in histologic sections, it is not surprising that diagnostic problems arise in aspiration cytology and needle core biopsy specimens obtained from these lesions. Nonetheless, there are cytologic features that suggest papillary carcinoma in such material. Papillary carcinomas tend to yield hypercellular specimens composed of papillary clusters that may have fibrovascular cores and dissociated single cells (49–51). Marked hypercellularity is encountered less often in the aspirate from a papilloma. Cellular pleomorphism, necrosis, and fragments with a cribriform pattern are features associated with papillary carcinoma. The cells tend to be low-to-tall columnar in papillomas and papillary carcinomas, but papillary carcinoma is more likely to be composed of cells with nuclear hyperchromasia and disorderly stratification. Signet-ring cells and extracellular mucin may be detected if the papillary carcinoma has mucinous differentiation. These features may be a clue to the diagnosis of spindle cell argyrophilic mucin-producing papillary carcinoma (52).

Infarction in papillomas may result in nuclear atypia and inflammation. Apocrine metaplasia, foamy histiocytes, and bipolar nuclei associated with myoepithelial cells are characteristic of a papilloma. Cohesive epithelial fragments and bipolar myoepithelial cells obtained from a papilloma may resemble the aspirate from a fibroadenoma. However, the epithelium from the latter lesion tends to be distributed in flat sheets rather than in three-dimensional groups, and there is no fibrovascular stroma within the epithelial groups. The epithelium from a fibroadenomas typically has a honeycomb appearance, but papillary hyperplasia of the fibroadenomatous epithelium may cause a more irregular cellular pattern.

The distinction between a papilloma and papillary carcinoma usually can be made with the tissue fragments obtained by needle core biopsy (53). Because carcinoma may only focally involve a papillary tumor, the absence of this element in a core biopsy specimen may simply be due to incomplete sampling of the lesion. It also should be noted that fragments of florid hyperplasia represented out of context in a core biopsy may suggest *in situ* carcinoma and that stromal samples containing entrapped epithelium from a benign sclerosing papillary lesion can mimic invasive carcinoma.

## PROGNOSIS AND TREATMENT

Whether cystic or solid, papillary carcinoma without invasion is a form of intraductal carcinoma. If completely resected surgically, these patients are virtually all cured by the procedure. Nonetheless, patients with apparently noninvasive papillary carcinoma are subject to the same very low risk of obscure invasion that occurs with other types of intraductal carcinoma. Consequently, axillary nodal metastases have been encountered in less than 1% of patients with "noninvasive" papillary carcinoma. In one series, three patients with no demonstrable invasion developed metastases, including one with involvement of axillary lymph nodes and two with negative axillary nodes who had systemic metastases detected 49 and 53 months after initial surgery (15).

Carter et al. (5) described 18 patients with noninvasive cystic papillary carcinoma who had simple mastectomies and 11 other patients who were treated by mastectomy with axillary dissection. None of the latter group had axillary metastases, and there were no recurrences. Sixteen patients remained alive after an average of 83 months; 13 died of causes other than breast carcinoma, having remained recurrence free for an average of 65 months. Eleven other patients studied by the same authors were treated by excisional biopsy alone. Three (27%) of the 11 had subsequent recurrences in the ipsilateral breast. Two were invasive lesions detected 3 and 6 years later. The third patient was found to have recurrent noninvasive papillary carcinoma 3 years after her initial excisional therapy. At the time of the report, there were no systemic recurrences. Six of the patients treated by excision survived disease free for an average of 10 years. Two additional patients were without recurrent breast carcinoma when they died of other causes 6 and 11 years after treatment by excisional biopsy alone. The series also included one woman treated with radiotherapy after excision of papillary intraductal carcinoma. She remained well 56 months later.

Invasive papillary carcinomas can be relatively large tumors if a bulky, cystic component is present, but invasion also is encountered in solid tumors and in lesions 3 cm or less in diameter. The frequency of axillary lymph node metastases encountered in patients with invasive papillary carcinoma is determined by the actual sizes of the invasive elements as well as the histologic and nuclear grade (1,2,4,15). When axillary nodal metastases occur, they usually do not involve more than three lymph nodes (2). The growth pattern of the primary tumor often is duplicated in metastatic foci. The prognosis of patients with invasive papillary carcinoma is reportedly very favorable, even in women who have axillary nodal metastases (2). When they occur, metastatic recurrences of invasive papillary carcinoma often become clinically apparent more than 5 years after diagnosis. These patients are subject to the same tendency to "late" recurrence as are women with mucinous carcinoma. Recurrence in the breast after underdiagnosis of a papillary carcinoma as a papilloma or after breast conservation therapy for a correctly diagnosed tumor typically occurs more than 3 years after initial treatment. Criteria for breast conservation therapy are similar to those employed for women with nonpapillary intraductal or invasive carcinoma.

## REFERENCES

1. Carter D. Intraductal papillary tumors of the breast. A study of 76 cases. *Cancer* 1977;39:1689–1692.
2. Fisher ER, Palekar AS, Redmond C, et al. Pathologic findings from the National Surgical Adjuvant Breast Project (Protocol No. 4). VI. Invasive papillary cancer. *Am J Clin Pathol* 1980;73:313–320.
3. Haagensen CD. *Diseases of the breast.* 2nd ed. Philadelphia: WB Saunders, 1971:528–544.
4. Foote FW Jr, Stewart FW. A histologic classification of carcinoma of the breast. *Surgery* 1946;19:74–99.
5. Carter D, Orr SL, Merino MJ. Intracystic papillary carcinoma of the breast after mastectomy, radiotherapy or excisional biopsy alone. *Cancer* 1983;52:14–19.
6. Bloodgood JC. Benign lesions of the female breast for which operation is not indicated. *JAMA* 1922;78:859–863.
7. Estes AC, Phillips C. Papilloma of lacteal duct. *Surg Gynecol Obstet* 1949;89:345–348.
8. Gray HK, Wood GA. Significance of mammary discharge in cases of papilloma of the breast. *Arch Surg* 1941;42:203–208.
9. Kilgore AR, Fleming R, Ramos N. The incidence of cancer with nipple discharge and the risk of cancer in the presence of papillary disease of the breast. *Surg Gynecol Obstet* 1953;96:649–660.
10. Stout AP. Diagnosis of benign, borderline and malignant lesions of the breast. Proceedings of the Second National Cancer Conference, 1952. Cincinnati: American Cancer Society, 1954:179–183.
11. Haagensen CD, Stout AP, Phillips JS. The papillary neoplasms of the breast. I. Benign intraductal papilloma. *Ann Surg* 1951;133:18–36.
12. Rosen PP. Arthur Purdy Stout and papilloma of the breast. Comments on the occasion of his 100th birthday. *Am J Surg Pathol* 1986;10[Suppl 1]:100–107.
13. Stout AP. The relationship of benign lesions of the breast to cancer. *J Natl Med Assoc* 1954;46:375–381.
14. Moore SW, Pearce J, Ring E. Intraductal papilloma of the breast. *Surg Gynecol Obstet* 1961;112:153–158.
15. Lefkowitz M, Lefkowitz W, Wargotz ES. Intraductal (intracystic) papillary carcinoma of the breast and its variants: a clinicopathological study of 77 cases. *Hum Pathol* 1994;25:802–809.
16. Schaefer G, Rosen PP, Lesser ML, et al. Breast carcinoma in elderly women: pathology prognosis and survival. *Pathol Annu* 1984;19[Pt 1]:195–219.
17. Rosen PP, Ashikari R, Thaler H, et al. A comparative study of some pathologic features of mammary carcinoma in Tokyo, Japan and New York, USA. *Cancer* 1977;39:429–434.
18. Tobin CE, Hendrix TM, Resnikoff LB, et al. Breast imaging case of the day. *Radiographics* 1996;16:720–722.
19. Hunter CE Jr, Sawyers JL. Intracystic papillary carcinoma of the breast. *South Med J* 1980;73:1484–1486.
20. Czernobilsky B. Intracystic carcinoma of the female breast. *Surg Gynecol Obstet* 1967;124:93–98.
21. Masood S, Barwick K. Estrogen receptor expression of the less common breast carcinomas. *Am J Clin Pathol* 1990;93:437.
22. Meyer JS, Bauer WC, Rao BR. Subpopulations of breast carcinoma defined by S-phase fraction, morphology and estrogen receptor content. *Lab Invest* 1978;39:225–235.

23. Tiltman AJ. DNA ploidy in papillary tumours of the breast. *S Afr Med J* 1989;75:379–380.
24. Estabrook A, Asch T, Gump F, et al. Mammographic features of intracystic papillary lesions. *Surg Gynecol Obstet* 1990;170:113–116.
25. Schneider JA. Invasive papillary breast carcinoma: mammographic and sonographic appearance. *Radiology* 1989;171:377–379.
26. McCulloch GL, Evans AJ, Yeoman L, et al. Radiological features of papillary carcinoma of the breast. *Clin Radiol* 1997;52:865–868.
27. Silva R, Ferrozi F, Paties C. Invasive papillary carcinoma in elderly women: sonographic and mammographic features. *AJR Am J Roentgenol* 1992;159:898.
28. Soo MS, Williford ME, Walsh R, et al. Papillary carcinoma of the breast: imaging findings. *AJR Am J Roentgenol* 1995;164:321–326.
29. Matsuo S, Eto T, Soejima H, et al. A case of intracystic carcinoma of the breast: the importance of measuring carcinoembryonic antigen in aspirated cystic fluid. *Breast Cancer Res Treat* 1993;28:41–44.
30. Inaji H, Koyama H, Motomura K, Simultaneous assay of erbB-2 protein and carcinoembryonic antigen in cyst fluid as an aid in diagnosing cystic lesions of the breast. *Breast Cancer* 1994;1:25–30.
31. Kraus FT, Neubecker RD. The differential diagnosis of papillary tumors of the breast. *Cancer* 1962;15:444–455.
32. Papotti M, Gugliotta P, Eusebi V, et al. Immunohistochemical analysis of benign and malignant papillary lesions of the breast. *Am J Surg Pathol* 1983;7:451–461.
33. Murad TM, Swaid S, Pritchett P. Malignant and benign papillary lesions of the breast. *Hum Pathol* 1977;8:379–390.
34. Papotti M, Gugliotta P, Ghiringhello B, et al. Association of breast carcinoma ad multiple intraductal papillomas: an histological and immunohistochemical investigation. *Histopathology* 1984;8:963–975.
35. Rosen PP, Oberman HA. Papillary carcinoma in tumors of the mammary gland. *Atlas of tumor pathology*. Fascicle 7, 3rd series. Washington, DC: Armed Forces Institute of Pathology, 1993:217.
36. Snyder WH, Chaffin L. Main duct papilloma of the breast. *Arch Surg* 1955;70:680–685.
37. Raju U, Vertes D. Breast papillomas with atypical ductal hyperplasia: a clinicopathologic study. *Hum Pathol* 1996;27:1231–1238.
38. Page DL, Salhany KE, Jensen RA, et al. Subsequent breast carcinoma risk after biopsy with atypia in a breast papilloma. *Cancer* 1996;78:258–266.
39. Ohuchi N, Abe R, Kasai M. Possible cancerous change in intraductal papillomas of the breast. A 3-D reconstruction study of 25 cases. *Cancer* 1984;54:605–611.
40. Ohuchi N, Abe R, Takahashi T, et al. Three-dimensional atypical structure in intraductal carcinoma differentiating from papilloma and papillomatosis of the breast. *Breast Cancer Res Treat* 1985; 5:57–68.
41. Saddik M, Lai R, Medeiros LJ, et al. Differential expression of cyclin D1 in breast papillary carcinomas and benign papillomas: an immunohistochemical study. *Arch Pathol Lab Med* 1999;123:152–156.
42. Cross AS, Azzopardi JG, Krausz T, et al. A morphologic and immunocytochemical study of a distinctive variant of ductal carcinoma *in situ* of the breast. *Histopathology* 1985;9:21–37.
43. Tsuda H, Uei Y, Fukutomi T, et al. Different incidence of loss of heterozygosity on chromosome 16q between intraductal papilloma and intracystic papillary carcinoma of the breast. *Jpn J Cancer Res* 1994;85:992–996.
44. Lininger RA, Zhuang Z, Man YG, et al. LOH at 16p13 detected in microdissected papillary neoplasms of the breast and their precursors. *Mod Pathol* 1997;10:22A.
45. Ahmed A. Ultrastructural aspects of human breast lesions. *Pathol Annu* 1980;15[Pt 2]:411–443.
46. Tsuchiya S, Takayama S, Higashi Y. Electron microscopy of intraductal papilloma of the breast. Ultrastructural comparison of papillary carcinoma with normal large duct. *Acta Pathol Jpn* 1983;33:97–112.
47. Youngson B, Cranor M, Rosen PP. Epithelial displacement in surgical breast specimens following needling procedures. *Am J Surg Pathol* 1994;18:896–903.
48. Rosen PP. Tumor emboli in intramammary lymphatics in breast carcinoma: pathologic criteria for diagnosis and clinical significance. *Pathol Annu* 1983;18[Pt 2]:215–232.
49. Bardales RH, Suhrland MJ, Stanley MW. Papillary neoplasms of the breast: fine-needle aspiration findings in cystic and solid cases. *Diagn Cytopathol* 1994;10:336–341.
50. Dawson AE, Mulford DK. Benign versus malignant papillary neoplasms of the breast. Diagnostic clues in fine needle aspiration cytology. *Acta Cytol* 1994;38:23–28.
51. Jeffrey PB, Ljung B-M. Benign and malignant papillary lesions of the breast. A cytomorphologic study. *Am J Clin Pathol* 1994;101:500–507.
52. Burgan AR, Frierson HF Jr, Fechner RE. Fine-needle aspiration cytology of spindle-cell argyrophilic mucin-producing carcinoma of the breast. *Diagn Cytopathol* 1996;14:238–242.
53. Rosen PP. *Breast pathology. Diagnosis by needle core biopsy*. Philadelphia: Lippincott, Williams & Wilkins 1999:21–42, 135–146.

# CHAPTER 17

# Medullary Carcinoma

Mammary carcinomas have been described as "medullary" for nearly a century. For approximately 50 years, however, the term was used clinically and pathologically for large, solid carcinomas with a papillary or fleshy gross appearance. Included in this group were tumors characterized by a marked lymphoid reaction and a favorable prognosis referred to as cystic neomammary carcinoma by Geschickter (1). At Memorial Hospital, these tumors were termed "bulky adenocarcinomas" until the name medullary carcinoma was proposed in the 1940s (2,3).

Medullary carcinoma is defined as a "well circumscribed carcinoma composed of poorly differentiated cells with scant stroma and prominent lymphoid infiltration" (4).

## CLINICAL PRESENTATION

Medullary carcinomas constitute less than 5% of tumors in most series (5–8), but frequencies as high as 7% have been reported (9–11). Studies of various racial groups indicate that medullary carcinoma is relatively more frequent among Japanese women in Japan than among white women in the United States (12–14). Medullary carcinoma has been reported to be relatively more common among black women in the United States than among whites (15–18), but a significant racial association has not been found in some series of cases from individual institutions (8,19,20).

Maternal breast carcinoma was reportedly more frequent among women with medullary carcinoma than among women with other types of carcinoma, whereas very few of their sisters had breast carcinoma (21). A detailed analysis of the family pedigrees of patients with medullary carcinoma did not reveal an increased risk for neoplastic disease, including breast carcinoma, when compared to the families of patients with tubular or invasive duct carcinoma (22).

Medullary carcinomas have a number of features in common with BRCA1-associated breast carcinomas, including relatively young age at diagnosis, poorly differentiated histology, lymphocytic infiltration, absence of hormone receptors, and frequent p53 alterations. A study of BRCA1-asso-

ciated breast carcinomas revealed that six (19%) of 32 tumors were true medullary carcinomas, which is a significantly higher frequency than observed among non–BRCA1-associated control tumors (23). BRCA1 nonsense mutations were found in two of 18 medullary carcinomas, seven times the frequency of these alterations in the general population. Malone et al. (24) reported finding BRCA1 mutations in five (23.8%) of 21 women with medullary carcinoma and in 17 (6%) of 285 of women with nonmedullary tumors. All patients included in the latter study underwent BRCA1 testing because of a family history of breast carcinoma and/or early onset of breast carcinoma.

Patients with medullary carcinoma tend to be relatively young and this type constitutes at least 10% of carcinomas diagnosed in women 35 years of age, or less. Moore and Foote (3) found that 59% of their patients were less than 50 years old. Others reported that 40% (10) and 60% (25) of patients were younger than 50 years and the mean age in several series ranged from 45 to 54 years (6,19,20,25). Medullary carcinoma is relatively uncommon in elderly patients (26), and it is rarely found in the male breast (7).

Early descriptions of medullary carcinoma referred to large, circumscribed tumors with a tendency to cystic degeneration (1,3). Ulceration of the skin and fixation to the chest wall have been reported with large tumors. Currently, medullary carcinomas tend to be smaller than 3 cm. Because they have circumscribed margins and a firm consistency, medullary carcinomas can be mistaken clinically and radiologically for fibroadenomas (7,27). Images obtained by ultrasound have not provided diagnostic criteria specific for medullary carcinoma (27). Kopans and Rubens (28) have emphasized that there are no radiologic criteria for distinguishing medullary from circumscribed nonmedullary carcinoma (Figs. 17.1 and 17.2).

The anatomic distribution of medullary carcinoma in the breast does not differ significantly from that of breast carcinomas in general. Medullary carcinoma arising in the axillary tail is difficult to distinguish from metastatic carcinoma in a lymph node (29). Medullary carcinoma is not especially

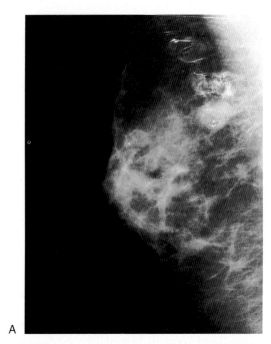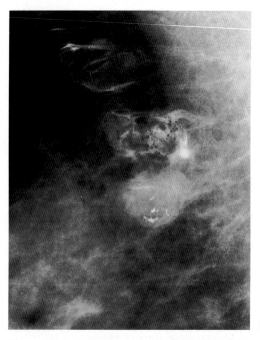

A                                                                                                                              B

**FIG. 17.1.** *Medullary carcinoma, mammography.* **A:** The tumor is an oval circumscribed mass. **B:** Dye injected into the breast for localization is present above the tumor, which contains coarse calcifications.

common among patients with bilateral mammary carcinoma. Bilateral carcinoma has been found in 3% to 18% of patients with medullary carcinoma (6,8,20,26,27,30). Synchronous or metachronous medullary carcinoma involving both breasts is very uncommon (6,20,26,30). Multicentricity, defined as microscopic foci of carcinoma outside the primary quadrant, is uncommon in patients with medullary carcinoma. It was found in 10% of 58 cases in one series (30) and in 8% in another study (8).

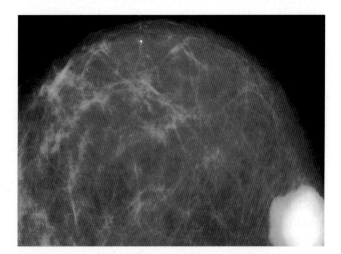

**FIG. 17.2.** *Circumscribed nonmedullary carcinoma, mammography.* Histologic examination of the circumscribed tumor revealed an infiltrating duct carcinoma with medullary features.

Ipsilateral axillary lymph nodes tend to be enlarged in medullary carcinoma patients, even when there are no nodal metastases. This phenomenon, which may complicate clinical staging (31), also can be encountered in patients with duct carcinomas that have medullary features (32). Microscopically, the lymph nodes have a lymphoplasmacytic infiltrate, germinal center hyperplasia, and frequently sinus histiocytosis. On average, the number of lymph nodes found grossly in an axillary dissection specimen from a patient with medullary or atypical medullary carcinoma is greater than for other types of carcinoma (32). This difference probably results from the greater ease of finding enlarged, hyperplastic lymph nodes.

The microscopic features of medullary carcinoma resemble those of lymphoepithelial carcinomas that arise at other sites. These and other characteristics have suggested that the Epstein-Barr virus might play a role in pathogenesis of medullary carcinoma. However, a study of ten tumors using immunohistochemistry, *in situ* hybridization, and the polymerase chain reaction failed to detect evidence of Epstein-Barr virus (33).

## GROSS PATHOLOGY

Early descriptions of medullary carcinoma emphasized large size, a characterization exemplified by the term "bulky carcinoma," which also was used for this tumor type. Presently, the size distribution of medullary carcinomas is not appreciably different from that of infiltrating duct carci-

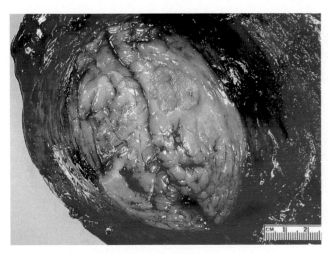

**FIG. 17.3.** *Medullary carcinoma, gross specimen.* The nodular tumor has a circumscribed border.

nomas, with a median size of 2 to 3 cm (9,20). A review of 524 consecutive patients with T1N0 and T1N1 breast carcinomas treated from 1964 to 1970 found that 2% of each group had medullary carcinoma (34,35).

When examined grossly, the typical intact medullary carcinoma is a moderately firm discrete tumor that is easily mistaken for a fibroadenoma (Fig. 17.3). A distinct margin outlines the tumor when bisected and distinguishes it from the surrounding breast tissue (Fig. 17.4). In larger lesions, particularly those that have prominent cystic areas, peripheral fibrosis may suggest encapsulation (Fig. 17.5). Some

small medullary carcinomas have poorly circumscribed borders on gross examination (19). Microscopically, the peripheral areas of ill-defined medullary carcinomas have an intense lymphoplasmacytic reaction that extends well beyond the immediate perimeter of the tumor into adjacent breast tissue. Consequently, gross circumscription is supportive of, but necessary for, a diagnosis of medullary carcinoma. Some nonmedullary infiltrating carcinomas are as well circumscribed as the typical medullary carcinoma (Fig. 17.6).

The cut surfaces of the fresh specimen and whole-mount histologic sections reveal that a medullary carcinoma has a lobulated or nodular internal structure (Fig. 17.7). Occasionally, one finds secondary nodules at the periphery of the main tumor, or it is possible to appreciate that the mass is composed of coalescent nodules (Fig. 17.8). The pale brown to gray tumor tissue is softer than the average breast carcinoma, and it tends to bulge above the surrounding parenchyma rather than having the retracted appearance of a typical invasive duct carcinoma. Hemorrhage and necrosis are not unusual features, even in medullary carcinomas smaller than 2 cm, but overall, the extent of necrosis is directly related to tumor size. The necrotic tissue sometimes has a grossly caseous, granular appearance. As the extent of necrosis increases, there is a greater likelihood that the tumor will develop cystic foci (Fig. 17.9). Prominent cystic degeneration usually is seen only in tumors larger than 5 cm (Fig. 17.10). Fragmented tumor in a cystic medullary carcinoma may be grossly indistinguishable from a cystic papillary carcinoma.

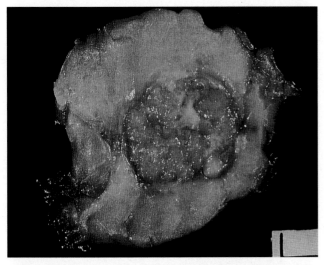

**FIG. 17.4.** *Medullary carcinoma, gross specimen.* The tumor protrudes above the surrounding tissue. The borders are circumscribed and the cut surfaces reveal internal nodularity. (From Rosen PP, Oberman HA. Tumors of the mammary gland. In: *Atlas of tumor pathology.* Washington, DC: Armed Forces Institute of Pathology, 1993, with permission.)

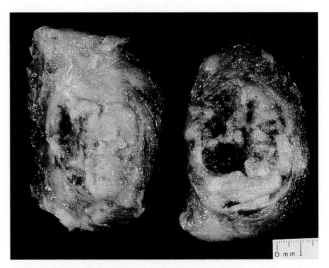

**FIG. 17.5.** *Medullary carcinoma, gross specimen.* Cystic degeneration is apparent. A pseudocapsule is evident at the lower border of the tumor. The tumor protrudes above the surrounding tissue and the internal structure is nodular. (From Ridolfi R, Rosen P, Port A, et al. Medullary carcinoma of the breast. A clinicopathologic study with 10 year follow-up. *Cancer* 1977;40:1365–1385, with permission.)

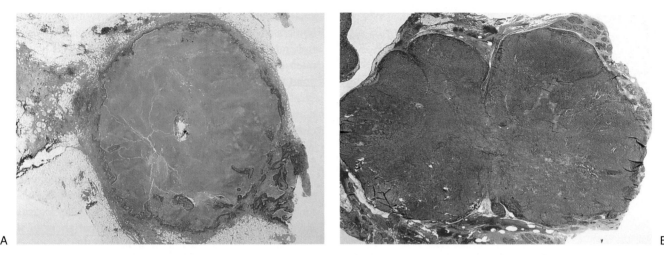

**FIG. 17.6.** *Circumscribed nonmedullary carcinomas.* Whole-mount histologic sections. **A:** Carcinoma with extensive central infarction and peripheral lymphocytic reaction. **B:** Bilobed diffuse infiltrating duct carcinoma with focal peripheral lymphocytic infiltration represented by the discontinuous, thin blue line at the border.

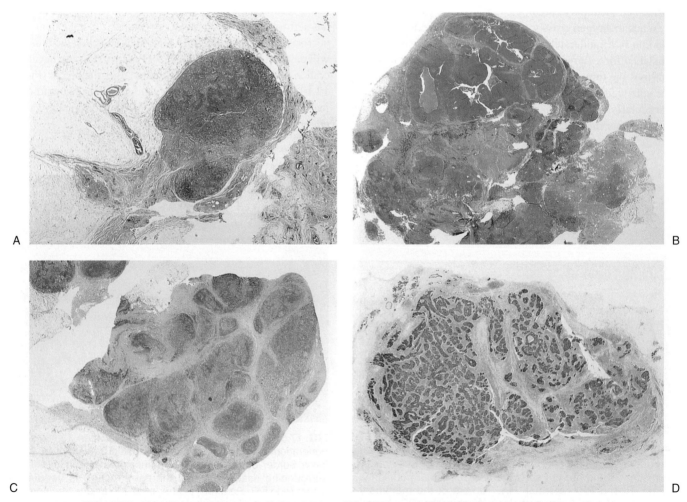

**FIG. 17.7.** *Medullary carcinoma, nodular structure.* Whole-mount histologic sections. **A–C:** Illustrations of varying complexity in the nodular structure of three different tumors. **D:** Epithelial areas within the nodules are stained brown by the immunoreaction for cytokeratin (anti-AE1/AE3, avidin-biotin).

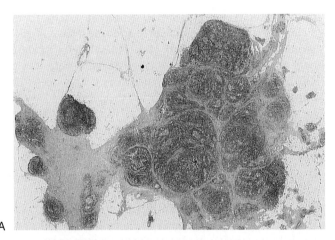

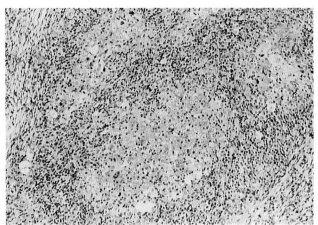

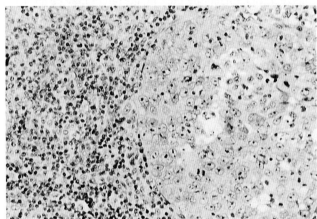

**FIG. 17.8.** *Medullary carcinoma, peripheral nodules.* **A:** In addition to multiple coalescent nodules forming the main tumor, smaller circumscribed nodules of tumor are evident on the *left*. **B,C:** Histologic appearance of carcinoma in one of the secondary tumor nodules on the *left* in **A** showing poorly differentiated carcinoma with a syncytial pattern and a lymphocytic reaction. Carcinoma merges with the lymphocytes in **B**, whereas in **C** the carcinoma is sharply circumscribed.

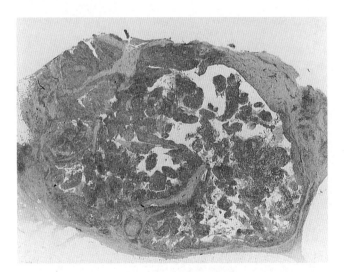

**FIG. 17.9.** *Medullary carcinoma, cystic degeneration.* The internal nodular structure is evident in areas of cystic degeneration in this whole-mount histologic section.

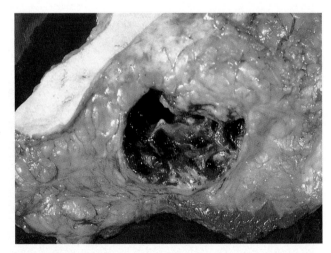

**FIG. 17.10.** *Medullary carcinoma, cystic.* Gross appearance of the tumor in a mastectomy specimen.

## MICROSCOPIC PATHOLOGY

It is necessary to adhere to strictly defined morphologic criteria if the diagnosis of medullary carcinoma is to be predictive of a relatively favorable prognosis (6,19). The gross appearance of a tumor may lead one to suspect medullary carcinoma, and occasionally this may be taken into consideration in deciding how to classify a lesion with "borderline" features. Ultimately, the diagnosis depends on the microscopic characteristics of the tumor. Overdiagnosis of medullary carcinoma has been reported in several reviews, usually the result of failure to limit the diagnosis to lesions that fulfill all diagnostic criteria (36,37).

Some investigators reported substantial interobserver and intraobserver variability in the diagnosis of medullary carcinoma (36,38). This has led to the suggestion that histologic criteria for the diagnosis be modified. However, the favorable prognosis attributed to true medullary carcinoma is not observed in cases classified according to modified criteria (36). Jensen et al. (39) compared three systems for defining medullary and atypical medullary carcinoma. The criteria set forth by Ridolfi et al. (19) proved to be more reliable for detecting survival differences between true medullary, atypical medullary, and nonmedullary carcinomas than the modified definitions set forth by Tavassoli (40) and Pedersen et al. (36). The specific diagnosis of medullary carcinoma will be improved by increased familiarity with, and strict adherence to, the diagnostic criteria already established. In doubtful situations, a tumor should be classified as a nonmedullary carcinoma.

Medullary carcinoma is defined by a constellation of histopathologic features that initially were described by Foote and Stewart (2) and Moore and Foote (3). A tumor should have all of the definitive characteristics to be classified as a medullary carcinoma. When most, but not all, of the needed components are present, the tumor may be termed an *atypical medullary carcinoma* or *infiltrating duct carcinoma with medullary features*. Definitive histopathologic features include the following: lymphoplasmacytic reaction, microscopic circumscription, growth in sheets (syncytial pattern), poorly differentiated nuclear grade, and high mitotic rate.

The *lymphoplasmacytic reaction* must involve the periph-

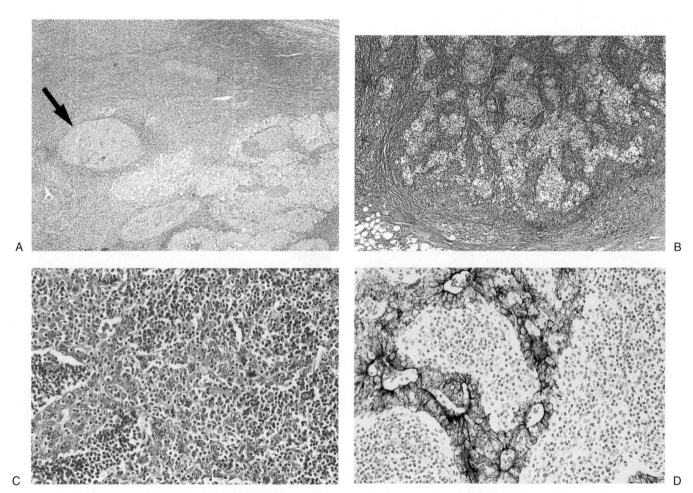

**FIG. 17.11.** *Medullary carcinoma, lymphoplasmacytic reaction.* **A:** Syncytial sheets of carcinoma cells surrounded by a diffuse lymphocytic reaction. The germinal center is an unusual occurrence *(arrow).* **B:** Lymphocytic reaction around groups of carcinoma cells in nodular aggregates. **C:** Lymphocytic reaction mingles with and obscures the carcinoma creating an appearance that resembles lymphoepithelioma. **D:** The carcinoma cells in **C** are highlighted with the cytokeratin immunostain (avidin-biotin).

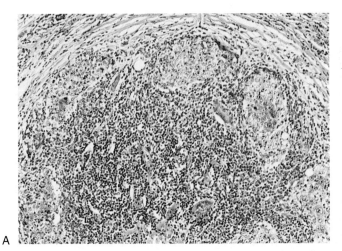 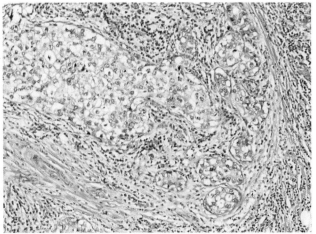

**FIG. 17.12.** *Medullary carcinoma, lobular extension.* **A:** Carcinoma cells have replaced most of the normal epithelium in this lobule at the periphery of a medullary carcinoma. A few clusters of dark nonneoplastic cells remain. A lymphocytic reaction is apparent in and around the lobule. **B:** Intraepithelial carcinoma in an intralobular ductule and in lobular glands with a lymphocytic reaction.

ery and be present diffusely in the substance of the tumor. In most medullary carcinomas, the internal lymphoplasmacytic infiltrate tends to be limited to fibrovascular stroma between syncytial zones of tumor cells. A minority of medullary carcinomas seem to be largely devoid of stroma, and the lymphoplasmacytic infiltrate mingles intimately with carcinoma cells (Fig. 17.11) (9). It can be difficult to distinguish this latter type of tumor from metastatic carcinoma in a lymph node. Peripherally, there may be some variation in the amount of lymphocytic reaction, but it should be at least moderately intense at the interface of the carcinoma with mammary parenchyma and in the adjacent tissue. In the usual case, the lymphoplasmacytic reaction encompasses surrounding ducts and lobules occupied by *in situ* carcinoma (Fig. 17.12). The reactive process also tends to involve more distant ducts and lobules that do not contain identifiable tumor cells (Fig. 17.13). These secondary peripheral alter-

ations are so common in medullary carcinoma that the diagnosis may be questioned when they are absent.

The lymphoplasmacytic infiltrate may be composed almost entirely of either lymphocytes or plasma cells, but most often there is a mixture of these cells (Fig. 17.14) (9). Intense lymphoplasmacytic infiltrates can occur as well in nonmedullary infiltrating duct carcinomas, but when plasma cells predominate, the tumor is more likely to be a medullary carcinoma. A few neutrophils, eosinophils, and monocytes can be found, especially when there is necrosis or cystic degeneration, but these are never the dominant cell types in a medullary carcinoma. Rarely, the lymphocytic infiltrate gives rise to germinal centers within and/or around the tumor (Fig. 17.15). Hence, the presence of germinal centers cannot be relied on as evidence that one is dealing with metastatic carcinoma in a lymph node.

*Microscopic circumscription* refers to the appearance of

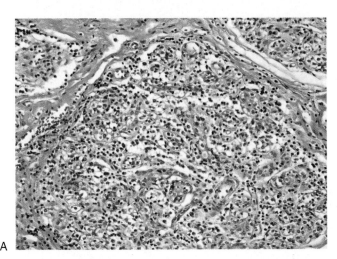 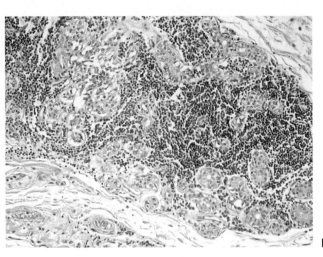

**FIG. 17.13.** *Medullary carcinoma, lobular lymphocytic reaction.* **A,B:** Lymphocytic reaction in lobules at the periphery of a medullary carcinoma. No carcinoma is evident.

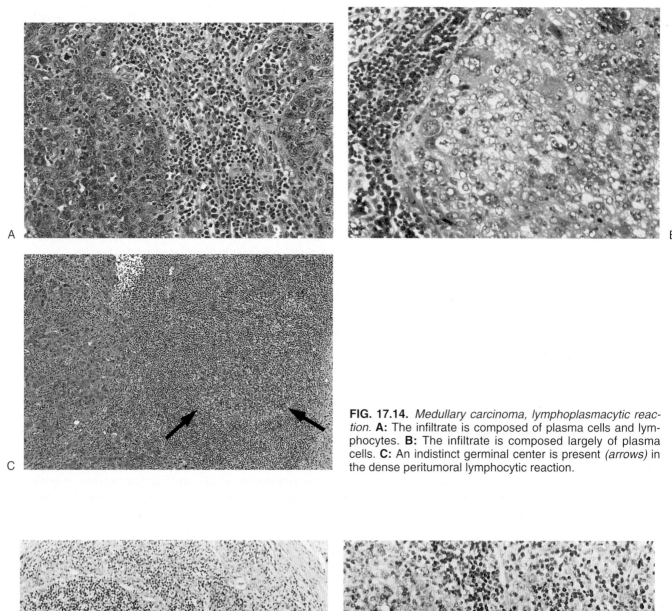

**FIG. 17.14.** *Medullary carcinoma, lymphoplasmacytic reaction.* **A:** The infiltrate is composed of plasma cells and lymphocytes. **B:** The infiltrate is composed largely of plasma cells. **C:** An indistinct germinal center is present *(arrows)* in the dense peritumoral lymphocytic reaction.

**FIG. 17.15.** *Medullary carcinoma, germinal center formation.* **A:** Germinal center is present in the dense lymphocytic reaction in the primary tumor. **B:** Infiltrating carcinoma with a syncytial structure next to the germinal center. *(continued)*

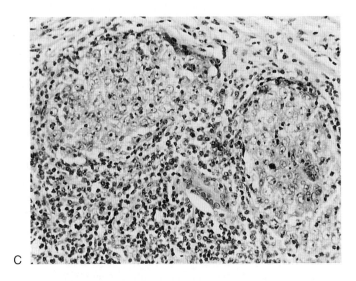

C

**FIG. 17.15.** *Continued.* **C:** *In situ* carcinoma in the epithelium of a lobule next to the tumor.

the border of the infiltrating carcinoma rather than the periphery of the surrounding lymphoplasmacytic reaction. In medullary carcinoma, the edge of the tumor should have a smooth, rounded contour that appears to push aside rather than infiltrate the breast parenchyma (Figs. 17.16 and 17.17). Consequently, glandular or fatty breast tissue should not be found within the main body of the invasive portion of the tumor. In assessing this feature, it is important to distinguish

between ducts, lobules, or islands of fat cells trapped in the surrounding lymphoplasmacytic reaction of medullary carcinoma and the same structures invaded by nonmedullary invasive carcinoma (Fig. 17.18). In the latter instance, the tumor typically lacks the cohesive syncytial structure of medullary carcinoma and the tumor cells tend to invade in trabecular, dendritic, or dispersed patterns.

A *syncytial pattern* requires that most of the tumor growth

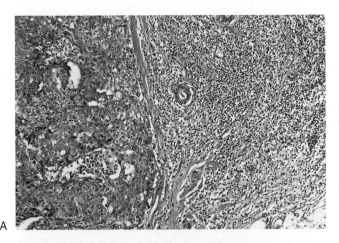

A

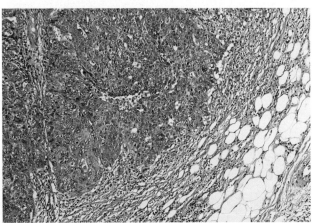

B

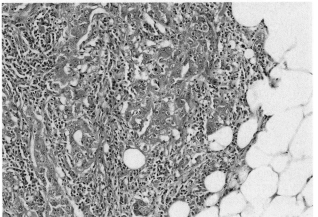

C

**FIG. 17.16.** *Medullary carcinoma, tumor border.* **A:** Carcinoma is confined to syncytial masses with a lymphocytic reaction at the tumor border. **B:** Carcinoma is confined to syncytial growth within the lymphocytic reaction which merges with the fat. **C:** This pattern of carcinoma and lymphocytes invading fat is not compatible with a diagnosis of medullary carcinoma.

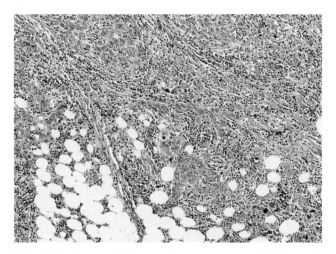

**FIG. 17.17.** *Nonmedullary carcinoma, tumor border.* Fat cells surrounded by carcinoma is a manifestation of invasive growth.

(variously defined as 75% or more of the histologically sampled areas) be arranged in broad irregular sheets or islands in which the borders of individual cells are indistinct (Fig. 17.19). The histology sometimes resembles a poorly differentiated epidermoid carcinoma (Fig. 17.20). This comparison is particularly apt because traces of epidermoid differentiation are not unusual in medullary carcinomas, and some tumors exhibit well-formed foci of squamous metaplasia. A tumor that is otherwise characteristic may be accepted as a medullary carcinoma if it has minor components of trabecular, glandular, alveolar, or papillary growth (Fig. 17.21). Such regions may have a diminished lymphoplasmacytic infiltrate and/or fibrosis and thus appear distinct from the medullary growth pattern. It has been reported that overall and relapse-free survival are directly related to the extent of the syncytial component (41). Although there was not a significant difference in outcome between patients with 75% and 90% syncy-

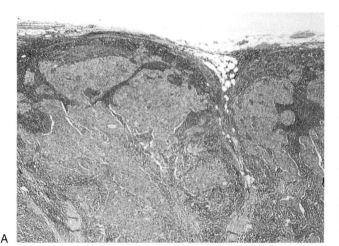
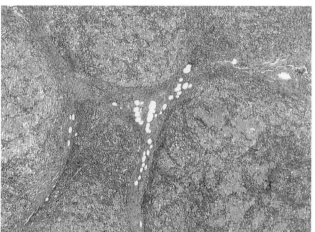

A                                    B

**FIG. 17.18.** *Medullary carcinoma, tumor border.* **A,B:** Fibrofatty stroma is trapped between the tumor nodules, but each nodule has a sharply circumscribed border.

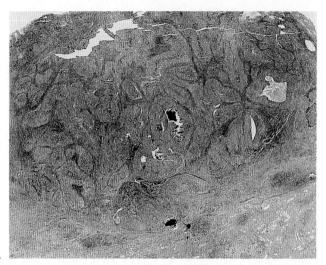
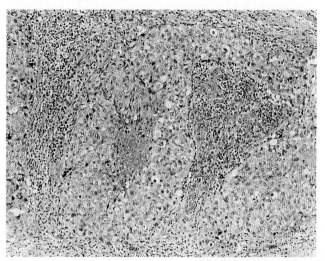

A                                    B

**FIG. 17.19.** *Medullary carcinoma, syncytial growth.* **A:** Syncytial growth in this medullary carcinoma has created a serpentine architecture. Dark calcifications have been formed in two foci of necrosis. **B:** Interlacing bands of carcinoma cells in a lymphoplasmacytic reaction. Focal necrosis is evident in the center of the carcinomatous epithelium.

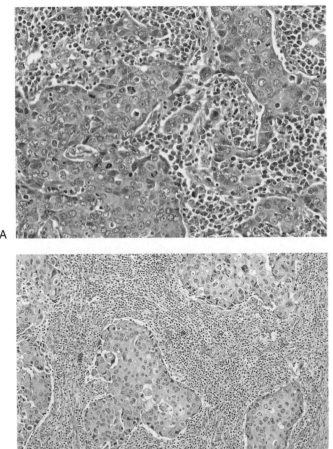

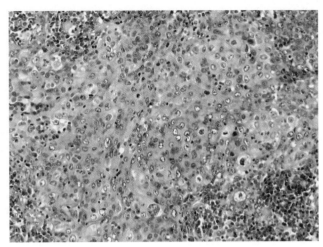

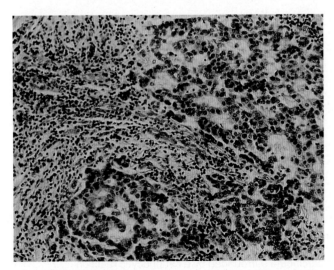

**FIG. 17.20.** *Medullary carcinoma, syncytial growth.* **A:** Carcinoma is distributed in sharply defined bands separated by stroma permeated predominantly by plasma cells. The cytoplasmic borders of individual cells are not seen. **B:** Diffuse cytoplasmic eosinophilia that hints at squamous differentiation (see Fig. 17.26A). **C:** Islands of syncytial carcinoma cells surrounded by lymphocytes.

tial growth, survival was diminished when less than 75% of a tumor was syncytial, with the difference most marked at or below the 50% level. These data substantiate the currently used requirement for at least a 75% syncytial component.

*Poorly differentiated nuclear grade* and *high mitotic rate* are interrelated characteristics of medullary carcinoma. Typically, the tumor cells have pleomorphic nuclei with coarse chromatin and prominent nucleoli (Fig. 17.22) (42,43). Pyknotic nuclei of degenerating cells are easily found, as are mitotic figures (Fig. 17.23).

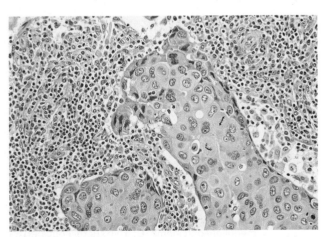

**FIG. 17.21.** *Medullary carcinoma, glandular differentiation.* Isolated foci of glandular differentiation such as this may be found in medullary carcinoma.

**FIG. 17.22.** *Medullary carcinoma, poorly differentiated nuclear grade.* This carcinoma has mitotic figures and pleomorphic nuclei with nucleoli.

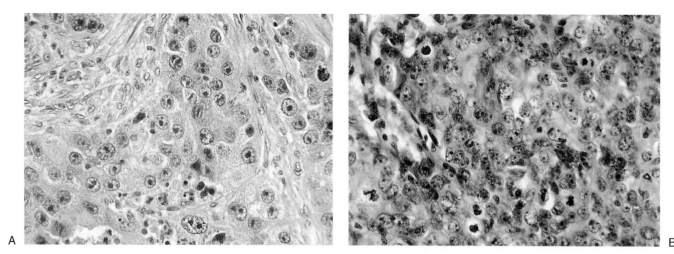

**FIG. 17.23.** *Medullary carcinoma, poorly differentiated nuclear grade.* **A:** Prominent nucleoli. **B:** Multiple nucleoli and numerous mitoses.

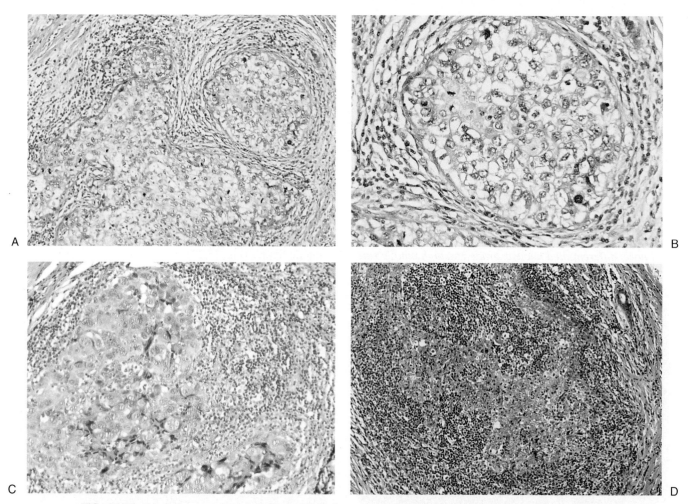

**FIG. 17.24.** *Medullary carcinoma, intraductal.* **A:** Intraductal carcinoma at the periphery of a medullary carcinoma. **B:** Enlarged view of **A** showing intraductal carcinoma that has the cytologic features of medullary carcinoma. **C:** This sharply outlined focus of carcinoma surrounded by a lymphocytic reaction was probably the site of intraductal carcinoma, but the basement membrane is no longer evident. **D:** At this stage, it is difficult to distinguish between intraductal and invasive carcinoma. Basement membrane components are not usually demonstrable with immunostains in such foci.

A number of other microscopic features may be found in some medullary carcinomas. The presence of one or more of these secondary histopathologic characteristics is helpful to confirm a diagnosis of medullary carcinoma, but none must be present to establish the diagnosis. These include the following: *in situ* carcinoma in ducts and lobules, squamous metaplasia, pseudosarcomatous metaplasia, and necrosis.

*Intraductal carcinoma* is found at the periphery of a substantial number of medullary carcinomas (Fig. 17.24). It also is not unusual for intraductal carcinoma to involve the epithelium of lobules (lobular extension of duct carcinoma), thereby creating foci of *in situ* carcinoma in lobules. These areas are so frequent that it is difficult to understand the origin of the oft repeated, undocumented contention that the *absence* of intraductal carcinoma is a diagnostic feature of medullary carcinoma. Foci of intraductal and intralobular carcinoma tend to be seen more frequently with increasing

tumor size, and they are accompanied by the same prominent mononuclear cell infiltrate that occurs in the main tumor. This reactive component can be so intense that it obscures the presence of subtle extension of duct carcinoma into lobular epithelium. Cytologically, these lobules contain cells with the same poorly differentiated nuclei as the invasive portion of the medullary carcinoma. The intraductal carcinoma often has a comedo or solid growth pattern, but only rarely contains calcifications.

Expansile growth of *in situ* carcinoma in ducts and lobules leads to the formation of secondary peripheral tumor nodules that have the appearance of small "satellite" medullary carcinomas (Fig. 17.25). Fat and mammary stroma may persist between nodules at the margin of the tumor. The presence of these marginal nodular foci and intervening stroma should not be interpreted as evidence of invasive growth. Coalescence of these enlarging nodules and their incorporation into

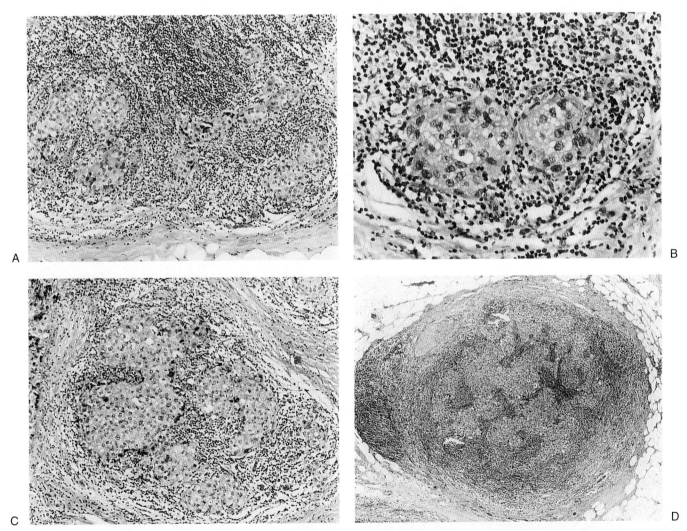

**FIG. 17.25.** *Medullary carcinoma, evolution of lobular extension to form a secondary nodule.* **A:** Intraepithelial carcinoma in a lobule adjacent to a medullary carcinoma. **B:** Magnified view of lobular glands depicted in the lower right corner of **A**. **C:** Expanded intralobular glands and ductules forming serpiginous nests of carcinoma cells with a syncytial arrangement. **D:** Fully developed secondary nodule formed by one or more expanded lobules like the one shown in **C**.

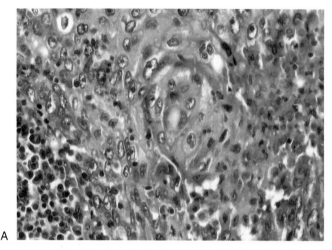 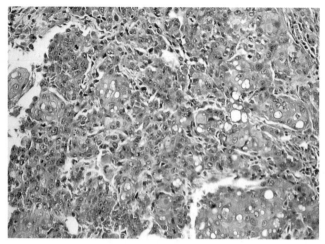

A

B

**FIG. 17.26.** *Medullary carcinoma, squamous metaplasia.* **A:** Poorly formed squamous pearl in the tumor depicted in Fig. 17.20B. **B:** Well-developed squamous metaplasia in another tumor.

the expanding main tumor mass is probably a factor in the rapid growth of medullary carcinomas in addition to a high mitotic rate. This process is responsible for the grossly nodular appearance of medullary carcinomas.

Rarely, one may encounter a lesion consisting only of intraductal carcinoma with the histologic features of *in situ* duct carcinoma found at the periphery of a medullary carcinoma. Typically, such foci have the poorly differentiated cytology that characterizes medullary carcinoma, a comedo growth pattern, and an intense lymphocytic reaction that can obscure the duct margins, thereby creating difficulty in evaluating the lesion for invasion. There is no definite proof that these lesions constitute an *in situ* form of medullary carcinoma, but this possibility can be inferred from uncommon examples of medullary carcinoma composed largely of intraductal carcinoma with only a minor invasive component.

*Metaplastic changes* occur in a minority of medullary carcinomas, and they usually involve only a part of the lesion. Squamous metaplasia has been found in 16% of medullary carcinomas (19). Osseous, cartilaginous, and spindle cell

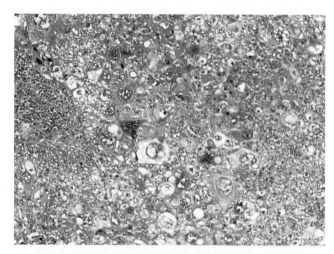

A

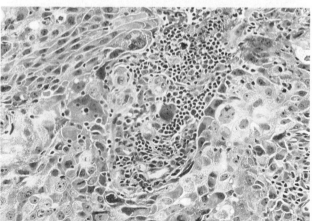

B

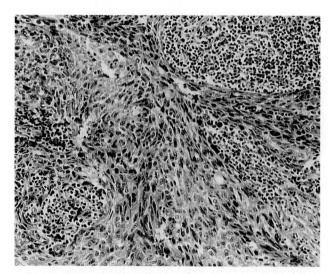

**FIG. 17.27.** *Medullary carcinoma, spindle cell change.* (From Ridolfi R, Rosen P, Port A, et al. Medullary carcinoma of the breast. A clinicopathologic study with 10 year follow-up. *Cancer* 1977;40:1365–1385, with permission.)

**FIG. 17.28.** *Medullary carcinoma, giant cells.* **A:** Many enlarged carcinoma cells have single or multiple cytologically atypical nuclei. **B:** Syncytial giant cells with bizarre hyperchromatic nuclei.

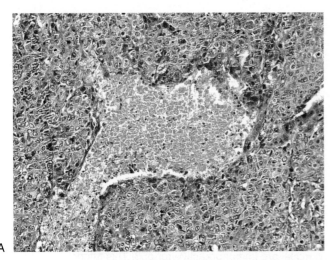

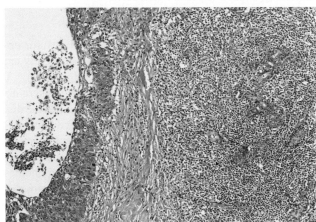

**FIG. 17.29.** *Medullary carcinoma, necrosis.* **A:** Comedonecrosis in a syncytial mass of carcinoma. **B:** Cystic degeneration resulting from extensive necrosis.

metaplasia are much less common (Figs. 17.26 and 17.27). It is not clear whether bizarre epithelial giant cell areas found in an otherwise typical medullary carcinoma represent a metaplastic variant or a degenerative change (Fig. 17.28).

*Necrosis* develops in medullary carcinomas, initially within zones of syncytial epithelial growth (Fig. 17.29). Expansion of these microscopic foci leads to the formation of small clefts and eventually to gross cystic areas. The pattern resembles the process of cystic degeneration sometimes seen in epidermoid carcinomas. Necrosis often is found in conjunction with squamous metaplasia in medullary carcinomas.

## ULTRASTRUCTURAL STUDIES

Electron microscopy has not yielded consistent findings in medullary carcinoma (44–46). This may be due to failure to adhere to rigorous diagnostic criteria in some cases, or it may reflect intrinsic variability in the tumors. The findings are not sufficiently specific to be regarded as diagnostic. However, some conclusions can be drawn. The tumor cells contain numerous organelles but no secretory vacuoles. Intracytoplasmic lumens lined by microvilli may be found, but they are present much less often than in other types of carcinoma. Myoepithelial cells are scant or absent, and there is little basal lamina (44). Desmosomes are found with varying frequency. Light and dark cells, differing in cytoplasmic density, have been described by most authors. Dark cells tend to have more organelles, especially rough endoplasmic reticulum (45). Migration of lymphocytes has been observed in the endothelium of vascular channels in tumor stroma. Cells containing tonofilaments may be evidence of squamous differentiation (45,47). Lloreta et al. (47) reported that medullary carcinomas with axillary lymph node metastases had 40% more desmosomes between tumor cells than tumors without nodal metastases and that metastatic tumors had a significantly higher proportion of cells with three or more nucleoli. Two studies failed to find distinctive ultrastructural differences between the tumor cells of medullary and atypical medullary carcinomas (45).

## IMMUNOHISTOCHEMISTRY

The immunohistochemical characteristics of the lymphoplasmacytic reaction in medullary carcinoma have been the subject of several studies (48–51). Immunoglobulin G (IgG) cells predominate in medullary carcinomas and in infiltrating duct carcinomas (49,50). Substantial numbers of immunoglobulin A (IgA) cells also may be found in nonmedullary infiltrating duct carcinomas and less often in medullary carcinomas (49). Immunoglobulin-containing cells in the lymphoplasmacytic infiltrate associated with normal breast tissue, benign tumors, and hyperplastic lesions tend to be of the IgA type (49,52). Data from one study suggest that there is an inverse relationship between the estrogen receptor and IgG content of breast carcinoma cytosols (53). One group of investigators reported an inverse relationship between estrogen receptor content determined by immunohistochemistry and biochemistry and the number of Leu-7–positive cells (51). The latter includes a subset of natural killer cells. Lymphocytes infiltrating medullary and nonmedullary carcinomas are predominantly peripheral T lymphocytes (48,53). There do not appear to be significant differences between medullary and infiltrating duct carcinomas in the distribution of antigenic phenotypes of lymphocytes (48,54). However, medullary and atypical medullary carcinomas are characterized by significantly increased numbers of activated cytotoxic lymphocytes that may play a role in prognosis (55).

Yazawa et al. (56) reported finding an exceptionally high frequency of human leukocyte antigen (HLA)-DR–positive lymphocytes in medullary carcinomas. There was correspondingly strong HLA-DR reactivity in the carcinoma cells. The authors speculated that HLA-DR expression was linked to the favorable prognosis of medullary carcinoma. These authors also found that nonmedullary carcinomas that expressed HLA-DR had a relatively better prognosis when compared with HLA-DR–negative tumors.

One immunohistochemical study of oncogene expression showed that the majority of medullary carcinomas exhibited

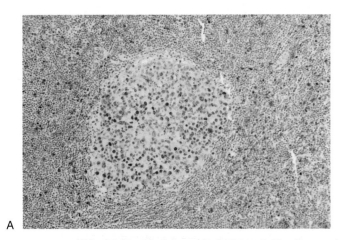 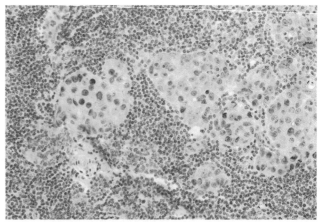

A                                                                                                        B

**FIG. 17.30.** *Medullary carcinoma, proliferative and oncogene markers.* **A:** High proliferative index indicated by nuclear reactivity for Ki67. **B:** Some tumor cell nuclei are immunoreactive for p53. This tumor had no reactivity for HER2/*neu* or hormone receptors (avidin-biotin).

nuclear expression of p53 and that membrane reactivity for HER2/*neu* usually was lacking (Fig. 17.30). Thus, the characteristic immunophenotype of medullary carcinoma was p53(+)/HER2/*neu*(−) (57). Other investigators detected p53 expression in 23 (46%) of 50 medullary carcinomas, a frequency that was not significantly different from nonmedullary carcinomas (44%) in the same study (58). Medullary carcinomas also had significantly higher apoptotic indices determined by the terminal deoxynucleotidyl transferase-mediated dUTP-biotin end labeling (TUNEL) method and higher proliferative indices demonstrated by Ki67 immunostaining (Fig. 17.30). Medullary carcinomas also exhibited significantly lower *bc1*-2 immunoreactivity. These observations suggested that the relatively favorable prognosis of medullary carcinoma might be due to "rapid cell turnover."

Vimentin expression was reported to be more frequent in medullary carcinomas and in duct carcinomas with medullary features than in ordinary invasive duct carcinomas (59). The presence or absence of vimentin did not prove to be prognostically significant. Immunoreactivity for epithelial membrane antigen and S-100 protein frequently are demonstrable in medullary carcinoma cells (Fig. 17.31).

The tumor cells usually are reactive for the cytokeratins AE1/AE3 and CAM5.2. Larsimont et al. (60) studied the distribution of keratin 19 in medullary and in nonmedullary carcinomas. Expression of keratin 19 was absent from 12 medullary carcinomas, whereas 23 of 29 high-grade nonmedullary carcinomas and all of 12 low-grade carcinomas were reactive. Other investigators found no significant difference in the expression of keratin 19 between medullary and poorly differentiated nonmedullary carcinomas (61,62).

## CYTOLOGY

The diagnosis of medullary carcinoma may be suggested by the findings in a fine needle aspiration smear (63), but it is impossible to distinguish classic medullary carcinoma from infiltrating duct carcinoma with medullary features using this method. The specimen usually is very cellular (Fig.

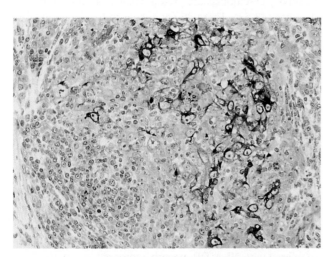

**FIG. 17.31.** *Medullary carcinoma, S-100 protein.* Many of tumor cells are S-100 positive (anti–S-100 protein, avidin-biotin).

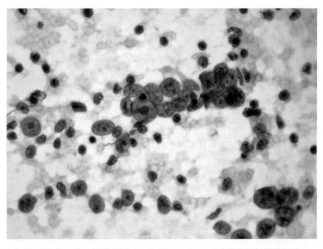

**FIG. 17.32.** *Medullary carcinoma, fine needle aspiration cytology.* Poorly differentiated carcinoma cells singly and in small groups with lymphocytes scattered in the background.

17.32). Large, poorly differentiated carcinoma cells are distributed individually and in sheets. The cells feature pleomorphic nuclei with prominent nucleoli. Numerous lymphocytes frequently admixed with plasma cells occupy much of the background. Hemorrhage and necrosis often are evident and are especially conspicuous when the tumor is cystic (64). Inflammatory debris from a cystic medullary carcinoma may obscure the degenerated tumor cells, leading to a mistaken diagnosis of abscess or infected cyst.

## GENETICS

Cytogenetic study has revealed the presence of trisomy 18 in a few medullary carcinomas (65,66), but this mutation also has been found in other types of breast carcinoma (67). Osin et al. (68) found BRCA1 mutations in six (25%) of 25 medullary carcinomas and in 6% of high-grade nonmedullary carcinomas.

## ATYPICAL MEDULLARY CARCINOMA

The term *atypical medullary carcinoma* was introduced in 1975 to describe carcinomas that have features generally suggestive of medullary carcinoma, but differ from this tumor in one or more major histologic characteristic (19,20). Most tumors in this category have a growth pattern that is at least 75% syncytial and some other histologic feature of medullary carcinoma. Structural variations that characterize atypical medullary carcinoma include (a) invasive growth at the periphery of the tumor, (b) diminished lymphoplasmacytic reaction, (c) well-differentiated nuclear cytology, (d) low frequency of mitoses, and (e) conspicuous glandular, trabecular, or papillary growth with fibrosis.

## PROGNOSIS AND TREATMENT

Overall, a high proportion of patients treated for medullary carcinoma survive without recurrence after treatment by modified or radical mastectomy. In the first description of the tumor, Moore and Foote (3) stated that only 11.5% of their patients with medullary carcinoma died of the tumor within 5 years. This favorable outcome was especially striking because 42% of the patients had axillary lymph node metastases. The series included nine women, each of whom had a single lymph node metastasis and survived disease-free for 5 years.

The results described by Richardson (10) several years later confirmed Moore and Foote's observations. The 5-year disease-free survival rate of their 99 patients was 78%, with death due to disease in only 10%. Ten-year follow-up was available for 47 patients. Overall survival in this subset was 64%, with only eight (17%) deaths due to breast cancer and nine (19%) deaths due to other causes. Axillary metastases occurred in 45% of the entire series, but these patients were found to have a much more favorable prognosis than stage II patients with ordinary types of breast carcinoma. In this series, the 20-year disease-free survival rate was 95% for stage I patients and 61% for stage II women (5).

Several later studies refined the diagnostic criteria for medullary carcinoma as described elsewhere in this chapter and confirmed the favorable prognosis of this type of tumor (8,19,20,69–71). In four of these series, pathologic review was carried out to classify all cases recorded as medullary carcinoma or as carcinoma with medullary features (8,19,20,70). As a result, fewer than 50% of the lesions were finally accepted as true medullary carcinomas; the remainder were diagnosed as atypical medullary or infiltrating duct carcinomas. Patients with medullary carcinoma proved to have a statistically significant more favorable prognosis than those in either of the other two groups (Fig. 17.33). Although the outcome of patients with atypical medullary carcinoma was slightly better than the prognosis of women with infiltrating duct carcinoma, the difference did not prove to be statistically significant in three of the series (8,19,20).

The major contribution of the term "atypical medullary carcinoma" has been to draw attention to the existence of a

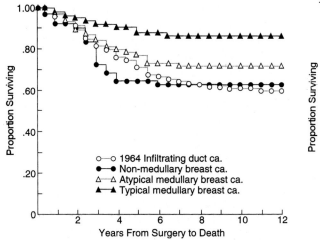

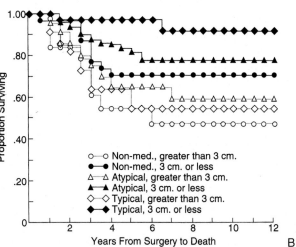

**FIG. 17.33.** *Medullary carcinoma, survival analysis.* **A:** The prognosis of patients with typical medullary carcinoma was significantly better than that of patients with three categories of nonmedullary carcinoma. **B:** Patients with medullary carcinomas 3 cm or less in diameter had the best prognosis.

subset of infiltrating duct carcinomas that may be misdiagnosed as medullary carcinoma. Failure to clearly distinguish medullary from atypical medullary carcinomas by applying rigorous diagnostic criteria undoubtedly has been an important factor in several studies that did not observe a favorable prognosis in medullary carcinoma patients overall or in those with stage II disease (6,72). The term "circumscribed carcinoma" is particularly misleading in this respect because it suggests that gross circumscription is the most important diagnostic feature without putting sufficient emphasis on microscopic criteria (73).

Patients with medullary carcinoma tend to have a lower overall frequency of axillary lymph node metastases than patients with atypical medullary or infiltrating duct carcinoma (8,19,20,70). When nodal metastases are present, they usually involve no more than three lymph nodes (8,19,20,70). Although stage II medullary carcinoma patients have a more favorable prognosis than equivalent patients with nonmedullary carcinoma, tumor size and nodal status are still significant determinants of disease-free survival (70). The prognosis of patients with node-negative medullary carcinoma is particularly favorable if the tumor is not larger than 3 cm in diameter, with a disease-free survival of 90% or better (19–21,74). The survival results for stage II, T1N1M0, medullary carcinoma also have been exceptionally good at 10 years (35) and 20 years (74) of follow-up. Patients whose tumors are larger than 3 cm or who have four or more involved lymph nodes have high recurrence rates that are not appreciably different from the recurrence rates of patients with infiltrating duct carcinoma.

Less than 10% of medullary carcinomas are estrogen and progesterone receptor positive when analyzed biochemically (75), an observation confirmed by immunohistochemical studies (76,77). This feature is consistent with clinical experience that metastatic medullary carcinoma is relatively unresponsive to endocrine therapy (78). As measured by thymidine incorporation (79) and flow cytometry (80,81), medullary carcinoma has one of the highest growth rates among breast carcinomas. Medullary carcinomas typically are aneuploid or polyploid (81,82). These observations are in agreement with patient descriptions of rapid growth of the primary tumor.

Recurrences tend to occur early in the clinical course of patients with medullary carcinoma, with very few women having recurrences 5 years or more after diagnosis (5,19,20,70). This phenomenon is observed equally in stage I and stage II patients. Most initial recurrences are systemic, but local recurrence has been observed in up to 25% of patients treated by modified or radical mastectomy. Survival after systemic recurrence tends to be brief, regardless of the site of the initial metastasis (3,19,20,70), although an occasional patient may benefit from resection of a solitary metastasis (20).

An examination of data from the Surveillance, Epidemiology and End Results (SEER) program has been undertaken to determine tumor-related survival and the likelihood of cure for patients with different histologic types of breast carcinoma (69). Analysis of 163,808 patients revealed 2,908 (3%) with stage I and 1,654 (2.4%) with stage II medullary carcinoma. Medullary carcinoma patients had relatively high "cured fractions" of 82% and 64% for stages I and II, respectively. The survival times after recurrence of 3 and 4 years for stages I and II, respectively, were relatively short when compared to other histologic types of carcinoma.

There is presently little reported experience with breast-conserving surgery and radiotherapy of medullary carcinoma (83–85). It has been suggested that this type of tumor may be radiosensitive (83). One group of 39 patients said to have medullary carcinoma was treated by radiotherapy to the breast after carcinoma was diagnosed only by needle biopsy (84). This series is not representative of medullary carcinomas in general, because virtually all of the patients had tumors larger than 3 cm and more than half were considered clinically to have positive axillary lymph nodes. In addition, needle biopsy specimens do not provide adequate material to distinguish accurately between medullary and atypical medullary carcinoma. Twenty-four had radiation alone, whereas 15 others also received adjuvant chemotherapy after radiation was given. Thirty-one patients were considered to have had complete regression of their tumors, whereas eight had persistent disease that was treated by surgery. Follow-up revealed two patients died of disease 3 and 31 months after recurrence, and four women were alive 6 to 30 months after recurrence. Overall, eight (20%) patients in this series died of metastatic carcinoma.

Combined data from two institutions included 27 women with medullary carcinoma treated by breast-conserving surgery and radiotherapy (84). The mammary recurrence rate was 4%, 5-year overall survival was 90%, and relapse-free survival was 92% at 5 years. A series of 1,008 patients treated by breast conservation with radiotherapy at Yale University included 17 women with medullary carcinoma (71). No medullary carcinoma patient developed a systemic recurrence, but there were five (29%) local breast recurrences after a median follow-up of nearly 17 years, with the longest interval to recurrence 18 years. The 10-year actuarial breast recurrence-free survival was lower for medullary carcinoma (75%) than for infiltrating duct carcinoma (85%).

Additional studies of patients treated by lumpectomy or quadrantectomy, and radiation for less advanced medullary carcinomas, will be necessary to judge the effectiveness of breast conservation in the management of this neoplasm.

## REFERENCES

1. Geschickter CF. *Diseases of the breast: diagnosis, pathology, treatment,* 2nd ed. Philadelphia: JB Lippincott, 1945:565–575.
2. Foote FW Jr, Stewart FW. A histologic classification of carcinoma of the breast. *Surgery* 1946;19:74–99.
3. Moore OS Jr, Foote FW Jr. The relatively favorable prognosis of medullary carcinoma of the breast. *Cancer* 1949;2:635–642.
4. World Health Organization. Histological typing of breast tumors. *Tumori* 1982;68:181–198.
5. Bloom HJG, Richardson WW, Fields JR. Host resistance and survival

in carcinoma of breast: a study of 104 cases of medullary carcinoma in a series of 1511 cases of breast cancer followed for 20 years. *BMJ* 1970;3:181–188.

6. Maier WP, Rosemond GP, Goldman LI, et al. A ten year study of medullary carcinoma of the breast. *Surg Gynecol Obstet* 1977; 144:695–698.

7. Markovitz P, Contesso G, Sarrazin D, et al. Le carcinome medullaire du sein. Étude clinique et anatomo-radiologique à propos de 56 observations. *Bull Cancer* 1970;57:517–526.

8. Rapin V, Contesso G, Mouriesse H, et al. Medullary carcinoma. A re-evaluation of 95 cases of breast cancer with inflammatory stroma. *Cancer* 1988;61:2503–2510.

9. Bassler R, Dittmann AM, Dittrich M. Mononuclear stromal reactions in mammary carcinoma with special reference to medullary carcinomas with a lymphoid infiltrate. Analysis of 108 cases. *Virchows Arch [A]* 1981;393:75–91.

10. Richardson WW. Medullary carcinoma of the breast. A distinctive tumor type with a relatively good prognosis following radical mastectomy. *Br J Cancer* 1956;10:415–423.

11. Rosen PP. The pathological classification of human mammary carcinoma: past, present and future. *Ann Clin Lab Sci* 1979;9:144–156.

12. Morrison AS, Black MM, Lowe CR, et al. Some international differences in histology and survival in breast cancer. *Int J Cancer* 1973;11:261–267.

13. Rosen PP, Ashikari R, Thaler H, et al. A comparative study of some pathologic features of mammary carcinoma in Tokyo, Japan and New York, USA. *Cancer* 1977;39:429–434.

14. Wynder EL, Kajitani T, Kuno J, et al. A comparison of survival rates between American and Japanese patients with breast cancer. *Surg Gynecol Obstet* 1963;117:196–200.

15. Berg JW, Robbins GF. The histologic epidemiology of breast cancer. In: *Breast cancer: early and late. Proceedings of the Annual Clinical Conference of MD Anderson Hospital and Tumor Institute.* Chicago: Year Book Medical Publishers, 1970:19–26.

16. Mittra NK, Rush BF, Verner E. A comparative study of breast cancer in the black and white populations of two inner-city hospitals. *J Surg Oncol* 1980;15:11–17.

17. Natarajan N, Nemoto T, Mettlin C, et al. Race related differences in breast cancer patients. Results of the 1982 national survey of breast cancer by the American College of Surgeons. *Cancer* 1985;56:1704–1709.

18. Owenby HE, Frederick J, Russo J, et al. Racial differences in breast cancer patients. *J Natl Cancer Inst* 1985;75:55–60.

19. Ridolfi R, Rosen P, Port A, et al. Medullary carcinoma of the breast. A clinicopathologic study with 10 year follow-up. *Cancer* 1977; 40:1365–1385.

20. Wargotz ES, Silverberg SG. Medullary carcinoma of the breast. A clinicopathologic study with appraisal of current diagnostic criteria. *Hum Pathol* 1988;19:1340–1346.

21. Rosen PP, Lesser ML, Senie RT, et al. Epidemiology of breast carcinoma. III. Relationship of family history to tumor type. *Cancer* 1982;50:171–179.

22. Burki N, Buser M, Emmons LR, et al. Malignancies in families of women with medullary, tubular and invasive ductal breast cancer. *Eur J Cancer* 1990;26:295–303.

23. Eisinger F, Jacquemier J, Charpin C, et al. Mutations at BRCA1: the medullary breast carcinoma revisited. *Cancer Res* 1998;58:1588–1592.

24. Malone KE, Daling JR, Ostrander EANC. BRCA1 and medullary breast cancer [Letter]. *JAMA* 1998;280:1227–1228.

25. Rosen PP, Lesser ML, Senie RT, et al. Epidemiology of breast carcinoma. IV. Age and histologic tumor type. *J Surg Oncol* 1982;19:44–47.

26. Rosen PP, Lesser ML, Kinne DW. Breast carcinoma at the extremes of age: a comparison of patients younger than 35 years and older than 75 years. *J Surg Oncol* 1985;28:90–96.

27. Meyer JE, Amin E, Lindfors KK, et al. Medullary carcinoma of the breast: mammographic and US appearance. *Radiology* 1989; 170:79–82.

28. Kopans DB, Rubens J. Medullary carcinoma of the breast. *Radiology* 1989;171:876.

29. Haupt HM, Rosen PP, Kinne DW. Breast carcinoma presenting with axillary lymph node metastasis: an analysis of specific histopathologic features. *Am J Surg Pathol* 1985;9:165–175.

30. Lesser ML, Rosen PP, Kinne DW. Multicentricity and bilaterality in invasive breast carcinoma. *Surgery* 1982;1:234–240.

31. Neuman ML, Homer MJ. Association of medullary carcinoma with reactive axillary adenopathy. *AJR Am J Roentgenol* 1996;167:185–186.

32. Rosen PP, Lesser ML, Kinne DW, et al. Discontinuous or "skip" metastases in breast carcinoma. *Ann Surg* 1983;197:276–283.

33. Lespagnard L, Cochaux P, Larsimont D, et al. Absence of Epstein-Barr virus in medullary carcinoma of the breast as demonstrated by immunophenotyping, in situ hybridization and polymerase chain reaction. *Am J Clin Pathol* 1995;103:449–452.

34. Rosen PP, Saigo PE, Braun DW Jr, et al. Predictors of recurrence in Stage 1 ($T_1N_0M_0$) breast carcinoma. *Ann Surg* 1981;193:15–25.

35. Rosen PP, Saigo PE, Braun DW Jr, et al. Prognosis in Stage II ($T_1N_1M_0$) breast cancer. *Ann Surg* 1981;194:576–584.

36. Pedersen LP, Holck S, Schiodt T, et al. Inter- and intraobserver variability in the histopathological diagnosis of medullary carcinoma of the breast, and its prognostic implications. *Breast Cancer Res Treat* 1989;14:91–99.

37. Rubens JR, Lewandrowski KB, Kopans DB, et al. Medullary carcinoma of the breast. Overdiagnosis of a prognostically favorable neoplasm. *Arch Surg* 1990;125:601–604.

38. Rigaud C, Theobald S, Noel P, et al. Medullary carcinoma of the breast. A multicenter study of its diagnostic consistency. *Arch Pathol Lab Med* 1993;117:1005–1008.

39. Jensen ML, Kiaer H, Andersen J, et al. Prognostic comparison of three classifications for medullary carcinomas of the breast. *Histopathology* 1997;30:523–532.

40. Tavassoli FA. Infiltrating carcinomas, common and familiar special types: medullary carcinoma. In: *Pathology of the breast*. Norwalk, CT: Appleton & Lange, 1992:333–339.

41. Pedersen L, Schiodt T, Holck S, et al. The prognostic importance of syncytial growth pattern in medullary carcinoma of the breast. *APMIS* 1990;98:921–926.

42. Black MM, Speer, FD. Nuclear structure in cancer tissues. *Surg Gynecol Obstet* 1957;105:97–102.

43. Bloom HJG, Richardson WW. Histological grading and prognosis in breast cancer. A study of 1049 cases, of which 359 have been followed 15 years. *Br J Cancer* 1957;11:359–377.

44. Ahmed A. The ultrastructure of medullary carcinoma of the breast. *Virchows Arch [A]* 1980;388:175–186.

45. Harris M, Lessells MM. The ultrastructure of medullary, atypical medullary and non-medullary carcinomas of the breast. *Histopathology* 1986;10:405–414.

46. Murad TM, Scarpelli DG. The ultrastructure of medullary and scirrhous mammary duct carcinoma. *Am J Pathol* 1967;50:335–360.

47. Lloreta J, Mariñoso ML, Corominas JM, et al. Medullary carcinoma of the breast: an ultrastructural morphometric study of nine cases. *Ultrastruct Pathol* 1997;21:499–507.

48. Ben-Ezra J, Sheibani K. Antigenic phenotype of the lymphocytic component of medullary carcinoma of the breast. *Cancer* 1987; 59:2037–2041.

49. Ito T, Saga S, Nagayoshi W, et al. Class distribution of immunoglobulin-containing plasma cells in the stroma of medullary carcinoma of breast. *Breast Cancer Res Treat* 1986;7:97–104.

50. Jacquemier J, Robert-Vague D, Torrente M, et al. Mise en evidence des immunoglobulines lymphoplasmocytaires et epitheliales dans les carcinomes infiltrants a stroma lymphoide et les carcinomes medullaries du sein. *Arch Anat Cytol Pathol* 1983;31:296–300.

51. Underwood JCE, Giri DD, Rooney N, et al. Immunophenotype of the lymphoid cell infiltrates in breast carcinomas of low estrogen receptor content. *Br J Cancer* 1987;56:744–746.

52. Sieinski W. Immunohistological patterns of immunoglobulins in dysplasia, benign neoplasms and carcinomas of the breast. *Tumori* 1980;66:699–711.

53. Winsten S, Tabachnick J, Young I. Immunoglobulin G (IgG) levels in breast tumour cytosols. *Am J Clin Pathol* 1985;83:364–366.

54. Gaffey MJ, Frierson, HF Jr, Mills SE, et al. Medullary carcinoma of the breast. Identification of lymphocyte subpopulations and their significance. *Mod Pathol* 1993;6:721–728.

55. Yakirevich E, Izhak OB, Rennert G, et al. Cytoxic phenotype of tumor infiltrating lymphocytes in medullary carcinoma of the breast. *Mod Pathol* 1999;12:1050–1056.

56. Yazawa T, Hioshi K, Ogata T. Frequent expression of HLA-DR antigen in medullary carcinoma of the breast. A possible reason for its prominent lymphocytic infiltration and favorable prognosis. *Appl Immunohistochem* 1993;1:289–296.

57. Rosen PP, Lesser ML, Arroyo CD, et al. Immunohistochemical detection of HER2/neu in patients with axillary lymph node negative breast carcinoma: a study of epidemiologic risk factors, histologic features and prognosis. *Cancer* 1995;75:1320–1326.

58. Kajiwara M, Toyoshima S, Yao T, et al. Apoptosis and cell proliferation in medullary carcinoma of the breast: a comparative study between medullary and non-medullary carcinoma using the TUNEL method and immunohistochemistry. *J Surg Pathol* 1999;70:209–216.

59. Holck S, Pedersen L, Schiodt T, et al. Vimentin expression in 98 breast cancers with medullary features and its prognostic significance. *Virchows Arch [A]* 1993;422:475–479.

60. Larsimont D, Lespagnard L, Degeyter M, et al. Medullary carcinoma of the breast: a tumour lacking keratin 19. *Histopathology* 1994; 24:549–552.

61. Dalal P, Shousha S. Keratin 19 in paraffin sections of medullary carcinoma and other benign and maglinant breast lesions. *Mod Pathol* 1995;8:413–416.

62. Jensen ML, Kiaer H, Melsen F. Medullary breast carcinoma vs. poorly differentiated ductal carcinoma: an immunohistochemical study with keratin 19 and oestrogen receptor staining. *Histopathology* 1996; 29:241–245.

63. Kline TS, Kannan V, Kline IK. Appraisal and cytomorphologic analysis of common carcinomas of the breast. *Diagn Cytopathol* 1985; 1:188–193.

64. Howell LP, Kline TS. Medullary carcinoma of the breast. An unusual cytologic finding in cyst fluid aspirates. *Cancer* 1990;65:277–282.

65. Bullerdiek J, Bonk U, Staats B, et al. Trisomy 18 as the first chromosome abnormality in a medullary breast cancer. *Cancer Genet Cytogenet* 1994;73:75–78.

66. Geleick D, Muller H, Matter A, et al. Cytogenetics of breast cancer. *Cancer Genet Cytogenet* 1990;46:217–218.

67. Pandis N, Heims S, Bardi G, et al. Chromosome analysis of 20 breast carcinomas: cytogenetic multiclonality and karyotype-pathologic correlations. *Genes Chromosomes Cancer* 1993;5:235–238.

68. Osin P, Crook T, Kote Jorai Z, et al. Analysis of BRCA1 gene function in medullary breast cancer. *Mod Pathol* 2000;13:43A.

69. Gamel JW, Meyer JS, Feuer E, et al. The impact of stage and histology on the long-term clinical course of 163,808 patients with breast carcinoma. *Cancer* 1996;77:459–464.

70. Reinfuss M, Stelmach A, Mitus J, et al. Typical medullary carcinoma of the breast: a clinical and pathological analysis of 52 cases. *J Surg Oncol* 1995;60:89–94.

71. Haffty BG, Perrotta PL, Ward B, et al. Conservatively treated breast cancer: outcome by histologic subtype. *Breast J* 1997;3:7–14.

72. Black CL, Morris DM, Goldman LI, et al. The significance of lymph node involvement in patients with medullary carcinoma of the breast. *Surg Gynecol Obstet* 1983;157:497–499.

73. Lane N, Goksel H, Salerno RA, et al. Clinicopathologic analysis of the surgical curability of breast cancers. A minimum 10 year study. *Ann Surg* 1961;153:483–498.

74. Rosen PP, Groshen S, Saigo PE, et al. A long-term follow-up study of survival in Stage I ($T_1N_0M_0$) and Stage II ($T_1N_1M_0$) breast carcinoma. *J Clin Oncol* 1989;7:355–366.

75. Rosen PP, Menendez-Botet CJ, Nisselbaum JS, et al. Pathological review of breast lesions analyzed for estrogen receptor protein. *Cancer Res* 1975;35:3187–3194.

76. Reiner A, Reiner G, Spona J, et al. Histopathologic characterization of human breast cancer in correlation with estrogen receptor status. A comparison of immunocytochemical and biochemical analysis. *Cancer* 1988;61:1149–1154.

77. Stegner HE, Jonat W, Maass H. Immunohistochemicher Nachweis nuklearer Ostrogenrezeptoren mit monoclonalen Antikorpern in verschiednen Typen des Mammakarzinoms. *Pathologe* 1986;7:156–163.

78. Patel JK, Nemoto T, Dao TL. Is medullary carcinoma of the breast hormone dependent? *J Surg Oncol* 1983;24:290–291.

79. Meyer JS, Friedman E, McCrate M, et al. Prediction of early course of breast carcinomas by thymidine labeling. *Cancer* 1983;51:1879–1886.

80. Meyer JS, Bauer WC, Rao BR. Subpopulations of breast carcinoma defined by S-phase fraction, morphology and estrogen receptor content. *Lab Invest* 1978;39:225–235.

81. Kallioniemi O-P, Blanco G, Alavaikko M, et al. Tumour DNA ploidy as an independent prognostic factor in breast cancer. *Br J Cancer* 1987;56:637–642.

82. McDivitt RW, Stone KR, Craig RB, et al. A proposed classification of breast cancer based on kinetic information derived from a comparison of risk factors in 168 primary operable breast cancers. *Cancer* 1986;57:269–276.

83. Vilcoq JR, Calle R, Ghossein NA. Radiosensitivity and radiocurability of medullary carcinoma of the breast [Abstract]. *Int J Radiat Oncol Biol Phys* 1980;6:1343–1344.

84. Fourquet A, Vilcoq JR, Zafrani B, et al. Medullary breast carcinoma, the role of radiotherapy as primary treatment. *Radiother Oncol* 1987;10:1–6.

85. Kurtz JM, Jacquemier J, Torhorst J, et al. Conservation therapy for breast cancers other than infiltrating ductal carcinoma. *Cancer* 1989;63:1630–1635.

# CHAPTER 18

# Carcinoma with Metaplasia

Because carcinoma of the breast arises from the mammary glandular epithelium, it usually exhibits the features of adenocarcinoma. However, in less than 5% of mammary adenocarcinomas, part or all of the carcinomatous epithelium is transformed into a nonglandular growth pattern by a process referred to as *metaplasia* (from the Greek *metaplasmos*), meaning the changing of one cell type into another.

The term metaplasia traditionally has been reserved for neoplasms that exhibit microscopic structural changes that diverge from glandular differentiation. In the breast, these phenotypic alterations represent the expression of genotypic properties not manifested in normal myoepithelial cells or glandular epithelial cells of the breast. This microscopic appearance may be a consequence of genetic alterations involving, in part, derepression of normally coded molecular mechanisms required for the production of proteins that contribute to the epithelial phenotype.

Increasing knowledge of the molecular control of cellular processes has served to reinforce our long-held perception that the histologic phenotype (or immunophenotype) of proliferating neoplastic cells is not always an accurate reflection of their histogenesis, or tissue of origin. What happens to any given cell in terms of histologic appearance or function (phenotype) is determined by how much the genetic keyboard is in or out of tune (mutated) and the nuances of how it is played (regulation of gene expression). Within this framework, there is considerable potential for plasticity of phenotypic expression that sometimes can be manifested in the "strange" structural variants encountered in neoplasms as well as more subtle differences in the appearances of tumors. Histologic phenotype (or immunophenotype) does not necessarily reflect "histogenesis." In some instances, the phenotype of cells in a tumor might actually mask the histogenesis of the neoplasm by the expression of "markers" not exhibited under "normal" conditions by the cells from which the tumor arose. In this respect, the molecular basis of neoplasia has cast a shadow over the histogenetic concept that seeks to link the histologic phenotype of each neoplasm to origin from a "primitive" or differentiated tissue with similar phenotypic or immunophenotypic characteristics.

In some mammary lesions, especially carcinomas, meta-plastic changes may be manifested by the formation of ectopic substances in sufficient quantity to be detectable. This form of metaplasia is typically recognized when an aberrant hormone is detected immunohistochemically. Corresponding structural metaplasia may be manifested in phenotypic morphologic patterns that, for example, resemble choriocarcinoma or carcinoid tumor (Fig. 18.1). These variants of metaplastic carcinoma are discussed in a separate chapter devoted to mammary carcinoma with endocrine differentiation. The discussion in this chapter is restricted to neoplasms with squamous, spindle cell, or heterologous (pseudosarcomatous) structural patterns.

Mammary glandular tissue is susceptible to metaplastic changes. An *in vitro* histologic study of human mammary gland explants revealed that the protein kinase C (PKC) inhibitor staurosporine is capable of inducing squamous metaplasia within 2 weeks of treatment (1). Other PKC inhibitors, such as tamoxifen and calphostin C, did not have this effect. The metaplastic epithelium expressed keratins 14 and 19, as well as glandular markers for human milk fat globulin-1 and mucin-1. Squamous metaplasia also occurred in untreated cultured explants from postmenopausal women, but not in untreated glands from premenopausal women.

Squamous metaplasia is found in the glandular epithelium of benign breast neoplasms such as papillomas and fibroadenomas, and it may be present in nonneoplastic epithelial proliferations such as cysts and gynecomastia. Reparative epithelium in ducts or lobules at a healing biopsy site may undergo squamous metaplasia (Fig. 18.2). Heterologous chondroid, adipose, or osseous metaplasia also are very rarely encountered in the stroma of fibroadenomas. Chondroid and osseous metaplasia in a sclerosing papilloma results in a lesion that resembles a mixed tumor of the salivary glands. In breast carcinomas, the extent of metaplasia varies from isolated microscopic foci in an otherwise typical mammary carcinoma to complete replacement of glandular growth by the metaplastic phenotype (Fig. 18.3).

The frequency of metaplastic change in mammary carcinoma probably is underreported because inconspicuous foci of such change are easily overlooked or ignored. This

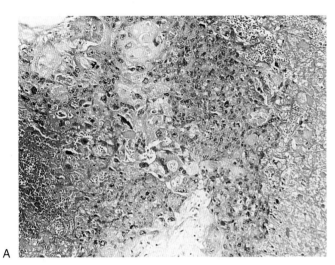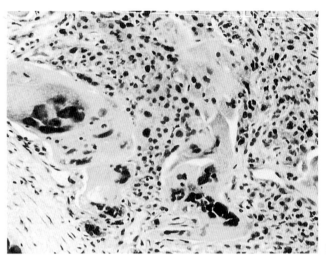

**FIG. 18.1.** *Metaplastic carcinoma, choriocarcinoma type.* **A:** High-grade metaplastic carcinoma with areas of hemorrhagic necrosis. **B:** Giant cells that resemble syncytiotrophoblast. The tumor was focally immunoreactive for human chorionic gonadotropin (HCG), and the serum HCG level was markedly elevated.

limitation applies especially to spindle and squamous metaplasia. Heterologous components, such as bone and cartilage, seem to engender greater interest, and they are more likely to be noted. Squamous metaplasia was reportedly present in 3.7% of 1,665 invasive carcinomas reviewed by Fisher et al. (2). Heterologous metaplasia was detected in 26 (0.2%) of 12,045 breast carcinomas in another study (3). Metaplastic carcinoma originates more often in poorly differentiated duct carcinomas, but it may be found rarely in other types of carcinoma, including invasive lobular carcinoma (Fig. 18.4) and papillary tumors (Fig. 18.5). Squamous metaplasia is found in up to 16% of medullary carcinomas (4). Medullary carcinoma with squamous metaplasia should be regarded as a variant of medullary carcinoma and excluded from the metaplastic carcinoma category because it has an exceptionally favorable prognosis that is a property of the underlying medullary carcinoma. Carcinomas with metaplasia usually have very low levels of estrogen and progesterone receptor,

and almost all have been classified as receptor negative when studied by biochemistry or immunohistochemistry (5,6).

The concept that heterologous metaplasia arises from changes in the neoplastic stroma has given way to the view that the metaplastic elements develop from altered epithelial and/or myoepithelial cells. Several lines of evidence support this conclusion. Histologic sections sometimes reveal direct transitions from epithelial to heterologous patterns. This is seen most readily where adenocarcinoma gives rise to squamous and spindle cell elements (Fig. 18.6). Electron microscopic studies have generally confirmed the epithelial origin of heterologous elements.

Experimental animal studies have proven the capacity of epithelial cells to undergo metaplastic change into a mesenchymal growth pattern. Mesenchymal conversion of epithelial tissues has been reported in normal embryogenesis (7), and similar alterations have been induced experimentally in mature epithelium (8). These alterations are accompanied by changes in the cytoskeleton of the metaplastic tissue and in the extracellular matrix (8,9). In one report, the

**FIG. 18.2.** *Squamous metaplasia in reparative epithelium.* Squamous metaplasia is present in the duct on the *left* in this healing biopsy site.

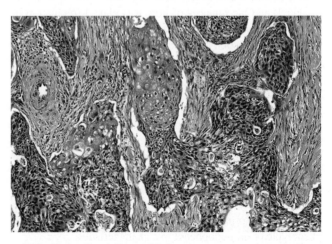

**FIG. 18.3.** *Carcinoma with focal squamous metaplasia.*

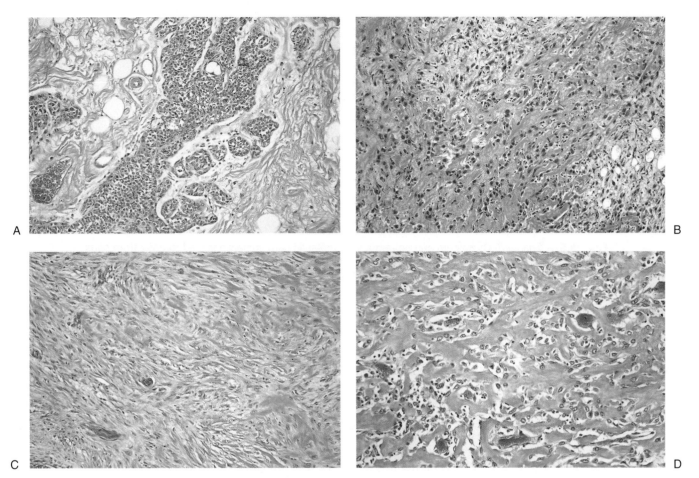

**FIG. 18.4.** *Metaplastic carcinoma, lobular.* All images are from the same specimen. **A:** *In situ* lobular carcinoma in a duct and lobular glands. **B:** Invasive lobular carcinoma, classic type. **C:** Spindle cell metaplastic carcinoma with focal squamous differentiation. **D:** Pseudoangiomatous metaplastic growth pattern.

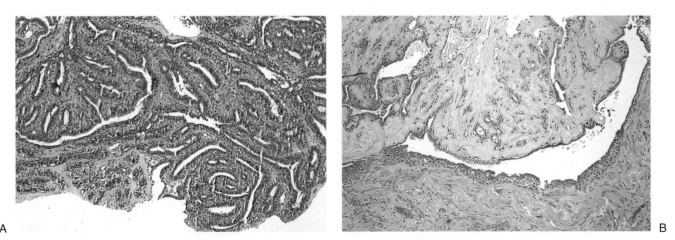

**FIG. 18.5.** *Metaplastic carcinoma arising in cystic papilloma.* All images are from the same patient. **A:** Needle core biopsy sample showing a papilloma at the site of an 8-mm mass. Surgical excision was not performed. Follow-up mammography revealed an enlarging lesion at the same site about 1 year later. **B:** Excised specimen contained a sclerotic cystic papilloma. *(continued)*

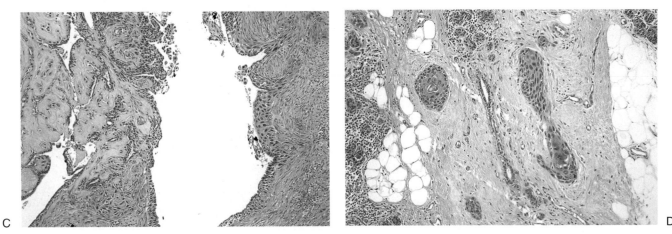

C

D

**FIG. 18.5.** *Continued.* **C:** Spindle and squamous metaplastic carcinoma appeared to arise from squamous differentiation of the surface epithelium of the cyst, shown here with underlying spindle cell carcinoma. **D:** Invasive squamous carcinoma surrounding the papillary lesion.

androgen-dependent Shionogi carcinoma 115 cell line was found to undergo cartilaginous metaplasia when grown under androgen-depleted conditions in mice (10). Various patterns of metaplasia were observed in a rat mammary epithelial cell line transfected with deoxyribonucleic acid (DNA) from another metastasizing rat mammary cell line (11). After transfection, the recipient cell line acquired the capacity to metastasize and exhibited squamous, spindle cell, and rhabdomyoblastic differentiation at the subcutaneous site of primary growth and in metastases. It was suggested that molecular changes associated with transfection resulted in activation of one or more differentiation-inducing genes. Loss of E-cadherin expression has been associated with metaplastic conversion of carcinoma cell lines from an epithelial to a spindle cell phenotype (12,13).

Confusing terminology used to describe these tumors reflects prevalent uncertainty about their histogenesis. Some lesions have been described as "mixed tumors," an unfortunate reference to tumors of the salivary glands that are predominantly benign (14). Others have referred to metaplastic

carcinomas as carcinosarcomas (15). The latter term is best reserved to describe malignant neoplasms in which the carcinomatous and sarcomatous elements can be traced separately to epithelial and mesenchymal origins, such as carcinoma arising in a malignant cystosarcoma.

The precise cell type that gives rise to metaplastic carcinoma remains uncertain. Cytogenetic and molecular studies have demonstrated clonality in the epithelial and pseudosarcomatous components of these tumors, a finding that indicates origin from a single stem cell (16,17). The concurrent presence of ordinary intraductal and invasive duct carcinoma in some tumors and transitions observed from these carcinomatous foci to metaplastic components has led to the conclusion that these neoplasms are derived from mammary glandular epithelial cells. Immunohistochemical studies that reveal coexpression of S-100, vimentin, and cytokeratin in components with epithelial and sarcomatoid phenotypes have been interpreted as evidence for the epithelial origin for both elements by some investigators (18). Others have pointed to these same observations as suggesting myoepithelial origin

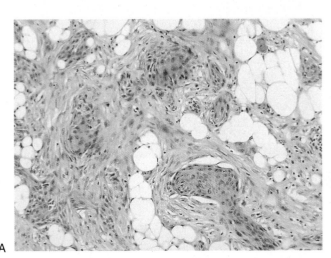

A

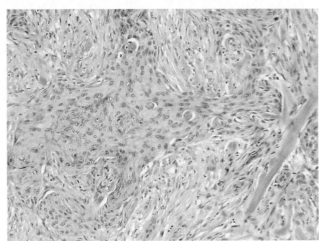

B

**FIG. 18.6.** *Metaplastic carcinoma, spindle and squamous.* **A:** Infiltrating carcinoma in fat showing transition from squamous to spindle cell metaplasia. **B:** Central stellate squamous area, less well differentiated than in **A**, blends imperceptibly with the surrounding spindle cell element.

(5,15). Squamous metaplasia of myoepithelial cells in a fibroadenoma was described by Raju (19), who found immunoreactivity for actin and vimentin in myoepithelial, and squamous metaplastic cells but not in normal epithelial cells (19). S-100 protein was demonstrated in epithelial, myoepithelial, and squamous metaplastic cells. Illustrations in this case report provide convincing evidence of transition from myoepithelial to squamous cells in the benign lesion. All of the immunohistochemical results presently available are consistent with epithelial or myoepithelial origin.

Immunohistochemical studies of nonmammary tumors with carcinomatous and sarcomatous components are relevant to this issue. Cytokeratin expression was observed in the sarcomatoid components of 37 sarcomatoid pulmonary carcinomas by Nakajima et al. (20). George et al. (21) reported concordant expression of a variety of epithelial and sarcomatous markers in both components in a series of female genital malignant müllerian mixed tumors. Biphasic growth patterns were observed in the majority of metastases. These observations led them to conclude that the epithelial and mesenchymal elements were derived from a common cell of origin. However, the authors could not determine if the neoplasms arose from a multipotential stem cell or if one

component gave rise to the other. Others concluded that müllerian mixed tumors are fundamentally epithelial neoplasms because all elements coexpress to some degree epithelial cytoskeletal markers (22).

## CLINICAL PRESENTATION

The range of age at diagnosis and the clinical features of metaplastic mammary carcinoma are not appreciably different from those of invasive mammary carcinoma generally (3,6,23–26). The first symptom is typically a palpable tumor. Large lesions can be complicated by fixation to the skin or chest wall and skin ulceration (26). There is no predilection for bilaterality, but one patient with bilateral metaplastic carcinoma has been described (3). The patient usually reports rapid growth and short duration prior to diagnosis (24). There are no specific features to the mammographic appearance of metaplastic carcinoma. The tumors tend to have circumscribed contours radiologically. Bone formation in tumors with osseous metaplasia may be detectable by mammography (27). Intense uptake of technetium 99m methylene diphosphonate (MDP) was observed in mammary carcinomas with osseous sarcomatoid metaplasia (Fig. 18.7) (27,28).

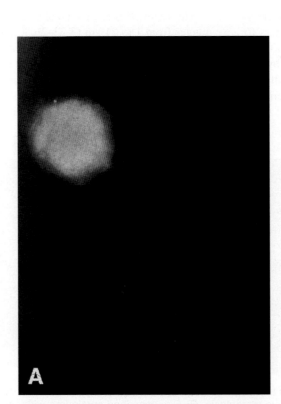
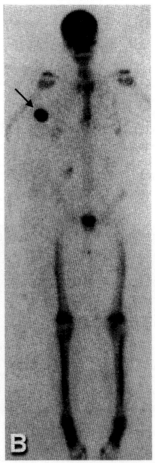

**FIG. 18.7.** *Metaplastic carcinoma with osseous sarcomatoid metaplasia, technetium scans.* **A:** The tumor is a dense mass on the mammogram. **B:** The technetium 99m methylene diphosphonate (MDP) scan shows uptake of radioactivity in the tumor in the right breast *(arrow). (continued)*

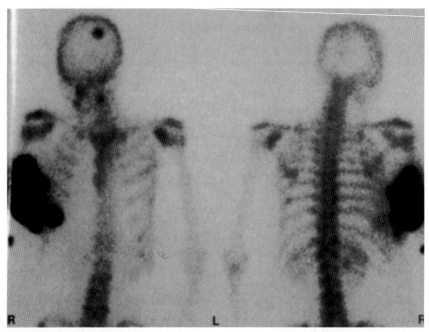

C R        L        R D

**FIG. 18.7.** *Continued.* Tumor is a large lobulated mass with radioactivity in the technetium 99m MDP scan in anterior (**C**) and posterior (**D**) views. A cranial metastasis is evident in the anterior view. **A** and **B** are a different patient then **C** and **D**. (**A,B** from Evans HA, Shaughnessy EA, Nikiforov YE. Infiltrating ductal carcinoma of the breast with osseous metaplasia: imaging findings with pathologic correlation. *AJR Am J Roentgenol* 1999;172:1420–1422, with permission. **C,D** from Pickhardt PJ, McDermott M. Intense uptake of technetium-99m-MDP in primary breast adenocarcinoma with sarcomatoid metaplasia. *J Nucl Med* 1997;38:528–530, with permission.)

Flow cytometric analysis of carcinomas with spindle cell metaplasia revealed aneuploidy or tetraploidy in six of eight tumors studied (29). The DNA indices differed between epithelial and mesenchymal areas in three of four tumors for which both components were sampled. Chao et al. (30) reported that five of six metaplastic carcinomas studied by flow cytometry were aneuploid (2), tetraploid (2), or multiploid (1). One tumor was diploid. The S-phase fraction determined for four tumors was 6.6%, 6.8%, 16.5%, and 27.5%.

## GROSS PATHOLOGY

The reported size of metaplastic mammary carcinomas ranges from 1 to 21 cm (3,23–26,30). The mean or median sizes (3 to 4 cm) reported in various series tend to be greater than that of ordinary carcinomas. The majority of tumors are described as firm to hard, nodular, and circumscribed, but some lesions have infiltrative borders (Fig. 18.8). Degenerated cystic areas can be encountered, especially in tumors

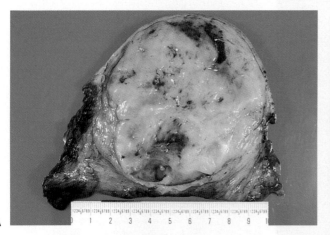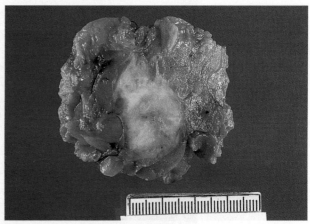

**FIG. 18.8.** *Metaplastic carcinoma, gross appearance.* **A:** Circumscribed fleshy tumor has a cystic area and hemorrhagic foci of angiosarcomatous metaplasia. **B:** Circumscribed carcinoma with spindle and squamous metaplasia that has a dense, fibrous-appearing cut surface.

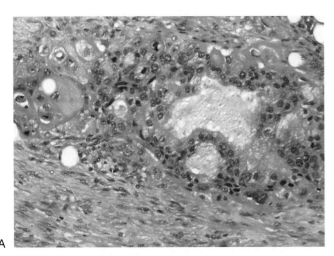
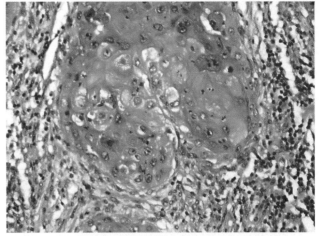

**FIG. 18.9.** *Metaplastic carcinoma, squamous type.* **A:** Direct conversion of the adenocarcinoma *(right)* to squamous differentiation *(left)*. **B:** Squamous metaplasia, moderately well differentiated, in an area of marked lymphoplasmacytic reaction from the tumor shown in **A**.

with squamous metaplasia (5,24). Some reports referred to such tumors as cholesteatomas of the breast (31).

## MICROSCOPIC PATHOLOGY

It has been customary to subdivide metaplastic carcinomas into two categories: squamous and heterologous or pseudosarcomatous metaplasia. These distinctions are somewhat arbitrary, because some tumors exhibit both types of growth. The most common combined configuration is the development of undifferentiated spindle cell areas, sometimes with a storiform pattern (26,32,33). Rarely, chondroid or osseous metaplasia is found to coexist with squamous metaplasia (29). An excellent description of such a complex tumor was reported in 1906 by Lecene (34).

Histologic sections of the excised tumor are required for definitive diagnosis of metaplastic carcinoma. A common pattern of metaplastic carcinoma is focal squamous metaplasia in an otherwise typical invasive duct carcinoma (Fig. 18.9). In unusual instances, the adenocarcinomatous component mingles with the metaplastic carcinomatous epithelium, sometimes with a pagetoid distribution (Fig. 18.10). The term "high-grade adenosquamous carcinoma" could be used for such lesions in contrast to "low-grade adenosquamous carcinoma," which is described elsewhere in this chapter.

When squamous metaplasia is the predominant pattern, a spectrum of differentiation may be found. Mature keratinizing epithelium, sometimes with keratohyalin granules, as well as adenocarcinoma, can be associated with transitions to spindle cell, pseudosarcomatous areas (Figs. 18.11–18.14).

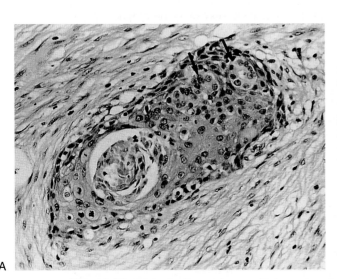
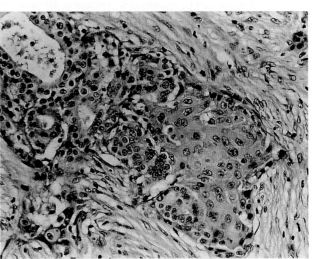

**FIG. 18.10.** *Metaplastic carcinoma, high-grade adenosquamous type.* **A:** Small carcinomatous glands *(arrows)* are embedded in this focus of metaplastic carcinoma. **B:** Adenosquamous carcinoma. *(continued)*

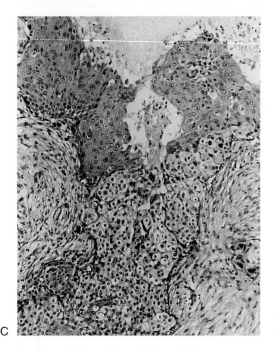

C

**FIG. 18.10.** *Continued.* **C:** Pagetoid spread of adenocarcinoma in metaplastic squamous carcinomatous epithelium.

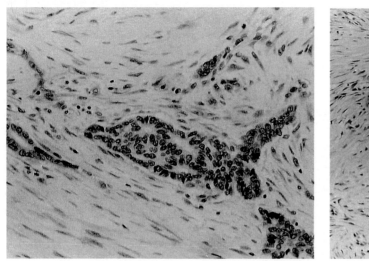

A

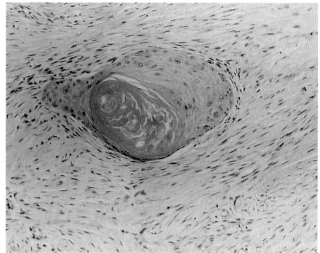

B

**FIG. 18.11.** *Metaplastic carcinoma, spindle and squamous type.* **A:** Well-differentiated adenocarcinoma surrounded by spindle cell carcinoma. **B:** Well-differentiated squamous element in the spindle cell carcinoma shown in **A.**

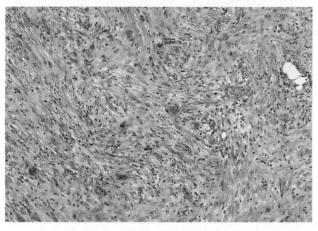

A

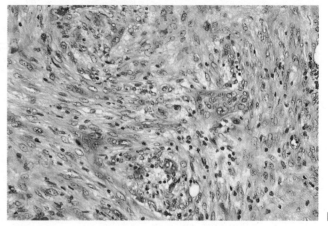

B

**FIG. 18.12.** *Metaplastic carcinoma, spindle and squamous type.* This specimen is a subareolar tumor that caused nipple retraction in an 84-year-old woman. **A,B:** Malignant spindle cell neoplasm has a storiform pattern and a sprinkling of lymphocytes. (*continued*)

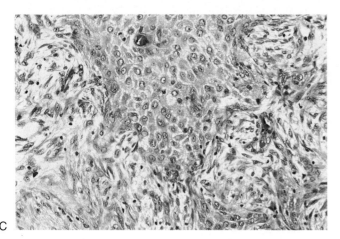

**FIG. 18.12.** *Continued.* **C:** Squamous differentiation in the carcinoma.

*Spindle cell carcinoma* of the breast is a subset of carcinomas with squamous metaplasia in which most or virtually all of the neoplasm has assumed this pseudosarcomatous growth pattern (24,33,35). At this extreme, the distinction between spindle cell carcinoma and primary sarcoma of the breast may be difficult. The neoplasm may be mistaken for fibromatosis, fibrosarcoma, or malignant fibrous histiocytoma because of the minimal epithelial component and a storiform growth pattern (Figs. 18.15 and 18.16) (26,29,32). Extensive sampling sometimes is necessary to identify areas of squamous differentiation in the tumor and to search for foci of intraductal or invasive adenocarcinoma that usually are located at the periphery. In a substantial number of cases, no epithelial elements are detected, and the diagnosis hinges on finding immunoreactivity for cytokeratin in the spindle cells. Because aberrant cytokeratin expression is rarely detected in primary mesenchymal neoplasms, reliance should not be placed only on cytokeratin reactivity. All histologic and clinical features must be taken into consideration when reaching a diagnosis in this circumstance.

An unusual variant of mammary carcinoma with spindle and squamous metaplasia has been characterized as *pseudoangiosarcomatous* or *acantholytic carcinoma* (36,37). This type of carcinoma also arises in the skin, lung, thyroid, oropharynx, and other sites. The acantholytic appearance is a consequence of the neoplastic epithelial component embedded

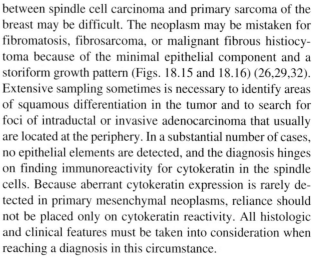

**FIG. 18.13.** *Metaplastic carcinoma, spindle and squamous type.* Small round groups of squamous cells *(arrows)* are the only evidence of epithelial differentiation in this spindle cell storiform neoplasm. Lymphocytes are scattered throughout the tumor.

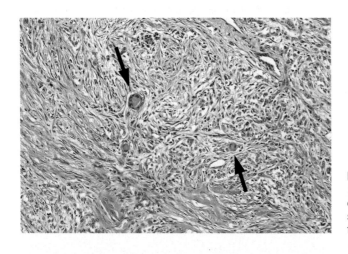

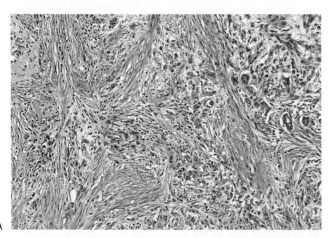

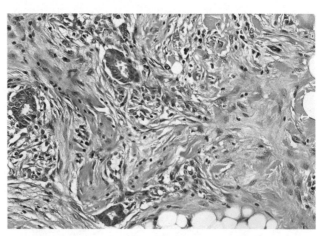

**FIG. 18.14.** *Metaplastic carcinoma, spindle cell type with adenocarcinoma.* **A:** Spindle cell neoplasm has a storiform pattern. Small carcinomatous glands are present *(upper right).* **B:** Well-differentiated adenocarcinoma in the spindle cell metaplastic carcinoma.

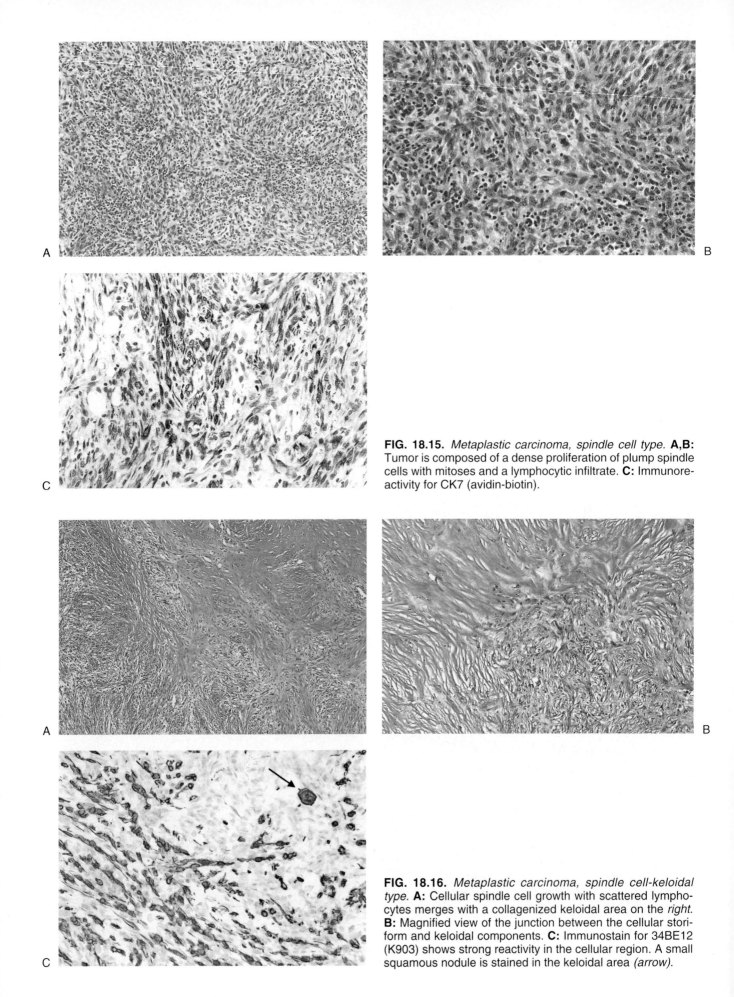

**FIG. 18.15.** *Metaplastic carcinoma, spindle cell type.* **A,B:** Tumor is composed of a dense proliferation of plump spindle cells with mitoses and a lymphocytic infiltrate. **C:** Immunoreactivity for CK7 (avidin-biotin).

**FIG. 18.16.** *Metaplastic carcinoma, spindle cell-keloidal type.* **A:** Cellular spindle cell growth with scattered lymphocytes merges with a collagenized keloidal area on the *right*. **B:** Magnified view of the junction between the cellular storiform and keloidal components. **C:** Immunostain for 34BE12 (K903) shows strong reactivity in the cellular region. A small squamous nodule is stained in the keloidal area *(arrow)*.

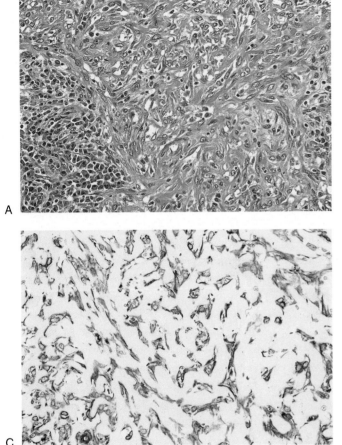

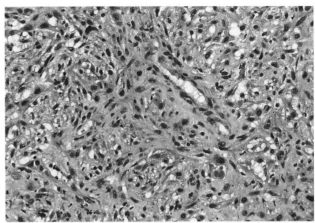

**FIG. 18.17.** *Metaplastic carcinoma, acantholytic.* **A,B:** Ill-defined spaces are formed in this relatively compact tumor. Note the collection of plasma cells in **A**. **C:** Immunostain for 34BE12 (K903) highlights the pseudoangiomatoid structure (avidin-biotin).

in abundant spindle cell stroma (Fig. 18.17). Degeneration of the epithelium results in a pseudovascular pattern of complex anastomosing spaces (Fig. 18.18) (38). Cells lining these spaces are immunoreactive for cytokeratin, and they do not stain for factor VIII or CD34, which characterize endothelial cells. Spindle cell and acantholytic variants of metaplastic carcinoma almost always are immunoreactive with the high–molecular-weight cytokeratin 34BE12 (K903), even when other keratin markers are negative.

A moderate round cell inflammatory reaction almost always is present in carcinomas with squamous and spindle cell metaplasia (Figs. 18.12, 18.14–18.16). This is such a characteristic feature that a diagnosis of metaplastic carcinoma should rarely be made when there is little or no inflammation. Sometimes the reaction is so prominent that it obscures the neoplastic nature of the process, leading to alternate diagnoses such as fasciitis or inflammatory pseudotumor. These latter lesions occur so infrequently in the breast that a tumor suggesting one or the other invariably proves to be metaplastic carcinoma.

*Heterologous metaplasia* is encountered most commonly as bone and/or cartilage. These foci, which may appear histologically benign or malignant, often coexist with poorly differentiated areas composed of round or spindle cells (Fig. 18.19). Rhabdomyoid, adipose, and angiosarcomatous metaplasia also have been encountered. In general, carcinomas with heterologous metaplasia tend to retain an epithelial component that may be glandular or squamous (Figs. 18.20 and 18.21). In a few cases, the lesion has been composed largely of undifferentiated spindle cell elements with scant heterologous components. The growth pattern in this setting tends to resemble malignant fibrous histiocytoma (Fig. 18.22) (29). Myxoid change, a common feature of these undifferentiated elements, also may be found in transitional zones between adenocarcinoma and chondroid metaplasia. Highly cellular areas resembling fibrosarcoma were described in nearly half of the cases in one series (3).

Metaplastic tumors that have multinucleated giant cells resembling osteoclasts are associated most frequently with osseous or cartilaginous metaplasia (1,3,24), but these cells can occur in spindle cell stroma without cartilaginous metaplasia (Fig. 18.23) (6). This variant of metaplastic carcinoma usually does not have the stromal hemorrhage and prominent adenocarcinoma typically found in carcinomas with osteoclast-like cells described in Chapter 25. Nonetheless, the existence of histologically benign osteoclast-like giant cells in both lesions suggests that they may be related. Osteoclast-like giant cells in metaplastic carcinomas are immunoreactive for vimentin and sometimes for histiocytic markers, but not for epithelial membrane antigen (EMA), cytokeratin, or S-100. On the other hand, cytokeratin immunoreactivity was found in the spindle cell mesenchymal component of 63% of

*text continues on p. 440*

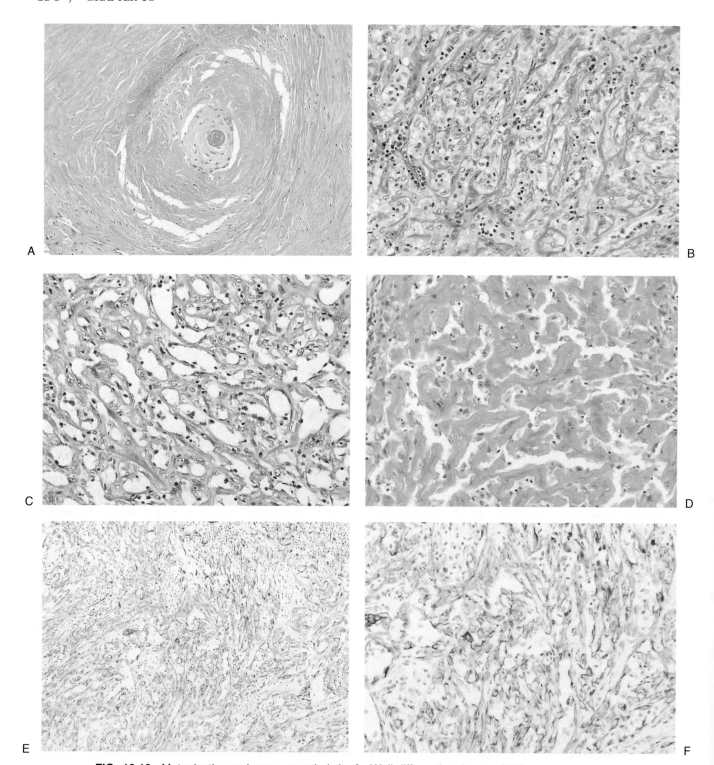

**FIG. 18.18.** *Metaplastic carcinoma, acantholytic.* **A:** Well-differentiated metaplastic squamous carcinoma surrounded by densely collagenous tissue that is part of the neoplastic process. **B:** Part of the tumor in which the carcinoma is arranged in a trabecular pattern. There is a sparse infiltrate of lymphocytes, and scattered degenerating tumor cells are represented by pyknotic nuclei. **C:** Extensive degeneration of the carcinoma resulting in an angiomatoid appearance. **D:** Dense stroma in angiomatoid metaplastic carcinoma. **E:** Diffuse immunoreactivity for cytokeratin (anti-AE1/AE3, avidin-biotin). **F:** Diffuse immunoreactivity for 34BE12 (avidin-biotin).

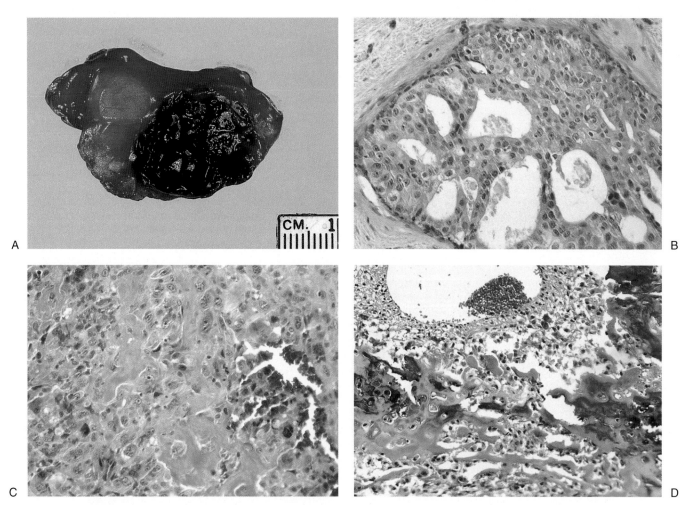

**FIG. 18.19.** *Metaplastic carcinoma, chondroosseous type.* **A:** Gross appearance of a tumor that is un-usually hemorrhagic. **B:** Cribriform intraductal carcinoma. **C:** Osteoid in an area of undifferentiated car-cinoma with hemorrhage. **D:** Neoplastic ossified cartilage and a dilated vascular space suggestive of telangiectatic osteosarcoma.

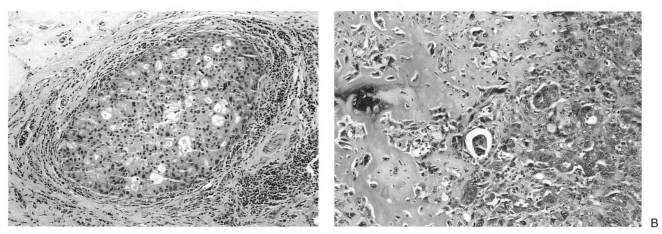

**FIG. 18.20.** *Metaplastic carcinoma, osseous type.* All images are from the same tumor in a 53-year-old woman. **A:** Intraductal carcinoma, apocrine cribriform type, with low nuclear grade. **B:** Osseous metaplasia (*left*) and poorly differentiated adenocarcinoma with undifferentiated spindle cell carcinoma. (*continued*)

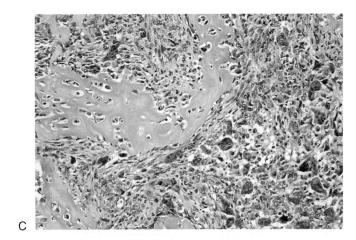

**FIG. 18.20.** *Continued.* **C:** Osseous metaplasia in spindle cell carcinoma with osteoclastic giant cells.

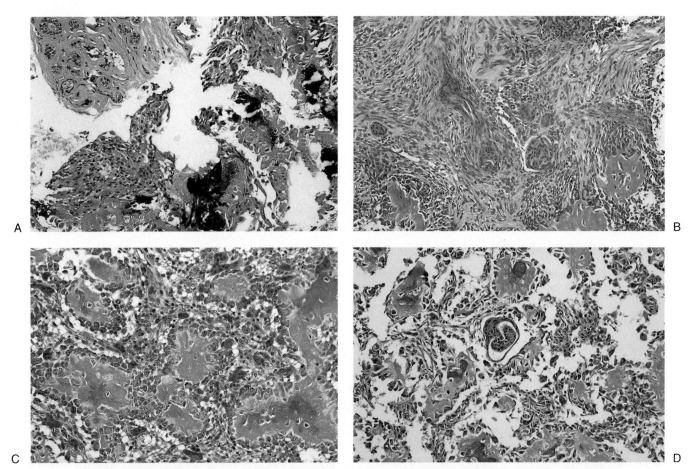

**FIG. 18.21.** *Metaplastic carcinoma, chondroosseous type.* **A:** Needle core biopsy showed fragments of osseous tissue and breast parenchyma. **B:** Spindle and squamous metaplasia were found at the core biopsy site in the excised specimen. Osseous differentiation is present *(below).* **C:** Bulk of the tumor consisted of ossifying osteoid with abundant osteoblasts and scattered osteoclastic cells. **D:** Isolated foci of adenosquamous differentiation were present in the osseous tissue. All images are from the same tumor.

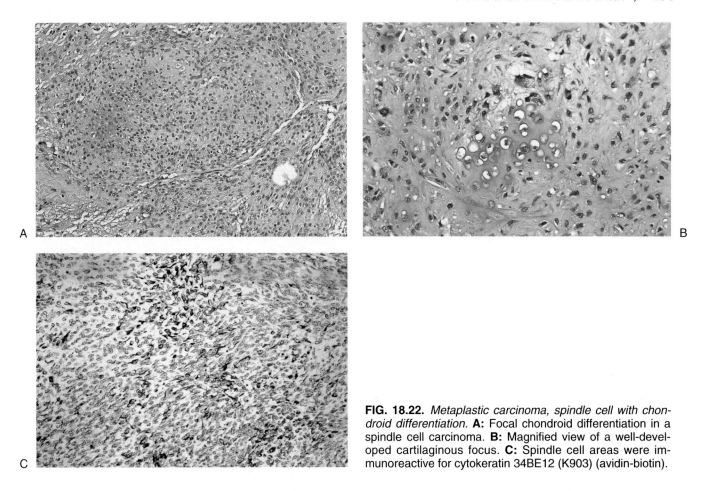

**FIG. 18.22.** *Metaplastic carcinoma, spindle cell with chondroid differentiation.* **A:** Focal chondroid differentiation in a spindle cell carcinoma. **B:** Magnified view of a well-developed cartilaginous focus. **C:** Spindle cell areas were immunoreactive for cytokeratin 34BE12 (K903) (avidin-biotin).

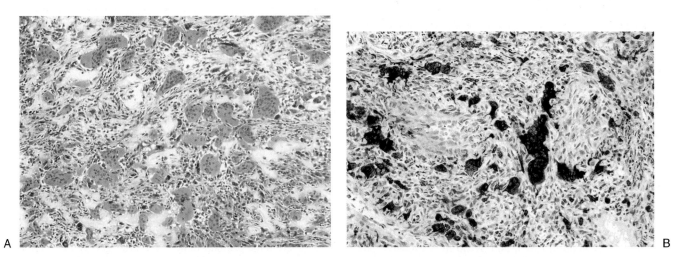

**FIG. 18.23.** *Metaplastic carcinoma with osteoclast-like giant cells.* **A:** Tumor did not exhibit cartilaginous and osseous differentiation. **B:** Giant cells and some stromal cells are immunoreactive for KP-1, a histiocytic marker (avidin-biotin).

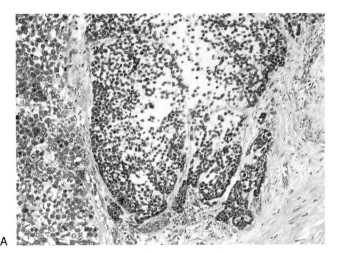
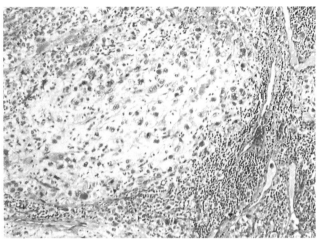

**FIG. 18.24.** *Metaplastic carcinoma, matrix-producing type.* **A:** Small focus of matrix formation emerging from poorly differentiated small cell carcinoma on the *left.* **B:** Metastatic matrix-producing carcinoma from the tumor shown in **A** in an axillary lymph node.

these tumors (6). Osteoclast-like giant cells may be found clustered around thin-walled vascular spaces in the primary tumor and in metastatic foci involving axillary lymph nodes and distant sites. Carcinomas with spindle cell metaplasia and osteoclast-like giant cells do not constitute a distinct category, and they should be included in the group of carcinomas with heterologous metaplasia.

*Matrix-producing carcinoma* (39) is a variant of heterologous metaplastic carcinoma composed of "overt carcinoma with direct transition to a cartilaginous and/or osseous stromal matrix without an intervening spindle cell zone or osteoclastic cells" (Fig. 18.24). The majority of the tumors are circumscribed or nodular, but occasional lesions have infiltrative borders. Ultrasound examination revealed a well-circumscribed nodular hypoechoic tumor that exhibited marginal enhancement on computed tomography with contrast (40).

Microscopically, the carcinomatous element in matrix-producing tumors usually is moderately to poorly differentiated adenocarcinoma, often with small cell features and infrequent foci of squamous or apocrine metaplasia (Fig. 18.25). Some tumors have components that resemble mucinous carcinoma (Fig. 18.26). Mucin positivity is demonstrated in the stroma, but chondroid-forming cells do not contain intracellular mucin. The chondroid matrix has histochemical properties of a sulfated acid mucopolysaccharide consistent with chondroitin sulfate. Carcinoma cells stain positively for keratin, EMA, and S-100 in adenocarcinoma areas (Fig. 18.27). The matrix-producing areas are strongly S-100 reactive but tend to be nonreactive for cytokeratin. A few tumors exhibit actin immunoreactivity, especially within metaplastic spindle cells, and actin myofilaments have been observed in the lesion by electron microscopy. Metastatic lesions usually have the same matrix-producing pattern as the primary tumor (Figs. 18.24 and 18.28).

Fine needle aspiration reveals cuboidal-to-oval tumor cells in a myxoid background (40). The matrix material stains pale green with the Papanicolaou stain and purple-red with the May-Giemsa stain. Tumor cells may be observed embedded in the matrix material.

Metastases derived from a metaplastic carcinoma can consist entirely of adenocarcinoma or entirely of metaplastic elements, or they may contain a mixture of these components (Figs. 18.24, 18.28, and 18.29). Tumors with squamous metaplasia often give rise to metastases with squamous differentiation in axillary lymph nodes and other sites. On the other hand, axillary lymph node metastases from some tumors with heterologous metaplasia are composed entirely of adenocarcinoma, or the axillary metastases consist mainly of heterologous elements. Heterologous elements are expressed with greater frequency in local recurrences on the chest wall and in visceral sites than in nodal metastases (Fig. 18.29) (3,24). Various combinations of epithelial and heterologous constituents have been described in separate metastases from one patient (3). There does not appear to be a consistent relationship between the type and the amount of heterologous elements in the primary tumor and their representation in metastases. When metaplastic foci occur in metastatic deposits, they usually duplicate at least some of the components found in the primary tumor. In one case, cutaneous metastases from a heterologous tumor with chondroid metaplasia grew entirely as chondrosarcoma (41). It is also possible for metaplastic changes to develop within metastases, although corresponding metaplasia may not be detected in the primary tumor even after generous sampling. This phenomenon was observed in a case reported by Chell et al. (42). The patient had a 2.2-cm primary carcinoma with chondroid metaplasia. Metastases in two axillary lymph nodes showed chondroid differentiation as well as focal squamous metaplasia that was not seen in the primary tumor. This case also is of interest because the patient developed a pulmonary metastasis with chondroid features.

Metaplastic carcinoma may be suspected in material obtained by fine needle aspiration if epithelial and metaplastic elements are present (43–47). When epithelial elements are

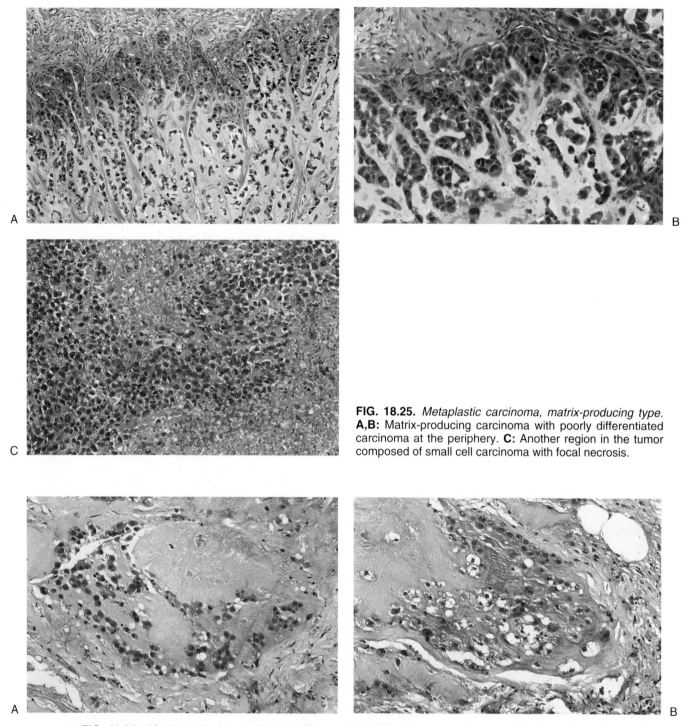

FIG. 18.25. *Metaplastic carcinoma, matrix-producing type.* **A,B:** Matrix-producing carcinoma with poorly differentiated carcinoma at the periphery. **C:** Another region in the tumor composed of small cell carcinoma with focal necrosis.

FIG. 18.26. *Matrix-producing carcinoma with mucinous appearance.* **A,B:** These areas lack a distinct rim of carcinoma cells and resemble invasive mucinous carcinoma.

not apparent in the aspirate, the material is likely to suggest a mesenchymal neoplasm (48–52). The diagnosis of metaplastic carcinoma can be entertained with greater confidence when distinct adenocarcinoma and either squamous or heterologous components can be identified. However, before rendering a definitive interpretation, careful consideration must be given to the differential diagnosis, which includes the following: papilloma, possibly infarcted, with squamous metaplasia; phyllodes tumor with epithelial hyperplasia; pri-

mary mammary sarcoma; and metastatic neoplasms. Osteoclastic-like giant cells may be found in the aspirate from a metaplastic carcinoma with heterologous metaplasia (53).

*Low-grade adenosquamous carcinoma* is an unusual variant of metaplastic duct carcinoma that is morphologically very similar to adenosquamous carcinoma of the skin (54). Four examples of mammary low-grade adenosquamous carcinoma have been reported under the diagnosis of syringomatous squamous tumors (55). Osteocartilaginous metaplasia

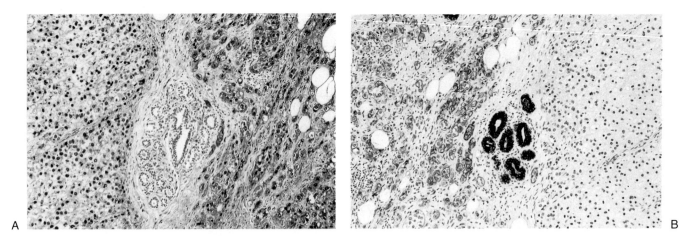

**FIG. 18.27.** *Matrix-producing carcinoma immunoreactivity.* **A:** Nuclear reactivity for S-100 protein in adenocarcinoma *(right)* and matrix-producing carcinoma *(left)*. Cytoplasmic reactivity is stronger in the adenocarcinoma area. **B:** Immunoreactivity for cytokeratin (AE1/AE3) is limited to adenocarcinoma *(left)* and a normal lobule *(center)*. No reactivity is present in matrix-producing carcinoma (*right*).

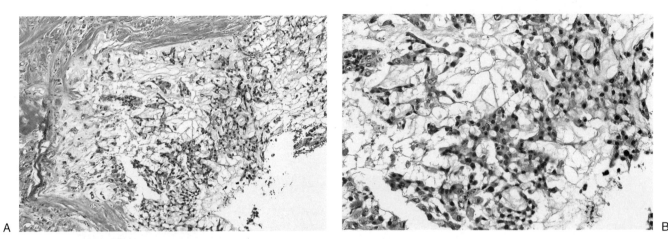

**FIG. 18.28.** *Matrix-producing carcinoma, chest wall recurrence.* **A,B:** Matrix-producing pattern resembles mucinous carcinoma.

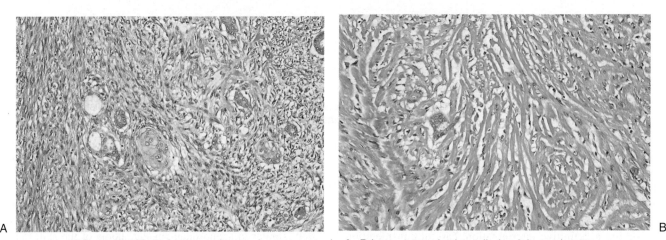

**FIG. 18.29.** *Metaplastic carcinoma, lung metastasis.* **A:** Primary tumor had small glandular and squamous foci in a storiform spindle cell background. **B:** Another area in the primary tumor with pseudoangiomatoid growth and a small focus of adenocarcinoma. (*continued*)

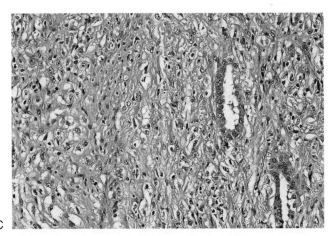

**FIG. 18.29.** *Continued.* **C:** Metastatic metaplastic carcinoma in the lung composed of cells similar to those shown in **A**. Two glandular structures are formed by residual benign alveolar epithelium of the lung.

has been seen in a minority of low-grade adenosquamous carcinomas. Intraductal carcinoma is variably present, but it may be difficult to distinguish from infiltrative areas.

These tumors typically are smaller than other varieties of metaplastic carcinoma (0.5 to 3.4 cm, average about 2.0 cm). They are hard, yellow-tan nodules with grossly ill-defined borders (Fig. 18.30). Microscopically, some tumors have a highly invasive, stellate growth pattern, whereas others are partly or entirely circumscribed (Fig. 18.31). The invasive carcinoma exhibits variable amounts of epidermoid differentiation in collagenous stroma (Figs. 18.32 and 18.33). A

tendency to grow between ducts and within lobules is seen throughout the tumor. It is not unusual to find a central area of radial sclerosing proliferation, such as a papilloma or sclerosing adenosis (Fig. 18.34). Association with adenomyoepitheliomatous proliferation has been reported (56,57). Some lesions appear to arise from radial sclerosing foci or adenomyoepitheliomas (Fig. 18.35).

Squamous metaplasia is found in varying patterns, including extensive epidermoid growth, syringoma-like differentiation, and inconspicuous squamous foci in predominantly glandular lesions (Figs. 18.31–18.33). Large keratinizing cysts are uncommon, but microcysts that may contain keratotic debris with calcification often are present. Osteocartilaginous foci have been encountered in primary tumors and in the chest wall recurrence of a tumor that did not have such heterologous expression in the primary lesion (Fig. 18.36). The tissue immediately around squamous foci often has a distinctive lamellar arrangement of spindle cells that merges with the epithelium (Figs. 18.31 and 18.32). Rarely, low-grade adenosquamous carcinoma shows transitions to conventional high-grade spindle cell and squamous sarcomatoid metaplastic carcinoma (55). The spindle cell stroma of low-grade adenosquamous carcinomas usually exhibits little or no cytokeratin reactivity (Fig. 18.37).

The diagnosis of low-grade adenosquamous carcinoma may be suggested by fine needle aspiration. Smears from low-grade adenosquamous carcinoma have low cellularity and small clusters containing uniform cells of small-to-medium size that tend to be oriented around a microlumen. Squamous metaplasia may be detected in the epithelial clusters,

*text continues on p. 449*

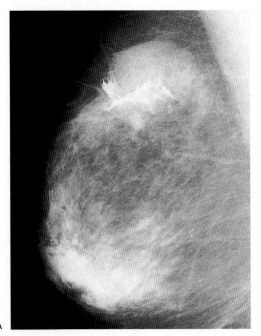
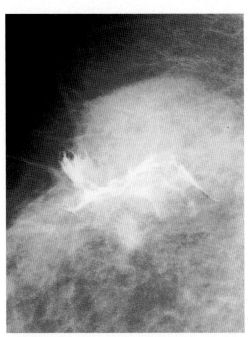

**FIG. 18.30.** *Low-grade adenosquamous carcinoma.* **A,B:** Tumor forms an oval stellate density with ill-defined borders in the upper half of the breast below the site of dye injected to localize the lesion. *(continued)*

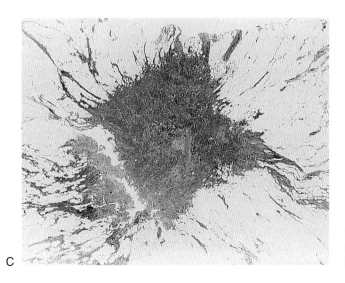

C

**FIG. 18.30.** *Continued.* **C:** Whole-mount histologic section of the low-grade adenosquamous carcinoma shown in the mammogram. The tumor has an infiltrating border.

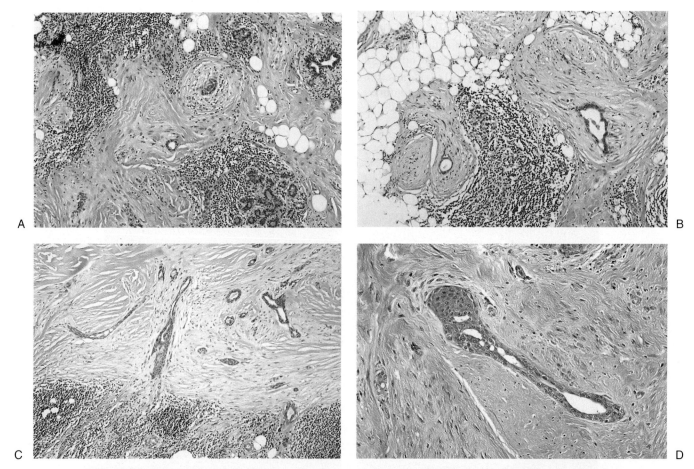

**FIG. 18.31.** *Low-grade adenosquamous carcinoma.* **A:** Tumor infiltrating breast stroma near a lobule *(below)* and duct *(upper right).* Note the character of the stroma around the neoplastic epithelium and the lymphocytic reaction. **B:** Carcinoma invading fat. **C:** A circumscribed low-grade adenosquamous carcinoma with dense collagenous stroma and peripheral lymphocytic reaction. **D:** Adenosquamous differentiation in the tumor shown in **C**.

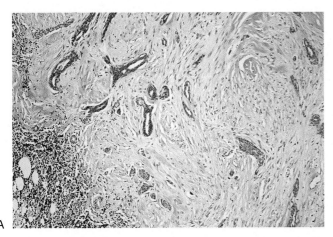
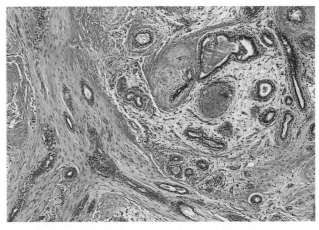

A

B

**FIG. 18.32.** *Low-grade adenosquamous carcinoma.* **A:** Prominent collagenized component typical of some of these tumors. Note the lymphocytic infiltrate at the border *(lower left)*. **B:** Magnified view of the tumor invading in and around a lobule. This focus is predominantly glandular with one squamous nodule.

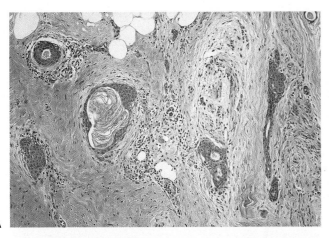
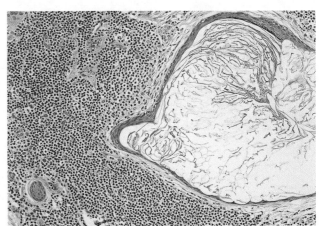

A

B

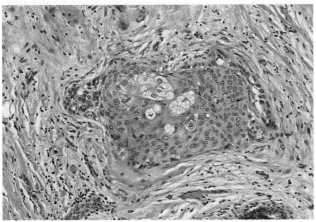

C

**FIG. 18.33.** *Low-grade adenosquamous carcinoma.* **A:** Various patterns of squamous differentiation. **B:** Marked cystic dilation of squamous epithelium with a dense lymphocytic reaction. **C:** Sebaceous metaplasia in the squamous epithelium.

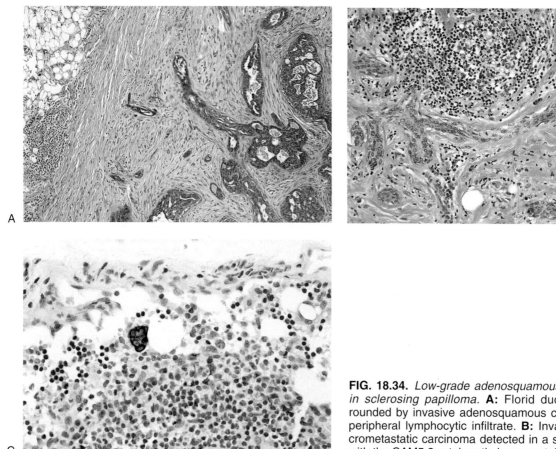

**FIG. 18.34.** *Low-grade adenosquamous carcinoma arising in sclerosing papilloma.* **A:** Florid duct hyperplasia surrounded by invasive adenosquamous carcinoma. Note the peripheral lymphocytic infiltrate. **B:** Invasive tumor. **C:** Micrometastatic carcinoma detected in a sentinel lymph node with the CAM5.2 cytokeratin immunostain (avidin-biotin).

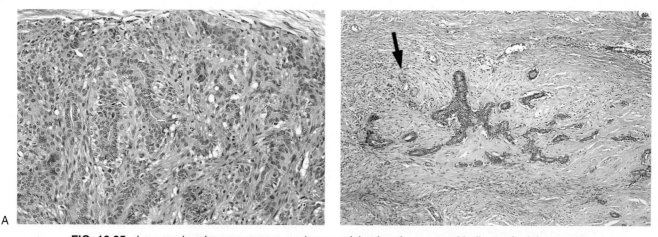

**FIG. 18.35.** *Low-grade adenosquamous carcinoma arising in adenomyoepithelioma.* **A:** Adenomyoepithelioma with florid epithelial and myoepithelial elements in an excisional biopsy. **B:** Recurrent tumor two years later at the site of the adenomyoepithelioma. The glandular elements (*arrow*) probably are remnants of the adenomyoepithelioma surrounded by dense collagenized tissue representing part of the low-grade adenosquamous carcinoma. *(continued)*

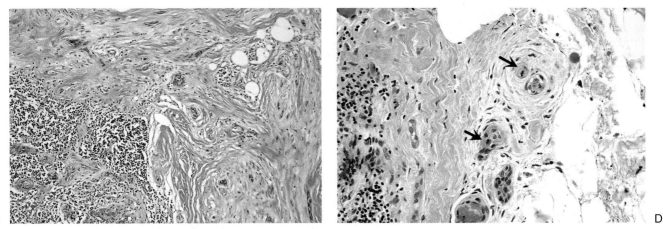

**FIG. 18.35.** *Continued.* **C:** Invasive low-grade adenosquamous carcinoma at the periphery of the lesion. **D:** Two mitotic figures are present *(arrows)*.

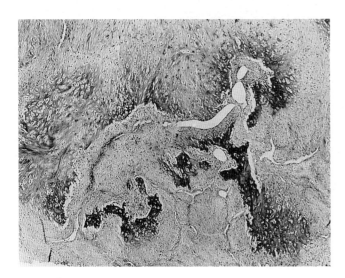

**FIG. 18.36.** *Low-grade adenosquamous carcinoma, recurrent.* Osteocartilaginous metaplasia in the recurrent lesion on the chest wall. The tumor was limited to soft tissue and had typical areas of low-grade adenosquamous carcinoma.

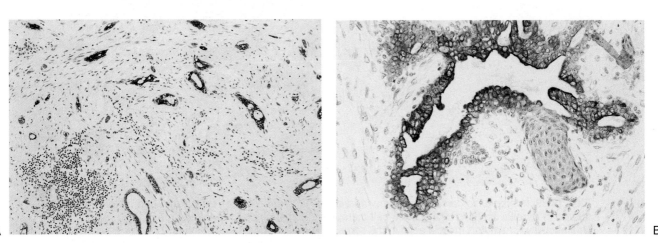

**FIG. 18.37.** *Low-grade adenosquamous carcinoma, immunoreactivity.* **A:** Staining for 34BE12, a cytokeratin marker, is limited to glandular elements, with no reactivity in the spindle cell areas. **B:** Immunoreactivity for cytokeratin CK7 is present in glandular but not in squamous epithelium (both avidin-biotin).

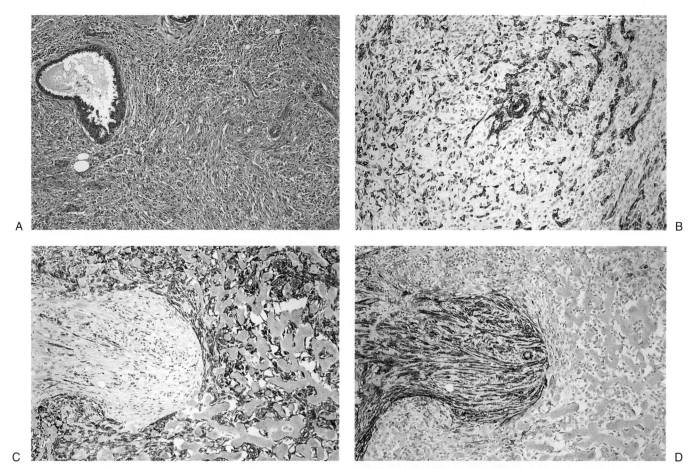

**FIG. 18.38.** *Metaplastic carcinoma, immunoreactivity.* **A:** Hyperplastic duct is surrounded by spindle cell metaplastic carcinoma. **B:** Immunoreactivity for cytokeratin AE1/AE3 is present in some but not all cells. **C:** Immunoreactivity for smooth muscle actin is shown surrounding a discrete largely nonreactive zone. **D:** Section parallel to **C** showing immunoreactivity for cytokeratin AE1/AE3 limited to the region that was minimally reactive for actin in **C** (all avidin-biotin).

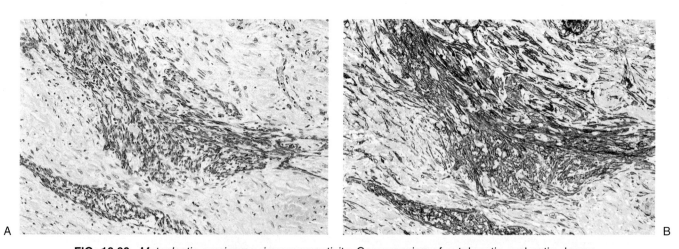

**FIG. 18.39.** *Metaplastic carcinoma, immunoreactivity.* Coexpression of cytokeratin and actin demonstrated in parallel sections of a spindle cell metaplastic carcinoma. **A:** Cytokeratin AE1/AE3 reactivity. **B:** Reactivity for smooth muscle actin in the same region as **A** (both avidin-biotin).

and bipolar spindle cells are present singly or in small bundles (58).

## IMMUNOHISTOCHEMISTRY AND ELECTRON MICROSCOPY

Immunohistochemical studies have attempted to elucidate the relationship between epithelial and heterologous elements in metaplastic carcinomas, but the reported results have been inconsistent. The usefulness of immunohistochemical markers is complicated by the reported coexpression of cytokeratin and vimentin in nonmetaplastic breast carcinomas (59). Some authors observed coexpression of epithelial (cytokeratin and EMA)- and mesenchymal (vimentin and actin)-associated markers in the spindle cell elements of metaplastic carcinomas (Figs. 18.38 and 18.39) (26,29,60,61). Others who failed to find coexpression reported vimentin reactivity in epithelial and spindle cells, but cytokeratin expression only in the epithelial elements (24,62). Cytokeratin and EMA have been reportedly positive in carcinomatous, spindle cell, and chondrosarcomatous elements in one case (61), whereas Wargotz and Norris (39) found keratin and EMA reactivity largely restricted to ep-

ithelial components and vimentin expression prominent only in chondroid areas. Others described EMA immunoreactivity in mesenchymal areas of 31% of heterologous carcinomas (29). There also has not been agreement on the distribution of carcinoembryonic antigen reactivity. Two studies reported negative results in the epithelial and spindle cell parts of the tumor (25,62), but other studies reported that both components exhibited focal carcinoembryonic antigen reactivity (61). S-100 has been reported to be positive (26,61) and negative (61) in spindle and epithelial elements.

Because of the varied and seemingly unpredictable cytokeratin immunoreactivity in these carcinomas, the workup of a tumor suspected to be metaplastic carcinoma requires the use of more than one reagent. The high–molecular-weight cytokeratin antibody K903 (34BE12) has been the reagent most often clearly immunoreactive in metaplastic carcinomas. Other cytokeratins that should be evaluated are CAM5.2, AE1/AE3, and CK7. In most tumors with one strongly reactive keratin reagent, careful inspection of slides immunostained for other cytokeratins will reveal isolated positive cells or small foci of reactivity in samples that appear to be nonimmunoreactive on cursory examination. This is an important corroborating observation (Fig. 18.40).

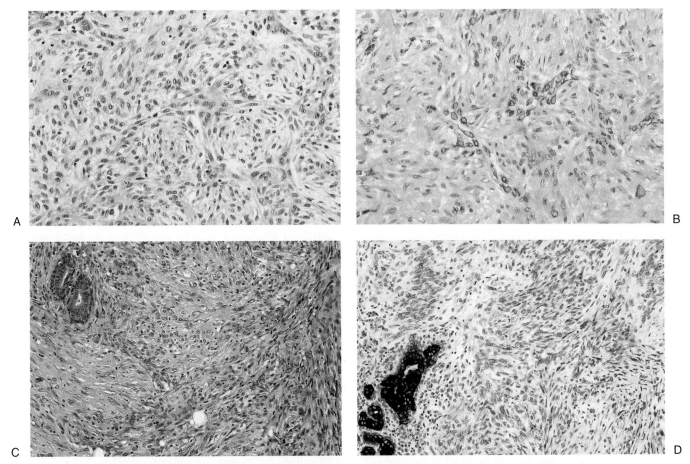

**FIG. 18.40.** *Metaplastic carcinoma, immunoreactivity.* **A:** Tumor has a storiform structure and a hint of angiomatoid growth. There is no CK7 reactivity in this region. **B:** CK7 immunostain highlights angiomatoid foci. **C:** Small ducts in spindle cell metaplastic carcinoma. **D:** Immunoreactivity for cytokeratin CK7 is stronger in the ducts than in the metaplastic carcinoma (all avidin-biotin).

Immunohistochemical studies for 34BE12, p53, retinoblastoma protein, HER2/*neu* (polyclonal), epidermal growth factor receptor, and cyclin D1 were performed on 18 metaplastic carcinomas with osteocartilaginous heterologous components (63). Positive staining was found as follows: 34BE12: 13 (72%), p53: 11 (61%), retinoblastoma protein: 12 (66%), HER2/*neu*: 2 (11%), epidermal growth factor receptor: 7 (38%), and cyclin D1: 5 (28%). Staining for 34BE12 was observed in the carcinomatous component in five (38%) of the neoplasms, in the metaplastic component in two (15%) cases, and in both elements in six (64%) cases. p53 staining was observed in the carcinomatous component exclusively in four (36%) of the 11 p53-positive tumors. Expression of these markers did not correlate with clinicopathologic features, such as patient age, tumor size, tumor type, relative proportion of metaplastic elements, and axillary nodal status, and was not predictive of disease-free survival.

CD44 is a cell adhesion receptor involved in cell–cell and cell–matrix interactions. It is strongly expressed in the basal layer of squamous epithelium and in normal glandular epithelium in various organs including the breast. Expression of CD44 has been observed in carcinomas of the breast (64) and other organs. Ylagan et al. (65) reported that CD44 and several of its variants were strongly and more extensively reactive with squamous than with glandular components of adenosquamous carcinomas. None of the tumors examined by these investigators originated in the breast. CD44 reactivity was most pronounced in low-grade tumors and tended to decrease with loss of differentiation. The role of CD44 as a diagnostic test for metaplastic breast carcinoma remains to be determined.

Many factors probably have contributed to the conflicting and variable published results with immunohistochemical markers. These include small numbers of cases available to most investigators, differing subtypes of tumors studied in this relatively heterogeneous group of neoplasms, the retrospective nature of the studies using paraffin blocks of differing age and quality of fixation, and the use of different reagents.

It is very likely that there also are intrinsic differences in the phenotypic expression of markers that reflect the variable nature of genetic alterations in individual tumors. Rather than a single pattern of cytoskeletal expression, these neoplasms appear to have a range of cytoskeletal phenotypes that express differing proportions and types of cytofilaments (Figs. 18.38 and 18.39).

Evidence to support this hypothesis can be found in studies of the relationship between vimentin and cytokeratin expression in breast carcinoma cell lines. Molecular study has disclosed vimentin expression in more than 50% of hormone-independent human breast carcinoma cell lines but not in hormone-dependent cell lines (66). Cytokeratin was diminished in vimentin-positive cell lines. Vimentin expression was absent from nontumorigenic human mammary epithelial cells, but it was present in a highly tumorigenic cell line (66). Acquisition of vimentin expression has been observed in some adriamycin-resistant MCF-7 cell lines (67). These altered cells were characterized by diminished keratin 19 expression and diminished cell adhesion mani-

fested by loss of expression of the adhesion molecule uvomorulin (E-cadherin) and reduced formation of cell junctions *in vitro*. Vimentin expression could be achieved by transfection of human vimentin complementary DNA into MCF-7 cells, but this did not result in phenotypic changes in the expression of keratins or cell adhesion molecules. Carcinoma cells with a mesenchymal phenotype expressing vimentin and lacking uvomorulin (E-cadherin) exhibited increased invasiveness and metastatic activity in nude mice (68). These observations suggest that vimentin expression may be a marker for metaplasia but that full expression of the fibroblastic or spindle cell phenotype is dependent on other genetic alterations.

The issue is complicated further by the fact that cytokeratin expression has been observed in a variety of primary mesenchymal spindle cell sarcomas (69,70). Cytokeratin expression can be induced in fetal mesenchymal cells under certain culture conditions (71) and in SV40-transformed fibroblasts (72).

Electron microscopy usually has supported the epithelial origin of heterologous elements by revealing that many ultrastructural characteristics are shared by the various cell types in the tumor. In most (2,3,73–76) but not all studies (77), the authors reported finding cells that had ultrastructural features intermediate between the epithelial and heterologous elements. Myoepithelial cells are present to a variable extent, occasionally constituting a significant part of the lesion (26,39).

## PROGNOSIS AND TREATMENT

Eight relatively large series of cases consisting of 22 (5), 26 (3,39), 27 (24), 30 (32), 34 (29), 40 (23), and 100 (26) cases have been reported with sufficient data to assess prognosis. When stratified by stage, the data indicate revealed declining survival with advancing stage (Table 18.1). Because of the rarity of metaplastic carcinomas and the relatively low frequency of axillary metastases, especially in patients with heterologous metaplastic tumors, it is difficult to assemble a sufficient number of cases to stratify them by major prognostic factors such as tumor size, nodal status, and pattern of metaplasia.

The frequency of positive axillary nodes associated with heterologous metaplastic carcinoma, including so-called matrix-producing tumors, ranges from 6% (39) to 31% (29). Disease-free survival, generally reported for 5 or more years of follow-up, ranges from 38% (3,23) to 67% (29).

Axillary lymph node metastases were reported in 0% (32), 6% (26), 11% (5), 13% (24), 14% (29), and 54% (23) of patients with squamous and spindle cell metaplasia. One study described a 5-year survival of 65% (23), whereas in another study, 25% of patients remained alive and disease free, 16% died of other causes, 8% were alive after recurrence, and 50% died of metastatic mammary carcinoma (24). Disease-free 5-year survival in a third series was 64% (5), and others reported that 86% of patients were alive and well (29).

The clinicopathologic features of 32 patients treated for metaplastic carcinomas with heterologous osteocartilagi-

**TABLE 18.1.** *Stage and prognosis in metaplastic mammary carcinoma*

| Reference | Type of metaplasia | No. of cases | (+) LN No. (%) | L&W No. (%) | AWD No. (%) | DOD No. (%) | DOC No. (%) |
|---|---|---|---|---|---|---|---|
| Oberman (24)[a] | Squamous/spindle | 12 | 1/8 (13) | 3 (25) | 1 (8) | 6 (50) | 2 (16) |
| | Heterologous | 15 | 1/11 (9) | 7 (47) | | 6 (40) | 2 (13) |
| Kaufman et al. (3)[b] | Heterologous | 26 | 5/20 (25) | 10 (38) | 1 (4) | 14 (54) | |
| | | | | Five-year survival 40% (stages I, II, III: 56%, 26%, 18%) | | | |
| Huvos et al. (23)[c] | Squamous/spindle | 24 | 13/2 (50) | Five-year survival 65% | | | |
| | Heterologous | 16 | 3/16 (19) | Five-year survival 38% | | | |
| Wargotz and Norris (5)[d] | Squamous | 22 | 2/19 (11) | 14 (64) | | 8 (36) | |
| Wargotz and Norris (39)[e] | Heterologous | 26 | 1/17 (6) | 17 (65) | 1 (4) | 8 (31) | |
| Wargotz et al. (26)[f,g] | Spindle | 100 | 3/7 (6) | 44 (44) | 12 (12) | 44 (44) | |

[a]Two cases of "pure" squamous carcinoma without spindle cell elements excluded.
[b]Follow-up available for 25 cases.
[c]Follow-up available for 33 cases.
[d]Spindle cell metaplasia in three cases; others pure squamous metaplasia.
[e]Cartilaginous and osseous.
[f]Seventy-two had infiltrating duct carcinoma, 11 were spindle/squamous, and 17 pure spindle.
[g]Recurrences in 56 cases; 44 patients without recurrence but deaths due to other causes not specified.
AWD, alive with disease; DOC, died of other causes; DOD, died of disease; LN, lymph node; L&W, living and well.

nous elements have been reported (63). Each neoplasm consisted of invasive adenocarcinoma accompanied by a cartilaginous and/or osseous component. The heterologous element consisted of cartilage in 10 neoplasms and was exclusively osteoid or bone in two neoplasms. The remaining 20 neoplasms contained a mixture of cartilaginous and osseous components. All patients were women with a mean age of 56 years. Twenty-four patients were treated by mastectomy and eight by local excision. Lymph node metastases were detected in 23% of the 26 patients who had an axillary dissection. Clinical follow-up was available for 29 (91%) of the 32 patients. Six (21%) patients developed a local recurrence or distant metastases within 2 years of initial treatment; four of these patients died of metastatic carcinoma. The overall 5-year survival rate was 60%. When compared with control patients with infiltrating duct carcinoma, the group with metaplastic carcinoma tended to have a more favorable prognosis after adjustment for nodal status and tumor size, although the difference was not statistically significant (Fig. 18.41). The prognosis of patients with metaplastic mammary carcinoma with heterologous osteocartilaginous elements is dependent on tumor stage at diagnosis.

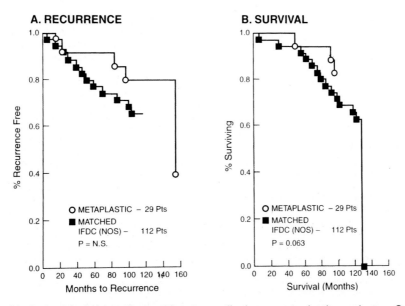

**FIG. 18.41.** *Survival analysis for patients with osteocartilaginous metaplastic carcinoma.* Comparison of time to recurrence **(A)** and survival **(B)** in patients with metaplastic carcinoma and stage-matched IFDC (NOS) patients. Patients with metaplastic carcinoma were compared to a cohort with invasive duct carcinoma matched for tumor stage. The two groups did not differ significantly in recurrence-free and overall survival (From Chhieng C, Cranor M, Lesser ME, et al. Metaplastic carcinoma of the breast with osteocartilaginous heterologous elements. *Am J Surg Pathol* 1998;22:188–194, with permission.)

Very few patients with low-grade adenosquamous carcinoma have developed metastases in axillary lymph nodes or systemic metastases. However, four of eight women treated initially by excisional biopsy had recurrences in the same breast requiring mastectomy 1 to 3.5 years later.

From the foregoing information, it appears that heterologous metaplasia probably does not have a negative impact on prognosis. Squamous metaplasia does not seem to influence prognosis, but extensive spindle cell metaplasia associated with squamous foci may have an adverse influence on outcome.

Prognostic data thus far have been based on patients treated by mastectomy, usually with axillary dissection. Mammary recurrence was reported in two of three patients after initial treatment by local excision for heterologous metaplastic carcinoma (3). A 53-year-old woman with a 2.0-cm heterologous metaplastic carcinoma was reportedly alive and well 3 years after lumpectomy and primary radiotherapy. Gobbi et al. (32) described 30 patients with spindle cell metaplastic carcinoma, including 17 who were treated by excisional surgery. Local recurrences in the breast were reported in eight patients, most of whom had limited excisions as their initial surgical therapy. The median time to breast recurrence was 15.5 months. The results of axillary dissection were available for 11 of the 30 patients, none of whom had nodal metastases.

The effect of primary irradiation and adjuvant chemotherapy on metaplastic carcinoma has not been determined. Chao et al. (30) reported on 14 women with spindle cell and heterologous metaplastic carcinomas treated in Taiwan. The median tumor size was 4.8 cm, and seven patients had axillary nodal metastases. Adjuvant chemotherapy was given to four of these women, and two had preoperative chemotherapy. Five of the seven patients died of metastatic breast carcinoma. Three node-negative patients had adjuvant chemotherapy and remained recurrence free. One of four node-negative patients not treated with adjuvant therapy developed metastatic carcinoma.

## REFERENCES

1. Heffelfinger SC, Miller MA, Gear R, et al. Staurosporine-induced versus spontaneous squamous metaplasia in pre- and postmenopausal breast tissue. *J Cell Physiol* 1998;176:245–254.
2. Fisher ER, Gregorio RM, Palekar AS, et al. Mucoepidermoid and squamous cell carcinomas of breast with reference to squamous metaplasia and giant cell tumors. *Am J Surg Pathol* 1984;7:15–27.
3. Kaufman MW, Marti JR, Gallager HS, et al. Carcinoma of the breast with pseudosarcomatous metaplasia. *Cancer* 1984;53:1908–1917.
4. Ridolfi R, Rosen PP, Port A, et al. Medullary carcinoma of the breast. A clinicopathologic study with 10 year follow-up. *Cancer* 1977; 40:1365–1385.
5. Wargotz ES, Norris HJ. Metaplastic carcinoma of the breast. IV. Squamous cell carcinoma of ductal origin. *Cancer* 1990;65:272–276.
6. Wargotz ES, Norris HJ. Metaplastic carcinomas of the breast. V. Metaplastic carcinoma with osteoclastic giant cells. *Hum Pathol* 1990;21: 1142–1150.
7. Hay ED. Extracellular matrix, cell skeletons, and embryonic development. *Am J Med Genet* 1989;34:14–29.
8. Greenburg G, Hay ED. Cytoskeleton and thyroglobulin expression change during transformation of thyroid epithelium to mesenchyme-like cells in vitro. *Dev Biol* 1988;102:605–622.
9. Boyer B, Tucker GC, Vallés AM, et al. Reversible transition towards a fibroblastic phenotype in a rat carcinoma cell line. *Int J Cancer (Suppl)* 1989;4:69–75.
10. Terada N, Yamamoto R, Uchida N, et al. Development of cartilage-like tissue from androgen-dependent Shionogi carcinoma 115 in androgen-depleted hosts. *Lab Invest* 1987;57:186–192.
11. Jamieson S, Rudland PS. Identification of metaplastic variants generated by transfection of a non-metastatic rat mammary epithelial cell line with DNA from a metastatic rat mammary cell line. *Am J Pathol* 1990;137:629–641.
12. Frixen UH, Behrens J, Sachs M, et al. E-cadherin–mediated cell-cell adhesion prevents invasiveness of human carcinoma cells. *J Cell Biol* 1991;113:173–185.
13. Navarro P, Gomez M, Pizzaro A, et al. A role for the E-cadherin cell-cell adhesion molecule during tumor progression of mouse epidermal carcinogenesis. *J Cell Biol* 1991;115:517–533.
14. Rottino A, Wilson K. Osseous, cartilaginous and mixed tumors of the human breast: a review of the literature. *Arch Surg* 1945;50:184–193.
15. Wargotz ES, Norris HJ. Metaplastic carcinomas of the breast. III. Carcinosarcoma. *Cancer* 1989;64:1490–1499.
16. Wada H, Enomoto T, Tsujimoto M, et al. Carcinosarcoma of the breast: molecular-biological study for analysis of histogenesis. *Hum Pathol* 1998;29:1324–1328.
17. Teixeira MR, Qvist H, Bohler PJ, et al. Cytogenetic analysis shows that carcinosarcomas of the breast are of monoclonal origin. *Genes Chromosomes Cancer* 1998;22:145–151.
18. Palmer JO, Ghiselli RW, McDivitt RW. Immunohistochemistry in the differential diagnosis of breast diseases. *Pathol Annu* 1990;25[Pt 2]:287–315.
19. Raju GC. The histological and immunohistochemical evidence of squamous metaplasia from the myoepithelial cells in the breast. *Histopathology* 1990;17:272–275.
20. Nakajima M, Kasai T, Hashimoto H, et al. Sarcomatoid carcinoma of the lung. A clinicopathologic study of 37 cases. *Cancer* 1999; 86:608–616.
21. George E, Manivel JC, Dehner LP, et al. Malignant mixed muellerian tumors: an immunohistochemical study of 7 cases with histogenetic considerations and clinical correlation. *Hum Pathol* 1991;22:215–223.
22. Bitterman P, Chun BK, Kurman RJ. The significance of epithelial differentiation in mixed mesodermal tumors of the uterus. A clinicopathologic and immunohistochemical study. *Am J Surg Pathol* 1990;14: 317–328.
23. Huvos AG, Lucas JC Jr, Foote FW Jr. Metaplastic breast carcinoma. *N Y State J Med* 1973;73:1078–1082.
24. Oberman HA. Metaplastic carcinoma of the breast. A clinicopathologic study of 29 patients. *Am J Surg Pathol* 1987;11:918–929.
25. Smith BH, Taylor HB. The occurrence of bone and cartilage in mammary tumors. *Am J Clin Pathol* 1969;51:610–618.
26. Wargotz ES, Deos PH, Norris HJ. Metaplastic carcinomas of the breast. II. Spindle cell carcinoma. *Hum Pathol* 1989;20:732–740.
27. Evans HA, Shaughnessy EA, Nikiforov YE. Infiltrating ductal carcinoma of the breast with osseous metaplasia: imaging findings with pathologic correlation. *AJR Am J Roentgenol* 1999;172:1420–1422.
28. Pickhardt PJ, McDermott M. Intense uptake of technetium-99m-MDP in primary breast adenocarcinoma with sarcomatoid metaplasia. *J Nucl Med* 1997;38:528–530.
29. Pitts WC, Rojas VA, Gaffey MJ, et al. Carcinomas with metaplasia and sarcomas of the breast. *Am J Clin Pathol* 1991;95:623–632.
30. Chao T-C, Wang C-S, Chen S-C, et al. Metaplastic carcinomas of the breast. *J Surg Oncol* 1999;71:220–225.
31. Stoerk O, Erdheim J. Über cholesteatomhältige Mammaaadenome. *Wien Klin Wochenschr* 1904;17:358–365.
32. Gobbi H, Simpson JF, Borowsky A, et al. Metaplastic breast tumors with a dominant fibromatosis-like phenotype have a high risk of local recurrence. *Cancer* 1999;85:2170–2182.
33. Gersell DJ, Katzenstein A-L. Spindle cell carcinoma of the breast. A clinicopathologic and ultrastructural study. *Hum Pathol* 1981;12: 550–561.
34. Lecene P. Les tumeurs mixtes du sein. *Rev Chir Paris* 1906;33: 434–439.
35. Bauer TW, Rostock RA, Eggleston JC, et al. Spindle cell carcinoma of the breast: four cases and review of the literature. *Hum Pathol* 1984;15:147–152.
36. Banerjee SS, Eyden BP, Wells S, et al. Pseudoangiosarcomatous carcinoma: a clinicopathological study of seven cases. *Histopathology* 1992;21:13–23.

37. Eusebi V, Lamovec J, Cattani MC, et al. Acantholytic variant of squamous cell carcinoma of the breast. *Am J Surg Pathol* 1986;10: 855–861.

38. Lamovec J, Kloboves-Prevodnik V. Teleangiectatic sarcomatoid carcinoma of the breast. *Tumori* 1992;78:283–286.

39. Wargotz ES, Norris HJ. Metaplastic carcinomas of the breast. I. Matrix-producing carcinoma. *Hum Pathol* 1989;20:628–636.

40. Murata T, Ihara S, Kato H, et al. Matrix-producing carcinoma of the breast: case report with radiographical and cytopathological features. *Pathol Int* 1998;48:824–828.

41. Sexton CW, White WL. Chondrosarcomatous cutaneous metastasis. A unique manifestation of sarcomatoid (metaplastic) breast carcinoma. *Am J Dermatopathol* 1996;18:538–542.

42. Chell SE, Nayar R, De Frias DV, et al. Metaplastic breast carcinoma metastatic to the lung mimicking a primary chondroid lesion: report of a case with cytohistologic correlation. *Ann Diagn Pathol* 1998;2: 173–180.

43. Cook SS, DeMay R. Adenocarcinoma of the breast with osseous metaplasia. Report of a case with needle aspiration cytology. *Acta Cytol* 1984;28:317–320.

44. Gal R, Gukovsky-Oren S, Lehman JM, et al. Cytodiagnosis of a spindle-cell tumor of the breast using antisera to epithelial membrane antigen. *Acta Cytol* 1987;31:317–321.

45. Stanley MW, Tani EM, Skoog L. Metaplastic carcinoma of the breast: fine needle aspiration of seven cases. *Diagn Cytopathol* 1989;5:22–28.

46. Kline TS, Kline IK. Metaplastic carcinoma of the breast. Diagnosis by aspiration biopsy cytology: report of two cases and literature review. *Diagn Cytopathol* 1990;6:63–67.

47. Castellà E, Gómez-Plaza MC, Urban A, et al. Fine-needle aspiration biopsy of metaplastic carcinoma of the breast: report of a case with abundant myxoid ground substance. *Diagn Cytopathol* 1996; 14:325–327.

48. Jebsen PW, Hagmar BM, Nesland JM. Metaplastic breast carcinoma. A diagnostic problem in fine needle aspiration biopsy. *Acta Cytol* 1991;35:396–402.

49. Pettinato G, Manivel JC, Petrella G, et al. Primary osteogenic sarcoma and osteogenic metaplastic carcinoma of the breast. Immunocytochemical identification in fine needle aspirates. *Acta Cytol* 1989; 35:620–626.

50. Nogueira M, André S, Mendonca E. Metaplastic carcinomas of the breast—fine needle aspiration (FNA) cytology findings. *Cytopathology* 1998;9:291–300.

51. Johnson TL, Kini SR. Metaplastic breast carcinoma: a cytohistologic and clinical study of 10 cases. *Diagn Cytopathol* 1996;14:226–232.

52. Gupta RK. Cytodiagnostic patterns of metaplastic breast carcinoma in aspiration samples: a study of 14 cases. *Diagn Cytopathol* 1999; 20:10–12.

53. Boccato P, Briani G, d'Atri C, et al. Spindle cell and cartilaginous metaplasia in a breast carcinoma with osteoclast-like stromal cells: a difficult fine needle aspiration diagnosis. *Acta Cytol* 1988;32:75–78.

54. Rosen PP, Ernsberger D. Low-grade adenosquamous carcinoma. A variant of metaplastic mammary carcinoma. *Am J Surg Pathol* 1987;11:351–358.

55. Suster S, Moran CA, Hurt MA. Syringomatous squamous tumors of the breast. *Cancer* 1991;67:2350–2355.

56. Van Hoeven KH, Drudis T, Cranor ML, et al. Low-grade adenosquamous carcinoma of the breast. A clinocopathologic study of 32 cases with ultrastructural analysis. *Am J Surg Pathol* 1993;17:248–258.

57. Foschini MP, Pizzicannella G, Peterse JL, et al. Adenomyoepithelioma of the breast associated with low-grade adenosquamous and sarcomatoid carcinomas. *Virchows Arch* 1995;427:243–250.

58. Ferrara G, Nappi O, Wick MR. Fine-needle aspiration cytology and immunohistology of low-grade adenosquamous carcinoma of the breast. *Diagn Cytopathol* 1999;20:13–18.

59. Raymond WA, Leong AS-Y. Co-expression of cytokeratin and vimentin intermediate filament proteins in benign and neoplastic breast epithelium. *J Pathol* 1989;157:299–306.

60. Ellis IO, Bell J, Ronan JE, et al. Immunocytochemical investigation of intermediate filament proteins and epithelial membrane antigen in spindle cell tumours of the breast. *J Pathol* 1988;154:157–165.

61. Santensanio G, Pascal RR, Bisceglia M, et al. Metaplastic breast carcinoma with epithelial phenotype of pseudosarcomatous components. *Arch Pathol Lab Med* 1988;112:82–85.

62. Meis JM, Ordone NG, Gallager HS. Sarcomatoid carcinoma of the breast: an immunohistochemical study of six cases. *Virchows Arch [A]* 1987;410:415–421.

63. Chhieng C, Cranor M, Lesser ME, et al. Metaplastic carcinoma of the breast with osteocartilaginous heterologous elements. *Am J Surg Pathol* 1998;22:188–194.

64. Kaufmann M, Heider KH, Sinn HP, et al. CD44 isoforms in prognosis of breast cancer. *Lancet* 1995;346:502.

65. Ylagan LR, Scholes J, Demopoulos R. CD44: a marker of squamous differentiation in adenosquamous neoplasms. *Arch Pathol Lab Med* 2000;124:212–215.

66. Sommers CL, Walker-Jones D, Heckford SE, et al. Vimentin rather than keratin expression in some hormone-independent breast cancer cell lines and in oncogene-transformed mammary epithelial cells. *Cancer Res* 1989;49:4258–4263.

67. Sommers CL, Heckford SE, Skerker JM, et al. Loss of epithelial markers and acquisition of vimentin expression in adriamycin- and vinblastine-resistant human breast cancer cell lines. *Cancer Res* 1992; 52:5190–5197.

68. Bae SW, Arand G, Azzam H, et al. Molecular and cellular analysis of basement membrane invasion by human breast cancer cells in Matrigel-based in vitro assays. *Breast Cancer Res Treat* 1993;24: 241–255.

69. Litzky LA, Brooks JJ. Cytokeratin immunoreactivity in malignant fibrous histiocytoma and spindle cell tumors: comparison between frozen and paraffin-embedded tissues. *Mod Pathol* 1992;5:30–34.

70. Weiss SW, Brathaeur GL, Morris PA. Postirradiation malignant fibrous histiocytoma expressing cytokeratin: implications for the immunodiagnosis of sarcomas. *Am J Surg Pathol* 1988;12:544–558.

71. Von Koskull H, Virtanen I. Induction of cytokeratin expression in human mesenchymal cells. *J Cell Physiol* 1987;133:321–329.

72. Knapp AC, Franke WW. Spontaneous losses of control of cytokeratin gene expression in transformed, non-epithelial human cells occurring at different levels of regulation. *Cell* 1989;59:67–79.

73. Battifora H. Spindle cell carcinoma. Ultrastructural evidence of squamous origin and collagen production by the tumor cells. *Cancer* 1976;37:2275–2282.

74. Gonzalez-Licea A, Yardley JH, Hartmann WH. Malignant tumor of the breast with bone formation. Studies by light and electron microscopy. *Cancer* 1967;20:1234–1247.

75. Kahn LB, Vys CJ, Dale J, et al. Carcinoma of the breast with metaplasia to chondrosarcoma: a light and electron microscopic study. *Histopathology* 1978;2:93–106.

76. Llombart-Bosch A, Peydro A. Malignant mixed osteogenic tumours of the breast. A ultrastructural study of two cases. *Virchows Arch [A]* 1975;366:1–4.

77. An T, Grathwohl M, Frable WJ. Breast carcinoma with osseous metaplasia: an electron microscopic study. *Am J Clin Pathol* 1983; 80:127–132.

# CHAPTER 19

# Squamous Carcinoma

Squamous carcinoma of the breast is a form of metaplastic carcinoma. The term should be restricted to lesions composed of keratinizing squamous carcinoma or one of its variant forms to distinguish these tumors from the usual examples of mammary carcinoma with squamous metaplasia. In practice, carcinomas in which more than 90% of the neoplasm is squamous have been classified under this heading. With thorough sampling, a ductal adenocarcinoma component can be detected in many cases, leaving a minority of pure squamous tumors that probably originate from squamous metaplasia (1). The earliest examples of squamous carcinoma were reported nearly a century ago (2,3).

Benign metaplastic squamous epithelium, the precursor to pure squamous carcinoma, occurs in the epithelium of cysts, in fibroadenomas, and in cystosarcomas. Cysts lined by metaplastic squamous epithelium can be found in fibroepithelial neoplasms (4). Squamous cysts also occur in gynecomastia, typically as isolated foci involving part of the epithelium of ducts that also exhibit papillary epithelial hyperplasia (5). Focal squamous metaplasia can occur in duct hyperplasia (Fig. 19.1), lobular hyperplasia (Fig. 19.2), and papillomas. In rare cases, the epithelium of multiple ducts in one portion of the breast can be altered by squamous metaplasia (6,7). Reddick et al. (6) studied squamous metaplasia in a papilloma by immunohistochemistry and electron microscopy, and they concluded that the metaplastic change originated in myoepithelial cells.

Diffuse squamous metaplasia of duct and lobular epithelium has been described in association with fat necrosis (8). Approximately 3 years after biopsy, the patient remained well (9). Squamous metaplasia can be found in other inflammatory or necrotizing lesions, such as infarcted adenomas (10), in inflamed cysts or other forms of mastitis, in infarcted papillomas (11), and in healing biopsy sites (Fig. 19.3). Cutaneous squamous epithelium displaced into the breast by needle core biopsy may persist in the healed tissues, resulting in the formation of an epidermal inclusion cyst (12). Metaplastic squamous epithelium may be embedded in the wall of an inflamed cyst, resulting in a pattern that is difficult to distinguish from invasive carcinoma. The diagnosis usu-ally hinges on careful evaluation of the cytologic appearance of the squamous epithelium. Squamous metaplasia of lactiferous ducts is important in the pathogenesis of subareolar abscesses (13).

Shousha described a $2 \times 2 \times 1$-cm multiloculated cyst lined largely by keratinizing stratified squamous epithelium obtained from the breast of a 70-year-old woman (14). Mucin-containing glandular cells also were present in the squamous epithelium individually and in small groups (Fig. 19.4).

Insulin enhances the development of squamous metaplasia in organ cultures of human breast tissue (15,16). Chemical carcinogens cause keratinizing metaplasia *in vitro* in murine mammary (17) and prostate glands (18). The primary mediator of benign squamous metaplasia in human breast epithelium may be cyclic adenine nucleotide (19). In one study, tissues obtained from patients in the early part of the menstrual cycle were less susceptible to induction of squamous metaplasia than specimens taken later in the cycle, an observation suggesting that progesterone and/or estrogen may influence the process (19).

## CLINICAL PRESENTATION

There are no clinical features that are specific for squamous carcinoma of the breast. The reported age at diagnosis, 31 to 83 years, is within the range of breast carcinoma generally (20,21). In one review, the average age of 20 patients was 57 years, and half were 60 years or older (20).

Primary squamous carcinomas have been found more often in the left breast (21). Fixation to the chest wall and invasion of the skin may complicate large tumors. Extension to the skin may make it difficult to distinguish between cutaneous origin and secondary skin involvement by a primary mammary lesion (22). When the bulk of the tumor is in the breast and the clinical history indicates a breast mass preceded skin ulceration, the lesion may be considered a mammary carcinoma. The tumors have indistinct or partially distinct margins on mammography, but no specific mammographic findings have been described (23,24). Calcifications

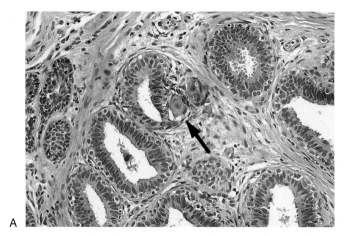
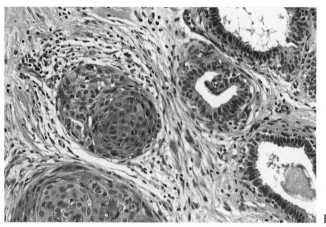

**FIG. 19.1.** *Squamous metaplasia in ducts.* **A:** Small focus of squamous differentiation in one of several ducts (*arrow*). **B:** Two ducts are fully involved by benign squamous epithelium.

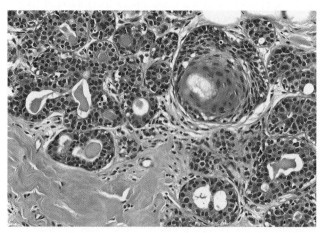

**FIG. 19.2.** *Squamous metaplasia in lobule.* Squamous differentiation is apparent in a lobular gland.

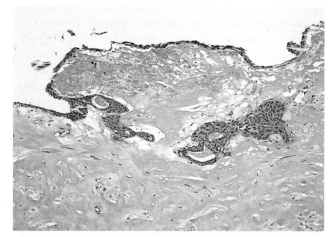

**FIG. 19.3.** *Squamous metaplasia in biopsy cavity.* Thin squamous epithelium lines the surface of this partially healed biopsy cavity, and squamous metaplasia arises from a duct in the underlying tissue.

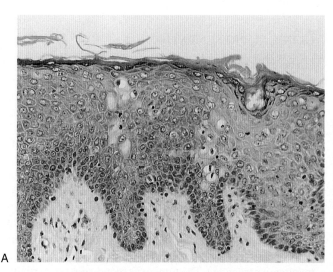
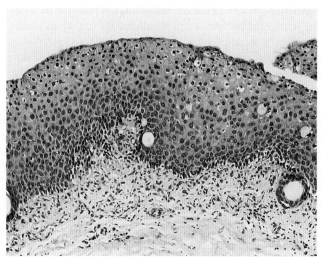

**FIG. 19.4.** *Squamous metaplasia in a cyst.* **A:** Superficial keratinizing cells in this benign metaplastic epithelium has keratohyalin granules. **B:** Squamous metaplasia with scattered clear cells and one residual gland on the *right.* *(continued)*

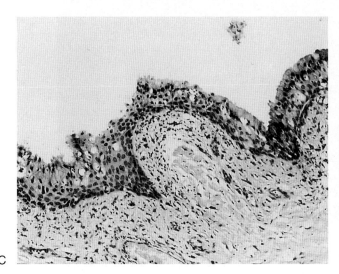

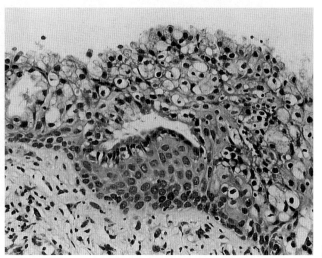

**FIG. 19.4.** *Continued.* **C:** Benign metaplastic squamous epithelium growing beneath residual glandular ductal epithelium. **D:** Glandular and squamous epithelium are seen merging. (Courtesy of Dr. S. Shousha.)

in necrotic squamous tissue sometimes can be seen radiographically. The cystic nature of the tumor usually is apparent on ultrasonography (1). Most of these tumors have been reported to be estrogen receptor negative (1,20,21). One lesion that was positive for estrogen and progesterone receptors had a diploid deoxyribonucleic acid content and a high S-phase fraction (25).

## GROSS PATHOLOGY

Squamous carcinomas tend to be somewhat larger than other types of breast carcinoma. Reported sizes vary from 1 to 10 cm, with nearly half of the tumors 5 cm or more in diameter. It is not unusual for the lesions to undergo cystic degeneration centrally (Fig. 19.5). This is especially common in tumors larger than 2 cm, in which the cavity is filled with necrotic squamous debris (25,26). The tumor tends to be softer and more granular when the lesion is composed largely of keratinizing epithelium. Extensive spindle cell metaplasia produces a firmer lesion.

## MICROSCOPIC PATHOLOGY

Before establishing a diagnosis of primary squamous carcinoma of the breast, it is necessary to exclude a metastasis from an extramammary primary (20,26,27). The most common sources of metastatic squamous carcinoma in the breast are the lung, uterine cervix, and urinary bladder. Although the patient may be known to have an extramammary primary clinically, this information sometimes is not given to the pathologist, especially if the other lesion was treated in the past and there is no active tumor apparent at the primary site.

Surgical biopsy is recommended to establish the diagnosis, but it is possible to recognize squamous carcinoma in an aspiration cytology specimen from the breast (1,25,26,28). The specimen obtained by fine needle aspiration usually does not present a diagnostic problem when atypical squamous cells are present (29). Anucleated and granular squamous cells are suggestive of an epidermal inclusion cyst, but they may be present in the aspirate from a well-differentiated mammary squamous carcinoma. The distinction between a

**FIG. 19.5.** *Squamous carcinoma.* **A:** Cystic tumor. The outer surface of the tissue has been colored with ink to demarcate the resection margin. *(continued)*

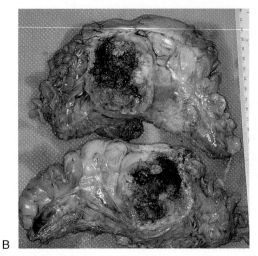

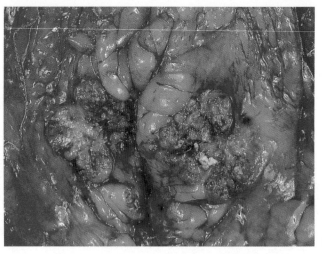

**FIG. 19.5.** *Continued.* **B:** Nodular foci of squamous carcinoma protrude into the lumen of this partly cystic tumor. (Courtesy of Dr. Roger Adlesberg.) **C:** Solid tumor with white foci of degenerated keratin.

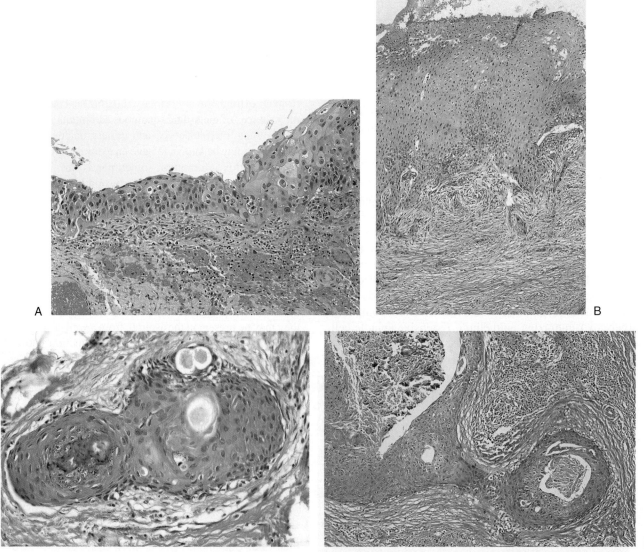

**FIG. 19.6.** *Squamous carcinoma* in situ. **A,B:** Carcinoma lining two cystic lesions. Superficial invasion is present at the deep surface of the epithelium in **B**. **C:** Intraductal carcinoma with keratohyalin granules. A small remnant of the duct lumen can be seen near the upper border. **D:** Cystic degeneration of intraductal carcinoma with calcified keratotic debris.

primary tumor and metastatic squamous carcinoma cannot be made in an aspiration cytology specimen, and this issue is unlikely to be resolved with a needle core biopsy unless intraductal carcinoma is included in the sample.

Microscopically, squamous carcinomas of the breast resemble similar carcinomas that arise in other sites. The *in situ* lesions tend to be differentiated sufficiently to keratinize, and keratohyalin granules may be seen in the neoplastic epithelium (Fig. 19.6). Ultrastructural and immunohistochemical studies have confirmed the squamous character of the tissue (30), but intracellular canaliculi seen ultrastructurally in some cells is evidence that glandular features may persist in some of these tumors.

Primary invasive squamous carcinoma of the breast can have varying appearances. A cytokeratin stain is useful for detecting superficial invasion in cystic lesions (Fig. 19.7). Cytoplasmic clearing occurs in some tumors (Fig. 19.8). Focal conversion of the squamous epithelial pattern to spindle cell pseudosarcomatous and acantholytic growth may be found in squamous carcinomas of the breast (Figs. 19.9 and 19.10) (31). Tumors classified as primary squamous carci-

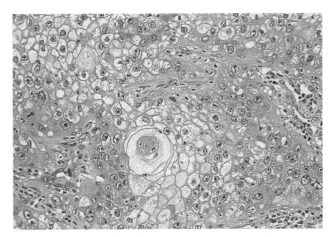

**FIG. 19.8.** *Squamous carcinoma, clear cell.*

noma of the breast are a variant of metaplastic carcinoma (see Chapter 18). They are distinguished from the diverse group of metaplastic carcinomas by origin from *in situ* squamous carcinoma in a cyst, ducts, or both. Spindle cell components may

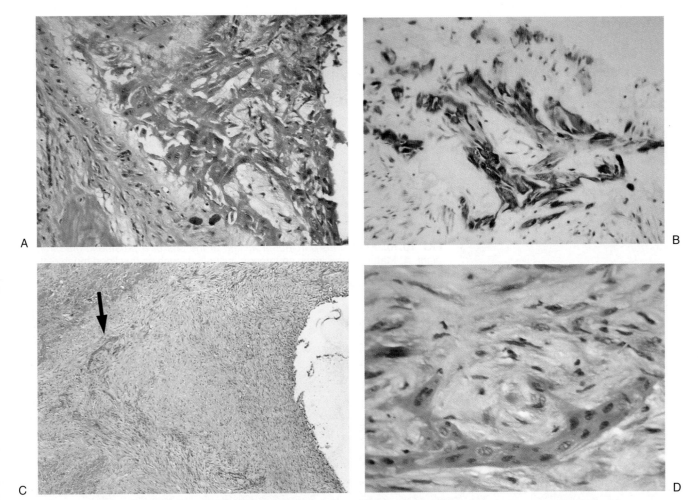

**FIG. 19.7.** *Squamous carcinoma, cystic.* **A:** Squamous carcinoma arising from the surface epithelium of a chronically inflamed cyst. **B:** The carcinoma is immunoreactive for cytokeratin (avidin-biotin). **C:** Invasive squamous carcinoma is present deep in the cyst wall (*arrow*). **D:** Magnified view of the invasive carcinoma at site marked by the *arrow* in **C.**

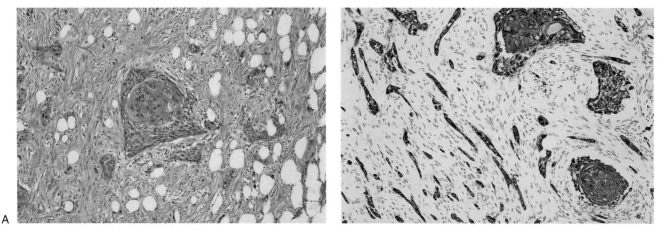

A                                                                                                    B

**FIG. 19.9.** *Squamous carcinoma, spindle cell.* **A:** Invasive keratinizing carcinoma surrounded by small nests of carcinoma cells in a spindle cell proliferation. **B:** Cytokeratin reactivity is demonstrated in spindle cells with the antibody K903 (34BE12) (avidin-biotin).

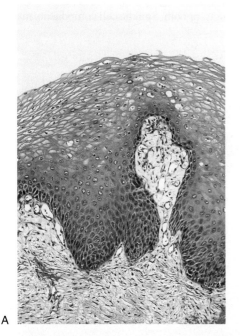

A

**FIG. 19.10.** *Squamous carcinoma arising at the site of a prosthetic breast implant.* **A:** Mature metaplastic squamous epithelium such as this lined much of the implant site. **B:** *In situ* squamous carcinoma overlying invasive carcinoma in fat necrosis. **C:** Acantholytic change in the invasive carcinoma.

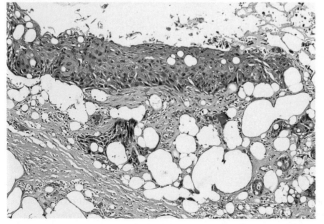

B

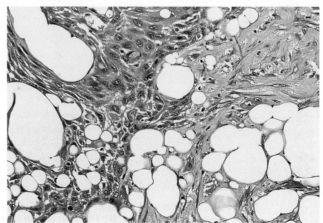

C

be obscured by the reactive stroma, and they are highlighted with cytokeratin stains such as 34BE12 (K903).

## TREATMENT AND PROGNOSIS

Information about the prognosis and follow-up of patients with squamous carcinoma tends to be variable or incomplete in reported cases. With few exceptions, the patients have been treated by mastectomy and axillary dissection, followed in some cases by postoperative radiotherapy or chemotherapy. One patient with a 2.5-cm cystic very well-differentiated squamous carcinoma was reportedly well 49 months after segmental resection of her lesion (26). Another patient developed local recurrence in the breast 13 months after local excision and radiotherapy (1).

Overall, the prognosis of patients with mammary squamous carcinoma does not appear to differ appreciably from that of patients with mammary adenocarcinoma of equal stage, especially when one considers the relatively large size of some of these tumors (31). The relationship of the growth pattern and degree of differentiation in squamous carcinomas to prognosis is uncertain. Some fatal lesions have had a prominent spindle cell component or necrosis and acantholytic features (31). However, metastases occur in the absence of these patterns.

In most patients, no axillary nodal metastases were found when an axillary dissection was performed. Among 19 women with negative axillary lymph nodes described in various published reports, eight were alive and free of disease 1 to 12 years later and two died of other causes 7 and 8 years after treatment. Six women who had negative axillary lymph nodes died of metastatic carcinoma 4 to 30 months after diagnosis. Two patients with axillary lymph node metastases died 6 and 17 months after treatment, whereas two others were alive and well after 16 months and 6 years of follow-up. One patient who presented with a stage III tumor that had clinical features of inflammatory carcinoma died of metastatic disease 5 months later. Local recurrence in the chest wall also has been reported.

## REFERENCES

1. Kokufu I, Yamamoto M, Fukuda K, et al. Squamous cell carcinoma of the breast: three case reports. *Breast Cancer* 1999;6:63–68.
2. Harrington S, Miller JM. Intramammary squamous-cell carcinoma. *Mayo Clin Proc* 1939;14:484–487.
3. Dalla Palma P, Prenti A. Squamous breast cancer; report of two cases and review of the literature. *Appl Pathol* 1983;1:14–24.
4. Salm R. Epidermoid metaplasia in mammary fibro-adenoma with formation of keratin cysts. *J Pathol Bacteriol* 1957;74:221–223.
5. Gottfried MD. Extensive squamous metaplasia in gynecomastia. *Arch Pathol Lab Med* 1986;110:971–973.
6. Reddick RS, Jennette C, Askin FB. Squamous metaplasia of the breast. An ultrastructural and immunologic evaluation. *Am J Clin Pathol* 1985;84:530–533.
7. Soderstrom K-O, Toikkanen S. Extensive squamous metaplasia simulating squamous cell carcinoma in benign breast papillomatosis. *Hum Pathol* 1983;14:1081–1082.
8. Hurt MA, Diaz-Arias AA, Rosenholtz MJ, et al. Posttraumatic lobular squamous metaplasia of breast. An unusual pseudocarcinomatous metaplasia resembling squamous (necrotizing) sialometaplasia of the salivary gland. *Mod Pathol* 1988;1:385–390.
9. Hurt MA, Diaz-Arias A. Personal communication.
10. Lucey JJ. Spontaneous infarction of the breast. *J Clin Pathol* 1975;28:937–943.
11. Flint A, Oberman HA. Infarction and squamous metaplasia of intraductal papilloma: a benign breast lesion that may simulate carcinoma. *Hum Pathol* 1984;15:764–767.
12. Davies JD, Nonni A, D'Costa HF. Mammary epidermoid inclusion cysts after wide-core needle biopsies. *Histopathology* 1997;31:549–551.
13. Habif DV, Perzin KH, Lipton R, et al. Subareolar abscess associated with squamous metaplasia of lactiferous ducts. *Am J Surg* 1970;119:523–526.
14. Shousha S. An unusual breast cyst. *Histopathology* 1989;14:423–425.
15. Van Bogaert LJ. Squamous metaplasia in human mammary epithelium in long-term organ culture. *Experientia (Basel)* 1977;33:1450–1451.
16. Elias JJ, Armstrong RC. Hyperplastic and metaplastic response of human mammary fibroadenoma and dysplasias in organ culture. *J Natl Cancer Inst* 1973;51:1341–1343.
17. Tonelli QT, Custer RP, Sorof S. Transformation of cultured mouse mammary glands by aromatic amines and amides and their derivatives. *Cancer Res* 1979;39:1784–1792.
18. Lasnitziki I. Precancerous changes induced by 20-methylcholanthrene in mouse prostates grown *in vitro. Br J Cancer* 1951;5:345–352.
19. Schaefer FV, Custer RP, Sorof S. Squamous metaplasia in human breast culture: induction by cyclic adenine nucleotide and prostaglandins and influence of menstrual cycle. *Cancer Res* 1983;43:279–286.
20. Rostock RA, Bauer TW, Eggleston JC. Primary squamous carcinoma of the breast: a review. *Breast* 1984;10:27–31.
21. Shousha S, James AH, Ferandez MD, et al. Squamous cell carcinoma of the breast. *Arch Pathol Lab Med* 1984;108:893–896.
22. Carnog JL, Mobini J, Steiger E, et al. Squamous carcinoma of the breast. *Am J Clin Pathol* 1971;55:410–417.
23. Tashjian J, Kuni CC, Bohn LE. Primary squamous cell carcinoma of the breast: mammographic findings. *J Can Assoc Radiol* 1989;40:228–229.
24. Samuels TH, Miller NA, Manchul LA, et al. Squamous cell carcinoma of the breast. *Can Assoc Radiol J* 1996;47:177–182.
25. Chen KTK. Fine needle aspiration cytology of squamous carcinoma of the breast. *Acta Cytol* 1990;34:664–668.
26. Leiman G. Squamous carcinoma of the breast: diagnosis by aspiration cytology. *Acta Cytol* 1982;26:201–209
27. Farrand R, LaVigne R, Lokich J, et al. Epidermoid carcinoma of the breast. *J Surg Oncol* 1979;12:207–211.
28. Lazarevic B, Katatikarn V, Marks RA. Primary squamous-cell carcinoma of the breast. Diagnosis by fine needle aspiration cytology. *Acta Cytol* 1984;28:321–324.
29. Motoyama T, Watanabe H. Extremely well differentiated squamous cell carcinoma of the breast. Report of a case with a comparative study of an epidermal cyst. *Acta Cytol* 1996;40:729–733.
30. Toikkanen S. Primary squamous cell carcinoma of the breast. *Cancer* 1981;48:1629–1632.
31. Eusebi V, Lamovec J, Cattani MG, et al. Acantholytic variant of squamous cell carcinoma of the breast. *Am J Surg Pathol* 1986;10:855–861.
31. Eggers JW, Chesney TMC. Squamous cell carcinoma of the breast: a clinicopathologic analysis of eight cases and review of the literature. *Hum Pathol* 1984;15:526–531.

# CHAPTER 20

# Mucinous Carcinoma

As described in the World Health Organization International Histological Classification of Tumours, mucinous carcinoma contains "large amounts of extracellular epithelial mucus, sufficient to be visible grossly, and recognizable microscopically surrounding and within tumour cells" (1). Other terms used to identify this tumor include gelatinous, colloid, mucous, and mucoid carcinoma.

The specific histologic appearance of mucinous carcinoma has been appreciated for more than 100 years (2–4). Some of the earliest descriptions commented on the slow growth rate and favorable prognosis of these tumors. The importance of distinguishing between pure mucinous tumors and those with a nonmucinous component was emphasized by Geschickter (5) in 1938. He noted that prognosis varied "with the amount of mucoid substance found" in the tumor. When the diagnosis is restricted to tumors consisting of pure or nearly pure mucinous carcinoma, not more than 2% of mammary carcinomas fall into this category (6–9). Focal mucinous differentiation may be found in up to 2% of other carcinomas. If this latter group also is classified as mucinous carcinoma, the reported frequency of tumor may be as high as 3.6% (7,10). However, as indicated later, carcinomas with mixed histologic patterns should not be included under the heading of mucinous carcinoma. They are best regarded as a subset of infiltrating duct carcinomas. The term infiltrating duct carcinoma with mucinous component or mucinous differentiation is preferable for the latter group of tumors. The term mixed mucinous carcinoma has also been used for these lesions.

Various criteria have been used to distinguish mucinous carcinoma from infiltrating duct carcinoma with mucinous differentiation. Pure mucinous carcinomas have been described as tumors that have no infiltrating duct carcinoma (11), tumors that were "virtually pure" (12), tumors with at least 50% growing in a mucinous pattern (13), and tumors in which extracellular mucin constituted at least 33% of the lesion (6). One author indicated that "these proportions were arbitrarily selected" (6). Criteria followed in this volume are set forth in the section on Microscopic Pathology.

## CLINICAL PRESENTATION

Mucinous carcinoma has been described to occur throughout most of the age range of breast carcinoma. Most studies have reported the mean age of women with mucinous carcinoma to be older than that of patients with nonmucinous carcinoma (7,8,14,15). Scopsi et al. (7) reported that a significantly greater proportion of women with mucinous carcinoma were older than 50 years than was the case among patients with carcinoma having focal mucinous differentiation or nonmucinous carcinoma. No significant difference in age distribution and the median age of women with pure and mixed mucinous carcinoma was found by Fentiman et al. (16). Analysis of patients at the extremes of the age distribution for breast carcinoma revealed a striking difference: mucinous carcinoma constituted about 7% of carcinomas in women 75 years or older and only 1% among those younger than 35 years (17).

The initial symptom is a breast mass in the majority of patients with pure mucinous carcinoma. Nipple discharge and pain are uncommon. Fixation to the skin and chest wall occurs with large lesions. Palpation reveals a soft to moderately firm lesion. Most mucinous carcinomas occur in the upper outer quadrant, and overall the anatomic distribution is not significantly different from that of other types of breast carcinoma. On reviewing patient records, one rarely finds mention of the "swish sign."

Only a minority of pure mucinous carcinomas have calcifications (18), and some of these are associated with a mucocele-like lesion (19). The tumor usually appears as a lobulated mass lesion on mammography (18). There are some radiologic correlates of the structure of mucinous carcinomas. Tumors with a high proportion of mucin production tend to be circumscribed or lobulated (Fig. 20.1) (20,21). These lesions are likely to have a slower growth rate, determined by comparing serial mammograms and a low frequency of axillary nodal metastases. Ductal carcinomas with mucinous differentiation typically have irregular margins mammographically due to fibrosis and an infiltrative growth pattern (22). A spiculated contour is associated with a lesser

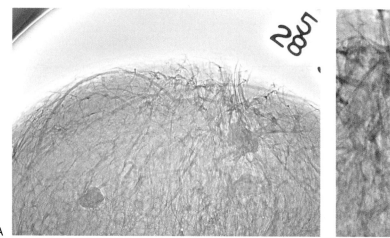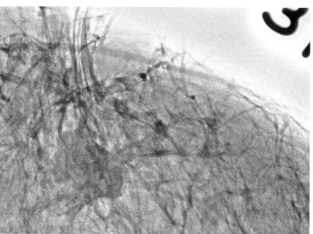

A                                                                                                                                B

**FIG. 20.1.** *Mucinous carcinoma, xerographic appearance.* **A:** Irregular nodular tumor in the upper central region is a mucinous carcinoma. Smaller, round tumor on the *left* is a fibroadenoma. **B:** Magnified view of the carcinoma. The technique used to produce these images is no longer used in clinical practice.

mucinous component and a higher frequency of lymph node metastases. Mammographically detected calcifications occur in about 40% of the tumors, involving the invasive portion of approximately 20% of mucinous carcinomas (22,23). Calcifications may be limited to associated intraductal carcinoma. The magnetic resonance imaging characteristics of mucinous carcinomas and fibroadenomas are not distinctively different (24,25).

The average duration of symptoms prior to biopsy and diagnosis tends to be 3 months or less, but some elderly patients who have large lesions may delay seeking treatment for considerably longer (13). One group of investigators observed that the majority of patients with tumors 4 cm or larger were older than 70 years (11). About 60% of pure mucinous carcinomas are estrogen receptor-positive when studied biochemically (26,27). Immunohistochemical studies have shown receptor activity in nearly 90% of cases (28). Similar patterns of estrogen receptor immunoreactivity were observed in nonargyrophilic and argyrophilic mucinous carcinomas and in mixed mucinous carcinomas (28).

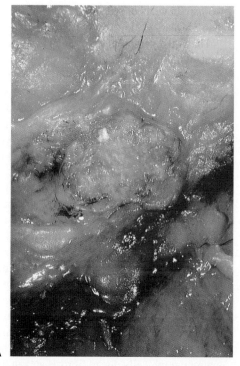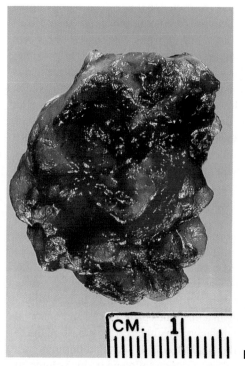

A                                                                                                                                B

**FIG. 20.2.** *Mucinous carcinoma, gross appearance.* **A:** Homogeneous tumor with a circumscribed lobulated contour. **B:** Tumor is composed of pale brown, gelatinous, partly cystic tissue.

## GROSS PATHOLOGY

Mucinous carcinomas have been described, ranging from less than 1 cm to more than 20 cm in diameter. Studies published prior to 1975 that stressed the relatively large size of mucinous carcinomas tend to support this perception, but with less extreme differences in size reported (13,29,30). A nationwide study of Danish breast cancer patients found that only 16% of mucinous carcinomas were larger than 5 cm (6). In a series from Finland, a greater proportion of mixed (48%) than of pure (22%) mucinous carcinomas were larger than 5 cm (8). A study from Japan stated that 53.6% of mucinous tumors were 2.0 cm or less (T1) and 37.8% were 2.1 to 5.0 cm (T2) (10). Fentiman et al. (16) reported that pure mucinous tumors were significantly smaller (mean 2.17 cm) than mixed mucinous tumors (mean, 3.25 cm). Diab et al. (15) did not find a significant difference in size between mucinous and nonmucinous carcinomas.

On palpation of the excised tumor, the consistency of mucinous carcinoma varies somewhat, depending on the amount of fibrous stroma in the lesion. When stroma is sparse, the tumor feels soft and gelatinous. The cut surface typically is moist and glistening, even in relatively fibrotic tumors (Fig. 20.2). Most mucinous carcinomas have a circumscribed gross margin that may be accentuated by a peripheral red-to-purple zone of congested parenchyma. Cystic degeneration has been reported in relatively large tumors.

## MICROSCOPIC PATHOLOGY

Mucinous carcinoma is characterized by the accumulation of abundant extracellular mucin around invasive tumor cells (Fig. 20.3). The relative proportions of secretion and neoplastic epithelium vary from one case to the next, but the distribution in any one tumor is fairly constant (Fig. 20.4). It may require multiple sections to detect carcinoma cells in a tumor composed almost entirely of extracellular mucin (Fig. 20.5). In one recent study, the proportion of extracellular

mucin in tumors classified as pure mucinous carcinomas varied from slightly less than 40% to 99.8%, with a mean of 83.5% ± 14.3% (10). Infiltrating duct carcinomas with a mucinous component had a lower mean proportion of extracellular mucin (68.3% ± 16.6%), with the distribution ranging from 32% to 97%. In practice, a carcinoma should not be classified as pure mucinous carcinoma if more than 10% of the invasive component is nonmucinous or if the nonmucinous invasive component is poorly differentiated cytologically (Figs. 20.6 and 20.7).

Pure mucinous carcinoma is a variant of invasive duct carcinoma. Intraductal carcinoma is found associated with 60% to 75% of the lesions, generally at the periphery (16). The intraductal component has any of the conventional patterns of intraductal carcinoma (cribriform, papillary, micropapillary, comedo). Occasionally, mucinous growth is evident in the intraductal component, and one can find transitions to the invasive carcinoma (Fig. 20.8). A minority of mucinous carcinomas does not have detectable intraductal carcinoma. These tend to be larger tumors, but rarely one encounters a pure mucinous carcinoma smaller than 2 cm with no apparent intraductal carcinoma.

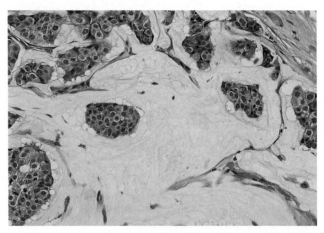

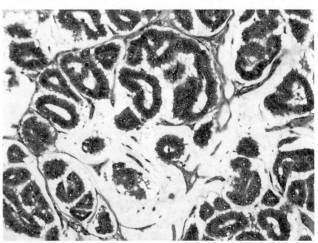

**FIG. 20.4.** *Mucinous carcinoma.* **A:** Moderately cellular carcinoma. Note the presence of capillaries in the mucin. **B:** Highly cellular carcinoma with a glandular pattern.

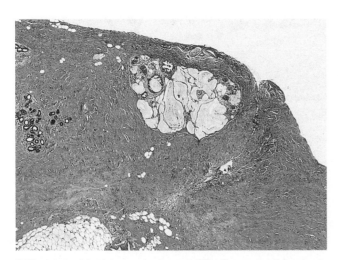

**FIG. 20.3.** *Mucinous carcinoma.* Whole-mount histologic section containing a 2-mm carcinoma.

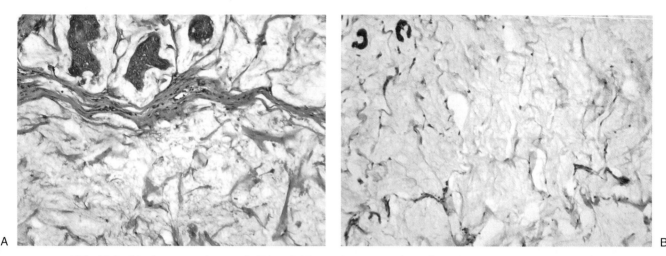

**FIG. 20.5.** *Mucinous carcinoma.* **A:** Part of this carcinoma consists of mucin devoid of neoplastic epithelium. Three clusters of carcinoma cells are present at the upper border. **B:** Instance of virtually acellular mucinous carcinoma with two clusters of tumor cells in the upper left corner.

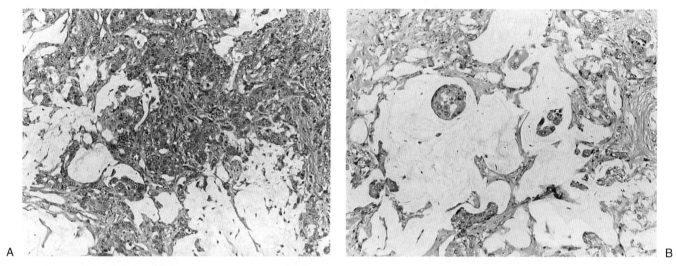

**FIG. 20.6.** *Infiltrating duct carcinoma with mucinous features.* **A:** Poorly differentiated infiltrating carcinoma above merging with mucinous carcinoma below. **B:** More conventional focus of mucinous carcinoma in the same tumor.

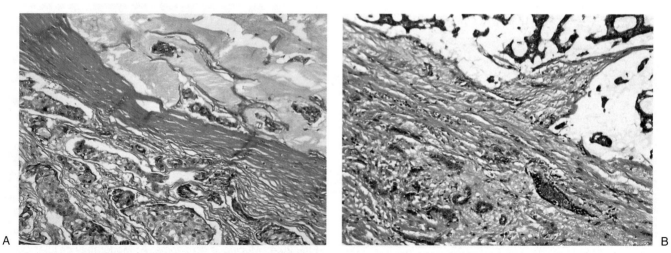

**FIG. 20.7.** *Infiltrating duct carcinoma with mucinous features.* **A,B:** Two infiltrating duct carcinomas that have limited, discrete areas of mucinous growth.

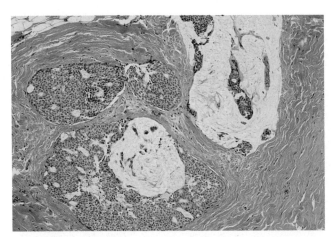

**FIG. 20.8.** *Mucinous carcinoma.* Duct containing intraductal carcinoma is distended with mucin in the lower center. Invasive mucinous carcinoma is present in the upper right area.

One of the most infrequent variants of this pattern is a cystic type of papillary mucinous carcinoma composed of multiple cysts distended by mucinous secretion and lined by micropapillary, papillary, and cribriform intraductal carcinoma (Fig. 20.9). Invasive areas in these tumors usually are mucinous, but sarcomatoid metaplasia also has been reported (31). Eleven patients with cystic papillary mucinous carcinoma described by Komaki et al. (10) had a relatively lower average age at diagnosis (41 years) than is typical for mucinous carcinoma. None of the patients had axillary nodal metastases when treated by mastectomy, and they remained disease free for an average of nearly 10 years. Mucinous carcinoma also may arise from solid papillary carcinoma (Fig. 20.10).

Capella et al. (32) presented criteria for the subclassification of mucinous carcinoma on the basis of the epithelial growth pattern and some associated features. They described two principal types (A and B) and an intermediate category (AB). By definition, at least 33% of each tumor consisted of extracellular mucin, but overall mucin was more abundant in type A than in type B lesions. Type A tumors had epithelium distributed in "trabeculae and ribbons or festoons." "Clumps" of cells, uncommon in type A tumors, were the characteristic growth pattern of type B lesions. Cribriform areas were seen in both types. Intracytoplasmic mucin was more abundant in type B lesions, and the cells in these tumors tended to have more granular cytoplasm than type A carcinomas. Cells with "foamy" cytoplasm were detected in a minority of type A tumors and in none of the type B group. Ten of 14 type B tumors contained argyrophilic granules detected with Grimelius and Bodian stains, whereas 15 type A tumors had no detectable argyrophilic granules (Fig. 20.11). A statistically significant difference was found in the age distribution of patients with type A and B lesions, with the former group tending to be younger at diagnosis. Type AB tumors, constituting 20% of the cases studied, were described as having "indeterminate" features or features "indicative of transitional forms between the two major groups," but little information was given about these cases. The authors concluded that type A lesions corresponded to carcinomas ordinarily regarded as classic pure mucinous carcinoma. It was recommended that type B tumors be regarded as a variant of mucinous carcinoma with endocrine differentiation.

Scopsi et al. (7) confirmed the common occurrence of argyrophilic granules in type B carcinomas. The presence or absence of argyrophilia was not significantly related to age, menstrual status, tumor size, or axillary nodal status. Classification as type A or B did not prove to be prognostically significant.

Tumor cells are arranged in a variety of patterns in mucinous carcinomas. Usually the epithelial pattern duplicates the structure of the associated intraductal carcinoma. These configurations include tumor cells in strands, alveolar nests, and papillary clusters, as well as larger sheets of cells that may have cribriform areas or focal comedonecrosis. Tubule and gland formation are uncommon. Calcifications are found

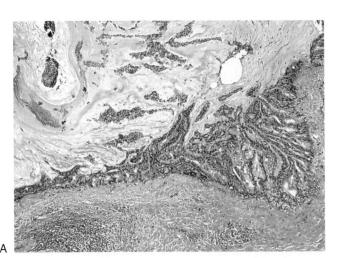

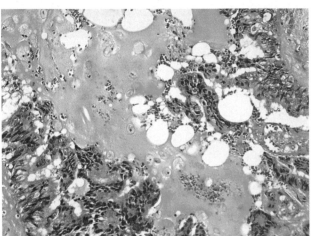

A B

**FIG. 20.9.** *Mucinous carcinoma, cystic papillary type.* **A,B:** Fronds of papillary carcinoma surround the cyst filled with mucinous carcinoma.

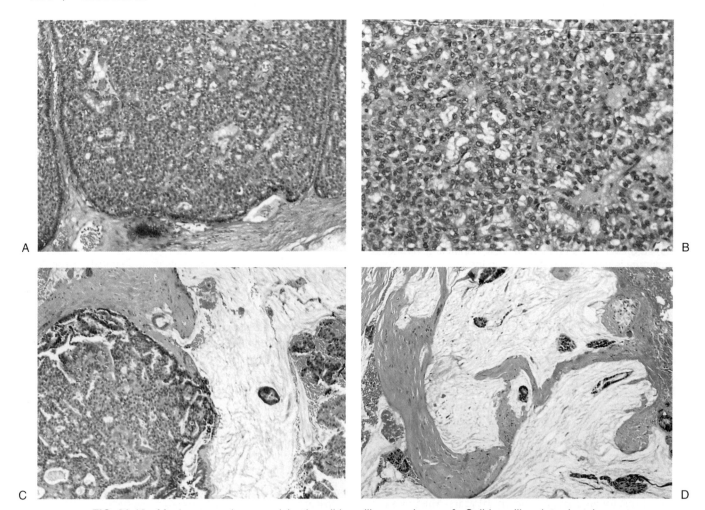

**FIG. 20.10.** *Mucinous carcinoma, arising in solid papillary carcinoma.* **A:** Solid papillary intraductal carcinoma. **B:** Mucin stained pale blue in this hematoxylin and eosin section is present in microlumens in the intraductal carcinoma. **C:** Transition between intraductal *(left)* and infiltrating *(right)* mucinous carcinoma. **D:** Mucinous carcinoma.

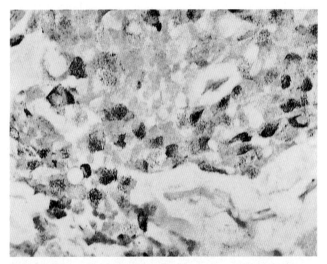

**FIG. 20.11.** *Mucinous carcinoma.* Clusters of fine black argyrophilic granules are demonstrated with the Grimelius stain in this island of solid carcinoma.

most often in mucinous carcinomas that have papillary or comedo patterns (Fig. 20.12).

The signet-ring cell variant of infiltrating lobular carcinoma rarely has an extracellular mucinous component. Lesions of this sort are best considered mucinous variants of infiltrating lobular carcinoma (33).

The margin of mucinous carcinoma is determined by the extent of the mucinous component, even if no epithelial cells are seen in such a peripheral zone (Fig. 20.13). The periphery is characterized by a pushing border in more than 70% of cases (21). Some of these tumors have irregular or knobby contours formed by protrusions of the neoplasm into the breast parenchyma (Fig. 20.14). When assessing the margins of excision, it is important to look for transected protrusions that may be obscured by cautery artifact or that blend with fat.

It is very difficult to recognize lymphatic tumor emboli in mucinous carcinoma. Clusters of carcinoma cells suspended in mucin often have an appearance that resembles intralymphatic carcinoma (Fig. 20.15). When the diagnosis

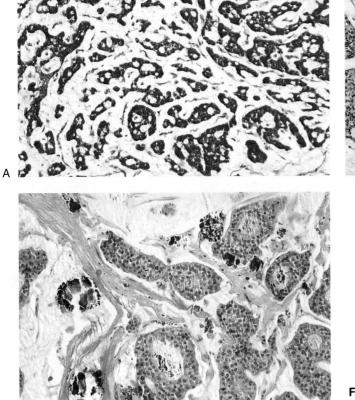

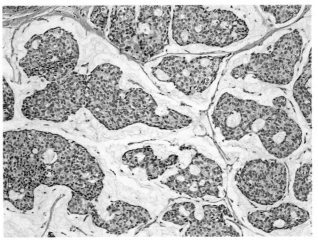

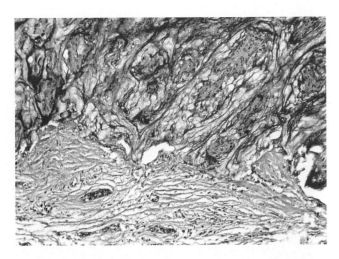

FIG. 20.12. *Mucinous carcinoma.* **A:** Trabecular pattern. **B:** Solid and cribriform pattern. **C:** Papillary carcinoma with calcifications.

FIG. 20.13. *Mucinous carcinoma.* Mucin stained a rose color with the mucicarmine stain has a sharp border. Clusters of carcinoma cells are present in the mucin.

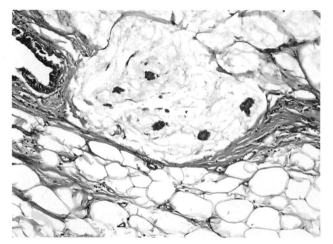

**FIG. 20.14.** *Mucinous carcinoma.* Knobby protrusion into fatty breast tissue.

of such foci is uncertain, a stain for mucin may be helpful because the material surrounding the carcinoma cells will be clearly stained in mucinous carcinoma, but it tends to be weakly reactive in lymphatic tumor emboli.

## MUCOCELE-LIKE TUMOR

The distinction between mucinous carcinoma and *mucocele-like tumor* is a challenging clinical and pathologic diagnostic problem (19). Some mucocele-like lesions of the breast present as palpable tumors that are well-circumscribed, lobulated lesions on mammography (Fig. 20.16). An increasing number of small, nonpalpable mucocele-like tumors has been detected by mammography alone. Ultrasonography shows a hypoechoic, round or lobulated tumor, sometimes with an ill-defined margin (34,35). Mammography reveals a nodular lesion with or without calcifications or clustered calcifications alone. Multiple aggregated cysts are

evident grossly containing viscous, often transparent, mucinous material (Fig. 20.17).

The mucocele-like tumor is composed of mucin-containing cysts that may rupture and discharge the secretion into the adjacent stroma (Fig. 20.18). The resultant picture resembles the mucocele of salivary gland origin commonly found in the oral cavity. The epithelium lining cysts in the typical mammary mucocele-like tumor is largely flat or low cuboidal, but low columnar and minor papillary elements may be present (Fig. 20.19). Detached epithelial cells are very rarely found in the secretion within cysts or when it is discharged into the stroma. Histiocytes and inflammatory cells may be present in the extruded mucin.

Ro et al. (36) described mucocele-like tumors that contained areas of atypical duct hyperplasia (Fig. 20.20), intraductal carcinoma, and focal invasive mucinous carcinoma. In several of the cases, calcifications detected mammographically were localized to the mucinous content of cysts in histologic sections. Identical results were obtained when

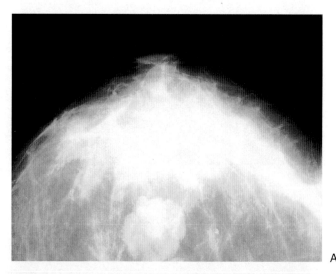

A

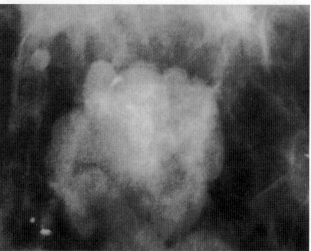

B

**FIG. 20.16.** *Mucocele-like tumor, mammographic appearance.* **A:** Lesion is a circumscribed, multinodular mass deep in the breast. **B:** Tumor is inhomogeneous.

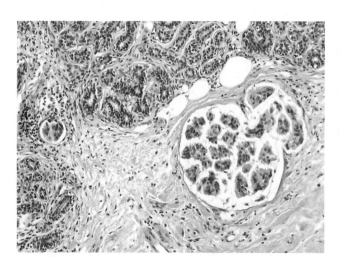

**FIG. 20.15.** *Mucinous carcinoma.* Discrete, sharply defined focus of invasive mucinous carcinoma that resembles tumor in a vascular space.

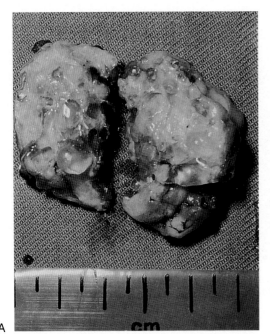
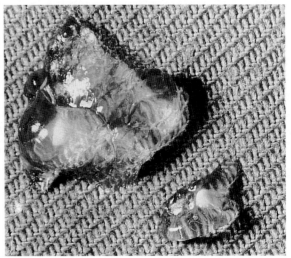

**FIG. 20.17.** *Mucocele-like tumor, gross appearance.* **A:** Tumor consists of many cysts. **B:** Masses of transparent gelatinous material from the tumor.

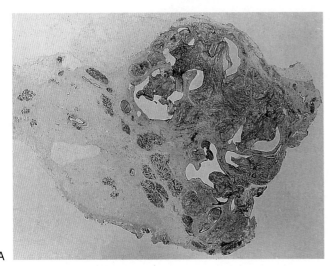
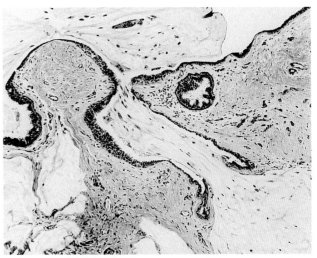

**FIG. 20.18.** *Mucocele-like tumor.* **A:** Whole-mount histologic section of a relatively small tumor. The dark oval foci to the left of the tumor are normal lobules. **B,C:** Two examples of ruptured cysts with mucin extruded into the surrounding stroma. Hyperplasia is evident in small ducts. Folding of epithelium toward the cyst of origin rather than into the stroma at the point of rupture is a typical finding. *(continued)*

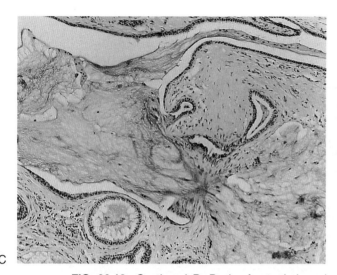

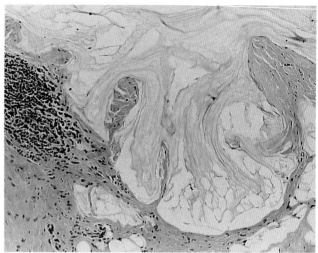

C

D

**FIG. 20.18.** *Continued.* **D:** Pools of extruded mucin in fibrous stroma with a focal lymphocytic reaction. (From Rosen PP. Mucocele-like tumors of the breast. *Am J Surg Pathol* 1986;10:464–469, with permission.)

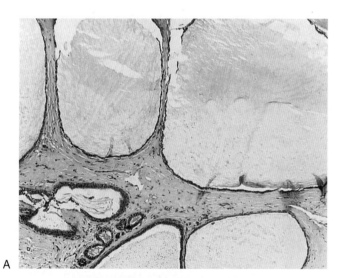

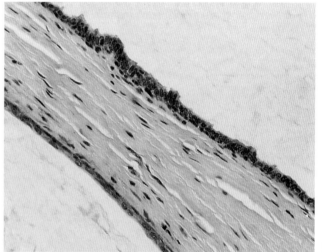

A

B

**FIG. 20.19.** *Mucocele-like tumor.* **A:** Cysts containing mucinous secretion lined by a thin epithelial layer. **B:** Flat and low cuboidal epithelium.

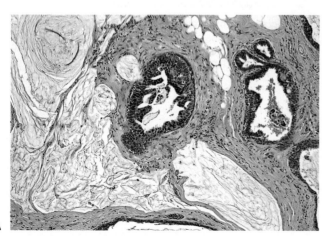

A

**FIG. 20.20.** *Mucocele-like tumor with ductal hyperplasia.* **A:** Two ducts with atypical micropapillary hyperplasia, partly surrounded by extravasated mucin. *(continued)*

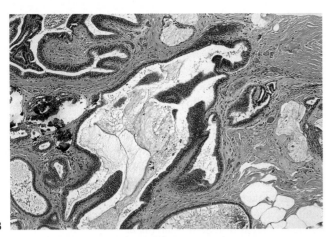

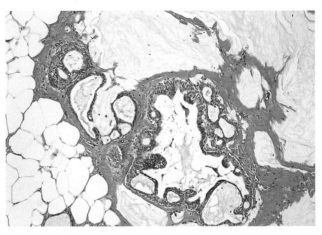

**FIG. 20.20.** *Continued.* **B:** Columnar cell hyperplasia with calcifications *(left)* and extravasated mucin *(right)*. **C:** Atypical micropapillary hyperplasia. Note mucin extravasation from the duct in the *left center.*

the secretion in mucinous carcinomas and in various mucocele-like tumors was studied immunohistochemically. The mucin in cysts and in the stroma was largely composed of neutral and nonsulfated acid-mucin (strongly positive with periodic acid-Schiff/diastase, mucicarmine, and Alcian blue at pH 2.7; weak to negative with Alcian blue at pH 0.9).

A mucocele-like tumor that originated in a cystic papilloma has been described (Fig. 20.21) (19). Mucocele-like le-

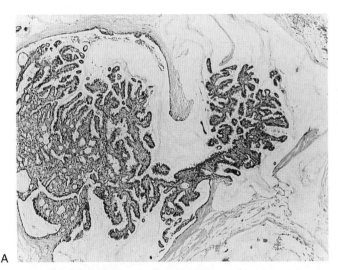

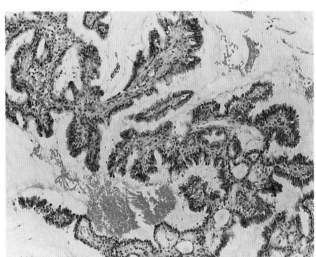

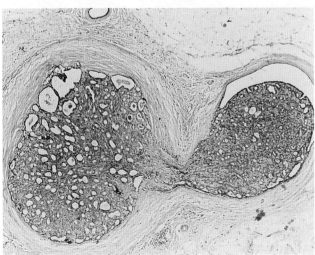

**FIG. 20.21.** *Mucocele-like tumor arising in a cystic papilloma.* **A:** Duct containing an intraductal papilloma has ruptured. Fragments of papilloma and mucin have been extruded. **B:** Papillary fronds have a thin layer of epithelium and fibrovascular stroma. **C:** Part of the lesion shown in **A** and **B** growing as a sclerosing papilloma. (From Rosen PP. Mucocele-like tumors of the breast. *Am J Surg Pathol* 1986;10:464–469, with permission.)

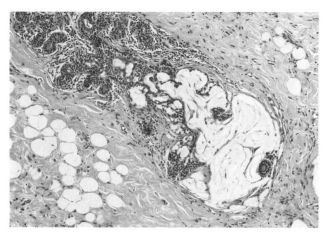

**FIG. 20.22.** *Mucocele-like lesion arising in a lobule.* Extravasated mucin arising from a terminal duct–lobular unit. This was an incidental finding in a biopsy performed for an unrelated lesion.

sions also can arise from lobules. This abnormality may be present as an incidental finding in a specimen obtained for an unrelated lesion, or it can be the source of a clinically detected tumor when multiple lobular foci become confluent (Figs. 20.22 and 20.23).

Kulka and Davies (37) described two mucocele-like tumors with atypical hyperplasia. In one case, the same breast harbored a separate nonmucinous invasive duct carcinoma.

Fisher and Millis (38) reported finding intraductal carcinoma and mucinous carcinoma 1 year after excision of a mucocele-like tumor with atypical hyperplasia. Yeoh et al. (35) summarized 13 patients with mucocele-like tumors, including seven with atypical duct hyperplasia. No recurrences were recorded with follow-up of 1 month to 3.8 years.

Evidence linking mucocele lesions to mucinous carcinoma was obtained by Weaver et al. (39). A review of 23 mucinous carcinomas revealed mucin-filled ducts without hyperplastic epithelium in 15 cases (65%), ductal hyperplasia in mucin-filled ducts in nine (39%), and atypical hyperplasia in mucin-filled ducts in five (22%) cases. The authors did not comment on the presence or absence of extravasated mucin in areas of mucin-filled ducts.

Hamele-Bena et al. (40) reviewed 49 examples of mucocele-like lesions. Four patients had bilateral tumors that were both benign in two cases and both carcinomatous in the other two patients. Overall, 25 of the lesions were classified as benign and 28 as carcinomatous. In 13 tumors, the carcinoma was entirely *in situ*, growing largely as micropapillary or focally cribriform intraductal carcinoma (Figs. 20.24 and 20.25). Twenty-five tumors had invasive carcinoma of the mucinous type (Fig. 20.26). The age range for the entire group was 24 to 79 years (mean, 48 years). There were no significant differences in the age distribution of patients with benign and malignant lesions. Malignant mucocele-like lesions tended to have coarse calcifications more often than

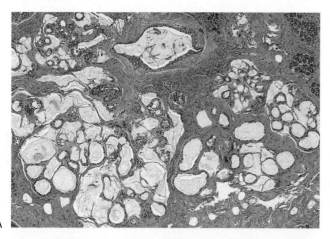

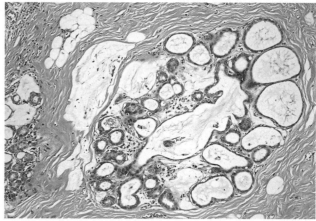

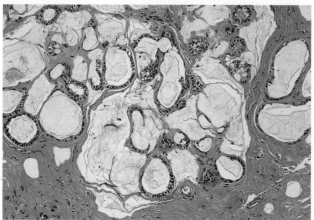

**FIG. 20.23.** *Mucocele-like tumor arising in lobules.* Three images from one specimen. **A:** Low-magnification view showing numerous lobular glands distended with mucin and extravasated mucin in the stroma. **B:** Early stage in the process. Mucin is present in lobular glands, an intralobular duct, and in adjacent stroma. **C:** Lobular architecture is substantially disrupted, and there is extensive mucin extravasation.

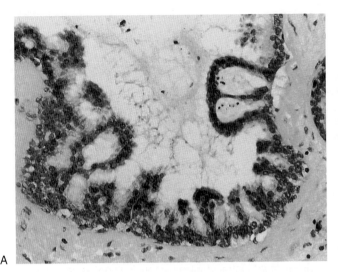
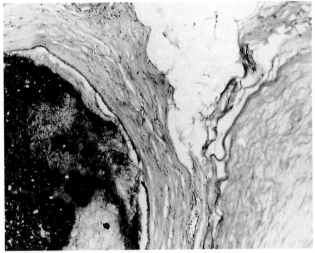

**FIG. 20.24.** *Mucocele-like tumor with intraductal carcinoma.* Both images are from the same case. **A:** Micropapillary intraductal carcinoma. **B:** Large, coarse calcification in a cyst next to extruded mucin.

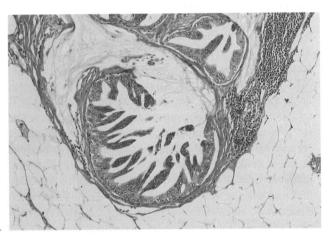
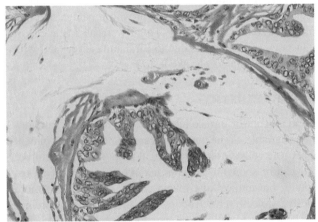

**FIG. 20.25.** *Mucocele-like tumor with intraductal carcinoma.* **A,B:** Micropapillary intraductal carcinoma with mucin extravasation. Carcinoma cells were not present in the extravasated mucin.

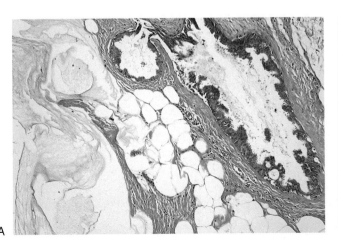
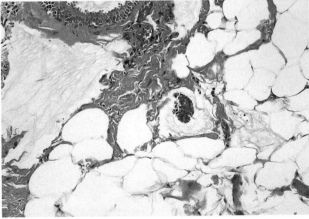

**FIG. 20.26.** *Mucocele-like tumor with mucinous carcinoma.* Both images are from the same specimen. **A:** Mucin in fat *(left)* and micropapillary intraductal carcinoma *(right).* **B:** Cluster of carcinoma cells in mucin surrounded by fat, representing invasive mucinous carcinoma.

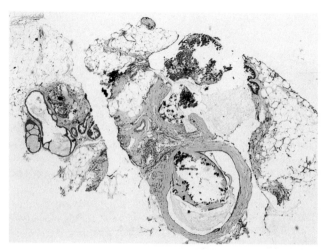

**FIG. 20.27.** *Mucocele-like lesion with intraductal carcinoma and calcifications.* Needle core biopsy specimen showing coarse calcifications and micropapillary carcinoma *(left)* (hematoxylin-phloxine-safranin stain).

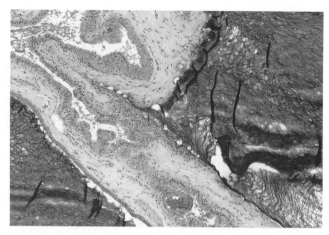

**FIG. 20.29.** *Mucocele-like tumor, mucicarmine stain.* Strong staining of mucin is seen in a cyst *(left)* and in extravasated mucin *(right).* Intracytoplasmic mucin is not apparent.

the benign tumors and therefore were detected more frequently by mammography (Figs. 20.27 and 20.28). Breast recurrences occurred in one patient with a benign and one with a carcinomatous lesion. There were no instances of metastases and no deaths due to carcinoma associated with carcinoma in a mucocele-like lesion.

## HISTOCHEMISTRY

The amount of intracellular mucin in mucinous carcinomas is variable. Some mucinous carcinomas have prominent signet-ring cells. Often only a small proportion of the tumor cells can be shown to contain mucin by histochemical procedures, but intracellular mucin can be demonstrated more readily by electron microscopy (41–44). Mucinous carcinomas contain acid and neutral mucopolysaccharides (45–47). Despite the abundant mucin present in mucocele-like tumors, intracellular mucin is not demonstrable unless there is associated carcinoma (Fig. 20.29).

The expression of mucin genes and their corresponding mucin glycoproteins differs in mucinous and nonmucinous carcinomas. Using immunohistochemistry and *in situ* hybridization, O'Connell et al. (48) found that mucinous carcinomas were characterized by increased MUC2 and MUC5 expression and decreased MUC1. Nonmucinous carcinomas featured increased MUC1 but no increases in MUC2 and MUC5. Tumors with mucinous and nonmucinous components exhibited MUC patterns corresponding to these respective elements. Hyperplasia and intraductal carcinoma from breasts with mucinous carcinoma also showed increased MUC2 and MUC5 expression, an observation interpreted as evidence of a field effect in these patients. Schmitt et al. (49) developed a monoclonal antibody to MUC5AC that was reactive with four (6%) of 66 nonmucinous ductal carcinomas, an observation suggesting that MUC5 expression is not specific for mucinous mammary carcinoma.

The finding of argyrophilic Grimelius-positive granules in mucinous carcinoma cells is a relatively recent observation (7,8,32,50,51). These structures, which have the ultrastruc-

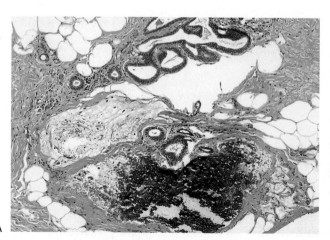

A

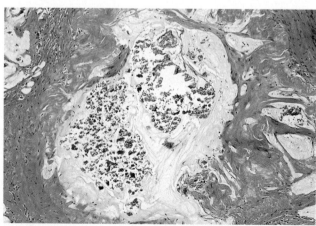

B

**FIG. 20.28.** *Mucocele-like tumor with calcifications.* Two different specimens are depicted. **A:** Coarse granular calcification in extravasated mucin associated with columnar cell hyperplasia. **B:** Loosely granular calcification in extravasated mucin.

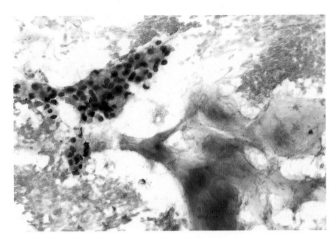

**FIG. 20.30.** *Mucinous carcinoma, cytologic appearance.* Irregular, cohesive cluster of carcinoma cells *(left)* and mucin *(right)* surrounded by red blood cells.

tural features of endocrine secretory granules, have been detected in 25% to 50% of mucinous carcinomas. Mucinous carcinomas that contain these granules tend to occur more frequently in elderly women. The tumors often grow in clumps, sheets, or trabeculae sometimes suggesting an endocrine growth pattern, the type B mucinous carcinoma with endocrine differentiation (32). Fentiman et al. (16) found Grimelius-positive staining more frequently in pure (25%) than in mixed mucinous carcinomas. The granules of some mucinous carcinomas contained immunohistochemically detectable serotonin (52) as well as somatostatin and gastrin (52). The tumors also were positive for neuron-specific enolase (NSE) (7,52). Scopsi et al. (7) reported finding NSE, synaptophysin, and chromogranins A and B in all of the argyrophilic mucinous carcinomas in their series. In the same study, they detected NSE reactivity in 75% and synaptophysin reactivity in 39% of nonargyrophilic, granin-negative tumors.

Immunoreactivity for S-100 and carcinoembryonic antigen (CEA) was found in almost all argyrophilic mucinous carcinomas by Coady et al. (45). About half of duct carcinomas with

mixed mucinous differentiation were CEA positive, but they were almost devoid of S-100. Nonargyrophilic pure mucinous carcinomas virtually all lacked S-100 and CEA. These authors also found abundant elastic fibers in the stroma of argyrophilic mucinous carcinomas, whereas these fibers were sparse or absent in the stroma of nonargyrophilic tumors. In three studies, the presence of argyrophilic granules was not prognostically significant in pure mucinous tumors or in infiltrating duct carcinomas with focal mucinous differentiation (6,7,45).

Nuclear reactivity for estrogen and progesterone receptors is found in 92% and 68%, respectively, of pure mucinous carcinomas (15).

Receptors for epidermal growth factor (EGFR), reportedly found in 30% to 40% of breast carcinomas, were absent from four mucinous carcinomas studied by Skoog et al. (53). Diab et al. (15) reported immunoreactivity for HER2/*neu* and EGFR in less than 5% of pure mucinous carcinomas.

## ELECTRON MICROSCOPY

Several types of cytoplasmic granules have been described ultrastructurally in mucinous carcinomas (42). Small (100 to 500 nm) and large (0.5 to 1.5 nm) dense-core granules were found in tumors that contained argyrophilic granules, and they were absent in almost all nonargyrophilic lesions. This observation appears to confirm the findings of Capella et al. (32). Tumor cells in mucinous carcinoma reportedly contain abundant cytoplasmic filaments with a perinuclear distribution (32,43). They also may exhibit luminal differentiation characterized by microvilli and well-formed intercellular junctions (42,43). Basal lamina and myoepithelial cells are absent (43).

## CYTOLOGY

The diagnosis of mucinous carcinoma may be suspected in material obtained by fine needle aspiration (54). Typically, the smears reveal tumor cells distributed singly or in small clusters in a background of mucin (Figs. 20.30 and 20.31). Attention must be given to distinguishing mucin

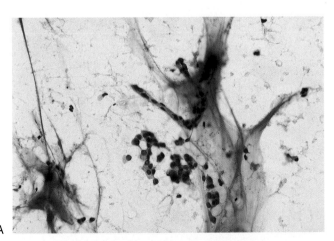

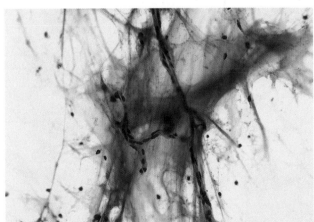

A          B

**FIG. 20.31.** *Mucinous carcinoma, cytologic appearance.* All images are from the same tumor. **A:** Fine needle aspiration sample showing disaggregated tumor cells associated with mucin. The U-shaped linear structure is a capillary. **B:** Another region in the same cytology specimen showing capillaries and mucin. *(continued)*

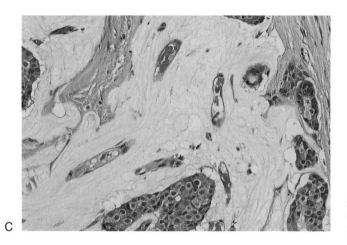

C

FIG. 20.31. *Continued.* **C:** Mucinous carcinoma subsequently excised consisted of clusters of carcinoma cells in mucin with capillaries.

from lysed blood, interstitial fluid, necrotic debris, or protein such as albumin used to coat slides. Occasionally, myxoid material from an edematous fibroadenoma results in an aspirate that resembles mucinous carcinoma (54,55). The finding of spindly stromal cell nuclei in the myxoid material is suggestive of a fibroadenoma. A mucicarmine stain may be useful to confirm the presence of true mucin. Mucinous material also can be present in cysts within fibroepithelial lesions, and the aspirated material that is mucicarmine positive may simulate mucinous carcinoma (56). Myxoid stroma associated with an inflammatory lesion, such as a suture granuloma, can be confused with mucin in an aspiration cytology specimen (57). The sample obtained by fine needle aspiration or needle core biopsy is not reliable for distinguishing between pure mucinous carcinoma and infiltrating duct carcinoma because of the limited nature of the sample. Mucin may be found in the aspirate from an infiltrating duct carcinoma with mucinous differentiation (58).

Difficulty also is encountered in the distinction between mucocele-like tumor and mucinous carcinoma (Fig. 20.32) (59,60). The aspirate from both tumors contains abundant extracellular mucin. Several studies have pointed out the lower cellular content, cellular cohesion, and lack of cytologic atypia in specimens from mucocele-like tumors (34,35,59).

## MORPHOMETRY AND FLOW CYTOMETRY

Morphometric study of needle aspirate specimens showed that the cells of mucinous carcinoma were significantly larger than cells obtained from fibroadenomas and infiltrating lobular carcinoma (61). On the other hand, they tended to be substantially smaller than cells of most duct carcinomas and of medullary carcinomas. No difference was observed between mucinous carcinoma and a small cell type of duct carcinoma.

The ploidy of mucinous carcinoma has been studied by flow cytometry. Pure mucinous carcinomas were reported to be diploid in 96% and 78% of cases, respectively (15,62). Only 42% (8/19) of duct carcinomas with mucinous differentiation were diploid, with the majority described as aneuploid (62). Diab et al. (15) reported that 83% of mucinous carcinomas had low S-phase, 10% were intermediate, and 7% were high.

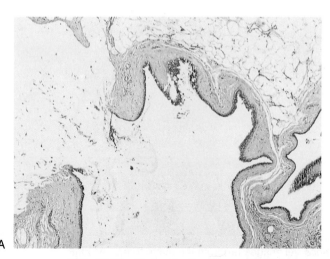

A

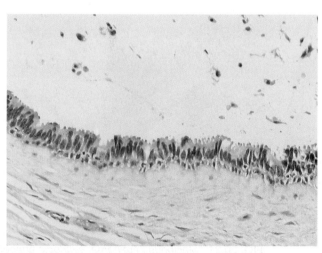

B

FIG. 20.32. *Mucocele-like tumor, cytologic appearance.* **A:** Ruptured cyst with extruded mucin *(upper left).* **B:** Columnar cell epithelium in the cyst with a myoepithelial cell layer. *(continued)*

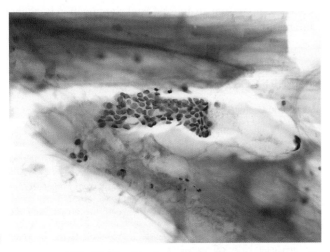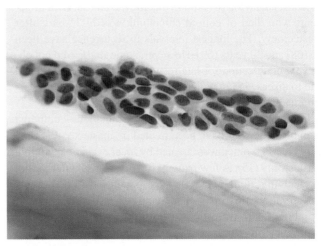

C                                               D

**FIG. 20.32.** *Continued.* **C,D:** Fine needle aspiration specimen with flat sheets of cytologically benign epithelial cells surrounded by mucin.

## PROGNOSIS AND TREATMENT

The relatively favorable prognosis commonly ascribed to mucinous carcinoma is supported by numerous studies (Table 20.1) (5,7,8,12,13,29,30,62). Because the tumor occurs infrequently, few investigators have been able to assemble substantial numbers of patients. Differences in the definition of the tumor and in reporting make it difficult to combine data from published series.

When compared with patients who have infiltrating duct carcinoma with a mucinous component and those who have infiltrating duct carcinoma, women with pure mucinous carcinoma had a better relapse-free survival 5 and 10 years after mastectomy (7,12–14,29,30,63,64). Pure mucinous carcinomas tend to be smaller than tumors with a mixed pattern, and these patients have a lower frequency of axillary lymph node metastases (6–8,10,12,13,64,65). In the past two decades, the reported frequency of negative axillary lymph nodes in patients with pure mucinous carcinoma ranged from

71% (13) to 97% (65) and 100% (21). Most series of patients with duct carcinoma with a mucinous component had at least 50% node-negative patients (7,10,13,50,64). In an exceptional study, only 28% of patients with these lesions had negative nodes (8).

Major prognostic factors that are relevant for most types of breast carcinoma also apply to pure mucinous carcinoma (8,12). Recurrence is least likely with smaller tumors and the absence of lymph node metastases. The presence of microcalcifications was associated with a relatively favorable outcome by Norris and Taylor (11).

Five-year survival rates after treatment of pure mucinous carcinoma by mastectomy have been 84% disease free (6), 86% alive (13), and 87% disease free (12). Norris and Taylor (11) reported an 80% 10-year survival. In their series, two of six patients with pure mucinous carcinoma who died of disease had a nonmucinous carcinoma of the opposite breast, which may have been responsible for the fatal outcome. Komaki et al. (10) reported a 90% 10-year survival rate for pure mucinous carcinoma (10). The 10-year survival rate for corresponding patients with infiltrating duct carcinoma with a mucinous component was 60%. In another series, the 15-year disease-free survival rates were 85% and 63% for pure mucinous and infiltrating duct carcinoma with a mucinous component, respectively (8). The "20-year cumulative corrected survival rate" for pure mucinous carcinoma was 79% ± 11% (8). Scopsi et al. (7) reported no deaths due to disease among 25 patients with node-negative pure mucinous carcinoma. In the same study, "there were no significant differences in overall survival rate" when node-positive patients with pure mucinous and nonmucinous carcinomas were compared. The long-term prognosis for small, node-negative pure mucinous carcinomas is exceptionally favorable; therefore, systemic adjuvant therapy usually is not indicated for tumors 3 cm or less (66).

Late systemic recurrences have been described after mastectomy in patients with mucinous carcinoma (5,14,29,

**TABLE 20.1.** *Prognosis of mucinous carcinoma*

| Follow-up period (yr) | Status | Type of mucinous carcinoma | | | |
| --- | --- | --- | --- | --- | --- |
| | | Pure | | Mixed | |
| | | No. | (%) | No. | (%) |
| 5 | NED | 35 | (85) | 19 | (83) |
| | DOD | 4 | (10) | 2 | (8) |
| | DOC | 2 | (5) | 2 | (8) |
| 10 | NED | 25 | (69) | 10 | (56) |
| | DOD | 6 | (17) | 5 | (28) |
| | DOC | 5 | (14) | 3 | (17) |
| 15 | NED | 19 | (58) | | |
| | DOD | 9 | (27) | | |
| | DOC | 5 | (15) | | |

DOC, died of other causes; DOD, died of disease; mixed, duct carcinoma with mucinous component; NED, no evidence of disease.

30,66,67). Clayton (67) found that the median survival of patients who died of colloid carcinoma was 11.3 years after mastectomy. The longest intervals to recurrence have been 25 (68) and 30 years (69). However, some studies did not observe a predilection for late recurrence (10,70) or late death due to disease (8) in women with small, pure mucinous carcinoma.

For the most part, patients with pure mucinous carcinoma in published series have been treated by mastectomy. Some very elderly women were treated by local excision or simple mastectomy (15). A few patients have done well after partial mastectomy alone (11), but most patients who had breast conservation treatment also received radiation therapy. Combined data from two institutions include 10 patients with mucinous carcinoma who have remained disease free after lumpectomy and radiotherapy with a median follow-up of 79 months (71).

A series of 1,008 women treated by breast conservation with radiotherapy at Yale University from 1970 to 1990 included 16 patients with mucinous carcinoma (72). After a median follow-up of 11.2 years, there were no breast recurrences. One patient developed a systemic recurrence 11 years after initial therapy.

Axillary or systemic metastases that arise from mucinous carcinoma of the breast usually have the histologic characteristics of the primary tumor. Axillary metastases from tumors with mixed histology usually resemble the nonmucinous component. Pure mucinous carcinomas also can have nonmucinous metastases (16). The distribution of sites of disseminated metastases does not differ from other types of

duct carcinoma, but an unusual fatal complication is cerebral infarction caused by mucin embolism (73,74).

## REFERENCES

1. World Health Organization. Histological typing of breast tumors. *Tumori* 1982;68:181–198.
2. Lange F. Der Gallertkrebs der Brustdruse. *Beitr Klin Chir* 1896;16:1–60.
3. Larey M. Tumeur gelatiniforme ou colloide de la mamelle. *Bull Soc Chir Paris* 1853;3:545.
4. Robinson RR. Gelatinous cancer of the breast. *Trans Pathol Soc Lond* 1852;4:275.
5. Geschickter CF. Gelatinous carcinoma of the breast. *Ann Surg* 1938;108:321–340.
6. Rasmussen BB, Rose C, Christensen I. Prognostic factors in primary mucinous breast carcinoma. *Am J Clin Pathol* 1987;87:155–160.
7. Scopsi L, Andreola S, Pilotti S, et al. Mucinous carcinoma of the breast. A clinicopathologic, histochemical and immunocytochemical study with special reference to neuroendocrine differentiation. *Am J Surg Pathol* 1994;18:702–711.
8. Toikkanen S, Kujari H. Pure and mixed mucinous carcinomas of the breast: a clinicopathologic analysis of 61 cases with long-term follow-up. *Hum Pathol* 1989;20:758–764.
9. Avisar E, Khan MA, Axelrod D, et al. Pure mucinous carcinoma of the breast: a clinicopathologic correlation study. *Ann Surg Oncol* 1998;5:447–451.
10. Komaki K, Sakamoto G, Sugano H, et al. Mucinous carcinoma of the breast in Japan. A prognostic analysis based on morphologic features. *Cancer* 1988;61:989–996.
11. Norris HJ, Taylor HB. Prognosis of mucinous (gelatinous) carcinoma of the breast. *Cancer* 1965;18:879–885.
12. Melamed MR, Robbins GF, Foote FW Jr. Prognostic significance of gelatinous mammary carcinoma. *Cancer* 1961;14:699–704.
13. Silverberg SG, Kay S, Chitale AR, et al. Colloid carcinoma of the breast. *Am J Clin Pathol* 1971;55:355–363.
14. Rosen PP, Wang T-Y. Colloid carcinoma of the breast. Analysis of 64 patients with long-term follow-up. *Am J Clin Pathol* 1980;73:30.
15. Diab SG, Clark GM, Osborne CK, et al. Tumor characteristics and clinical outcome of tubular and mucinous breast carcinomas. *J Clin Oncol* 1999;17:1442–1448.
16. Fentiman IS, Millis RR, Smith P, et al. Mucoid breast carcinomas: histology and prognosis. *Br J Cancer* 1997;75:1061–1065.
17. Rosen PP, Lesser ML, Kinne DW. Breast carcinoma at the extremes of age: a comparison of patients younger than 35 years and older than 75 years. *J Surg Oncol* 1985;28:90–96.
18. Cardenosa G, Doudna C, Eklund GW. Mucinous (colloid) breast cancer: clinical and mammographic findings in 10 patients. *AJR Am J Roentgenol* 1994;162:1077–1079.
19. Rosen PP. Mucocele-like tumors of the breast. *Am J Surg Pathol* 1986;10:464–469.
20. Conant EF, Dillon RL, Palazzo J, et al. Imaging findings in mucin-containing carcinomas of the breast: correlation with pathologic features. *AJR Am J Roentgenol* 1994;163:821–824.
21. Goodman DNF, Boutross-Tadross O, Jong RA. Mammographic features of pure mucinous carcinoma of the breast with pathological correlation. *Can Assoc Radiol J* 1995;46:296–301.
22. Wilson TE, Helvie MA, Oberman HA, et al. Pure and mixed mucinous carcinoma of the breast: pathologic basis for differences in mammographic appearance. *AJR Am J Roentgenol* 1995;165:285–289.
23. Ruggieri AM, Scola FH, Schepps B, et al. Mucinous carcinoma of the breast: mammographic findings. *Breast Dis* 1995;8:353–361.
24. Miller RW, Harris SE. Mucinous carcinoma of the breast: potential false-negative MR imaging interpretation. *AJR Am J Roentgenol* 1996;167:539–540.
25. Orel S, Schnall M, Livolsi V, et al. Suspicious breast lesions: MR imaging with radiologic-pathologic correlation. *Radiology* 1994;190:485–493.

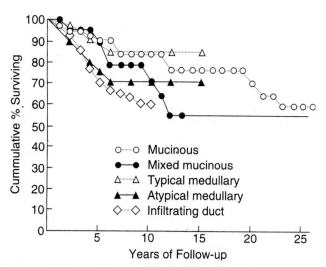

**FIG. 20.33.** *Mucinous carcinoma, survival analysis.* Life-table analysis of survival comparing patients with mucinous, medullary, and duct carcinoma, not stratified by stage at diagnosis. Patients with mucinous and medullary carcinoma had equally favorable survival rates for 10 years of follow-up. Note the progressive decline in survival for mucinous carcinoma patients after 10 years.

26. Lesser ML, Rosen PP, Senie RT, et al. Estrogen and progesterone receptors in breast carcinoma: correlations with epidemiology and pathology. *Cancer* 1981;48:229–309.

27. Rosen PP, Menendez-Botet CJ, Senie RT, et al. Estrogen in receptor protein (ERP) and the histopathology of human mammary carcinoma. In: McGuire WL, ed. *Hormones, receptors and breast cancer.* New York: Raven Press, 1978:71–83.

28. Shousha S, Coady AT, Stamp T, et al. Oestrogen receptors in mucinous carcinoma of the breast: an immunohistochemical study using paraffin wax sections. *J Clin Pathol* 1989;42:902–905.

29. Lee BJ, Hauser H, Pack GT. Gelatinous carcinoma of the breast. *Surg Gynecol Obstet* 1934;59:841–857.

30. Wulsin JH, Schreiber JT. Improved prognosis in certain patterns of carcinoma of the breast. *Arch Surg* 1962;85:791–800.

31. Koenig C, Tavassoli FA. Mucinous cystadenocarcinoma of the breast. *Am J Surg Pathol* 1998;22:698–703.

32. Capella C, Eusebi V, Mann B, et al. Endocrine differentiation in mucoid carcinoma of the breast. *Histopathology* 1980;4:613–630.

33. Steinbrecher JS, Silverberg SG. Signet ring cell carcinoma of the breast. The mucinous variant of infiltrating lobular carcinoma. *Cancer* 1976;37;828–840.

34. Kim Y, Takatsuka Y, Morino H. Mucocele-like tumor of the breast: a case report and assessment of aspirated cytological specimens. *Breast Cancer* 1998;5:317–320.

35. Yeoh GP, Cheung PS, Chan KW. Fine-needle aspiration cytology of mucocelelike tumors of the breast. *Am J Surg Pathol* 1999;23:552–559.

36. Ro JY, Sneige N, Sahin AA, et al. Mucocele-like tumor of the breast associated with atypical duct hyperplasia or mucinous carcinoma. A clinicopathologic study of seven cases. *Arch Pathol Lab Med* 1991;115:137–140.

37. Kulka J, Davies JD. Mucocele-like tumours: more associations and possibly ductal carcinoma *in situ?* *Histopathology* 1993;22:511–512.

38. Fisher CJ, Millis RR. A mucocele-like tumour of the breast associated with both atypicaly ductal hyperplasia and mucoid carcinoma. *Histopathology* 1992;23:69–71.

39. Weaver MG, Abdul-Karim FW, Al-Kaisi N. Mucinous lesions of the breast. A pathologic continuum. *Pathol Res Proc* 1993;189:873–876.

40. Hamele-Bena D, Cranor ML, Rosen PP. Mammary mucocele-like lesions (MLL): benign and malignant. *Am J Surg Pathol* 1996;20:1081–1085.

41. Ahmed A. Electron-microscopic observations of scirrhous and mucin-producing carcinomas of the breast. *J Pathol* 1974;112:177–181.

42. Ferguson DJP, Anderson TJ, Wells CA, et al. An ultrastructural study of mucoid carcinoma of the breast: variability of cytoplasmic features. *Histopathology* 1986;10:1219–1230.

43. Jao W, Lau IO, Chowdhury LN, et al. Ultrastructural aspects of mucinous (colloid) breast carcinoma. *Diagn Gynecol Obstet* 1980;2:83–92.

44. Harris M, Vasudev KS, Anfield C, et al. Mucin producing carcinomas of the breast: ultrastructural observations. *Histopathology* 1978;2:177–188.

45. Coady AT, Shousha S, Dawson PM, et al. Mucinous carcinoma of the breast: further characterization of its three subtypes. *Histopathology* 1989;15:617–626.

46. Tellem M, Nedwick A, Amenta PS, et al. Mucin-producing carcinoma of the breast: tissue culture, histochemical and electron microscopic study. *Cancer* 1966;19:573–584.

47. Walker RA. Mucoid carcinomas of the breast: a study using mucin histochemistry and peanut lectin. *Histopathology* 1982;6:571–579.

48. O'Connell JT, Shao Z-M, Drori E, et al. Altered mucin expression is a field change that accompanies mucinous (colloid) breast carcinoma histogenesis. *Hum Pathol* 1998;29:1517–1523.

49. Schmitt FC, Pereira M, Reis C. MUC5 expression in breast carcinomas. *Hum Pathol* 1999;30:1270.

50. Fetissof F, Dubois MP, Arbeille-Brassart B, et al. Argyrophilic cells in mammary carcinoma. *Hum Pathol* 1983;14:127–134.

51. Rasmussen BB, Rosen C, Thorpe SM, et al. Argyrophilic cells in 202 human mucinous breast carcinomas. Relation to histopathologic and clinical features. *Am J Clin Pathol* 1985;84:737–740.

52. Hull MT, Warfel KA. Mucinous breast carcinomas with abundant intracytoplasmic mucin and neuroendocrine features: light microscopic, immunohistochemical and ultrastructural study. *Ultrastruct Pathol* 1987;11:29–38.

53. Skoog L, Macias A, Azavedo E, et al. Receptors for EGF and oestradiol and thymidine-kinase activity in different histological subgroups of human mammary carcinomas. *Br J Cancer* 1986;54:271–276.

54. Gupta RK, McHutchison AGR, Simpson JS, et al. Value of fine needle aspiration cytology of the breast, with an emphasis on the cytodiagnosis of colloid carcinoma. *Acta Cytol* 1991;35:703–709.

55. Matsuda M, Wada A, Nagumo S, et al. Pitfalls in fine needle aspiration cytology of breast tumors. A report of two cases. *Acta Cytol* 1993;37:247–251.

56. Simsir A, Tsang P, Greenebaum E. Additional mimics of mucinous mammary carcinoma: fibroepithelial lesions. *Am J Clin Pathol* 1998;109:169–172.

57. Maygarden SJ, Novotny DB, Johnson DE, et al. Fine-needle aspiration cytology of suture granulomas of the breast: a potential pitfall in the cytologic diagnosis of recurrent breast cancer. *Diagn Cytopathol* 1994;10:175–179.

58. Stanley MW, Tani EM, Skoog L. Mucinous breast carcinoma and mixed mucinous-infiltrating ductal carcinoma: a comparative cytologic study. *Diagn Cytopathol* 1989;5:134–138.

59. Bhargava V, Miller TR, Cohen MB. Mucocele-like tumors of the breast. Cytologic findings in two cases. *Am J Clin Pathol* 1991;95:875–877.

60. Komaki K, Sakamoto G, Sugano H, et al. The morphologic feature of mucinous leakage appearing in low papillary carcinoma of the breast. *Hum Pathol* 1991;22:231–236.

61. Duane GB, Kanter MH, Branigan T, et al. A morphologic and morphometric study of cells from colloid carcinoma of the breast obtained by fine needle aspiration. *Acta Cytol* 1987;31:742–750.

62. Toikkanen S, Eerola E, Ekfors TO. Pure and mixed mucinous breast carcinomas: DNA stemline and prognosis. *J Clin Pathol* 1988;41:300–303.

63. Veronesi U, Gennari L. Il carcinoma gelatinoso della mammella. *Tumori* 1960;46:119–155.

64. Andre S, Cunha F, Bernardo M, et al. Mucinous carcinoma of the breast: a pathologic study of 82 cases. *J Surg Oncol* 1995;58:162–167.

65. Rasmussen BB. Human mucinous carcinomas and their lymph node metastases. A histological review of 247 cases. *Pathol Res Pract* 1985;180:377–382.

66. Rosen PP, Groshen S, Kinne DW. Survival and prognostic factors in node-negative breast cancer: results of long-term follow-up studies. In: *Proceedings of Consensus Development Conference on Treatment of Early-Stage Conference on Treatment of Early-Stage Breast Cancer, JNCI, Monograph 11.* Bethesda, MD: National Institutes of Health, 1992.

67. Clayton F. Pure mucinous carcinomas of breast: morphologic features and prognostic correlates. *Hum Pathol* 1986;17:34–38.

68. Lee M, Terry R. Surgical treatment of carcinomas of the breast. I. Pathological findings and pattern of relapse. *J Surg Oncol* 1983;23:11–15.

69. Scharnhorst D, Huntrakoon M. Mucinous carcinoma of the breast: recurrence 30 years after mastectomy. *South Med J* 1981;81:656–657.

70. Rosen PP, Groshen S, Saigo PE, et al. A long-term follow-up study of survival in Stage I ($T_1N_0M_0$) and Stage II ($T_1N_1M_0$) breast carcinoma. *J Clin Oncol* 1989;7:355–366.

71. Kurtz JM, Jacquemier J, Torhorst J, et al. Conservation therapy for breast cancers other than infiltrating ductal carcinoma. *Cancer* 1989;63:1630–1635.

72. Haffty BG, Perrotta PL, Ward B, et al. Conservatively treated breast cancer: outcome by histologic subtype. *Breast J* 1997;3:7–14.

73. Deck JHN, Lee MA. Mucin embolism to cerebral arteries. A fatal complication of carcinoma of breast. *Can J Neurol Sci* 1978;5:327–330.

74. Towfighi J, Simmonds MA, Davidson EA. Mucin and fat emboli in mucinous carcinoma. Cause of hemorrhagic cerebral infarcts. *Arch Pathol Lab Med* 1983;107:646–649.

# CHAPTER 21

# Apocrine Carcinoma

Apocrine glands are a normal constituent of the skin, where they may give rise to cutaneous apocrine carcinoma (1–3). Mammary carcinoma also can exhibit apocrine features. Because apocrine glands are morphologically and functionally different from sweat glands, carcinomas that exhibit apocrine differentiation should not be referred to as *sweat gland carcinoma* (4). According to Hamperl, "The term sweat gland carcinoma of the human breast should be abolished since there exists no proof that they really occur" (5). Secretory *(juvenile)* carcinoma is a morphologically and clinically distinct neoplastic process that is not part of the spectrum of apocrine carcinoma.

Rarely, tumors conventionally classified as apocrine are probably true oncocytic neoplasms characterized by abundant mitochondria at the ultrastructural level. Damiani et al. described three oncocytic carcinomas of the breast that were strongly immunoreactive with an antimitochondrial antibody but not for gross cystic disease fluid protein-15 (GCDFP-15), which is invariably reactive with apocrine cells (6). The term *oncocytic carcinoma* should be reserved for lesions with the appropriate immunohistochemical and ultrastructural characteristics.

Cells with functional apocrine characteristics have been detected in fetal breast tissue (7). This observation suggests that apocrine differentiation occurs in a subset of normal mammary glandular cells and that the apocrine proliferative lesions found in the adult breast may arise by expansion of this constituent rather than through metaplastic alteration of nonapocrine cells. Benign apocrine change can be found in lobular glands and in cysts, where it frequently has a papillary configuration (Fig. 21.1). Apocrine metaplasia is prone to develop mammographically detectable calcium oxalate calcifications (Fig. 21.2). Calcium oxalate deposits are associated with benign apocrine lesions and only rarely occur in apocrine carcinoma.

It is likely that most apocrine carcinomas arise from pre-existing benign apocrine epithelium rather than *de novo*. Two observations support this conclusion. Although apocrine epithelium is commonly found in adult female breast tissue excised for various reasons, it is particularly abundant and often atypical in the breasts of women with apocrine carcinoma. Transitions from atypical hyperplastic apocrine lesions to carcinoma are evident in some but not all examples of apocrine carcinoma (8–10). The fact that a cell line derived from an apocrine carcinoma retained apocrine characteristics *in vitro* may be regarded as further evidence that such carcinomas represent a morphologically distinct tumor variant (11).

The frequency of apocrine carcinoma in published series reportedly ranges from less than 1% (12,13) to about 4% (14). This variability is probably the result of inconsistent diagnostic criteria and variations in the way cases were identified. Apocrine traits are present in a greater proportion of mammary carcinomas, but the term should be reserved for neoplasms in which all or nearly all the epithelium has apocrine cytologic features. When so described, fewer than 1% of breast carcinomas can be classified as apocrine carcinomas. Some carcinomas described under the term *histiocytoid* are variants of lobular carcinoma with apocrine differentiation (14,15).

## CLINICAL PRESENTATION

There are no striking differences in the clinical or mammographic features of patients with apocrine and nonapocrine duct carcinomas (16). In rare instances, the mammogram in a patient with extensive intraductal apocrine carcinoma displays diffuse "mixed form" linear and punctate calcifications "characterized by a strikingly wild, chaotic appearance with profuse deposition of calcium" (17). Whereas some reports suggest that apocrine carcinoma is associated with postmenopausal or elderly women (12), most researchers have observed no difference in the age distribution of patients with apocrine and nonapocrine duct carcinomas. The reported age range is from 19 to 86 years.

Patients who have invasive apocrine carcinoma usually present with a mass. Pain, Paget's disease, nipple discharge, and other symptoms are relatively uncommon initial mani-

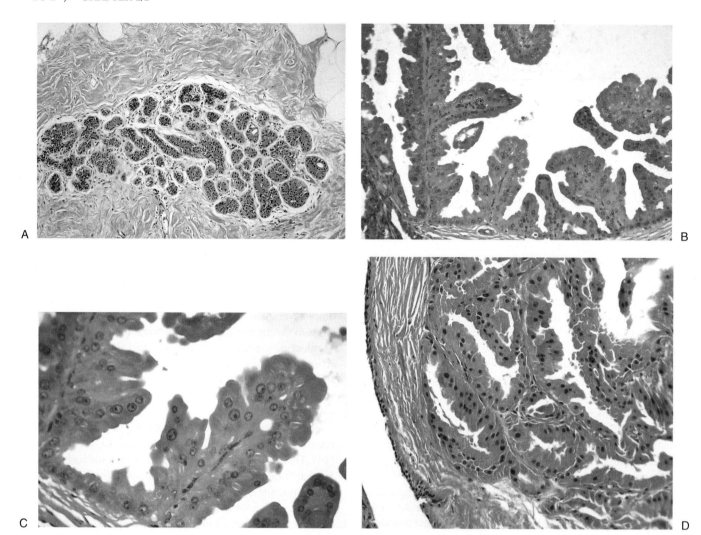

**FIG. 21.1.** *Aprocrine metaplasia.* **A:** Apocrine metaplasia in a lobule. **B,C:** Cystic papillary apocrine metaplasia. Fibrovascular stroma is present in the papillary structures. Nuclei are basally oriented and relatively evenly spaced. **D:** Complex apocrine metaplasia.

festations. Occasionally, intraductal carcinoma is sufficiently abundant to form a mass, but more often apocrine intraductal carcinoma is detected by mammography (Fig.

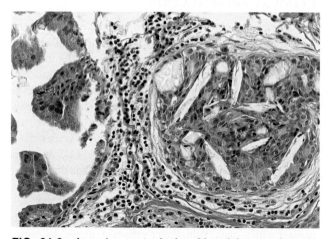

**FIG. 21.2.** *Apocrine metaplasia with calcium oxalate deposits.* Crystalline calcium oxalate deposits are shown in a hyperplastic duct next to papillary apocrine metaplasia.

21.3). Compared with other types of breast carcinoma, the distribution of sites of apocrine carcinoma is not unusual, with most of the lesions located in the upper outer quadrant. The stage at diagnosis of apocrine carcinoma does not differ appreciably from that of nonapocrine carcinomas.

The frequency of bilaterality in patients who have apocrine carcinoma in one breast is not exceptional. An occasional patient has nonapocrine carcinoma in her contralateral breast (18). Bilateral apocrine carcinomas are uncommon. Schmitt et al. studied simultaneous bilateral apocrine carcinomas found in a 74-year-old patient and demonstrated that they were independent primary tumors (19). The right breast contained a 4-cm invasive carcinoma with metastases in three axillary lymph nodes. This tumor was immunoreactive for p53 but not for c-*erb*B-2 and exhibited p53 mutation by polymerase chain reaction (PCR)-SSCP. The left breast carcinoma measured 3 cm and had no axillary lymph node metastases. It was not immunoreactive for p53, and no p53 mutation was detected. The left breast tumor was immunoreactive for c-*erb*B-2. Data on risk factors for carcinoma, such as family history, are limited. Six patients in one

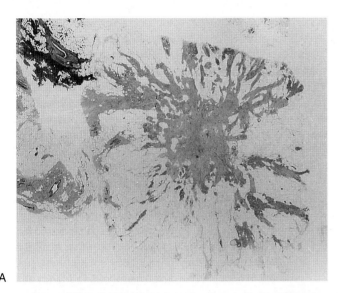

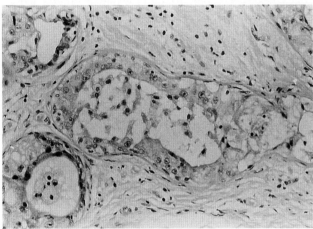

**FIG. 21.3.** *Apocrine carcinoma.* **A:** A whole-mount histologic section of a stellate lesion detected by mammography. Hemorrhage due to needle localization is evident in the upper left-hand corner. **B:** The ducts contain apocrine intraductal carcinoma with cytoplasmic clearing.

series gave a negative family history for breast carcinoma (12).

Hormone receptor analyses of apocrine carcinomas have yielded conflicting results. In one series, six tumors were estrogen receptor (ER)- and progesterone receptor (PR)-negative, despite the fact that all of the patients were postmenopausal (12). Others found that most of the tumors were ER- or PR-positive [ER(+) PR(+): 2; ER(+) PR(−): 1; ER(−) PR(+): 1; ER(+) PR not done: 2; ER(−) only: 1] (14). Androgen receptors were positive in 22% of tumors that were analyzed (20). When studied by immunohistochemistry, 98% of 102 apocrine lesions, including benign conditions and carcinomas, were ER- and PR-negative (21); in the latter series, androgen receptors were present in 94% of benign lesions and 72% of carcinomas with apocrine differentiation.

*In vitro* studies have demonstrated enhanced metabolism of testosterone precursors by apocrine carcinomas compared with other types of breast carcinoma (20). The growth of cutaneous apocrine glands can be stimulated by androgens (22), and some androgen metabolites are concentrated in apocrine secretions (23).

Ploidy in apocrine lesions has been evaluated in Feulgen-stained sections by image analysis. A diploid DNA content was found in benign apocrine metaplasia, atypical apocrine metaplasia, and orderly, low-grade forms of intraductal carcinoma (24,25). Ploidy correlated with grade; as a consequence, almost all poorly differentiated apocrine carcinomas were aneuploid (25). If the study yields a diploid DNA content, ploidy analysis is not useful for distinguishing between proliferative lesions with atypical apocrine metaplasia and apocrine carcinoma. Apocrine lesions with an aneuploid DNA content are most likely to be carcinoma.

Apocrine carcinoma of the male breast has been described but is uncommon (26). One unusual apocrine male mammary carcinoma had a glandular architecture and psammoma bodies.

## GROSS PATHOLOGY

No gross morphologic features are particularly associated with apocrine carcinoma. Invasive carcinomas are firm to hard tumors that usually have infiltrating borders. The bisected tumor is generally gray or white. The tan–brown color associated with some cellular benign apocrine lesions is generally not evident in apocrine carcinomas. Exceptional tumors are grossly cystic or have a medullary appearance (Fig. 21.4). Comedonecrosis can be found in intraductal lesions.

## MICROSCOPIC PATHOLOGY

The distinguishing histologic feature of apocrine carcinoma is the cytologic appearance of the tumor cells. Lee et al. (4) pointed out more than 50 years ago that apocrine

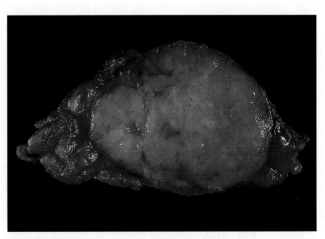

**FIG. 21.4.** *Apocrine carcinoma, gross appearance.* This invasive carcinoma has a well defined border and a fleshy or medullary-appearing cut surface.

carcinomas "have much the same structure as other mammary carcinomata, e.g., we find that the bulky adenocarcinomata, the comedocarcinomata, the papillary, intraductal and intracystic carcinomata, the carcinoma simplex, and even scirrhous carcinomata of the breast are represented in this group." Attention has been drawn recently to a variant of lobular carcinoma that exhibited apocrine features. Apocrine differentiation also has been noted in a mucinous carcinoma (14), in duct carcinomas with tubular features (12,27), and in medullary carcinoma (28).

The most important consideration in establishing a diagnosis of apocrine carcinoma is the determination that the lesion has a structural growth pattern customarily associated with a nonapocrine form of mammary carcinoma. This factor is particularly significant when evaluating cytologically atypical apocrine components in lesions such as sclerosing adenosis or sclerosing papillomatosis (radial scar). Carter and Rosen described sclerosing breast lesions with atypical

apocrine epithelium that were characterized by nuclear atypia, varying degrees of cytoplasmic clearing, and rare mitoses (29) (Figs. 21.5 and 21.6). The distinction from carcinoma was based in most cases on the absence of sufficient epithelial proliferation to produce the characteristic growth patterns of intraductal carcinoma. Rarely, cytologic features are so abnormal that a diagnosis of carcinoma is indicated in the absence of a characteristic *in situ* carcinomatous structure.

Others have attempted to distinguish atypical apocrine lesions on the basis of extent as well as cytologic and structural criteria. Tavassoli and Norris considered apocrine ductal lesions that occupied an area of less than 2 mm, regardless of cytologic and structural features, to be atypical apocrine hyperplasia (30). Larger histologically identical foci qualified as apocrine intraductal carcinoma. They applied the same size criterion to nonapocrine duct hyperplasia. O'Malley and colleagues used a combination of cytologic criteria and le-

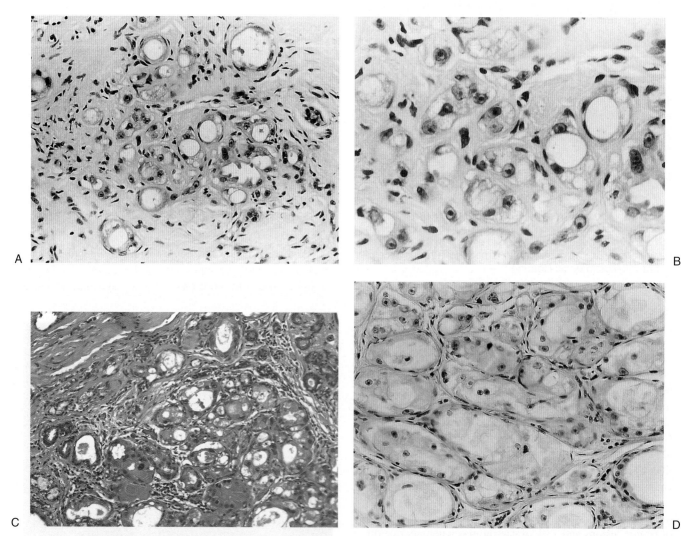

**FIG. 21.5.** *Apocrine lesions in sclerosing adenosis.* **A:** Atypical apocrine metaplasia in sclerosing adenosis. The glands are not enlarged and cellularity is not increased. **B:** Magnified view of **A** showing cytologic features. **C:** Marked cytologic atypia and glandular expansion with cytoplasmic clearing. **D:** Enlarged glands in sclerosing adenosis occupied by apocrine carcinoma. Cytoplasmic clearing is evident.

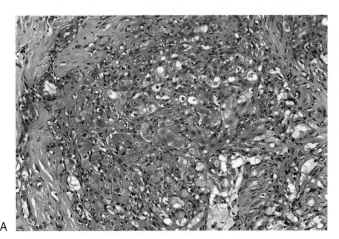
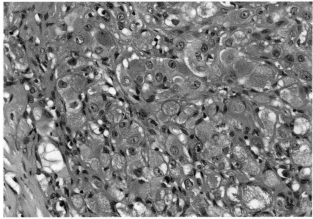

**FIG. 21.6.** *Apocrine carcinoma in sclerosing adenosis.* **A,B:** This unusual lesion features large cells with pleomorphic nuclei and basophilic intracytoplasmic mucin vacuoles.

sional diameter to define a "borderline" group of apocrine lesions (31). Foci with borderline cytologic features were considered to be apocrine intraductal carcinoma if larger than 8 mm. Lesions with cytologic features of carcinoma were termed *apocrine intraductal carcinoma,* regardless of size; but those smaller than 4 mm were referred to as *limited.* Borderline, or atypical, apocrine hyperplasias were proliferative foci smaller than 8 mm with nuclear atypia lacking the characteristic irregular nuclear membranes, coarse chromatin, and large, often multiple nucleoli of apocrine carcinoma (see Chapters 9 and 13).

The 2-mm size criterion of Tavassoli and Norris was described by the authors as "arbitrary" (30), and the 4- to 8-mm criteria of O'Malley et al. was stated by these authors to "require follow-up studies for linkage . . . to clinical outcomes" (31). The precision of such measurements is highly unreliable. A cluster of closely connected duct cross-sections with little intervening stroma could occupy an area smaller than 2 mm, leading to a diagnosis of atypical apocrine hyperplasia on the basis of the 2-mm "rule," whereas the same group of duct sections separated by more stroma would encompass an area greater than 2 mm and qualify as intraductal carcinoma.

The architecture of apocrine intraductal carcinoma is similar to that commonly found in nonapocrine intraductal carcinomas, including comedo, micropapillary, solid, and cribriform patterns (Figs. 21.7–21.10). Calcifications may be seen in the affected ducts. Periductal fibrosis and inflammation are common reactive changes around the ducts. "Foamy" histiocytes may be a prominent feature of the reactive process (32). They should not be mistaken for invasive carcinoma cells. In some cases, intraductal apocrine carcinoma arises in complex papillary lesions in which there is also a benign hyperplastic component. In one instance, a 4-cm cystic papillary apocrine intraductal carcinoma manifested with skin ulceration (33).

Extension of intraductal apocrine carcinoma into the epithelium of lobules is frequently present in these lesions

(Fig. 21.11). Apocrine intraductal carcinoma growing extensively in sclerosing adenosis may simulate an invasive carcinoma, an issue usually resolved by immunostains for actin and cytokeratin performed individually or in combination (13).

Cytologic features that characterize intraductal and invasive apocrine carcinomas are manifested in the nuclei and in the cytoplasm. Nuclear grade can be determined within the spectrum of cytologic features found in apocrine carcinoma. The nuclei are enlarged and pleomorphic compared with the nuclei of benign apocrine cells. They contain nucleoli that are typically prominent and usually eosinophilic, although they occasionally exhibit basophilia. Nuclear membranes tend to be hyperchromatic and irregular. Low-grade nuclei are usually darker with more dense chromatin and slightly pleomorphic compared with nuclei in benign apocrine lesions. Nucleoli are variably present and are not conspicuous (Fig. 21.7). High nuclear grade features have diverse appearances (Figs. 21.9 and 21.12). Nuclei are strikingly enlarged with one or more macronucleoli. Other apocrine carcinomas with high nuclear grade have pleomorphic, deeply basophilic nuclei in which little or no internal structure can be discerned; in other instances, the chromatin is coarse. In these cells, nucleoli usually are obscured by the dense hyperchromatic chromatin.

In most cases, the cytoplasm exhibits eosinophilia that may be homogeneous or granular. Cytoplasmic vacuolization or clearing are features associated with atypical apocrine proliferations, and they are usually most prominent in apocrine carcinomas. Some apocrine carcinomas, especially the clear cell variant, attract an intense lymphocytic or lymphoplasmacytic reaction (Fig. 21.13). The cytologic features of such a lesion may suggest that the tumor is metastatic, possibly in a lymph node, from a renal carcinoma. Rarely, the mononuclear infiltrate may obscure the carcinoma, especially when there is an accompanying granulomatous reaction. An immunohistochemical stain for cytokeratin can be

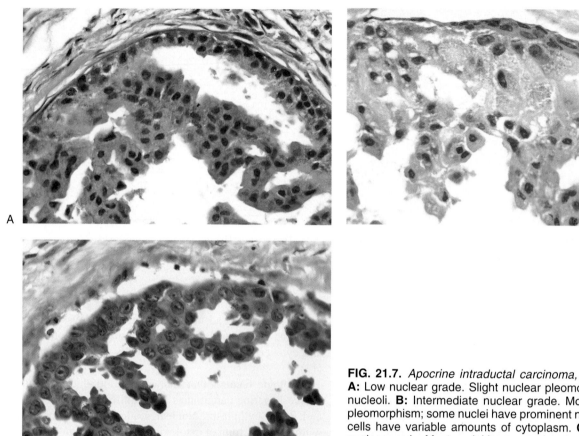

**FIG. 21.7.** *Apocrine intraductal carcinoma, micropapillary.*
**A:** Low nuclear grade. Slight nuclear pleomorphism and no nucleoli. **B:** Intermediate nuclear grade. Moderate nuclear pleomorphism; some nuclei have prominent nucleoli, and the cells have variable amounts of cytoplasm. **C:** Intermediate nuclear grade. Most nuclei have prominent, pleomorphic nucleoli.

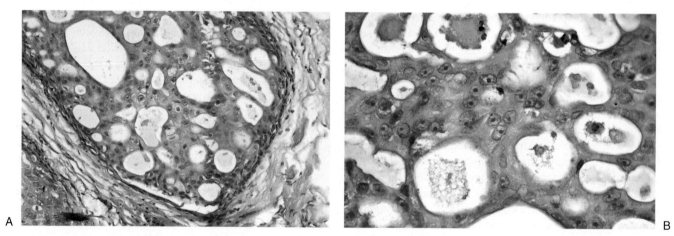

**FIG. 21.8.** *Apocrine intraductal carcinoma, cribriform.* **A,B:** Intermediate nuclear grade. Some nuclei have prominent nucleoli.

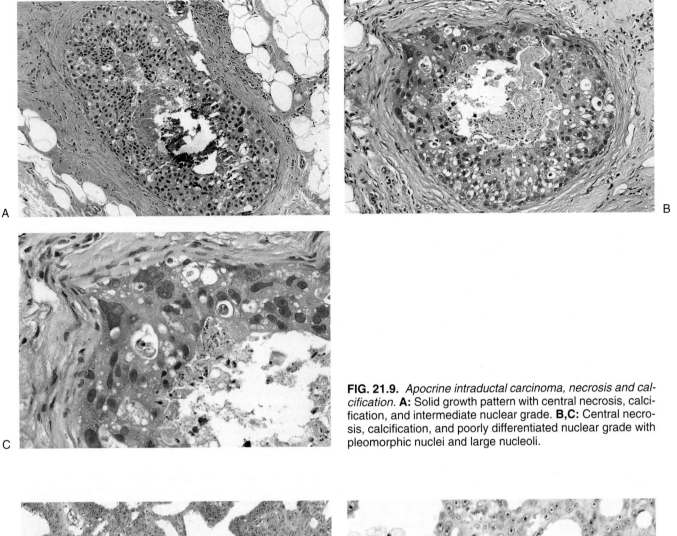

**FIG. 21.9.** *Apocrine intraductal carcinoma, necrosis and cal-cification.* **A:** Solid growth pattern with central necrosis, calci-fication, and intermediate nuclear grade. **B,C:** Central necro-sis, calcification, and poorly differentiated nuclear grade with pleomorphic nuclei and large nucleoli.

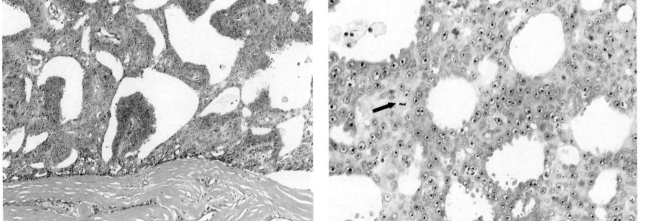

**FIG. 21.10.** *Apocrine carcinoma, cystic papillary type.* **A:** Papillary fronds of papillary apocrine carci-noma are shown attached to the wall of the cystic tumor. **B:** A cribriform area in the papillary carcinoma. The *arrow* indicates a mitotic figure.

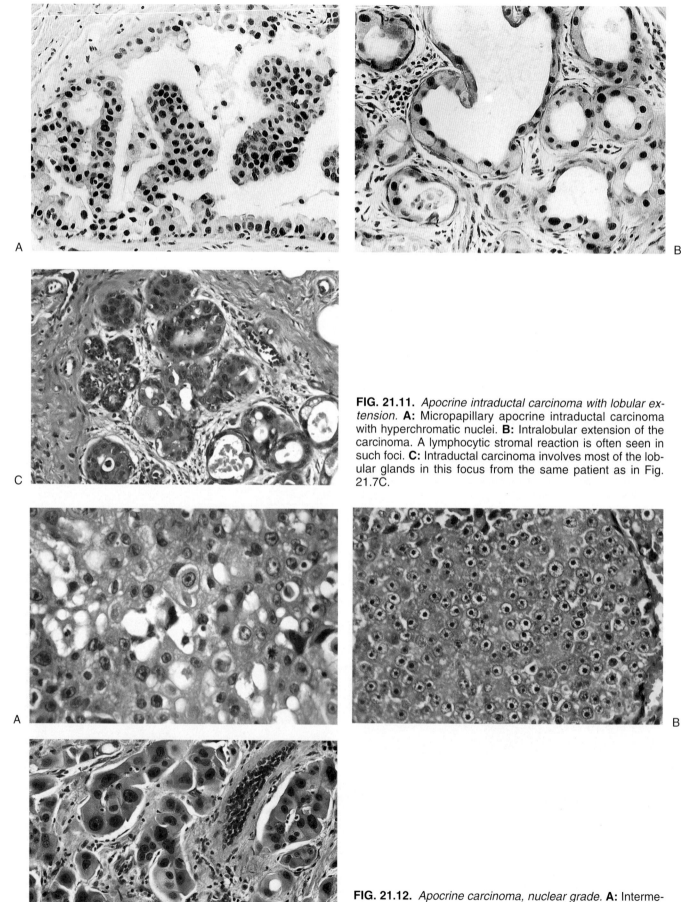

**FIG. 21.11.** *Apocrine intraductal carcinoma with lobular extension.* **A:** Micropapillary apocrine intraductal carcinoma with hyperchromatic nuclei. **B:** Intralobular extension of the carcinoma. A lymphocytic stromal reaction is often seen in such foci. **C:** Intraductal carcinoma involves most of the lobular glands in this focus from the same patient as in Fig. 21.7C.

**FIG. 21.12.** *Apocrine carcinoma, nuclear grade.* **A:** Intermediate nuclear grade. Nuclei and nucleoli are generally round and variable in size. **B:** High nuclear grade with large nucleoli. **C:** High nuclear grade large hyperchromatic pleomorphic nuclei. Dense chromatin obscures nucleoli.

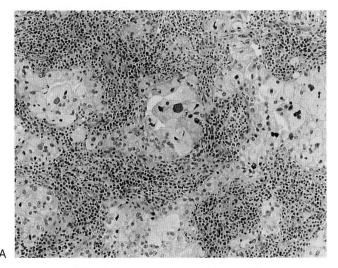
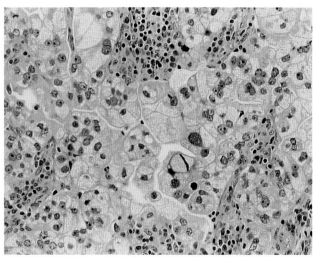

A

B

**FIG. 21.13.** *Apocrine carcinoma with lymphocytic reaction.* **A:** Islands of infiltrating apocrine carcinoma surrounded by a lymphoplasmacytic infiltrate. **B:** The carcinoma cells have pleomorphic nuclei and abundant finely granular cytoplasm.

used to highlight the presence of epithelial elements in such tumors (Fig. 21.14). The apocrine character of these lesions can be established by immunohistochemistry and electron microscopy, but in most instances the presence of an *in situ* component is sufficient to make a diagnosis of mammary carcinoma.

Infiltrating apocrine carcinomas may have any of the usual growth patterns of infiltrating duct carcinoma, but they

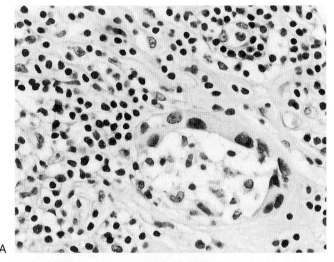
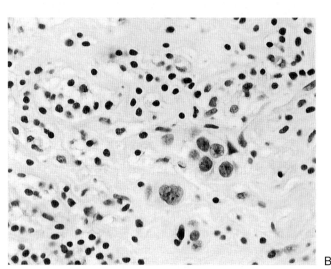

A

B

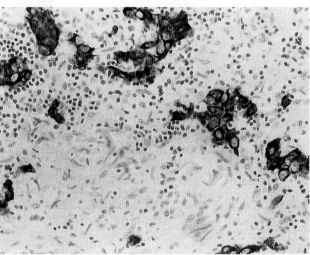

C

**FIG. 21.14.** *Apocrine carcinoma with a granulomatous reaction.* **A:** A lymphocytic reaction is present around a carcinomatous gland. **B:** A cluster of carcinoma cells is shown in the reactive background. **C:** Carcinoma cells immunoreactive for cytokeratin are highlighted in the inflammatory reaction. A granuloma is shown in the lower part of the picture (anti-CAM5.2, avidin-biotin).

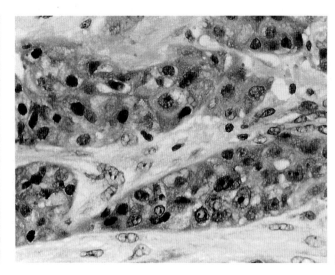

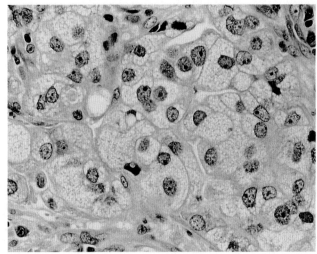

FIG. 21.15. *Apocrine carcinoma, infiltrating.* **A:** A gland-forming pattern in which some carcinoma cells have prominent nucleoli. **B:** Trabecular carcinoma with pleomorphic nuclei and vacuolated cytoplasm. **C:** Carcinoma with solid growth composed of large cells with finely granular pale cytoplasm.

tend to be structurally poorly differentiated (Figs. 21.12 and 21.15). An uncommon variant of invasive solid histiocytoid apocrine carcinoma is composed of large polygonal cells with abundant foamy or eosinophilic cytoplasm (Fig. 21.16) (34). The presence of GGDFP has been demonstrated in these lesions by immunohistochemistry and by *in situ* hybridization (34). There is insufficient follow-up information to define the prognosis of this type of apocrine carcinoma. Invasive apocrine carcinoma in dense collagenous stroma may be difficult to identify and could be mistaken for a granular cell tumor (Fig. 21.17).

There is evidence that invasive apocrine carcinomas are prone to develop lymphatic tumor emboli. A review of patients with recurrent mammary carcinoma that grew in an inflammatory pattern at the time of recurrence revealed that a substantial proportion (33%) of the primary tumors were apocrine carcinomas (35). When examined retrospectively, most of the primary lesions also had peritumoral lymphatic tumor emboli. These data were biased somewhat by the fact that the study was undertaken initially to examine inflammatory carcinoma patients, but it is notable that apocrine carcinoma, an uncommon tumor, was relatively more frequent

than expected among patients who experienced recurrent carcinoma with an inflammatory pattern.

Others also have commented on vascular or lymphatic invasion in apocrine carcinoma. This feature was not specifically studied in the series of 19 apocrine carcinomas de-

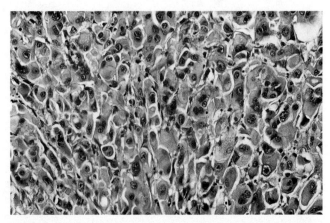

FIG. 21.16. *Apocrine carcinoma, histiocytoid.* Large, poorly cohesive tumor cells with abundant dense cytoplasm and darkly stained pleomorphic nuclei.

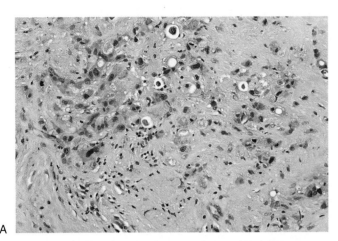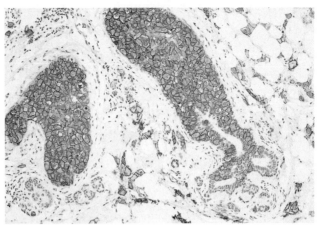

**FIG. 21.17.** *Apocrine carcinoma, invasive.* **A:** The carcinoma cells are obscured by the collagenous stroma. **B:** Solid intraductal carcinoma as well as the surrounding invasive carcinoma exhibited strong membrane reactivity for HER2/*neu* (avidin-biotin).

scribed by Frable and Kay, but they noted vascular invasion in one tumor (18). D'Amore et al. found dermal invasion in 7 of 34 (21%) of their cases, and in four (12%), associated lymphatic invasion was found within the breast (36). Matsuo et al. detected lymphatic tumor emboli in three of eight (38%) invasive apocrine carcinomas (13).

## CYTOLOGY

The finding of atypical apocrine cells in a fine needle aspirate may suggest a diagnosis of apocrine carcinoma (37). Specimens obtained from apocrine carcinoma tend to be highly cellular with marked nuclear pleomorphism, large nucleoli, and cellular debris (38); however, caution should be exercised in the evaluation of such findings, especially when the aspirate is obtained from a mammographically detected nonpalpable lesion. Apocrine metaplasia in sclerosing adenosis and radial scars, which are likely to be identified in this fashion, may be cytologically atypical (29).

## ELECTRON MICROSCOPY, IMMUNOHISTOCHEMISTRY, AND MOLECULAR PATHOLOGY

At the ultrastructural level, the cells of apocrine carcinoma contain abundant organelles, including mitochondria varying in size (39) and often having incomplete cristae and varying numbers of osmiophilic secretory granules (10,12,14). Many tumor cells also contain empty vesicles of about the same size as the osmiophilic granules.

Immunohistochemical studies may be used to confirm the diagnostic impression of apocrine differentiation in some cases, but they are usually not essential to establish the diagnosis of apocrine carcinoma. Cutaneous and mammary apocrine carcinomas have similar immunohistochemical features. In most cases, the tumor cells contain diastase-resistant periodic acid-Schiff–positive granules, which are also stained with toluidine blue and appear red with the trichrome stain. Cytoplasmic iron granules, a feature of benign apocrine cells, are variably present in apocrine carcinomas. Occasional cells may contain mucicarmine-positive secretion, but most tumors are negative for mucin and alphalactalbumin (40,41). In exceptional cases, there can be extensive intracytoplasmic mucin accumulation, resulting in numerous, sometimes substantially enlarged signet-ring-type cells (Fig. 21.18).

Apocrine carcinomas tend to be immunoreactive for carcinoembryonic antigen (CEA) (32). They are usually negative for S-100 and are always reactive for cytokeratins. Benign and malignant apocrine cells are strongly immunoreactive for prolactin-inducible protein (PIP)/GCDFP-15. GCDFP-15 was detected in 55% of carcinomas, including 75% of those with apocrine histologic features, 70% of intraductal carcinomas, and 90% of infiltrating lobular carcinomas that had signet-ring cell features (12,14). Positive GCDFP-15 staining was found in only 23% of carcinomas that did not have apocrine features and in 5% of medullary carcinomas. PIP/GCDFP-15 mRNA detected by *in situ* hybridization is a more precise method for establishing apocrine differentiation than is immunohistochemistry (42,43). Immunostaining for GCDFP-15 has not been a useful predictor of prognosis (44).

Zinc alpha 2-glycoprotein is a marker of apocrine differentiation detectable by immunohistochemistry (45). Using a polyclonal rabbit antibody, Bundred et al. (46) found that 36% of carcinomas were positive, with most nonreactive (45%) or minimally reactive (19%). Immunoreactivity for this manifestation of apocrine differentiation was not significantly correlated with tumor size, nodal status, grade, or hormone receptor expression in the carcinoma; however, carcinomas with zinc alpha 2-glycoprotein expression had a significantly reduced survival and disease-free interval. It is unfortunate that the authors did not report on the correlation between zinc alpha 2-glycoprotein immunoreactivity and the expression of apocrine differentiation as described by conventional histological criteria.

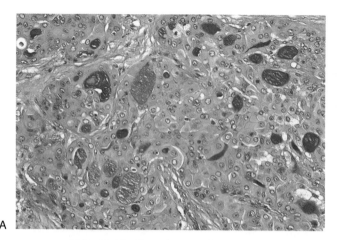
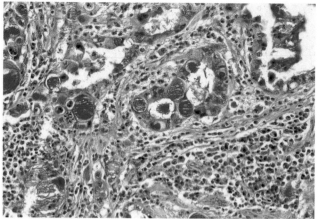

A

B

**FIG. 21.18.** *Apocrine carcinoma with mucin.* **A:** Prominent basophilic mucin in present in glandular spaces and in tumor cells. **B:** Intracytoplasmic mucin is stained magenta with the mucicarmine stain in this gland-forming invasive apocrine carcinoma.

Benign proliferative apocrine lesions almost always express androgen receptors, which are detectable by immunohistochemistry (47). Conversely, benign apocrine lesions are typically negative for ERs and PRs. The distribution of androgen receptors in apocrine carcinomas has not been well characterized.

Compared with benign apocrine proliferative lesions, apocrine carcinomas have been more frequently Ki67 positive and have a significantly higher Ki67 labeling index (48). Reactivity for p53 was demonstrated in 68.2% of apocrine carcinomas but not in any benign apocrine proliferation. Carcinomas with poorly differentiated nuclear grade were more likely to be p53 positive. There was a lower frequency of p53 reactivity in invasive than in intraductal carcinomas. Moriya et al. also reported finding reactivity for p21 and p27 in 36.8% and 66.7%, respectively, of benign apocrine lesions and in 63.6% and 52.4% of carcinomas (48).

A study of microdissected apocrine lesions revealed loss of heterozygosity (LOH) in about a third of the samples of apocrine carcinoma at one of several marker sites, including VHL (3p25.5), TP53(17p13), NB(1p35-36), and TSC2/PKD/(16p13) (49). LOH was detected in 36%, 33%, 32%, and 30% of cases, respectively, at these loci. LOH occurred more frequently in invasive than in intraductal lesions. No LOH was found in apocrine hyperplasias.

## TREATMENT AND PROGNOSIS

Several investigators have examined the prognosis of apocrine mammary carcinoma. Lee et al. (4) reviewed 81 patients treated for "sweat gland" carcinoma and concluded that they did not differ clinically or in prognosis from "the general group of mammary cancers." Frable and Kay (18) compared 18 apocrine carcinoma patients with 34 matched controls and found no significant differences in survival between the two groups. A similar approach was used by d'Amore et al. in an analysis of 34 cases (36) and by Abati et al. (27) who investigated 17 women with invasive apocrine

carcinoma. Both of the latter series revealed no statistically significant differences between apocrine and nonapocrine cases in recurrence free or in overall survival (Fig. 21.19).

Patients with intraductal apocrine carcinoma have generally had the same clinical course as women with nonapocrine intraductal carcinoma. In one study (27), 33 of 55 (60%) patients were treated by mastectomy, whereas 22 (40%) had only an excisional biopsy. Recurrences occurred in the breast in three of 20 (15%) who had excisional biopsies alone but not in two others who had excision and radiotherapy. When treated by mastectomy, one patient whose lesion appeared to be entirely intraductal had axillary metastases at the time of mastectomy and later died of systemic disease. All other patients with apocrine intraductal carcinoma remained disease free at last follow-up.

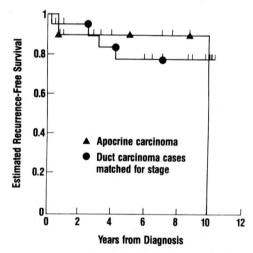

**FIG. 21.19.** *Apocrine carcinoma, survival analysis.* Compared with patients with duct carcinomas matched for stage, women with apocrine carcinoma do not have a significantly different recurrence-free survival. (From Abati AD, Kimmel M, Rosen PP. Apocrine mammary carcinoma: a clinicopathologic study of 72 patients. *Am J Clin Pathol* 1990;94:371–377, with permission.)

The prognosis of apocrine carcinoma, whether intraductal or invasive, is determined mainly by conventional prognostic factors such as grade, tumor size, and nodal status (4,18, 27,36). Apocrine differentiation should be mentioned as a descriptive feature of the lesion, but presently it does not seem to be an important determinant of prognosis or of treatment. Biopsies of the conserved breast after radiotherapy are difficult to interpret in women with apocrine carcinoma because the treatment results in severe cytologic changes that resemble apocrine carcinoma in nonneoplastic apocrine epithelium. The observation that androgen metabolism is altered in apocrine carcinoma cells may prove therapeutically useful in the future.

# REFERENCES

1. Nishikawa Y, Tokusashi Y, Saito Y, et al. A case of apocrine adenocarcinoma associated with hamartomatous apocrine gland hyperplasia of both axillae. *Am J Surg Pathol* 1994;18:832–836.
2. Patie C, Taccagni GL, Papotti M, et al. Apocrine carcinoma of the skin: a clinicopathologic, immunocytochemical and ultrastructural study. *Cancer* 1993;71:375–381.
3. Pelosi G, Martignoni G, Bonetti F. Intraductal carcinoma of mammary-type apocrine epithelium arising within a papillary hydradenoma of the vulva. *Arch Pathol Lab Med* 1991;115:1249–1254.
4. Lee BJ, Pack GT, Scharnagel I. Sweat gland cancer of the breast. *Surg Gynecol Obstet* 1933;54:975–996.
5. Hamperl H. The so-called sweat gland carcinoma of the human breast: a review. *Z Krebsforsch* 1977;88:105–199.
6. Damiani S, Eusebi V, Losi L, et al. Oncocytic carcinoma (malignant oncocytoma) of the breast. *Am J Surg Pathol* 1998;22:221–230.
7. Viacava P, Naccarato AG, Bevilacqua G. Apocrine epithelium of the breast: does it result from metaplasia? *Virchows Arch* 1997;431:205–209.
8. Foote FW Jr, Stewart FW. A histologic classification of carcinoma of the breast. *Surgery* 1946;19:74–99.
9. Higginson JF, McDonald JR. Apocrine tissue, chronic cystic mastitis and sweat gland carcinoma of the breast. *Surg Gynecol Obstet* 1949;88:1–10.
10. Yates AJ, Ahmed A. Apocrine carcinoma and apocrine metaplasia. *Histopathology* 1988;13:228–231.
11. Shivas AA, Hunt CT. Cultural characteristics of an apocrine variant of human mammary carcinoma. *Clin Oncol* 1979;5:299–303.
12. Mossler J, Barton TK, Brinkhous AD, et al. Apocrine differentiation in human mammary carcinoma. *Cancer* 1980;46:2463–2471.
13. Matsuo K, Fukutomi T, Tsuda H, et al. Apocrine carcinoma of the breast: clinicopathological analysis and histological subclassification of 12 cases. *Breast Cancer* 1998;5:279–284.
14. Eusebi V, Betts C, Haagensen DE, et al. Apocrine differentiation in lobular carcinoma of the breast: a morphologic, immunologic and ultrastructural study. *Hum Pathol* 1984;15:134–140.
15. Walford N, Velden JT. Histiocytoid breast carcinoma: an apocrine variant of lobular carcinoma. *Histopathology* 1989;14:515–522.
16. Gilles R, Lasnik A, Guinebretière J-M, et al. Apocrine carcinoma: clinical and mammographic features. *Radiology* 1994;190:495–497.
17. Kopans DB, Nguyen PL, Koerner FC, et al. Mixed form, diffusely scattered calcifications in breast cancer with apocrine features. *Radiology* 1990;177:807–811.
18. Frable WJ, Kay S. Carcinoma of the breast: histologic and clinical features of apocrine tumors. *Cancer* 1968;21:56–763.
19. Schmitt FC, Soares R, Seruca R. Bilateral apocrine carcinoma of the breast. Molecular and immunocytochemical evidence for two independent primary tumours. *Virchows Arch* 1998;433:505–509.
20. Miller WR, Telford J, Dixon JM, et al. Androgen metabolism and apocrine differentiation in human breast cancer. *Breast Cancer Res Treat* 1985;5:67–73.
21. Tavassoli FA, Purcell CA, Bratthauer GL, et al. Androgen receptor expression along with loss of bcl-2, ER, and PR expression in benign and malignant apocrine lesions of the breast: implications for therapy. *Breast J* 1996;2:261–269.
22. Wales NAM, Ebling FJ. The control of apocrine glands of the rabbit by steroid hormones. *J Endocrinol* 1971;51:763–770.
23. Labows JN, Preti G, Hoelzle E, et al. Steroid analysis of human apocrine secretion. *Steroids* 1979;34:249–258.
24. DePotter CR, Pratt MM, Slavin RE, et al. Feulgen DNA content and mitotic activity in proliferative breast disease: a comparison with ductal carcinoma *in situ*. *Histopathology* 1987;11:1307–1319.
25. Raju U, Zarbo RJ, Kubus J, et al. The histologic spectrum of apocrine breast proliferations: a comparative study of morphology and DNA content by image analysis. *Hum Pathol* 1993;24:173–181.
26. Bryant J. Male breast cancer: a case of apocrine carcinoma with psammoma bodies. *Hum Pathol* 1981;12:751–753.
27. Abati AD, Kimmel M, Rosen PP. Apocrine mammary carcinoma: a clinicopathologic study of 72 patients. *Am J Clin Pathol* 1990; 94:371–377.
28. Burt AD, Seywright MM, George WD. Mixed apocrine-medullary carcinoma of the breast. *Acta Cytol* 1987;31:322–324.
29. Carter D, Rosen PP. Atypical apocrine metaplasia in sclerosing lesions of the beast: a study of 51 patients. *Mod Pathol* 1991;4:1–5.
30. Tavassoli FA, Norris HJ. Intraductal apocrine carcinoma: a clinicopathologic study of 37 cases. *Mod Pathol* 1994;7:813–818.
31. O'Malley FP, Page DL, Nelson EH, et al. Ductal carcinoma in situ of the breast with apocrine cytology: definition of a borderline category. *Hum Pathol* 1994;25:164–168.
32. Shousha S, Bull TB, Southall PJ, et al. Apocrine carcinoma of the breast containing foam cells. An electron microscopic and immunohistochemical study. *Histopathology* 1987;11:611–620.
33. Kenwright DN, Gaskell D, Wakefield L, et al. Apocrine ductal carcinoma in situ of the breast presenting as a chronic abscess. *Aust N Z J Surg* 1998;68:72–75.
34. Eusebi V, Foschini MP, Bussolati G, et al. Myoblastomatoid (histiocytoid) carcinoma of the breast: a type of apocrine carcinoma. *Am J Surg Pathol* 1995;19:553–562.
35. Robbins GF, Shah J, Rosen P, et al. Inflammatory carcinoma of the breast. *Surg Clin North Am* 1974;54:801–810.
36. d'Amore ESG, Terrier-Lacombe MJ, Travagli JP, et al. Invasive apocrine carcinoma of the breast: a long term follow-up study of 34 cases. *Breast Cancer Res Treat* 1988;12:37–44.
37. Johnson TL, Kini SR. The significance of atypical apocrine cells in fine-needle aspirates of the breast. *Diagn Cytopathol* 1989;5:248–254.
38. Yoshida K, Inoue M, Furuta S, et al. Apocrine carcinoma vs. apocrine metaplasia with atypia of the breast. Use of aspiration biopsy cytology. *Acta Cytol* 1996;40:247–251.
39. Roddy HJ, Silverberg SG. Ultrastructural analysis of apocrine carcinoma of the human breast. *Ultrastruct Pathol* 1980;1:385–393.
40. Bussolati G, Cattani MG, Gugliotta P, et al. Morphologic and functional aspects of apocrine metaplasia in dysplastic and neoplastic breast tissue. *Ann NY Acad Sci* 1986;464:262–274.
41. Eisenberg BL, Bagnall JW, Harding CT. Histiocytoid carcinoma—a variant of breast cancer. *J Surg Oncol* 1986;31:271–274.
42. Pagani A, Sapino A, Eusebi V, et al. PIP/GCDFP-15 gene expression and apocrine differentiation in carcinomas of the breast. *Virchows Arch* 1994;425:459–465.
43. Eusebi V, Damiani S, Losi L, et al. Apocrine differentiation in breast epithelium. *Adv Anat Pathol* 1997;4:139–155.
44. Mazoujian G, Bodian C, Haagensen DE Jr, et al. Expression of GCDFP-15 in breast carcinomas: relationship to pathologic and clinical factors. *Cancer* 1989;63:2156–2161.
45. Bundred NJ, Miller WR, Walker RA. An immunohistochemical study of the tissue distribution of the breast cyst fluid protein, zinc alpha 2-glycoprotein. *Histopathology* 1987;11:603–610.
46. Bundred NJ, Walker RA, Everington D, et al. Is apocrine differentiation in breast carcinoma of prognostic significance? *Br J Cancer* 1990;62:113–117.
47. Selim AA, Wells CA. Immunohistochemical localisation of androgen receptor in apocrine metaplasia and apocrine adenosis of the breast: relation to oestrogen and progesterone receptors. *J Clin Pathol* 1999;52:838–841.
48. Moriya T, Sakamoto K, Sasano H, et al. Immunohistochemical analysis of Ki-67, p53, p21, and p27 in benign and malignant apocrine lesions of the breast: its correlation to histologic findings in 43 cases. *Mod Pathol* 2000;13:13–18.
49. Lininger RA, Zhuang Z, Man YG, et al. Loss of heterozygosity is detected in chromosomes 1p35-36(NB), 3p25(VHL), 16p13 (TSC2/PKD1), and 17p13(TP53) in microdissected apocrine carcinomas of the breast. *Mod Pathol* 1999;12:1083–1089.

# CHAPTER 22

# Mammary Carcinoma with Endocrine Features

Some mammary carcinomas are able to synthesize hormones not considered to be normal products of the breast. This capacity to produce ectopic hormones may be considered endocrine or biochemical metaplasia. Such tumors have been found to contain peptide hormones, including human chorionic gonadotrophin (HCG) (1), calcitonin (2), and epinephrine (3). These substances are detectable not only by biochemical analysis but also by immunohistochemical study of the tumor tissue.

In a few unusual instances, the microscopic growth pattern simulates the structure of nonmammary neoplasms that commonly contain the ectopic substance, resulting in coincidence of the biochemical and structural phenotypes. A striking example of this phenomenon is mammary carcinoma with choriocarcinomatous differentiation (1,4). In these mammary carcinomas, areas that microscopically have the appearance of syncytiotrophoblast and cytotrophoblast are strongly reactive for the $\beta$-subunit of HCG. Carcinomas of the breast and other organs that exhibit structural choriocarcinomatous metaplasia have an aggressive clinical course, often resulting in recurrence and death from disease.

Isolated carcinoma cells that are reactive immunohistologically for $\alpha$- and $\beta$-HCG can be found in 5% to 21% of ordinary infiltrating duct carcinomas that do not exhibit choriocarcinomatous metaplasia (5). The reactive cells are otherwise morphologically indistinguishable microscopically from surrounding carcinoma cells that are not immunoreactive for HCG. The presence of these occasional HCG-positive cells does not appear to have prognostic significance, and no functional effects have been described (5).

A more frequent form of biochemical and structural metaplasia occurs in mammary carcinomas that contain argyrophilic cytoplasmic granules detected by light microscopy. The procedures most commonly used to demonstrate argyrophilic granules rely on reactions in which ammoniacal silver is reduced to particulate metallic silver that can be visualized with the light microscope (6). Argentaffin granules, typically found in midgut carcinoid tumors, contain endogenous-reducing substances. In the argyrophil reaction (e.g., Grimelius stain), an exogenous reducing agent is added be-

cause some granules do not contain endogenous reducing substances. Because most cells with either argentaffin or argyrophilic granules are visualized with the argyrophil reaction, this is the preferable procedure. Breast neoplasms that contain argyrophilic granules have been argentaffin-negative (7,8). Argyrophilic mammary carcinomas are a heterogeneous group of neoplasms that have been referred to as *mammary carcinomas* with endocrine features. This term also has been applied to carcinomas with an endocrine growth pattern, even when argyrophilic granules were not demonstrable.

The reported frequency of argyrophilia in female mammary carcinomas varies from 3% to 25% (9). No systematic study of the frequency of argyrophilic granules in male breast carcinomas has been reported, but a few descriptions of argyrophil-positive tumors in men have been published (10).

## CLINICAL PRESENTATION

There are no specific clinical features associated with mammary carcinomas that exhibit structural or histochemical evidence of endocrine differentiation. Because most of the lesions are invasive carcinomas, most patients present with a palpable tumor. The tumors may be detected in any part of the breast, but the most common location is the upper outer quadrant. Systemic evidence of ectopic hormonal secretion has been absent in all but a few cases of patients described as having symptoms attributable to ectopic adrenocorticotrophic hormone (ACTH) (11), parathormone (12), calcitonin (2), and epinephrine (3) produced by breast carcinomas.

Argyrophilia has been identified in breast carcinomas throughout the age distribution of the disease, ranging from patients in their early thirties to women in their late eighties (7,13,14). Men with argyrophilic carcinomas have been 71 to 83 years old.

## GROSS PATHOLOGY

Argyrophilic mammary carcinomas have not exhibited specific gross pathologic features (Fig. 22.1). The invasive

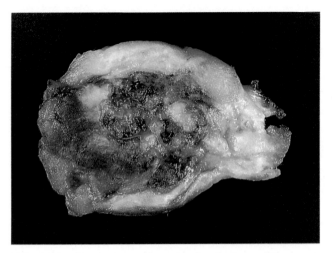

**FIG. 22.1.** *Carcinoma with endocrine features.* The carcinoma is a circumscribed mass with focal hemorrhage probably resulting from a prior surgical biopsy.

tumors generally measure 1 to 5 cm in diameter, with most between 1.5 and 3.0 cm. The tumors are likely to be grossly circumscribed, and rarely multiple foci of carcinoma were described in the breast.

## MICROSCOPIC PATHOLOGY

Many of the tumors are infiltrating duct carcinomas, with varying degrees of differentiation (Figs. 22.2 and 22.3). Argyrophilic cells can be found in the intraductal as well as the invasive portion of these tumors (8,14), and in metastatic deposits originating from such tumors. Argyrophilic intraductal carcinomas tend to have a distinctive solid papillary or organoid growth pattern (8,15), whereas conventional cribriform and comedo intraductal carcinomas are typically nonargyrophilic (15). Neurosecretory granules can be detected in some tumors by electron microscopy (7,16,17).

In several studies, the proportion of invasive mucinous

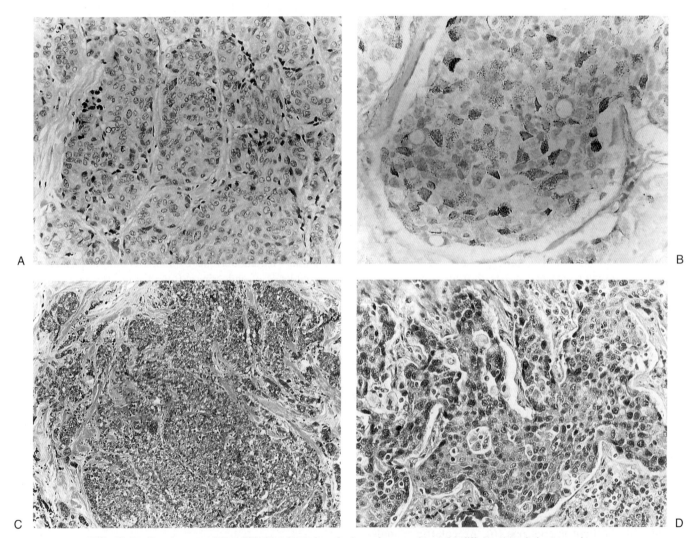

**FIG. 22.2.** *Carcinoma with endocrine features.* **A:** Invasive moderately differentiated duct carcinoma with an alveolar growth pattern. **B:** The Grimelius stain reveals fine black granules in the cytoplasm of carcinoma cells. **C:** Poorly differentiated invasive duct carcinoma that was strongly Grimelius positive is shown. **D:** The tumor cells in **C** have dense, finely granular cytoplasm.

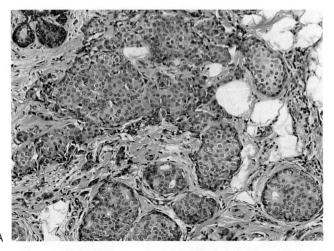

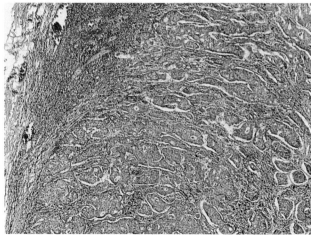

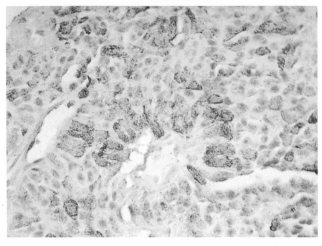

FIG. 22.3. *Carcinoma with endocrine features.* **A:** Moderately differentiated invasive duct carcinoma with small, round nuclei and characteristic deeply staining cytoplasm. **B:** Metastatic carcinoma in an axillary lymph node with an endocrine growth pattern and stroma with hemosiderin. **C:** A positive Grimelius reaction in the carcinoma shown in **A**.

carcinomas with argyrophilia ranged from 8% to 80% (7,16,18). The reported frequency of argyrophilic infiltrating duct carcinomas varied from 15% (7) to 71% (17), and, among infiltrating lobular carcinomas, 50% (7) to 100% (17) have reportedly been argyrophilic. Carcinomas with neuroendocrine differentiation rarely have areas that resemble Merkel's cell carcinoma, expressing immunoreactivity for cytokeratin, synaptophysin, chromogranin A, calcitonin, and neuron-specific enolase (19).

Some argyrophilic carcinomas have endocrine growth patterns that resemble carcinoid tumors originating in other organs (Fig. 22.4). Recognition of this structural similarity led to a search for argyrophilic granules in mammary carcinomas. The term *primary carcinoid tumor of the breast* was introduced in 1977 by Cubilla and Woodruff to characterize a group of neoplasms that they regarded as "a new pathologic entity" (14). Although they failed to detect argyrophilic granules in normal breast epithelium, Cubilla and Woodruff concluded that the primary mammary carcinoid was a neuroendocrine neoplasm of the breast derived from argyrophil cells of neural crest origin, presumed to have migrated to mammary ducts. This concept has not been substantiated by other investigators, and the term *primary carcinoid tumor of the breast* is no longer used.

Not all carcinomas with an endocrine growth pattern contain argyrophilic cells, and it has not been possible to demonstrate polypeptide hormones or biogenic amines in most argyrophilic carcinomas (7,16,20). Some argyrophilic mammary carcinomas are microscopically indistinguishable from argyrophil-negative mammary carcinomas. Despite the efforts of many investigators to find progenitor argyrophilic cells in normal mammary duct epithelium, such cells have rarely been detected, and then only in small numbers, leaving doubt as to the specificity of these observations (18,21,22). No neuroendocrine cells were detected in human fetal and adult breasts studied by immunohistochemistry and electron microscopy (23).

Sapino et al. studied the cytologic features of mammary carcinomas with neuroendocrine differentiation (24). The tumors were characterized by cell clusters with rigid borders, isolated cells with a plasmacytoid appearance, and peripheral chromogranin-positive cytoplasmic granules, which were demonstrated using the Giemsa stain. Neuroendocrine carcinomas with mucinous differentiation exhibited less cytoplasmic granularity.

In 1982, Clayton et al. reported that most argyrophilic carcinomas they studied were also reactive for lactalbumin (20). Intracytoplasmic localization of argyrophilia and

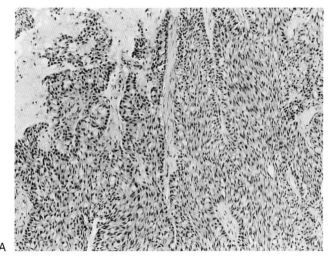

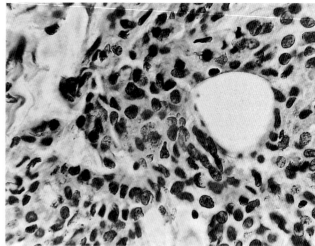

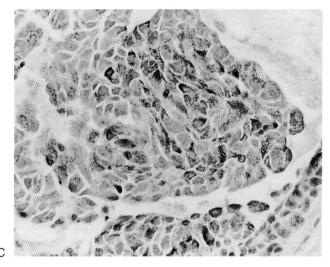

**FIG. 22.4.** *Carcinoma with endocrine features.* **A:** This invasive duct carcinoma has an endocrine growth pattern that includes signet-ring cells and spindle-shaped nuclei. **B:** The carcinoma cells are cytologically low grade. **C:** Fine black granules in the cytoplasm are shown; these are indicative of a positive Grimelius reaction.

lactalbumin showed a similar tendency to apical cytoplasmic staining in carcinomas as well as in lactating breast tissue. They concluded that argyrophilia might be evidence of lactational differentiation because "the secretory granules appear to contain milk secretory product rather than neuroendocrine polypeptides." This conclusion was later rejected by Bussolati et al., who reported that the apparent immunoreactivity for α-lactalbumin found in argyrophilic carcinomas by Clayton et al. and others was the result of a contaminant in the antibody preparation that had an affinity for endocrine cells (25).

The foregoing observations led most investigators to conclude that neoplasms with argyrophilic granules do not constitute a specific histopathologic category of mammary carcinoma. Although the idea of a primary mammary carcinoid tumor now has been largely discredited, it is apparent that there is a group of mammary carcinomas capable of producing ectopic endocrine substances and that some mammary carcinomas also have a neuroendocrine phenotype histologically.

It is also important to recognize that metastases in the breast from a carcinoid that arose at another site might be mistaken for a primary mammary tumor (26,27). The finding of an *in situ* component provides convincing evidence of breast origin.

## PROGNOSIS AND TREATMENT

When they are recognized, argyrophilic breast tumors should be diagnosed as *mammary carcinomas with endocrine features.* If ectopic hormones are detected, they should be specified as, for example, *infiltrating duct carcinoma with endocrine features, argyrophil- and ACTH-positive.* The recognition of these tumors is necessary to define more fully their clinical characteristics. Although it appears that the stage at diagnosis is the major determinant of prognosis, there have been no case-controlled studies comparing patients who have mammary carcinoma with endocrine differentiation to age- and stage-matched control groups. In one study, patients with argyrophilic mucinous carcinomas were more likely to have axillary nodal metastases (48%) than those with Grimelius-negative tumors (26%), and they also had a higher frequency of recurrence and death from breast carcinoma (65% versus 33%) (28).

Currently, it appears that the choice of primary treatment for mammary carcinomas with endocrine features should be determined by conventional clinical and pathologic criteria. Until further information becomes available, neither ectopic hormone production nor endocrine differentiation have been proven to be factors that critically influence the prognosis or treatment of patients with mammary carcinoma.

## REFERENCES

1. Saigo PE, Rosen PP. Mammary carcinoma with "choriocarcinomatous" features. *Am J Surg Pathol* 1981;5:773–778.
2. Coombes RC, Easty GC, Detre SI, et al. Secretion of immunoreactive calcitonin by human breast carcinomas. *BMJ* 1975;4:197–199.
3. Kaneko H, Hojo H, Ishikawa S, et al. Norepinephrine-producing tumors of bilateral breasts: a case report. *Cancer* 1978;41:2002–2007.
4. Green DM. Mucoid carcinoma of the breast with choriocarcinoma in its metastases. *Histopathology* 1990;16:504–506.
5. Lee AK, Rosen PP, DeLellis RA, et al. Tumor marker expression in breast carcinomas and relationship to prognosis: an immunohistochemical study. *Am J Clin Pathol* 1985;84:687–696.
6. Smith DM Jr, Haggitt RC. A comparative study of generic stains for carcinoid secretory granules. *Am J Surg Pathol* 1983;7:61–63.
7. Fetissof F, Dubois MP, Arbeille-Brassart B, et al. Argyrophilic cells in mammary carcinoma. *Hum Pathol* 1983;14:127–134.
8. Partanen S, Syrjanen J. Argyrophilic cells in carcinoma of the female breast. *Virchows Arch* 1981;391:45–51.
9. Nesland JM, Holm R, Johannessen JV. A study of different markers for neuroendocrine differentiation in breast carcinomas. *Pathol Res Pract* 1986;181:524–530.
10. Gill IS. Carcinoid tumour of the male breast. *J R Soc Med* 1990;83:401.
11. Woodard BH, Eisenbarth G, Wallace NR, et al. Adrenocorticotropin production by a mammary carcinoma. *Cancer* 1981;47:1823–1827.
12. Mavligit GM, Cohen JL, Sherwood LM. Ectopic production of parathyroid hormone by carcinoma of the breast. *N Engl J Med* 1971;285:154–156.
13. Azzopardi JG, Muretto P, Goddeeris P, et al. Carcinoid tumors of the breast: the morphological spectrum of argyrophil carcinomas. *Histopathology* 1982;6:549–569.
14. Cubilla AL, Woodruff JM. Primary carcinoid tumor of the breast: A report of eight patients. *Am J Surg Pathol* 1977;1:283–292.
15. Cross AS, Azzopardi JG, Krausz T, et al. A morphological and immunocytochemical study of a distinctive variant of ductal carcinoma in situ of the breast. *Histopathology* 1985;9:21–37.
16. Min K-W. Argyrophilia in breast carcinomas: histochemical, ultrastructural and immunocytochemical study. *Lab Invest* 1983;48:58A–59A.
17. Nesland JM, Memoli VA, Holm R, et al. Breast carcinomas with neuroendocrine differentiation. *Ultrastruct Pathol* 1985;8:225–240.
18. Fisher ER, Palekar AS. Solid and mucinous varieties of so-called mammary carcinoid tumors. *Am J Clin Pathol* 1979;72:909–916.
19. Fukunaga M. Neuroendocrine carcinoma of the breast with Merkel cell carcinoma-like features. *Pathol Int* 1998;48:557–561.
20. Clayton F, Sibley RK, Ordonez NG, et al. Argyrophilic breast carcinomas: evidence of lactational differentiation. *Am J Surg Pathol* 1982;6:323–333.
21. Bussolati G, Gugliotta P, Sapino A, et al. Chromogranin-reactive endocrine cells in argyrophilic carcinomas ("carcinoids") and normal tissue of the breast. *Am J Pathol* 1985;120:186–192.
22. Feyrter F, Hartmann G. Uber die carcinoide wachsform des Carcinoma mammae, inbesondere das Carcinoma solidum (gelatinosum) mammae. *Frankf Z Pathol* 1963;73:24–35.
23. Viacava P, Castagna M, Bevilacqua G. Absence of neuroendocrine cells in fetal and adult mammary gland: are neuroendocrine breast tumours real neuroendocrine tumours? *The Breast* 1995;4:143–146.
24. Sapino A, Papotti M, Pietribiasi F, et al. Diagnostic cytological features of neuroendocrine differentiated carcinoma of the breast. *Virchows Arch* 1998;433:217–222.
25. Bussolati G, Papotti M, Sapino A, et al. Endocrine markers in argyrophilic carcinomas of the breast. *Am J Surg Pathol* 1987;11:248–256.
26. Kashlan RB, Powell RW, Nolting SF. Carcinoid and other tumors metastatic to the breast. *J Surg Oncol* 1982;20:25–30.
27. Ordonez NG, Manning JT Jr, Raymond K. Argentaffin endocrine carcinoma (carcinoid) of the pancreas with concomitant breast metastasis: an immunohistochemical and electron microscopic study. *Hum Pathol* 1985;16:746–751.
28. Rasmussen BB, Rose C, Thorpe SM, et al. Argyrophilic cells in 202 human mucinous breast carcinomas: relation to histopathologic and clinical features. *Am J Clin Pathol* 1985;84:737–740.

# CHAPTER 23

# Small Cell (Oat Cell) Carcinoma

Carcinomas that resemble oat cell carcinoma of the lung can occur in extrapulmonary sites (1). Small cell (oat cell) carcinoma is one of the most uncommon variants of breast carcinoma. The diagnosis of primary small cell mammary carcinoma can be made with confidence only if a nonmammary site is excluded clinically or if an *in situ* component can be demonstrated histologically. These criteria have not been met in all published descriptions of this rare neoplasm.

A small cell carcinoma originating in the breast is illustrated in Fig. 23.1. Cribriform intraductal carcinoma at the primary site was composed of the same small cell type as the invasive lesion. Immunohistochemical studies revealed that the small tumor cells were immunoreactive for cytokeratin (CAM5.2) and for synaptophysin. In another instance, small cell carcinoma was part of a dimorphic intraductal carcinoma (Fig. 23.2). The small tumor cells were cytokeratin positive (CAM5.2) and variably stained with 34BE12. The large tumor cells showed traces of squamous metaplasia and were strongly stained for 34BE12 but negative for CAM5.2. Most small cell carcinomas have an intraductal component composed of cells with poorly differentiated nuclear grade (Fig. 23.3). The invasive component is typically solid with focal necrosis, but a neuroendocrine architecture sometimes is encountered (Fig. 23.4). Rarely, small cell (oat cell) carcinoma arises from *in situ* and infiltrating lobular carcinoma (Fig. 23.5).

Abrupt juxtaposition of small cell and other adenocarcinoma elements, without transitional phases, is not unusual in dimorphic small cell carcinoma. Fukunaga and Ushigome described a 56-year-old woman with a 13-cm ulcerating tumor, 90% of which was small cell type (2). These investigators reported that the "small cell and ductal carcinomatous lesions were mixed but there was no transition from the ordinary ductal to small cell carcinoma." In this case, the single lymph node metastasis was small cell type, and the intraductal component had various growth patterns composed of large carcinoma cells. Various growth patterns occur in dimorphic small cell carcinomas, including focal squamous differentiation (Fig. 23.6) and gland formation (Fig. 23.7).

The diagnosis of a palpable 4-cm small cell carcinoma of the breast by fine needle aspiration, not confirmed by histopathology, was reported by Sebenik et al. (3). Mammography revealed a lobulated tumor with smooth, ill-defined margins and two secondary 1-cm nodules. Extensive clinical workup revealed no evidence of an extramammary tumor. Treatment with VP-16 and cisplatin resulted in marked clinical regression of the tumor. No lesions were seen on mammography 2 months after diagnosis, and no tumor was found in a lumpectomy specimen. The patient then received radiotherapy to the breast. She was alive and well 33 months after diagnosis.

The cytologic specimens from small cell carcinoma tend to be cellular, with dispersed and clustered small cells approximately twice the size of lymphocytes (4,5). There is minimal cellular or nuclear pleomorphism. Nuclear molding is a conspicuous feature (4). The cytologic specimens exhibit "squash" artifact, typically found in small cell carcinomas resulting from disruption of nuclei. Primary and metastatic lesions are not distinguishable cytologically.

No consistent pattern of immunoreactivity for neuroendocrine markers has been seen in mammary small cell carcinoma. The tumors are almost always reactive for cytokeratin (AE1/AE3, CAM5.2, or CK7) and neuron-specific enolase (NSE). Most are also positive with one or more other indicators of neuroendocrine differentiation, such as the Grimelius stain, synaptophysin, chromogranin (A or B), gastrin-releasing peptide (bombesin), serotonin, and Leu7 (6). *In situ* hybridization has been used to demonstrate chromogranin A and B mRNA (6). Electron microscopy has detected neurosecretory granules with variable appearances in several cases (6,7).

The origin of small cell carcinoma in the breast is uncertain in some published cases. One described a 52-year-old woman with a large mammary tumor and clinically involved axillary lymph nodes (8). Lesions in the liver at the time of diagnosis were considered to be metastatic, and bone metastases were also detected clinically. No intraductal carcinoma was identified. A modified Grimelius stain was negative for

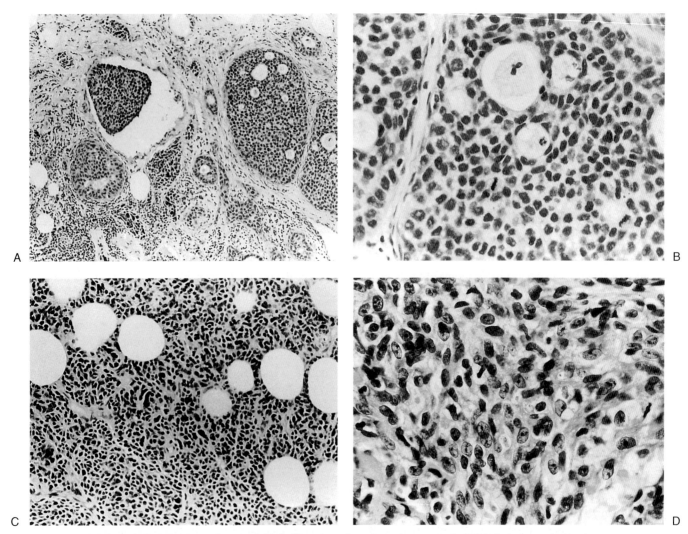

A
B
C
D

**FIG. 23.1.** *Small cell carcinoma.* **A:** Cribriform intraductal carcinoma on the *right* is surrounded by invasive carcinoma partly of the small cell type. The cluster of tumor cells in a space is a shrinkage artifact rather than lymphatic invasion. **B:** The cribriform carcinoma is composed of small cells with hyperchromatic nuclei. **C:** Invasive small cell carcinoma is shown. **D:** A magnified view of the carcinoma cells.

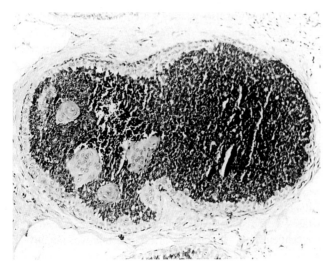

**FIG. 23.2.** *Small cell carcinoma.* This dimorphic intraductal carcinoma has pale-staining clusters of large cells with squamous metaplasia.

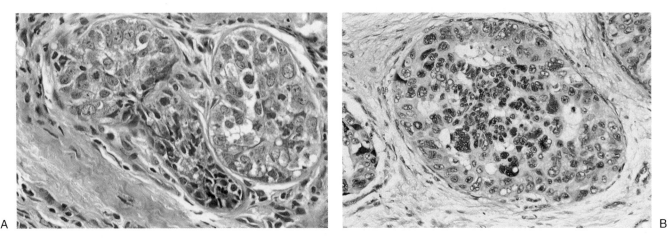

**FIG. 23.3.** *Small cell carcinoma.* **A:** Intraductal carcinoma solid type with poorly differentiated nuclear grade and focal transition to small cell carcinoma. **B:** Intraductal carcinoma with cribriform structure, poorly differentiated nuclear grade, and central transition to small cell carcinoma.

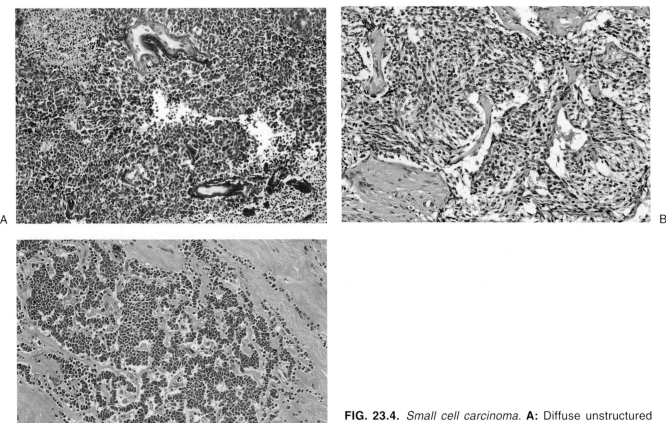

**FIG. 23.4.** *Small cell carcinoma.* **A:** Diffuse unstructured small cell carcinoma with focal necrosis and basophilic deposits around blood vessels. **B:** Organoid groups of cells. **C:** Trabecular, neuroendocrine architecture.

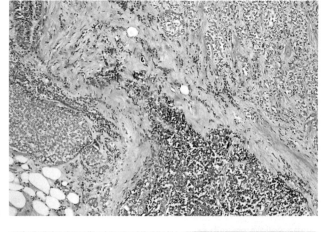

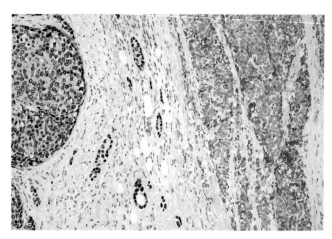

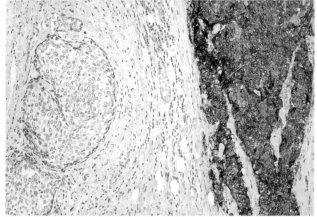

**FIG. 23.5.** *Small cell carcinoma with invasive tubulolobular carcinoma.* **A:** Small cell carcinoma in the lower center is surrounded by *in situ (left)* and invasive *(right)* lobular carcinoma. **B:** *In situ* lobular carcinoma *(left)* and invasive tubulolobular carcinoma *(center)* display nuclear immunoreactivity for estrogen receptor. Small cell carcinoma *(right)* is nonreactive (avidin-biotin). **C:** Chromogranin immunoreactivity is diffusely present in small cell carcinoma *(right)* and absent in lobular carcinoma *(left)* (avidin-biotin).

argyrophilic granules, but scattered neurosecretory granules were detected by electron microscopy. No autopsy was performed to rule out a nonmammary primary. Another article documents a 68-year-old woman with a 4-cm small cell carcinoma that was estrogen and progesterone receptor-negative (9). The patient died with widespread metastases 21 months after diagnosis. No intraductal carcinoma was

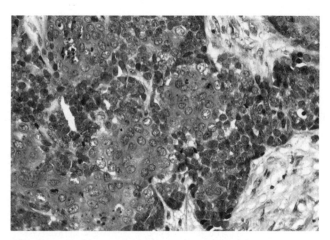

**FIG. 23.6.** *Small cell carcinoma, squamoid dimorphic structure.* Discrete clusters of cells with poorly differentiated squamous appearance surrounded by small cell carcinoma.

detected. The tumor was negative with the Grimelius stain but immunoreactive for chromogranin and NSE and weakly for cytokeratin. A nonmammary primary site cannot be excluded in these patients.

There are numerous reports of metastatic nonmammary small cell (oat cell) carcinoma in the breast (4,10,11). In most cases, the existence of an extramammary primary was previously documented in the lung or other site, such as the uterine cervix (4); however, the mammary metastasis may be the first manifestation of an occult pulmonary oat cell carcinoma. Metastatic neoplasms affecting the breast are discussed in Chapter 36.

The largest published series of primary mammary small cell carcinomas was reported by Shin et al. (12). The patients ranged in age from 43 to 70 years. Two patients had prior cutaneous malignant melanoma, and one had lobular carcinoma *in situ* in an earlier biopsy of the breast where small cell carcinoma developed. Tumor size ranged from 1.3 to 5.0 cm (mean, 2.6 cm). Dimorphic histologic features were present in four tumors. In three cases, a component of poorly differentiated invasive carcinoma with lobular and glandular features was found. The fourth patient had invasive lobular carcinoma. *In situ* ductal carcinoma was found in seven tumors. All small cell carcinomas were immunoreactive for cytokeratin and *bcl*-2 and negative for HER2/*neu*. Five were immunoreactive for estrogen and progesterone receptors

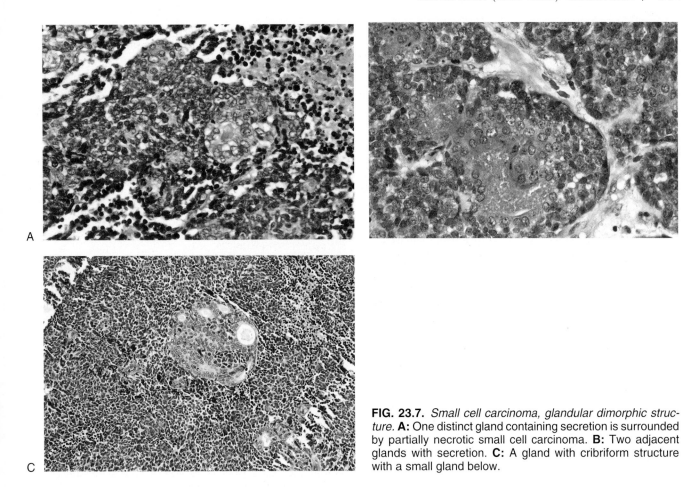

**FIG. 23.7.** *Small cell carcinoma, glandular dimorphic structure.* **A:** One distinct gland containing secretion is surrounded by partially necrotic small cell carcinoma. **B:** Two adjacent glands with secretion. **C:** A gland with cribriform structure with a small gland below.

(Fig. 23.8). Neuroendocrine markers were detected with variable expression. Six of the nine tumors were reactive for chromogranin, synaptophysin, or peptide hormones, including four that were positive for chromogranin and synaptophysin as well as two positive for chromogranin and gastrin-releasing peptide.

Several articles described "small cell carcinoma" of the male breast (7,13–15). On the basis of the illustrations and histologic descriptions provided, most of these appear to be examples of other types of carcinoma, possibly infiltrating lobular carcinoma (8,14,15). Jundt et al. described a 52-year-old man with small cell (oat cell) carcinoma in the breast and

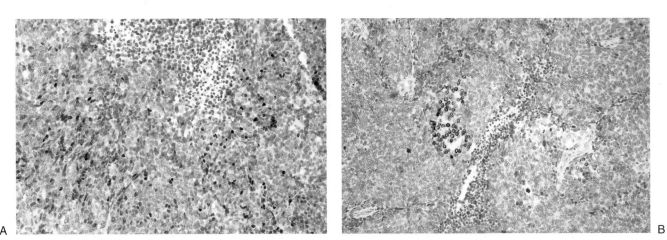

**FIG. 23.8.** *Small cell carcinoma, hormone receptors.* **A:** The tumor displays heterogeneous nuclear reactivity for progesterone receptor. **B:** Nuclear reactivity for estrogen receptor limited to the glandular dimorphic component (avidin-biotin). Some tumors also display nuclear reactivity for estrogen receptor in small cell areas.

axillary lymph nodes (7). The histologic appearance was that of an oat cell carcinoma, and the tumor cells were immunoreactive for NSE. *In situ* carcinoma was not detected. Electron microscopy revealed desmosomes and cytoplasmic granules with neuroendocrine features. No nonmammary primary was detected by clinical evaluation.

## TREATMENT AND PROGNOSIS

Some patients with mammary small cell carcinoma have had relatively large tumors with axillary lymph node metastases and an unfavorable prognosis; however, one woman with a 10-cm tumor and a single axillary lymph node metastasis was reportedly well 4 years after treatment by mastectomy alone (2). Mammary small cell carcinoma has been responsive to chemotherapy used for similar tumors at other sites, such as VP-16 and cisplatin (3). Neoadjuvant chemotherapy resulted in decreased primary tumor size in a 60-year-old woman who presented with an 8-cm tumor and grossly involved axillary nodes, but residual tumor was found in the breast and axilla at mastectomy. The patient developed metastatic carcinoma six months after surgery (16).

Treatment and follow-up information for nine patients described in reports up to 1999 were summarized by Shin et al. (12). Six of the patients had axillary lymph node metastases, and seven underwent mastectomy. Four patients died of small cell carcinoma, two died of other causes, and three were alive without recurrence. In the series of nine new cases reported by Shin et al., three women had axillary lymph node metastases (12). Mastectomy was performed in three cases, whereas six had lumpectomy with radiation or chemotherapy or both. After follow-up of 3 to 35 months, two patients had developed metastatic tumor, and all were alive. These more recent results suggest that the prognosis for relatively early stage small cell carcinoma may be more favorable than suggested by earlier reports based on patients with more advanced disease at diagnosis. Chemotherapy and radiation appear to improve local and systemic control of the small cell carcinoma.

## REFERENCES

1. Levenson RM, Ihde DC, Matthew MJ. Small cell carcinoma presenting as an extrapulmonary neoplasm: sites of origin and response to chemotherapy. *J Natl Cancer Inst* 1981;67:607–612.
2. Fukunaga M, Ushigome S. Small cell (oat cell) carcinoma of the breast. *Pathol Int* 1998;48:744–748.
3. Sebenik M, Nair SG, Hamati HF. Primary small cell anaplastic carcinoma of the breast diagnosed by fine needle aspiration cytology: a case report. *Acta Cytol* 1998;42:1199–1203.
4. Ali SZ, Miller BT. Small cell neuroendocrine carcinoma: cytologic findings in a breast aspirate [letter]. *Acta Cytol* 1997;41:1237–1240.
5. Fiorella RM, Kragel PJ, Shariff A, et al. Fine-needle aspiration of well differentiated small-cell duct carcinoma of the breast. *Diagn Cytopathol* 1997;16:226–229.
6. Papotti M, Gherardi G, Eusebi V, et al. Primary oat cell (neuroendocrine) carcinoma of the breast: report of four cases. *Virchows Arch* 1992;420:103–108.
7. Jundt G, Schulz A, Heitz PhU, et al. Small cell neuroendocrine (oat cell) carcinoma of the male breast. Immunocytochemical and ultrastructural investigations. *Virchows Arch* 1984;404:213–221.
8. Wade PM Jr, Mills SE, Read M, et al. Small cell neuroendocrine (oat cell) carcinoma of the breast. *Cancer* 1983;52:121–125.
9. Francois A, Chatikhine VA, Chevallier B, et al. Neuroendocrine primary small cell carcinoma of the breast: report of a case and review of the literature. *Am J Clin Oncol* 1995;18:133–138.
10. Deeley TJ. Secondary deposits in the breast. *Br J Cancer* 1965;19:738–743.
11. Hadju SI, Urban JA. Cancers metastatic to the breast. *Cancer* 1972;29:1691–1696.
12. Shin SJ, DeLellis RA, Ying L, et al. Small cell carcinoma of the breast: a clinicopathologic and immunohistochemical study of nine patients. *Am J Surg Pathol* 2000;24:1231–1238.
13. Giffler RF, Kay S. Small cell carcinoma of the male mammary gland. A tumor resembling infiltrating lobular carcinoma. *Am J Clin Pathol* 1976;66:715–722.
14. Wolff M, Reinis MS. Breast cancer in the male: clinicopathological study of 40 patients and review of the literature. In: Fenoglio CM, Wolff M, eds. *Progress in surgical pathology.* New York: Masson Publishing, 1981:77–109.
15. Yogore III MG, Sahgal S. Small cell carcinoma of the male breast: report of a case. *Cancer* 1977;39:1748–1751.
16. Samli B, Celik S, Evrensel T, et al. Primary neuroendocrine small cell carcinoma of the breast. *Arch Pathol Lab Med* 2000;124:296–298.

# CHAPTER 24

# Secretory Carcinoma

Many of the histologic patterns of breast carcinoma that occur in adults also have been reported in patients younger than 20 years of age (1). Juvenile or secretory carcinoma is found often in children, but most cases have been reported in adults (2) (Fig. 24.1). The term *secretory* is therefore preferable to *juvenile*. The microscopic appearance of the lesion is the same regardless of patient age.

## CLINICAL PRESENTATION

Secretory carcinoma was first fully described in 1966 by McDivitt and Stewart in a report on seven patients whose ages ranged from 3 to 15 years, averaging 9 years (3). Six years later, Oberman and Stephens reported secretory carcinoma diagnosed in two women whose ages were 25 and 56 years (4). Oberman subsequently described four more examples in adult women 22 to 73 years of age (5). More than 40 adult cases now have been described (6–10), and numerous single case reports of secretory carcinoma in children have appeared (11–18), including lesions detected in girls 5 years of age or younger (13,16,18,19) as well as boys 6 (20) and 9 (21) years old. There is a dearth of cases of secretory carcinoma in girls 10 to 15 years of age.

With three exceptions, affected males have been younger than 10 years (22–25). Secretory carcinoma was reported in a 24-year-old man who was treated by simple mastectomy and axillary radiation (22). Twenty years later, the patient developed an axillary mass regarded as recurrent carcinoma, and within a year he died of systemic metastases. A biopsy of a metastatic lesion confirmed that it was secretory carcinoma. Secretory carcinoma in a 20-year-old man was diagnosed by aspiration cytology (24). The tumor was immunoreactive for carcinoembryonic antigen, α-lactalbumin, and vimentin. The tumor cells were diploid when analyzed by flow cytometry.

Secretory carcinoma can occur in any part of the breast. Subareolar lesions have been associated with nipple discharge, but in most cases, the patient has a painless, circumscribed mass that may be present for 1 year or longer before a biopsy is performed (5,13,16,18). A subareolar tumor is most common in prepubertal patients and in male patients because the breast tissue of these patients is localized in this region. Mammography usually reveals a discrete, solitary tumor with irregular borders (10). In one case, multiple tumors were detected by mammography and confirmed by needle biopsy sampling to be secretory carcinoma in a 35-year-old woman (9). The mastectomy specimen contained "multiple firm nodules ranging from 0.5 to 1.2 cm." There were no axillary lymph node metastases.

No clinical evidence of a hormonal abnormality has been described that would explain the secretory properties of the tumor, and secretory carcinoma has not been associated with pregnancy. Estrogen receptors were negative in most tumors examined by biochemistry or immunohistochemistry (6,10,13,17,20,23,25–28). Five tumors were estrogen receptor-positive (6,20,23). Seven carcinomas were progesterone receptor-positive (17,20,23), and four were negative for progesterone receptors (10,23,26,27). Five tumors studied by flow cytometry were diploid or near diploid with a low S-phase (23,27).

Molecular analysis of 10 secretory carcinomas revealed a p53 mutation in only one tumor (10%) from a 25-year-old woman (28). This was a lower frequency of p53 mutation than the 35% to 50% occurrence in invasive duct carcinomas. Loss of heterozygosity (LOH) was not detected at 17p13 in secretory carcinomas, whereas LOH was present at this locus in 46% of invasive duct carcinomas studied by these investigators. No significant differences in LOH were found between secretory and invasive duct carcinomas at 12 other chromosomal regions analyzed.

Associated breast conditions have been described in a few cases. Secretory carcinoma may have developed in gynecomastia in a 23-year-old man who had a small antecedent nodule in his breast since the age of 2 years that was interpreted clinically as gynecomastia (29). One patient was pregnant when she noted a tumor that proved to be secretory carcinoma, but a biopsy was not performed until 4 years later (26). Coexistence of juvenile papillomatosis and secretory carcinoma has been described (13,30,31,32); however, the

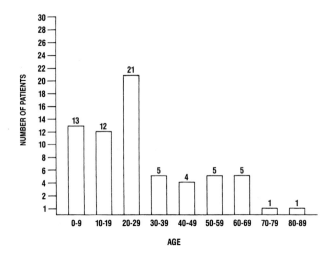

**FIG. 24.1.** *Secretory carcinoma, age distribution.* The data were based on published case reports. (From Rosen PP, Cranor ML. Secretory carcinoma of the breast. *Arch Pathol Lab Med* 1991;115:141–144, with permission.)

evidence for juvenile papillomatosis is not convincing in all instances. For example, Tokunaga et al. described a 13-year-old girl who had secretory carcinoma in one breast that ultimately proved fatal (32). At autopsy, a proliferative lesion was found in the contralateral breast. The diagnosis given to the contralateral breast abnormality was "juvenile cystic papillomatosis," but the illustration provided shows a lesion more appropriately termed juvenile papillary duct hyperplasia. A second case presented by these investigators as a secretory carcinoma in "juvenile papillomatosis" appears from the illustrations to be cystic transformation of secretory carcinoma.

## GROSS PATHOLOGY

Grossly, secretory carcinoma is usually a circumscribed, firm mass that may be lobulated (Fig. 24.2). Rarely, the tumor has infiltrative margins. Various colors have been mentioned, usually a shade of white to gray or of tan to yellow.

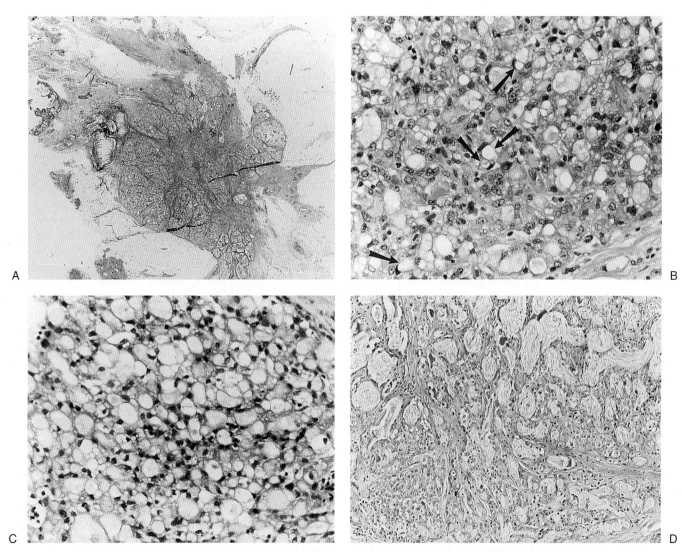

**FIG. 24.2.** *Secretory carcinoma.* **A:** This whole-mount histologic section demonstrates the lobulated partly stellate structure of a tumor that had varied histologic patterns. **B:** Microlumens and "bubbly" cytoplasm with signet-ring cells *(arrows).* **C:** Markedly vacuolated cells. **D:** An unusual mucinous pattern.

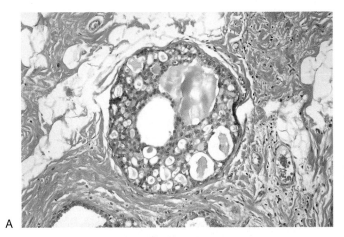 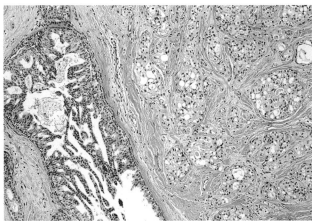

**FIG. 24.3.** *Secretory carcinoma, intraductal.* **A:** Solid growth with secretory carcinoma structure. **B:** Papillary and micropapillary carcinoma next to invasive secretory carcinoma.

The tumors tend to be 3 cm or smaller in diameter, with larger lesions up to 12 cm found mainly in adults.

## MICROSCOPIC PATHOLOGY

As a form of ductal carcinoma, secretory carcinoma has an intraductal component that can exhibit some of the growth patterns associated with more conventional types of duct carcinoma. The intraductal carcinoma sometimes extends beyond the confines of the grossly evident tumor, and multifocal gross lesions were described in two cases (9,16). Most commonly, the intraductal carcinoma is papillary or cribriform (Fig. 24.3). Solid foci and, rarely, comedonecrosis also may be found. These features are carried over into the structure of the invasive components, which tend to be relatively compact, with papillary, microcystic, and glandular patterns (Fig. 24.4). Gross lobulation is usually the result of fibrous septae distributed in the lesion (Fig. 24.5). Microcalcifications are rarely seen in the neoplastic glands or in the stroma. The borders of the carcinoma usually are circumscribed microscopically, but invasion is sometimes present (Fig. 24.6).

The tumor cells, glands, and microcystic spaces contain abundant secretion, which is usually pale pink or amphophilic with hematoxylin and eosin. It is often vacuolated or "bubbly," reacting variably for mucin and with the periodic acid-Schiff reaction. In microcystic areas, the secretion resembles the material that accumulates in cystic hypersecretory lesions (Fig. 24.4B). Strong positive staining has been reported for α-lactalbumin (20,23,33) as well as S-100 protein (20,23) and carcinoembryonic antigen (polyclonal) (20). No reactivity was observed for gross cystic disease fluid protein or for monoclonal carcinoembryonic antigen (20). The vacuoles correspond to intracytoplasmic lumens noted ultrastructurally (25,33). Ultrastructurally, secretion, sometimes in membrane-bound vacuoles, can be found within the cytoplasm of tumor cells and in intracytoplasmic lumina.

The tumor consists of cells with pale-to-clear, pink, or amphophilic cytoplasm and small, round, cytologically low-grade nuclei (Fig. 24.7). Part or most of the lesion can have more granular or eosinophilic cytoplasm and the nuclear cytology of apocrine differentiation (34) (Fig. 24.8). Rarely, secretory features are obscured by apocrine cytology and solid growth (Fig. 24.9).

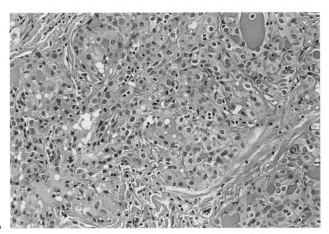 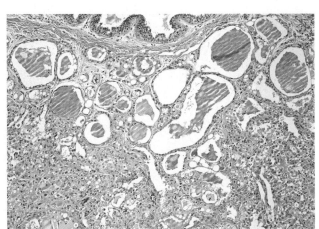

**FIG. 24.4.** *Secretory carcinoma, growth patterns.* Samples shown in **A–C** are from a 20-year-old woman. **A:** Solid growth with focal microlumen formation *(left)*. **B:** A microcystic area. *(continued)*

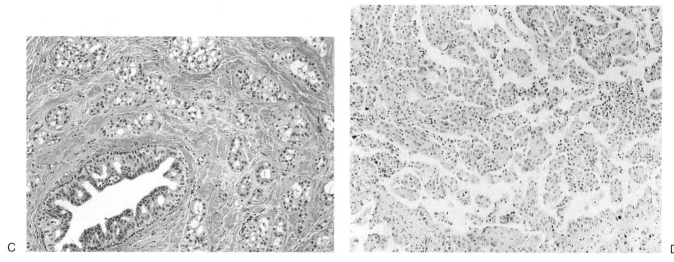

C

D

**FIG. 24.4.** *Continued.* **C:** Part of this tumor has a tubular structure. Atypical duct hyperplasia is also present *(left).* **D:** Papillary growth. (From Rosen PP, Cranor ML. Secretory carcinoma of the breast. *Arch Pathol Lab Med* 1991;115:141–144, with permission.)

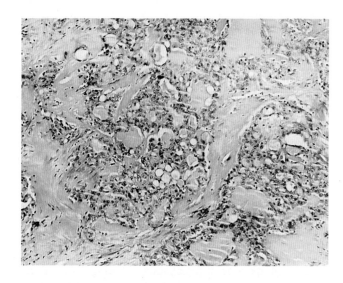

**FIG. 24.5.** *Secretory carcinoma, stromal fibrosis.*

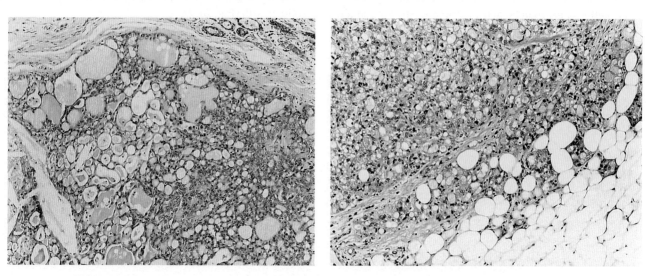

A

B

**FIG. 24.6.** *Secretory carcinoma, tumor border.* **A:** A circumscribed border. **B:** An invasive border.

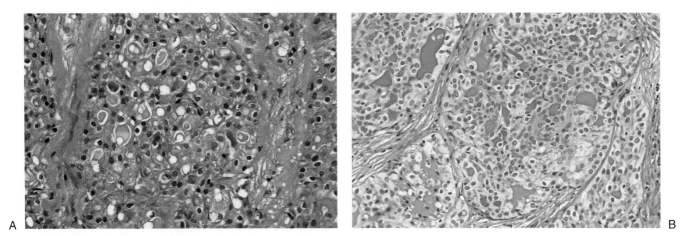

**FIG. 24.7.** *Secretory carcinoma.* **A:** This tumor from a 69-year-old woman has a solid structure with small microlumens and dense secretion. Nuclei are small, round, and uniform without visible nucleoli. **B:** This tumor from a 5-year-old girl has a fenestrated structure. Nuclei are round to oval.

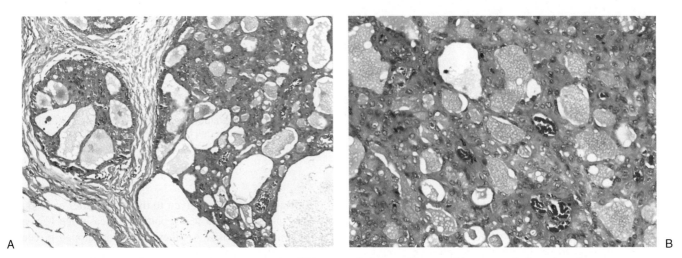

**FIG. 24.8.** *Secretory carcinoma, apocrine.* This tumor is from a 64-year-old woman. **A:** Intraductal carcinoma is present on the *left*. **B:** The tumor cells have apocrine features.

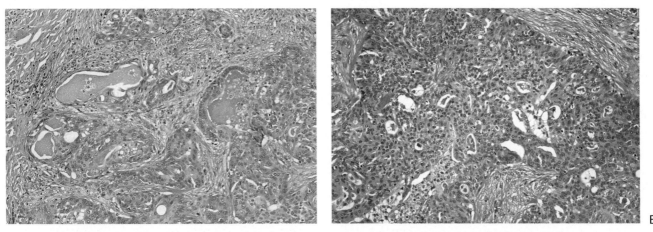

**FIG. 24.9.** *Secretory carcinoma, apocrine and solid.* This tumor from a 16-year-old boy produced an axillary lymph node metastasis. **A:** Secretory activity is seen at the invasive tumor border. **B:** A solid area with apocrine cytoplasm and irregular microlumens containing sparse secretion. *(continued)*

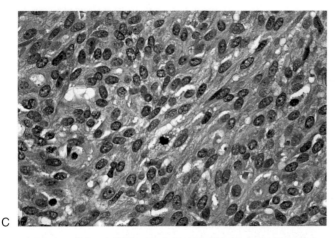

C

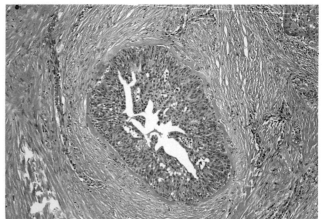

D

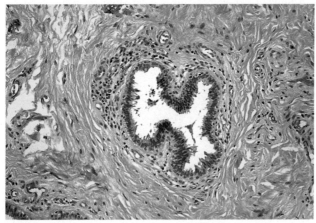

E

**FIG. 24.9.** *Continued.* **C:** Magnified view of carcinoma cells exhibiting moderate pleomorphism, and a mitosis in the center. **D:** Intraductal carcinoma with scant secretory differentiation. **E:** Mild columnar cell hyperplasia in the surrounding gynecomastia.

Cytoplasmic vacuolization may suggest a diagnosis of secretory carcinoma in a fine needle aspiration cytology specimen (6,28,34,35). Signet-ring cell forms can be present. The tumor cells tend to be distributed in cohesive groups or sheets. In most cases, the nuclei are small and round to oval with inconspicuous nucleoli. Scattered atypical cells, sometimes with prominent nuclei, are encountered in lesions with apocrine features. "Grape like clusters of mucous globular structures" are a distinctive feature of secretory carcinoma in a cytology preparation (36,37). These consist of rounded, homogeneous masses of mucoid material with adherent sheets of tumor cells. The mucoid material has a purple or violet color with the crystal violet stain.

**PROGNOSIS AND TREATMENT**

In most patients, secretory carcinoma has a low-grade clinical course resulting in an exceptionally favorable prognosis. Most children and adults have been treated by mastectomy. A few have been free of disease 7 to 15 years after excisional biopsy (3,4), which in one case was followed by radiotherapy (17). Recurrence on the chest wall in residual breast tissue has been reported 8 years after modified radical mastectomy (27). A 4-year-old girl developed local recurrence in the scar of a mastectomy 8 months postoperatively

(18). Radiotherapy was given to the region after excisional biopsy, and the patient was reportedly disease free 11 years after initial diagnosis. Another patient developed a recurrence in the breast 21 years after an initial excision performed when the patient was 4 years of age (4).

Axillary metastases have been described, but they rarely involve more than three lymph nodes (2,11,12,14,22,23, 26,28) (Fig. 24.10). Some patients with positive lymph nodes have been more than 20 years of age (2,8,14,22, 23,26), but the risk of nodal involvement is at least as great in children because a recent literature review found positive nodes in 5 of 18 (27%) childhood cases, and among the six children in the series with lymph mode dissections, three (50%) had positive nodes (14). Recurrence in the breast after excisional surgery has been described by several investigators (2–4,11,16,22,38). In one case, axillary metastases were first evident when a local recurrence was found 7 years after local excision of the primary from a 19-year-old patient. Patients with axillary metastases have been reported to be well as long as 6 years after primary therapy, but the finding of multiple involved lymph nodes may be a harbinger of systemic metastases.

Surgical biopsy is usually necessary for the diagnosis of secretory carcinoma, although the lesion may be suspected in a fine needle aspiration or core biopsy specimen (6,9,35).

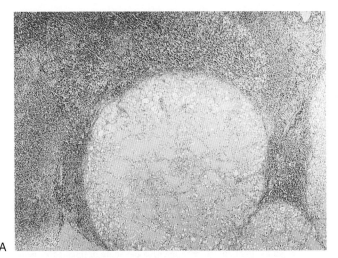

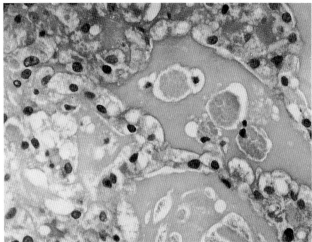

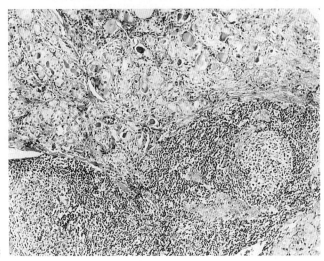

**FIG. 24.10.** *Metastatic secretory carcinoma.* The patient was 31 years old. **A:** Round areas of metastatic carcinoma are present in a lymph node. **B:** A magnified view of the metastatic carcinoma in **A** showing low-grade nuclei and characteristic secretion. **C:** A lymph node metastasis with microlumens in another case.

Local excision is the preferred initial treatment in children found to have secretory carcinoma (8). Consideration should be given to preserving the breast bud in prepubertal patients. Unfortunately, this cannot always be accomplished, and breast development may be impaired or abolished. In postmenarcheal children, wide local excision may suffice for small lesions, but quadrantectomy can be necessary to obtain negative margins around larger tumors. Axillary dissection is indicated if clinical examination suggests nodal involvement; however, clinical examination is not always a good guide to the appropriateness of axillary dissection in children because most lymph node metastases in these patients were not palpable. Sentinel lymph node mapping may be an effective method for assessing the axilla in patients with secretory carcinoma.

No evidence has been found that radiation therapy is beneficial in adults after excisional biopsy, and radiation may inhibit normal breast development if it is administered to the premenarchal or developing breast. Because few patients have received systemic adjuvant therapy (25), it is not possible to judge the effectiveness of this treatment in children and adults with secretory carcinoma.

## REFERENCES

1. Ashikari H, Jun MY, Farrow JH, et al. Breast carcinoma in children and adolescents. *Clin Bull* 1977;7:55–62.
2. Tournemaine N, Audouin AF, Anguill C, et al. Le carcinome secretoire juvenile: cinq nouveaux cas chez des femmes d'age adulte. *Arch Anat Cytol Pathol* 1986;34:146–151.
3. McDivitt RW, Stewart FW. Breast carcinoma in children. *JAMA* 1966;195:388–390.
4. Oberman HA, Stephens PJ. Carcinoma of the breast in childhood. *Cancer* 1972;30:420–474.
5. Oberman HA. Secretory carcinoma of the breast in adults. *Am J Surg Pathol* 1980;4:465–470.
6. Dominguez F, Riera JR, Junco P, et al. Secretory carcinoma of the breast. Report of a case with diagnosis by fine needle aspiration. *Acta Cytol* 1992;36:507–510.
7. Gupta RK, Lallu SD, Fauck R, et al. Needle aspiration cytology, immunocytochemistry, and electron microscopy in a rare case of secretory carcinoma of the breast in an elderly woman. *Diagn Cytopathol* 1992;8:388–391.
8. Rosen PP, Cranor ML. Secretory carcinoma of the breast. *Arch Pathol Lab Med* 1991;115:141–144.
9. Beatty SM, Orel SG, Kim P, et al. Multicentric secretory carcinoma of the breast in a 35-year-old woman: mammographic appearance and the use of core biopsy in preoperative management. *Breast J* 1998;4: 200–203.
10. Siegel JR, Karcnik TJ, Hertz MB, et al. Secretory carcinoma of the breast. *Breast J* 1999;5:204–207.

11. Botta G, Fessia L, Ghiringhello B. Juvenile milk protein secreting carcinoma. *Virchows Arch* 1982;395:145–152.

12. Byrne MP, Fahey MM, Gooselaw JG. Breast cancer with axillary metastasis in an 8-1/2 year old girl. *Cancer* 1972;31:726–728.

13. Ferguson TB Jr, McCarty KS Jr, Filston HC. Juvenile secretory carcinoma and juvenile papillomatosis: diagnosis and treatment. *J Pediatr Surg* 1987;22:637–639.

14. Karl SR, Ballantine TVN, Zaino R. Juvenile secretory carcinoma of the breast. *J Pediatr Surg* 1985;20:368–371.

15. Masse SR, Rioux A, Beauchesne C. Juvenile carcinoma of the breast. *Hum Pathol* 1981;12:1044–1046.

16. Romdhane KB, Ayed B, Labbane N, et al. Carcinome secretant juvenile du sein. A propos d'une observation chez une fille de 4 ans. *Ann Pathol* 1987;3:227–230.

17. Serour F, Gilad A, Kopolovic J, et al. Secretory breast cancer in childhood and adolescence: report of a case and review of the literature. *Med Pediatr Oncol* 1992;20:341–344.

18. Longo OA, Mosto A, Moran JCH, et al. Breast carcinoma in childhood and adolescence: case report and review of the literature. *Breast J* 1999;5:65–69.

19. Tanimura A, Konaka K. Carcinoma of the breast in a 5 year old girl. *Acta Pathol Jpn* 1980;30:157–160.

20. Hartman AW, Magrish P. Carcinoma of breast in children. Case report: six-year-old boy with adenocarcinoma. *Ann Surg* 1955;141:792–797.

21. Titus J, Sillar RW, Fenton LE. Secretory breast carcinoma in a 9-year-old boy. *Aust N Z J Surg* 2000;70:144–146.

22. Krausz T, Jenkins D, Grontoft O, et al. Secretory carcinoma of the breast in adults; emphasis on late recurrence and metastasis. *Histopathology* 1989;14:25–36.

23. Lamovec J, Bracko M. Secretory carcinoma of the breast: light microscopical, immunohistochemical and flow cytometric study. *Mod Pathol* 1994;7:475–479.

24. Pohar-Marinsek Z, Golouh R. Secretory breast carcinoma in a man diagnosed by fine needle aspiration biopsy. A case report. *Acta Cytol* 1994;38:446–450.

25. Yildirim E, Turhan N, Pak I, et al. Secretory breast carcinoma in a boy. *Eur J Surg Oncol* 1999;25:98–99.

26. Abe R, Masuda T. Secretory carcinoma of the breast in a Japanese woman. *Jpn J Surg* 1986;16:52–55.

27. Mies C. Recurrent secretory carcinoma in residual mammary tissue after mastectomy. *Am J Surg Pathol* 1993;17:715–721.

28. Maitra A, Tavassoli FA, Albores-Saavedra J, et al. Molecular abnormalities associated with secretory carcinomas of the breast. *Hum Pathol* 1999;30:1435–1440.

29. Roth JA, Discafani C, O'Malley M. Secretory breast carcinoma in a man. *Am J Surg Pathol* 1988;12:150–154.

30. Nonomura A, Kimura A, Mizukami Y, et al. Secretory carcinoma of the breast associated with juvenile papillomatosis in a 12-year-old girl. A case report. *Acta Cytol* 1995;39:569–576.

31. Rosen PP, Holmes G, Lesser ML, et al. Juvenile papillomatosis and breast carcinoma. *Cancer* 1985;55:1345–1352.

32. Tokunaga M, Wakimoto J, Muramoto Y, et al. Juvenile secretory carcinoma and juvenile papillomatosis. *Jpn J Clin Oncol* 1986;15:457–465.

33. Akhtar M, Robinson C, Ali MA, et al. Secretory carcinoma of the breast in adults: light and electron microscopic study of three cases with review of the literature. *Cancer* 1983;51:2245–2254.

34. Nguyen G-K. Aspiration biopsy cytology of secretory carcinoma of the breast. *Diagn Cytopathol* 1987;3:234–237.

35. d'Amore ESG, Maisto L, Gatteschi MB, et al. Secretory carcinoma of the breast. Report of a case with fine needle aspiration biopsy. *Acta Cytol* 1986;30:309–312.

36. de la Cruz Mera A, de la Cruz Mera E, Leston JS, et al. Secretory carcinoma of the breast [Letter]. *Acta Cytol* 1994;38:968–969.

37. Shinagawa T, Tadokoro M, Kitamura H, et al. Secretory carcinoma of the breast. Correlation of aspiration cytology and histology. *Acta Cytol* 1994;38:909–914.

38. Sullivan JJ, Magee JJ, Donald KJ. Secretory (juvenile) carcinoma of the breast. *Pathology* 1977;9:341–346.

# CHAPTER 25

# Mammary Carcinoma with Osteoclast-like Giant Cells

Carcinomas containing osteoclast-like multinucleated giant cells arise in many organs, including the breast, lung, pancreas, small intestine, and thyroid gland. Similar giant cells also have been found in noncarcinomatous tumors, such as uterine leiomyosarcoma (1) and intestinal carcinoid (2). Fewer than 100 examples of this type of breast carcinoma have been reported since the first series was published in 1979 (3). They constituted 0.5% to 1.2% of breast carcinomas in two reviews of at least 500 consecutively treated carcinomas (4,5).

## CLINICAL PRESENTATION

Despite the unusual histologic properties of these tumors, the clinical features are similar to those of breast carcinoma generally. Patients range in age from 28 to 88 years. The average age at diagnosis in three recent reviews was 53 years (3,5,6). Typically, the patient presents with a palpable tumor in the upper outer quadrant, but the lesion has been found in all quadrants. Multifocal lesions in more than one quadrant were described clinically in one case (7). On mammography and ultrasonography, the well-circumscribed margin of most tumors suggests a benign lesion such as a cyst or fibroadenoma (5,8).

## GROSS PATHOLOGY

The tumors are usually well defined, fleshy, firm lesions. Reported diameters range from 0.5 to 10 cm, with most measuring 3 cm or less. The gross appearance of most tumors is quite striking. When bisected, the dark brown or red–brown tumor tissue tends to bulge slightly above the surrounding breast parenchyma, from which it may be separated by a rounded, discrete margin (Fig. 25.1). Tumors with ill-defined margins and multinodular tumors have been described (7,9). The color may suggest heavily pigmented, metastatic malignant melanoma, but it tends to be brown rather than black. Tumors with relatively few osteoclast-like giant cells or with little hemorrhage may be tan or white. The gross appearance is not specific for this neoplasm because hemorrhagic papillary or nonmedullary circumscribed carcinomas that lack giant

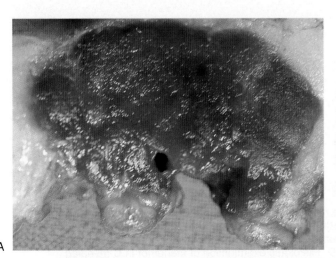
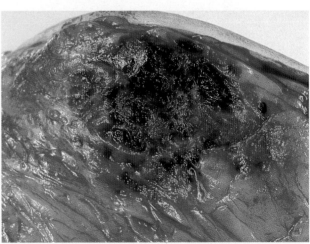

A          B

**FIG. 25.1.** *Mammary carcinoma with osteoclast-like giant cells, gross.* **A,B:** The tumors are usually well circumscribed and chocolate-brown or red-brown. *(continued)*

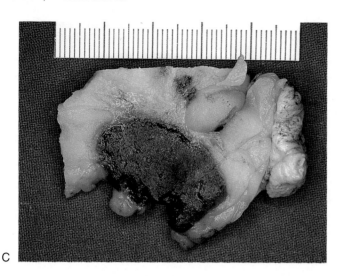

**FIG. 25.1.** *Continued.* **C:** The tumor shown in **A** retains the dark brown color after fixation in formalin.

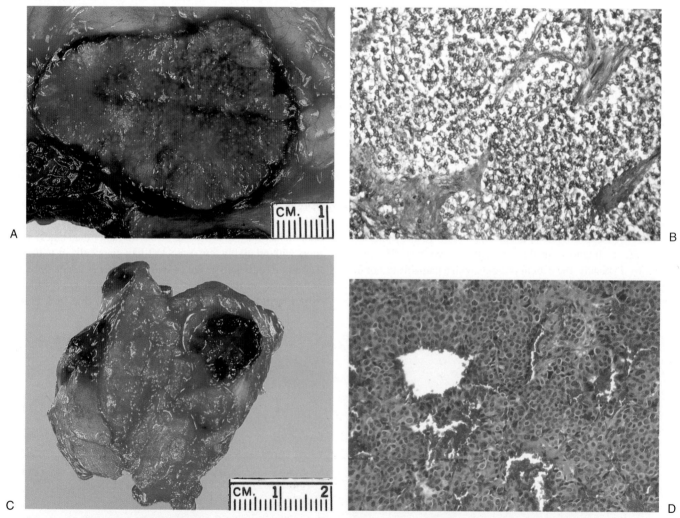

**FIG. 25.2.** *Mammary carcinomas that grossly resemble carcinoma with osteoclast-like giant cells.* **A:** A circumscribed, bulging tumor with a hyperemic border and red mottled surface. **B:** The tumor in **A** was a poorly differentiated carcinoma with stromal hemorrhage and no giant cells. **C:** The gross appearance of a bisected, circumscribed, dark red carcinoma. **D:** Histologic examination of the tumor in **C** revealed a solid papillary carcinoma with stromal hemorrhage and lacking giant cells. Endocrine differentiation was evidenced by positive Grimelius and chromogranin stains and confirmed by electron microscopy.

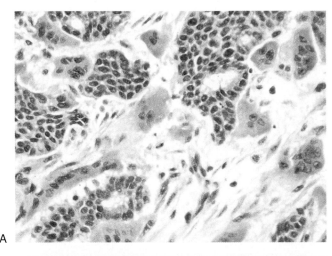

A

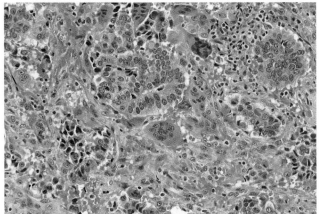

B

**FIG. 25.3.** *Carcinoma with osteoclast-like giant cells.* **A:** Multinucleated giant cells close to carcinomatous glands. The absence of stromal hemorrhage is unusual. **B:** Large multinucleated giant cells in the stroma mingle with lymphocytes, red blood cells, and stromal cells. **C:** One stellate osteoclast-like giant cell is shown in the center (*arrow*). The stroma contains hemosiderin, lymphocytes, and plasma cells. Several shrunken osteoclast-like giant cells are also present.

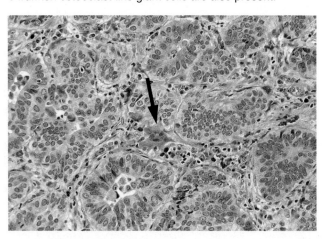

C

cells microscopically may be indistinguishable grossly from carcinomas with osteoclast-like giant cells (Fig. 25.2).

## MICROSCOPIC PATHOLOGY

Most of these lesions are moderately or poorly differentiated invasive duct carcinomas (Fig. 25.3). A cribriform growth pattern is present relatively more often than occurs among duct carcinomas generally (Fig. 25.4). Uncommon examples of well-differentiated or tubular (4,9) (Fig. 25.5), infiltrating lobular (3,8) (Fig. 25.6), squamous (10), papillary (3) (Fig. 25.7), apocrine (Fig. 25.8), mucinous (6) (Fig. 25.9), and metaplastic (9) carcinomas with osteoclast-like giant cells have been reported. Rarely, the carcinoma has a glandular pattern reminiscent of infiltrating colonic carcinoma (Fig. 25.10). Osteoclast-like giant cells can be

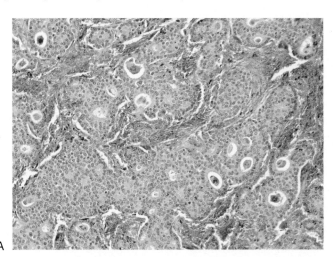

A

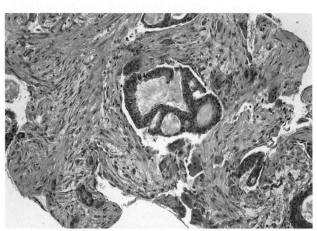

B

**FIG. 25.4.** *Carcinoma with osteoclast-like giant cells, cribriform.* **A:** Diffuse stromal hemorrhage with hemosiderin obscures the osteoclast-like giant cells. **B:** A needle core biopsy sample with numerous osteoclast-like giant cells and cribriform duct carcinoma.

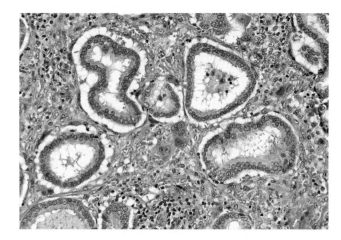

**FIG. 25.5.** *Carcinoma with osteoclast-like giant cells, well differentiated.*

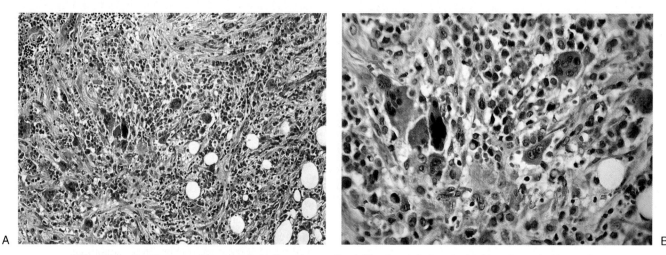

A

B

**FIG. 25.6.** *Carcinoma with osteoclast-like giant cells, infiltrating lobular.* **A:** Multinucleated giant cells mingle with the carcinoma cells. **B:** Extravasated red blood cells, signet-ring carcinoma cells, and giant cells are shown.

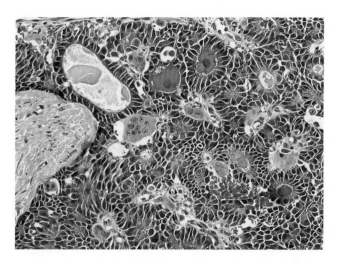

**FIG. 25.7.** *Carcinoma with osteoclast-like giant cells, solid papillary.*

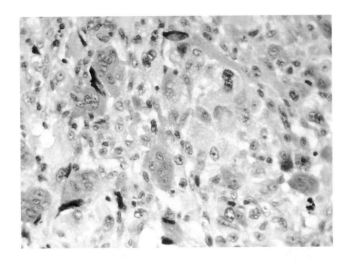

**FIG. 25.8.** *Carcinoma with osteoclast-like giant cells, apocrine.* The giant cells mingle with apocrine carcinoma cells which have prominent nucleoli.

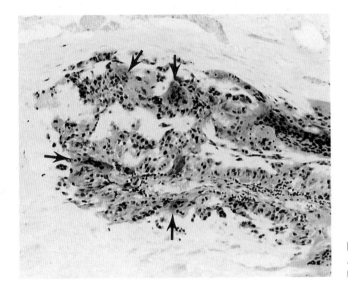

**FIG. 25.9.** *Carcinoma with osteoclast-like giant cells, mucinous.* Giant cells *(arrows)* are hidden in this island of carcinoma surrounded by mucin.

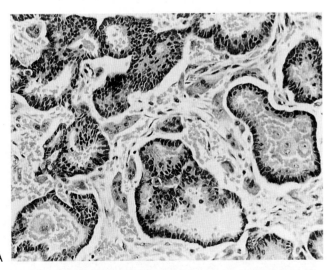

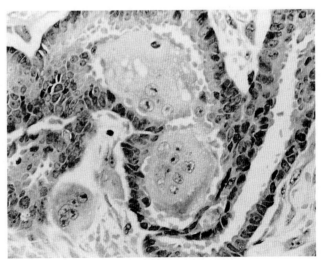

A                                                                                                              B

**FIG. 25.10.** *Carcinoma with osteoclast-like giant cells, colonic type.* **A:** Infiltrating adenocarcinoma glands in stroma containing giant cells and red blood cells. **B:** Giant cells in the lumen of a carcinomatous gland and in the stroma.

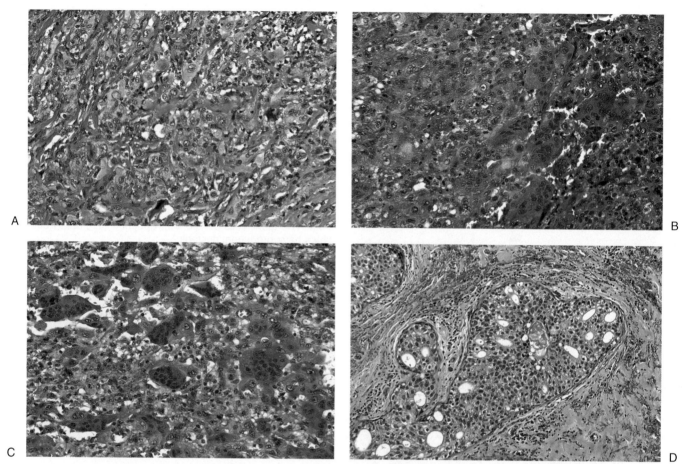

**FIG. 25.11.** *Carcinoma with osteoclast-like giant cells, anaplastic.* **A:** Giant cells are not evident in this part of the tumor. **B:** Osteoclast-like giant cells are difficult to distinguish from carcinoma cells in this region. **C:** Numerous osteoclast-like giant cells where carcinoma is inconspicuous. **D:** Cribriform intraductal carcinoma.

encountered in anaplastic carcinomas, which are probably variants of metaplastic carcinoma (Fig. 25.11). When present, intraductal carcinoma has the appearance of one of the conventional variants, usually cribriform, solid, or papillary. Osteoclast-like giant cells are not always present in the associated intraductal carcinoma (Fig. 25.11), and rarely, osteoclast-like giant cells are found in intraductal carcinoma in the absence of an invasive lesion (Fig. 25.12).

The giant cells are usually close to the edges of invasive carcinomatous glands or in intervening stroma, and they may be found in the glandular lumens (Figs. 25.3, 25.7, 25.9, and 25.10). Evidence of recent and past hemorrhage consisting of extravasated erythrocytes and hemosiderin is present in the vascular stroma in most cases (Figs. 25.3, 25.5, and 25.6). Erythrophagocytosis by the giant cells is uncommon, and they contain little hemosiderin that is detectable by light microscopy. Fibroblastic reaction, collagenization, and lymphocytic infiltration are variably present (Figs. 25.3, 25.4, and 25.13).

The diagnosis of mammary carcinoma with osteoclast-like giant cells may be suggested by the findings in a fine needle aspiration specimen (7,8,11–14). The slides show a

cellular aspirate containing inflammatory cells, erythrocytes, and tumor cells intermixed with osteoclast-like giant cells. The giant cells contain a variable number of small, regular nuclei, but they do not exhibit phagocytosis of red blood

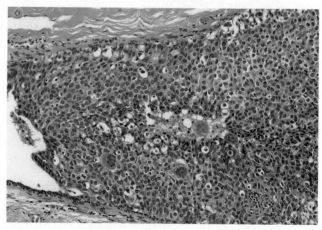

**FIG. 25.12.** *Osteoclast-like giant cells in intraductal carcinoma.*

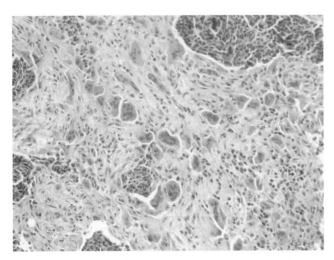

**FIG. 25.13.** *Carcinoma with osteoclast-like giant cells.* This abundant stromal fibrosis is unusual. A lymphoplasmacytic infiltration is present but hemorrhage and hemosiderin are lacking.

cells or cellular debris. The distinction between osteoclast-like giant cells and multinucleated tumor giant cells may be difficult in an aspiration cytology specimen (15,16). Infiltrating lobular carcinoma with osteoclast-like giant cells can be recognized in a fine needle cytology specimen if the giant cells are found among small, disaggregated tumor cells with signet-ring features (8) (Fig. 25.14).

It has been postulated that one or more substances produced by the neoplastic cells in these tumors induce the formation of the giant cells and that the same process is in some way responsible for the accompanying angiogenesis and hemorrhage (3,6). In experimental studies, the angiogenesis associated with mammary carcinoma has not been accompanied by osteoclast-like giant cells (17). The formation of giant cells from blood monocytes incubated *in vitro* with hu-

man breast carcinoma cells has been ascribed to viruses presumably carried by the monocytes (18). Jimi et al. demonstrated *in vitro* that multinucleation and functional osteoclastic differentiation of stromal cells could be induced by interleukin-1 (IL-1) (19).

Inconspicuous and infrequent metaplastic foci with spindle cells and squamous or osseous features have been described in tumors that were otherwise typical examples of mammary carcinoma with osteoclast-like giant cells (3,9). Mammary carcinoma with osteoclast-like giant cells may be a variant of metaplastic mammary carcinoma, but it is inappropriate to separate these tumors until the clinicopathologic characteristics of the lesion have been better defined. Osteoclast-like giant cells are found in examples of metaplastic carcinoma that contain areas of osseous and cartilaginous differentiation (13,20).

The differential diagnosis includes some noncarcinomatous lesions. Megakaryocytes in myeloid metaplasia in the breast might be mistaken for osteoclast-like giant cells, but these lesions have abundant myeloid elements in various stages of maturation, a feature not found in carcinomas with osteoclast-like giant cells (21). Granulomatous foci in inflammatory conditions such as sarcoidosis or coexistent with carcinoma also contain giant cells (22,23) (Fig. 25.15). Because mammary carcinoma with osteoclast-like giant cells does not have a granulomatous pattern, the distinction from sarcoid or tuberculoid reactions can be made without difficulty in histologic sections (see Chapters 3 and 4). The osteoclastic-like giant cells found in mammary carcinoma do not resemble multinucleated stromal giant cells, which are an incidental finding in breast tissue from patients with benign conditions or carcinoma, usually not at the site of the lesion (Fig. 25.16). Multinucleated stromal giant cells may be found in the stroma of fibroepithelial tumors (Chapter 8).

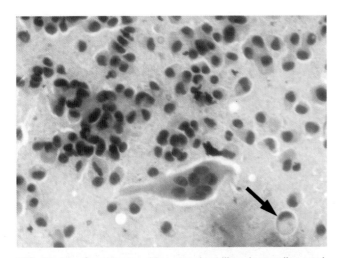

**FIG. 25.14.** *Carcinoma with osteoclast-like giant cells, cytology.* A fine needle aspiration smear showing infiltrating lobular carcinoma with an osteoclast-like giant cell. Note the signet-ring cell in the lower right corner *(arrow)*.

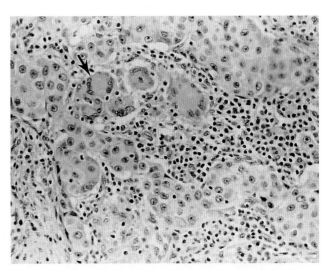

**FIG. 25.15.** *Carcinoma with a granulomatous reaction.* Langhans-type giant cells *(arrow)* and a lymphocytic infiltrate distinguish this pattern from carcinoma with osteoclast-like giant cells. Epithelioid granulomas, which usually are present, are not shown here.

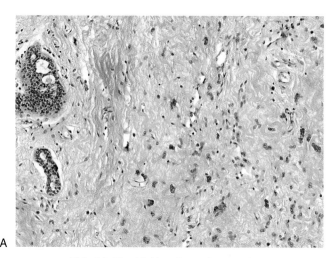
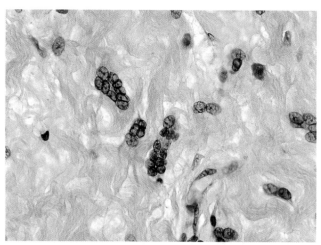

A                                                                                                                                                                B

**FIG. 25.16.** *Multinucleated stromal giant cells.* **A:** These giant cells are localized in the stroma, unassociated with epithelial components. **B:** Multiple overlapping nuclei and inconspicuous cytoplasm are characteristic features.

## ULTRASTRUCTURE AND IMMUNOHISTOCHEMISTRY

Electron microscopic and immunohistochemical studies have shown conclusively that the giant cells have no epithelial features and that they are of mesenchymal origin (5,6,9,14,23–28) (Fig. 25.17). Athanasou et al. (25) carried out *in vitro* functional studies with osteoclast-like giant cells isolated from a mammary carcinoma. When incubated with bone slices, the giant cells were stimulated by parathormone, but not by calcitonin, to cause bone resorption. Immunohistochemical studies revealed that the giant cells expressed human leukocyte antigen DR locus (HLA-DR) and Fc receptors. They also were stained by a variety of antibodies that react with macrophages and osteoclasts. These investigators

concluded that the giant cells are a specific type of macrophage with osteoclastic functional capability.

At the ultrastructural level, the cytoplasm of osteoclast-like giant cells contains many organelles, including mitochondria, endoplasmic reticulum, ribosomes, relatively few lysosomes, and occasional hemosiderin granules (5,6, 24,29). Absence of factor VIII and *Ulex* activity from osteoclast-like giant cells suggests they are not of endothelial origin (6,24,29). Strong acid phosphatase reactivity (4,6,26), staining for histiocytic markers such as $\alpha_1$-antitrypsin, KP-1 (CD68) (Fig. 25.18), and lysozyme in some (8,14), but not all, tumors (29), an absence of alkaline phosphatase staining, and other histochemical features (6) are consistent with the morphologic similarity to histiocytic cells or osteoclasts of bone (26). The carcinoma cells in these tumors are immunoreactive with various cytokeratins (CK7, AE1/AE3,

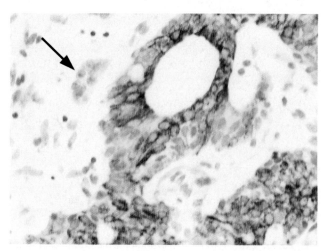

**FIG. 25.17.** *Carcinoma with osteoclast-like giant cells.* The carcinoma cells are immunoreactive for cytokeratin, but the osteoclast-like giant cell *(arrow)* is not stained (anti-AE1/AE3, avidin-biotin).

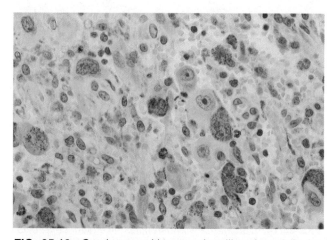

**FIG. 25.18.** *Carcinoma with osteoclast-like giant cells.* Immunoreactivity for KP1(CD68) is evident in the osteoclast-like giant cells but not in carcinoma cells (avidin-biotin).

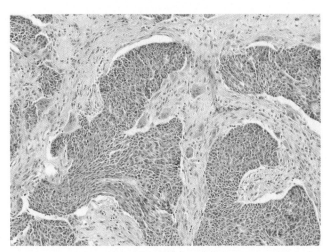

**FIG. 25.19.** *Carcinoma with osteoclast-like giant cells, metastatic.* Osteoclast-like giant cells are present in the stroma of metastatic carcinoma in the liver.

CAM5.2), epithelial membrane antigen, and variably for carcinoembryonic antigen (6,8).

## PROGNOSIS AND TREATMENT

Axillary lymph node metastases have been reported in approximately a third of cases. Local recurrence (5,9) and systemic metastases in the eye, liver, and other organs have been described (3,9). Osteoclast-like giant cells are found in some, but not all, metastases in axillary lymph nodes or other sites (3,5,30) (Fig. 25.19). The presence of osteoclast-like giant cells within intralymphatic carcinomatous emboli suggests that these stromal cells can be transported to regional lymph nodes and to distant metastases (Fig. 25.20). It is also possible that osteoclast-like giant cell formation is induced by metastases, possibly through a mechanism such as IL-1 secretion (19).

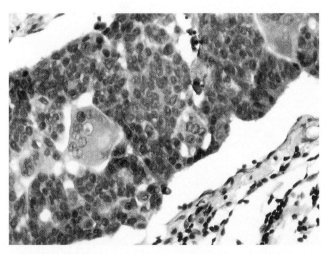

**FIG. 25.20.** *Carcinoma with osteoclast-like giant cells.* Carcinoma with giant cells in a dilated lymphatic channel.

Nearly two-thirds of patients have been reported to be alive and well, with follow-up rarely reaching beyond five years (4,9). The tumors have had low levels of estrogen receptor, but many had remarkably high progesterone receptors (5,9,11). Primary treatment usually has been mastectomy with axillary dissection. Data on lumpectomy with primary radiotherapy and adjuvant systemic therapy for this neoplasm are only anecdotal, but presently it appears appropriate to use the same treatment criteria as for invasive mammary carcinoma generally.

## REFERENCES

1. Darby A, Papadaki L, Beilby JOW. An unusual leiomyosarcoma of the uterus containing osteoclast-like cells. *Cancer* 1975;36:495–504.
2. Alpers CE, Beckstead JH. Malignant neuroendocrine tumor of the jejunum with osteoclast-like giant cells. Enzyme histochemistry distinguishes tumor cells from giant cells. *Am J Surg Pathol* 1985;9:57–64.
3. Agnantis NT, Rosen PP. Mammary carcinoma with osteoclast-like giant cells. *Am J Clin Pathol* 1979;72:383–389.
4. Ichijima K, Kobashi Y, Ueda Y, et al. Breast cancer with reactive multinucleated giant cells: report of three cases. *Acta Pathol Jpn* 1986; 36:449–457.
5. Holland R, Van Haelst VJGM. Mammary carcinoma with osteoclast-like giant cells. Additional observations on six cases. *Cancer* 1984;53:1963–1973.
6. Nielsen BB, Kiaer HW. Carcinoma of the breast with stromal multinucleated cells. *Histopathology* 1985;9:183–193.
7. Shabb NS, Tawil A, Mufarrij A, et al. Mammary carcinoma with osteoclastlike giant cells cytologically mimicking benign breast disease: a case report. *Acta Cytol* 1997;41:1284–1288.
8. Takahashi T, Moriki T, Hiroi M, et al. Invasive lobular carcinoma of the breast with osteoclastlike giant cells: a case report. *Acta Cytol* 1998;42:734–741.
9. Tavassoli FA, Norris HJ. Breast carcinoma with osteoclast-like giant cells. *Arch Pathol Lab Med* 1986;110:636–639.
10. Fisher ER, Gregorio RM, Palekar AS, et al. Mucoepidermoid and squamous cell carcinomas of breast with reference to squamous metaplasia and giant cell tumors. *Am J Surg Pathol* 1983;7:15–27.
11. Bertrand G, Bidabe M-Cl, Bertrand AF. Le carcinome mammaire a stroma reaction giganto-cellulare. *Arch Anat Cytol Pathol* 1982;30:5–9.
12. Volpe R, Carbone A, Nicalo G, et al. Cytology of the breast carcinoma with osteoclastlike giant cells. *Acta Cytol* 1981;27:184–187.
13. Boccato P, Briani G, d'Atri C, et al. Spindle cell and cartilaginous metaplasia in breast carcinoma with osteoclast-like stromal cells: a difficult fine needle aspiration diagnosis. *Acta Cytol* 1988;32:75–78.
14. Phillipson J, Ostrzega N. Fine needle aspiration of invasive cribriform carcinoma with benign osteoclastlike giant cells of histiocytic origin: a case report. *Acta Cytol* 1994;38:479–482.
15. Douglas-Jones AG, Barr WT. Breast carcinoma with tumor giant cells: report of a case with fine needle aspiration cytology. *Acta Cytol* 1989;33:109–114.
16. Gupta RK, Holloway LJ, Wakefield SJ, et al. Fine needle aspiration cytology, immunocytochemistry and electron microscopy in a rare case of carcinoma of the breast with malignant epithelial giant cells. *Acta Cytol* 1991;35:412–416.
17. Gullino PM. Natural history of breast cancer. Progression from hyperplasia to neoplasia as predicted by angiogenesis. *Cancer* 1977; 39:2697–2703.
18. Al-Sumidaie AM, Leinster SJ, Jenkins SA. Transformation of blood monocytes to giant cells in vitro from patients with breast cancer. *Br J Surg* 1986;73:839–842.
19. Jimi E, Nakamura I, Duong LT, et al. Interleukin 1 induces multinucleation and bone-resorbing activity of osteoclasts in the absence of osteoblasts/stromal cells. *Exp Cell Res* 1999;247:84–93.
20. Wargotz ES, Norris HJ. Metaplastic carcinomas of the breast: V. Metaplastic carcinoma with osteoclastic giant cells. *Hum Pathol* 1990;21:1142–1150.
21. Brooks JJ, Krugman DT, Damjanov I. Myeloid metaplasia presenting as a breast mass. *Am J Surg Pathol* 1980;4:281–285.

22. Bassler R, Birke F. Histopathology of tumour associated sarcoid-like stromal reaction in breast cancer: an analysis of 5 cases with immunohistochemical investigations. *Virchows Arch* 1988;412:231–239.

23. Oberman HA. Invasive carcinoma of the breast with granulomatous response. *Am J Clin Pathol* 1987;88:718–721.

24. McMahon RFT, Ahmed A, Connoly CF. Breast carcinoma with stromal multinucleated giant cells: a light microscopic, histochemical and ultrastructural study. *J Pathol* 1986;150:175–179.

25. Athanasou NA, Wells CA, Quinn J, et al. The origin and nature of stromal osteoclast-like multinucleated giant cells in breast carcinoma: implications for tumor osteolysis and macrophage biology. *Br J Cancer* 1989;59:491–498.

26. Chilose M, Bonetti F, Menestrina F, et al. Breast carcinoma with stromal multinucleated giant cells [Letter]. *J Pathol* 1987;152:55–57.

27. Factor FM, Biempica L, Ratner I, et al. Carcinoma of the breast with multinucleated reactive stromal giant cells: a light and electron microscopic study of two cases. *Virchows Arch* 1977;374:1–12.

28. Sugano I, Nagao K, Kondo Y, et al. Cytologic and ultrastructural studies of a rare breast carcinoma with osteoclast-like giant cells. *Cancer* 1983;52:74–78.

29. Viacava P, Naccarato AG, Nardini V, et al. Breast carcinoma with osteoclast-like giant cells: immunohistochemical and ultrastructural study of a case and review of the literature. *Tumori* 1995;81:135–141.

30. Levin A, Rywlin AM, Tachmes P. Carcinoma of the breast with stromal epulis-like giant cells. *South Med J* 1981;74:889–891.

# CHAPTER 26

# Cystic Hypersecretory Carcinoma and Cystic Hypersecretory Hyperplasia

This variant of duct carcinoma, first described in 1984 (1), deserves separate discussion because of its unusual pathologic features. Most cases have been intraductal carcinomas. A benign proliferative lesion that resembles cystic hypersecretory carcinoma has been termed *cystic hypersecretory hyperplasia* (2). About 30 cystic hypersecretory lesions have been reported (3).

The reported age distribution of cystic hypersecretory carcinoma is similar to that of breast carcinoma generally, with the youngest patient aged 34 years and the oldest thus far reported at 79 years. The mean age in the largest series was 56 years (2). The presenting symptom usually has been a mass or other palpable abnormality. Mammography in one case revealed a prominent ductal pattern and an irregular density in the breast (4). Mammography in another patient with a 2-cm palpable tumor revealed two tumors (5). A "large tumor filling the upper outer quadrant" had "massive calcification" on mammography in a 50-year-old woman (6). Among 11 tumors studied biochemically, eight had negative levels of estrogen and progesterone receptors, and two specimens were positive for both receptors.

## GROSS PATHOLOGY

The tumors have measured from 1 to 10 cm in diameter. The lesion is firm but not usually hard. It is visibly distinct from the surrounding breast parenchyma but not sharply demarcated. The distinctive gross feature of cystic hypersecretory carcinoma is the presence of numerous cysts within the lesion (Fig. 26.1). Many of these tumors are a shade of brown or gray–brown, which reflects the cyst contents. The cysts vary considerably in size, with some measuring up to 1.5 cm. Secretion within cysts has been described as sticky, mucinous, gelatinous, or as resembling thyroid colloid.

Although cystic hypersecretory lesions have a distinctive gross appearance, it usually is not possible to distinguish cystic hypersecretory carcinoma from cystic hypersecretory hyperplasia grossly. Both processes have essentially the same gross patterns and distribution of cysts. An invasive component associated with cystic hypersecretory carcinoma usually produces a distinct, solid mass.

## MICROSCOPIC PATHOLOGY

Microscopically, all cystic hypersecretory lesions have cysts that contain eosinophilic secretion that bears a striking resemblance to thyroid colloid (Fig. 26.2). The secretion is homogeneous and usually virtually acellular. It often retracts from the surrounding epithelium, with a smooth or scalloped margin reflecting the extent of epithelial proliferation. Defects in the secretion sometimes consist of folds, linear cracks, or small punched-out holes (Fig. 26.3). Necrosis and calcifications ordinarily are not seen; histiocytes are rarely present in the secretion (Fig. 26.4). There are no appreciable differences in the character of the secretion in cystic hypersecretory carcinoma and cystic hypersecretory hyperplasia. Positive reactions for carcinoembryonic antigen, α-lactalbumin, periodic acid-Schiff, and mucin have been observed in the cyst contents, which are consistently negative for thyroglobulin. Disruption of cysts results in spillage of cyst contents, eliciting an intense inflammatory reaction consisting of lymphocytes and histiocytes.

Many of the cysts in cystic hypersecretory lesions are lined by inconspicuous flat cells or a single layer of cuboidal or columnar cells (Figs. 26.3 and 26.4). When this is the only epithelial pattern, the lesion is cystic hypersecretory hyperplasia (2). Generally, the cells in such lesions have uniform cytologically bland nuclei and scant cytoplasm. Atypical features in this setting are epithelial crowding, hyperchromasia, rare mitotic figures and enlargement of nuclei, which may contain nucleoli. Epithelial crowding of cells in cystic hypersecretory hyperplasia may result in atypical hyperplasia (Fig. 26.5).

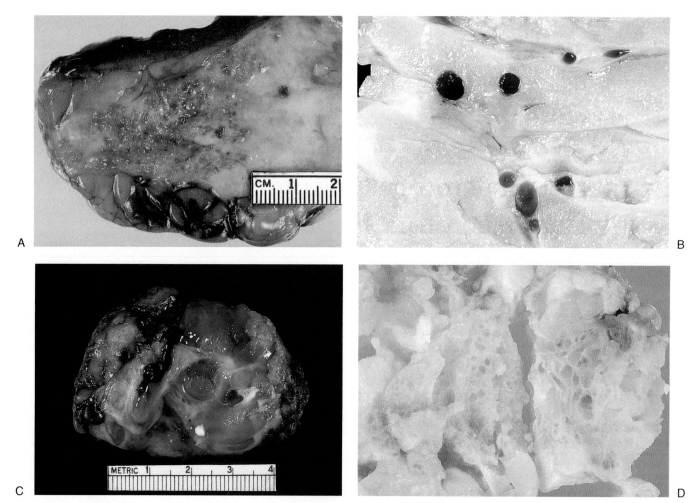

**FIG. 26.1.** *Cystic hypersecretory carcinoma.* **A:** The lesion is a discrete but not circumscribed mass with many cysts. **B:** Cysts filled with tan secretion that resembles thyroid colloid. **C:** Some of the cysts are larger than 1.0 cm. **D:** A fixed specimen that has been dissected to reveal numerous cysts.

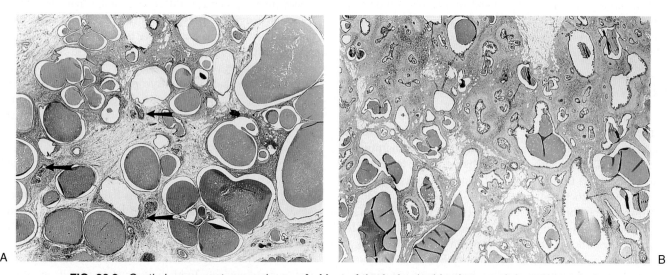

**FIG. 26.2.** *Cystic hypersecretory carcinoma.* **A:** Most of the lesion in this photograph is composed of cysts lined by flat epithelium characteristic of cystic hypersecretory hyperplasia. A few ducts with micropapillary intraductal carcinoma are present *(arrows).* **B:** Many ducts and cysts in this lesion contain micropapillary intraductal carcinoma.

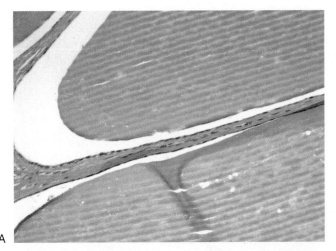

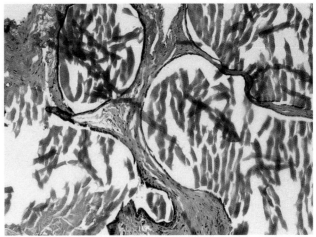

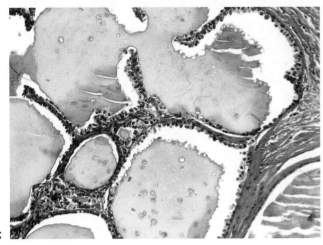

FIG. 26.3. *Cystic hypersecretory hyperplasia.* **A:** These cysts are lined by flat epithelium. Note the wavy appearance and retraction of the secretion. **B:** This secretion displays exaggerated cracks as a result of fragmentation during histologic preparation. **C:** The hyperplastic epithelium has a hobnail appearance. Note the scalloped edges of the retracted secretion.

In cystic hypersecretory carcinoma, the epithelium of some cysts and ducts grows as micropapillary intraductal carcinoma (Fig. 26.6). In any one case, a spectrum of epithelial patterns is encountered, ranging from short, knobby epithelial tufts to complex branching fronds that may extend across the duct lumen (Fig. 26.7). The so-called Roman arch,

or bridging pattern, which is commonly seen in other forms of micropapillary carcinoma, however, is uncommon in these lesions. Ducts with intraductal carcinoma may not contain secretion.

Cytologically, the cells that constitute this type of carcinoma usually have crowded and overlapping hyperchromatic nuclei and sparse cytoplasm. The nuclear grade is most often intermediate to poorly differentiated. High-grade lesions exhibit more pronounced mitotic activity. There is no secretion within the cytoplasm, but frayed, irregular cell borders and apical cytoplasmic blebs are consistent with some degree of secretory activity in most foci of intraductal carcinoma.

Lobules in and around the lesional areas in women with cystic hypersecretory lesions often exhibit hypersecretory change that includes the accumulation of secretion (Fig. 26.8). This lobular abnormality may occur as an isolated finding in the absence of a fully developed cystic hypersecretory lesion, an observation that suggests that the process may originate in such foci.

Cystic hypersecretory hyperplasia sometimes coexists with pregnancy-like hyperplasia, and aspects of the two conditions seem to overlap when this occurs. Consequently, secretion with characteristics associated with a cystic hyper-

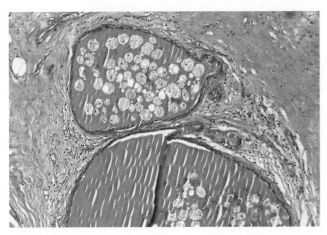

FIG. 26.4. *Cystic hypersecretory hyperplasia with histiocytes.*

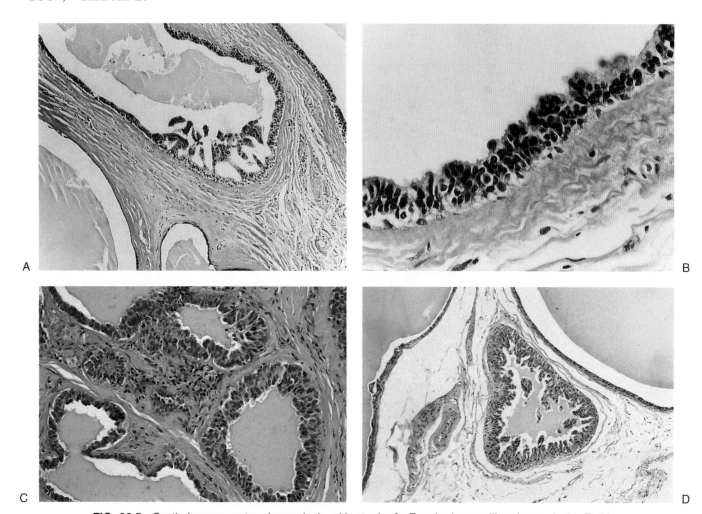

**FIG. 26.5.** *Cystic hypersecretory hyperplasia with atypia.* **A:** Focal micropapillary hyperplasia. **B:** Hyperplasia with nuclear crowding and hyperchromasia. **C:** Marked epithelial crowding with loss of basal polarity in an example of marked atypia in cystic hypersecretory hyperplasia. **D:** Atypical micropapillary hyperplasia in a cystic hypersecretory lesion.

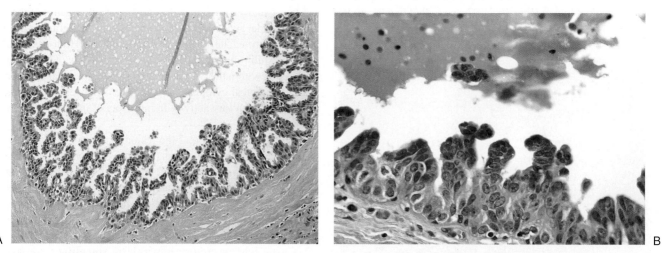

**FIG. 26.6.** *Cystic hypersecretory carcinoma.* **A,B:** Intraductal cystic hypersecretory carcinoma, micropapillary. *(continued)*

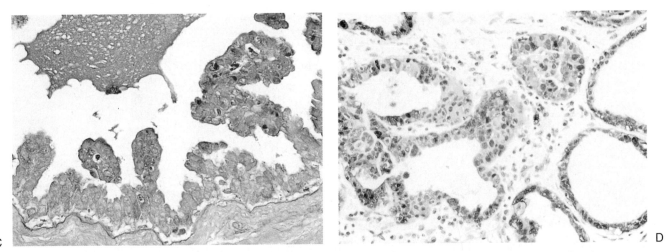

**FIG. 26.6.** *Continued.* **C:** A positive reaction with the periodic acid-Schiff (PAS) reagent that persisted after diastase treatment in cystic hypersecretory carcinoma. (PAS-disastase). **D:** Immunoreactivity for S-100 in the cytoplasm and nuclei of cells in cystic hypersecretory hyperplasia is shown (avidin-biotin).

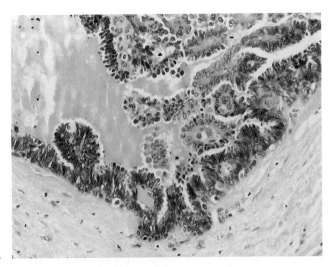

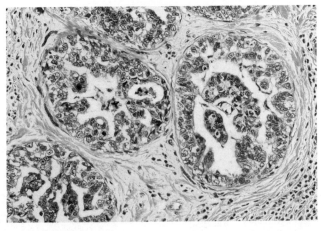

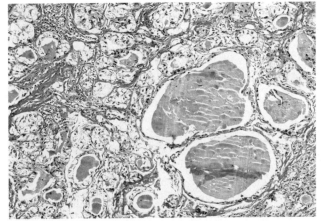

**FIG. 26.7.** *Cystic hypersecretory intraductal carcinoma.* **A:** An unusual papillary growth pattern in which the carcinomatous fronds contain fibrovascular stroma. **B:** Micropapillary intraductal carcinoma with high nuclear grade. **C:** An unusual clear cell lesion with microglandular growth. *(continued)*

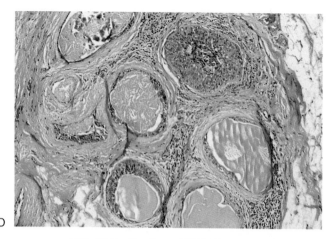

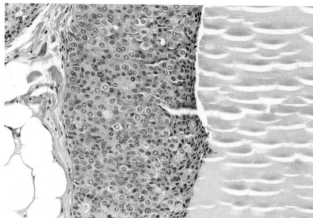

**FIG. 26.7.** *Continued.* **D,E:** Two examples of solid intraductal carcinoma with cystic hypersecretory secretion.

secretory lesion may be found in glands formed by epithelium with the appearance of pregnancy-like hyperplasia. This convergence usually is marked by cytologic and structural atypia that may be severe. Rarely, the proliferative and

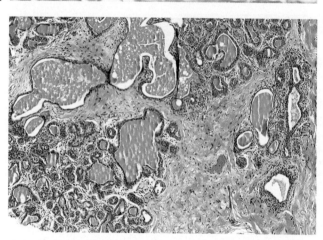

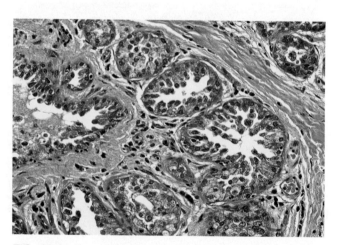

**FIG. 26.8.** *Hypersecretory change in lobules.* The illustrations present lobular changes in patients with cystic hypersecretory carcinoma. **A:** The lobular glands contain small amounts of retracted secretion. **B:** Lobular glands and ducts dilated with secretion that exhibits typical pock marks and parallel cracks.

cytologic abnormalities warrant a diagnosis of cystic hypersecretory carcinoma, which has features of pregnancy-like change with especially pronounced cytoplasmic vacuolization (Fig. 26.9). See Chapter 1 for additional information about pregnancy-like hyperplasia.

Invasive cystic hypersecretory carcinoma consists of cystic hypersecretory intraductal carcinoma accompanied by an invasive component. Most invasive carcinomas thus far encountered in this setting have been poorly differentiated duct carcinomas with a solid growth pattern (Fig. 26.10). Nuclei of invasive carcinoma cells may have a clear vacuolated appearance similar to the pattern observed in papillary thyroid carcinoma. Lymphatic tumor emboli may be present in the vicinity of the invasive tumor. Light microscopy has disclosed little or no secretory activity within the cells. Metastatic foci in the axillary lymph nodes of two patients had cystic foci that contained eosinophilic secretion (2). In one case, metastatic carcinoma involved 12 of 28 lymph nodes (5).

One patient had a separate invasive lobular carcinoma in a breast which harbored cystic hypersecretory carcinoma

**FIG. 26.9.** *Pregnancy-like hyperplasia.* This intralobular lesion lacks cystic hypersecretory secretion. Note the vacuolated cytoplasm and apical nuclear extrusion. The florid micropapillary structure seen here is atypical and may coexist with cystic hypersecretory intraductal carcinoma.

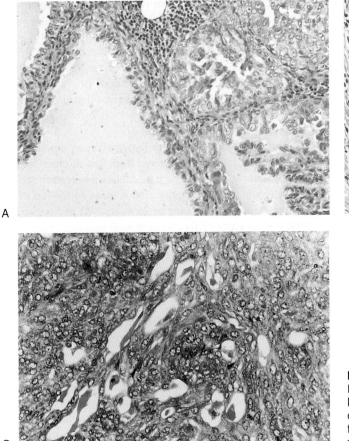

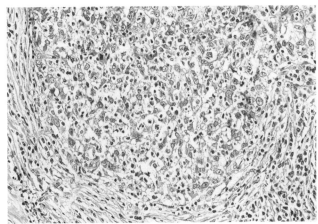

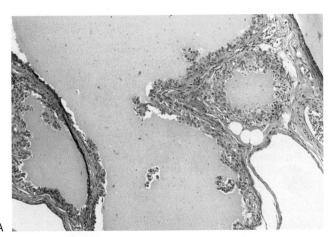

**FIG. 26.10.** *Cystic hypersecretory carcinoma, invasive.* **A:** Intraductal cystic hypersecretory micropapillary carcinoma. Note the vesicular nuclei. **B:** Poorly differentiated invasive ductal carcinoma with a lymphocytic infiltrate in the stroma from the same specimen as **A**. **C:** Magnified view of the invasive component in another case showing vesicular nuclei.

(Fig. 26.11). Another patient developed invasive lobular carcinoma of the contralateral breast 10 years after ipsilateral mastectomy for invasive cystic hypersecretory carcinoma (3).

Electron microscopy has been performed in two cases (2,5). The involved ductules were lined by epithelial cells surrounded by myoepithelial cells. Ductular epithelial cells were largely devoid of surface microvilli. No polarization of secretory vesicles or inclusions was seen. Large secretory granules that contained sparse, fine granular material were limited to the basal cytoplasm. Ductular lumens contained amorphous or finely granular material. These ultrastructural findings differ appreciably from those seen in secretory carcinoma, which features abundant intracytoplasmic secretory granules as well as intracytoplasmic glandular lumens. Mucinous carcinoma also differs ultrastructurally from cystic

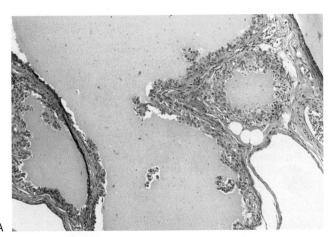

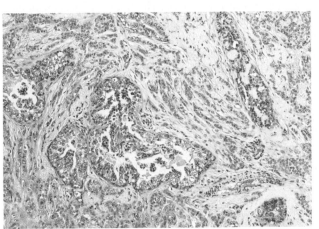

**FIG. 26.11.** *Cystic hypersecretory carcinoma and invasive lobular carcinoma.* **A:** Cystic hypersecretory micropapillary intraductal carcinoma. **B:** Another area in the tumor where papillary intraductal carcinoma is surrounded and partly overgrown by invasive lobular carcinoma.

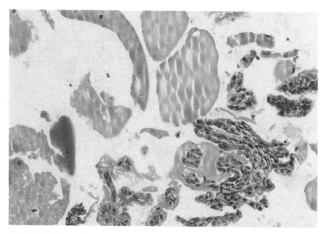

**FIG. 26.12.** *Cystic hypersecretory carcinoma, fine needle aspiration.* The specimen consists of dislodged secretion with characteristic cracks and fragments of papillary carcinomatous epithelium.

hypersecretory carcinoma in having abundant extracellular mucin and intracytoplasmic mucinogen granules.

Cystic hypersecretory lesions can be diagnosed in a fine needle aspiration specimen if the secretion is recognized (4,5,7). The secretory material forms dense masses that duplicate the appearance of this material in histologic sections (Fig. 26.12). Epithelial cells in clusters and individually may be found amidst the secretory material. Lesions with intraductal carcinoma usually produce papillary clusters of tumor cells in a fine needle aspiration specimen.

## PROGNOSIS AND TREATMENT

Excisional biopsy is required for definitive diagnosis and especially to distinguish cystic hypersecretory hyperplasia from cystic hypersecretory carcinoma. On more than one occasion, an incompletely excised lesion has been misclassified as "cystic disease" (1,4), with the true nature of the process becoming apparent when the lesion recurred.

Little is known about the clinical course of this uncommon type of breast carcinoma. The finding of areas with the typical features of cystic hypersecretory hyperplasia, sometimes with atypia, associated with cystic hypersecretory carcinoma suggests that these processes are related, but convincing evidence of progression through these stages has not yet been presented. Review of prior biopsies from women later found to have cystic hypersecretory carcinoma has disclosed various lesions, including seemingly unrelated common proliferative changes, cystic hypersecretory hyperplasia, and cystic hypersecretory carcinoma. Follow-up of eight patients with cystic hypersecretory hyperplasia revealed subsequent breast carcinoma in two cases. One women developed a fatal contralateral invasive duct carcinoma that lacked cystic hypersecretory features. The other patient had intraductal carcinoma separate from cystic hypersecretory hyperplasia in a biopsy and residual cystic hypersecretory hyperplasia in the mastectomy specimen. Bogomoletz described a 55-year-old woman who was well without recurrence 6 years after excisional biopsy of a 7-cm example of cystic hypersecretory hyperplasia (8).

The clinical course of cystic hypersecretory intraductal carcinoma thus far has not differed from that of other forms of intraductal carcinoma. There have been no recurrences in women treated by mastectomy after a mean follow-up of 8 years, extending in one case to 23 years. All had negative lymph nodes. Three of five women with invasive cystic hypersecretory carcinoma had metastases in axillary lymph nodes. One patient had locally advanced or inflammatory carcinoma at diagnosis. Thus far, the only reported death from cystic hypersecretory carcinoma occurred in this patient.

Therapeutic options for patients with cystic hypersecretory carcinoma are similar to those available to women with other forms of duct carcinoma. Mastectomy has proven curative for women with intraductal lesions. Too few patients have been treated by lumpectomy and radiotherapy to assess this type of treatment. When invasive carcinoma is present, axillary dissection or sentinel lymph node mapping should be performed. Adjuvant chemotherapy should be added for stage II patients, and it may be considered for stage I patients in view of the poorly differentiated character of the invasive tumors thus far encountered.

## REFERENCES

1. Rosen PP, Scott M. Cystic hypersecretory duct carcinoma of the breast. *Am J Surg Pathol* 1984;8:31–41.
2. Guerry P, Erlandson RA, Rosen PP. Cystic hypersecretory hyperplasia and cystic hypersecretory duct carcinoma of the breast: pathology, therapy and follow-up of 39 patients. *Cancer* 1988;61:1611–1620.
3. Herrmann ME, McClatchey KD, Siziopikou KP. Invasive cystic hypersecretory ductal carcinoma of the breast: a case report and review of the literature. *Arch Pathol Lab Med* 1999;123:1108–1110.
4. Colandrea JM, Shmookler BM, O'Dowd GJ, et al. Cystic hypersecretory duct carcinoma of the breast: report of a case with fine needle aspiration. *Arch Pathol Lab Med* 1988;112:560–563.
5. Lee W-Y, Cheng L, Chang T-W. Diagnosing invasive cystic hypersecretory duct carcinoma of the breast with fine needle aspiration cytology: a case report. *Acta Cytol* 1999;43:273–276.
6. Cserni G, Virágh S. Immunohistochemical and ultrastructural analysis of a mammary cystic hypersecretory carcinoma. *Pathol Oncol Res* 1997;3:287–292.
7. Kim M-K, Kwon G-Y, Gong G-Y. Fine needle aspiration cytology of cystic hypersecretory carcinoma of the breast: a case report. *Acta Cytol* 1997;41:892–896.
8. Bogomoletz W-V. Hyperplasia hypersécrétoire kystique du sein: un diagnostic rare en pathologie mammaire. *Ann Pathol* 1994;14:131–132.

# CHAPTER 27

# Adenoid Cystic Carcinoma

The term *cylindroma,* used interchangeably with *adenoid cystic carcinoma,* was proposed by Billroth, who concluded that the tumor was composed of entwined cylinders of stroma and epithelial cells. Ewing (1) mentioned adenoid cystic carcinoma of the salivary glands, and this term was applied in 1945 to tumors of the breast by Geschickter to refer to lesions he classified as adenocystic basal cell carcinoma (2). Three examples of mammary adenoid cystic carcinoma were cited by Foote and Stewart in 1946 (3). Two decades later, Galloway et al. at the Mayo Clinic described the first series of cases and reviewed twelve others previously reported (4).

## CLINICAL FEATURES

Adenoid cystic carcinoma occurs in adult women throughout the age distribution of mammary carcinoma, with patients between 25 and 80 years of age (4–11). The mean age varies from 50 to 63 years. Isolated cases have been encountered in men and in children (12,13) (Fig. 27.1). Cutaneous adenoid cystic carcinoma has been reported in the periareolar region of a 35-year-old man (14).

The left and right breasts are equally affected, and there is no predilection for adenoid cystic carcinoma to develop bilaterally. Other types of carcinoma may develop in the contralateral breast (6,9,10,15), or in rare instances, another type of carcinoma may be found in the same breast (7).

Adenoid cystic carcinoma usually presents as a palpable, discrete, firm mass. Although calcifications develop in these tumors, few have been detected by mammography, and in some cases the mammogram was reportedly negative (10,15). Mammography of clinically palpable tumors reveals a well-defined lobulated mass or an ill-defined lesion (15,16). Magnetic resonance imaging (MRI) revealed an unusual pattern of enhancement in one case (17). Pain or tenderness described in a minority of cases has not been particularly correlated with the finding of perineural invasion histologically. Skin dimpling, ulceration, or peau d'orange have been reported in patients with superficial or large lesions. Nipple discharge is rarely an initial symptom (10), de-

spite the fact that adenoid cystic carcinoma occurs with disproportionately high frequency centrally or in the subareolar part of the breast (15).

Most patients report that their tumor was detected shortly before seeking medical attention, but intervals of 9 (10,15), 10 (13), and 15 (4) years have been described. The median duration in one series was 24 months, and six tumors were present for a year or longer before diagnosis (10).

Few examples of adenoid cystic carcinoma have been examined biochemically for hormone receptors, and most tumors have been described as hormone receptor negative (11,18,19). In one report, four of six lesions were negative for estrogen or progesterone receptors or both, one tumor was positive for estrogen (15 fmol) and progesterone (17 fmol) receptors, and one was positive for progesterone (19 fmol) and negative for estrogen receptors (10). The latter two were low-grade lesions with no special distinguishing morphologic features. Eleven tumors examined by immunohistochemistry were reported to be negative for estrogen and progesterone receptors (15,20).

## GROSS PATHOLOGY

Gross size of the lesions has varied from less than 1 cm to 12 cm (4,5,9,10). Most are between 1 and 3 cm. Tumors with low-grade histologic features tend to be smaller (0.5–2.8 cm; mean, 1.6 cm) than high-grade tumors (1.5–8.0 cm; mean, 3.5 cm).

Most adenoid cystic carcinomas are circumscribed or nodular grossly. Small cystic areas are not unusual, especially in lesions smaller than 5 cm (Fig. 27.2). Larger tumors may have areas of gross cystic degeneration (3,4,10) (Fig. 27.3). The lesions have been variously described as gray, pale yellow, tan, and pink.

## MICROSCOPIC PATHOLOGY

Despite their well-defined gross borders, about 50% of adenoid cystic carcinomas have an invasive growth pattern microscopically in which the tumor invades the surrounding

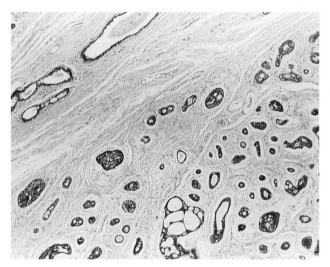

**FIG. 27.1.** *Adenoid cystic carcinoma, child.* This tumor arose in the breast of a 13-year-old boy. Juvenile breast ducts are visible in the *upper left* corner.

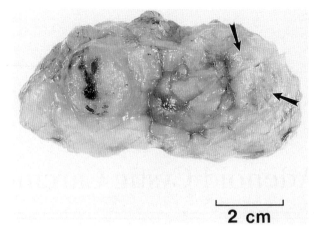

**FIG. 27.2.** *Adenoid cystic carcinoma, gross appearance.* The circumscribed tumor has a central cavity on the *left* in this bisected specimen. Part of the tumor on the *right* is indistinct *(arrows).*

breast parenchyma beyond the central grossly apparent nodule (10) (Fig. 27.4). Microcystic areas formed by the coalescent spaces in dilated glands are seen in about 25% of tumors. When sufficiently large, these spaces can be appreciated grossly (Fig. 27.5). Invasion around nerves (perineural invasion) is found in a minority of tumors. Lymphatic tumor emboli are extremely uncommon (10). Shrinkage artifacts occur relatively often in adenoid cystic carcinoma and may be mistaken for lymphatic tumor emboli. Shrinkage tends to be more pronounced in fibrotic portions of the tumor (Fig. 27.6).

It is usually difficult to detect an *in situ* component, but in a minority of low-grade adenoid cystic carcinomas, there may be conspicuous lobular and duct involvement (Fig. 27.7). This type of intraductal carcinoma can be responsible for local recurrence (Fig. 27.8).

Adenoid cystic carcinoma consists of a mixture of proliferating glands (adenoid component) and stromal or basement membrane elements ("pseudoglandular" or cylindromatous component) (Fig. 27.9). These components are rarely distributed homogeneously in a given tumor (Fig. 27.10). Some areas consist of only the adenoid elements, creating a close resemblance to cribriform carcinoma (21). Abundant stromal material in other parts of the tumor produces a pattern that may be mistaken for scirrhous carcinoma (Fig. 27.11). As a result of this intratumoral heterogeneity, adenoid cystic carcinoma may be difficult to recognize in a needle biopsy specimen unless a characteristic sample has been obtained. Adenoid cystic carcinoma can be diagnosed in a fine needle aspiration specimen if adenoid glandular clusters and nodules of cylindromatous material are present (Fig. 27.12) (19,22,23). Inspissated secretion and stromal

*Text continues on p. 541.*

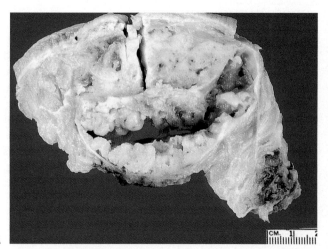

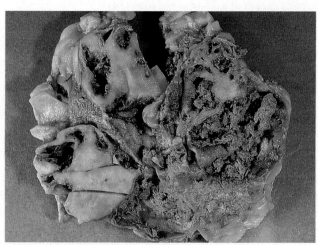

**FIG. 27.3.** *Adenoid cystic carcinoma, cystic.* **A:** Mastectomy specimen with a large partly cystic tumor that occupied most of the breast. **B:** Extensive cystic degeneration developed in this tumor. Some solid areas remain.

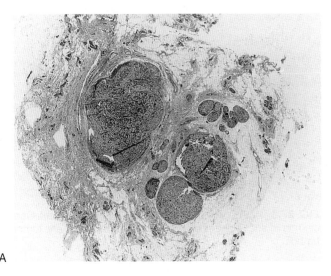

A

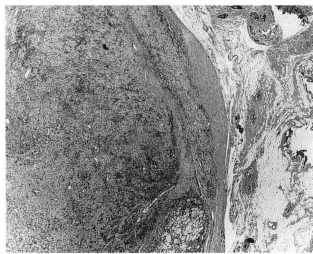

B

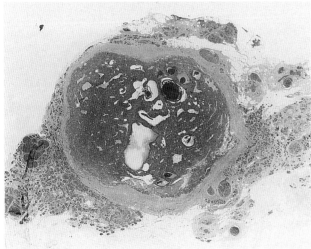

C

**FIG. 27.4.** *Adenoid cystic carcinoma.* **A:** A whole-mount histologic section of an adenoid cystic carcinoma composed of aggregated circumscribed nodules with no stromal invasion beyond the grossly evident tumor. **B:** The border of this circumscribed tumor appears to be encapsulated. **C:** A whole-mount histologic section that demonstrated a circumscribed central tumor nodule surrounded by areas of carcinoma with an invasive pattern. (**A,C** from Rosen PP. Adenoid cystic carcinoma of the breast: a morphologically heterogeneous neoplasm. *Pathol Annu* 1989;24:237–254, with permission.)

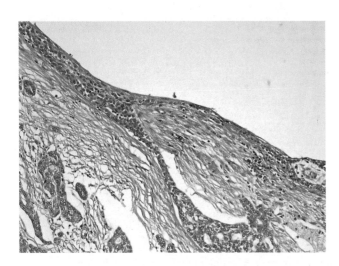

**FIG. 27.5.** *Adenoid cystic carcinoma, cystic.* The cyst cavity is lined by neoplastic epithelium with superficial squamous differentiation.

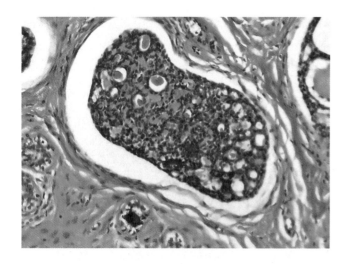

**FIG. 27.6.** *Adenoid cystic carcinoma, shrinkage artifact.* Carcinoma in such spaces may be mistaken for lymphatic tumor emboli.

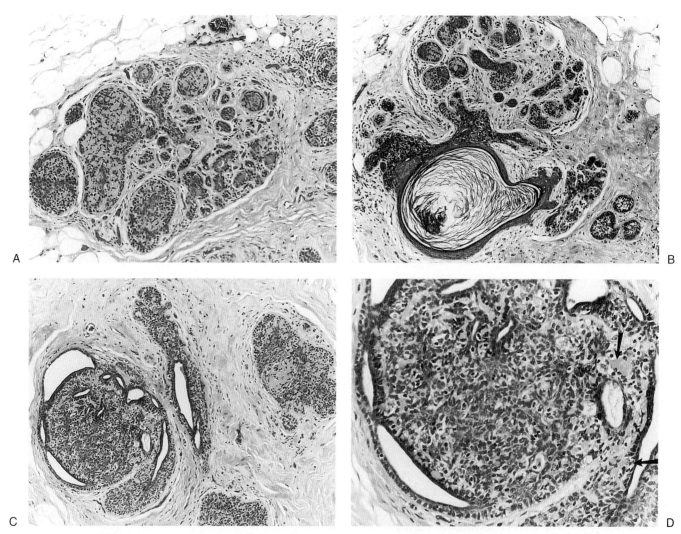

**FIG. 27.7.** *Adenoid cystic carcinoma, lobular and duct involvement.* **A:** Intralobular carcinoma with conspicuous cylindromatous differentiation. **B:** Squamous differentiation in a lobule. **C:** Predominantly adenomyoepithelial structure in ducts. **D:** Enlarged view of adenomyoepithelial differentiation in a duct with traces of cylindromatous differentiation *(arrows).* (**B,C** From Rosen PP. Adenoid cystic carcinoma of the breast: a morphologically heterogeneous neoplasm. *Pathol Annu* 1989;24:237–254, with permission.)

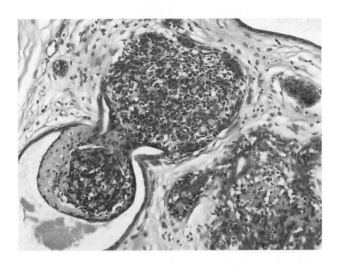

**Fig. 27.8.** *Adenoid cystic carcinoma, intraductal.* Intraductal carcinoma found in a reexcision specimen.

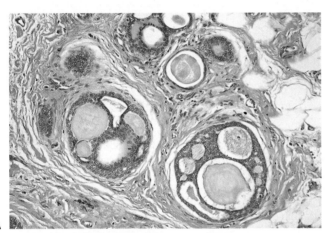

A

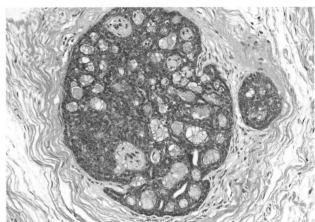

B

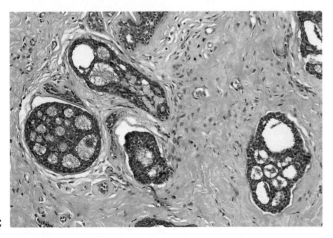

C

**FIG. 27.9.** *Adenoid cystic carcinoma.* **A:** Invasive tumor with conspicuous solid, pink cylindromatous nodules and glandular spaces with basophilic secretion. **B:** Isolated nuclei of myoepithelial cells are attached to cylindromatous nodules in the *upper center*. Note the basophilic degeneration of some cylindromatous nodules. **C:** This focus is predominantly cribriform with a minor cylindromatous component in the upper left gland.

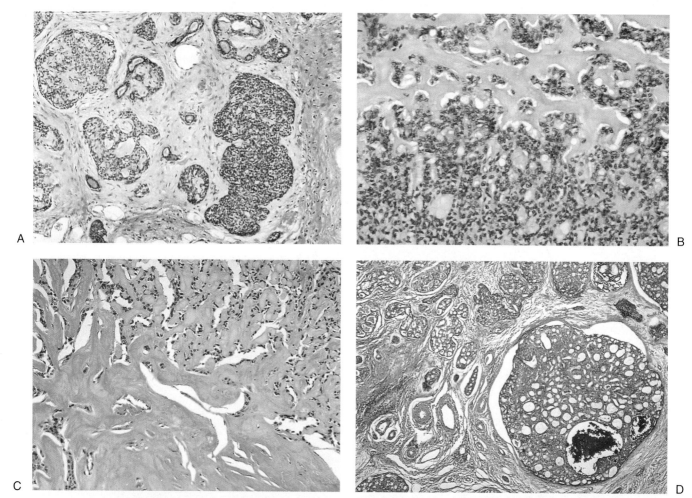

**FIG. 27.10.** *Adenoid cystic carcinoma, structural heterogeneity.* **A:** This microscopic field displays typical *(left)* and solid *(right)* growth patterns. **B:** An area of solid growth below and a striking cylindromatous component above. **C:** Dense amyloid-like stroma with residual cylindromatous nodules visible in the *upper right* area. The cellular constituent is almost entirely myoepithelial. **D:** A prominent cribriform element and, at the *upper border*, a more conventional adenoid cystic element.

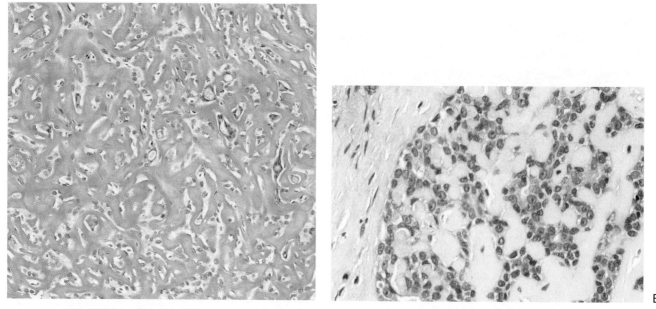

**FIG. 27.11.** *Adenoid cystic carcinoma.* **A:** Overgrowth of cylindromatous material leaving sparse glands. This tumor resembles pseudoangiomatous stromal hyperplasia. A needle core biopsy sample could be mistaken for invasive lobular or scirrhous carcinoma. **B:** Excessive cylindromatous material in a circumscribed tumor nodule.

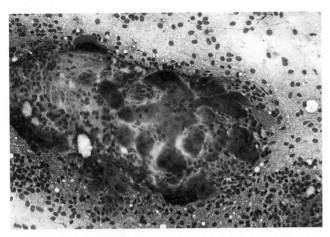

**FIG. 27.12.** *Adenoid cystic carcinoma, aspiration cytology.* This fine needle aspiration specimen shows eosinophilic nodules of cylindromatous material surrounded by myoepithelial cells.

fragments from benign lesions or other forms of carcinoma may resemble cylindromatous material (24). The differential diagnosis of a cytologic preparation from an adenoid cystic carcinoma is collagenous spherulosis.

A variety of microscopic growth patterns found in adenoid cystic carcinoma of the salivary glands (25) also may be present when this type of tumor occurs in the breast (10,26,27). These configurations have been described as cribriform, solid, tubular, reticular (trabecular), and basaloid (Figs. 27.13 and 27. 14). Sebaceous differentiation was found in 14% of adenoid cystic carcinomas (Fig. 27.15), and a substantial number of the tumors have foci of adenosquamous differentiation (28). Adenomyoepitheliomatous and syringomatous areas are further evidence of structural diversity (29) (Fig. 27.16). Ductular structures that resemble the intercalated ducts in salivary glands and salivary gland tumors are also present in mammary adenoid cystic carcinomas (Fig. 27.17).

Ro et al. suggested that adenoid cystic carcinomas be stratified into three grades on the basis of the proportion of solid growth within the lesion (I, no solid elements; II, <30% solid; III, > 30% solid) (27). In high-grade lesions (grade III), tumor cells are poorly differentiated, often with sparse cytoplasm, relatively large, hyperchromatic nuclei, and mitoses (Fig. 27.18). Intraductal carcinoma sometimes is seen in high-grade tumors (Fig. 27.19). Areas of cribriform and

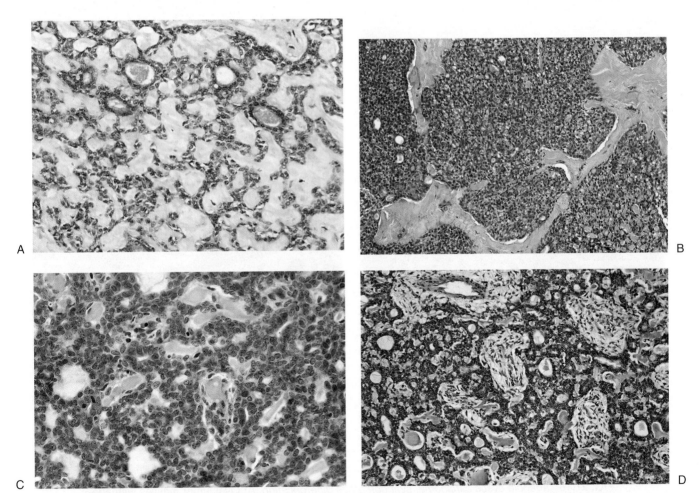

**FIG. 27.13.** *Adenoid cystic carcinoma, reticular and solid patterns.* **A:** Small glands remain in this predominantly myoepithelial proliferation. **B:** Solid growth. **C:** Magnified view of solid lesion showing numerous cylindromatous nodules. **D:** Solid growth pattern with fibrovascular stroma. This appearance resembles solid papillary carcinoma.

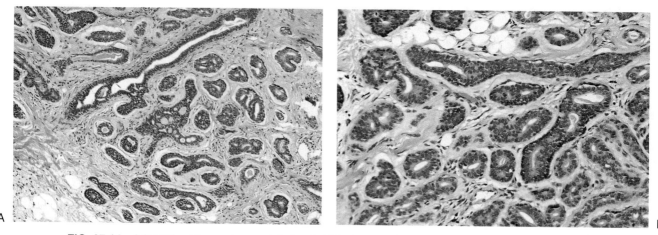

**FIG. 27.14.** *Adenoid cystic carcinoma, tubular.* **A:** Tubular growth surrounds a central tumor focus with cylindromatous nodules and a benign duct. **B:** Pure tubular growth in the same tumor.

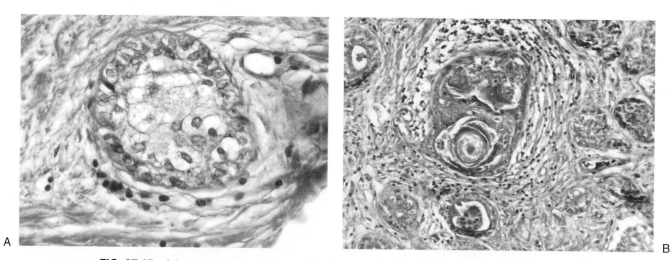

**FIG. 27.15.** *Adenoid cystic carcinoma.* **A:** Sebaceous metaplasia. **B:** Squamous metaplasia.

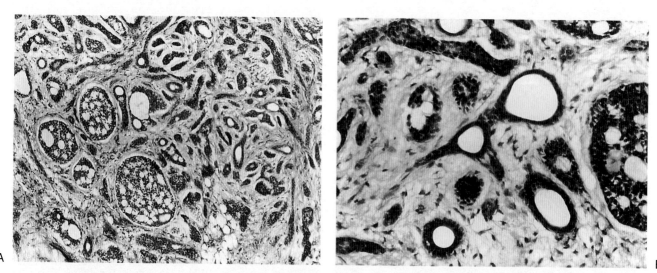

**FIG. 27.16.** *Adenoid cystic carcinoma, syringomatous differentiation.* **A:** Oval tumor masses with adenoid cystic differentiation are surrounded by swirling syringomatous elements. **B:** Syringomatous glands next to adenoid cystic tumor on the *right* border. (**A** from Rosen PP. Adenoid cystic carcinoma of the breast: a morphologically heterogeneous neoplasm. *Pathol Annu* 1989;24:237–254, with permission.)

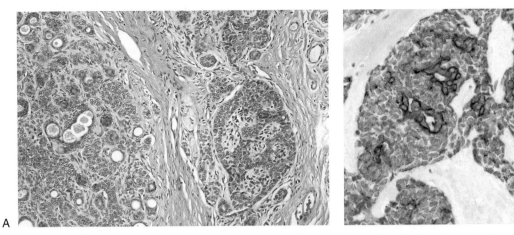

**FIG. 27.17.** *Adenoid cystic carcinoma, ductular differentiation.* **A:** Ductular structures which resemble intercalated salivary gland ducts with darkly stained cytoplasm and nuclei are present in this tumor. **B:** Ductules are immunoreactive with the cytokeratin antibody 34BE12 (K903) (avidin-biotin).

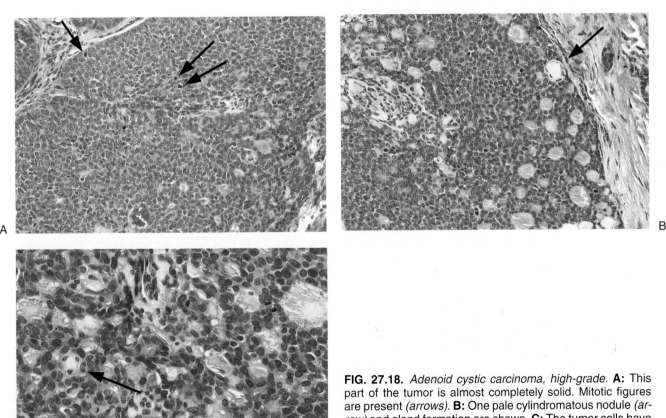

**FIG. 27.18.** *Adenoid cystic carcinoma, high-grade.* **A:** This part of the tumor is almost completely solid. Mitotic figures are present *(arrows)*. **B:** One pale cylindromatous nodule *(arrow)* and gland formation are shown. **C:** The tumor cells have small nucleoli. Mitotic figures are present. One cylindromatous nodule encircled by myoepithelial cells is evident *(arrow)*.

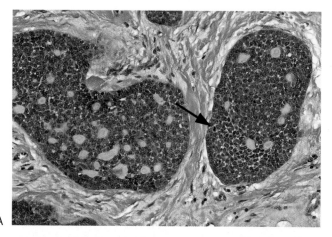

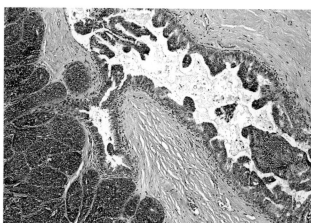

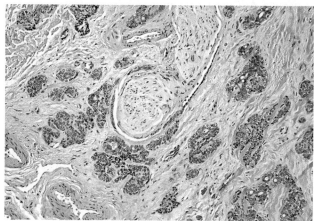

**FIG. 27.19.** *Adenoid cystic carcinoma, high-grade.* **A:** Solid tumor nests containing cylindromatous nodules and mitotic activity *(arrow).* **B:** Intraductal carcinoma *(right)* next to invasive high-grade adenoid cystic carcinoma is composed of the same tumor cells. **C:** Perineural invasion.

nearly confluent solid growth as well as typical adenoid cystic components are sometimes present in a single tumor. Prominent basaloid features are seen in some cases (Fig. 27.20). High-grade tumors with sparse glandular and cylindromatous areas can be mistaken for small cell carcinoma (Fig. 27.21).

High-grade lesions do not differ from low-grade tumors in regard to patient age, laterality, duration prior to treatment,

hormone receptors, or in the likelihood of finding residual tumor in a mastectomy specimen (10). Ro et al. found that tumors with a solid component (grades II and III) tended to be larger than those without a solid element (grade I) and that tumors with a solid element were more likely to have recurrences (27). In their series, the only patient who developed

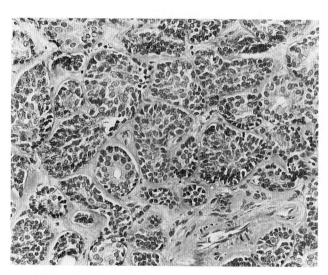

**FIG. 27.20.** *Adenoid cystic carcinoma, basaloid.*

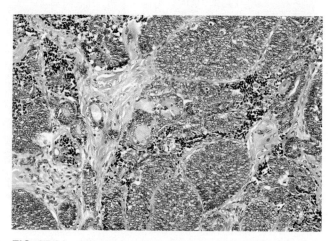

**FIG. 27.21.** *Adenoid cystic carcinoma, high grade.* Cylindromatous nodules are present in this tumor. Note the zones of tumor disruption with darkly staining cells. A limited sample of this tumor could be interpreted as small cell carcinoma with "crush artefact."

metastatic adenoid cystic carcinoma had a grade III lesion. Others have reported that the Ki67 labeling index obtained by using the MIB1 antibody was greater in high-grade than in low-grade tumors, but proliferative activity was not significantly related to tumor grade or mitotic rate (30). Two patients described by Santamaria et al. with high-grade adenoid cystic carcinoma treated by modified radical mastectomy did not have axillary nodal metastases (15).

Some conventional forms of mammary carcinoma may be diagnosed incorrectly as adenoid cystic carcinoma (4,21,31). In one review (31), about half of the cases recorded by the Connecticut Tumor Registry as adenoid cystic carcinoma had been misclassified. Most of the errors resulted from including duct carcinomas with a prominent cribriform component. Problems also were encountered in distinguishing adenoid cystic from papillary and mucinous carcinomas. These mistakes can be avoided by strict adherence to the diagnostic criteria for adenoid cystic carcinoma, especially the

requirement that there be a cylindromatous component. Because cribriform areas may be found in an adenoid cystic carcinoma, their presence does not exclude this diagnosis if other diagnostic components are present.

Adenoid cystic carcinoma with an organoid structure formed by adipose tissue and myofibroblastic proliferation is an extremely unusual variant of this neoplasm (Fig. 27.22).

Collagenous spherulosis is a structural pattern in some benign duct proliferations that must be considered in the differential diagnosis of adenoid cystic carcinoma (32). It combines benign gland formation and spherules of basement membrane components containing myoepithelial cells surrounded by epithelial cells in a combination that mimics adenoid cystic carcinoma (Fig. 27.23). The spherules contain elastin, periodic acid-Schiff (PAS)–positive material, and type IV collagen (33,34). Collagenous spherulosis occurs most often in ducts involved by hyperplasia, but it also can develop in papillomas and sclerosing adenosis.

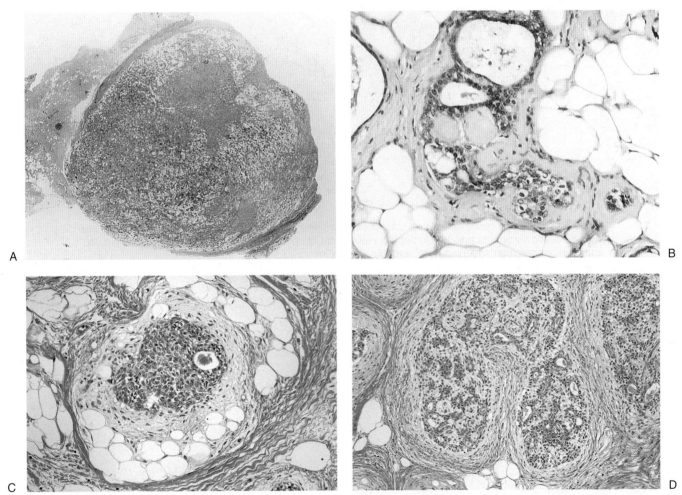

**FIG. 27.22.** *Adenoid cystic carcinoma with unusual stromal differentiation.* **A:** This whole-mount histologic section shows a circumscribed tumor in which the pale areas consist of fat. **B:** Adenoid cystic carcinoma surrounded by fat. **C:** A lobulated nest of tumor in an organoid structure surrounded by fat and collagen. Cells clustered around the glandular structure are probably neoplastic myoepithelial cells, whereas the peripheral spindle cells may be myofibroblastic. The circumscribed appearance of the tumor and internal organoid structure composed of adipose tissue and collagen suggests that these are intrinsic constituents of the tumor. **D:** Organoid tumor clusters showing glandular differentiation.

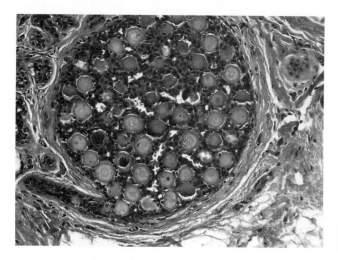

**FIG. 27.23.** *Collagenous spherulosis.* Note the concentric layers and central rings in some spherules.

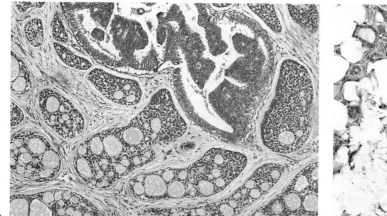

A

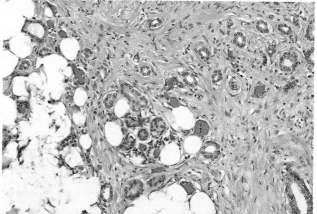

B

**FIG. 27.24.** *Adenoid cystic carcinoma and tubular carcinoma.* **A:** The primary tumor in this patient was adenoid cystic carcinoma adjacent to papillary intraductal carcinoma. **B:** The breast also harbored a separate tubular carcinoma, shown here, and lobular carcinoma *in situ.*

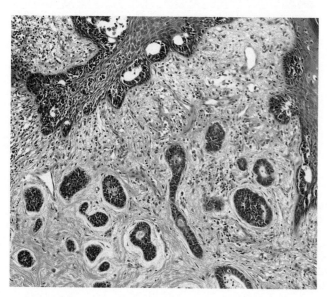

**FIG. 27.25.** *Paget's disease and adenoid cystic carcinoma.* Carcinoma glands are apparent in the epidermis overlying adenoid cystic carcinoma, which was confined to the nipple.

The breast that harbors adenoid cystic carcinoma also can be the site of one or more other types of carcinoma. I encountered one patient who had a separate concurrent apocrine intraductal carcinoma and lobular carcinoma *in situ* (Fig. 27.24). Rarely, adenoid cystic carcinoma arising in the nipple can be associated with Paget's disease (Fig. 27.25). The differential diagnosis of adenoid cystic carcinoma in the nipple includes other types of carcinoma as well as syringomatous adenoma, which does not produce Paget's disease.

## HISTOCHEMISTRY, ELECTRON MICROSCOPY, AND CYTOLOGY

Before it was appreciated that the cylindromatous component is composed of basal lamina material, this element was often referred to as a *pseudoglandular structure,* but this term is no longer appropriate. It is usually not necessary to resort to electron microscopy to distinguish between glands and cylindromatous structures. Histochemical stains such as mucicarmine or Alcian blue ordinarily identify the secretion within glands. The structural polarity of the glandular cells can be demonstrated with immunostains for fodrin, E-cadherin and β-catenin (35). Laminin and fibronectin, noncollagenous glycoproteins associated with basal lamina, and type IV collagen can be demonstrated by immunohistochemistry in the cylindromatous elements (18,35,36). Production of laminin and type IV collagen by a salivary gland adenoid cystic carcinoma has been demonstrated in xenografts grown in nude mice (37). Cells cultured from salivary gland adenoid cystic carcinoma produce laminin, fibronectin, chondroitin sulfate proteoglycan, and type IV collagen, which are demonstrable in the culture matrix as well as at the cell surface (38). Fibronectin and laminin may be found in the basement membranes of ducts that contain intraductal cribriform carcinoma but neither is seen within the tumor itself (36).

Cheng et al. (39) examined the distribution of type IV collagen, laminin, heparin sulfate proteoglycan, and entactin, components of normal basement membrane, in adenoid cystic carcinoma. The cylindromatous component within nests of carcinoma cells and basement membrane surrounding these groups of cells was strongly reactive for each of these molecules. These investigators concluded that the cells of adenoid cystic carcinoma produce, have an affinity for, and may require basement membrane components. They speculated that this characteristic provides an explanation for the ability of this carcinoma to invade around nerves and blood vessels, which are basement membrane-rich tissues.

Vimentin-positive cells in adenoid cystic carcinomas have been referred to as *myoepithelium-like* (18) or *basaloid* cells (19). A low proliferative rate was found in one tumor studied immunohistochemically with the Ki67 antibody (18). When studied by flow cytometry, four adenoid cystic carcinomas were diploid (20). Three of the tumors that had a low proliferative rate and did not express p53 protein occurred in women with negative axillary lymph nodes. The fourth tumor had a high proliferative rate, p53 expression, and axillary nodal metastases. Adenoid cystic carcinomas of the breast and salivary glands reportedly have similar immunohistochemical profiles (18). Mutations of the p53 gene occur more frequently in high-grade than in nonhigh-grade foci of adenoid cystic carcinoma (40).

The differential diagnosis of high-grade adenoid cystic carcinoma sometimes includes small cell carcinoma. A study of basaloid, small cell, and adenoid cystic carcinomas of the oropharynx revealed some interesting immunophenotypic differences (41). Immunoreactivity for high-molecular-weight keratin detected with the antibody 34BE12 was present in virtually all basaloid and adenoid cystic carcinomas and absent from small cell carcinomas. Other cytokeratin antibodies were equally immunoreactive in all three tumor types. Actin immunoreactivity was observed in most adenoid cystic carcinomas but was absent from basaloid and small cell carcinomas. Neuroendocrine markers were undetectable in virtually all basaloid and adenoid cystic carcinomas and variably expressed in small cell carcinoma. Vimentin was detected in 93% of adenoid cystic carcinomas, 80% of small cell carcinomas, and 35% of basaloid carcinomas.

KIT, a transmembrane tyrosine kinase receptor encoded by the protooncogene c-*kit* located on chromosome 4(q11-12), is involved in the regulation of cell growth. Altered KIT expression has been detected in breast carcinomas, but this has not been studied specifically in adenoid cystic carcinoma of the breast. Although KIT is not detectable by immunohistochemistry in normal salivary glands, a study of 30 adenoid cystic carcinomas of the salivary glands revealed expression in 90% of the tumors (42). KIT expression was significantly more extensive in high-grade tumors. It remains to be determined whether a similar pattern of KIT reactivity will be found in mammary adenoid cystic carcinomas.

Electron microscopic studies have revealed the same diverse cell types in mammary adenoid cystic carcinoma that are encountered in adenoid cystic carcinoma arising from salivary glands and other organs (43). In addition to populations of epithelial and myoepithelial cells (7,11,13), the tumors contain varying numbers of basaloid cells (11,28) as well as cells exhibiting sebaceous and adenosquamous differentiation (28).

Fine needle aspiration cytology yields variably cellular specimens in which the most significant finding is clusters of epithelial cells oriented around solid spheres of basement membrane material (44). Glandular spaces also may be present accompanied by bipolar spindle cells (Fig. 27.12). Similar findings may be encountered in a sample from collagenous spherulosis.

## PROGNOSIS AND TREATMENT

Currently, data on the prognosis of adenoid cystic carcinoma are based mainly on published reports of patients treated surgically, usually by mastectomy (4–13,27,31).

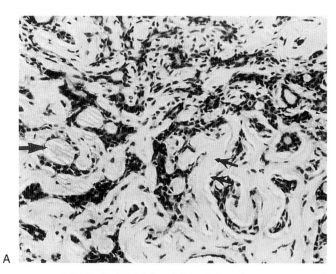
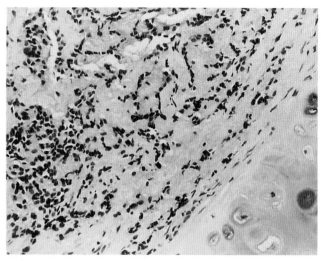

A

B

**FIG. 27.26.** *Adenoid cystic carcinoma, metastatic.* **A:** The primary tumor in the breast had glandular *(large arrow)* and cylindromatous *(small arrows)* elements. This was a histologically low-grade tumor. **B:** Metastatic adenoid cystic carcinoma in the lung next to bronchial cartilage.

Mastectomy has been curative in virtually all cases. Chest wall recurrence was reported after simple mastectomy in one case (45), and there have been a few isolated instances of systemic metastases after mastectomy (9,22,46–48). All patients with metastases have had pulmonary involvement (Fig. 27.26), with recurrences in the lung being detected as late as 6 years (46,49), 8 years (22), 9 years (48), 10 years (9), and 12 years (46,47) after initial treatment. All of these patients had negative axillary lymph nodes. Axillary metastases were present at mastectomy in two other cases (27,50). Each of these patients had pulmonary metastases, and both reportedly died of metastatic mammary adenoid cystic carcinoma. One of these women had a locally advanced, ulcerated, 10-cm tumor that had been present for at least 10 years (50). Other sites of metastases include bone (27), the liver (27), the brain (26,47), and the kidney (46).

Recurrence in the breast has been described after treatment by local excision alone (5,9,13,27,30,48,51), with the interval to recurrence varying from less than 1 year to more than 20 years. Negative axillary lymph nodes were found in three cases when an axillary dissection was performed, and the tumor reportedly was controlled by surgery in all seven cases of local recurrence in the breast.

Although most adenoid cystic carcinomas are nodular and appear grossly circumscribed, this may be misleading because about 50% of the tumors extend microscopically into the surrounding breast as *in situ* or invasive carcinoma (30). Multinodular tumors sometimes have inapparent small nodular foci beyond the grossly evident tumor. Lesions with these microscopically invasive features are prone to local recurrence when treated by excisional biopsy and are best managed by wide reexcision in most cases if mastectomy is not performed (10).

The treatment of adenoid cystic carcinoma will depend on the circumstances in a given case. Small circumscribed tumors that lack microscopic invasion beyond the gross tumor may be treated by excision alone, an approach that might not be feasible if a tumor is located superficially in the subareolar region. Wide excision or quadrantectomy is indicated for relatively large lesions and for tumors that have an invasive growth pattern. Radiotherapy may be used to supplement excisional surgery when there is concern about the margins, but there is presently too little experience to judge the effectiveness of radiation in treating this type of carcinoma (30). Mastectomy is curative in virtually all cases when the axillary lymph nodes prove to be negative, and it is recommended for invasive lesions when a cosmetically satisfactory excision is not possible, especially when the tumor has a high-grade pattern. A low axillary dissection or sentinel lymph node mapping should be performed if the clinical examination suggests lymph node involvement, if the breast contains another type of invasive carcinoma, for high-grade adenoid cystic lesions, and for tumors larger than 3 cm. Systemic adjuvant chemotherapy is recommended for patients with axillary lymph metastases and may be considered in patients with high-grade lesions or if the tumor is larger than 3 cm.

## REFERENCES

1. Ewing J. Epithelial tumors of the salivary gland. In: *Neoplastic diseases*, 3rd ed. Philadelphia: WB Saunders, 1919:780.
2. Geschickter CF. In: *Diseases of the breast: diagnosis, pathology, treatment*, 2nd ed. Philadelphia: JB Lippincott, 1945:824.
3. Foote FW Jr, Stewart FW. A histologic classification of carcinoma of the breast. *Surgery* 1946;19:74–99.
4. Galloway JR, Woolner LB, Clagett OT. Adenoid cystic carcinoma of the breast. *Surg Gynecol Obstet* 1966;122:1289–1294.
5. Cavanzo FJ, Taylor HB. Adenoid cystic carcinoma of the breast: an analysis of 21 cases. *Cancer* 1969;24:740–745.
6. Friedman BA, Oberman HA. Adenoid cystic carcinoma of the breast. *Am J Clin Pathol* 1970;54:1–14.
7. Koss LG, Brannan CD, Ashikari R. Histologic and ultrastructural features of adenoid cystic carcinoma of the breast. *Cancer* 1970;26:1271–1279.
8. Lerner AG, Molnar JJ, Adam YG. Adenoid cystic carcinoma of the breast. *Am J Surg* 1974;127:585–587.

9. Peters GN, Wolff M. Adenoid cystic carcinoma of the breast; report of 11 new cases. *Cancer* 1982;52:680–686.

10. Rosen PP. Adenoid cystic carcinoma of the breast: a morphologically heterogeneous neoplasm. *Pathol Annu* 1989;24:237–254.

11. Zaloudek C, Oertel YC, Orenstein JM. Adenoid cystic carcinoma of the breast. *Am J Clin Pathol* 1984;81:297–307.

12. Hjorth S, Magnusson PH, Blomquite P. Adenoid cystic carcinoma of the breast. *Acta Chir Scand* 1977;143:155–158.

13. Quizilbash AH, Patterson MC, Oliveira KF. Adenoid cystic carcinoma of the breast. *Arch Pathol Lab Med* 1977;101:302–306.

14. Hollingsworth AB, Iezzoni JC. Primary cutaneous adenoid cystic carcinoma of the male breast: a case report and review of the literature. *Breast Dis* 1994;7:213–218.

15. Santamaria G, Velasco M, Zanon G, et al. Adenoid cystic carcinoma of the breast: mammographic appearance and pathologic correlation. *AJR Am J Roentgenol* 1998;171:1679–1683.

16. Bourke AG, Metcalf C, Wylie EJ. Mammographic features of adenoid cystic carcinoma. *Australas Radiol* 1994;38:324–325.

17. Tsuboi N, Ogawa Y, Inomata T, et al. Dynamic MR appearance of adenoid cystic carcinoma of the breast in a 67-year-old female. *Radiat Med* 1998;16:225–228.

18. Düe W, Herbst H, Loy V, et al. Characterization of adenoid cystic carcinoma of the breast by immunohistology. *J Clin Pathol* 1989;42:470–476.

19. Lamovec J, Uskrasovec M, Zidar A, et al. Adenoid cystic carcinomas of the breast: a histologic, cytologic and immunohistochemical study. *Semin Diagn Pathol* 1989;6:153–164.

20. Pastolero G, Hanna W, Zbieranowski I, et al. Proliferative activity and p53 expression in adenoid cystic carcinoma of the breast. *Mod Pathol* 1996;9:215–219.

21. Harris M. Pseudoadenoid cystic carcinoma of the breast. *Arch Pathol Lab Med* 1977;101:307–309.

22. Nayer HR. Cylindroma of the breast with pulmonary metastases. *Dis Chest* 1957;31:324–327.

23. Oertel YC, Goldblum LI. Fine needle aspiration of the breast. Diagnostic criteria. *Pathol Ann* 1983;18(Part 1):375–407.

24. Stanley MW, Tani EM, Rutquist L-E, et al. Adenoid cystic carcinoma of the breast: diagnosis by fine-needle aspiration. *Diagn Cytopathol* 1993;9:184–187.

25. Azumi N, Battifora H. The cellular composition of adenoid cystic carcinoma. An immunohistochemical study. *Cancer* 1987;60:1589–1598.

26. Orenstein JM, Dardick I, van Nostrand AWP. Ultrastructural similarities of adenoid cystic carcinoma and pleomorphic adenoma. *Histopathology* 1985;9:623–638.

27. Ro JY, Silva EG, Gallager HS. Adenoid cystic carcinoma of the breast. *Hum Pathol* 1987;18:1276–1281.

28. Tavassoli FA, Norris HJ. Mammary adenoid cystic carcinoma with sebaceous differentiation: a morphologic study of the cell types. *Arch Pathol Lab Med* 1986;110:1045–1053.

29. Van Dorpe J, De Pauw A, Moerman P. Adenoid cystic carcinoma arising in an adenomyoepithelioma of the breast. *Virchows Arch* 1998;432:119–122.

30. Kleer CG, Oberman HA. Adenoid cystic carcinoma of the breast: value of histologic grading and proliferative activity. *Am J Surg Pathol* 1998;22:569–575.

31. Sumpio BE, Jennings TA, Merino MJ, et al. Adenoid cystic carcinoma of the breast: data from the Connecticut Tumor Registry and a review of the literature. *Ann Surg* 1987;205:295–301.

32. Clement PB, Young RH, Azzopardi JG. Collagenous spherulosis of the breast. *Am J Surg Pathol* 1987;11:411–417.

33. Clement PB. Collagenous spherulosis [Letter]. *Am J Surg Pathol* 1987;11:907.

34. Grignon DJ, Ro JY, MacKay BN, et al. Collagenous spherulosis of the breast: immunohistochemical and ultrastructural studies. *Am J Clin Pathol* 1989;91:386–392.

35. Kasami M, Olson SJ, Simpson JF, et al. Maintenance of polarity and a dual cell population in adenoid cystic carcinoma of the breast: an immunohistochemical study. *Histopathology* 1998;32:232–238.

36. d'Ardenne AJ, Kirkpatrick P, Wells CA, et al. Laminin and fibronectin in adenoid cystic carcinoma. *J Clin Pathol* 1986;39:138–144.

37. Barsky SH, Layfield L, Varki N, et al. Two human tumors with high basement membrane-producing potential. *Cancer* 1988;61:1798–1806.

38. Sobue M, Takeuchi J, Niwa M, et al. Establishment of a cell line producing basement membrane components from an adenoid cystic carcinoma of the human salivary gland. *Virchows Arch* 1989;57:203–208.

39. Cheng J, Saku T, Okabe H, et al. Basement membranes in adenoid cystic carcinoma. An immunohistochemical study. *Cancer* 1992;69:2631–2640.

40. Yamamoto Y, Wistuba II, Kishimoto Y, et al. DNA analysis at p53 locus in adenoid cystic carcinoma: comparison of molecular study and p53 immunostaining. *Pathol Int* 1998;48:273–280.

41. Morice WG, Ferreiro JA. Distinction of basaloid squamous cell carcinoma from adenoid cystic and small cell undifferentiated carcinoma by immunohistochemistry. *Hum Pathol* 1998;29:609–612.

42. Holst VA, Marshall CE, Moskaluk CA, et al. KIT protein expression and analysis of c-kit gene mutation in adenoid cystic carcinoma. *Mod Pathol* 1999;12:956–960.

43. Lawrence JB, Mazur MT. Adenoid cystic carcinoma. A comparative pathologic study of tumors in salivary gland, breast, lung and cervix. *Hum Pathol* 1982;13:916–924.

44. Gupta RK, Green C, Naran S, et al. Fine-needle aspiration cytology of adenoid cystic carcinoma of the breast. *Diag Cytopathol* 1999;20:82–84.

45. Wilson WB, Spell JP. Adenoid cystic carcinoma of breast: a case of recurrence and regional metastasis. *Ann Surg* 1967;166:861–864.

46. Herzberg AJ, Bossen EH, Walter PJ. Adenoid cystic carcinoma of the breast metastatic to the kidney: a clinically symptomatic lesion requiring surgical management. *Cancer* 1991;68:1015–1020.

47. Koller M, Ram Z, Findler G, et al. Brain metastasis: a rare manifestation of adenoid cystic carcinoma of the breast. *Surg Neurol* 1986;70:470–472.

48. Lim SK, Kovi J, Warner OG. Adenoid cystic carcinoma of breast with metastasis: a case report and review of the literature. *J Natl Med Assoc* 1979;71:329–330.

49. Eisner B. Adenoid cystic carcinoma of the breast. *Pathol Eur* 1970;3:357–364.

50. Wells CA, Nicoll S, Ferguson DJP. Adenoid cystic carcinoma of the breast: a case with axillary lymph node metastasis. *Histopathology* 1986;10:415–424.

51. Lusted D. Structural and growth patterns of adenoid cystic carcinoma of breast. *Am J Clin Pathol* 1970;54:419–425.

# CHAPTER 28

# Cribriform Carcinoma

Invasive carcinomas with a cribriform pattern are termed *classic cribriform carcinomas.* Some of these tumors have cribriform and tubular components. The diagnosis of mixed invasive cribriform carcinoma has been reserved for tumors in which less than 50% of the lesion has a cribriform pattern and the remainder of the tumor is composed of nontubular, less well-differentiated areas.

Three major studies of cribriform carcinoma have been published. Page et al. found 35 classic (4%) and 16 mixed (2%) cribriform carcinomas among 1,003 invasive breast carcinomas treated at the University of Edinburgh in a 10-year period (1). Venable et al. reviewed 1,087 primary breast carcinomas at the George Washington University and reported that 32 (3%) were pure or largely cribriform (classic) carcinomas and that 30 (3%) were mixed cribriform carcinomas in which fewer than 50% of the lesion had a cribriform pattern (2). Marzullo et al. found three pure and two mixed cases in a series of 1,759 infiltrating carcinomas, representing 0.3% of the entire group (3).

Cribriform carcinoma is a well-differentiated variant of invasive duct carcinoma. Because the information thus far available is limited, it has not been possible to determine whether cribriform carcinoma should be regarded as a low-grade variant of invasive duct carcinoma or whether it would be better considered a specific subtype of carcinoma. For the present, it is appropriate to use a diagnosis of invasive duct carcinoma, cribriform type, to identify these lesions for further study.

## CLINICAL PRESENTATION

One of the reported patients was a man (1–4). The female patients ranged in age from 7 to 91 years. Page et al. found that patients with classic cribriform carcinoma tended to be younger and to have smaller tumors than women with mixed lesions (1). On the other hand, three patients with pure tumors in another series were 70 to 90 years old (3). A mammographic study of eight cases revealed spiculated masses measuring 20 to 35 mm in four of the patients (5). Two of these lesions contained a few punctate calcifications. Four other tumors were not visualized radiographically.

Venable et al. reported that 16 classic and mixed cribriform carcinomas were estrogen receptor positive and that 11 (69%) of the tumors were also progesterone receptor-positive (2). There was no appreciable difference in progesterone receptor positivity between classic and mixed cribriform tumors. Marzullo et al. reported that one of two pure and two mixed tumors were positive for estrogen receptors, but only one of the two pure tumors was positive for progesterone receptors and all four tumors were MIB1 positive (3).

## GROSS PATHOLOGY

No specific gross pathologic features have been noted. Data from two studies suggested that a small but distinct proportion of cribriform carcinomas occur as multifocal lesions (1,3). In one study, 7 of 35 (20%) patients with classic and 1 of 16 (6%) patients with a mixed cribriform carcinoma had grossly apparent multifocal invasive foci in the affected breast (1). One patient studied by Marzullo et al. had two lesions measuring 1.6 and 0.4 cm in the same breast (3).

## MICROSCOPIC PATHOLOGY

The invasive component of cribriform carcinoma exhibits the same sieve-like growth pattern that characterizes conventional cribriform intraductal carcinoma (Fig. 28.1). The rounded and angular masses of uniform, well-differentiated tumor cells are embedded in variable amounts of collagenous stroma. Sharply outlined round or oval glandular spaces are distributed throughout these tumor aggregates, creating a fenestrated appearance. Perineural invasion is rarely found in this low-grade type of carcinoma (Fig. 28.2). Mucin-positive secretion is present in varying amounts within these lumens (4), and they may contain microcalcifications (6). The tumor cells do not contain argyrophilic granules when examined with the Grimelius stain (1). Electron microscopy reveals luminal differentiation of tumor cells, which have microvilli and are joined by tight junctions (4,6). Only a few scattered remnants of basal lamina are present, and myoepithelial cells are not demonstrable with an actin

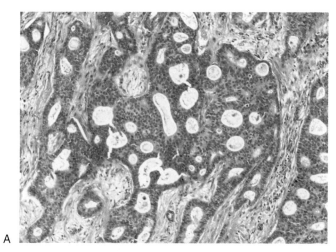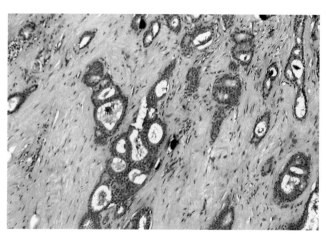

**FIG. 28.1.** *Cribriform carcinoma.* **A:** Invasive carcinoma with a cribriform growth pattern. **B:** This tumor displays stromal fibrosis and some tubular glands. Calcifications are present.

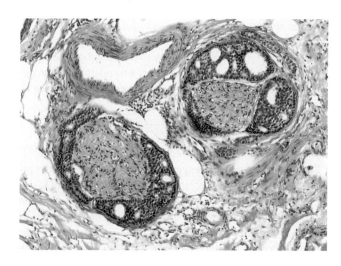

**FIG. 28.2.** *Cribriform carcinoma, perineural invasion.*

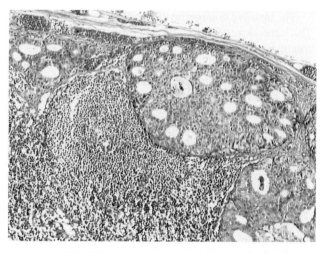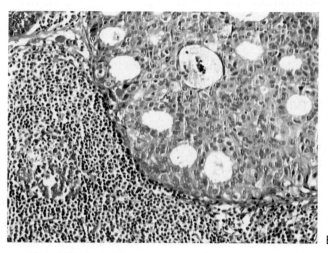

**FIG. 28.3.** *Cribriform carcinoma, metastatic.* **A:** Metastatic cribriform carcinoma in an axillary lymph node. **B:** The rigid growth pattern resembles cribriform intraductal carcinoma.

immunostain. Neurosecretory-type granules have not been found by electron microscopy (2,4).

In addition to the cribriform structure, some tumors have areas of tubular growth that comstitute up to 50% of the lesion in a minority of cases (1,2). Page et al. found tubular areas in 6 of 35 classic tumors (17%) (1). The intraductal component has a cribriform pattern in most but not all classic cribriform carcinomas. When present, nodal metastases from classic tumors usually also have a cribriform structure, whereas metastases derived from mixed tumors are more likely to have a noncribriform pattern (Fig. 28.3) (1,2).

Cribriform carcinoma should be distinguished morphologically from adenoid cystic carcinoma. Cribriform growth produces a fenestrated structural pattern that lacks the cylindromatous components composed of basal lamina material characteristic of adenoid cystic carcinoma. Cribriform areas, however, may be found in adenoid cystic carcinomas in which gland formation is prominent. Although the term *adenocystic* has been applied to such lesions (7), they are part of the spectrum of adenoid cystic carcinoma (8).

The diagnosis of tubular carcinoma should be reserved for tumors in which almost the entire lesion has a tubular structure. The glands of classic tubular carcinoma, which have rounded or angular contours, are lined by neoplastic cells arranged in a single cell layer. Papillary proliferation or bridging of the gland lumens rarely occurs in tubular carcinoma glands, although the intraductal component of tubular carcinoma typically has a micropapillary or cribriform structure. An invasive carcinoma with tubular elements in which most of the invasive neoplasm has a cribriform pattern should be classified as a *cribriform* rather than as a *tubular carcinoma*.

## TREATMENT AND PROGNOSIS

Most reported patients have been treated by mastectomy and axillary dissection (1,2). Two studies concluded that patients with classic cribriform carcinoma were less likely to develop axillary lymph node metastases than women with mixed cribriform (1) or ordinary invasive duct carcinoma (2). The data are not definitive because the groups compared were not standardized for tumor size or type of surgical treatment. Page et al. reported that patients with mixed cribriform carcinomas had nodal metastases more often (4 of 16, 25%) than those with classical tumors (1). In their series, however, the average size of classic tumors (3.1 cm) was less than that of tumors with a mixed cribriform pattern (4.2 cm). Venable et al. also did not stratify their cribriform and noncribriform cases for nodal status and tumor size (2). They also apparently included in their analysis patients treated without axillary dissection or for whom surgical therapy was unknown.

No deaths attributable to classic cribriform carcinoma occurred among 34 patients studied by Page et al. with follow-up of 10 to 21 years (1). One of these patients was alive with recurrent classic cribriform carcinoma, and another died of metastases from a contralateral carcinoma. Among 16 women with mixed cribriform carcinoma with an average follow-up of 12.5 years, six deaths resulted from the breast carcinoma. Venable et al. reported a disease-free survival of 100% among 45 patients with classical cribriform carcinoma followed for 1 to 5 years (2). In this series, follow-up information was unavailable for 17 other patients. With follow-up of 6 years or less, Marzullo reported that three patients with pure and two with mixed tumors were disease free (3).

The foregoing data suggest that pure invasive cribriform carcinoma has a relatively favorable prognosis and a low frequency of axillary nodal metastases. If adequate excision can be performed, breast-conservation therapy would appear feasible, although published data are presently largely based on mastectomy. In the absence of axillary nodal metastases, systemic adjuvant therapy is probably not warranted for tumors 1 cm or smaller unless there are specific unfavorable findings such as lymphatic tumor emboli.

## REFERENCES

1. Page DL, Dixon JM, Anderson TJ, et al. Invasive cribriform carcinoma of the breast. *Histopathology* 1983;7:525–536.
2. Venable JG, Schwartz AM, Silverberg SG. Infiltrating cribriform carcinoma of the breast: a distinctive clinicopathologic entity. *Hum Pathol* 1990;21:333–338.
3. Marzullo F, Zito FA, Marzullo A, et al. Infiltrating cribriform carcinoma of the breast: a clinico-pathologic and immunohistochemical study of 5 cases. *Eur J Gynaecol Oncol* 1996;17:228–231.
4. Wells CA, Ferguson DJP. Ultrastructural and immunocytochemical study of a case of invasive cribriform breast carcinoma. *J Clin Pathol* 1988;41:17–20.
5. Stutz JA, Evans AJ, Pinder S, et al. The radiological appearances of invasive cribriform carcinoma of the breast. *Clin Radiol* 1994;49:693–695.
6. Shousha S, Schoenfeld A, Moss J, et al. Light and electron microscopic study of an invasive cribriform carcinoma with extensive microcalcification developing in a breast with silicone augmentation. *Ultrastruct Pathol* 1994;18:519–523.
7. Fisher ER, Gregorio RM, Fisher B. The pathology of invasive breast cancer: a syllabus derived from findings of the National Surgical Adjuvant Breast Project (Protocol No. 4). *Cancer* 1975;36:1–84.
8. Rosen PP. Adenoid cystic carcinoma of the breast: a morphologically heterogeneous neoplasm. *Pathol Annu* 1989;24:237–254.

# CHAPTER 29

# Lipid-rich Carcinoma

Only a few examples of this rare variant of infiltrating duct carcinoma have been described (1–9). It is composed of cells that contain abundant lipid, which is extracted when the tissue is processed for histologic sections, leaving vacuolated cytoplasm (Fig. 29.1). Extraction of the cytoplasm also occurs in glycogen-rich carcinoma and in some apocrine carcinomas (5). Cells with clear, vacuolated cytoplasm also have been found in benign breast lesions (10) and in occult mammary carcinomas that present with axillary lymph node metastases (11). The tumor cells in lipid-rich carcinoma have small, dark nuclei. The presence of lipid can be demonstrated in frozen sections of fresh tissue, by electron microscopy, or in tissue prepared by processes that preserve cytoplasmic lipids. In cytologic specimens, the tumor cells have vacuolated or clear cytoplasm that appears foamy (6,8). Nuclei are round or slightly oval with finely granular chromatin.

The disease was first described by Aboumrad et al. in a case report (1). Subsequently, these investigators found one other example among 100 breast carcinomas and estimated the frequency of lipid-rich carcinoma to be 1%. Ramos and Taylor described 13 cases that had the growth pattern of lipid-rich carcinoma in routine histologic sections, but they were able to demonstrate lipid in only four cases that were available as unfixed specimens (2). The other nine were identified retrospectively among 900 tumors on the basis of histologic pattern alone. Eleven of the 12 patients treated by radical mastectomy had axillary lymph node metastases. Follow-up revealed that six patients died of metastatic carcinoma, and two were alive with recurrence. The remainder were alive and recurrence free; most had follow-up of less than 2 years.

One tumor was positive for progesterone receptor but negative for estrogen receptor, and it contained abundant sudanophilic cytoplasmic lipid (7). The cells were also immunoreactive for epithelial membrane antigen, cytokeratin, and α-lactalbumin. Membrane-bound cytoplasmic lipid droplets were seen on electron microscopy. Lipid-rich carcinoma in the breast of a 55-year-old man had high levels of estrogen and progesterone receptors (7). Varga et al. described a lipid-rich carcinoma with focal chondroid metaplasia (9). The tumor was estrogen receptor-negative, and fewer

than 10% of the tumor cells had nuclear progesterone receptor reactivity. The tumor cells were immunoreactive for cytokeratin, S-100, and vimentin.

Tsubura et al. described an unusual variant of lipid-secreting carcinoma in patients who were treated with neuroleptic

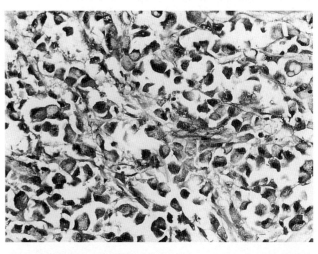

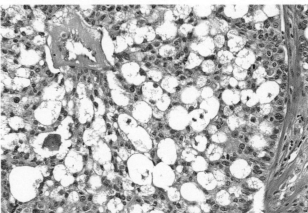

**FIG. 29.1.** *Lipid-rich carcinoma.* **A:** Marked cytoplasmic clearing is evident. The tumor cells were strongly sudanophilic in frozen sections. **B:** Intraductal carcinoma. (Courtesy of Frank Braza, M.D.).

drugs for severe psychiatric disorders (3). One effect of these medications is prolactin release, resulting in increased fatty acid synthetase activity and milk protein synthesis, often manifested clinically by galactorrhea. Benign, focal, pregnancy-like changes have been attributed to neuroleptic drugs (12). Two of 13 breast carcinomas identified by Tsubura et al. were lipid-secreting and strongly immunoreactive for alphalactalbumin, properties not exhibited by the other 11 tumors (3). The lipid-rich carcinomas had a growth pattern similar to that of pregnancy-like change in *in situ* areas. Large, pleomorphic carcinoma cells arranged in an alveolar pattern had a "hobnail" appearance. The luminal borders of these cells exhibited apocrine-type cytoplasmic blebs and extrusion of hyperchromatic pleomorphic nuclei. Cytoplasmic clearing was more evident in the solid, diffusely invasive component, with little gland formation. Both patients had axillary lymph node metastases. The dispersed growth pattern and cytologic features of axillary metastases may suggest metastatic malignant melanoma or a histiocytic form of malignant lymphoma (11).

Additional studies of more patients will be required to determine whether lipid-rich tumors constitute a morphologically and clinically distinctive type of carcinoma.

## REFERENCES

1. Aboumrad MH, Horn RC, Fine G. Lipid-secreting mammary carcinoma: report of a case associated with Paget's disease of the nipple. *Cancer* 1963;16:521–525.
2. Ramos CV, Taylor HB. Lipid-rich carcinoma of the breast: a clinicopathologic analysis of 13 examples. *Cancer* 1974;33:812–819.
3. Tsubura A, Hatano T, Murata A, et al. Breast carcinoma in patients receiving neuroleptic therapy: morphologic and clinicopathologic features of thirteen cases. *Acta Pathol Jpn* 1991;7:494–499.
4. Van Bogaert L-J, Maldague P. Histologic variants of lipid-secreting carcinoma of the breast. *Virchows Arch* 1977;375:345–353.
5. Dina R, Eusebi V. Clear cell tumors of the breast. *Semin Diagn Pathol* 1997;14:175–182.
6. Aida Y, Takeuchi E, Shinagawa T, et al. Fine needle aspiration cytology of lipid-secreting carcinoma of the breast: a case report. *Acta Cytol* 1993;37:547–551.
7. Mazzella FM, Sieber SC, Braza F. Ductal carcinoma of male breast with prominent lipid-rich component. *Pathology* 1995;27:280–283.
8. Lapey JD. Lipid-rich mammary carcinoma: diagnosis by cytology. Case report. *Acta Cytol* 1977;21:120–122.
9. Varga Z, Robl C, Spycher M, et al. Metaplastic lipid-rich carcinoma of the breast. *Pathol Int* 1998;48:912–916.
10. Barwick KW, Kashgarian M, Rosen PP. "Clear-cell" change within duct and lobular epithelium of the human breast. *Pathol Annu* 1982;17:319–328.
11. Haupt HM, Rosen PP, Kinne DW. Breast carcinoma presenting with axillary node metastases: an analysis of specific histologic features. *Am J Surg Pathol* 1985;9:165–176.
12. Kiaer HW, Andersen JA. Focal pregnancy-like changes in the breast. *Acta Pathol Microbiol Scand* 1977;85:931–941.

# CHAPTER 30

# Glycogen-rich Carcinoma

Carcinomas that accumulate abundant glycogen arise in many organs, including the lungs, endometrium, cervix, ovary, and salivary glands (1). Extraction of the water-soluble glycogen during histologic processing causes the cytoplasm to have a clear, vacuolated appearance in routine sections. In one series, 3% of 1,555 carcinomas were classified as clear cell, glycogen-rich carcinomas (2). These investigators were able to find intracytoplasmic glycogen in 58% of nonclear-cell carcinomas. Others reported that the glycogen-rich clear cell variant of duct carcinoma accounted for fewer than 1% of mammary duct carcinomas (3). Fewer than 50 examples have been described since the first case was reported in 1981 (4).

## CLINICAL PRESENTATION

The patients, who ranged in age from 35 to 78 years, presented with a mass that was sometimes accompanied by skin dimpling, nipple retraction, or pain. Most tumors have measured between 2 and 5 cm, with the largest lesion reported to be 10 cm clinically (5). Intraductal and invasive lesions may be detected by mammography (4–6). Hormone receptor analysis revealed that about 50% of tumors were estrogen receptor-positive, but all lesions studied have been negative for progesterone receptor (4–8). When analyzed by flow cytometry, the tumors have been nondiploid (8,9).

## GROSS PATHOLOGY

No specific gross features have been identified (6). An intraductal papillary component was noted grossly in one case (4).

## MICROSCOPIC PATHOLOGY

The lesions have basic structural features of intraductal carcinoma alone or of intraductal and infiltrating duct carcinoma. The intraductal component that is identified in most cases has compact solid, comedo, cribriform, or papillary growth patterns (6). Clear cell intraductal carcinoma is typically present (Fig. 30.1). In invasive areas, the tumor cells form cords, solid nests, or papillary structures (Fig. 30.2). A linear pattern consisting of strands of cells and resembling invasive lobular carcinoma may be seen, and clear cell glycogen-rich variants of tubular and medullary carcinoma have been noted (2). Lymphatic tumor emboli and perineural invasion have been reported. Patches of necrosis often occur in large tumors. Mitotic figures are easily identified in some cases.

In tissue sections, the tumor cells tend to have sharply defined borders and polygonal rather than rounded contours. The cytoplasm is clear and less often finely granular or foamy. The central or eccentrically placed nuclei are hyperchromatic, sometimes exhibiting clumped chromatin and nucleoli. Mitotic figures are infrequent. The histologic appearance of the primary tumor is duplicated in the metastases. The differential diagnosis includes apocrine and lipid-rich carcinomas of the breast and metastatic clear cell renal carcinoma. Apocrine features are identified focally in most of the tumors, and it has been suggested that glycogen-rich carcinoma may be a variant of apocrine carcinoma (6). Foamy, vacuolated cytoplasm is seen in the tumor cells in fine needle aspiration cytology specimens (8).

The cytoplasm gives a positive, diastase-labile reaction with the periodic acid-Schiff stain (Figs. 30.1 and 30.2). Cells are only focally Alcian blue or mucicarmine positive (3,5,8), and the oil red O stain for lipid is negative (5). In one case, the tumor cells were immunoreactive for carcinoembryonic antigen, cytokeratin, and epithelial membrane antigen but negative for α-lactalbumin, desmin, and vimentin (5). Others reported no immunoreactivity for actin and S-100 and on this basis, excluded myoepithelial origin for the clear cells (6). Many glycogen-rich carcinomas are estrogen-receptor-positive (Fig. 30.2.)

At the electron microscopy level, the tumor cells contain non-membrane-bound glycogen as well as smaller amounts of glycogen intermixed with cytoplasmic organelles (10). Clusters of tumor cells are surrounded by a basal lamina, and basal lamina is present underlying cells in papillary areas. Poorly formed lumens were found between and occasionally within tumor cells (5,7).

557

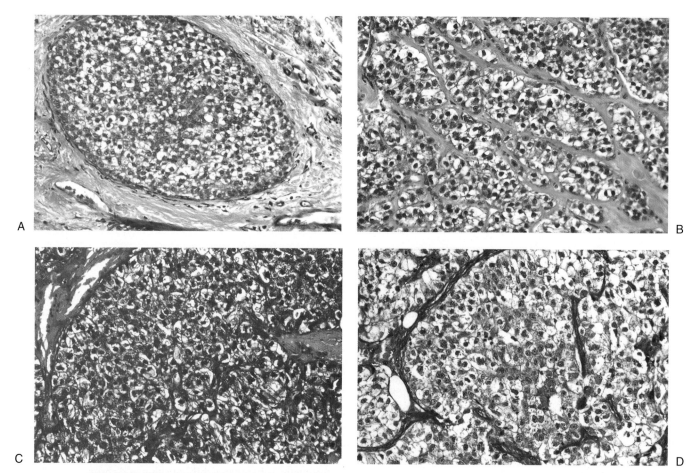

**FIG. 30.1.** *Glycogen-rich carcinoma.* **A,B:** Intraductal and invasive carcinoma composed of cells with clear cytoplasm and small, dark, punctate nuclei. **C:** The tumor is strongly positive with the periodic acid-Schiff (PAS) reaction. **D:** After treatment with diastase, PAS reactivity is almost entirely abolished. The same pattern of PAS staining occurred in the intraductal carcinoma.

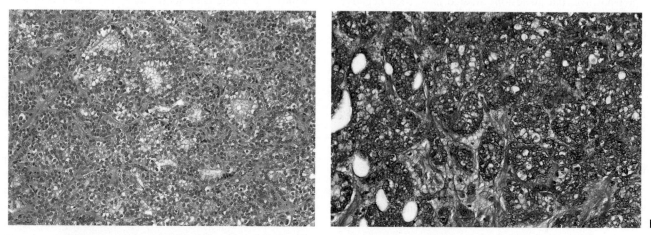

**FIG. 30.2.** *Glycogen-rich carcinoma.* **A:** This tumor has moderate cytoplasmic clearing and a gland-forming structure. **B:** Periodic acid-Schiff (PAS) reactivity is strong. (*continued*)

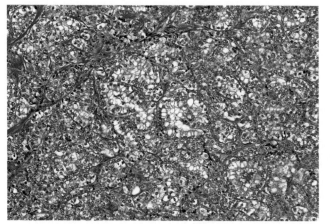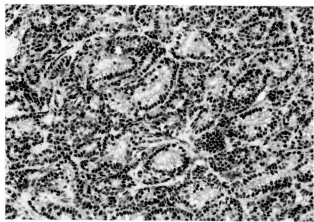

C                                                                                              D

**FIG. 30.2.** *Continued.* **C:** PAS reactivity is abolished by diastase treatment. **D:** Strong nuclear reactivity for estrogen receptor is present (avidin-biotin immunoperoxidase).

## TREATMENT AND PROGNOSIS

With rare exceptions, invasive glycogen-rich carcinoma has been treated by mastectomy and axillary dissection. About 30% of the reported patients had metastatic tumor in their axillary lymph nodes. In one series, 50% of the patients treated by mastectomy died of metastatic mammary carcinoma 1 to 175 months (median, 15 months) after diagnosis, and one patient was alive with recurrent carcinoma 36 months after local excision and lymph node dissection (3). Except for one woman who underwent simple mastectomy without axillary dissection, all patients with recurrent or fatal carcinoma had axillary nodal metastases. Others found axillary nodal metastases in five of six cases, and these five patients died of metastatic carcinoma. The single woman with negative lymph nodes died of intercurrent disease without recurrence (9). Hayes et al. reported that three of eight patients with follow-up information died of metastatic carcinoma (6). These data suggest that the prognosis of patients with glycogen-rich mammary carcinoma is not particularly favorable and that it may be similar to or worse than ordinary invasive duct when compared on a stage-matched basis (2,6).

## REFERENCES

1. Mohamed AH, Cherrick HM. Glycogen-rich adenocarcinoma of minor salivary glands. A light and electron microscopic study. *Cancer* 1975;36:1057–1066.
2. Fisher ER, Tavares J, Bulatao IS, et al. Glycogen-rich, clear cell breast cancer: with comments concerning other clear cell variants. *Hum Pathol* 1985;16:1085–1090.
3. Hull MT, Warfel KA. Glycogen-rich clear cell carcinomas of the breast. A clinicopathologic and ultrastructural study. *Am J Surg Pathol* 1986;10:553–559.
4. Hull MT, Priest JB, Broadie TA, et al. Glycogen-rich clear cell carcinoma of the breast: a light and electron microscopic study. *Cancer* 1981;48:2003–2009.
5. Sorensen FB, Paulsen SM. Glycogen-rich clear cell carcinoma of the breast: a solid variant with mucus: a light microscopic, immunohistochemical and ultrastructural study of a case. *Histopathology* 1987;11:857–869.
6. Hayes MM, Seidman JD, Ashton MA. Glycogen-rich clear cell carcinoma of the breast: a clinicopathologic study of 21 cases. *Am J Surg Pathol* 1995;19:904–911.
7. Benisch B, Peison B, Newman R, et al. Solid glycogen-rich clear cell carcinoma of the breast (a light and ultrastructural study). *Am J Clin Pathol* 1983;79:243–245.
8. Kern SB, Andera L. Cytology of glycogen-rich (clear cell) carcinoma of the breast: a report of two cases. *Acta Cytol* 1997;41:556–560.
9. Toikkanen S, Joensuu H. Glycogen-rich clear cell carcinoma of the breast: a clinicopathologic and flow cytometric study. *Hum Pathol* 1991;22:81–83.
10. Alexiev BA. Glycogen-rich clear cell carcinoma of the breast: report of a case with fine-needle aspiration cytology and immunocytochemical and ultrastructural studies. *Diagn Cytopathol* 1994;12:62–66.

# CHAPTER 31

# Invasive Micropapillary Carcinoma

Invasive micropapillary carcinoma is a morphologically distinctive form of duct carcinoma in which the tumor cells are arranged in morule-like clusters. Fisher et al. referred to this configuration as an "exfoliative appearance" (1). This growth pattern may be found throughout the lesion (pure invasive micropapillary carcinoma) or as part of an otherwise conventional invasive duct carcinoma (mixed invasive micropapillary carcinoma). Luna-Moré et al. found micropapillary differentiation in 27 of 986 (2.7%) consecutive breast carcinomas (2). In 15 of the tumors, the micropapillary component occupied more than 50% of the lesion. Pure invasive micropapillary carcinoma was found in 21 of 1,287 (1.7%) of tumors reviewed by Paterakos et al. (3).

## CLINICAL PRESENTATION

The reported age at diagnosis ranges from 36 to 81 years (4,5). The median age in two studies was 54 and 62 years, respectively (2,4). The mean age in two reports was 50 and 58 years (3,5). Patients with more than 50% micropapillary carcinoma tend to be older than patients with focal involvement (2). Most patients present with a palpable mass, but an occasional lesion has been detected mammographically as a density or as a result of microcalcifications (4,5). Rarely, an entire small nonpalpable invasive micropapillary carcinoma may be removed by a needle core biopsy. The distribution of tumors in terms of laterality and location in the breast does not differ significantly from that of ordinary invasive duct carcinomas (2,5). Presentation as an "axillary mass" was described in one case and in the subareolar region in three cases (5).

## GROSS PATHOLOGY

Tumor size ranged from 0.3 to 3.0 cm, with a median of 1.5 cm in one series (4). Others described larger lesions with a mean size of 4.9 cm, including 14.8% T1, 51.8% T2, and 33.3% T3 tumors (2). Two previously unreported examples that measured less than 5 mm have been seen by the author. Tumors with more than 50% of micropapillary growth tend to be larger (mean size, 6 cm) than those with a lesser amount of this pattern (mean size,

3.5 cm). Gross descriptions of the tumors do not suggest any specific features.

## MICROSCOPIC PATHOLOGY

The carcinoma cells are cuboidal to columnar, containing finely granular or dense eosinophilic cytoplasm. Nuclear grade is usually intermediate to poorly differentiated, and mitotic activity is greater in more high-grade lesions. Paterakos et al. reported that invasive micropapillary carcinomas had a significantly greater proportion of high-grade features and a higher mitotic rate (3). The tumor cells are arranged in small clusters that may have a serrated outer border. A central lumen is usually present, but solid groups also occur (Fig. 31.1). Uncommon variants feature microcystic dilatation of lumens within cell clusters (Fig. 31.2) or apocrine differentiation (Fig. 31.3). A clear space defined by intervening stroma consisting of dense fibrocollagenous tissue or a more delicate network of reticular tissue surrounds each tumor cell cluster. In some instances, a lymphoid infiltrate may permeate the stroma. The sponge-like pattern of spaces filled by tumor cell clusters occurs in metastatic lesions as well as in primary tumors. The spaces generally appear to be empty, but in some instances mucinous material has been demonstrated with special stains (2). Myxoid stroma has been noted in a minority of cases (4). Microcalcifications are variably present in the tumor cell clusters, and they can have a psammomatous appearance (Fig. 31.3).

Luna-Moré et al. studied the distribution of several prognostic markers in invasive micropapillary carcinoma detected by immunohistochemistry (6). Immunoreactivity was present as follows: estrogen receptor (73%), progesterone receptor (45%), HER2/*neu* (36%), p53 (12%), and *bcl*-2 (70%). Others reported that 75% of invasive micropapillary carcinomas were immunoreactive for p53, all were HER2/*neu* positive, and loss of heterozygosity for 17p13.1 was found in 80% of these tumors (7). Compared with a large series of invasive duct carcinoma, invasive micropapillary carcinomas were HER2/*neu* positive significantly more often (3).

The tumor cells are immunoreactive for epithelial membrane antigen, which stains the cell membranes at the periphery of the clusters and the borders of lumens within the

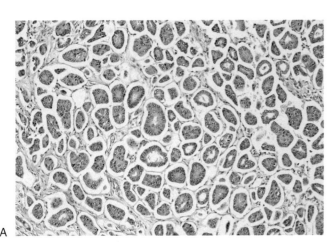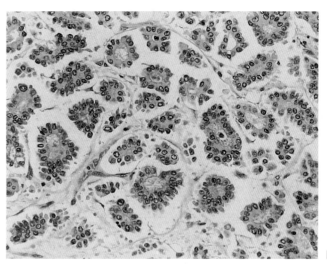

**FIG. 31.1.** *Invasive micropapillary carcinoma.* **A:** Morule-like clusters of tumor cells within spaces defined by a network of loose fibrocollagenous stroma. **B:** Small lumens are present in the carcinomatous glands, which have serrated outer borders.

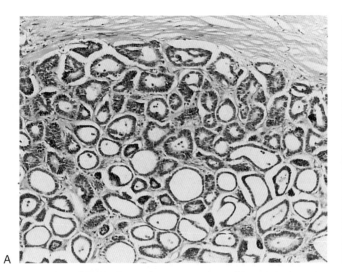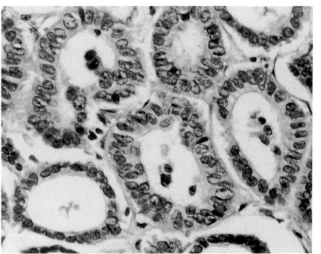

**FIG. 31.2.** *Invasive micropapillary carcinoma.* **A:** This aggregate of carcinomatous glands bears a superficial resemblance to adenosis. Spaces are present around some glands. **B:** Microlumens are evident within the glands. Periglandular spaces are less conspicuous in this configuration than in Fig. 31.1.

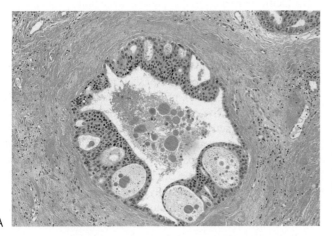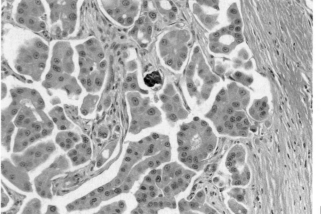

**FIG. 31.3.** *Invasive micropapillary carcinoma, apocrine.* **A:** Intraductal apocrine carcinoma with peripheral arcades. **B:** Invasive micropapillary apocrine carcinoma with calcification.

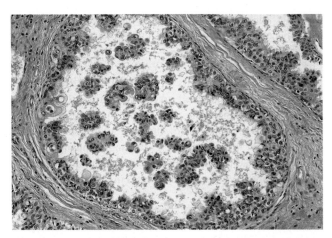

**FIG. 31.4.** *Invasive micropapillary carcinoma, intraductal carcinoma.* Micropapillary structure and poorly differentiated nuclear grade are evident.

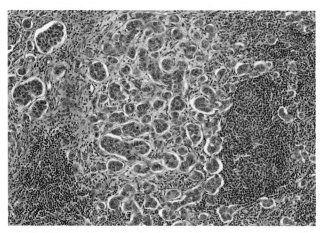

**FIG. 31.6.** *Invasive micropapillary carcinoma, lymph node metastasis.* Note the fibrosis around nests of tumor cells, a frequent occurrence at metastatic sites.

clusters (2). Microvilli have been demonstrated on these same cell surfaces by electron microscopy, suggesting that cells at the periphery are oriented as though the spaces around the tumor cell clusters were glandular lumens (2). This has been referred to as an *inside-out growth pattern* (8).

Lymphatic invasion was reportedly present in 72.7% of cases in one series (6) and in nearly 50% by others (5). These may be overestimates because it is difficult to identify true lymphatic tumor emboli in the vicinity of the primary tumor, which has the intrinsic capacity to grow in a sponge-like pattern. When convincing evidence of lymphatic emboli is encountered, the intravascular tumor cells are arranged in the same papillary clusters that characterize the invasive part of the tumor.

Intraductal carcinoma, which is detected in most cases, is micropapillary, sometimes with cribriform elements, in cases of pure micropapillary carcinoma (Fig. 31.4). Comedo intraductal carcinoma usually is seen in tumors with an invasive nonmicropapillary component. Cells in the intraductal carcinoma have poorly differentiated hyperchromatic nuclei rather

than the bland nuclear cytology usually associated with micropapillary intraductal carcinoma. Necrosis and calcification often are found in intraductal foci. Invasive nonmicropapillary elements tend to be poorly differentiated. Associated mucinous carcinoma has been described (Fig. 31.5) (5).

The differential diagnosis of invasive micropapillary carcinoma includes primary mucinous carcinoma and metastatic serous ovarian carcinoma. Mucinous carcinoma features abundant extracellular mucin, which is absent from invasive micropapillary carcinoma. Tumor cell clusters in mucinous carcinoma usually have a smooth rather than a serrated periphery. The presence of an intraductal component serves to exclude metastatic ovarian carcinoma, which typically has readily identified lymphatic tumor emboli in the breast and psammoma bodies.

The diagnosis of invasive micropapillary carcinoma may be suggested by a fine needle aspiration specimen containing round, oval, or angular three-dimensional clusters of neoplastic cells lacking fibrovascular cores (9). Dispersed, discohesive "inside out" clusters of tumor cells also may be pre-

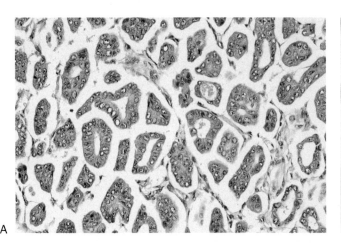

A

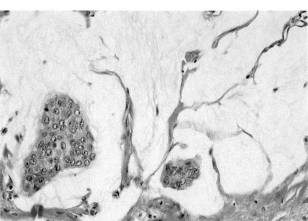

B

**FIG. 31.5.** *Invasive micropapillary and mucinous carcinoma.* This tumor had a mixed growth pattern. **A:** Invasive micropapillary carcinoma. **B:** Mucinous carcinoma.

sent (10). This cytologic pattern is likely to be duplicated in a specimen from metastatic invasive micropapillary carcinoma (Fig. 31.6).

## TREATMENT AND PROGNOSIS

Most patients described in published reports have been treated by mastectomy and axillary dissection. In one report, all patients had axillary lymph node metastases (2). Data were incomplete in a second report, but three of nine patients had confirmed metastases in axillary lymph nodes. Middleton et al. reported that 36% were "stage II," 57% "stage III," and 7% "stage IV" (5). I have seen cases of mammographically detected nonpalpable micropapillary carcinoma with no axillary nodal metastases.

Information about the clinical course of invasive micropapillary carcinoma is limited. In one series, 50% of the patients died of disease (2). A second study reported one patient with a local recurrence 2.8 years after mastectomy and four patients who were alive 3.4 to 4.7 years after mastectomy (4). Patients with nonpalpable tumors detected by mammography may be candidates for breast-conservation with radiotherapy. Chest-wall radiation would be prudent for large tumors in view of the apparent proclivity for local recurrence after mastectomy. Middleton et al. reported that 9 of 14 patients developed recurrences in the skin and chest wall following mastectomy with a mean time to recurrence of 24 months (5). Among 10 patients with follow-up, five died of breast cancer 3 to 12 years after diagnosis, and five were alive for 1 to 8 years. Compared with patients with nonmicropapillary invasive carcinoma, patients with invasive micropapillary carcinoma had a significantly shorter disease-free and overall survival after a median follow-up of 13.8 years (3). After stratification for the number of lymph nodes involved and other prognostic factors in multivariate analysis, invasive micropapillary carcinoma had survival rates similar to nonmicropapillary invasive duct carcinomas.

Presently, mastectomy with axillary dissection would be preferable to breast conservation in most cases. Adjuvant chemotherapy is indicated when there are axillary lymph node metastases and in the absence of lymph node metastases for tumors larger than 1.0 cm. Invasive micropapillary carcinomas smaller than 1.0 cm are exceedingly unusual. The decision to give adjuvant systemic treatment in this latter situation will depend on the circumstances in the individual case.

## REFERENCES

1. Fisher ER, Palekar AS, Redmond C, et al. Pathologic findings from the National Surgical Adjuvant Breast Project (Protocol No. 4): VI. Invasive papillary cancer. *Am J Clin Pathol* 1980;73:313–322.
2. Luna-Moré S, Gonzalez B, Acedo C, et al. Invasive micropapillary carcinoma of the breast: a new special type of invasive mammary carcinoma. *Pathol Res Pract* 1994;190:668–674.
3. Paterakos M, Watkin WG, Edgerton SM, et al. Invasive micropapillary carcinoma of the breast: a prognostic study. *Hum Pathol* 1999;30:1459–1463.
4. Siriaunkgul S, Tavassoli FA. Invasive micropapillary carcinoma of the breast. *Mod Pathol* 1993;6:660–662.
5. Middleton LP, Tressera F, Sobel ME, et al. Infiltrating micropapillary carcinoma of the breast. *Mod Pathol* 1999;12:499–504.
6. Luna-Moré S, de los Santos F, Breton JJ, et al. Estrogen and progesterone receptors, c-erbB-2, p53, and BCL-2 in thirty-three invasive micropapillary breast carcinomas. *Pathol Res Pract* 1996;192:27–32.
7. Merino MJ, Albuquerque A, Bryant B, et al. Genetic changes in chromosome 17p in aggressive variants of breast cancer. *Mod Pathol* 1997;10:23A.
8. Petersen JL. Breast carcinoma with an unexpected inside out growth pattern, rotation of polarisation associated with angioinvasion. *Pathol Res Pract* 1993;189:780.
9. Khurana KK, Wilbur D, Dawson AE. Fine needle aspiration cytology of invasive micropapillary carcinoma of the breast: a report of two cases. *Acta Cytol* 1997;41:1394–1398.
10. Wong S-I, Cheung H, Tse GMK. Fine needle aspiration cytology of invasive micropapillary carcinoma of the breast. *Acta Cytol* 2000;44:1085–1089.

# CHAPTER 32

# Paget's Disease of the Nipple

In 1874, Sir James Paget (1) described "an eruption on the nipple and areola: with characteristics of 'ordinary chronic eczema' or 'psoriasis'." He observed that "cancer of the mammary gland has followed within at the most two years" and that "the formation of cancer has not in any case taken place first in the diseased part of the skin. It has always been in the substance of the mammary gland." The cancers that occurred in these patients followed the clinical course of other cases without Paget's disease and showed "nothing which might not be written in the ordinary history of cancer of the breast."

Paget did not describe the histopathology of this condition; however, he inferred from his clinical observations "that a superficial disease induces in the structures beneath it, in the course of many months, such degeneracy as makes them apt to become the seats of cancer." To support this conclusion, he referred to the development of carcinoma of the penis, tongue, and lip after "chronic soreness or irritation."

The existence of extramammary Paget's disease was recognized before the end of the nineteenth century, by which time the characteristic histologic features of the disease had been reported (2,3). Thin studied a series of specimens in the pathological museum of the British Medical Association and concluded that "this malignant dermatitis has neither the symptoms nor the pathological anatomy of any known skin disease" (2). He described the histopathologic features of breast carcinoma in Paget's disease and illustrated the "blocking up of the lactiferous ducts in the affection by newly formed cancerous epithelium [which] may break through the wall of the duct into the connective tissue of the nipple." Thin interpreted his observations as indicating that secretions emerging from the mammary ducts injured the epidermis and that this process induced the underlying carcinoma. Although histologic, electron microscopic, and immunohistochemical data have been put forward to support the view that Paget's disease is a neoplasm derived from altered epidermal keratinocytes (4,5), this is no longer considered to be the histogenesis of the condition.

The concept that Paget's disease represents the spread of carcinoma cells into the epidermis from an underlying mammary adenocarcinoma was first advanced in 1904 by Jacobaeus based on histologic study of three cases (Fig. 32.1) (6). He concluded that "Paget's disease is a carcinoma from its inception, derived from the glandular epithelium of the lactiferous ducts." He also noted that extension through the duct system provided a mechanism for the development of Paget's disease in association with a carcinoma located deep within the breast. These observations were confirmed in 1927 by Muir (7), who also described the phenomenon of "secondary" Paget's disease, which occurs when an invasive primary carcinoma of the breast extending directly into the epidermis is accompanied by the intraepidermal spread of Paget's cells. Secondary Paget's disease also has been described in the skin at sites of adenocarcinoma metastatic from the breast (8) and other organs.

Considerable histochemical data support the evidence from anatomic and histopathologic studies that Paget's cells are derived from an underlying adenocarcinoma. In particular, the distribution of carcinoembryonic antigen (CEA) immunoreactive protein (9–11), casein (12), milk-fat globule membrane antigens (13,14), cytokeratins (15–17), and estrogen receptors (18) are all indicative of a glandular origin.

The discontinuous distribution of Paget's cells in the nipple epidermis is a fascinating and unexplained phenomenon which suggests that Paget's cells are able to move within the epidermis. Evidence in support of this possibility has been obtained as a result of studies that demonstrated that normal epidermal cells produce heregulin-alpha, a motility factor (18a). Paget's cells express heregulin receptors including HER2/*neu*. It has been suggested that binding of heregulin and HER2/*neu* receptors exerts a chemotactic effect on Paget's cells, resulting in their migration into the epidermis (18a).

## CLINICAL PRESENTATION

Paget's disease shows no predilection for any age group. The age range in several large series (15,19–21) consisting of 508 patients was 26 to 88 years. Changes caused by Paget's disease may be limited to the nipple or extend to the

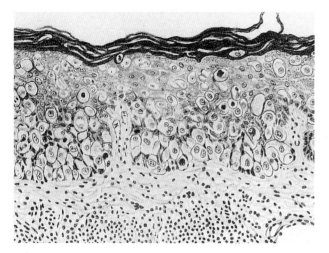

**FIG. 32.1.** *Paget's disease.* The lesion illustrated by Jacobaeus shows the characteristic features, including a dermal lymphocytic infiltrate. Paget's cells are aggregated in the deep epidermis and scattered in the superficial epidermis. The cells have abundant pale cytoplasm, and nucleoli are evident in the nuclei. (From Jacobaeus HC. Paget's disease und sein Verhültniss zum Milchdrüsenkarzinom. *Virchows Arch* 1904;178:124–142, with permission.)

areola, and in advanced cases the lesion also involves the skin surrounding the areola (Fig. 32.2). Complaints of pain or itching are frequent. Early changes include scaling and redness, which may be mistaken for eczema or some other inflammatory condition. Consequently, a delay of 6 to 12 months, during which time the syumptoms are treated topically, is not uncommon before biopsy. The inflammatory component may be improved by topical treatment, a result that masks the underlying condition and contributes to delay. Ulceration, crusting, and serous or bloody discharge characterize more advanced cases.

A number of mammographic abnormalities may be found in the breast with Paget's disease (22). Lesions anywhere in the breast may be indicative of a separate distant coexistent carcinoma. In the nipple–subareolar region, the significant findings include thickening of the nipple, an underlying mass possibly with nipple retraction, and calcifications. Patients with clinically apparent Paget's disease tend to have radiologic findings in the nipple–subareolar region. When Paget's disease is not evident clinically, mammography more often discloses lesions away from the nipple region; however, mammography is not always a reliable procedure

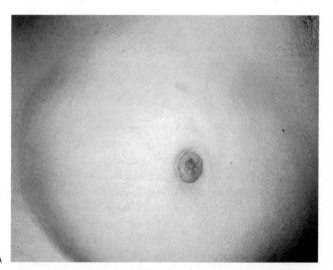

A

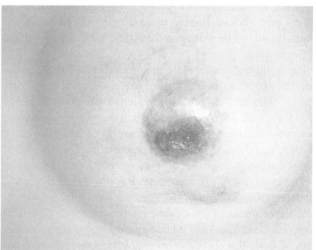

B

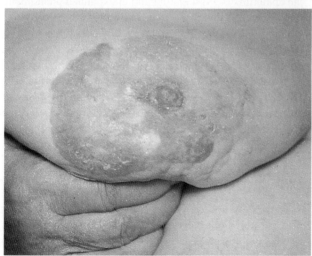

C

**FIG. 32.2.** *Paget's disease, clinical.* **A:** The appearance of a lesion limited to the nipple surface. **B:** Paget's disease extending to the areola. Note skin dimpling in the 6 o'clock radius. **C:** Paget's disease extending to the skin of the breast. Skin dimpling is present in the 5 o'clock radius.

for detecting Paget's disease. In one study of 25 breasts that proved to have Paget's disease on pathologic examination of a mastectomy, only three of the cases (12%) had nipple abnormalities on mammography (23). Among 14 patients in the series with clinical evidence of Paget's disease, mammography identified an underlying tumor in six (43%).

Paget's disease occurs in 1% to 2% of female patients with mammary carcinoma. Most of these women have a clinically evident nipple lesion, but 10% to 28% of cases of Paget's disease are detected only in histologic sections of the nipple removed at mastectomy, having caused no clinical abnormality. Paget's disease has been observed in a nipple 8 years after subcutaneous mastectomy for fibrocystic disease (24). No clinical or epidemiologic factors are known to predispose patients to develop Paget's disease. A 35-year-old patient who had systemic scleroderma involving the skin of the breast with coexistent Paget's disease has been described (25).

Fifty percent to 60% of patients have a palpable tumor in the breast that exhibits Paget's disease. In one study, the mean age of women with a tumor (49 years) was significantly less than that of women without a tumor (58 years) (20). An invasive carcinoma was detected in more than 75% to 90% of women who had Paget's disease accompanied by a tumor (15,19,26), and 45% to 66% reportedly had axillary lymph node metastases (15,19,20,26). In the absence of a clinically apparent tumor, invasive carcinoma occurs in no more than 40% of cases, and axillary metastases have been reported in 5% to 13% of cases (15,19,20,26).

Fewer than 1% of reported cases of Paget's disease have been found in men (27). Fewer than 5% of male breast carcinomas are complicated by Paget's disease, despite the fact that almost all carcinomas of the male breast are centrally located (28). Paget's disease of the male breast exhibits the same cytokeratin reactivity as the lesion in women (29). Paget's disease has been found associated with breast carcinoma developing in males who had Klinefelter's syndrome (30).

## GROSS PATHOLOGY

The gross pathologic changes of Paget's disease on the surface of the resected nipple duplicate those observed clinically. Occasionally, enlarged lactiferous ducts can be detected if the nipple and underlying breast are examined carefully. Clinically palpable tumors have no specific gross pathologic features. A small percentage of women who present with Paget's disease and have no tumor detected on clinical examination are found to have a grossly evident invasive carcinoma in the resected breast (31).

Most studies of Paget's disease give little information about the distribution of underlying carcinoma in the breast. Intraductal carcinoma usually can be found in at least one lactiferous duct. An invasive tumor, if present, tends to be central, but instances of peripherally placed tumors have been recorded (31). Chaudary et al. reported that 45% of palpable invasive carcinomas associated with Paget's disease in their series were located in the upper, outer quadrant (15).

## MICROSCOPIC PATHOLOGY

The diagnosis of Paget's disease can be made from a wedge biopsy, a superficial "shave" biopsy of epidermis, or punch biopsy. The wedge biopsy is most likely to yield a diagnosis because the epidermis is adequately represented and this type of specimen is likely to include a section of lactiferous duct. The shave biopsy is less likely to contain a sufficient number of Paget's cells because these specimens sometimes consist largely of superficial keratinized debris or inflammatory exudate. Although a punch biopsy will include the underlying stroma and possibly part of a duct, there is frequently little epidermis to study. None of these procedures is always successful, however, and it is sometimes necessary to take a second biopsy or excise the nipple. The detection of Paget's cells in the epidermis in a biopsy that appears to contain a nipple adenoma is indicative of an associated carcinoma even if the portion of adenoma seen in the biopsy appears benign (32).

It may be possible to recognize carcinoma cells cytologically in an imprint or scraping from the nipple surface, but this material is not suitable for the specific diagnosis of Paget's disease. Estrogen receptor (ER) activity has been demonstrated in Paget's cells in cytologic specimens obtained by scraping the nipple with a scalpel (18). The underlying carcinomas exhibited estrogen receptor activity similar to that seen in the cytologic specimens. Immunohistochemical detection of estrogen receptor is not a reliable basis for the diagnosis of Paget's disease because the underlying carcinomas tend to be poorly differentiated and receptor negative. ER-positive cells may be present in an imprint or scrape cytologic sample from the ulcerated surface of benign florid papillomatosis.

The characteristic histopathologic feature of this condition is the presence of adenocarcinoma cells (Paget's cells) in the keratinizing epithelium of the nipple epidermis (Fig. 32.3). These cells occur singly in superficial epidermal layers. They are more likely to form clusters in the basal portions of the epidermis and have a distribution similar to that of junctional melanocytes. The resemblance to melanoma is enhanced if the carcinoma cells take up melanin pigment released by epidermal cells (33,34). Isolated Paget's cells appear to lie in vacuoles within the epidermis. The cytoplasm is usually pale or clear, and it may contain mucin secretion vacuoles. Nuclei of Paget's cells tend to have prominent nucleoli.

Other microscopic aspects of Paget's disease sometimes obscure the lesion and may interfere with the diagnosis. Hyperplasia and hyperkeratosis of the epidermis occur to some degree, and this occasionally is severe enough to suggest pseudoepitheliomatous hyperplasia (Fig. 32.4). The superficial dermal stroma of the nipple usually is infiltrated by a moderate to marked lymphocytic reaction. When ulceration denudes the affected epithelium, a biopsy of the exposed stroma will reveal only the underlying inflammatory reaction. Unless this misleading appearance is recognized, the

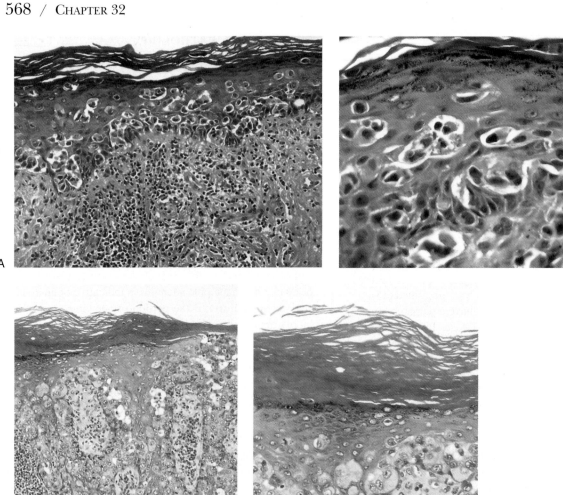

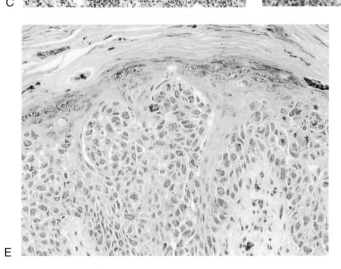

**FIG. 32.3.** *Paget's disease.* **A:** Carcinoma cells form a band in the deep epidermis, and they are scattered individually throughout the squamous epithelium. **B:** The lacunar arrangement of carcinoma cells is commonly seen in Paget's disease. **C:** An extensive infiltrate with involvement largely concentrated in the deep epidermis. Lacunae are not conspicuous in this instance. **D:** The tumor cells have abundant pale cytoplasm, pleomorphic nuclei, and prominent nucleoli. **E:** Granules of dark brown melanin pigment are present in some Paget's cells.

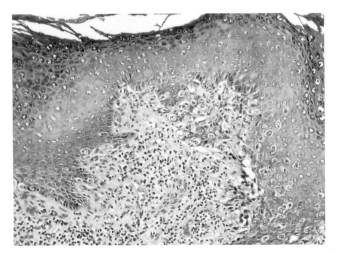

**FIG. 32.4.** *Paget's disease.* Paget's cells are obscured in this somewhat tangential section of hyperplastic epidermis. Note the dermal lymphocytic infiltrate, which is often present.

biopsy findings may reinforce an erroneous clinical diagnosis of an inflammatory condition. It is therefore important to state in the pathological report whether epidermal tissue is present. Absence of epidermis is an indication for rebiopsy.

An associated carcinoma has been found in the breast or the nipple in more than 95% of the hundreds of cases of Paget's disease described in the literature. These have virtually all been duct carcinomas, with or without an invasive component. Rarely, these have been specialized forms of ductal carcinoma (e.g., papillary or medullary) (19) or duct carcinoma arising in florid papillomatosis (adenoma) of the nipple (32). Although the extension of cells from lobular carcinoma *in situ* to the epithelium of ducts within the breast, referred to as *pagetoid spread,* may resemble Paget's disease, this process rarely involves the major lactiferous ducts and only very rarely spreads to the keratinizing epidermis of the nipple (Fig. 32.5). Decreased expression of E-cadherin occurs around lobular carcinoma cells involving the nipple epidermis as Paget's disease.

Paget's disease can be encountered at sites of squamous metaplasia in the breast (Fig. 32.6). Secondary Paget's disease is involvement of the epidermis over cutaneous metastases anywhere on the body or when a primary carcinoma extends up to the skin (Fig. 32.7).

Intraductal carcinoma associated with Paget's disease characteristically has a comedo or solid growth pattern. Foci of cribriform and papillary duct carcinoma also may be

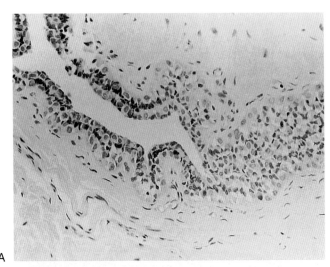

A

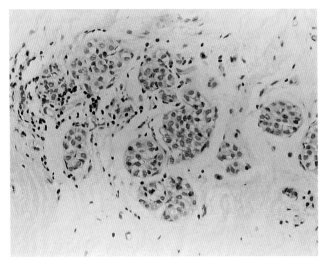

B

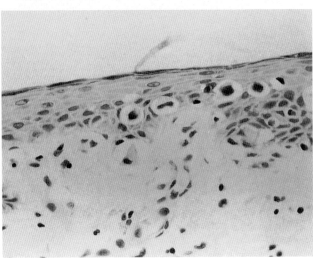

C

**FIG. 32.5.** *Paget's disease associated with lobular carcinoma.* **A:** *In situ* carcinoma with pagetoid spread in a large lactiferous duct. **B:** Lobular carcinoma *in situ* in a lobule. **C:** Paget's disease of the nipple epidermis in the same specimen as **A** and **B.**

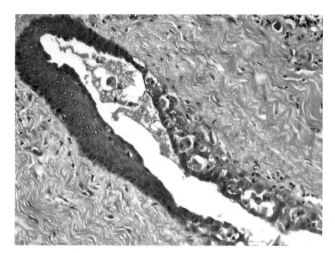

**FIG. 32.6.** *Paget's disease in squamous metaplasia.* Paget's disease extending from nearby intraductal carcinoma involves the metaplastic squamous epithelium of this cyst within the breast parenchyma.

found as part of the process somewhere in the breast, but the lactiferous ducts directly connected to Paget's disease contain comedocarcinoma in most cases. Cribriform or papillary carcinomas are found in about 10%, and about 40% have mixed types of intraductal carcinoma (35). Because comedocarcinoma frequently contains calcifications, the underlying intraductal lesion may be detectable by mammography. In a series reported by Chaudary et al., 25 of 32 (78%) mastectomy specimens had intraductal carcinoma beyond the subareolar area, and in eight of these patients multicentric invasive foci were found (15). Intraductal carcinoma was limited to subareolar ducts in only two cases.

Invasive carcinoma associated with Paget's disease does not have a specific histopathologic pattern. It is typically a poorly differentiated, solid, invasive carcinoma that arises from affected ducts within the underlying breast paren-

chyma. Rarely, invasive carcinoma may develop from a superficial or terminal portion of a lactiferous duct close to the site of Paget's disease. In exceptional cases, invasion appears to arise directly from Paget's disease in the epidermis growing downward into the nipple, there being no other carcinoma elsewhere in the nipple and breast (Fig. 32.8).

Failure to detect an underlying carcinoma in a small number of cases has been used as an argument to support the concept that Paget's disease arises directly from keratinocytes of the epidermis. In most of these rare instances, the carcinomas associated with Paget's disease arise from ductal epithelium at or near the squamocolumnar junction, with growth limited to upward spread as Paget's disease (Fig. 32.9). Mai et al. studied the distribution of intraductal carcinoma in 19 nipples with Paget's disease by a serial section technique (35a). A minority of specimens had intraductal carcinoma limited to superficial portions of lactiferous ducts. Rarely, a segment of benign duct was found between the intraductal carcinoma in a lactiferous duct and carcinoma in the underlying breast. Origin of carcinoma from adnexal glands in the nipple is also theoretically possible (Fig. 32.10). The claim that no underlying carcinoma was detectable in the breasts of patients treated only by excisional biopsy of the nipple is unwarranted because the entire breast was not examined (36).

Because Paget's cells are by their nature entrapped among nonneoplastic squamous cells in the epidermis, it is difficult to determine the flow cytometric features of this neoplastic population. One group of investigators has described a method for isolating Paget's cells from the epidermis in a biopsy of the nipple (37). The tumor cells obtained from a patient with a 7-year history of Paget's disease were said to have a normal ploidy distribution.

The histologic differential diagnosis in a biopsy for suspected Paget's disease includes inflammatory conditions of the skin, clear cell change in epidermal cells, Toker cells

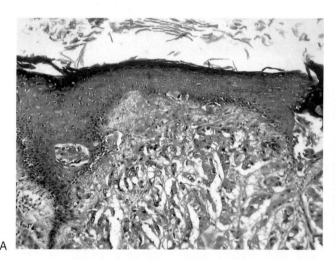
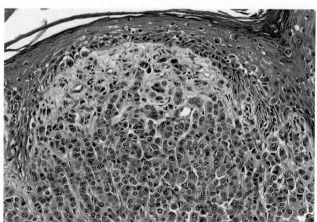

**FIG. 32.7.** *Paget's disease, secondary.* **A:** Invasive duct carcinoma, apocrine-type, invading into the skin from the underlying breast, with Paget's disease in the epidermis. **B:** Invasive pleomorphic lobular carcinoma in the nipple with overlying secondary Paget's disease.

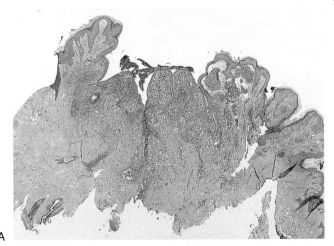
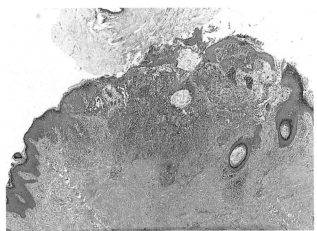
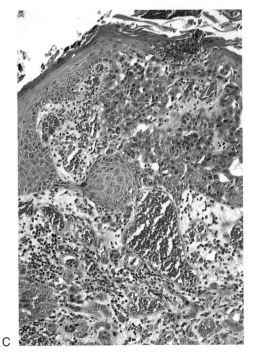

**FIG. 32.8.** *Paget's disease giving rise to invasive carcinoma of nipple.* **A,B:** Specimens from two different patients showing invasive duct carcinoma arising from lactiferous ducts near the surface of the nipple with Paget's disease at the lateral borders. No carcinoma was found in the remainder of either breast. **C:** Florid Paget's disease above gives rise to invasive carcinoma below in **B**.

(38), florid papillomatosis of nipple ducts or nipple adenoma (32), malignant melanoma (39), and such extremely uncommon lesions as squamous or basal cell carcinoma (40), and syringomatous adenoma (41). With an adequate sample, most of these lesions can be readily distinguished from Paget's disease (42,42a).

Clear cells in the epidermis constitute a nonneoplastic alteration of keratinocytes (Fig. 32.11). The change tends to occur in the basal or midepidermis, with isolated cells also distributed in more superficial and deep layers (Fig. 32.12). These cells have small, inconspicuous nuclei, and in extreme cases consist largely of a vacuole that appears empty on routine sections (Fig. 32.13). Mucin and other secretory substances detectable in Paget's cells are absent (42).

Toker cells are a subset of benign clear cells found in the nipple epidermis (38). These cells tend to be distributed around the nipple duct orifices singly or in small groups, a pattern that suggests origin from nonneoplastic lactiferous duct epithelium. As discussed later in this chapter, Toker cells are immunoreactive with CK7, which was previously considered to be specific for Paget's disease. This reagent can detect Toker cells in histologically normal nipples from breasts not known to harbor carcinoma and lacking demonstrable intraductal carcinoma in lactiferous ducts (42b). These recent observations have raised concern about the diagnosis of Paget's disease based solely on CK7 reactivity in the absence of cytologically characteristic Paget's cells and corroborating immunohistochemical/histochemical studies, and failure to identify carcinoma in the breast or lactiferous ducts. Toker cell hyperplasia was reportedly present in association with Paget's disease limited to the areola in the absence of a demonstrable carcinoma in the breast (42c). Neoplastic transformation of Toker cells, if they are of mammary duct origin, could account for some rare examples of Paget's

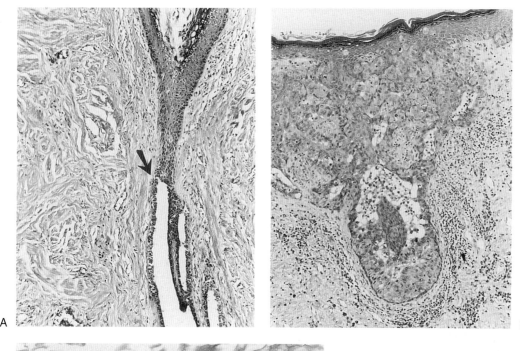

A
B

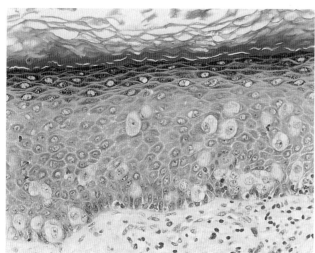

C

**FIG. 32.9.** *Paget's disease and intraductal carcinoma of a terminal lactiferous duct.* **A:** A section of a terminal lactiferous duct in which there is squamous metaplasia of the distal duct epithelium. Clear cell change is present in squamous cells. The *arrow* points to the squamocolumnar junction. **B:** Intraductal carcinoma in a terminal lactiferous duct in continuity with overlying Paget's disease. The primary intraductal carcinoma in this case was limited to ducts in the superficial part of the nipple. **C:** Paget's cells in the epidermis of the specimen in **B**.

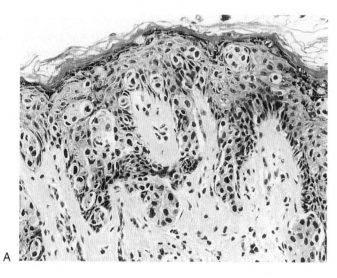

A

**FIG. 32.10.** *Paget's disease involving adnexal glands in the nipple.* **A:** Paget's disease with slight pseudoepitheliomatous hyperplasia of the epidermis. *(continued)*

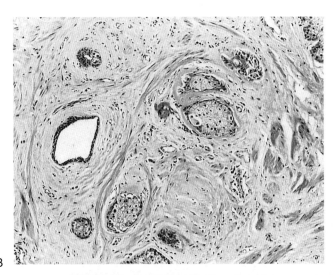

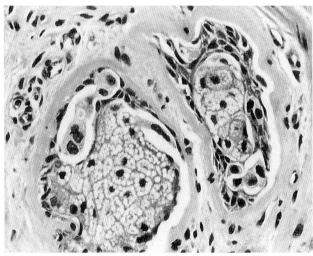

**FIG. 32.10.** *Continued.* **B:** Paget's cells are present in the epithelium of sebaceous glands and a sweat gland duct. Also present are the dilated duct of a gland of Montgomery and bundles of subareolar smooth-muscle cells. **C:** A magnified view of a sebaceous gland with Paget's cells.

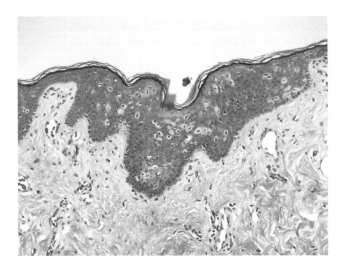

**FIG. 32.11.** *Clear cell change in the nipple epidermis.* Epidermal cells with clear cytoplasm are distributed mainly in the midepidermis.

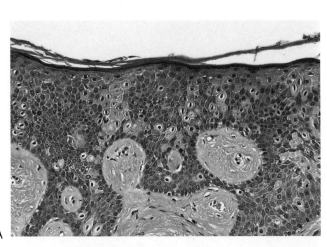

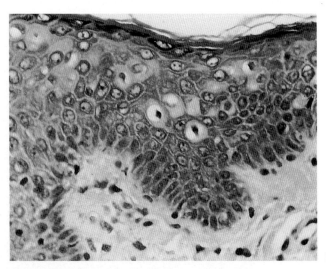

**FIG. 32.12.** *Clear cell change.* **A:** Alterations in squamous cells leading to clear cell change are evident. The process has a patchy distribution. Many of the cells in the affected areas display cytoplasmic pallor. **B:** Clear cell change appears to arise in cells with cytoplasmic pallor.

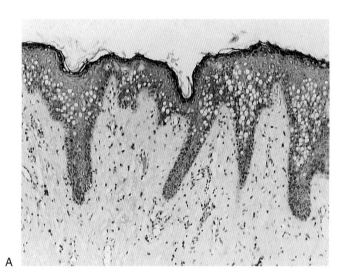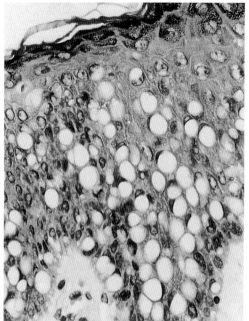

A

B

**FIG. 32.13.** *Clear cell change, vacuolated.* **A:** Marked vacuolization is evident in the midepidermis, largely sparing the deep layer. **B:** Vacuolated epidermal cells with eccentric nuclei resemble signet-ring cells.

disease without demonstrated underlying carcinoma, or for the discontinuous distribution of Paget's cells (42d).

Malignant melanoma has been found to arise in the areola, but melanoma of the nipple proper, and especially the surface of the nipple, is exceedingly rare (Fig. 32.14) (39). The histopathologic distinction between malignant melanoma and Paget's disease may be exceedingly difficult in limited biopsy material. Routine cytologic features of the tumor cells and their distribution in the epidermis may be identical. Some melanomas are devoid of pigment, whereas Paget's cells can incorporate melanin from epidermal cells, and in many cases Paget's cells do not contain mucin.

## IMMUNOHISTOCHEMISTRY

Using a panel of monoclonal antibodies, it is possible to distinguish Paget's disease from malignant melanoma and Bowen's disease (43) (Table 32.1).Hormone receptor reactivity in the nuclei of Paget's cells reflects the reactivity of the underlying carcinoma. Since nearly 50% of mammary carcinomas are nonreactive for one or both of these markers, a negative result does not exclude a diagnosis of Paget's disease. Paget's disease often is estrogen- and progesterone-receptor-negative, because the underlying carcinomas tend to be poorly differentiated. About 50% of extramammary

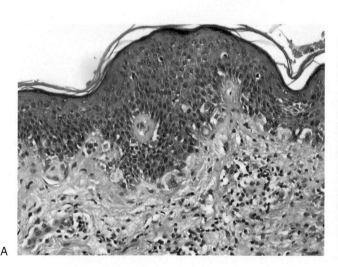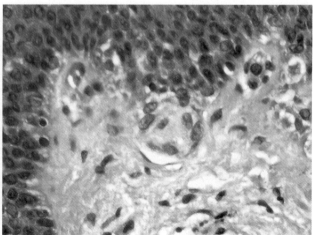

A

B

**FIG. 32.14.** *Malignant melanoma of the nipple.* **A:** The neoplastic junctional melanocytes resemble Paget's cells. There is a mild dermal lymphocytic infiltrate. **B:** A nest of junctional cells. *(continued)*

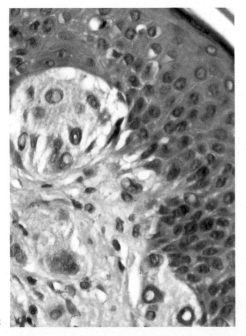

C

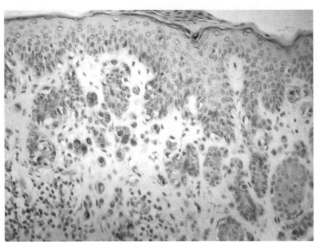

D

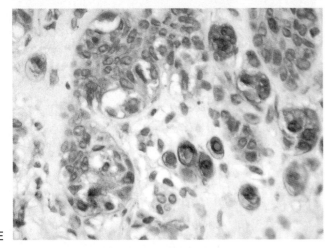

E

FIG. 32.14. *Continued.* **C:** Junctional cells with nuclear vacuoles, a feature of malignant melanoma not typically seen in Paget's disease. **D:** Melanoma cells are highlighted in the epidermis and dermis by this immunostain for S-100. **E:** Nuclear vacuoles can be seen in S-100-positive cells (avidin-biotin).

**TABLE 32.1.** *Reactivity of antibodies*

| Monoclonal antibody | Paget's disease | Bowen's disease | Malignant melanoma |
|---|---|---|---|
| S-100 | ± | − | + |
| HMB45 | − | − | + |
| CEA | ± | − | − |
| EMA | + | − | − |
| HMFG | + | − | − |
| CAM5.2 | + | − | − |
| CK7 | + | − | − |
| CK20 | − | + | − |
| ER | ± | − | − |
| HER2/*neu* | ± | − | − |

CEA, carcinoembryonic antigen; CK, cytokeratin; EMA, epithelial membrane antigen; ER, estrogen receptor; HMFG, human milk-fat globule.

Paget's disease specimens display nuclear reactivity for androgen receptor, and these carcinomas lack reactivity for nuclear estrogen and progesterone receptors (43a).

The immunohistochemical demonstration of estrogen receptor in the nuclei of Paget's cells will exclude melanoma. Paget's cells were reportedly negative for S-100 in two studies (11,44) but were positive for S-100 in 18% of lesions in a third series (45). S-100 and HMB45 are positive in virtually all melanomas. Paget's disease is HMB45 negative. The finding of immunoreactive CEA has proven to be a widely available useful procedure because this is present in many mammary carcinomas. Paget's cells were reportedly positive with a polyclonal anti-CEA, but negative with a monoclonal anti-CEA, in one study (13). Ordonez et al., using a different commercially available monoclonal anti-CEA reagent, reported that all eight examples of Paget's disease they studied were immunoreactive (11).

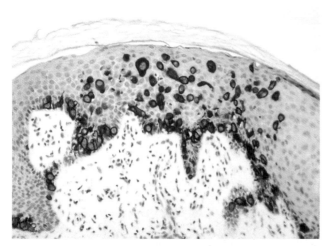

**FIG. 32.15.** *Paget's disease.* Paget's cells are highlighted by this immunostain for low-molecular-weight cytokeratin (anti-CAM5.2; avidin-biotin).

The neoplastic cells in Paget's disease have histochemical and immunohistochemical properties in common with adenocarcinomas growing within the breast. They are positive for epithelial membrane antigen (EMA) and human milk-fat globule (11,13,46). Paget's cells are reactive with monoclonal antibodies against low-molecular-weight cytokeratin (11,15,17,46) (Fig. 32.15), and they typically are not reactive with antibodies to high-molecular-weight cytokeratins that stain the neoplastic cells of epidermoid carcinoma or Bowen's disease (11,17). Paget's cells are immunoreactive for CK7 in nearly all cases and are not reactive for CK20 (47,48). Absence of CK7 reactivity in Paget's cells is usually associated with lack of CK7 reactivity in the underlying carcinoma (42b). This pattern differs from extramammary Paget's disease, which exhibits immunoreactivity for CK20 as well as CK7 (48). Merkel cells and some epidermal clear

cells also have been reported to be CK7-positive (48).

Immunoreactivity for the *ras* oncogene protein product p21 has been demonstrated in mammary and extramammary Paget's disease (49). Strong immunoreactivity for the HER2/*neu* oncoprotein has been detected in 79% to 100% of mammary Paget's disease samples studied (50–52) and in 0% to 40% of cases of extramammary Paget's disease (51–53) (Fig. 32.16). Most breast lesions have underlying comedo or solid forms of intraductal carcinoma, which is frequently HER2/*neu* positive (50,54).

Immunostains are useful for confirming the presence of carcinoma in cytologic specimens obtained by scraping the nipple surface (55). Benign proliferative lesions, such as

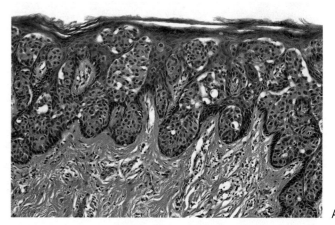

A

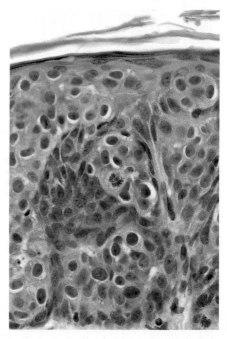

B

**FIG. 32.17.** *Paget's disease, mucin positive.* **A:** Paget's disease fills most of the epidermis. **B:** Intracytoplasmic mucin appears pink with the mucicarmine stain. This relatively weak and sparse pattern of staining is typical.

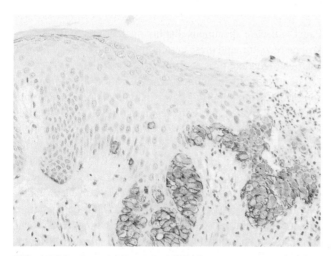

**FIG. 32.16.** *Paget's disease, HER2/*neu. Membrane staining for the Her2/*neu* protein highlights Paget's cells in the epidermis (avidin-biotin).

florid papillomatosis and inflammatory conditions that simulate Paget's disease, initially may be sampled by scrape cytology. Atypical epithelial cells and some inflammatory cells in such preparations may suggest Paget's disease (56).

Before the availability of monoclonal antibodies, it was necessary to rely on routine histochemical stains for mucin to assist in diagnosing Paget's disease. These procedures, especially mucicarmine and Alcian blue/periodic acid-Schiff stains, are still useful because they are readily available and easy to perform (Fig. 32.17). Because few examples of Paget's disease have numerous mucin-positive cells and because, in at least 25% of cases, no mucin-positive cells are detectable, a negative result with these procedures does not rule out Paget's disease.

## PROGNOSIS AND TREATMENT

Paget's disease is a manifestation of mammary duct carcinoma. The prognosis of patients who have Paget's disease is determined by the extent of the associated carcinoma (19–21,26,57). Paget's disease without an underlying mass is usually an indication of noninvasive ductal carcinoma or a small invasive tumor. Such patients treated by modified or radical mastectomy have a reported 10-year survival of 82% to 100% (19–21). For those proven to have only intraductal carcinoma, a 100% cure rate at 10 years has been achieved with mastectomy (19). The 10-year survival of node-negative patients who present with Paget's disease and a palpable invasive tumor is reported to be nearly 70% (19,20). The outcome is less favorable when there are axillary metastases, but the prognosis is somewhat better for women who present without a palpable tumor and nodal metastases, possibly reflecting the smaller size of the primary lesions (57).

Some patients with Paget's disease, especially those without a palpable tumor or extensive disease demonstrated by mammography, may be candidates for breast-conservation therapy. Lagios et al. described five patients treated by excision of the nipple–areola complex without radiation (36). One of these patients initially had partial resection of the nipple followed by complete excision when she had recurrent Paget's disease 12 months later. Patients chosen for this treatment had no clinical or radiologic evidence of disease beyond the nipple. They remained well for 30 to 69 months (average, 50 months). Dixon et al. reported a 40% local recurrence rate with less than 2 years of follow-up in patients treated only by complete resection of the nipple–areolar complex and central breast tissue (58).

In 1969, Rissanen and Holsti described eight patients treated with limited surgery and radiotherapy (57). Three of the eight developed recurrences, and one woman ultimately died of breast carcinoma. A more recent report described three recurrences among 20 patients after a median follow-up of 90 months (range, 15 months to 20 years) (59). Two recurrences were found within 2 years, and the third occurred about 4 years after treatment. All recurrences were in

the form of Paget's disease, and the lesions were controlled by mastectomy. In a third series, primary radiotherapy was effective when Paget's disease was not associated with a palpable tumor or mammographic abnormality (60). Three of 19 patients developed invasive recurrent carcinoma 4 to 6 years after treatment, but the others remained well from 1 to 13 years later. Recurrent carcinoma was detected in six of seven women who had an abnormal mammogram or palpable tumor. Most recurrences in the latter group included Paget's disease as well as invasive carcinoma. Blakeley et al. described a patient who developed a 9-mm invasive recurrent carcinoma in the breast at the site of a wide nipple excision performed 8 months previously for Paget's disease (61). The initial mammogram showed no evidence of a parenchymal lesion. Pierce et al. analyzed 30 women who had breast conservation therapy with radiotherapy for Paget's disease (62). Surgery varied from biopsy only to complete resection of the nipple–areolar complex with underlying breast tissue. The 5- and 8-year actuarial estimates of local failure in the breast alone were 9% and 16%, respectively. Three of the five recurrences in the breast occurred after complete resections, and two were in women with partial resections. The median time to local failure was 69 months.

Treatment of Paget's disease of the male breast by radiotherapy also has been reported (63). Clinically unapparent, occult Paget's disease has been responsible for recurrence in the breast after limited resection and primary radiotherapy administered for carcinoma discovered in another part of the breast (64–67).

## REFERENCES

1. Paget J. On disease of the mammary areola preceding cancer of the mammary gland. *St Bartholomew's Hospital Report* 1874;10:87–89.
2. Thin G. Malignant papillary dermatitis of the nipple and the breast-tumours with which it is found associated. *BMJ* 1881;1:760–763, 798–801.
3. Darier J, Couillaud P. Sur un cas de maladie de Paget de la region perineoanale et scrotale. *Societe Francaise de Dermatologie et de Syphiligraphie* 1893;4:25–31.
4. Willis RA. In: *Pathology of tumors*, 3rd ed. Washington, DC: Butterworth, 1960;247.
5. Nagle RB, Lucas DO, McDaniel KM, et al. Paget's cells. New evidence linking mammary and extramammary Paget cells to a common cell phenotype. *Am J Clin Pathol* 1985;83:431–438.
6. Jacobaeus HC. Paget's disease und sein Verhültniss zum Milchdrüsenkarzinom. *Virchows Arch* 1904;178:124–142.
7. Muir R. Paget's disease of the nipple and its relationships. *J Pathol Bacteriol* 1927;30:451–471.
8. Greenwood SM, Minkowitz S. Paget's disease in metastatic breast carcinoma. *Arch Dermatol* 1971;104:312–315.
9. Kuhajda FP, Offutt LE, Mendelsohn G. The distribution of carcinoembryonic antigen in breast carcinoma: diagnostic and prognostic implications. *Cancer* 1983;52:1257–1264.
10. Mariani-Costantini R, Andreola S, et al. Tumour-associated antigens in mammary and extramammary Paget's disease. *Virchows Arch* 1985;405:333–340.
11. Ordonez NG, Awalt H, Mackay B. Mammary and extramammary Paget's disease: an immunocytochemical and ultrastructural study. *Cancer* 1987;59:1173–1183.
12. Bussolati G, Pich A, Alfani V. Immunofluorescence detection of casein in human mammary dysplastic and neoplastic tissues. *Virchows Arch* 1975;365:15–21.

13. Vanstapel M-J, Gatter KC, DeWolf-Peeters C, et al. Immunohisto-chemical study of mammary and extra-mammary Paget's disease. *Histopathology* 1984;8:1013–1023.

14. Imam A, Yoshida SO, Taylor CR. Distinguishing tumour cells of mammary from extramammary Paget's disease using antibodies to two different glycoproteins from human milk-fat-globule membrane. *Br J Cancer* 1988;58:373–378.

15. Chaudary MA, Millis RR, Lane EB, et al. Paget's disease of the nipple: a ten-year review including clinical, pathological and immunohisto-chemical findings. *Breast Cancer Res Treat* 1986;8:139–146.

16. Kariniemi A-L, Ramaekers F, Lehto VP, et al. Paget cells express cy-tokeratins typical of glandular epithelia. *Br J Dermatol* 1985; 112:179–183.

17. Shah KD, Tabibzadeh SS, Gerber MA. Immunohistochemical distinction of Paget's diseases from Bowen's disease and superficial spreading melanoma with the use of monoclonal cytokeratin antibodies. *Am J Clin Pathol* 1987;88:689–695.

18. Tani EM, Skoog L. Immunocytochemical detection of estrogen receptors in mammary Paget cells. *Acta Cytol* 1988;23:825–828.

18a. Schelfhout VRJ, Coene ED, Delaey B, et al. Pathogenesis of Paget's disease: epidermal heregulin-alpha, motility factor, and HER receptor family. *J Natl Cancer Inst* 2000;92:622–628.

19. Ashikari R, Park K, Huvos AG, et al. Paget's disease of the breast. *Cancer* 1970;26:680–685.

20. Kister SJ, Haagensen CD. Paget's disease of the breast. *Am J Surg* 1970;119:606–609.

21. Salvadori B, Fariselli G, Saccozzi R. Analysis of 100 cases of Paget's disease of the breast. *Tumori* 1976;62:529–536.

22. Ikeda DM, Helvie MA, Frank TS, et al. Paget disease of the nipple: radiologic-pathologic correlation. *Radiology* 1993;189:89–94.

23. Stomper PC, Penetrante RB, Carson WE. Sensitivity of mammography on patients with Paget's disease of the nipple. *Breast Dis* 1995; 8:173–178.

24. Mendez-Fernandez MA, Henly WS, Geis RC, et al. Paget's disease of the breast after subcutaneous mastectomy and reconstruction with a silicone prosthesis. *Plast Reconstr Surg* 1980;65:683–685.

25. Suster S, Ronnen M, Huszar M, et al. Paget's disease of the breast with underlying carcinoma arising in systemic scleroderma. *J Dermatol Surg Oncol* 1988;14:648–650.

26. Kollmorgen DR, Varanasi JS, Edge SB, et al. Paget's disease of the breast: a 33-year experience. *J Am Coll Surg* 1998;187:171–177.

27. Gupta S, Khanna NN, Khanna S, et al. Paget's disease of the male breast: a clinicopathologic study and a collective review. *J Surg Oncol* 1983;22:151–156.

28. Heller KS, Rosen PP, Schottenfeld D, et al. Male breast cancer: a clinicopathologic study of 97 cases. *Ann Surg* 1978;188:60–65.

29. Muretto P, Polizzi V, Staccioli MP. Paget's disease in gynecomastia: immunohistochemical study of a case. *Tumori* 1988;74:183–190.

30. Moshakis V, Fordyce MJ, Griffiths JD. Klinefelter's syndrome associated with breast carcinoma and Paget's disease of the nipple. *Clin Oncol* 1983;9:257–261.

31. Sievers DB, Huvos AG, Beattie EJ Jr, et al. Paget's disease of the nipple. *Mem Hosp Clin Bull* 1973;3:141–145.

32. Rosen PP, Caicco J. Florid papillomatosis of the nipple: a study of 51 patients including nine having mammary carcinoma. *Am J Surg Pathol* 1986;10:87–101.

33. Azzopardi JG, Eusebi V. Melanocyte colonization and pigmentation of breast carcinoma. *Histopathology* 1977;1:21–30.

34. Culberson JD, Horn RC Jr. Paget's disease of the nipple: a review of 25 cases with special reference to melanin pigmentation of Paget cells. *Arch Surg* 1956;72:224–231.

35. Vielh P, Validire P, Kheirallah S, et al. Paget's disease of the nipple without clinically and radiologically detectable breast tumor: histochemical and immunohistochemical study of 44 cases. *Pathol Res Pract* 1993;189:150–155.

35a. Mai K, Yazdi HM, Perkins DG. Mammary Paget's disease: evidence of diverse origin of the disease with a subgroup of Paget's disease developing from the superficial portion of lactiferous duct and a discontinuous pattern of tumor spread. *Pathol Int* 1999;49:956–961.

36. Lagios MD, Westdahl PR, Rose MR, et al. Paget's disease of the nipple: alternative management in cases without or with minimal extent of underlying breast carcinoma. *Cancer* 1984;54:545–551.

37. Mori O, Hachisuka H, Nakano S, et al. A case of mammary Paget's disease without an underlying carcinoma: microscopic analysis of the DNA content of Paget cells. *J Dermatol* 1994;21:160–165.

38. Toker C. Clear cells in nipple epidermis. *Cancer* 1979;25:601–610.

39. Papachristou DN, Kinne DW, Rosen PP, et al. Cutaneous melanoma of the breast. *Surgery* 1979;85:322–328.

40. Sauven P, Roberts A. Basal cell carcinoma of the nipple. *J R Soc Med* 1983;76:699–701.

41. Rosen PP. Syringomatous adenoma of the nipple. *Am J Surg Pathol* 1983;7:739–745.

42. Kohler S, Rouse RV, Smoller BR. The differential diagnosis of page-toid cells in the epidermis. *Mod Pathol* 1998;11:79–92.

42a. Lloyd J, Flanagan AM. Mammary and extramammary Paget's disease. *J Clin Pathol* 2000;53:742–749.

42b. Yao D, Hoda S, Ying L, et al. Intraepidermal cytokeratin-7 immunoreactive cells in non-neoplastic nipples represent intraepithelial extension of lactiferous duct cells. *Mod Pathol* 2001;14:42A.

42c. van der Putte SCJ, Toonstra J, Hennipman A. Mammary Paget's disease confined to the areola and associated with multifocal Toker cell hyperplasia. *Am J Dermatopathol* 1995;4:678–683.

42d. Mai KT. Morphological evidence for field effect as a mechanism for tumour spread in mammary Paget's disease. *Histopathology* 1999;35: 567–576.

43. Reed W, Oppedal BR, Larsen TE. Immunohistology is valuable in distinguishing superficial spreading melanoma. *Histopathology* 1990;16: 583–588.

43a. Diaz de Leon E, Carcangiu ML, Preito VG, et al. Extramammary Paget disease is characterized by the consistent lack of estrogen and progesterone receptors but frequently expresses androgen receptor. *Am J Clin Pathol* 2000;113:572–575.

44. Wood WS, Hegedus C. Mammary Paget's disease and intraductal carcinoma: histologic, histochemical and immunocytochemical comparison. *Am J Dermatopathol* 1988;10:183–188.

45. Gillett CE, Bobrow LG, Millis RR. S-100 protein in human mammary tissue—immunoreactivity in breast carcinoma, including Paget's disease of the nipple, and value as a marker of myoepithelial cells. *J Pathol* 1990;160:19–24.

46. Jones RR, Spaull J, Gusterson B. The histogenesis of mammary and extramammary Paget's disease. *Histopathology* 1989;14:409–416.

47. Smith KJ, Tuur S, Corvette D, et al. Cytokeratin 7 staining in mammary and extramammary Paget's disease. *Mod Pathol* 1997;10:1069–1074.

48. Lundquist K, Kohler S, Rouse RV. Intraepidermal cytokeratin 7 expression is not restricted to Paget cells but is also seen in Toker cells and Merkel cells. *Am J Surg Pathol* 1999;23:212–219.

49. Mori O, Hachisuka H, Nakano S, et al. Expression of ras p21 in mammary and extramammary Paget's disease. *Arch Pathol Lab Med* 1990;114:858–861.

50. Gusterson BA, Machin LG, Gullick WJ, et al. Immunohistochemical distribution of c-erbB-2 in infiltrating and *in situ* breast cancer. *Int J Cancer* 1988;42:842–846.

51. Wolber RA, Dupuis BA, Wick MR. Expression of C-erbB-2 oncoprotein in mammary and extramammary Paget's disease. *Am J Clin Pathol* 1991;96:243–247.

52. Meissner K, Rivire A, Haupt G, et al. Study of neu-protein expression in mammary Paget's disease with and without underlying breast carcinoma and in extramammary Paget's disease. *Am J Pathol* 1990;137:1305–1309.

53. Keatings L, Sinclair J, Wright C, et al. c-erbB-2 oncoprotein expression in mammary and extramammary Paget's disease: an immunohisto-chemical study. *Histopathology* 1990;17:243–247.

54. van de Vijver MJ, Peterse JL, Mooi WJ, et al. Neu-protein overexpression in breast cancer: association with comedo-type ductal carcinoma *in situ* and limited prognostic value in Stage II breast cancer. *N Engl J Med* 1988;319:1239–1245.

55. Lucarotti ME, Dunn JM, Webb AJ. Scrape cytology in the diagnosis of Paget's disease of the breast. *Cytopathology* 1994;5:301–305.

56. Kobayashi TK, Ueda M, Nishino T, et al. Scrape cytology of *Pemphigus vulgaris* of the nipple, a mimicker of Paget's disease. *Diagn Cytopathol* 1997;16:156–159.

57. Rissanen PM, Holsti P. Paget's disease of the breast: the influence of the presence or absence of an underlying palpable tumor on the prognosis and on the choice of treatment. *Oncology* 1969;23:209–216.

58. Dixon AR, Galea MH, Ellis IO, et al. Paget's disease of the nipple. *Br J Surg* 1991;78:722–723.

59. Fourquet A, Campana F, Vielh P, et al. Paget's disease of the nipple without detectable breast tumor: conservative management with radiation therapy. *Int J Radiat Oncol Biol Phys* 1987;13:1463–1465.

60. Stockdale AD, White WF, Brierley JD, et al. Radiotherapy for Paget's disease of the nipple: a conservative alternative. *Lancet* 1989;II:664–666.

61. Blakeley S, Fornage BD, Rapini RP, et al. Ductal carcinoma after conservative management of Paget's disease of the breast: a case report. *Breast Dis* 1994;7:361–366.

62. Pierce LJ, Haffty BG, Solin LJ, et al. The conservative management of Paget's disease of the breast with radiotherapy. *Cancer* 1997;80: 1065–1072.

63. Verniers D, Van den Bogaert W, van der Schueren E, et al. Paget's disease of the male breast treated by radiotherapy. *Br J Radiol* 1991; 64:1062–1064.

64. Markopoulos C, Gazet JC. Paget's disease of the nipple occurring after conservative management of early breast cancer. *Eur J Surg Oncol* 1988;14:77–78.

65. Menzies D, Barr L, Ellis H. Paget's disease of the nipple occurring after wide local excision and radiotherapy for carcinoma of the breast. *Eur J Surg Oncol* 1989;15:271–273.

66. Plowman PN, Gilmore OJA, Curling M, et al. Paget's disease of the nipple occurring after conservation management of early infiltrating breast cancer. *Br J Surg* 1986;73:45.

67. Schnitt SJ, Connolly JL, Recht A, et al. Breast relapse following primary radiation therapy for early breast cancer. II. Detection, pathologic features and prognostic significance. *Int J Radiat Oncol Biol Phys* 1985;11:1277–1284.

# CHAPTER 33

# Lobular Carcinoma *In Situ* and Atypical Lobular Hyperplasia

## LOBULAR CARCINOMA *IN SITU*

Two papers published in 1941 established lobular carcinoma *in situ* (LCIS) as a distinct morphologic entity. Muir's description appeared in an overview of the earliest stages of mammary carcinoma (1). Lesions were subdivided according to whether carcinoma appeared to originate in ducts or lobules *(acini)*. Muir found that it may be difficult to prove origin from the lobular epithelium in some cases:

> The question is complicated by the fact that when malignant cells are present within them they may not have developed *in situ*. Intra-acinous carcinoma is often merely the result of the spread of cancer cells from terminal ducts in which the malignant process has started (1).

Among his illustrations of "intra-acinous" carcinoma are some with histologic patterns that might be regarded today as ductal in type, thus constituting a condition now recognized as extension of duct carcinoma into lobules. One picture showed the typical features of LCIS (Fig. 33.1).

Foote and Stewart introduced the term LCIS to describe "a disease of small lobular ducts and lobules" (2) (Fig. 33.2). They commented on almost all the important clinical and pathologic features of the disease including the following:

1. The inconspicuous character of LCIS, which cannot be detected by palpation or gross pathologic examination: "There is no way in which a clinical diagnosis of lobular carcinoma *in situ* can be made. . . . There is no way by which it can be recognized grossly."
2. Multicentricity: "This lesion occurs in multiple lobules. . . . It is always a disease of multiple foci."
3. Origin from the terminal duct–lobular complex or from terminal ducts.
4. Pagetoid extension in ducts and the rarity of true Paget's disease: "Isolated cells or groups of cells . . . in the terminal lobular duct . . . recall certain features of Paget's disease and we have designated them Pagetoid cells. The

clinical entity, Paget's disease, has not been encountered in this group of cases."
5. Signet-ring cells as a feature of LCIS: "the formation of central mucoid globules."
6. Association with a distinctive type of infiltrating carcinoma: "When the tumor infiltrates, it is apt to do so in a peculiar fashion which permits one, after some experience, to recognize the high probability of such origin."
7. Coexistence of LCIS with other patterns of carcinoma, including association with ordinary duct carcinoma and tubular carcinoma.
8. The tendency of infiltrating lobular carcinoma to grow around ducts and lobules, sometimes described as a *targetoid growth pattern.*
9. The desmoplastic stromal reaction in infiltrating lobular carcinoma.

Because LCIS is a microscopic lesion that does not form a palpable tumor, the incidence of the disease is unknown. When it occurs alone in patients in whom a biopsy is performed, LCIS constitutes 1% to 6% of mammary carcinomas and 30% to 50% of noninvasive carcinomas (3,4). In retrospective reviews, each involving several thousand "benign" breast specimens, the frequency of LCIS was 1.5% (5), 1.4% (6), 0.6% (7), and 0.5% (8). A review of nearly 10,000 breast biopsies without other neoplastic lesions performed from 1960 through 1979 revealed that the annual frequency of LCIS or lobular neoplasia ranged from 1.2% to 4.3%, averaging 2.7% (9).

An autopsy study of breasts from 83 elderly hospitalized women revealed LCIS in three of these women, or 3.6% (10). This relatively small series, which included six women previously known to have breast carcinoma, cannot be regarded as generally representative. Nielsen et al. examined breasts from young women, many of whom died unexpectedly, including only one with previously diagnosed breast carcinoma, and they found LCIS in 4 of 110 (3.6%) cases (11). Three other autopsy studies, comprising a total of

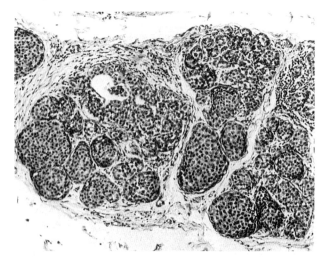

**FIG. 33.1.** *Lobular carcinoma* in situ. A photograph of a intra-acinous carcinoma published by Muir in 1941. (From Muir R. The evolution of carcinoma of the mamma. *J Pathol Bacteriol* 1941;52:155–172, with permission.)

more than 300 women, failed to detect any examples of LCIS (12–14).

## Clinical Presentation

Typically, LCIS is discovered coincidentally in breast tissue removed for proliferative lesions that cause a mass or in apparently normal tissue surrounding a benign tumor such as a fibroadenoma. Mammography has not been an effective method for detecting LCIS in most cases and cannot be depended on to assess the multicentricity or bilaterality of the disease (15,16). Only 4 of 50 patients with LCIS described in a report on the Breast Cancer Diagnosis Demonstration Pro-

jects had calcifications in LCIS seen on pathology examination (17). Benign processes are usually the site of mammographic abnormalities that lead to a biopsy in which LCIS is detected. Calcifications are infrequently formed in LCIS, but they occur commonly in coexisting lesions such as sclerosing adenosis, columnar cell hyperplasia (18), atrophic lobules and ducts (19–21), and collagenous spherulosis. The calcifications tend to be poorly defined with low density in mammograms (19). An exceptional situation exists in infrequent instances of florid LCIS, which can cause marked expansion of ducts and lobules. This condition is often extensive, sometimes partially involving sclerosing adenosis. Necrosis and calcification occur in such LCIS with a pattern and distribution more commonly encountered in intraductal carcinoma. The resultant appearance on mammography is likely to be interpreted as suggesting intraductal carcinoma (21a). The histologic diagnosis of these lesions is sometimes controversial. As discussed later in this chapter, the most compelling evidence supporting classification of these cases as LCIS is that they have the cytologic appearance typical of LCIS, the presence of coexistent classic LCIS in virtually all cases, association with invasive lobular carcinoma of the classic type, and absence of E-cadherin immunoreactivity (see figures in front of book).

Haagensen and colleagues (22,23) reported that LCIS is largely a disease of premenopausal women and speculated that spontaneous regression of LCIS occurred during the menopause. Later, Haagensen et al. (9,24) noted that 10% to 12% of LCIS patients were postmenopausal, and Gump urged caution in concluding that LCIS regresses after the menopause (25). Rosen et al. reported that up to 25% of LCIS patients are postmenopausal (26).

The relationship of LCIS to exogenous estrogens was studied in a consecutive series of 59 patients with LCIS and 190 controls treated consecutively for duct carcinoma (26).

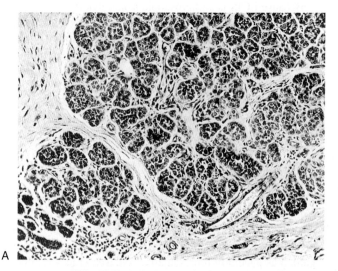

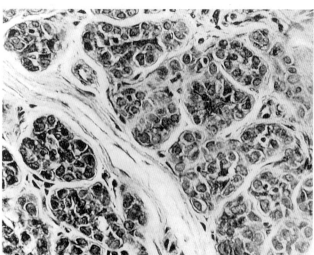

A                                                                              B

**FIG. 33.2.** *Lobular carcinoma* in situ. **A:** The lesion depicted by Foote and Stewart in 1941. Part of the lobule in the *lower left corner* is not involved by carcinoma. **B:** A magnified view of the lesion in **A** demonstrating a homogeneous population of carcinoma cells with some loss of cohesion. (From Foote FW Jr, Stewart FW. Lobular carcinoma *in situ:* a rare form of mammary cancer. *Am J Pathol* 1941;17:491–496, with permission.)

Exogenous estrogen use was reported by 29% of LCIS patients and 35% of women with duct carcinoma. Most exogenous estrogen use occurred more than 1 year before diagnosis. Among the older women with LCIS only in the series, five had been postmenopausal for 11 to 29 years. Only one of these five women had used exogenous hormones. Documented use of exogenous hormones was slightly more frequent in postmenopausal patients with duct carcinoma than it was among those with LCIS. These data confirmed prior studies indicating that LCIS occurred in postmenopausal women and that the presence of LCIS was not related to exogenous estrogenic hormones in most women found to have this lesion after the menopause (27–29).

The age distribution of LCIS is similar to that of most other forms of mammary carcinoma. It occurs infrequently as an isolated lesion in women younger than 35 years or older than 75 years of age. LCIS arising in bilateral mammary "hypertrophy" was reported in a 15-year-old girl (30). In different studies, the average age at diagnosis of LCIS ranged from 44 to 54 years. In a consecutive series of more than 1,000 patients treated for breast carcinoma, the mean age of women with LCIS (53 years) was younger but not significantly different from the mean age of patients who had infiltrating duct carcinoma (57 years) (31).

Documentation of bilaterality in many reported series is uncertain because few surgeons have routinely performed biopsies on the contralateral breast or performed bilateral mastectomy for this disease. Involvement of both breasts by LCIS was described in 1959 by Barnes, who documented two patients treated by bilateral mastectomy (32). Newman found that 6 of 26 patients (23%) with LCIS had bilateral disease (33). Bilaterality among 18 women who actually had a contralateral biopsy was 33%. In 1965, Benfield et al. reported that two of five women with LCIS who underwent a subsequent contralateral biopsy had LCIS in the opposite breast (34). Lewison and Finney found bilateral disease in 7 of 15 women (46%) who had tissue from both breasts examined (28), and bilateral LCIS was found in 25 of 84 LCIS patients (30%) with specimens from both breasts studied by Haagensen (9).

Urban systematically performed contralateral biopsies for all types of breast carcinoma and reported finding concurrent contralateral LCIS in 9 of 22 biopsied patients (40%) (35). In addition, one woman had concurrent contralateral invasive carcinoma. Thus, 45% of patients with an opposite breast available for biopsy were found to have contralateral carcinoma. Among nine patients with LCIS studied by Donegan and Perez-Mesa, two had been treated previously for contralateral carcinoma (36). *In situ* carcinoma was found in the opposite breast of three of the other seven patients (43%). Subsequently, Erdreich et al. reported bilaterality in 12 of 31 women (39%) who had LCIS in one breast, but they did not specify the histologic type of contralateral disease (37).

Ringberg et al. studied 73 contralateral subcutaneous mastectomy specimens obtained from patients with unilateral carcinoma (38). Forty-three of the patients had ipsilateral intraepithelial carcinoma, including 16 with LCIS. Contralateral LCIS was found in 11 of the 16 (69%), intraductal carcinoma in three (19%), and invasive carcinoma in one case (6%). There were also four women whose initial diagnosis had been intraductal carcinoma plus LCIS. Three had LCIS in the contralateral breast. Sunshine et al. reported that 21 of 36 (67%) women with LCIS treated by bilateral mastectomy had LCIS in their opposite breast (39).

Data on bilaterality in LCIS are presented in Table 33.1. The 59 women with LCIS represent 4.5% of patients with breast carcinoma treated from mid-1976 to early 1979. Coincidental contralateral pathologic breast status was known for 43 patients (73%), a proportion substantially greater than for women with intraductal carcinoma. This difference reflects the tendency at the time to perform contralateral biopsies more often in patients with LCIS. Among the 43 women with LCIS for whom the status of the opposite breast was known, the distribution of contralateral findings was as follows: benign, 18 of 43 (42%); previous contralateral carcinoma treated by mastectomy, 9 of 43 (21%); and concurrent contralateral carcinoma, 16 of 43 (37%). Concurrent biopsy of the opposite breast was performed in the 34 women with an intact contralateral breast, revealing carcinoma in 16 (47%).

**TABLE 33.1.** *Bilaterality in patients with* in situ *carcinoma[a]*

| Primary diagnosis in one breast[d] | Status of opposite breast[b] | | | | | | | | | |
|---|---|---|---|---|---|---|---|---|---|---|
| | Benign | | Carcinoma[c] | | | | No biopsy | | Total cases | |
| | | | Prior | | Concurrent | | | | | |
| | No. of patients | % | No. of patients | % | No. of patients | % | No. of patients | % | No. of patients | % |
| Intraductal | 25 | 39 | 5 | 8 | 4 | 6 | 30 | 47 | 64 | 52 |
| LCIS | 18 | 31 | 9 | 15 | 16 | 27 | 16 | 27 | 59 | 48 |
| Total | 43 | 35 | 14 | 11 | 20 | 16 | 46 | 37 | 123 | |

LCIS, lobular carcinoma *in situ*.
[a] *p* <0.004 for the entire table. *p* <0.02 when cases not biopsied were excluded.
[b] Status of opposite breast determined by biopsy or mastectomy.
[c] Includes LCIS.
[d] Primary diagnosis based on pathologic examination of a mastectomy specimen.

**TABLE 33.2.** *Frequency of bilaterality associated with selected histologic types of invasive breast carcinoma*

| Histologic type of tumor[a] | Bilaterality | | | | | |
| --- | --- | --- | --- | --- | --- | --- |
| | Yes | | No | | Total | |
| | No. of patients | % | No. of patients | % | No. of patients | % |
| Infiltrating duct | 82 | 22 | 285 | 78 | 367 | 72 |
| Infiltrating duct and LCIS | 30 | 57 | 23 | 43 | 53 | 10 |
| Infiltrating lobular | 12 | 28 | 31 | 72 | 43 | 8 |
| Medullary | 3 | 12 | 23 | 88 | 26 | 5 |
| Atypical medullary | 2 | 10 | 19 | 90 | 21 | 4 |
| Total | 129 | 25 | 381 | 75 | 510[b] | |

LCIS, lobular carcinoma *in situ.*

[a] Based on 880 women treated for invasive carcinoma of one breast (40). The tumor type listed describes the dominant (ipsilateral) lesion. If bilateral carcinomas were simultaneously detected, criteria to assign one lesion as ipsilateral were as follows: (1) With bilateral invasive carcinoma, the larger tumor was considered ipsilateral; (2) With invasive disease in one breast and contralateral *in situ*, the breast with invasion was considered ipsilateral.

[b] The 510 patients shown in this table were all women with one of the five histologic types of ipsilateral tumor listed. All had a confirmed contralateral biopsy or mastectomy. Contralateral diagnoses subsequent to treatment of the ipsilateral tumor are not included.

The foregoing data on bilaterality of LCIS provide compelling evidence that both breasts frequently are affected by the disease, often at the same time, but it has not been shown that all women with LCIS always have bilateral disease. When the ipsilateral breast contains only LCIS, contralateral LCIS will be found in approximately 40% of breasts on which biopsies have been performed. When contralateral mastectomy has been performed, bilateral LCIS can be demonstrated in two-thirds of patients. It seems likely that some women with LCIS do not have simultaneous bilaterality and may never have both breasts affected by LCIS or any other form of mammary carcinoma.

The finding of LCIS coexisting with invasive carcinoma also implies a substantial risk of bilaterality. Data shown in Table 33.2 are drawn from a study of the relationship of bilaterality and multicentricity (40). An infiltrating duct carcinoma was found in 420 patients, including 53 (13%) who had coexistent LCIS in the same breast. Bilaterality was found in 57% of women with both lesions, in 22% with infiltrating duct carcinoma alone, and in 28% with infiltrating

lobular carcinoma (p<0.01). Because coexistent LCIS usually was not detected in a frozen section at the time of operation for the ipsilateral carcinoma, this was not a factor in the selection of patients for contralateral biopsy. Medullary carcinoma and carcinomas with medullary features were rarely associated with bilaterality.

Table 33.3 summarizes the relationship between the histologic type of carcinoma in the ipsilateral and contralateral breast. Lobular carcinoma, most often *in situ*, was more likely to be found in the contralateral breast when the ipsilateral breast also had lobular carcinoma.

Multicentricity and bilaterality are interrelated characteristics of mammary carcinoma. Types of carcinoma associated with a high frequency of bilaterality are also more likely to occur as multicentric foci in the affected breast. The reported frequency of multicentricity is influenced by sampling techniques, but virtually all investigators have reached the same conclusion about LCIS as that reached by Foote and Stewart, that "this lesion occurs in multiple lobules" (2). Multicentric foci of carcinoma have been found in 60% to 85% of patients undergoing mastectomy for LCIS

**TABLE 33.3.** *Relationship between ipsilateral tumor type and type of carcinoma in the contralateral breast[a]*

| Type of invasive ipsilateral carcinoma | Contralateral breast | | | | | |
| --- | --- | --- | --- | --- | --- | --- |
| | Ductal | | Lobular | | Total | |
| | No. of Patients | % | No. of Patients | % | No. of Patients | % |
| Infiltrating duct | 58 | 81 | 14 | 19 | 72 | 62 |
| Infiltrating duct and LCIS | 10 | 37 | 17 | 63 | 27 | 23 |
| Infiltrating lobular | 2 | 17 | 10 | 83 | 12 | 10 |
| Medullary and atypical medullary | 4 | 80 | 1 | 20 | 5 | 4 |
| Total | 74 | 64 | 42 | 36 | 116 | |

LCIS, lobular carcinoma *in situ.*

[a] p < 0.001 (Fisher exact test) for infiltrating duct vs. infiltrating duct and LCIS vs. infiltrating lobular.

Based on Lesser ML, Rosen PP, Kinne DW. Multicentricity and bilaterality in invasive breast carcinoma. *Surgery* 1982;91:234–240, with permission.

**TABLE 33.4.** *Findings at mastectomy after biopsy diagnosis of lobular carcinoma* in situ

| | | | Mastectomy findings | | | | | |
| | | | Carcinoma | | | | No carcinoma | |
| | | | Intraepithelial | | Invasive | | | |
| Biopsy diagnosis | | No. of pts | No. of pts | % | No. of pts | % | No. of pts | % |
|---|---|---|---|---|---|---|---|---|
| Rosen et al. (93) | LCIS | 50 | 30 | 60 | 2 | 4 | 18 | 36 |
| Carter and Smith (45) | LCIS | 49 | 31 | 63 | 3 | 6 | 15 | 31 |
| Shah et al. (44) | LCIS | 40 | 26 | 65 | 2 | 5 | 12 | 30 |

LCIS, lobular carcinoma *in situ.*

(26,28,41–43). Benfield et al. noted that residual carcinoma was present in 39 of 44 mastectomies (89%) for LCIS described in the literature before 1965 (34). A retrospective review of mastectomy specimens by Shah et al. revealed that 26 of 40 breasts (65%) removed for LCIS had multicentric *in situ* carcinoma that was LCIS in 93% and intraductal in 7% (44). Carter and Smith found *in situ* carcinoma in 31 of 49 mastectomies (63%) performed for LCIS (45). Occult, clinically unsuspected invasive carcinoma has been detected in 4% to 6% of breasts removed after a biopsy showed only LCIS (26,44,45) (Table 33.4). Invasive carcinoma was present in 4 of 38 mastectomy and mammoplasty specimens (11%) obtained 2 years after a biopsy diagnosis of LCIS, and intraductal carcinoma was found in a fifth specimen (46).

### Gross Pathology

By itself, LCIS does not result in a grossly apparent pathologic alteration in breast tissue, but the tissue that harbors LCIS often appears abnormal as a result of coexisting proliferative changes. The gross description often records nodular lesions, such as fibroadenomas, areas of firm or hard tissue, or cysts. None of these visible or palpable abnormalities is attributable to LCIS. In patients with florid and extensive LCIS, the cut surface of the breast tissue may have a faintly granular appearance when viewed with tangential light because the affected lobules are sufficiently enlarged to be visible.

### Microscopic Pathology

The microscopic anatomic distribution of LCIS in lobules and terminal ducts and alterations in the morphology of these structures influence the histopathologic appearance of LCIS in any given case. Foote and Stewart observed that LCIS arises from the terminal ducts in the postmenopausal atrophic breast, whereas in premenopausal women, LCIS is distributed in the terminal duct–lobular complex (2).

In the typical lobular form, a population of neoplastic cells replaces the normal epithelium of acini and intralobular ductules (Fig. 33.3). The abnormal cells may be sufficiently numerous to cause expansion of these structures as well as enlargement of the entire lobule compared with uninvolved lobules in the adjacent breast (Figs. 33.4 and 33.5). Lobular

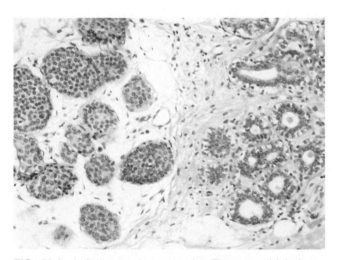

**FIG. 33.3.** *Lobular carcinoma* in situ. The normal lobule on the *right* is about the same size as the lobule on the left with *in situ* carcinoma. Neoplastic cells fill the lobular glands, which are larger than uninvolved glands on the *right.*

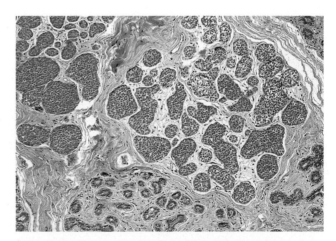

**FIG. 33.4.** *Lobular carcinoma* in situ (LCIS), *glandular distension.* The enlarged lobular glands have filled most of the intralobular stroma. Note the variable size of glands with LCIS and the uninvolved lobule below.

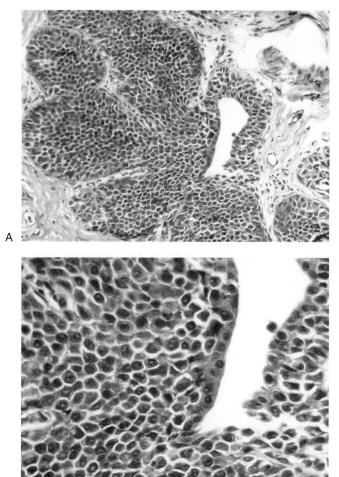

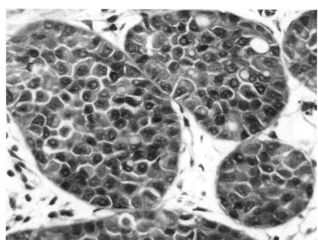

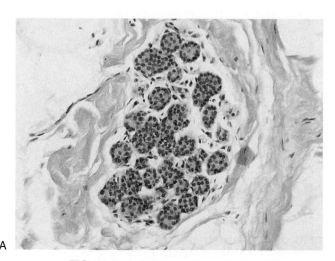

**FIG. 33.5.** *Lobular carcinoma* in situ, *marked glandular distension.* **A:** Carcinoma involves the lobular glands and a terminal duct. **B:** Carcinoma in lobular glands with loss of cohesion. Some cells have intracytoplasmic lumens. **C:** Carcinoma in the duct beneath persisting benign duct epithelium. Loss of cohesion is evident.

enlargement is not, however, an absolute diagnostic criterion (Fig. 33.6). Foote and Stewart found that "large lobules, small lobules . . . and hyalinized lobules may all assume this pattern. Occasionally, only part of a lobule is involved and a sharp line of division between normal epithelium and carcinoma *in situ* is seen . . . distension of the lobule does not as-

sume marked proportions prior to infiltration. . ." (2) (Figs. 33.7 and 33.8). Myoepithelial cells may persist in LCIS, especially when there is relatively little glandular enlargement (Fig. 33.7).

There is no universal yardstick that permits accurate evaluation of what constitutes lobular distension. Comparison of

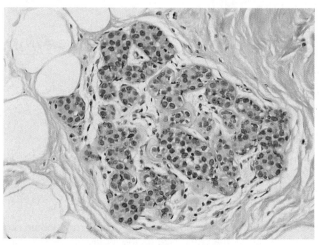

**FIG. 33.6.** *Lobular carcinoma* in situ *without glandular distension.* **A,B:** Two examples of *in situ* carcinoma in which the lobular glands are not enlarged. *(continued)*

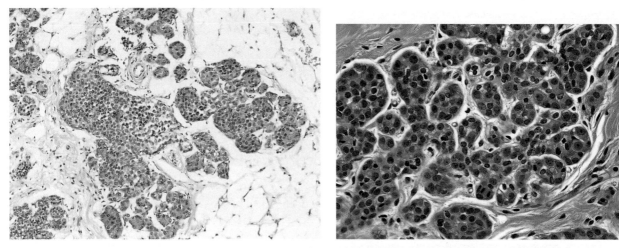

**FIG. 33.6.** *Continued.* **C,D:** *In situ* carcinoma fills the terminal duct and adjacent lobular glands.

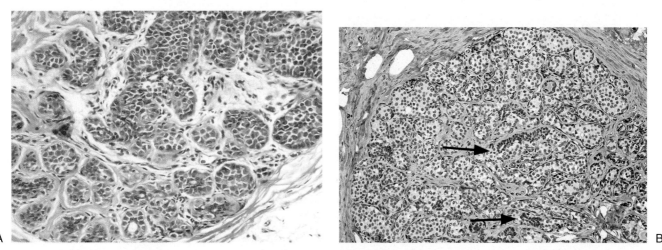

**FIG. 33.7.** *Lobular carcinoma* in situ. **A:** *In situ* carcinoma involves lobular glands on the *right* but spares the glands in the *lower left corner*. This image from a contemporary case is quite similar to the one published by Foote and Stewart, shown in Fig. 33.2. **B:** The immunostain for smooth-muscle myosin heavy chain highlights inconspicuous, attenuated myoepithelial cells in this lesion. Clusters of dark cells are residual nonneoplastic lobular epithelium *(arrows)* (avidin-biotin).

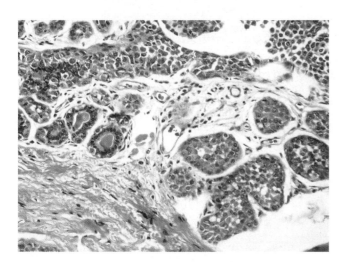

**FIG. 33.8.** *Lobular carcinoma* in situ, *partial lobular involvement.* Carcinoma involves lobular glands on the *right* and an intralobular ductule *above*. Pagetoid spread is seen in lobular glands on the *left*.

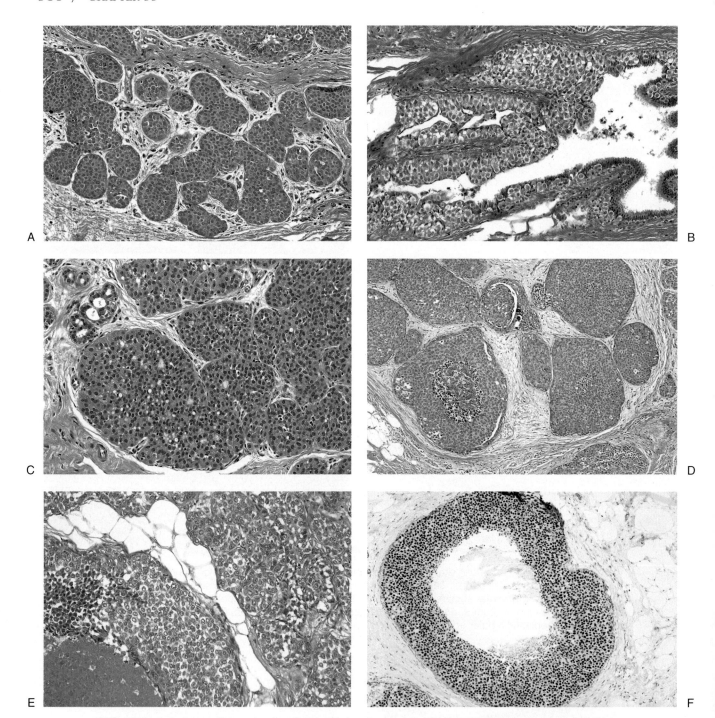

**FIG. 33.9.** *Lobular carcinoma* in situ, *florid with focal necrosis.* All images are from a single specimen. **A:** Well-developed lobular carcinoma *in situ* (LCIS). **B:** Pagetoid spread of LCIS. **C:** Enlargement of lobular glands. **D:** Florid enlargement of lobular glands with focal necrosis and small calcifications *(upper center).* Note the persistence of lobular stroma around the *in situ* carcinoma. **E:** Magnified view showing identical cells in a lobule *(right)* and a duct with necrosis. **F:** Surviving epithelium around the necrotic center in a duct shows strong nuclear immunoreactivity for estrogen receptor. *(continued)*

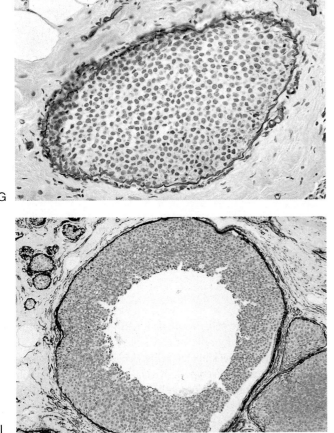

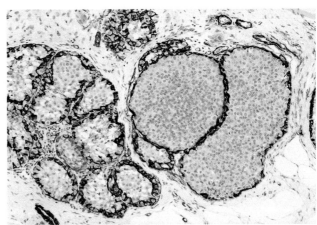

**FIG. 33.9.** *Continued.* **G:** The intact basement membrane of a duct demonstrated with the immunostain for laminin. **H:** Preserved myoepithelial cells are highlighted in a lobule comparable to **C** by the immunostain for smooth-muscle myosin heavy chain. **I:** Myoepithelial cells are highlighted by the smooth muscle actin immunostain. The duct is expanded by lobular carcinoma *in situ* with necrosis (all immunostains avidin-biotin).

adjacent involved and uninvolved lobules in a given case is a recommended approach, but in practice it becomes readily apparent that lobular diameters vary considerably within a given breast and from case to case. In one study, there was a slight, but not statistically significant, trend for a greater risk of subsequent carcinoma when distension was minimal (6). Others found a slight increase in the risk of subsequent carcinoma in patients with maximal distention but did not regard the difference as significant (9). If the diagnosis of LCIS is to be meaningful because it identifies a lesion associated with a substantial risk of later carcinoma, then lobular distension cannot be regarded as an important diagnostic criterion in lesions that have reached an acceptable qualitative level of cytologic abnormality. An important exception to this circumstance is florid LCIS, in which extreme ductal and lobular enlargement occurs, often with necrosis and calcification (Fig. 33.9). These cases should be examined carefully for evidence of microinvasion, which can be obscured by the stromal reaction. Absence of E-cadherin reactivity distinguishes florid LCIS in ducts from intraductal carcinoma of the small cell type (see figures in front of book).

Quantitative factors have been included by some investigators among the diagnostic criteria for LCIS. The question of how much lobular involvement is necessary for the diagnosis of LCIS as a marker of risk remains unanswered. Some

researchers required a finding of at least two lobules exhibiting diagnostic features (47). Others concluded that one fully affected lobule was sufficient evidence for the diagnosis (6,24). The latter position was based on the observation that the number of affected lobules in a biopsy did not prove to be related to the risk of subsequent carcinoma among patients not treated by mastectomy (6). In particular, there was no significant difference in risk between patients with one or with two affected lobules. This finding was not unexpected because a sampling error may misrepresent the extent of LCIS. As a consequence, there appears to be no logical reason for drawing a distinction between one and two involved lobules as the basis for a diagnosis of LCIS.

Partial involvement of one or more lobules is not an uncommon finding in a patient whose biopsy also contains many completely affected lobules. Glandular lumens persist in unaffected portions of a partially involved lobule, or the lumen may remain when glandular cells have been displaced but not destroyed as a consequence of pagetoid spread of LCIS cells within a lobule (Figs. 33.7 and 33.8). In some biopsies, the only evidence of a neoplastic lobular proliferation is one lobule in which some, but not all, of the acini are involved. The significance of such minimal evidence has not been determined. It has been suggested arbitrarily that at least 50% (48) or 75% (4) of one lobule in a biopsy be

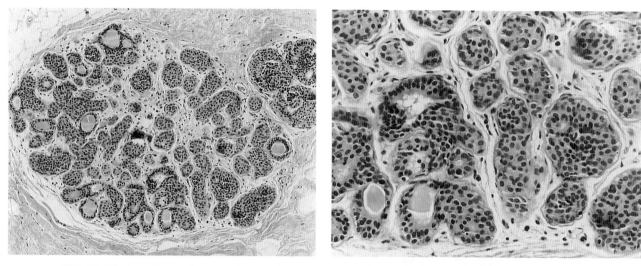

**FIG. 33.10.** *Lobular carcinoma* in situ, *partial lobular involvement.* **A,B:** *In situ* carcinoma involves about 80% of the lobular glands. A calcification is present in the center of the lobule on the *left.*

involved to establish a diagnosis of LCIS and that specimens with lesser lesions be included in the category of atypical lobular hyperplasia.

A complete absence of spaces or lumens is not necessary for a diagnosis of LCIS (Fig. 33.10). Loss of cohesion is a characteristic of neoplastic cells in LCIS, although this is not always readily apparent in acini filled and expanded by the process. When loss of cohesion is prominent and the neoplastic cells have a dissociated distribution, spaces may be created between them that can be mistaken for glandular lumens. Degenerative changes also may disrupt the cellular composition of LCIS (Fig. 33.11). In these situations, the neoplastic cells are not arranged in the polarized fashion that characterizes nonneoplastic cells persisting around true glandular lumens.

The neoplastic cells in classical LCIS have been described as having scant cytoplasm and small, round, cytologically bland nuclei that lack nucleoli (Fig. 33.12). This cytologic pattern was referred to as type A by Haagensen et al. (24). In some instances, cytologic pleomorphism may be encountered, and the more varied cells have been classified as type B or pleomorphic LCIS (6,24) (Fig. 33.13). Type A cells tend to have a diploid DNA content, whereas type B cells are largely hyperdiploid (49). Type B cells have more abundant cytoplasm than cells classified as type A and larger more pleomorphic nuclei that sometimes have nucleoli. Some examples of LCIS have both cell types (Fig. 33.14) (see figures in front of book).

The presence of intracytoplasmic mucin secretion favors a diagnosis of LCIS. Intracytoplasmic mucinous secretion is frequently present in at least some cells in LCIS (50,51).

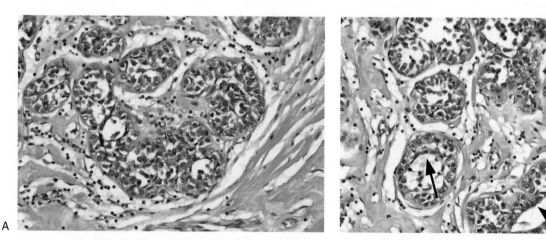

**FIG. 33.11.** *Lobular carcinoma* in situ. **A:** Spaces created among carcinoma cells shown here due to loss of cohesion should not be mistaken for glandular lumens. **B:** Flattened residual epithelial cells encircle persisting true lumens in glands involved by pagetoid *in situ* carcinoma *(arrows).* Spaces in some glands *(upper left)* are the result of cellular discohesion.

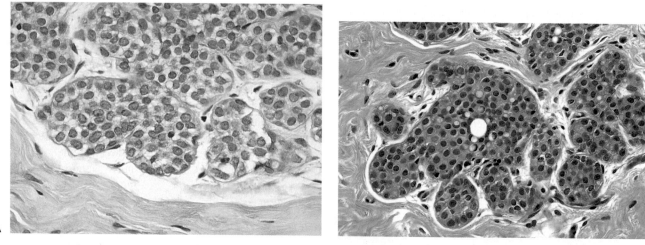

**FIG. 33.12.** *Lobular carcinoma* in situ, *small cell classic type.* **A:** Classic *in situ* lobular carcinoma. **B:** Classic *in situ* lobular carcinoma with signet-ring cells.

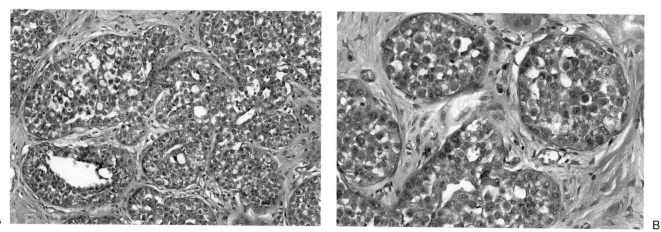

**FIG. 33.13.** *Lobular carcinoma* in situ, large cell pleomorphic type. **A,B:** The tumor cells display discohesive growth. Pleomorphic nuclei have nucleoli.

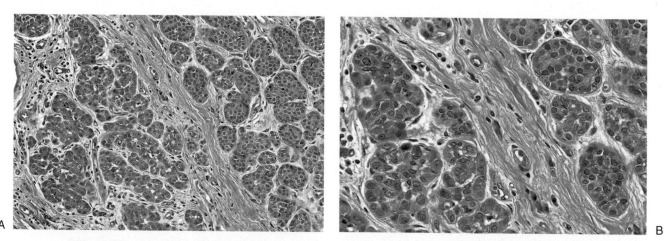

**FIG. 33.14.** *Lobular carcinoma* in situ, *classic and pleomorphic types.* **A,B:** Classic *(right)* and pleomorphic *(left)* types are present in this biopsy.

Mucin is often an inconspicuous feature that must be demonstrated and highlighted with a stain such as mucicarmine or Alcian blue–periodic acid-Schiff (PAS) (51) (Fig. 33.15). The mucin may be present diffusely in the cytoplasm, but more often it is limited to vacuoles that contain condensed globules of secretion, resulting in a targetoid appearance. An extreme manifestation of this phenomenon is the formation of signet-ring cells in which a distended cytoplasmic vacuole causes the nucleus to be eccentric and compressed into a crescentic shape (52) (Figs. 33.16 and 33.17). The signet-ring cells in LCIS and infiltrating lobular carcinoma are sim-

ilar cytologically (Fig. 33.18). Degenerative changes in the cytoplasm of LCIS cells and in the epithelium of hyperplastic lobules may produce cytoplasmic defects that resemble vacuoles, but intracytoplasmic mucin is not detectable in these cells (Figs. 33.11 and 33.13). Intracytoplasmic mucin is not demonstrable in the epithelial cells of a normal lobule, but it may be present in the glandular lumen (Fig. 33.19). It is important to distinguish between mucin in true intracytoplasmic vacuoles and mucin demonstrated in small pockets of the lobular lumen, which reside between epithelial cells in hyperplastic lobules. Casein and other secretory products,

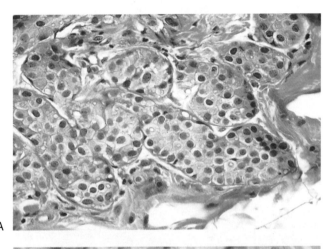

A

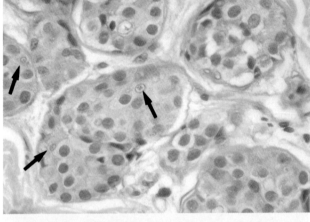

B

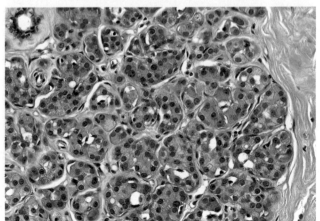

C

**FIG. 33.15.** *Lobular carcinoma* in situ, *intracytoplasmic mucin.* **A:** Punctate cytoplasmic vacuoles are evident in this lesion. **B:** The mucicarmine stain demonstrates mucin (*arrows*). **C:** Intracytoplasmic mucin stains blue with the Alcian blue reaction. **D:** Signet-ring cells in florid lobular carcinoma *in situ* with necrosis. **E:** Basophilia is evidence of diffuse cytoplasmic mucin in this example of *in situ* lobular carcinoma.

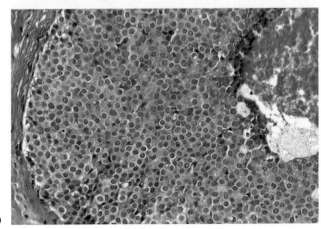

D

E

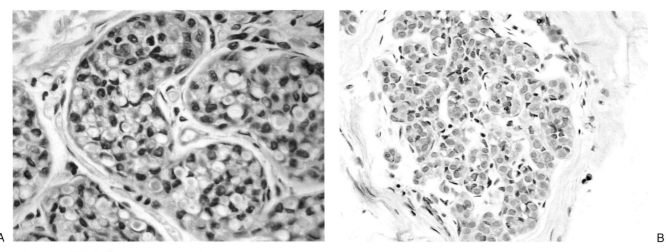

A                         B

**FIG. 33.16.** *Lobular carcinoma* in situ, *signet-ring cells.* **A:** Large cytoplasmic vacuoles and eccentric nuclei characterize signet-ring cells. **B:** Mucin is highlighted by the mucicarmine stain.

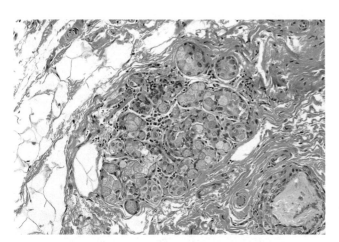

**FIG. 33.17.** *Lobular carcinoma* in situ, *signet-ring cells.* An example of extreme signet-ring cell formation is shown.

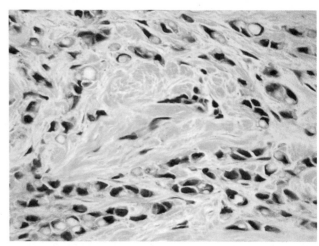

**FIG. 33.18.** *Invasive lobular carcinoma with signet-ring cells.* This specimen is from the patient shown in Fig. 33.16.

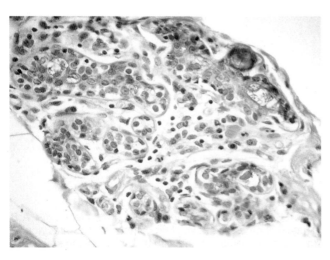

**FIG. 33.19.** *Normal lobule, mucicarmine stain.* Mucin in the glandular lumens is stained. There is no intracytoplasmic mucin.

such as carcinoembryonic antigen, are also concentrated in the lobular secretion (53). Because intracytoplasmic mucin vacuoles are uncommon in the cells of ductal carcinoma and are virtually absent in hyperplastic lesions of duct or lobular epithelium, their presence is an important, but not a necessary, criterion for the diagnosis of LCIS (50–52).

A diagnosis of LCIS may be suspected in a fine needle aspiration specimen if signet-ring cells are identified associated with detached fragments of lobular epithelium (so-called lobular casts) but the samples are usually so sparsely cellular that a positive diagnosis is not always possible (54).

Several uncommon cytologic features also may be found in LCIS. Cytoplasmic pallor or clear cell change, more often encountered in nonneoplastic, hyperplastic lobules, occurs rarely in LCIS (55). Clear cell LCIS is composed of cells with abundant intracytoplasmic mucin (Fig. 33.20). Apocrine metaplasia has been described in LCIS (56). Mucin within LCIS cells that have undergone apocrine change is usually evident as cytoplasmic amphophilia or basophilia (Fig. 33.17). Another cytologic appearance seen largely in atrophic lobules and terminal ducts of postmenopausal women features cells with dark eosinophilic to basophilic cytoplasm and deeply basophilic eccentric nuclei. This appearance is probably the result of cytoplasmic condensation associated with loss of co-

hesion and shrinkage of cells. These cells resemble rhabdomyoblasts and have been referred to as the *myoid form* of LCIS (Fig. 33.21). Similar cells are found in the corresponding infiltrating lobular carcinoma, which may be of the pleomorphic variety (Fig. 33.22). Myoid lobular carcinoma cells frequently have intracytoplasmic mucin. In another variant, the cells of LCIS have a mosaic or "fried egg" appearance that results from the presence of distinct cell borders between the cells and prominent, round, centrally placed nuclei surrounded by pale cytoplasm (Fig. 33.23). Intracytoplasmic mucin vacuoles usually can be found in this type of lobular carcinoma. Weak E-cadherin activity can be found outlining the cells of the mosaic type of LCIS. This observation is consistent with the cohesive appearance of these lesions.

Typically, LCIS involves intralobular and extralobular or terminal ductules as well as acinar units within the lobule. Extralobular LCIS involving the epithelium of ducts and ductules occurs in 65% to 75% of patients (9,56–58) (Fig. 33.24). In postmenopausal patients with atrophic lobules, duct involvement may be the only manifestation of LCIS (9,23) (Fig. 33.25). Haagensen reported that the lobular phase, alone or in combination with ductal LCIS, was found in 95% of premenopausal and 53% of postmenopausal women (9). Quantitatively, there was no significant differ-

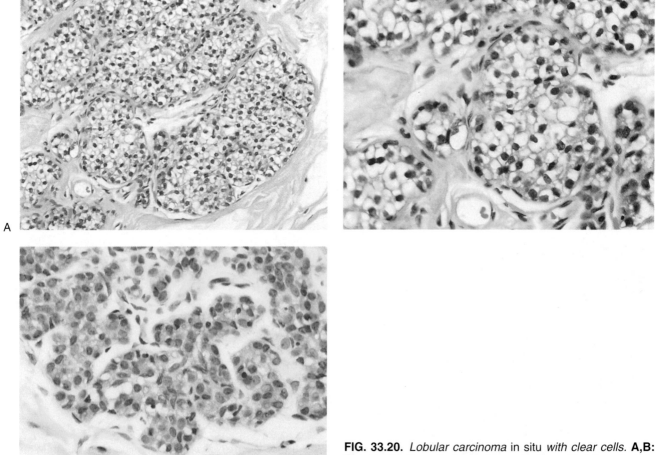

**FIG. 33.20.** *Lobular carcinoma* in situ *with clear cells.* **A,B:** The carcinoma cells have clear cytoplasm. **C:** Intracytoplasmic mucin is demonstrated with the mucicarmine stain.

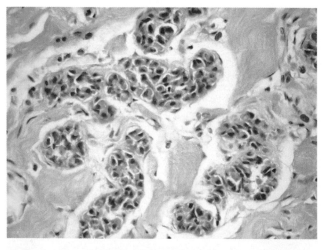

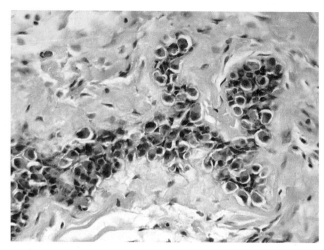

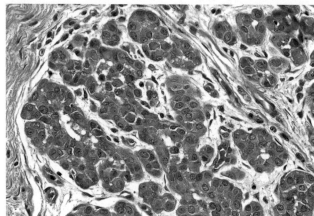

**FIG. 33.21.** *Lobular carcinoma* in situ *with myoid pleomorphic cells.* **A,B:** The carcinoma cells have deeply stained, dense cytoplasm and irregular contours. Loss of cohesion is conspicuous. **C:** Another example of myoid lobular carcinoma *in situ* composed of pleomorphic carcinoma cells.

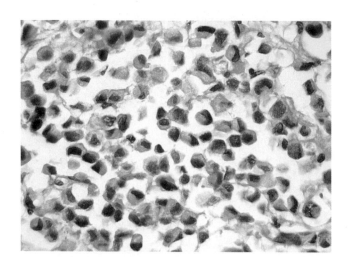

**FIG. 33.22.** *Invasive lobular carcinoma with myoid cells.* Many cells have eccentric nuclei. It is usually possible to demonstrate intracytoplasmic mucin in such cells.

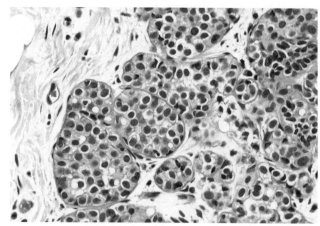

**FIG. 33.23.** *Lobular carcinoma* in situ, *mosaic type.* The cells have distinct cell borders and central nuclei. A few signet-ring cells are present.

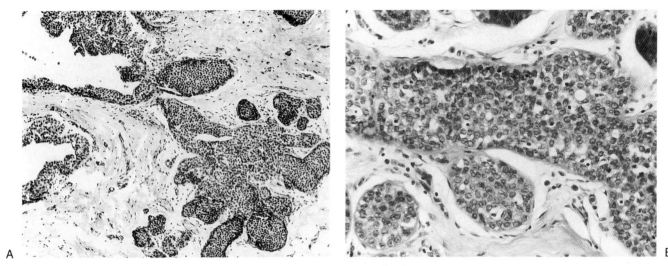

**FIG. 33.24.** *Lobular carcinoma* in situ *with duct extension.* **A:** *In situ* carcinoma involving extralobular duct. **B:** *In situ* carcinoma in an intralobular ductule.

ence between premenopausal and postmenopausal women with respect to the average amount of duct or lobular LCIS. Page found no striking age difference between patients who did or did not have ductal involvement by LCIS (59).

The irregular configuration of some ductules affected by LCIS has been described as saw-toothed or as resembling a cloverleaf. Clusters of LCIS cells beneath the nonneoplastic ductal epithelium form buds around the periphery of the duct protruding outward (Fig. 33.26). The neoplastic cells are distributed continuously or discontinuously along the ductal system, undermining and ultimately displacing the normal ductal epithelium. When this occurs, the normal glandular epithelium sometimes persists, having been elevated and pushed toward the lumen (Fig. 33.27). The myoepithelial layer is preserved to a variable extent, and it may require an immunostain for actin to confirm that it is present. In some instances, iso-

lated LCIS cells also may be found singly or in small groups within the epithelium of lobules and ducts in a pattern that resembles Paget's disease of the nipple (Figs. 33.28 and 33.29).

These intraepithelial growth patterns have been referred to as *pagetoid spread* because of presumed growth of the neoplastic cells, originating in lobules, into the ductal epithelium. In postmenopausal women, the cloverleaf pattern sometimes appears to arise *de novo* in ducts rather than by pagetoid spread. The occurrence of this microscopic structural alteration in isolated large ducts, including those in the subareolar region, suggests that they retain the capacity for lobular differentiation (60). This provides an explanation for finding LCIS or atypical lobular hyperplasia in breast biopsies without a classic lobular component. Paget's disease of the squamous surface of the nipple is not a feature of LCIS except in rare instances when there is involvement of lactiferous ducts.

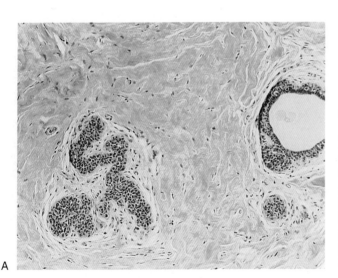
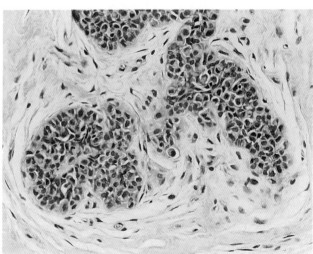

**FIG. 33.25.** *Lobular carcinoma* in situ, *postmenopausal.* **A:** *In situ* carcinoma fills an atrophic lobular ductule. There is pagetoid involvement of a small duct. **B:** The carcinoma cells have myoid features and exhibit characteristic loss of cohesion.

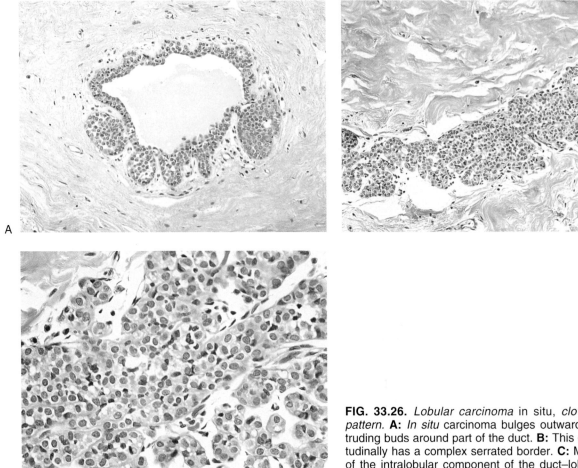

**FIG. 33.26.** *Lobular carcinoma* in situ, *cloverleaf ductal pattern.* **A:** *In situ* carcinoma bulges outward forming protruding buds around part of the duct. **B:** This duct cut longitudinally has a complex serrated border. **C:** Magnified view of the intralobular component of the duct–lobular complex shown in **B**.

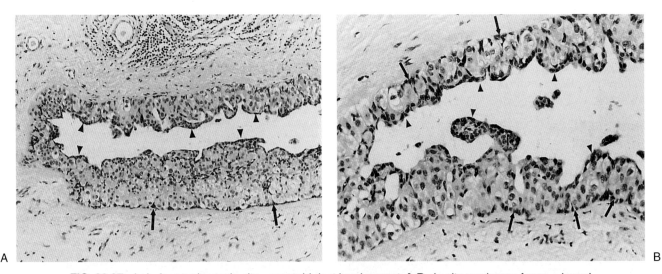

**FIG. 33.27.** *Lobular carcinoma* in situ, *pagetoid duct involvement.* **A,B:** *In situ* carcinoma forms a broad layer between attenuated normal epithelial cells that outline the lumen *(arrowheads)* and myoepithelial cells at the periphery *(arrows)*.

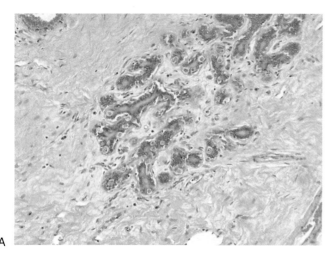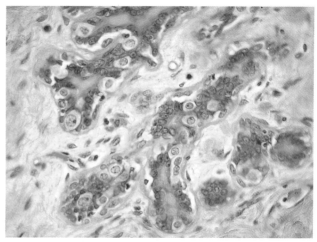

A                                                                                                                    B

**FIG. 33.28.** *Lobular carcinoma* in situ, *pagetoid lobular involvement.* **A,B:** Isolated carcinoma cells in the epithelium of a lobule. The findings shown here are not diagnostic, but may indicate the presence of LCIS elsewhere in the specimen.

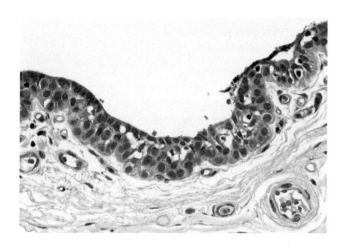

**FIG. 33.29.** *Lobular carcinoma* in situ, *pagetoid duct involvement.* An attenuated layer of nonneoplastic ductal cells overlies pagetoid lobular carcinoma *in situ.*

An unusual pattern of ductal involvement occurs when LCIS develops in ducts altered by collagenous spherulosis (61) (Fig. 33.30). This configuration mimics cribriform intraductal carcinoma (Fig. 33.31); however, myoepithelial cells outline spherule material, which should be distinguished

from the true microlumens of cribriform carcinoma. The carcinoma cells in such foci display loss of cohesion and intracytoplasmic vacuoles characteristic of lobular carcinoma.

Two abnormalities in benign epithelium must be considered in the differential diagnosis of pagetoid change: histio-

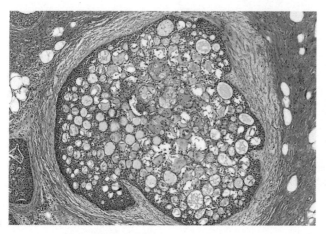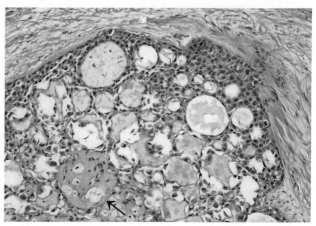

A                                                                                                                    B

**FIG. 33.30.** *Lobular carcinoma* in situ *in collagenous spherulosis.* **A,B:** Neoplastic cells outline the degenerative spherules in this example of collagenous spherulosis in an intraductal papilloma. *(continued)*

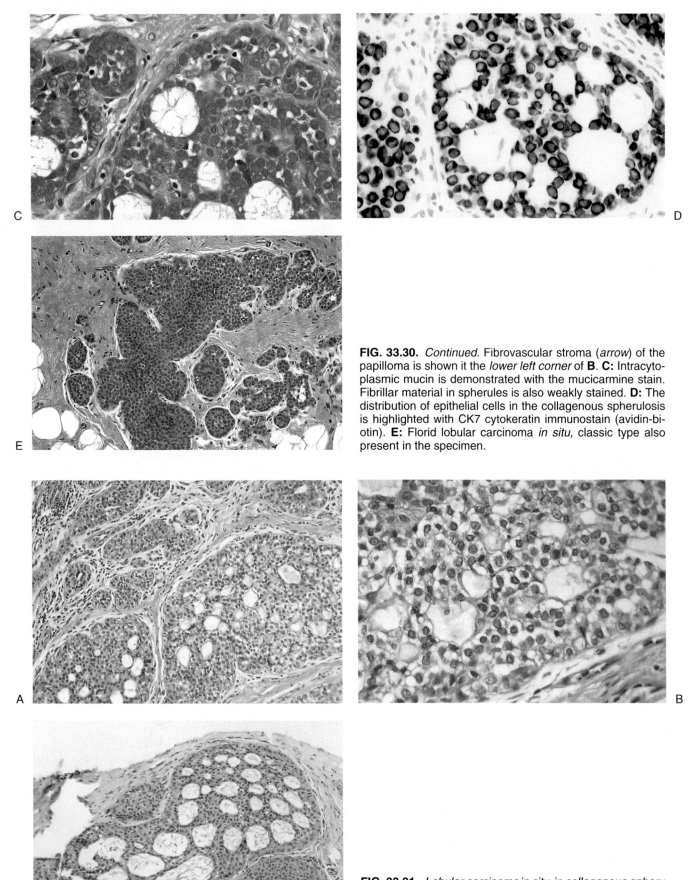

**FIG. 33.30.** *Continued.* Fibrovascular stroma (*arrow*) of the papilloma is shown it the *lower left corner* of **B**. **C:** Intracytoplasmic mucin is demonstrated with the mucicarmine stain. Fibrillar material in spherules is also weakly stained. **D:** The distribution of epithelial cells in the collagenous spherulosis is highlighted with CK7 cytokeratin immunostain (avidin-biotin). **E:** Florid lobular carcinoma *in situ,* classic type also present in the specimen.

**FIG. 33.31.** *Lobular carcinoma* in situ *in collagenous spherulosis.* **A,B:** These images were incorrectly labelled as "lobular carcinoma *in situ* and intraductal carcinoma," cribriform type in the prior edition of this book. **C:** This image was incorrectly labeled as "cribriform intraductal carcinoma" in the previous edition of this book.

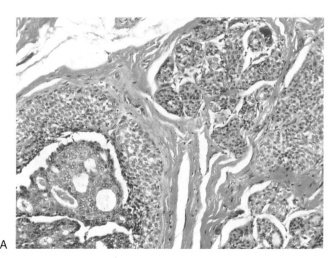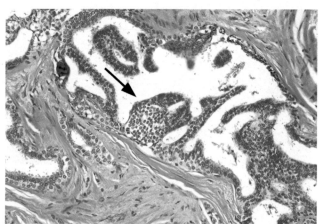

A                                                                                      B

**FIG. 33.32.** *Lobular carcinoma* in situ *merging with intraductal carcinoma.* **A:** Cribriform intraductal carcinoma fills the duct lumen on the *left* surrounded by lobular carcinoma *in situ,* which is also present on the *right* in the adjacent lobule. **B:** A focus of lobular carcinoma *in situ (arrow)* is present in this duct with micropapillary intraductal carcinoma.

cytes in the epithelium and myoepithelial cell hyperplasia. When examined at high magnification, intraepithelial histiocytes are found to have abundant foamy cytoplasm, sometimes with lipofuscin or hemosiderin pigment, and small dark nuclei. Intracytoplasmic mucin is absent from histiocytes, and the histiocytes are not immunoreactive for cytokeratin or actin. The overlying nonneoplastic epithelium is attenuated and flattened over intraepithelial histiocytes and pagetoid spread of LCIS. Intraepithelial histiocytes may be relatively sparse, or they may form a continuous layer one or more cells thick.

Myoepithelial hyperplasia is more likely to be mistaken for pagetoid spread of LCIS than is the presence of intraepithelial histiocytes. Epithelioid myoepithelial cells have pale cytoplasm. Hyperplastic myoepithelial cells tend to be distributed in a single layer, however, causing less attenuation of the overlying epithelium than pagetoid change. Some myoid immunohistochemical properties are usually retained in myoepithelial hyperplasia. The smooth-muscle myosin heavy chain immunostain is particularly useful for high-

lighting myoepithelial cells. Myoepithelial cells persisting in ducts with pagetoid LCIS and overlying duct epithelial cells are E-cadherin positive. These two cell types are responsible for discontinuous E-cadherin reactivity in LCIS lesions.

An unusual neoplastic proliferation is the coexistence of LCIS and intraductal carcinoma in a single duct. Such foci may have LCIS with a saw-toothed or cloverleaf configuration at the periphery of a duct in which ductal epithelium is carcinomatous and fills the lumen with a cytologically different population of cells growing as cribriform, papillary, or comedo intraductal carcinoma (Fig. 33.32). LCIS involving ducts that harbor apocrine intraductal carcinoma is another variant of such a combined lesion (Fig. 33.33).

Usually, LCIS arises within lobules and ductules that are not deformed by other conditions; however, lobular tissue previously altered by various benign proliferative processes also may be the site of LCIS. LCIS has been encountered in fibroadenomas, a mammary hamartoma (62), papillomas (Fig. 33.34), radial sclerosing lesions (Fig. 33.35), and sclerosing adenosis (Fig. 33.36). The diagnosis of LCIS under

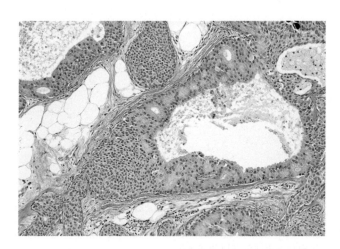

**FIG. 33.33.** *Lobular carcinoma* in situ *in apocrine intraductal carcinoma.* Lobular carcinoma *in situ,* classic type, coexists with apocrine intraductal carcinoma.

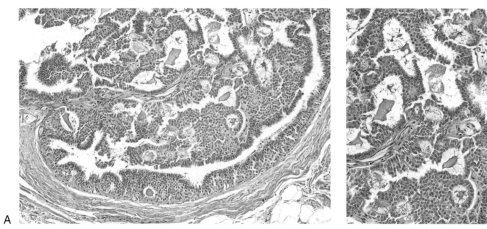
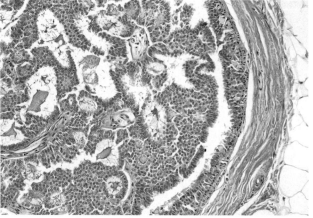

**FIG. 33.34.** *Lobular carcinoma* in situ *in a papilloma.* **A,B:** *In situ* lobular carcinoma has a pagetoid distribution in this papilloma.

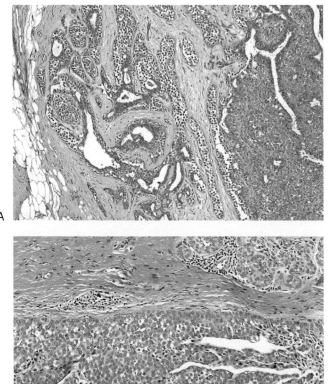
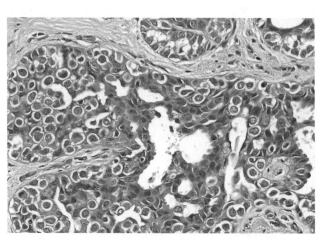

**FIG. 33.35.** *Lobular carcinoma* in situ *in radial sclerosing lesions.* **A:** Part of a sclerosing lesion with florid adenosis and *in situ* lobular carcinoma is shown *(right).* Marked discohesion of *in situ* lobular carcinoma is apparent *(left).* **B:** Pagetoid lobular carcinoma *in situ.* **C:** Part of the lesion where the ductal epithelium has been reduced to a thin layer of cells that outlines slender remnants of the duct lumen.

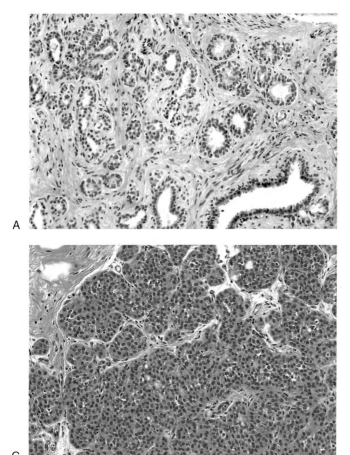

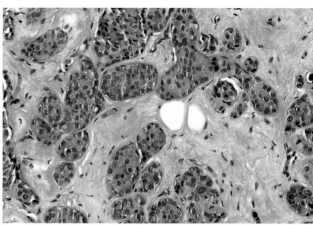

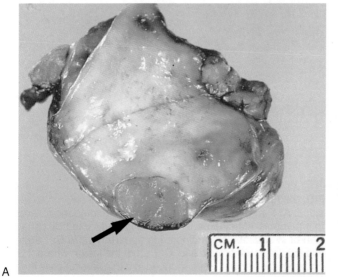

**FIG. 33.36.** *Lobular carcinoma* in situ *in sclerosing adenosis.* **A:** Sclerosing adenosis with preserved lobular gland lumens. **B:** Lobular carcinoma *in situ* fills the lobular glands. Myoepithelial cell hyperplasia is not present in this example, and consequently individual glands remain discrete. **C:** The neoplastic proliferation is nearly confluent in this lesion.

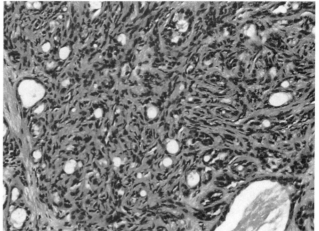

**FIG. 33.37.** *Lobular carcinoma* in situ *in sclerosing adenosis.* **A:** The gross appearance of the tan, oval adenosis tumor at the lower edge of the specimen *(arrow)* gave no indication that it harbored lobular carcinoma *in situ.* **B:** Sclerosing adenosis in the tumor shown in **A**. *(continued)*

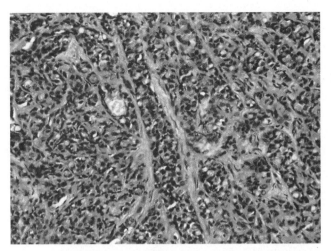

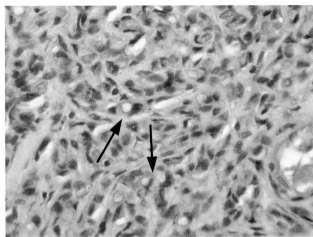

C

D

**FIG. 33.37.** *Continued.* **C:** Lobular carcinoma *in situ* in the sclerosing adenosis. **D:** Intracytoplasmic mucin in the lobular carcinoma *in situ (arrows).*

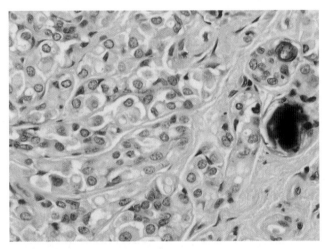

**FIG. 33.38.** *Lobular carcinoma* in situ, *sclerosing adenosis.* Signet-ring cells are present in this lesion with a microcalcification.

these circumstances rests largely on the identification of the appropriate cytologic features. The demonstration of intracytoplasmic mucin droplets is especially helpful for distinguishing florid adenosis from adenosis with LCIS (Figs. 33.37 and 33.38). LCIS in tubular adenosis has a striking histologic appearance (Fig. 33.39).

The lobular configuration is radically distorted in sclerosing lesions, and as a result it is difficult to exclude invasion when LCIS occurs in such foci (63) (Figs. 33.40 and 33.41). Careful inspection usually reveals the underlying adenosis pattern in which glandular units are surrounded by a basement membrane, myoepithelial cells, and stroma (Fig. 33.42). These elements can be highlighted with the reticulin stain and by the immunohistochemical demonstration of laminin, type IV collagen, and actin (Fig. 33.43). Attenuated, spindle-shaped myoepithelial cells in sclerosing adenosis usually persist and may be accentuated when the lesion is

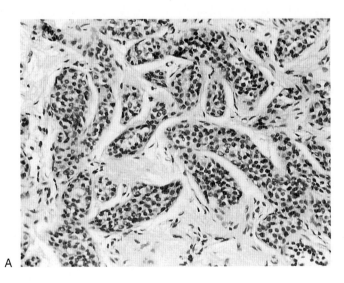

A

**FIG. 33.39.** *Lobular carcinoma* in situ, *tubular adenosis.* **A:** *In situ* carcinoma fills glands in tubular adenosis. *(continued)*

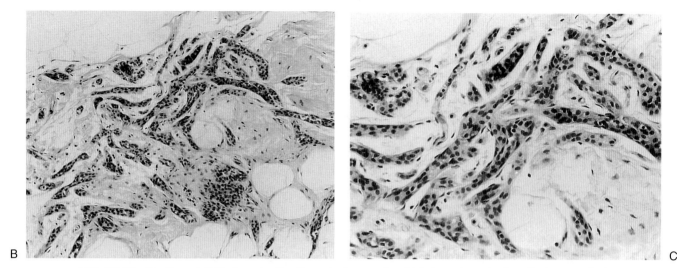

**FIG. 33.39.** *Continued.* **B,C:** A markedly attenuated example of tubular adenosis classified as atypical lobular hyperplasia.

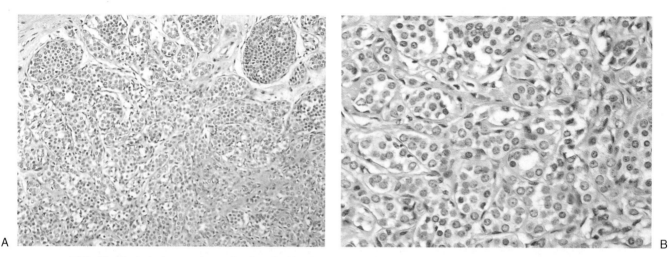

**FIG. 33.40.** *Lobular carcinoma* in situ, *florid sclerosing adenosis.* **A:** The underlying adenosis structure is obscured in the center of the lesion. **B:** At higher magnification, closely approximated adenosis glands are apparent.

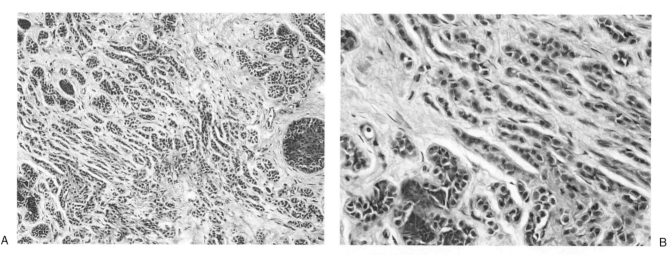

**FIG. 33.41.** *Lobular carcinoma* in situ *in sclerosing adenosis.* **A,B:** The lesion is composed of myoid carcinoma cells. Pagetoid spread is evident in the lobule in the *lower left corner* (hematoxylin-phloxine-safranin).

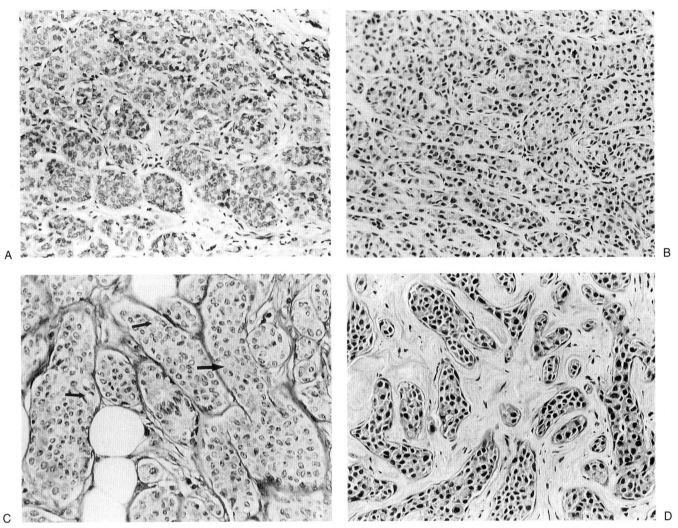

**FIG. 33.42.** *Lobular carcinoma* in situ *in sclerosing adenosis.* Four different structural patterns are represented. **A:** A compact lesion with fully developed *in situ* carcinoma in the round glands in the lower half of the picture. **B:** *In situ* carcinoma with conspicuous signet-ring cells. **C:** Adenosis glands separated by distinct basement membranes. A few cells have intracytoplasmic lumens *(arrows).* **D:** Lobular carcinoma *in situ* with myoid features in a radial sclerosing lesion. Note the loss of cohesion among the carcinoma cells.

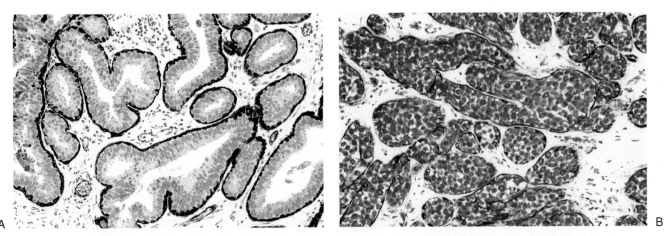

**FIG. 33.43.** *Lobular carcinoma* in situ *in sclerosing adenosis, immunohistochemistry.* **A:** Myoepithelial cells in florid sclerosing adenosis are highlighted with the smooth-muscle myosin heavy chain immunostain. **B:** Double immunolabeling demonstrates cytokeratin AE1/AE3 positive lobular carcinoma *in situ (red)* and smooth-muscle actin positive myoepithelial cells *(brown).* The *in situ* carcinoma is confined within the boundaries of the myoepithelial cells. *(continued)*

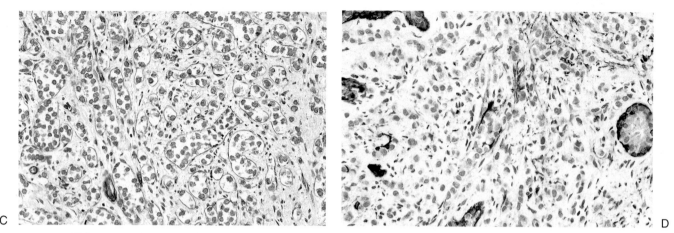

**FIG. 33.43.** *Continued.* **C:** An attenuated laminin layer demonstrates basement membrane material surrounding the epithelial cells. **D:** Immunoreactivity for smooth-muscle myosin heavy chain was incomplete or absent in the lesion shown in **C**, but invasion was not diagnosed because of persistent basement membranes. (**A,C,D**, avidin-biotin; **B**, Courtesy S. Hoda, M.D.; alkaline phosphatase and avidin-biotin).

colonized by LCIS (64). Myofibroblastic proliferation in the stroma can obscure myoepithelial cells in sclerosing adenosis. The smooth-muscle myosin heavy chain antibody stains myoepithelial cells preferentially and is useful in this situation. Invasion is difficult to identify when the neoplastic cells remain confined to the configuration of sclerosing adenosis. The diagnosis of invasion when there is LCIS in a sclerosing lesion is based on the finding of carcinoma cells in the stroma in the absence of actin-positive cells and basement membrane components (Fig. 33.43). The appearance of invasive foci outside sclerosing adenosis is no different from that of invasive lobular carcinoma in the absence of a sclerosing lesion (Fig. 33.44). For additional discussion of LCIS in sclerosing adenosis, see Chapter 7.

Most lobules are surrounded by fibrous stroma, but infrequently lobules are distributed in mammary adipose tissue. Lobules in fat are subject to the same pathologic alterations that occur in parenchymal lobules, including the development of sclerosing adenosis and LCIS. These conditions may resemble invasive carcinoma. Important distinguishing features of LCIS in fat are the presence of well-circumscribed glands containing LCIS, basement membrane components, and myoepithelial cells (Figs. 33.45 and 33.46). The lobular glandular pattern is lost when infiltrating lobular carcinoma involves fat (Fig. 33.47).

### Microinvasion

The term *microinvasion* is applied to an invasive lesion measuring less than 1 mm ($T1_{mic}$). Invasive foci 1 mm or larger are described by the diameter measured in the histologic section. This definition of microinvasion is the same as has been recommend for ductal carcinoma (see Chapter 13).

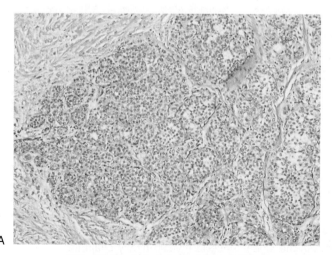
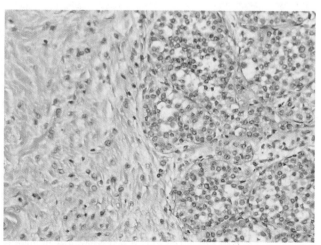

**FIG. 33.44.** *Lobular carcinoma* in situ *in sclerosing adenosis, microinvasive.* **A:** Florid *in situ* lesion in sclerosing adenosis. **B:** Individual carcinoma cells in the stroma adjacent to *in situ* carcinoma. This invasive focus was present near the left border of the lesion shown in **A**.

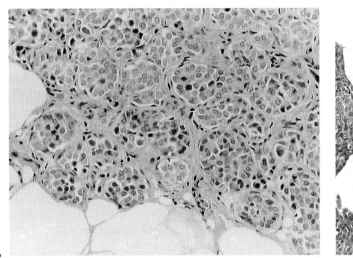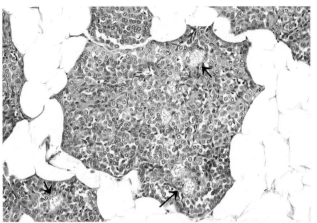

**FIG. 33.45.** *Lobular carcinoma* in situ *in fat.* **A:** No fibrous stroma separates the *in situ* carcinoma from fat. **B:** Lobular carcinoma *in situ* in collagenous spherulosis surrounded by fat. *Arrows* indicate spherules.

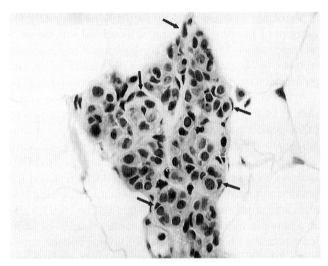

**FIG. 33.46.** *Lobular carcinoma* in situ *in fat.* A basement membrane and myoepithelial cells with crescentic nuclei *(arrows)* are present around most groups of carcinoma cells.

Small and microinvasive foci are characterized by carcinoma cells distributed singly or in slender cords within the stroma (Figs. 33.44 and 33.48) (65). One clue to the presence of these obscure invasive foci is slightly increased stromal cellularity, which may contain activated myofibroblasts and lymphocytes as well as carcinoma cells. Microinvasion should be looked for, especially when the specimen contains florid LCIS with marked enlargement of duct–lobular structures accompanied by necrosis and calcification. Subtle irregularities of lobular gland borders suggesting disruption of the basement membrane are also of particular concern. More than one microinvasive focus may be present in a biopsy (65). Microinvasion usually is detected close to a focus of LCIS in lobular glands or ductal extension, but rarely there is no contiguous *in situ* carcinoma. When LCIS or atypical lobular hyperplasia is identified in a needle core or surgical breast biopsy, the tissue should be examined thoroughly and carefully for foci of invasive lobular carcinoma.

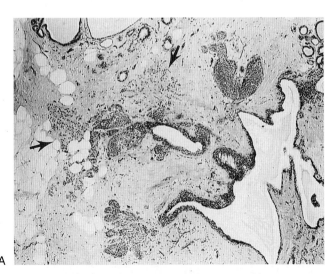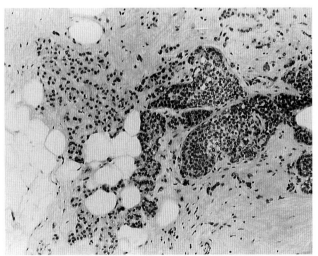

**FIG. 33.47.** *Lobular carcinoma invading fat.* **A:** Lobular carcinoma *in situ* is present in three ducts branching from a large lactiferous duct. Invasive lobular carcinoma is distributed around the middle duct *(arrows).* **B:** Invasive lobular carcinoma with a linear growth pattern around fat cells and in the fibrous stroma.

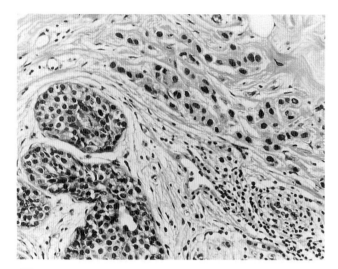

**FIG. 33.48.** *Lobular carcinoma* in situ *and microinvasive lobular carcinoma, classic type.* Histologically identical cells are present in both components.

Because small numbers of classic invasive lobular carcinoma cells may be difficult to distinguish from inflammatory or stromal cells, immunohistochemistry is often helpful in these cases. Cytokeratin immunostains are especially useful to highlight carcinoma cells in the stroma. Double immunostaining for actin as well as cytokeratin has been recommended to detect small or microinvasive foci of lobular carcinoma in sclerosing lesions (Fig. 33.43) (66). Also see Chapter 34 for information about microinvasive and invasive lobular carcinoma.

### *Electron Microscopy*

Electron microscopic studies have documented the origin of LCIS from lobular epithelial cells (67,68). Intracytoplasmic lumina lined by microvilli are seen ultrastructurally in the typical case. Myoepithelial cells have been demonstrated

in LCIS by electron microscopy and by immunohistochemistry (69). The distribution of these cells tends to be disordered in LCIS, and they are less numerous or absent when LCIS is associated with invasive lobular carcinoma (69). Protrusion of LCIS cells through the basement membrane, a phenomenon described by Ozzello (67), seems uncommon. Discontinuity of basement membranes in LCIS was demonstrated histochemically by Andersen, who noted that gaps could be detected not only in the basement membranes of lobules with LCIS, but also in normal lobules (70).

### Immunohistochemistry and Molecular Genetics

Usually, LCIS exhibits nuclear immunoreactivity for estrogen and progesterone receptors (71–73). Reactivity is more likely to be present in classic lesions with low nuclear grade than in cases of *in situ* pleomorphic lobular carcinoma.

Membrane immunoreactivity for HER2/*neu* is rarely detected in LCIS and when present, is associated with the pleomorphic variety (71,74,75). Overexpression of p53 is not detectable by immunohistochemistry in classic LCIS and proliferation estimated by MIB1 nuclear reactivity is low (71).

Vos et al. and Moll et al. found loss of E-cadherin expression in LCIS (76,77). Vos et al. studied two examples of LCIS associated with infiltrating lobular carcinoma. Immunohistochemistry revealed an absence of E-cadherin staining in both components. Loss of heterozygosity (LOH) analysis on microdissected samples of LCIS revealed the same point mutations as were present in the infiltrating lobular carcinoma from the same patient. LOH on 16q22.1 was also found in four of five microdissected samples of LCIS from patients who did not have infiltrating lobular carcinoma. Despite the high frequency of somatic E-cadherin mutations in LCIS, germline E-cadherin mutations have not been detected in these patients (77a). This observation indicates that susceptibility to LCIS is unlikely to be linked to constitutional mutations in the E-cadherin gene.

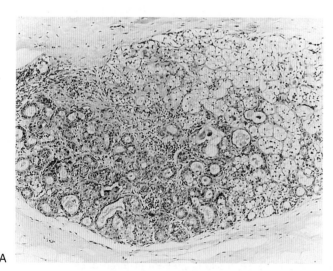

A

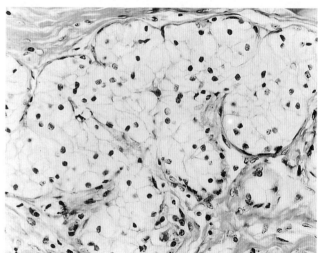

B

**FIG. 33.49.** *Clear cell change.* **A:** Cells in about 40% of the lobular glands show clear cell change. **B:** Lobular cells with clear cytoplasm and small dark nuclei. (*continued*)

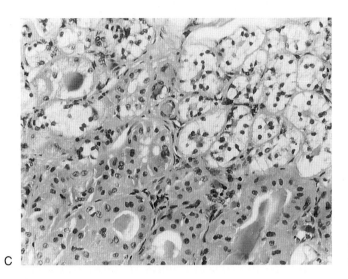

**FIG. 33.49.** *Continued.* **C:** Apocrine metaplasia is evident in the glands below an area of clear cell change.

Several other studies confirmed the absence or weak expression of E-cadherin in lobular carcinomas (78–80). Acs et al. reported complete absence of E-cadherin expression in 96% of *in situ* and invasive lobular carcinomas; one lesion had weak staining in both components (78). Ioffe et al. also found E-cadherin to be absent from most atypical lobular lesions (79). E-cadherin expression was absent when LCIS involved ducts, including cases with pleomorphic cytology (80). On the other hand, lesions in ducts with cytologic features of LCIS but some architectural aspects of ductal carcinoma, such as a microacinar pattern, exhibited variable E-cadherin staining, with only 33% reported to be E-cadherin negative (80). Each of the foregoing studies reported that E-cadherin reactivity was present in all the intraductal carcinomas examined (78–80). Ioffe et al. reported E-cadherin reactivity in all benign and atypical duct proliferations in their study (79).

These data support the recommendation in this chapter that florid ductal lesions with cytologic features of LCIS belong in this diagnostic category, even if they have necrosis and calcification. As noted elsewhere in this discussion, patients with this pattern of LCIS may be predisposed to have microinvasion and might require treatment customarily recommended for intraductal carcinoma. E-cadherin is a useful marker for distinguishing between ductal and lobular carcinoma lesions. This can be especially helpful when carcinoma *in situ* involves terminal duct–lobular units and the differential diagnosis lies between LCIS and ductal carcinoma involving lobules. E-cadherin immunoreactivity is totally absent from virtually all examples of classical and pleomorphic LCIS. Mosaic LCIS is also an exceptional variant in which there may be distinct but weak E-cadherin reactivity consistent with the cohesive appearance of these lesions. Discontinuous, attenuated E-cadherin reactivity associated with persisting epithelial and myoepithelial cells occurs when there is pagetoid LCIS in ducts and lobules as well as in atypical lobule hyperplasia. Finally, there appears to be a form of *in situ* carcinoma, possibly derived from terminal ductule cells, in which weak, attenuated, and discontinuous E-cadherin reactivity seems to

be intrinsic to the lesion. Until studies have more fully characterized the latter lesion, I have tended to classify it as ductal carcinoma (see figures in front of book).

Molecular analysis has been carried out to detect LOH on samples of LCIS and atypical lobular hyperplasia isolated by microdissection (81). The investigators found LOH at chromosome 11q13 in 33% of evaluable cases. The frequency of LOH was higher (50%) in LCIS associated with infiltrating lobular carcinoma than in LCIS without an invasive component (11%). LOH at 11q13 was detected in 2 of 19 (10%) samples of atypical lobular hyperplasias and in 9 of 22 (41%) infiltrating lobular carcinomas. These researchers concluded that the presence of LOH at 11q13 in LCIS might be a marker for increased risk for developing invasive carcinoma subsequently.

## Differential Diagnosis

The differential diagnosis of LCIS encompasses a number of proliferative changes affecting terminal ducts and lobules. These include pregnancy-like or "pseudolactational" hyperplasia, clear cell change, apocrine metaplasia, and atypical lobular hyperplasia. Pregnancy-like hyperplasia occurs in premenopausal women who are not pregnant and in postmenopausal women. The cells may have vacuolated cytoplasm, apical apocrine tufts, and hyperchromatic, atypical nuclei. Clear cell change that occurs in premenopausal and postmenopausal women may be a variant of apocrine metaplasia because the two are sometimes combined in a single lobule (Fig. 33.49). These lobular proliferative changes are discussed and illustrated in Chapter 1.

Apocrine metaplasia in lobular hyperplasia is manifested by cytoplasmic eosinophilia (Fig. 33.50). The orderly cellular distribution of this alteration is usually distinguishable from LCIS with cytoplasmic eosinophilia, lobular involvement by pleomorphic LCIS, and lobular extension of apocrine intraductal carcinoma (Fig. 33.51). Difficulty making these distinctions may be encountered in limited samples obtained by needle core biopsy.

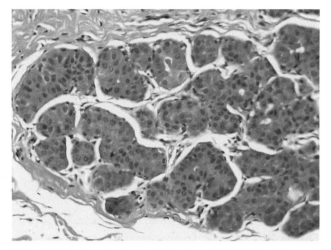

FIG. 33.50. *Apocrine metaplasia in a lobule.* Note the small punctate nuclei that are distributed in a fairly regular pattern around the periphery of the glands.

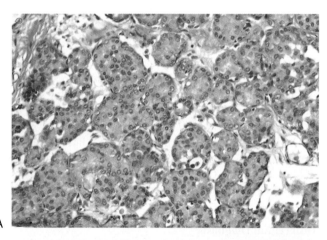

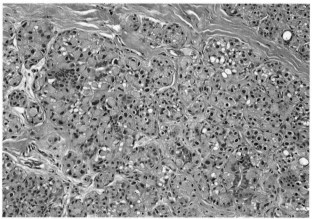

FIG. 33.51. *Carcinoma with apocrine differentiation in lobules.* **A:** Lobular carcinoma *in situ* with apocrine features. There is insufficient nuclear pleomorphism to qualify as pleomorphic *in situ* lobular carcinoma. **B:** Pleomorphic *in situ* lobular carcinoma. Note nuclear pleomorphism. Many cells have abundant diffuse intracytoplasmic mucin resulting in eccentric, crescentic nuclei and intracytoplasmic vacuoles.

The distinction between LCIS and solid small cell ductal carcinoma involving medium-sized ducts is difficult. Subtle clues that characterize this type of intraductal carcinoma are the presence of small distinct or poorly formed micracinar spaces, small capillaries in the epithelial proliferation, and a tendency to columnar orientation of cells at the periphery of the lesion. When it is present, E-cadherin reactivity highlights microacini and capillaries, as well as the peripheral orientation of cells in intraductal carcinoma. In my experience, these subtle attributes of intraductal carcinoma have been absent from E-cadherin negative LCIS in ducts.

## ATYPICAL LOBULAR HYPERPLASIA

### Clinical Presentation

No specific clinical features are associated with the diagnosis of atypical lobular hyperplasia. The clinical

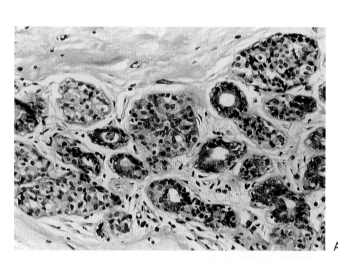

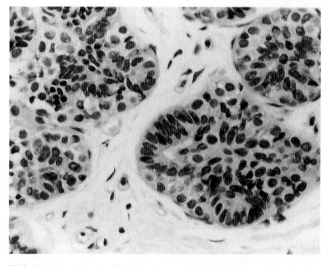

FIG. 33.52. *Atypical lobular hyperplasia.* **A:** Partial lobular involvement with evidence of pagetoid spread. This was the only affected lobule, and less than 75% of it was involved. **B:** Pagetoid spread of atypical cells in lobular glands in another case. Residual nonneoplastic lobular epithelium composed of columnar cells is evident.

indications for biopsy are the same as those that lead to the detection of LCIS: a palpable lesion or a mammographic abnormality. Atypical lobular hyperplasia is usually an incidental finding that is not specifically associated with the abnormality that prompted the diagnostic procedure. In one series of atypical lesions discovered in mammography-directed biopsies, only one of 11 cases (9%) of atypical lobular hyperplasia was at the site of the radiographic abnormality (82). On the other hand, 20 of 42 cases (48%) of atypical duct hyperplasia in this series were at the site of the mammographic lesion.

## Pathology

The glandular proliferation in atypical lobular hyperplasia has some features of LCIS, but they are not sufficiently developed to qualify for the latter diagnosis. As with atypical duct hyperplasia and intraductal carcinoma, no universally accepted criteria have been established for the precise distinction between atypical lobular hyperplasia and LCIS. Qualitative and quantitative factors must be considered.

Quantitative criteria for the diagnosis of LCIS discussed in the foregoing section influence the distribution of cases classified as atypical lobular hyperplasia. Most investigators have recommended that lesions that are quantitatively below the level of LCIS be classified as atypical lobular hyperplasia. As discussed in the foregoing section, some authors have diagnosed atypical lobular hyperplasia if the diagnostic lobular change involved less than 50% of one lobule or if less than one complete lobule was affected. The distinction proposed here, which is admittedly arbitrary, is to render a diagnosis of atypical lobular hyperplasia if less than 75% of a lobule shows the features of LCIS (Figs. 33.52 and 33.53). Rarely, the distinction may be made solely on this quantitative basis. More often, qualitative criteria also are considered.

Qualitatively, atypical lobular hyperplasia is characterized by the presence, within one or more lobules, of abnormal cells similar to those found in LCIS. In the least conspicuous configuration, these cells replace some of the normal lobular glandular epithelium, effacing the lumens (Fig. 33.54). Acinar units are small at this proliferative level (Fig. 33.55). As the process evolves, the accumulation of a greater number of these cells causes progressive acinar ex-

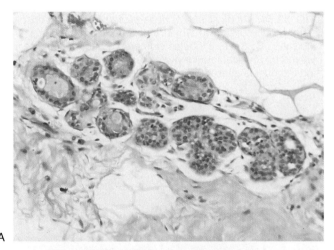

A

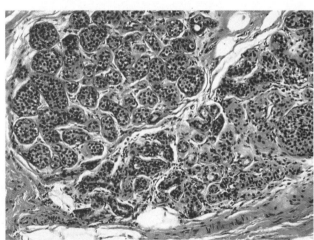

B

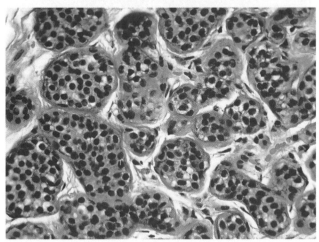

C

**FIG. 33.53.** *Atypical lobular hyperplasia.* **A:** A lobule in which less than 50% of the glandular epithelium is replaced by atypical cells. **B,C:** Approximately 60% of this lobule shows changes compatible with lobular carcinoma *in situ*.

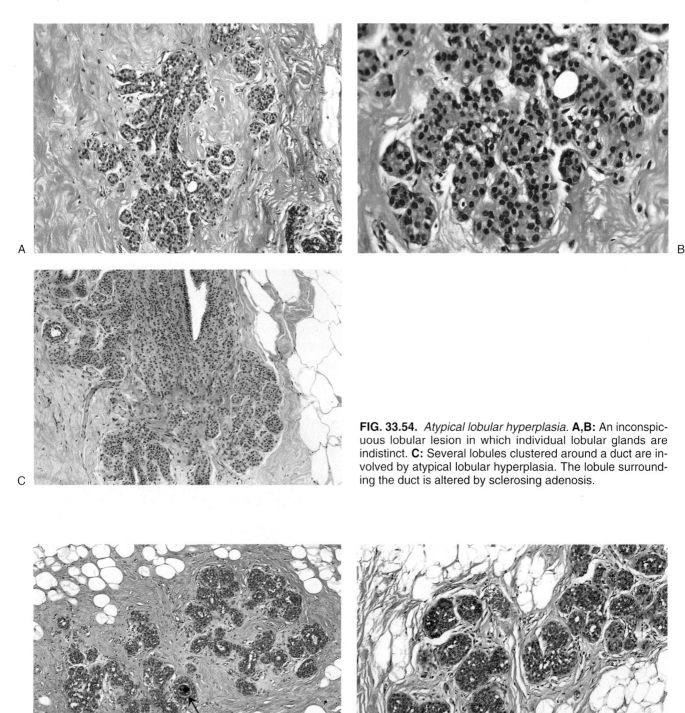

**FIG. 33.54.** *Atypical lobular hyperplasia.* **A,B:** An inconspicuous lobular lesion in which individual lobular glands are indistinct. **C:** Several lobules clustered around a duct are involved by atypical lobular hyperplasia. The lobule surrounding the duct is altered by sclerosing adenosis.

**FIG. 33.55.** *Atypical lobular hyperplasia.* **A,B:** Acinar glands are small. Note the cellular proliferation. Loss of cohesion is not evident. *Arrow* in **A** indicates a calcification.

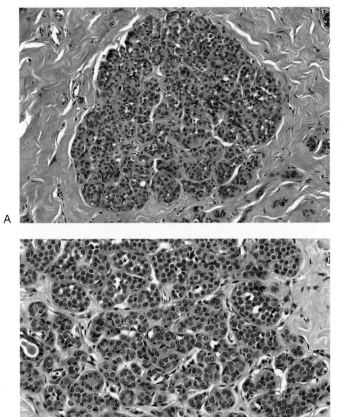

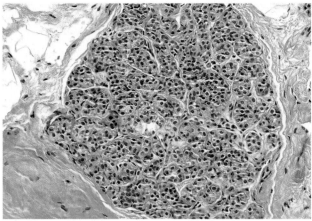

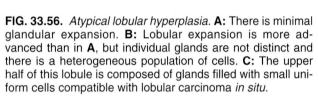

**FIG. 33.56.** *Atypical lobular hyperplasia.* **A:** There is minimal glandular expansion. **B:** Lobular expansion is more advanced than in **A**, but individual glands are not distinct and there is a heterogeneous population of cells. **C:** The upper half of this lobule is composed of glands filled with small uniform cells compatible with lobular carcinoma *in situ.*

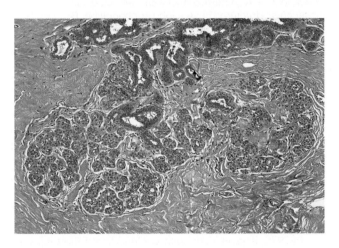

**FIG. 33.57.** *Atypical lobular hyperplasia, borderline.* The acinar glands are not well defined.

pansion, but the borders of individual acinar units and intralobular ductules remain indistinct (Fig. 33.56). Clear delineation of intralobular acinar units filled by the abnormal cell population is an important feature that distinguishes LCIS from atypical lobular hyperplasia. In LCIS there is accumulation of enough homogeneous neoplastic cells to cause the individual glands to have a distinct round or oval

configuration (Fig. 33.57). The cells in atypical lobular hyperplasia usually lack intracytoplasmic mucin and loss of cohesion is minimal or absent.

Similar criteria apply to the diagnosis of lobular proliferations that involve the terminal duct structures. These alterations tend to occur around rather than in the duct lumen, creating the cloverleaf pattern (Fig. 33.58). The lumen of

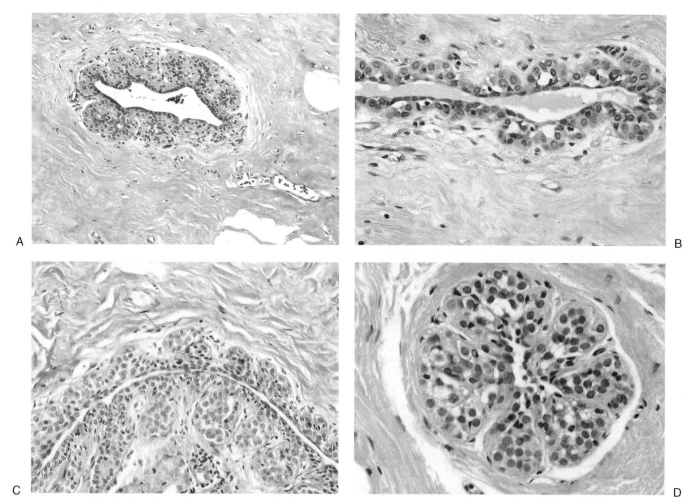

**FIG. 33.58.** *Atypical lobular hyperplasia in ducts, cloverleaf pattern.* **A:** A normal duct with a serrated contour created by abortive ductule formation. The resultant saccular structures have a lobular phenotype. **B:** Minimal atypical lobular hyperplasia in a duct cut longitudinally. **C:** More complex atypical lobular hyperplasia involving a duct. **D:** The cloverleaf pattern of atypical lobular hyperplasia in a duct cut transversely.

such a duct is usually clearly defined by a distinct layer of cuboidal ductal cells. Protruding outward from the lumen are circumferential pockets or outpouchings, which may be open, in continuity with the main duct lumen, or filled to a variable degree by atypical cells (Fig. 33.59). When such ducts are cut tangentially, the outpouchings have a parallel distribution described as a saw-toothed appearance. Atypical lobular hyperplasia of ductules is diagnosed when the cellular proliferation in the outpouchings is insufficient to cause them to appear as individual, distinct knobs protruding around the duct. In this situation, the outpouchings are sometimes inhabited by a mixture of normal and neoplastic cells. Atypical lobular hyperplasia of terminal ducts may also occur in a solid form that develops when the neoplastic growth is distributed in the duct lumen (Fig. 33.60). Atypical lobular hyperplasia in ducts should be distinguished from duct hyperplasia involving terminal ducts or uncoiled lobules (Fig. 33.61) and duct hyperplasia extending into terminal duct–lobular units (Fig. 33.62). E-cadherin expression is usually manifested by discontinuous, weak, or absent reactivity in atypical lobular hyperplasia involving ducts.

### Prognosis

Estimates of the risk for subsequent carcinoma in women with atypical lobular hyperplasia are clouded by the absence of a clear definition for this lesion. Some investigators who did not distinguish between atypical lobular hyperplasia and LCIS have reported relative risk estimates for both lesions under the heading of *lobular neoplasia* (24,83). Data describing the follow-up of patients with LCIS and atypical lobular hyperplasia are summarized in Table 33.5.

In 1978, Page et al. published a long-term follow-up study of patients with proliferative lesions that included atypical lobular hyperplasia identified in a retrospective review (84). The diagnosis of atypical lobular hyperplasia was

> reserved for atypical epithelium involving lobular units which approaches in appearance that accepted as LCIS. Loss of evidence of a 2-cell population above the basement membrane, near obliteration of lumens in 50% of the involved structures and modest distention of the ductules are necessary criteria. The cells have a small-to-moderate amount of clear cytoplasm and tend to have a regular relationship to

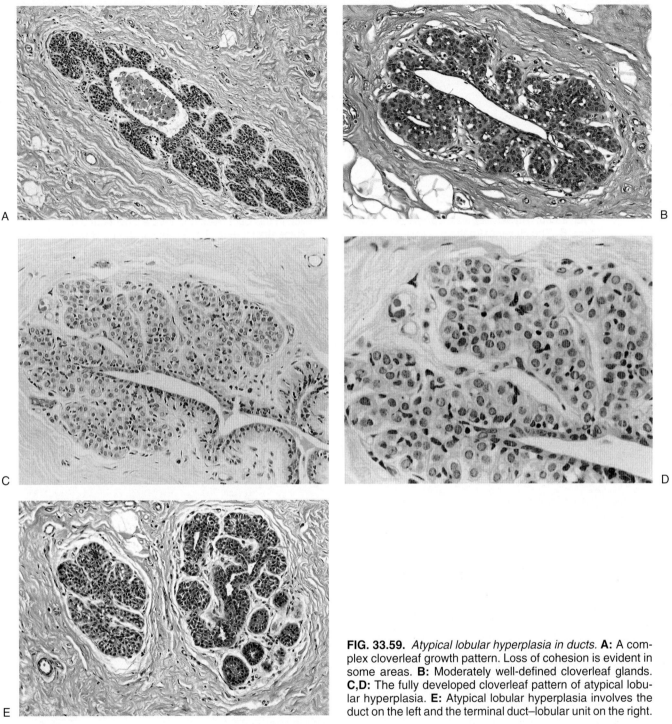

**FIG. 33.59.** *Atypical lobular hyperplasia in ducts.* **A:** A complex cloverleaf growth pattern. Loss of cohesion is evident in some areas. **B:** Moderately well-defined cloverleaf glands. **C,D:** The fully developed cloverleaf pattern of atypical lobular hyperplasia. **E:** Atypical lobular hyperplasia involves the duct on the left and the terminal duct–lobular unit on the right.

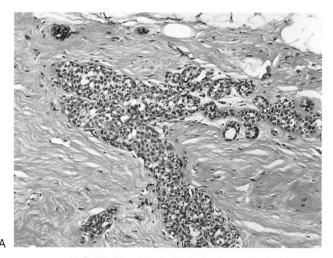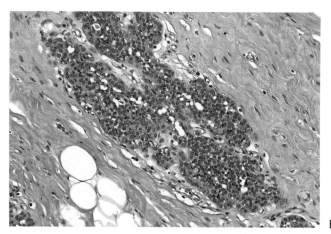

**FIG. 33.60.** *Atypical lobular hyperplasia in ducts.* **A:** Growth in this duct does not have a cloverleaf pattern. **B:** The cloverleaf pattern is obscured by cells that fill the duct lumen. The lesions in **A** and **B** border on *in situ* carcinoma.

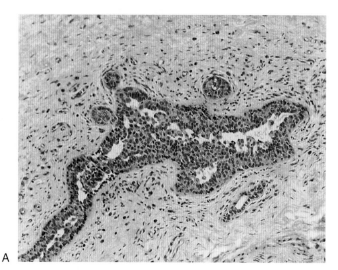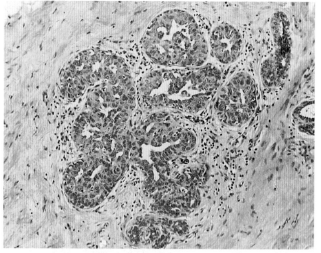

**FIG. 33.61.** *Duct hyperplasia with lobular extension.* **A:** Hyperplasia with a papillary pattern in a duct. **B:** Papillary duct hyperplasia in an uncoiled lobule from the same patient as **A**.

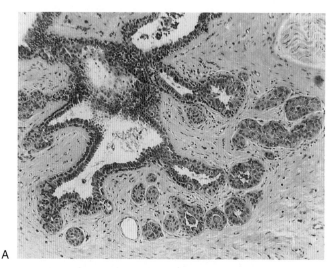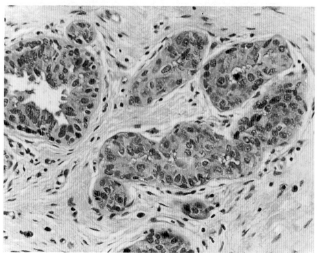

**FIG. 33.62.** *Duct hyperplasia with lobular extension.* **A,B:** Columnar cell hyperplastic epithelium forms a thin layer around the duct and extends into contiguous lobular glands.

**TABLE 33.5.** *The risk of subsequent carcinoma in patients with "untreated" LCIS or ALH*

| Source | Average age (yr) | No. of patients | % LCIS or ALH | % CA | RR |
|---|---|---|---|---|---|
| Andersen (5) | 46 | 47 | 1.5 LCIS | 21.3 | 12.0 |
| Rosen et al. (6) | 45 | 99 | 1.3 LCIS[a] | 36.4[b] | 9.0[b] |
| Haagensen et al. (24) | 46 | 211 | 3.8 LN[c] | 17.0 | 7.2 |
| Page et al. (8) | 45 | 44 | 0.5 LCIS | 23 | 9.0 |
| Bodian et al. (83) | 43 | 99 | 5.5 LN[c] | 24 | 5.7 |
| Page et al. (84) | 46 | 33 | 3.5 ALH | 12 | 4.0 |
| Page et al. (85) | 46 | 126 | 1.6 ALH | 12.6 | 4.2 |

ALH, atypical lobular hyperplasia; % CA, percent subsequent carcinoma; LCIS, lobular carcinoma *in situ*; RR, relative risk of subsequent carcinoma when compared with specified age-matched controls.

[a] Based on 99 cases identified.
[b] Based on 84 cases with follow-up.
[c] Diagnosis of lobular neoplasia (LN) included unspecified proportions of LCIS and of ALH.

each other. Nuclei are rounded similar to each other, and hyperchromatic (84).

On the basis of this definition, atypical lobular hyperplasia was diagnosed in 33 of 925 women (3.6%), four of whom later developed carcinoma. The relative risk for subsequent carcinoma was 4.0 compared with the expected frequency of subsequent carcinoma in age-matched controls. The relative risk was significantly higher (6.06) among women 31 to 45 years of age than in those older than 45 years (3.17) when atypical lobular hyperplasia was diagnosed.

A second follow-up study by Page et al. of patients with atypical lobular hyperplasia detected in a retrospective review of benign breast biopsies was published in 1985 (85). The definition of atypical lobular hyperplasia was similar to the one put forth in 1978. Atypical lobular hyperplasia was found in 126 of 10,542 biopsies (1.6%) examined, and 16 (12.6%) of these women later developed invasive breast carcinoma. Subsequent carcinomas were ipsilateral in 69% of the cases. The interval to subsequent carcinoma averaged 11.9 years (range, 4.6–21.9 years). Compared with age-matched controls in the Third National Cancer Survey, the overall relative risk for subsequent carcinoma in women with atypical lobular hyperplasia was 4.2 [95% confidence interval (CI), 2.6–6.9]. The risk was higher in those with a family history of breast carcinoma in a female, first-degree relative (8.4; 95% CI, 3.5–20) than in those with no affected first-degree relatives (3.5; 95% CI, 1.9–6.2). Eighty-seven percent of patients with atypical lobular hyperplasia were 31 to 55 years of age, and all subsequent carcinomas occurred in women initially identified in this age range. The relative risk was higher (6.4; 95% CI, 3.6–11) among those who were 46 to 55 years old when atypical lobular hyperplasia was diagnosed than among women 31 to 45 years old (2.7; 95% CI, 1.0–7.2). The overall relative risk for women with atypical lobular hyperplasia as well as the relative risks with or without a positive family history of breast carcinoma was similar to the relative risks associated with atypical ductal hyperplasia among women stratified in similar categories.

In a subsequent analysis of the same series of patients, Page et al. described the significance of ductal involvement

as a marker of breast carcinoma risk when associated with atypical lobular hyperplasia (59). Ductal involvement was present in 47 of 125 patients (37.6%) with atypical lobular hyperplasia, and another 66 women had only ductal involvement by atypical lobular hyperplasia. Thus, most (58.4%) patients with ductal involvement did not have an appreciable lobular component. Compared with age-matched control women in the Third National Cancer Survey, the relative risk for subsequent carcinoma was higher among those with atypical lobular hyperplasia accompanied by ductal involvement (6.8; 95% CI, 3.6–13) than when ductal involvement was absent (2.7; 95% CI, 1.2–5.9). The relative risk (2.1; 95% CI, 0.78–5.6) of subsequent carcinoma was not significantly increased over expected in women whose only manifestation of atypical lobular hyperplasia was limited to ducts.

### Lobular Carcinoma *In Situ* or Lobular Neoplasia

The term *lobular neoplasia* was introduced largely to alter the treatment of LCIS by removing the word *carcinoma* from the diagnosis (9). This strategy may have been useful in an era when breast-conserving therapy was not common for any form of breast carcinoma. Breast-conserving therapy is now widely accepted for most types of carcinoma; therefore, this rationale for using lobular neoplasia as a diagnostic term no longer exists.

Lobular neoplasia refers to the spectrum of lobular proliferative lesions, including mild atypia, atypical hyperplasia with partial lobular involvement, and fully developed LCIS involving one or more lobules. Advocates of lobular neoplasia point to differing criteria for the diagnosis of LCIS. An additional argument put forth in favor of using the diagnosis of lobular neoplasia is that atypical lobular hyperplasia and LCIS both are associated with an increased risk for subsequent breast carcinoma.

The spectrum of lesions encompassed by lobular neoplasia is so broad as to render it a misleading and useless diagnostic term. In clinical practice, the use of this term creates a situation in which a single diagnosis does not discriminate between the patient with a minimal proliferative lesion that might be only mildly atypical hyperplasia and a patient who has fully developed florid LCIS. The argument that it is sometimes difficult to classify borderline cases or that there is no consensus on diagnostic criteria does not justify a failure to distinguish between patients with lesions that are identifiable histologically in most cases. Furthermore, this line of reasoning does not provide a clear definition of lesions to be included in the lobular neoplasia category at the level of a atypical lobular hyperplasia. Consequently, the term *lobular neoplasia* suffers from one of the flaws it was intended to address. Although it obviates the need to make a distinction between atypical lobular hyperplasia and LCIS, the diagnosis of lobular neoplasia still requires separating ordinary lobular hyperplasia from a neoplastic proliferation in lobules.

Data purporting to demonstrate that atypical lobular hyperplasia and LCIS are associated with similar risks for subsequent carcinoma are at best tenuous. The difficulty in accepting these results lies in the lack of uniform diagnostic criteria. If the risk of subsequent carcinoma is higher for patients with LCIS, then inclusion of patients with atypical lobular hyperplasia among them would lower the risk for this combined group. Conversely, classifying patients with LCIS as having atypical lobular hyperplasia would inflate the risk for the latter diagnosis.

The foregoing discussion provides a rationale for continuing to discriminate between atypical lobular hyperplasia and LCIS and to eschew the term *lobular neoplasia* in clinical practice. Although this distinction may be difficult in individual cases, most often the diagnosis can be made by adhering to an established set of criteria such as those set forth in this chapter. Further studies that use immunohistochemistry and molecular techniques may help in refining these criteria by relating these biologic properties to breast carcinoma risk. The term *lobular neoplasia* disguises our limitations and creates a false sense of specificity for the patient and clinician. The range of morphologic changes covered by lobular neoplasia is broad, making this diagnosis one of the least specific in breast pathology and one that is not recommended.

## Risk for Developing Subsequent Invasive Carcinoma

In their original paper, Foote and Stewart anticipated the most controversial aspect of LCIS, the risk that subsequent invasive carcinoma might develop if the breast harboring LCIS were not removed at the time of initial diagnosis. They commented:

> It has been forcibly impressed upon us that a breast in which this process occurs in the slightest degree constitutes an extreme hazard. Whereas it is not clinical cancer until infiltration occurs, it is always a disease of multiple foci. . . . In our first case, local excision revealed this process and we were unfortunately not aware of its significance. Within the space of a few months the patient had infiltrating cancer with axillary metastases and now has skeletal dissemination. It is our feeling that simple mastectomy is essential, with further procedures dependent on finding the least evidence of infiltration (2).

The rapid clinical progression of disease in this case suggests that invasion had probably occurred when LCIS was diagnosed but it was not represented in the biopsy.

Several case reports followed more than a decade later. Godwin described a patient who died of ipsilateral invasive lobular carcinoma that developed 12 years after a biopsy that contained LCIS had been interpreted as "cystic disease" (86). Two additional articles described the development of carcinoma in the ipsilateral (87) and contralateral (22,87) breast after a biopsy contained LCIS. The risk associated with residual breast tissue after mastectomy was documented by Newman in a report which described a patient treated for LCIS (29). Four years after a mastectomy, a mass in the inferior aspect of the scar was found to contain residual breast tissue with *in situ* and infiltrating lobular carcinoma.

Several papers subsequently described small selected groups of patients with LCIS and reported that most women not treated by mastectomy remained well. Benfield et al. cited five patients treated by partial mastectomy who remained well up to 11 years after a biopsy showed LCIS (34). A similar outcome was recorded by Lewison and Finney, who reported on three patients 3 to 10 years after biopsy (28). Giordano et al. traced 19 patients who did not undergo mastectomy for LCIS (88). Two had invasive carcinomas in the ipsilateral breast at 3 and 5 years subsequently treated by mastectomy. Thirteen patients remained well an average of 11.7 years (7–21 years) after biopsy. In other studies, subsequent ipsilateral carcinoma was reported in 6% and 16% of women after a median follow-up of 7 and 10 years, respectively (89,90).

Retrospective pathology studies were undertaken in the 1970s and 1980s to identify consecutive series of patients with LCIS not treated by mastectomy (Table 33.5). Wheeler et al. found 30 examples of LCIS among 4,898 breast biopsies performed at the University of Pennsylvania from 1948 to 1960 (7). They added another eight cases diagnosed between 1960 and 1963 to this series but did not review all biopsies for the latter interval. Immediate ipsilateral mastectomy had been performed in 13 of 38 women (34%) in the study group, leaving 25 women for follow-up of the breast in which the diagnosis of LCIS was initially made. The mean follow-up was 17.5 years. Subsequently, one patient developed ipsilateral invasive lobular carcinoma (1 of 25, or 4%). Subsequent invasive duct carcinoma of the opposite breast was found in 3 of 32 patients (9.7%) with a contralateral breast available for follow-up. One significant weakness in this study is that nearly one-third of patients were treated by mastectomy, suggesting a selection bias in the group not treated surgically.

Another series of cases was studied in Denmark by Andersen (5). Slides of 3,299 breast specimens obtained from 1942 to 1961 were reviewed, yielding 52 patients who had had LCIS. Five had been treated previously for contralateral invasive breast carcinoma. Ipsilateral mastectomy was performed for LCIS in six cases. After an average follow-up of

15 years, invasive carcinoma was detected in 8 of 46 patients (17.4%) with an ipsilateral breast available for study. The average interval to subsequent ipsilateral carcinoma was 9 years (range, 1–22 years). Four contralateral carcinomas (4 of 47, or 8.5%) were found an average of 13 years (range, 7 to 24 years) after biopsy. The total burden of contralateral carcinoma (9 of 25, or 17.3%) was essentially the same as for ipsilateral disease. A retrospective review by Harvey and Fechner of 879 breast biopsies originally reported as benign yielded 24 patients with previously undiagnosed LCIS (91). After a median follow-up of 8 years, one patient developed invasive lobular carcinoma in the ipsilateral breast.

Two comprehensive investigations of LCIS undertaken at Columbia Presbyterian Medical Center (CPMC) and Memorial Sloan-Kettering Cancer Center (MSKCC) appeared in 1978. The CPMC study was based on a retrospective review of histologic sections of 5,560 breast biopsies performed from 1930 to 1972 (24). A total of 211 patients were found to have lesions diagnosed as lobular neoplasia unassociated with invasive carcinoma, resulting in an incidence of 3.8% for lobular neoplasia. The term *lobular neoplasia* is used here with specific reference to data from the CPMC series. This distinction is made because lobular neoplasia as used by these researchers includes lesions ordinarily diagnosed as atypical lobular hyperplasia as well as LCIS. None of the patients was treated by mastectomy. Follow-up was obtained for 210 women, averaging 14 years (range, 1–42 years).

Prior or subsequent carcinoma exclusive of LCIS was identified in 36, or 17.1%, of the patients, including three with bilateral carcinoma. The number of carcinomas in the contralateral breast was nearly the same as in the ipsilateral breast. The incidence rate for subsequent breast carcinoma was seven times more than expected compared with Connecticut State Cancer Registry data. After 15 years of follow-up, the cumulative probabilities for subsequent carcinoma were 10% and 9% in the ipsilateral and contralateral breast, respectively. During the follow-up interval of 16 to 25 years, the risk for ipsilateral carcinoma reached 22%. For the contralateral breast, the risk increased to 15% by 25 years. Data were presented that suggested that a family history of breast carcinoma in a first-degree female relative contributed to increase the risk of carcinoma subsequent to "lobular neoplasia." It was recommended that patients with "lobular neoplasia" enter into follow-up by palpation every 4 months rather than have treatment by mastectomy.

Data from CPMC were updated by Haagensen, who extended the series to 1977 thereby including 297 patients with "lobular neoplasia" (9). The average follow-up was 16.3 years, including 82 patients (27.6%) with more than 20 years' follow-up. Subsequent carcinoma was found in 53 of 285 patients (18.6%). Compared with data from the state of Connecticut, the ratio of observed to expected or relative risk for developing subsequent carcinoma was 5.9. The cumulative probability of subsequent ipsilateral carcinoma increased with longer follow-up from 8% at 6 to 10 years, to 12% at 11 to 15 years, and to 19% at 25 years. A similar

trend was observed for contralateral carcinoma, which increased in frequency from 7% at 6 to 10 years, to 8% at 11 to 15 years, to 14% at 25 years, and to 23% at 35 years. Axillary dissection was performed in the treatment of 54 subsequent carcinomas. Lymph node metastases were found in 26% of these cases. Eleven of 53 patients (20.8%) with subsequent carcinoma died of metastatic carcinoma, and at last follow-up two others (3.7%) were alive with systemic metastases.

A third retrospective analysis of cases from CPMC was reported by Bodian et al. in 1993 (83). This series, based entirely on patients treated by Haagensen, included 99 women with lesions classified on review as "lobular neoplasia"/LCIS among 1,799 women analyzed in a follow-up study of proliferative breast disease. LCIS was not distinguished from atypical lobular hyperplasia in reporting the results of the follow-up. After an average follow-up of 21 years, 24 women (24%) developed subsequent breast carcinoma other than LCIS. Compared with controls from the Connecticut Tumor Registry, the expected relative risk for subsequent carcinoma was 5.7 (95% CI, 3.8–8.5), similar to that in the 1986 report from the same institution.

A further analysis of the CPMC series published in 1996 comprised 236 women with a median follow-up of 18 years (92). The probability of developing subsequent carcinoma was 1 in 3, or 5.4 times the rate in the general population (95% CI, 4.2–7.0). The relative risk was elevated for more than 20 years after the diagnosis of LCIS and increased from 4.9 (95% CI, 3.7–6.4) for women with LCIS in one biopsy to 16.1 (95% CI, 6.9–31.8) for women with LCIS in a second biopsy.

The MSKCC study was based on a systematic review of 8,609 breast biopsies performed between 1940 and 1950 (6). Included were all specimens in which there was a diagnosis other than carcinoma. Sixty-four examples of previously unrecognized LCIS were found. During the same period, there were also 53 cases in which the original diagnosis had been LCIS. The incidence of LCIS was therefore 1.3% among biopsies that did not contain intraductal or invasive carcinoma. Eighteen patients with LCIS were excluded from subsequent analysis because incomplete identifying information precluded follow-up.

Follow-up averaging 24 years was obtained for 84 of the 99 study patients with LCIS, and it was found that 32 patients (38%) were treated at some time for mammary carcinoma other than the LCIS diagnosed in the biopsy under consideration. Subsequent ipsilateral carcinoma was diagnosed in 12 patients (14%), and seven other patients (8%) had bilateral carcinomas. Twelve patients (14%) had only contralateral carcinoma, including three who had had treatment of contralateral carcinoma prior to the biopsy in which LCIS was found. Laterality was not known for one subsequent carcinoma. Thirty-nine patients (46%) who remained alive had had no breast carcinoma other than the original LCIS. Thirteen other patients (25%) with no evidence of breast carcinoma died of other causes.

The average age at the diagnosis of subsequent ipsilateral carcinoma was 59 years, and for subsequent contralateral carcinoma, it was 62 years. The intervals between the diagnosis of LCIS and carcinoma of the ipsilateral breast varied from 2 to 31 years and from 3 to 30 years in the contralateral breast. In the ipsilateral breast, 6 of 19 (32%) of subsequent carcinomas were diagnosed 20 years or longer after LCIS. Forty-four percent of subsequent contralateral carcinomas (7 of 16) were not detected for at least 20 years after diagnosis of LCIS. Thirty-eight percent of all patients with subsequent carcinoma did not have evidence of the disease until at least 20 years after LCIS was found. The hazard rate for the subsequent development of carcinoma increased annually over a period of 25 years after the diagnosis of LCIS.

Infiltrating duct carcinoma was the most common type of carcinoma to develop after LCIS (Fig. 33.63). Infiltrating lobular carcinoma was encountered in eight ipsilateral and five contralateral breasts. All but five of the breasts contained invasive carcinoma. Three of these five patients had bilateral carcinoma and were treated at some time for inva-

sive carcinoma of one breast. A patient who had only intraductal carcinoma and another with subsequent LCIS were the only women whose carcinoma, found subsequent to the biopsy with LCIS, was not invasive.

Subsequent carcinomas were treated by mastectomy. Lymph node status was known for 13 ipsilateral and 15 contralateral breasts with carcinoma. Axillary metastases were found in seven (54%) ipsilateral and in seven (47%) contralateral axillary dissections. Sixteen of the 32 patients (50%) with subsequent breast carcinoma died of their disease. Six of these women died of carcinoma of the ipsilateral breast, and five died of carcinoma in the contralateral breast. Among the four patients with bilateral carcinoma, the fatal lesion was judged on the basis of size and nodal status to be ipsilateral in two and contralateral in one. In one case of bilateral carcinoma, it was not possible to ascertain which breast was primarily involved, and the fatal lesion was recorded as bilateral. In an additional case, laterality of the fatal primary carcinoma was not known. The average length of survival of patients who died of breast carcinoma was 4

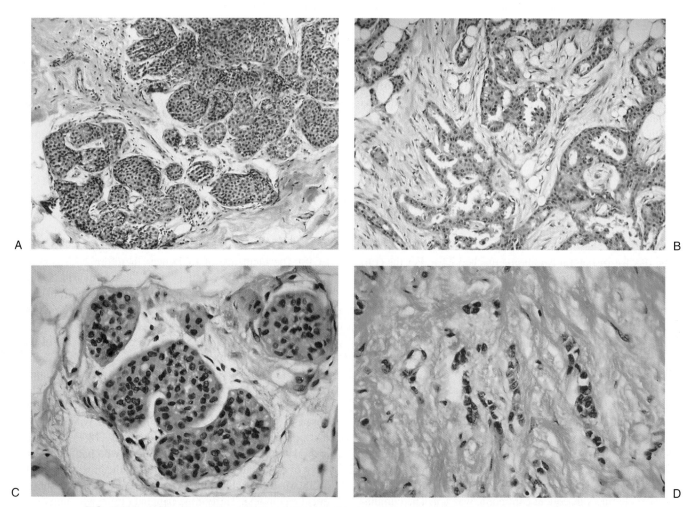

**FIG. 33.63.** *Infiltrating duct carcinoma subsequent to lobular carcinoma* in situ. **A:** Lobular carcinoma *in situ* of the right breast in a biopsy performed in 1948. No other treatment was given. **B:** Infiltrating duct carcinoma detected as a palpable tumor in the right breast in 1977. **C,D:** The mastectomy specimen also had *in situ* and invasive lobular carcinoma.

years following the diagnosis of subsequent invasive carcinoma. In 10 of 13 fatal cases (77%) for which nodal status could be determined, there were axillary metastases. Compared with an age-matched control population identified in the Connecticut State Tumor Registry, LCIS patients had nine times the expected frequency of subsequent carcinoma ($p<0.001$). Deaths from breast carcinoma, of which there were 16, were 10.7 times more frequent than expected.

Clinical and pathologic factors were examined in the CPMC and MSKCC studies to identify patients with a significantly greater likelihood of developing invasive carcinoma after LCIS. Subsequent carcinoma was more frequent among women with a family history of breast cancer and among nulliparous patients. These factors are known to increase the risk of carcinoma for all women, whether they have LCIS or not.

No study thus far has identified a reliable pathologic predictor of increased risk for the subsequent development of carcinoma after LCIS has been diagnosed. The risk of subsequent carcinoma was not related to the number of lobules with LCIS in the original biopsy. Whereas the CPMC and MSKCC reports described a greater risk in patients with LCIS that contained both small (type A) and large (type B) cells compared to LCIS with either cell type alone, LCIS of the mixed cell type was infrequent. In a later analysis, Haagensen reported a substantially increased risk (17.9 times expected) associated with LCIS composed of "hyperchromatic closely packed cells," but this pattern was encountered in only 13 (4.5%) of their cases"—too few on which to base any conclusions" (9). In both series, about 25% of carcinomas that arose in patients with LCIS were classified as infiltrating lobular carcinomas.

One additional long-term follow-up study should be noted (8). This series consisted of 48 patients with LCIS found in a retrospective review of 10,542 benign breast biopsies, an incidence of 0.5%. Follow-up averaging 19 years was available for 39 patients, nine (23%) of whom had subsequent invasive breast carcinoma. Compared with a normal control population, the overall relative risk of subsequent invasive breast carcinoma was 6.9, and the relative risk was 10.8 compared with that in women who had nonproliferative changes in a breast biopsy. After 15 years of follow-up, the relative risk was 8.0, and the absolute risk was 17%. In this study, the risk for developing subsequent carcinoma was not affected by a family history of invasive breast carcinoma.

### Risk of Having Concurrent Invasive Carcinoma

To determine whether finding LCIS in a biopsy accurately reflects the extent of carcinoma in the breast, a series of 121 consecutively treated patients was analyzed (93). In each case, paraffin sections of a breast biopsy revealed intraepithelial carcinoma. The series included 53 women with LCIS. Comparison of the findings at mastectomy with those in the biopsy is shown in Table 33.5, which includes data from two other reports (44,45). In these studies, 4% to 6% of

women were found to have invasive carcinoma in the breast after a biopsy showed only LCIS. Multifocal intraepithelial carcinoma was usually the same type seen in the biopsy. In patients whose biopsy showed LCIS, 93% of the intraepithelial carcinoma at mastectomy was also LCIS, and 7% was classified as intraductal. The two invasive carcinomas were ductal and lobular, respectively. Others have reported a higher frequency of carcinoma detected in mastectomy and mammoplasty specimens obtained within 2 years of a biopsy diagnosis of LCIS. Invasive carcinoma was found in 4 of 38 cases (11%), and in another case the specimen contained intraductal carcinoma (46).

When axillary metastases are the first evidence of breast carcinoma, a small occult invasive tumor is usually found in the breast. In a few unusual cases, the only identifiable neoplastic lesion has been *in situ* carcinoma insofar as could be determined by light microscopy. One study described four women who presented with metastatic mammary carcinoma in one or more axillary lymph nodes in whom the only carcinoma demonstrable at mastectomy was LCIS (94). The absence of demonstrable invasion in these unusual cases is probably due to incomplete sampling or failure to recognize microinvasive foci.

## CLINICAL MANAGEMENT OF LCIS AND ATYPICAL LOBULAR HYPERPLASIA

Presently, clinical follow-up is recommended when the diagnosis is atypical lobular hyperplasia and for most patients with LCIS. Tamoxifen may be indicated (95). Biopsy of the opposite breast may be performed if there are clinical indications. The patient should be informed of the treatment options and the potential consequences or risks of each.

The clinical follow-up of patients with atypical lobular hyperplasia and LCIS is a lifetime undertaking in view of the extended risk for late-occurring carcinomas. The possibility that an antiestrogen such as tamoxifen might inhibit the evolution of atypical lobular hyperplasia or LCIS was proposed in 1978 (6). It was later noted that patients receiving tamoxifen as adjuvant therapy following invasive carcinoma had a lower than expected frequency of contralateral carcinoma (96–99). A recent clinical trial used tamoxifen in patients with markers of a high breast carcinoma risk including women with LCIS (95,99). After 5 years of treatment with tamoxifen, women with LCIS had a 56% reduction in the risk of developing subsequent invasive carcinoma (95).

It remains to be seen whether lifetime mortality from subsequent invasive carcinoma can be reduced by close clinical surveillance and preventive intervention with antiestrogens. In the event that subsequent carcinomas were 1 cm or smaller in diameter when detected, data from the Surveillance, Epidemiology, and End Results (SEER) Program (100) and other sources (101) indicate that axillary metastases would be found in 13% to 16% of cases. In the one series with no systematic follow-up of LCIS patients, about 50% had nodal metastases when carcinoma was later detected, whereas in a more carefully followed series axillary metastases were present in 26%, and nearly 25% later developed systematic metastases. It is unlikely that even with the most careful clinical follow-up, all later invasive carcinomas would be found before axillary or systemic metastases had occurred.

Several studies published after 1990 have assessed prospectively the follow-up of patients with LCIS after biopsy or wide excision alone. Ciatto et al. described the status of 60 women with an average follow-up of 5.3 years (102). Ipsilateral invasive carcinoma was detected subsequently in 5 of 37 (14%) who did not have a mastectomy, and two others were found to have persistent LCIS. The intervals to subsequent invasive carcinoma were 5, 13, 20, 49, and 63 months. Three of the five invasive carcinomas were of the lobular variety. The relative risk for subsequent carcinoma based on age-specific incidence and years of follow-up for the 37 patients was 36 (95% CI, 11.6–83.3). Three of the five patients with subsequent invasive ipsilateral carcinoma developed metastases and died 6, 7, and 8 years after the initial diagnosis of LCIS. Two patients had metachronous contralateral carcinoma. On the basis of these results, these researchers concluded that "the present study does not provide definitive evidence to recommend total mastectomy as the standard treatment of LCIS . . . [but] . . . when limited surgery is adopted as the standard treatment of LCIS, careful follow-up of the ipsilateral and contralateral breast is mandatory" (102).

The National Surgical Adjuvant Breast Project Protocol B-17 randomized patients to receive or not receive radiotherapy after lumpectomy (103). Included were 182 patients with LCIS whose only treatment was the diagnostic lumpectomy with a standardized follow-up program of mammography and clinical examination. After a mean prospective follow-up of 5 years, 13 patients developed subsequent carcinoma in the ipsilateral breast and four in the contralateral breast, including one case of bilateral disease. All but one of the subsequent ipsilateral lesions were detected by mammography. All subsequent ipsilateral carcinomas were in the same quadrant as the original biopsy, which suggested that the LCIS was a precursor to invasive carcinoma as well as a marker for risk. Subsequent ipsilateral carcinomas were invasive lobular (n = 4), intraductal (n = 4) and lobular carcinoma *in situ* (n = 5). Two subsequent contralateral carcinomas were invasive (lobular and mucinous types, respectively), and two were intraductal and *in situ* lobular, respectively. No patient had axillary nodal metastases. All initial LCIS cases were diploid, were HER2/*neu* negative, and had a low S-phase. The risk of developing subsequent carcinoma within the follow-up period was significantly related to the following: degree of distention of affected lobules, which was greatest in cases with maximal distention; and cell size, which was maximal in cases with both small and large cells (types A and B). Factors not significantly associated with subsequent carcinoma risk were the number of affected lobules, the presence of duct extension, intralesional calcification, the presence of signet-ring cells, mitoses, histiocytoid differentiation, and loss of cohe-

sion in the initial LCIS. The results of this relatively short-term prospective follow-up are largely consistent with prior retrospective studies with respect to the lack of correlation between most morphologic features and the risk for subsequent carcinoma. Extended follow-up will be needed to assess the long-term overall cancer risk in both breasts and survival in this series of patients.

The only report of a population-based prospective study of LCIS was provided by the Danish Breast Cancer Cooperative Group (104). The series included 69 women with LCIS and 19 with LCIS and intraductal carcinoma entered into a nationwide program from 1982 through 1987. All patients underwent excisional biopsy, including two cases diagnosed in reduction mammoplasty specimens. After a median follow-up of 61 months, 15 patients (17%) were found to have subsequent intraductal or invasive carcinoma in the ipsilateral breast. Eight invasive, one intraductal, and four combined LCIS–intraductal carcinomas occurred in breasts with prior LCIS. Two subsequent carcinomas in patients with initial LCIS–intraductal carcinoma were of the same type. The median interval to detection of all subsequent carcinomas was 18 months (range, 6–42) and for invasive carcinomas 22.5 months (range, 7–42). The frequency of subsequent carcinomas was significantly higher (12 of 50, 24%) when there were 10 or more lobules with LCIS in the initial biopsy than if fewer than 10 lobules were affected (3 of 38, 8%). Nuclear size also proved to be a significant predictor: subsequent carcinoma in 8 of 26 (31%) with large nuclei and in 7 of 62 (11%) with small nuclei. The median size of invasive carcinomas was 10 mm. Axillary metastases were found in two patients with subsequent invasive carcinoma. At the time of the report, no patient had a systemic recurrence, and no deaths occurred from breast carcinoma. Compared with a reference control population, the frequency of subsequent invasive carcinoma was 11 times greater than expected (95% CI, 4.8–21.7) *Despite careful surveillance, these investigators noted that all eight subsequent invasive carcinomas presented as palpable tumors. The failure of mammography to detect an invasive carcinoma in five of seven women studied was attributed to the youth of the women (35–52 years) at the time of recurrence. These investigators offered no treatment recommendations.*

## LCIS in Needle Core Biopsy

Until recently, follow-up studies of LCIS have consisted of patients who were biopsied for palpable clinical abnormalities in which LCIS was an incidental finding. Although LCIS infrequently causes a mammographic abnormality that leads to biopsy, it may be discovered in biopsies performed for nonpalpable lesions detected by mammography. Little information is available about this latter group. Zurrida et al. reported the follow-up of 157 patients who had LCIS detected in a biopsy performed for a mammographic or palpable lesion (105). The ipsilateral breast was conserved in 135 cases, and no patient had a bilateral mastectomy. After a mean follow-up of 5 years, eight patients had developed invasive carcinoma. Two patients had asynchronous bilateral carcinomas, and six patients had unilateral tumors (two ipsilateral, four contralateral). The observed rate of carcinoma in the ipsilateral breast (4 carcinomas/639 years at risk = 0.00625) was significantly ($p<0.05$) greater than the expected rate (0.98 carcinomas/639 years = 0.00152), resulting in a risk ratio of 4.1 (95% CI, 1.1–10.5). The person-years at risk for carcinomas in either breast was 865, with an expected rate of 0.0015, an observed rate of 0.00925 (8/865), and a risk-ratio of 5.93 (95% CI, 2.6–11.7). Unfortunately, the data were not analyzed in terms of the original indication for biopsy (mammography versus palpable lesion).

A small subset of patients with LCIS have the most florid form of the disease, which results in extreme glandular enlargement, necrosis, and calcification (see figures in front of book). This uncommon manifestation of LCIS can be detected by mammography, and the images may suggest intraductal carcinoma.

The management of a patient with LCIS in a mammographically directed needle core biopsy is a relatively recent concern. Liberman et al. found LCIS as the only neoplastic lesion in 16 (1.2%) of 1,315 consecutive needle core biopsies (106). Other significant proliferative lesions in the core biopsies with LCIS included "radial scar" in three cases and atypical ductal hyperplasia in two cases. Subsequent excision revealed intraductal carcinoma in the region of the LCIS in two cases and infiltrating carcinoma in a third. Florid LCIS involving markedly expanded ducts was present in two core biopsies; subsequent surgery revealed intraductal carcinoma in one case and invasive carcinoma in the other. Atypical duct hyperplasia accompanied LCIS in another core biopsy that was followed by intraductal carcinoma at surgery. These researchers concluded that surgical biopsy should be performed when a core biopsy contains LCIS accompanied by a "high-risk" proliferative lesion, when florid LCIS is present resembling intraductal carcinoma or if there is discordance between histologic and imaging findings.

A larger series of patients with LCIS and atypical lobular hyperplasia diagnosed in needle core biopsies performed for mammographic indications was reported by Lechner et al. (107). This multiinstitutional study of 32,424 biopsies revealed 89 (0.3%) examples of LCIS and 154 (0.5%) instances of atypical lobular hyperplasia. Surgical biopsies were performed on 58 (65%) of the LCIS lesions, yielding the following: invasive lobular carcinoma in 8 (14%), invasive duct carcinoma in 2 (3%), tubular carcinoma in 8 (14%), intraductal carcinoma in 2 (3%), LCIS in 23 (40%), atypical duct hyperplasia in 2 (3%), atypical lobular hyperplasia in 4 (7%) and various benign findings in 8 (14%). Surgical biopsies performed in 84 cases after atypical lobular hyperplasia was diagnosed in a needle core biopsy yielded invasive lobular carcinoma in 2 (2%), invasive duct carcinoma in 3 (4%), intraductal carcinoma in 4 (5%), LCIS in 18 (21%), atypical duct hyperplasia in 18 (21%), atypical lobular hyperplasia in 13 (15%), and various benign findings in 32 (38%).

The foregoing studies provide compelling evidence to in-dicate that surgical biopsy usually should be performed after a needle core biopsy diagnosis of LCIS; this is also appropriate for some patients with atypical lobular hyperplasia. When the surgical specimen does not detect invasive or intraductal carcinoma, the patient may be a candidate for antiestrogen therapy.

The role of mammography as an adjunct to physical examination in the follow-up of LCIS is unresolved. Mammography is able to identify benign lesions such as sclerosing adenosis, which may coexist with LCIS, but it is much less effective for finding LCIS (20). The most important role of mammography in the follow-up of a patient with LCIS is to detect invasive carcinoma or intraductal carcinoma at a stage when they are most amenable to cure. As noted by Ottesen et al., mammography may be less reliable for the follow-up of premenopausal women with dense glandular breasts (104). Ultrasound examination is an important adjunct to mammography in this setting. The role of magnetic resonance imaging in the follow-up of women with LCIS or atypical lobular hyperplasia remains to be determined.

When follow-up is recommended, it must be with the understanding that the patient accepts the responsibilities involved. Medical facilities must be provided for follow-up. An optimum practical schedule for repeated clinical examinations is yet to be devised.

## Mastectomy

Total mastectomy is the preferred operation if a mastectomy is to be performed. This procedure preserves the pectoral musculature and fold, thereby assisting reconstruction. Subcutaneous mastectomy, whether unilateral or bilateral, may leave an appreciable amount of breast tissue, especially if the nipple is preserved, because lobules occur in the nipple (60).

Conclusions regarding bilateral risk have been based largely on retrospective studies described already in which only the breast that harbored LCIS had been biopsied. The status of the opposite breast in these cases was unknown. Bilaterality of LCIS occurs frequently, but it is unproven that it occurs in every patient. Among patients with LCIS in one breast who undergo a contralateral biopsy, about one-third are found to have LCIS in the opposite breast. Biopsy of the opposite breast should be considered before performing a contralateral mastectomy if there are any clinical abnormalities in the other breast. The biopsy should be a substantial one to provide adequate material for histologic examination. Clinical features, genetic predisposition to breast carcinoma, and psychological factors must be weighed before bilateral mastectomy is performed (108).

## Radiation and Chemotherapy

Lobular carcinoma *in situ* that appears histologically unaffected by radiation has been observed in mastectomies from patients with recurrent carcinoma following lumpectomy and irradiation for intraductal or invasive carcinoma. Atrophy of radiated normal lobules is invariably seen in the same specimens. This observation suggests that LCIS is not a radiosensitive disease. No systematic study of radiation therapy for LCIS alone has been undertaken. Cutuli et al. described 17 women with LCIS who received whole-breast radiotherapy between 1980 and 1992 (109). Surgery consisted of quadrantectomy (4 patients) or lumpectomy (13 patients). Two patients also had intraductal carcinoma measuring less than a millimeter. Two patients underwent contralateral mastectomy for infiltrating lobular carcinoma. In addition to biopsy and radiation, 12 patients received tamoxifen. During follow-up with a median of 88 months, one patient developed contralateral infiltrating carcinoma. No recurrences were detected in the ipsilateral breast or at another site.

The presence of LCIS in conjunction with various types of invasive carcinoma does not appear to influence the outcome of patients treated with radiotherapy and breast conservation. Moran and Haffty studied 46 patients who had LCIS associated with invasive carcinoma (110). Invasive lobular carcinoma was present in 27 (59%), and the remaining 19 (41%) had ductal carcinoma. Compared with 973 patients who had invasive ductal or invasive lobular carcinoma without LCIS, there was no statistically significant difference in overall survival, distant disease-free actuarial survival, or breast recurrence-free survival after 5 and 10 years of follow-up. In a subsequent study, Abner et al. also reported that the presence or absence of coexistent LCIS did not significantly influence local control or survival in women with invasive ductal, invasive lobular, or mixed duct–lobular carcinomas (111).

## CONCLUDING COMMENT

It is evident from the foregoing discussion that LCIS is a morphologically and clinically heterogeneous disease. The concept that LCIS is simply a "marker" lesion has been widely promulgated. The impression created by this idea is that LCIS is a proliferative abnormality associated with an increased risk for the development of breast carcinoma; but, in contrast to intraductal carcinoma, LCIS does not progress to invasive carcinoma. This misperception is unfortunate. Data extensively set forth in this chapter and in Chapter 34 on invasive lobular carcinoma document the relationship between the two conditions. It appears that progression to the invasive phenotype is less frequent and that on average takes longer than is the case for intraductal carcinoma. LCIS and intraductal carcinoma coexist in a substantial number of patients. It is not surprising that such patients develop invasive ductal carcinoma more frequently than they develop invasive lobular carcinoma. This phenomenon most likely reflects differences in the rates of progression of the two diseases. The earlier appearance of the invasive ductal lesion results in treatment before the *in situ* lobular lesion has had an opportunity to evolve into invasive lobular carcinoma.

Lobular carcinoma *in situ* is a heterogeneous disease cytologically and structurally. The relationship of these differ-

ences to prognosis or to the risk of progression has not been well characterized. Perhaps the greatest challenge to regarding LCIS as a "marker" lesion has come from the recent recognition of the extremely florid variant of LCIS characterized by marked gland expansion with a tendency to necrosis and calcification. Contrary to the widely held perception that LCIS is not detected by mammography except as an incidental lesion, the florid form of LCIS is likely to manifest with calcifications and a pattern that resembles intraductal carcinoma. The paradigm of LCIS as an incidental "marker" lesion does not fit well with this clinical presentation and the histopathologic findings. Additional study of this lesion is needed, especially with clinical correlation. Based on admittedly anecdotal observations, including a number of instances of coincidental microinvasive lobular carcinoma, it is my opinion that this florid form of LCIS might best be treated as if it were intraductal carcinoma, at least with respect to local control in the conserved breast.

The most fruitful studies of LCIS in the future most likely will involve the investigation of microdissected samples of selected lesions for molecular and genetic changes. The methodologies presently available examine tissues for LOH at specific loci and determine whether there has been a loss or gain in genetic information by comparative genomic hybridization. Substantial information already has been acquired about intraductal carcinoma by this approach, and it is likely to be productive for LCIS. The higher frequency of LOH at 11q13 in LCIS associated with invasive lobular carcinoma than in LCIS alone suggests that detectable differences exist (81). The results of these studies may prove especially useful in view of the current trend to treat LCIS with the antiestrogen tamoxifen and possibly other agents. Further molecular characterization of LCIS is likely to provide a basis in the future for the selective treatment of subgroups of patients with this heterogeneous disease.

## REFERENCES

1. Muir R. The evolution of carcinoma of the mamma. *J Pathol Bacteriol* 1941;52:155–172.
2. Foote FW Jr, Stewart FW. Lobular carcinoma in situ: a rare form of mammary cancer. *Am J Pathol* 1941;17:491–496.
3. Rosen PP. The pathological classification of human mammary carcinoma: past, present and future. *Ann Clin Lab Sci* 1979;9:144–156.
4. Rosen PP. Lobular carcinoma *in situ* and intraductal carcinoma of the breast. In: McDivitt RW, Oberman HA, Ozzello L, et al., eds. *The breast.* Baltimore: Williams & Wilkins, 1984:59–105.
5. Andersen J. Lobular carcinoma *in situ:* a long-term follow-up in 52 cases. *Acta Pathol Microbiol Scand Sect A* 1974;82:519–533.
6. Rosen PP, Lieberman PH, Braun DW Jr, et al. Lobular carcinoma *in situ* of the breast: detailed analysis of 99 patients with average follow-up of 24 years. *Am J Surg Pathol* 1978;2:225–251.
7. Wheeler JE, Enterline HT, Roseman J, et al. Lobular carcinoma *in situ* of the breast: long term follow-up. *Cancer* 1974;34:554–563.
8. Page DL, Kidd TE Jr, Dupont WD, et al. Lobular neoplasia of the breast: higher risk for subsequent invasive cancer predicted by more extensive disease. *Hum Pathol* 1991;22:1232–1239.
9. Haagensen CD. Lobular neoplasia (lobular carcinoma *in situ*) In: *Diseases of the breast*, 3rd ed. Philadelphia: WB Saunders, 1986:192.
10. Nielsen M, Jensen J, Andersen J. Precancerous and cancerous breast lesions during lifetime and at autopsy. *Cancer* 1984;54:612–615.
11. Nielsen M, Thomsen JL, Primdahl L, et al. Breast cancer and atypia

among young and middle-aged women: a study of 110 medicolegal autopsies. *Br J Cancer* 1987;56:814–819.

12. Alpers CE, Wellings SR. The prevalence of carcinoma *in situ* in normal and cancer associated breasts. *Hum Pathol* 1985;16:796–807.

13. Frantz VK, Pickren JW, Melcher GW, et al. Incidence of chronic cystic disease in so-called normal breasts: a study based on 225 postmortem examinations. *Cancer* 1951;4:762–783.

14. Kramer WM, Rush BF Jr. Mammary duct proliferation in the elderly. *Cancer* 1973;31:130–137.

15. Mackarem G, Yacoub LK, Lee AKC, et al. Effects of screening on detection of lobular carcinoma *in situ* of the breast: nonspecificity of mammography and physical examination. *Breast Disease* 1994;7: 339–345.

16. Morris DM, Walker AP, Cocker DC. Lack of efficacy of xeromammography in preoperatively detecting lobular carcinoma *in situ* of the breast. *Breast Cancer Res Treat* 1982;1:365–368.

17. Beahrs O, Shapiro S, Smart C. Report of the working group to review the National Cancer Institute—American Cancer Society Breast Cancer Demonstration Projects. *J Natl Cancer Inst* 1979;62:640–708.

18. Rosen PP. Columnar cell hyperplasia is associated with lobular carcinoma *in situ* and tubular carcinoma. *Am J Surg Pathol* 1999;23:1561.

19. Hermann G, Keller R, Tartter P, et al. Lobular carcinoma *in situ* as nonpalpable breast lesion: mammographic features and pathologic correlation. *Breast Dis* 1993;6:269–276.

20. Hutter RVP, Snyder RE, Lucas J, et al. Clinical and pathologic correlation with mammographic findings in lobular carcinoma *in situ*. *Cancer* 1969;23:826–839.

21. Pope TL Jr, Fechner RE, Wilhelm MC, et al. Lobular carcinoma *in situ* of the breast: mammographic features. *Radiology* 1988;168:63–66.

21a. Sapino A, Frigerio A, Peterse JL, et al. Mammographically detected in situ lobular carcinomas of the breast. *Virchow Arch* 2000;436: 421–430.

22. Haagensen CD. Lobular carcinoma of the breast: a precancerous lesion? *Clin Obstet Gynecol* 1962;5:1093–1101.

23. Haagensen CD, Lane N, Lattes R. Neoplastic proliferation of the epithelium of the mammary lobules: adenosis, lobular neoplasia and small cell carcinoma. *Surg Clin North Am* 1972;52:497–524.

24. Haagensen CD, Lane N, Lattes R, et al. Lobular neoplasia (so-called lobular carcinoma *in situ*) of the breast. *Cancer* 1978;42:737–769.

25. Gump FE. Lobular carcinoma *in situ*: pathology and treatment. *Surg Clin North Am* 1990;70:873–883.

26. Rosen PP, Senie R, Ashikari R, et al. Age, menstrual status, and exogenous hormone usage in patients with lobular carcinoma *in situ* (LCIS). *Surgery* 1979;85:219–224.

27. Dall'Olmo CA, Ponka JL, Horn RC Jr, et al. Lobular carcinoma *in situ*: are we too radical in its treatment? *Arch Surg* 1975;110:537–542.

28. Lewison EF, Finney GG Jr. Lobular carcinoma *in situ* of the breast. *Surg Gynecol Obstet* 1968;126:1280–1286.

29. Newman W. Lobular carcinoma of the female breast: report of 73 cases. *Ann Surg* 1966;164:305–314.

30. Ackerman BL, Otis C, Stueber K. Lobular carcinoma *in situ* in a 15-year-old girl: a case report and review of the literature. *Plast Reconst Surg* 1994;94:714–718.

31. Rosen PP, Lesser ML, Senie RT, et al. Epidemiology of breast carcinoma IV: age and histologic tumor type. *J Surg Oncol* 1982;19:44–47.

32. Barnes JP. Bilateral lobular carcinoma *in situ* of the breast. Report of two cases. *Texas State J Med* 1959;55:581–584.

33. Newman W. *In situ* lobular carcinoma of the breast. *Ann Surg* 1963;151:591–599.

34. Benfield JR, Jacobson M, Warner NE. *In situ* lobular carcinoma of the breast. *Arch Surg* 1965;91:130–135.

35. Urban JA. Biopsy of the "normal" breast in treating breast cancer. *Surg Clin North Am* 1969;49:291–301.

36. Donegan WL, Perez-Mesa CM. Lobular carcinoma—an indication for elective biopsy of the second breast. *Ann Surg* 1972;176:178–187.

37. Erdreich LS, Asal NR, Hoge AF. Morphologic types of breast cancer: age, bilaterality and family history. *South Med J* 1980;73:28–32.

38. Ringberg A, Palmer B, Linell F. The contralateral breast at reconstructive surgery after breast cancer operation—a histological study. *Breast Cancer Res Treat* 1982;2:151–161.

39. Sunshine JA, Moseley HS, Fletcher WS, et al. Breast carcinoma *in situ*. A retrospective review of 112 cases with minimum 10 year follow-up. *Am J Surg* 1985;150:44–51.

40. Lesser ML, Rosen PP, Kinne DW. Multicentricity and bilaterality in invasive breast carcinoma. *Surgery* 1982;91:234–240.

41. Andersen JA. Multicentric and bilateral appearance of lobular carcinoma *in situ* of the breast. *Acta Pathol Microbiol Scand A* 1974;82:730–734.

42. Farrow JH. Current concepts in the detection and treatment of the earliest of the early breast cancers. *Cancer* 1970;25:458–479.

43. Warner NE. Lobular carcinoma of the breast. *Cancer* 1969;23: 840–846.

44. Shah JP, Rosen PP, Robbins GF. Pitfalls of local excision in the treatment of carcinoma of the breast. *Surg Gynecol Obstet* 1973;136: 721–725.

45. Carter D, Smith AL. Carcinoma *in situ* of the breast. *Cancer* 1977;40:1189–1193.

46. Tulusan AH, Egger H, Schneider ML, et al. A contribution to the natural history of breast cancer. IV. Lobular carcinoma *in situ* and its relation to breast cancer. *Arch Gynecol* 1982;231:219–226.

47. Hutter RVP, Foote FW Jr, Farrow JH. *In situ* lobular carcinoma of the female breast, 1939–1968. In: *Breast cancer, early and late.* Chicago: Year Book Medical Publishers, 1970:201–236.

48. Page DL, Anderson TJ. *Diagnostic histopathology of the breast.* New York: Churchill Livingstone, 1987.

49. Zippel HH, Hematsch HJ, Kunze WP. Morphometric and cytophotometric investigations of lobular neoplasia of the breast with ductal involvement. *J Cancer Res Clin Oncol* 1979;93:265–274.

50. Andersen JA, Vendelhoe ML. Cytoplasmic mucous globules in lobular carcinoma *in situ*: diagnosis and prognosis. *Am J Surg Pathol* 1981;5:251–255.

51. Gad A, Azzopardi JG. Lobular carcinoma of the breast: a special variant of mucin secreting carcinoma. *J Clin Pathol* 1975;28:711–716.

52. Breslow A, Brancaccio ME. Intracellular mucin production by lobular carcinoma cells. *Arch Pathol Lab Med* 1976;100:620–621.

53. Eusebi V, Pich A, Macchiorlatti E, et al. Morphofunctional differentiation in lobular carcinoma of the breast. *Histopathology* 1977;1: 301–314.

54. Salhany KE, Page DL. Fine-needle aspiration of mammary lobular carcinoma *in situ* and atypical lobular hyperplasia. *Am J Clin Pathol* 1989;92:22–26.

55. Barwick K, Kashgarian M, Rosen PP. "Clear cell" change within duct and lobular epithelium of the human breast *Pathol Annu* 1982;17(Part 1):319–328.

56. Eusebi V, Betts C, Haagensen DE, et al. Apocrine differentiation in lobular carcinoma of the breast: a morphologic, immunologic and ultrastructural study. *Hum Pathol* 1984;15:134–140.

57. Andersen JA. Lobular carcinoma *in situ* of the breast with ductal involvement: frequency and possible influence on prognosis. *Acta Pathol Microbiol Scand A* 1974;82:655–662.

58. Fechner RE. Epithelial alterations in extralobular ducts of breasts with lobular carcinoma. *Arch Pathol* 1972;93:164–171.

59. Page DL, Dupont WD, Rogers LW. Ductal involvement by cells of atypical lobular hyperplasia in the breast: a long-term follow-up study of cancer risk. *Hum Pathol* 1988;19:201–207.

60. Rosen PP, Tench W. Lobules in the nipple: frequency and significance for breast cancer treatment. *Pathol Annu* 1985;20(Part 2):317–322.

61. Sgroi D, Koerner FC. Involvement of collagenous spherulosis by lobular carcinoma *in situ*: potential confusion with cribriform ductal carcinoma *in situ*. *Am J Surg Pathol* 1995;19:1366–1370.

62. Coyne J, Hobbs FM, Boggis C, et al. Lobular carcinoma in a mammary hamartoma. *J Clin Pathol* 1992;45:936–937.

63. Fechner RE. Lobular carcinoma *in situ* in sclerosing adenosis. A potential source of confusion with invasive carcinoma. *Am J Surg Pathol* 1981;5:233–239.

64. Oberman HA, Markey BA. Noninvasive carcinoma of the breast presenting in adenosis. *Mod Pathol* 1991;4:31–35.

65. Nemoto T, Castillo N, Tsukada Y, et al. Lobular carcinoma *in situ* with microinvasion. *J Surg Oncol* 1998;67:41–46.

66. Prasad ML, Hyjek E, Giri DD, et al. Double immunolabeling with cytokeratin and smooth-muscle actin in confirming early invasive carcinoma of breast. *Am J Surg Pathol* 1999;23:176–181.

67. Ozzello L. Ultrastructure of intra-epithelial carcinomas of the breast. *Cancer* 1971;28:1508–1515.

68. Tobon H, Price HM. Lobular carcinoma *in situ*: some ultrastructural observations. *Cancer* 1972;30:1082–1091.

69. Bussolati G. Actin-rich (myoepithelial) cells in lobular carcinoma *in situ* of the breast. *Virchows Arch* 1980;32:165–176.

70. Andersen JA. The basement membrane and lobular carcinoma *in situ* of the breast: a light microscopical study. *Acta Pathol Microbiol Scand A* 1975;83:245–250.

71. Rudas M, Neumayer R, Gnant MF, et al. p53 protein expression, cell proliferation and steroid hormone receptors in ductal and lobular *in situ* carcinomas of the breast. *Eur J Cancer* 1997;33:39–44.

72. Bur ME, Zimarowski MJ, Schnitt SJ, et al. Estrogen receptor immunohistochemistry in carcinoma *in situ* of the breast. *Cancer* 1992;69:1174–1181.

73. Pallis L, Wilking N, Cedermark B, et al. Receptors for estrogen and progesterone in breast carcinoma *in situ*. *Anticancer Res* 1992;12:2113–2115.

74. Ramachandra S, Machin L, Ashley S, et al. Immunohistochemical distribution of c-erbB-2 in *in situ* breast carcinoma—a detailed morphological analysis. *J Pathol* 1990;161:7–14.

75. Somerville JE, Clarke LA, Biggart JD. c-erbB-2 overexpression and histological type of *in situ* and invasive breast carcinoma. *J Clin Pathol* 1992;45:16–20.

76. Vos CB, Cleton-Jansen AM, Berx G, et al. E-cadherin inactivation in lobular carcinoma *in situ* of the breast: an early event in tumorigenesis. *Br J Cancer* 1997;76:1131–1133.

77. Moll R, Mitze M, Frixen UH, et al. Differential loss of E-cadherin expression in infiltrating ductal and lobular breast carcinomas. *Am J Pathol* 1993;143:1731–1742.

77a. Rahman N, Stone JG, Coleman G, et al. Lobular carcinoma in situ of the breast is not caused by constitutional mutations in the E-cadherin gene. *Br J Cancer* 2000;82:568–570.

78. Acs G, Lawton TJ, Livolsi VA, et al. Differential expression of E-cadherin in ductal and lobular carcinoma of the breast. *Mod Pathol* 2000;13:17A.

79. Ioffe O, Silverberg SG, Simsir A. Lobular lesions of the breast: immunohistochemical profile and comparison with ductal proliferations. *Mod Pathol* 2000;13:23A.

80. Jacobs TW, Pliss N, Kouria G, et al. Carcinomas in situ (CIS) of the breast with indeterminate features: role of E-cadherin (e-cad) staining in categorization. *Mod Pathol* 2000;13:23A.

81. Nayar R, Zhuang Z, Merino MJ, et al. Loss of heterozygosity on chromosome 11q13 in lobular lesions of the breast using tissue microdissection and polymerase chain reaction. *Hum Pathol* 1996;28:277–282.

82. Helvie MA, Hessler C, Frank TS, et al. Atypical hyperplasia of the breast: mammographic appearance and histologic correlation. *Radiology* 1991;179:759–764.

83. Bodian CA, Perzin KH, Lattes R, et al. Prognostic significance of benign proliferative breast disease. *Cancer* 1993;71:3896–3907.

84. Page DL, Van der Zwaag R, Rogers LW, et al. Relation between component parts of fibrocystic disease complex and breast cancer. *J Natl Cancer Inst* 1978;61:1055–1063.

85. Page DL, Dupont WD, Rogers LW, et al. Atypical hyperplastic lesions of the female breast. A long-term follow-up study. *Cancer* 1985;55:2698–2708.

86. Godwin JT. Chronology of lobular carcinoma of the breast. *Cancer* 1952;5:259–266.

87. Miller HW Jr, Kay S. Infiltrating lobular carcinoma of the female mammary gland. *Surg Gynecol Obstet* 1956;102:661–667.

88. Giordano JM, Klopp CT. Lobular carcinoma *in situ:* incidence and treatment. *Cancer* 1973;31:105–109.

89. Carson W, Sanchez-Forgach E, Stomper P, et al. Lobular carcinoma *in situ:* observation without surgery as an appropriate therapy. *Ann Surg Oncol* 1994;1:141–146.

90. Singletary SE. Lobular carcinoma *in situ* of the breast: a 31-year experience at the University of Texas M.D. Anderson Cancer Center. *Breast Dis* 1994;7:157–163.

91. Harvey DG, Fechner RE. Atypical lobular and papillary lesions of the breast: a follow-up study of 30 cases. *South Med J* 1978;71:361–364.

92. Bodian CA, Perzin KH, Lattes R. Lobular neoplasia. Long term risk of breast cancer and relation to other factors. *Cancer* 1996;78:1024–1034.

93. Rosen PP, Senie R, Schottenfeld D, et al. Noninvasive breast carcinoma: frequency of unsuspected invasion and implication for treatment. *Ann Surg* 1979;189:98–103.

94. Rosen PP. Axillary lymph node metastases in patients with occult non-invasive breast carcinoma. *Cancer* 1980;46:1298–1306.

95. Fisher B, Costantino JP, Wickerham DL, et al. Tamoxifen for prevention of breast cancer: report of the National Surgical Adjuvant Breast and Bowel Project P-1 Study. *J Natl Cancer Inst* 1998;90:1371–1388.

96. Baum M, Brinkley DM, Dossett JA, et al. Control trial of tamoxifen and adjuvant agent in management of early breast cancer. *Lancet* 1983;1:257–269.

97. Nayfield SG, Karp JE, Ford LG, et al. Potential role of tamoxifen in prevention of breast cancer. *J Natl Cancer Inst* 1991;83:1450–1459.

98. Rutqvist LE, Cedermark B, Glas U, et al. Contralateral primary tumors in breast cancer patients in a randomized trial of adjuvant tamoxifen therapy. *J Natl Cancer Inst* 1991;83:1299–1306.

99. Powles TJ, Hardy JR, Ashley SE, et al. Chemoprevention of breast cancer. *Breast Cancer Res Treat* 1989;14:23–31.

100. Smart CR, Myers MH, Gloeckler LA. Implications from SEER data on breast cancer management. *Cancer* 1978;41:787–789.

101. Rosen PP, Saigo PE, Braun DW Jr. Predictors of recurrence in Stage I (T1N0M0) breast carcinoma. *Ann Surg* 1981;193:15–31.

102. Ciatto S, Cataliotti C, Cardona G, et al. Risk of infiltrating breast cancer subsequent to lobular carcinoma *in situ*. *Tumori* 1992;78:244–246.

103. Fisher ER, Costantino J, Fisher B, et al., for the National Surgical Adjuvant Breast and Bowel Project Collaborating Investigators. Pathologic findings from the National Surgical Adjuvant Breast Project (NSABP) Protocol B-17: five-year observations concerning lobular carcinoma *in situ*. *Cancer* 1996;78:1403–1416.

104. Ottesen GL, Graversen HP, Blichert-Toft M, et al. Lobular carcinoma *in situ* of the female breast: short-term results of a prospective nationwide study. *Am J Surg Pathol* 1993;17:14–21.

105. Zurrida S, Bartoli C, Galimberti V, et al. Interpretation of the risk associated with the unexpected finding of lobular carcinoma *in situ*. *Ann Surg Oncol* 1996;3:57–61.

106. Liberman L, Sama M, Susnik B, et al. Lobular carcinoma *in situ* at percutaneous breast biopsy: surgical biopsy findings. *AJR Am J Roentgenol* 1999;173:291–299.

107. Lechner MD, Park SL, Jackman RJ, et al. Lobular carcinoma *in situ* and atypical lobular hyperplasia at percutaneous biopsy with surgical correlation: a multi-instiutitonal study. *Radiology* 1999;213:106.

108. Osborne MP, Borgen PI. Atypical ductal and lobular hyperplasia and breast cancer risk. *Surg Oncol Clin N Am* 1993;2:1–11.

109. Cutuli B, Jaeck D, Renaud R, et al. Lobular carcinoma *in situ* of the breast: results of a radiosurgical conservative treatment. *Oncol Rep* 1998;5:1531–1533.

110. Moran M, Haffty BG. Lobular carcinoma *in situ* as a component of breast cancer: the long-term outcome in patients treated with breast-conservation therapy. *Int J Radiat Oncol Biol Phys* 1998;40:353–358.

111. Abner AL, Connolly JL, Recht A, et al. The relation between the presence and extent of lobular carcinoma *in situ* and the risk of local recurrence for patients with infiltrating carcinoma of the breast treated with conservative surgery and radiation therapy. *Cancer* 2000;88:1072–1077.

# CHAPTER 34

# Invasive Lobular Carcinoma

The term *lobular carcinoma* became fully established in 1941 with the publication of the classic paper on lobular carcinoma *in situ* (LCIS) by Foote and Stewart (1). They stated that ". . . when the tumor infiltrates, it is apt to do so in a peculiar fashion which permits one, after some experience, to recognize the high probability of such origin." An associated desmoplastic stromal reaction, linear arrangement of the carcinoma cells and their tendency to grow in a circumferential fashion around ducts and lobules (targetoid growth) were "peculiar" diagnostic features emphasized by Foote and Stewart. They also observed that although concurrent LCIS carcinoma was not found in every case, the histologic pattern was distinctive enough to be considered a specific histologic type of invasive carcinoma that arose from the lobular and terminal duct epithelium.

When the diagnosis is based strictly on the criteria of Foote and Stewart, invasive lobular carcinoma usually constitutes 5% or less of carcinomas in most series. Newman reviewed 1,396 carcinomas treated over a 17-year period and found that 5% could be classified as invasive lobular carcinoma (2). A review of more than 4,000 carcinomas treated at the Mayo Clinic revealed that 3.2% were invasive lobular carcinomas (3). An analysis of more than 21,000 breast carcinomas diagnosed in the United States from 1969 to 1971 found 3% classified as infiltrating lobular (4). A review of 362 carcinomas in a study from Japan yielded 21 (5.8%) invasive lobular carcinomas (5). As less restrictive diagnostic criteria have been advocated, the frequency of invasive lobular carcinoma reportedly has been as high as 10% to 14% of invasive carcinomas (6–8). A review of population-based cancer registry data from the United States found that the incidence rates of invasive lobular carcinoma increased steadily after 1977, whereas the incidence rates for ductal carcinoma have remained level since 1987 (8a). The increased incidence of invasive lobular carcinoma was limited to women older than 50 years.

## CLINICAL FEATURES

Invasive lobular carcinoma occurs throughout virtually the entire age range of breast carcinoma in adult women (age range, 28–86 years). Most studies placed the median age at diagnosis between 45 and 56 years (2,3,6,9–12). At the extremes of the age distribution of breast carcinoma (13), invasive lobular carcinoma is relatively more common among women older than 75 years (11%) than in women 35 years or younger. In an analysis of the age distribution of patients with various types of breast carcinoma, the mean ages of women with invasive lobular and invasive duct carcinoma were both 57 years (14).

Differences have been reported in the age distributions of the classic and variant forms of invasive lobular carcinoma. Three studies found that patients with classic invasive lobular carcinoma tended to be younger than those with variant types of invasive lobular carcinoma (5,6,10). A fourth study reported that patients with variant tumors had a lower median age at diagnosis (47 years) than those with classic lesions (53 years) (12).

An exceptional case of invasive lobular carcinoma occurring in a woman seropositive for human immunodeficiency virus (HIV) has been described (15). In this case report, tumor progression was observed despite a CD4 count greater than 500/mm$^3$. Other case reports of breast carcinoma in HIV-positive women have described a variety of histologic tumor types. The evidence for an association between tumor type, clinical course, and immunodeficiency in these patients is inconclusive (16–18).

The presenting symptom in most cases is a mass with ill-defined margins, but in some cases, the only evidence of the neoplasm is vague thickening or fine, diffuse nodularity. Large lesions are more likely to cause skin retraction or fixation, but these signs can be encountered with small superficial tumors. Paget's disease of the nipple ordinarily is not caused by invasive lobular carcinoma, but it can develop secondarily when a centrally located tumor extends directly to the epidermis of the nipple.

Invasive lobular carcinoma is not prone to form calcifications, but calcifications may be present coincidentally in benign proliferative lesions such as sclerosing adenosis (19) or when there is florid LCIS in ducts with necrosis and calcification. Several investigators reported a lower frequency of calcifications detected by mammography in invasive lobular carcinomas than in duct carcinomas (20–23). In a screening situation, invasive lobular carcinoma was more likely to be diagnosed during intervals between examinations than by the actual screening examination (24). The mammographic estimate of tumor size tends to be less than the grossly measured size in a significant proportion of cases (25) and magnetic resonance imaging (MRI) has been helpful for determining tumor size in these patients (26). Rodenko et al. found that MRI was more effective than mammography for determining the extent of the primary invasive lobular carcinoma in a significant proportion of cases, but the presence of metastatic carcinoma in axillary lymph nodes was not detected in four cases that were examined (27).

In some cases, invasive lobular carcinoma has been associated with a decrease in breast size on mammography, although no change in size was perceived clinically (28). On clinical examination, these patients tend to have thickening rather than a discrete mass. These findings correspond to diffuse invasive carcinoma in the breast.

On sonography, 60.5% of invasive lobular carcinomas produced "a heterogeneous hypoechoic mass with angular or ill-defined margins and posterior acoustic shadowing" (29). The remaining tumors had various other sonographic characteristics, including 12% that were "sonographically invisible." The sensitivity of sonography for tumors measuring less than 1 cm was 85.7%. Classic invasive lobular carcinoma tended to produce "focal shadowing without a discrete mass," whereas tumors with pleomorphic histology were seen as "a shadowing mass." Tumors of the alveolar, solid, and signet-ring variety most often were manifested as a "lobulated, well circumscribed mass" (29). Ultrasonography has been useful for detecting multifocal and multicentric invasive lobular carcinoma (30), and in one study it was more accurate than mammography for predicting tumor size (31).

A comparison between mammograms of invasive lobular and other types of carcinoma revealed that lobular carcinomas more often are spiculated and more often are associated with retraction of the nipple or skin (22,32). The most common mammographic manifestations of invasive lobular carcinoma were asymmetric, ill-defined, or irregular, spiculated masses (20,22,33). Carcinomas with mixed lobular and duct features tended to have mammographic features intermediate between the groups. In one study, 46% of mammograms from patients who ultimately proved to have invasive lobular carcinoma initially were reported to be negative (21), but others reported that mammograms were negative in 7% of cases (32). The absence of well-defined margins, and in some cases, a tendency to form multiple small nodules throughout the breast are features that may hinder the radiologic detection of invasive lobular carcinoma and may lead to a false-negative diagnosis. Patients with a spiculated mass are less likely to have residual carcinoma when reexcision is performed than are those with ill-defined or asymmetric lesions (33).

Mendelson et al. described five mammographic patterns that they found associated with invasive lobular carcinoma (19). These included asymmetric density without defined margins, dense spiculated mass, dense breast without a distinct tumor, microcalcifications, and a discrete round mass. Asymmetric, ill-defined density was the most common pattern. It was concluded that invasive lobular carcinoma did not produce a specific or characteristic mammographic appearance. Mitnick et al. did not find a significant difference in average tumor size among lesions with differing mammographic appearances (32). The average size of the tumors was 1.2 cm. Invasive lobular carcinomas were relatively more frequent among interval carcinomas recorded in a breast cancer screening program than in the screening-detected group (34). Retrospective analysis revealed that a disproportionate number of these lesions had been "missed" in the screening process.

Patients with invasive lobular carcinoma are generally considered to have a relatively high frequency of bilateral carcinoma compared with women who have other types of carcinoma (35). The reported relative risk for contralateral carcinoma in women with invasive lobular carcinoma compared with that of women with breast carcinoma generally or women with ductal carcinoma alone ranged from 1.6 [95% confidence interval (CI), 0.7–3.6] to 2.0 (95% CI, 0.8–8.4) in three studies (35–38). The wide range of overall bilaterality that has been described (6%–47%) has been influenced by how the data have been tabulated. Prior and concurrent contralateral carcinomas were present in 6% to 28% of cases (2,3,10,11,39–41). The reported incidence of subsequent contralateral carcinoma ranges from 1.0 (39,42) to 2.38 (43) per 100 women per year, or 0.7% per patient-year of follow-up (44). Lee et al. estimated the frequency of subsequent contralateral carcinoma to be 10% after 10 years of follow-up (45). Some evidence has been presented to show that the frequency of bilaterality is higher in patients with classic invasive lobular carcinoma than in patients with variant subtypes (43). Follow-up studies described subsequent contralateral carcinoma in 4% to 14% of patients previously treated for invasive lobular carcinoma (9,39,41). A lobular component was found in the majority of synchronous or metachronous contralateral carcinomas, and at least 50% of these have been invasive (11,39,40,42). Hislop et al. found that patients with stage II infiltrating lobular carcinoma were more likely to develop contralateral carcinoma subsequently than those who have had negative lymph nodes (42). In a retrospective study, Babiera et al. found contralateral carcinoma consisting of LCIS in 3 of 18 (17%) contralateral prophylactic mastectomies and subsequent invasive carcinoma in 3 of 115 (3%) remaining contralateral breasts (46).

In one series, random concurrent contralateral biopsies in 108 patients revealed intraductal carcinoma in 6% and invasive carcinoma in 10% of patients (47). Biopsies performed for clinical indications in an additional 22 cases yielded intraductal carcinoma in 5% and invasive carcinoma in 32%. The probability of detecting contralateral invasive carcinoma was significantly greater in women who had multicentric invasive carcinoma in the ipsilateral breast or if there were ipsilateral lymph node metastases. Substantially different observations were reported by Cody, who compared the results of routine contralateral biopsy in 58 women with invasive lobular and 733 with invasive ductal carcinoma (48). None of the lobular carcinoma patients had invasive contralateral carcinoma, whereas contralateral invasive carcinoma was detected in 13 (1.8%) of the ductal group. Contralateral intraductal carcinoma was found more often in women with ipsilateral lobular (5.2%) than in those with ipsilateral invasive ductal (1.1%) carcinoma.

Early studies suggested that invasive lobular carcinoma was exceptionally estrogen receptor rich (49), but this was not substantiated in a subsequent analysis of a larger group of patients (50). Particularly high levels of estrogen receptor were found in the alveolar variant of invasive lobular carcinoma, with amounts ranging from 336 to 1,495 fmol/mg of cytosol protein (43,51). Most of these lesions also had high levels of progesterone receptors. Immunohistochemical methods have reportedly detected estrogen receptors in most invasive lobular carcinomas, including classic and variant types (52). Heterogeneous immunoreactivity for estrogen receptor can be present. Decreased or absent immunoreactivity for estrogen or progesterone receptors has been reported in pleomorphic invasive lobular carcinoma (52).

## GROSS PATHOLOGY

The size of invasive lobular carcinoma ranges from occult, grossly inapparent lesions of microscopic dimensions to tumors that diffusely involve the entire breast. The median and average sizes of measurable tumors are not significantly different from the dimensions of invasive duct carcinomas.

Typically, invasive lobular carcinoma forms a firm to hard tumor with irregular borders. The edges of the lesion may be appreciated more easily by palpation than by inspection because the margin may blend imperceptibly with the surrounding parenchyma. Cyst formation, hemorrhage, necrosis, or grossly visible calcification in the form of "chalky streaks" are generally not present. Most tumors are gray or white, with a scirrhous or fibrous appearance. Cellular variants of invasive lobular carcinoma are sometimes described as tan.

In some cases, the excised specimen may not be visibly abnormal and only slightly firm to palpation, although substantial involvement by tumor is evident microscopically. This situation was vividly described by Foote and Stewart:

> On some occasions the gross specimens can be quite confusing and misleading. These episodes usually come about at the time of operation when a locally excised specimen of breast tissue is sent in for frozen section diagnosis. Such a specimen may present no distinctly visible lesion and yet contain a palpable area of peculiar induration, the precise limits of which are vague. Such lesions can cause difficulty in frozen section diagnosis. . . After the diagnosis of cancer is made it is well to be prepared for querulousness from the operating surgeon who understandably would like to be op-

erating for something more finite than indistinct induration (53).

Another gross manifestation of invasive lobular carcinoma is the formation of numerous, fine, hard nodules that feel like tiny pebbles or grains of sand in the breast parenchyma. These foci mimic the appearance of sclerosing adenosis grossly and microscopically. Indistinct foci of induration or minute nodules may be the only gross evidence of carcinoma in a contralateral breast biopsy specimen when the opposite breast was deemed not to be affected by clinical examination.

## MICROSCOPIC PATHOLOGY

Foote and Stewart summarized their definition of the microscopic characteristics of invasive lobular carcinoma 5 years after they commented on the lesion in their paper on LCIS. On this second occasion, they emphasized the following:

> The infiltrating portions of lobular carcinoma typically reveal thread-like strands of tumor cells rather loosely dispersed throughout a fibrous stroma. After infiltration has occurred there is no tendency for the cells to simulate atypical lobules. Sheet-like growth is distinctly uncharacteristic. . . . Great cellularity in the primary tumor is unusual but there are occasional cases in which this does occur (53).

At the cytologic level, the tumor cells were described as "small or medium-sized," "rather uniform in their staining properties," and as exhibiting relatively little "irregularity." Because of the small size of the carcinoma cells and the extremely dense cellularity sometimes encountered in lymph node metastases, Foote and Stewart cautioned against mistaking such metastases for lymphoma. They noted that the presence of "central mucoid globules" in the tumor cells was a helpful diagnostic feature (1).

Foote and Stewart's description of invasive lobular carcinoma has been widely accepted as defining the classic pattern of this type of carcinoma, and most subsequent clinicopathologic studies adhere closely to this definition. Newman's study published in 1966 described the first large series of cases (2). After reviewing histologic sections of 142 tumors that had features of invasive lobular carcinoma, he determined that 73 could be regarded as "pure" because they exhibited largely or entirely a "single cell pattern" of growth. He excluded cases in which there was a prominent duct-forming component or the growth pattern was not largely linear.

Several growth patterns may be encountered in lesions classified as classic invasive lobular carcinoma. The tumor cells exhibit a lack of cohesion. The most prominent manifestation of this property in the two-dimensional plane of a histologic section is a tendency to form slender strands of cells arranged in a linear fashion (Figs. 34.1 and 34.2). For the most part, the strands are no more than one or two cells across. Broader bands of cells constitute trabecular invasive lobular carcinoma (Fig. 34.3).

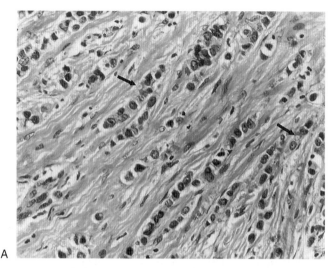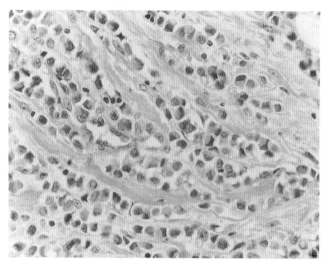

A                                                                                  B

**FIG. 34.1.** *Invasive lobular carcinoma, classic type.* Linear growth and loss of cohesion are illustrated. **A:** Strands of carcinoma one or two cells across are shown. A few cytoplasmic mucin vacuoles are present *(arrows).* (From Rosen PP, Oberman HA. Tumors of the mammary gland. In: *Atlas of tumor pathology.* Washington, DC: Armed Forces Institute of Pathology, 1993, with permission.) **B:** These carcinoma cells have pale cytoplasm, but distinct cytoplasmic vacuoles are not evident.

Some tumors feature a growth pattern in which the tumor cells are arranged around ducts and lobules in a concentric fashion (Figs. 34.4 and 34.5). This distribution can have a bull's eye or "targetoid" appearance. Inflammatory cells distributed around ducts may mimic the targetoid pattern of invasive lobular carcinoma, and this phenomenon can present a notable diagnostic problem, especially in a frozen section or in a needle core biopsy (54).

Invasive lobular carcinoma is accompanied only rarely by a notable lymphocytic reaction (Fig. 34.6). In exceptional cases, an intense lymphoid infiltrate with germinal centers is encountered, which may suggest a diagnosis of coexistent lymphocytic mastopathy (55) (Fig.34.7). A lymphoplasmacytic reaction is found relatively more often in the solid and alveolar variants than in classic invasive lobular carcinoma. Granulomatous inflammation is unusual in invasive lobular

carcinoma (Fig. 34.8). An infiltrating lobular carcinoma with marked lymphocytic reaction was described in a case report as lymphoepithelioma-like carcinoma (55a).

In a minority of cases, the linear strand-forming pattern is not conspicuous, and the tumor cells tend to grow mainly in small dispersed, disorderly foci. This type of invasive growth does not produce a discrete mass and is largely found in patients with little or no gross evidence of invasive carcinoma. The small tumor cells in such occult microinvasive foci may be mistaken for lymphocytes or plasma cells when a section is examined at low magnification (Figs. 34.9 and 34.10). The interlobular stroma should be carefully studied for cryptic foci of invasion in biopsies from patients with LCIS (Figs. 34.10–34.12).

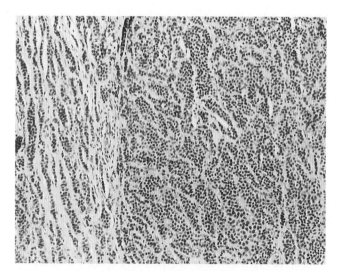

**FIG. 34.3.** *Invasive lobular carcinoma, trabecular type.* The classic structure on the *left* contrasts with the trabecular pattern on the *right.*

**FIG. 34.2.** *Invasive lobular carcinoma, classic type.* The small carcinoma cells are arranged in slender strands.

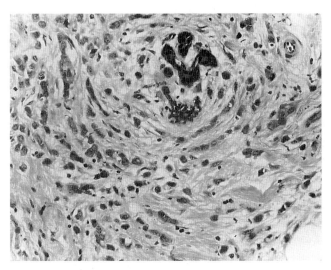

**FIG. 34.4.** *Invasive lobular carcinoma.* Circumferential infiltration around an atrophic lobule is shown.

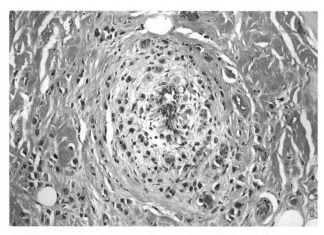

**FIG. 34.5.** *Invasive lobular carcinoma, periductal.* Concentric infiltration around a duct is shown.

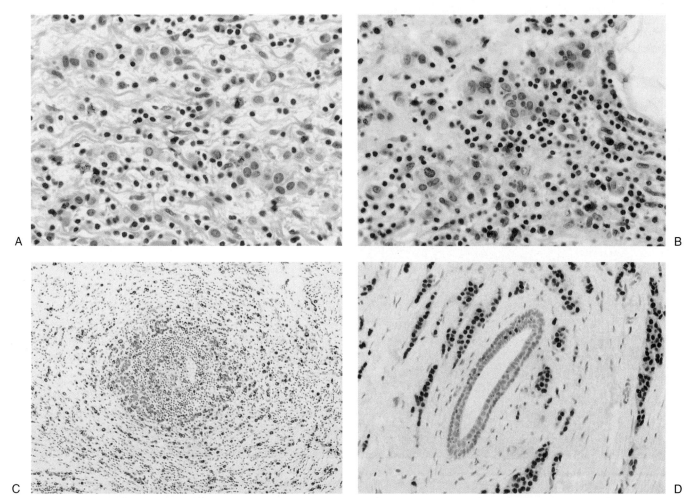

**FIG. 34.6.** *Invasive lobular carcinoma, lymphocytic reaction.* **A:** Carcinoma cells that might be mistaken for histiocytes are distributed among lymphocytes. **B:** Intracytoplasmic mucin within carcinoma cells is stained red with the mucicarmine stain. **C:** The carcinoma cells distributed circumferentially in the lymphocytic reaction around an atrophic duct are highlighted by a cytokeratin immunostain for AE1/AE3 (avidin-biotin). **D:** Nuclear immunoreactivity for estrogen receptor is shown in carcinoma around a duct (avidin-biotin).

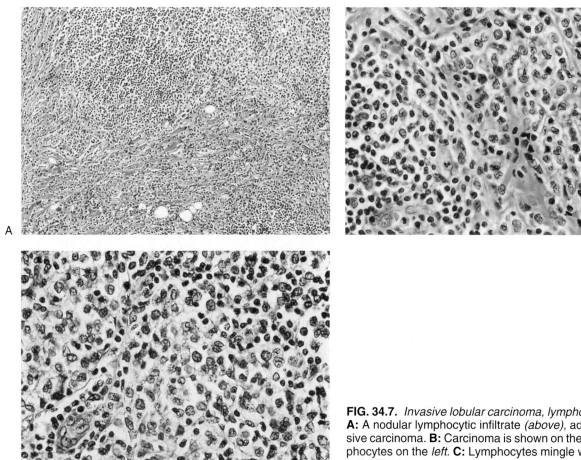

**FIG. 34.7.** *Invasive lobular carcinoma, lymphocytic reaction.* **A:** A nodular lymphocytic infiltrate *(above)*, adjacent to invasive carcinoma. **B:** Carcinoma is shown on the *right* with lymphocytes on the *left*. **C:** Lymphocytes mingle with carcinoma cells. The lymphocytes are only slightly smaller than the carcinoma cells.

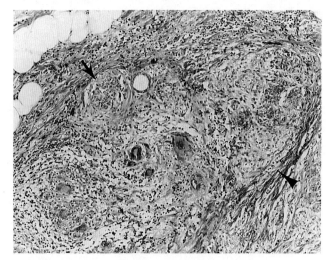

**FIG. 34.8.** *Invasive lobular carcinoma, granulomatous reaction.* Residual lobular carcinoma *in situ* on the left *(arrow)* and invasive lobular carcinoma on the right *(arrowhead)* with intervening granulomatous inflammation.

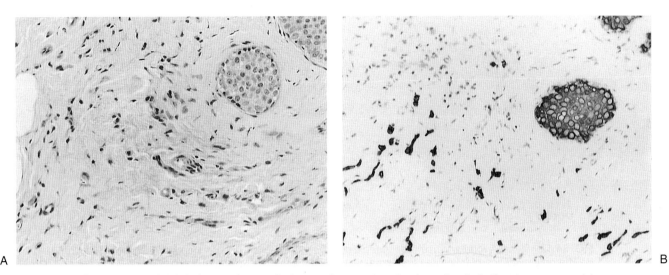

**FIG. 34.9.** *Invasive lobular carcinoma.* **A:** Inconspicuous strands of small cells in the stroma around *in situ* lobular carcinoma. **B:** Invasive carcinoma is highlighted with the cytokeratin immunostain for AE1/AE3 (avidin-biotin).

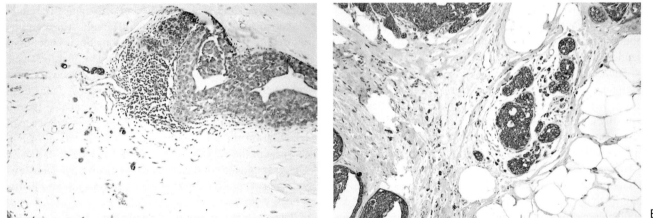

**FIG. 34.10.** *Invasive lobular carcinoma, occult.* **A:** The CK7 cytokeratin immunostain reveals pagetoid *in situ* lobular carcinoma in a duct, focal periductal lymphocytic reaction and a few invasive carcinoma cells in the stroma *(left).* **B:** Invasive lobular carcinoma in the perilobular and interlobular stroma is highlighted with the AE1/AE3 cytokeratin immunostain. *In situ* lobular carcinoma is also present (avidin-biotin).

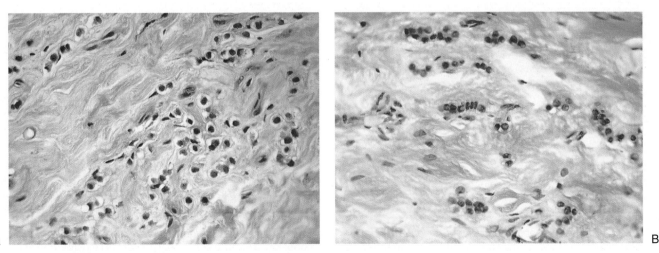

**FIG. 34.11.** *Invasive lobular carcinoma, dispersed.* **A,B:** These ill-defined foci of inconspicuous invasive carcinoma cells can be mistaken for inflammatory cells dispersed in collagenous stroma.

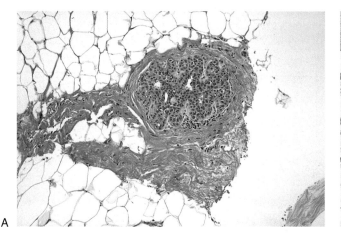
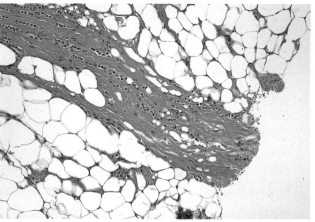

A

B

**FIG. 34.12.** *Invasive lobular carcinoma, needle core biopsy.* **A:** *In situ* lobular carcinoma in a small duct. **B:** The only evidence of invasive carcinoma was this small focus in collagenous stroma near the edge of one core sample.

It is quite unusual to encounter an invasive carcinoma in which 100% of the microscopic fields fulfill the foregoing histologic criteria for classic invasive lobular carcinoma. Many of the tumors composed largely of classic invasive lobular carcinoma have minor components in which the identical cells exhibit other growth patterns. This situation led Richter et al. to limit the diagnosis of invasive lobular carcinoma to tumors in which at least 70% had a "single-file" growth pattern, and this quantitative criterion has been generally accepted (3). The diversity of growth patterns is a factor that contributes to problems in reproducible diagnosis reported with invasive lobular carcinoma (56,57).

Tumors with the cytologic features of invasive lobular carcinoma in which there are substantial elements of nonlinear growth have been referred to as *variant* forms of invasive lobular carcinoma. Trabecular (Fig. 34.3), alveolar (Fig. 34.13), and solid (Fig. 34.14) variants have been described, extending the diagnosis of invasive lobular carcinoma to a

larger group of tumors in the last decade. Fechner described six carcinomas in which the confluent growth pattern, characterized as solid, was composed of cells typically found in classic invasive lobular carcinoma. The cells were "arranged in irregularly shaped solid nests . . . sometimes in continuity with a single file pattern of cytologically identical cells" (12). Sometimes these confluent or solid groups of tumor cells were distributed in circumscribed, rounded masses that could be appreciated not only microscopically but also grossly. No significant differences were observed in age distribution or in tumor size between women with classic and those with the solid variant of invasive lobular carcinoma. Others found the solid pattern in 9 of 22 invasive lobular carcinomas (41%) (58). Coexistent LCIS was detected in 10 of 22 cases (45%).

Twenty-four examples of tubulolobular carcinoma were found among 1,665 tumors in the National Surgical Adjuvant Breast Project (NSABP) series reviewed by Fisher et al.

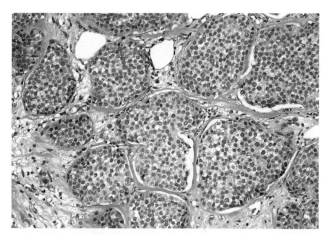
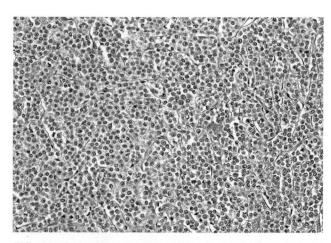

**FIG. 34.13.** *Invasive lobular carcinoma, alveolar type.* Discrete, alveolar groups of carcinoma cells are separated by thin bands of fibrous stroma. The cells have uniform, round central nuclei.

**FIG. 34.14.** *Invasive lobular carcinoma, solid type.* Loss of cohesion, a feature commonly present in invasive lobular carcinoma, is illustrated in this solid area. Slender strands of stroma are present.

(59). These lesions, which constituted 1.4% of the series, were composed of small tubules as well as cords of tumor cells growing in the linear arrangement of classic invasive lobular carcinoma. Because it had many features intermediate between classic invasive lobular and tubular carcinoma, including a less favorable prognosis than tubular carcinoma, these researchers concluded that tubulolobular carcinoma should be regarded as a separate variant of invasive lobular carcinoma. Illustrations and a discussion of tubuolobular carcinoma can be found in Chapter 15.

Trabecular and alveolar variants of invasive lobular carcinoma were described in 1979 (7). The definition of the trabecular structure provided is unclear, and these researchers stated that "there is a wide overlap between the Indian-file appearance and the one-cell-thick trabeculae." About 50% of tumors had trabeculae of one cell thickness, whereas only 10% had trabeculae of three cell thickness. To be meaningful, the term probably should be restricted to tumors with prominent bands two or more cells broad. Usually, the trabecular pattern is found in association with other variants, and the tumors are classified as *mixed*. The alveolar pattern was defined as "a more-or-less globular aggregate of 20 or more cells, as seen in two planes, the cells being similar to those seen in other parts of the tumour" (7). The fact that many examples of classic invasive lobular carcinoma have minor components of alveolar, tubular, trabecular, or solid growth is evidence that supports classifying neoplasms that express these features more prominently as variants of invasive lobular carcinoma.

A major problem in attempts to define and compare the so-called variant forms of invasive lobular carcinoma has been the rarity of this entire group of tumors and the relatively small numbers of the several variant lesions. A series of 230 patients with stage I and II invasive lobular carcinoma included 176 women with classic lesions and 54 (23%) with variant growth patterns (10). Except for a younger age at diagnosis of classic invasive lobular carcinoma, no clinical differences were found when patients with classic and variant lesions were compared. Women with classic invasive lobular carcinoma had significantly more frequent ductular extension and exhibited a stronger trend to multicentricity manifested by greater frequencies of bilaterality as well as gross and microscopic multifocality.

The reported frequency of finding LCIS in association with invasive lobular carcinoma of the classic type varies considerably. Newman found LCIS in 72 of 73 (98%) cases (2). DiCostanzo et al. detected LCIS associated with 65% of 176 examples of classic invasive lobular carcinoma and in 57% of 54 variant tumors (10). In other smaller series of classic invasive lobular carcinoma, an LCIS component was found in 31% (60), 45% (58), and 87% (6) of the cases. In the latter series, proliferative lesions described as atypical lobular hyperplasia and LCIS were grouped together. These investigators also reported finding LCIS in association with 56% of 72 variant types of invasive lobular carcinoma (6). Martinez and Azzopardi studied 38 invasive lobular carcino-

mas, including lesions characterized as tubular and solid variants (7). LCIS was present in 86% of the specimens.

The cytology of cells that constitute invasive lobular carcinoma has received considerable attention. All the cytologic appearances found in LCIS also may be present in invasive lobular carcinoma. Classic invasive lobular carcinoma consists of small, uniform cells with round nuclei and inconspicuous nucleoli. A variable proportion of cells have intracytoplasmic lumina containing sialomucins demonstrable with the mucicarmine and Alcian blue stains (61,62) (Fig. 34.15). When the secretion is prominent, the cells have a signet-ring configuration (Figs. 34.15 and 34.16). With the aforementioned stains, it is often possible to demonstrate small amounts of secretion in non–signet-ring cells. Most so-called signet-ring cell carcinomas are forms of invasive lobular carcinoma (8,10,61–64), but similar cells also are found in invasive duct carcinomas (65–67).

Some invasive lobular carcinomas consist entirely or in part of cells larger than classic invasive lobular carcinoma with relatively abundant, eosinophilic cytoplasm (Fig.

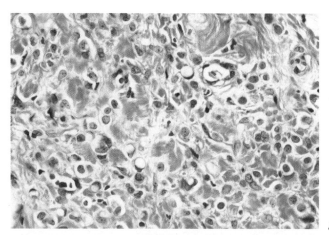

A

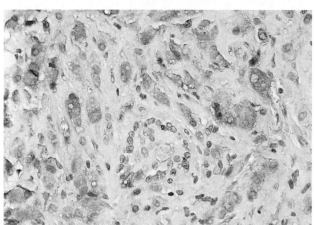

B

**FIG. 34.15.** *Invasive lobular carcinoma with mucin secretion.* **A:** Some of the carcinoma cells have large cytoplasmic vacuoles. **B:** The mucin is stained red with the mucicarmine stain. The carcinoma cells are distributed concentrically around a duct (avidin-biotin).

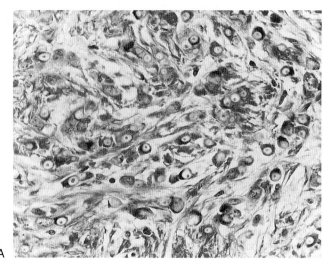 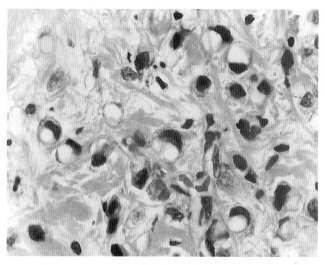

A                                                                                    B

**FIG. 34.16.** *Invasive lobular carcinoma, signet-ring cells.* **A:** Many of the cytoplasmic vacuoles contain dots of condensed secretion. **B:** Signet-ring cells with eccentric, semilunar nuclei and transparent cytoplasmic vacuoles. (**B**, From Rosen PP, Oberman HA. Tumors of the mammary gland. In: *Atlas of tumor pathology.* Washington, DC: Armed Forces Institute of Pathology, 1993, with permission.)

34.17). The nucleus in some examples is pleomorphic, hyperchromatic, and eccentric with a distinct nucleolus creating a plasmacytoid appearance (Fig. 34.18). These cells have been referred to variously as *myoid* (10), *histiocytoid* (68–70), and *pleomorphic lobular carcinoma* (71,72) (Figs. 34.18 and 34.19). Eusebi et al. emphasized the presence of apocrine differentiation in pleomorphic invasive lobular carcinoma and concluded that these patients have an especially aggressive clinical course because nine of ten patients in their series developed recurrences (71). Each of these nine patients had nodal metastases at the time of diagnosis. Apocrine differentiation also was noted by other researchers, who

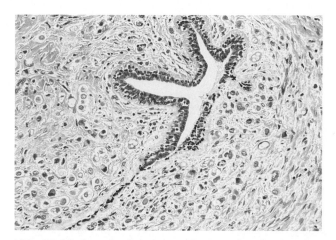

**FIG. 34.17.** *Invasive lobular carcinoma, pleomorphic.* The carcinoma cells with relatively abundant eosinophilic cytoplasm are arranged around a duct in a somewhat haphazard distribution. Cells with cytoplasmic vacuoles are most conspicuous in the *lower left corner.* The carcinoma cells have a "histiocytoid" appearance.

drew attention to transitions between classic and pleomorphic patterns in the *in situ* components (70,73) (see figures in front of book). Pleomorphic invasive lobular carcinomas are immunoreactive for gross cystic disease fluid protein 15 (GCDFP-15), a marker of apocrine differentiation (52,74).

Other evidence that pleomorphic lobular carcinoma is a variant of lobular carcinoma includes pagetoid *in situ* ductal involvement with a "cloverleaf" pattern, the frequent presence of intracytoplasmic mucin, a linear invasive growth pattern, and coexistent classic invasive lobular carcinoma in some instances. It should be borne in mind that an uncommon variant of invasive apocrine duct carcinoma is composed of dispersed pleomorphic tumor cells, sometimes with linear growth that results from distribution of the carcinoma in stroma altered by pseudoangiomatous stromal hyperplasia. Intraductal carcinoma, typically solid with necrosis and lobular extension, is usually present, and there is no *in situ* element with lobular features.

Middleton et al. found *in situ* lobular carcinoma in 25 of 38 (66%) examples of pleomorphic invasive lobular carcinoma, including 17 in which the *in situ* component also had pleomorphic cytology (74a). The frequencies of marker immunoreactivity in the invasive carcinoma were: estrogen receptor, 67%; GCDFP-15, 71%; HER2/*neu*, 81%; p53, 48%.

Perineural invasion is uncommon in invasive lobular carcinoma but may occur when the lesion is extensive (Fig. 34.20). Lymphatic tumor emboli also are rarely found in this type of carcinoma, and in some situations, shrinkage artefacts may simulate carcinoma in lymphatic spaces. True lymphatic tumor emboli usually consist of small clusters of tumor cells or isolated cells.

Morphopoulous et al. studied the extent of angiogenesis in invasive lobular carcinoma by immunohistochemistry using the factor VIII-related antibody (75). Microvessel density

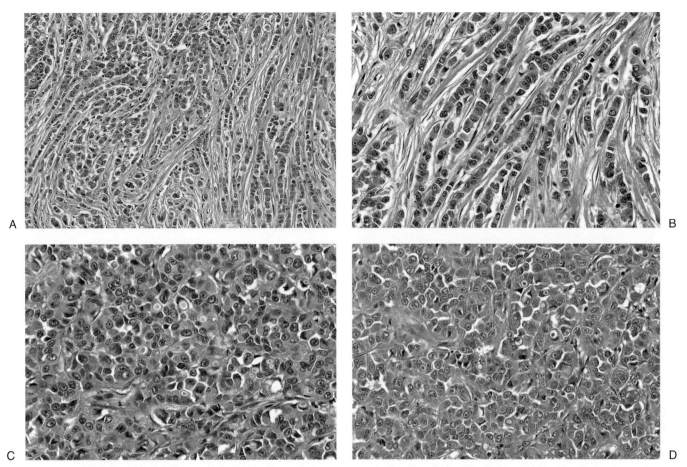

**FIG. 34.18.** *Invasive lobular carcinoma, pleomorphic.* **A,B:** The invasive carcinoma cells have dense, "myoid" cytoplasm and nuclei with punctate nucleoli. Linear growth typical for invasive lobular carcinoma is shown. **C:** Pleomorphic invasive lobular carcinoma with solid growth and signet-ring cells. **D:** Intracytoplasmic mucin is demonstrated by the mucicarmine stain in the tumor shown in **C**.

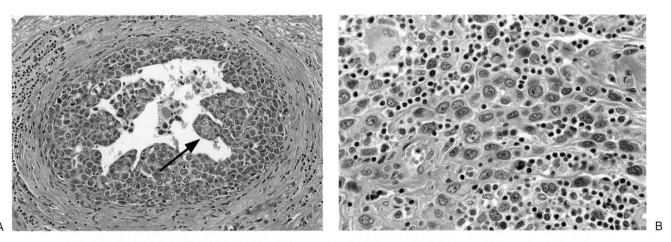

**FIG. 34.19.** *Invasive lobular carcinoma, pleomorphic.* **A:** Pleomorphic lobular carcinoma *in situ* is present in this duct. Some cells have cytoplasmic vacuoles *(arrow).* **B:** Invasive pleomorphic lobular carcinoma accompanied by lymphocytes and multinucleated histiocytes *(upper left).* The tumor cells have a histiocytoid appearance. Both images are from the same specimen.

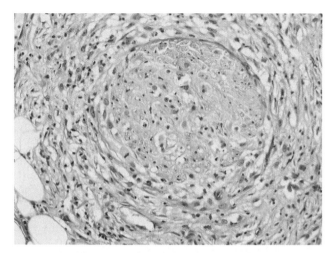

**FIG. 34.20.** *Invasive lobular carcinoma, perineural invasion.* Carcinoma cells are distributed concentrically around and invade a nerve.

was not significantly related to age, menopausal status, tumor size, histologic subtype of the lesion, or lymph node involvement. Microvessel density was not a predictor of overall survival or of relapse-free survival.

## IMMUNOHISTOCHEMISTRY AND HISTOCHEMISTRY

A substantial number of invasive lobular carcinomas have some reactivity for carcinoebryonic antigen (76–78). The intensity of reactivity tends to be correlated with mucin secretion and is most pronounced in tumors with the most prominent signet-ring cell features (Fig. 34.15). Variable reactivity for α-lactalbumin also has been reported in invasive lobular carcinomas, with the proportion of positive tumors varying from 19% to 100% (76,77,79). Casein-positive cells have been found in most lobular carcinomas, but reactivity may be limited to only a few cells (62).

Immunoreactivity for GCDFP-15 occurs in a substantial proportion of invasive lobular carcinomas, predominantly those with pleomorphic and signet-ring cytology (52,71, 80–82). The HER2/*neu* gene product is rarely detected immunohistochemically in classical *in situ* or invasive lobular carcinoma (83), but is present in most invasive pleomorphic lobular carcinomas (74a). Compared with infiltrating duct carcinoma, classic invasive lobular carcinoma is more often cathepsin-D positive, but it is typically negative for p53 protein and vimentin (84). Nuclear reactivity for p53 has been detected in most examples of pleomorphic invasive lobular carcinoma (52).

Immunohistochemical analyses of the expression of epidermal growth factor receptor (EGFR) in invasive lobular carcinoma have not produced consistent results. One report stated that "EGF-R positive cases were much less common in invasive lobular than in invasive duct carcinoma," a difference that was statistically significant (85). Others also reported a lower frequency of EGFR positivity in invasive lob-

ular than in invasive duct carcinoma, but the difference was not statistically significant (86). A third investigation stated that "no significant relationship was observed between EGFR tumor content and . . . histological type" (87).

Grimelius-positive cells have been described in a minority of invasive lobular carcinomas, generally in tumors with a variant growth pattern (76). Chromogranin immunoreactivity has been detected in classic and pleomorphic invasive lobular carcinomas, generally in 5% or less of the tumor cells (52). Dense-core granules of a "neurosecretory" type also have been detected by electron microscopy (76,88). In view of this finding and the coexistence of the two tumor types in some cases, it has been suggested that small cell (oat cell) neuroendocrine carcinoma of the breast may be a variant of invasive lobular carcinoma (89,90) (see Chapter 23).

Immunohistochemical studies of the stroma in invasive lobular carcinoma yielded some interesting observations. Fibronectin is a noncollagenous glycoprotein associated with basement membranes as well as interstitial collagen. Increased fibronectin typically is found in the stroma of most malignant tumors (91,92). Coincidental with a decrease in other basement membrane constituents, such as laminin and type IV collagen, loss of fibronectin also has been observed immediately around tumor cells (93,94). Fibronectin is reportedly strikingly decreased in invasive lobular carcinomas, especially in tumors with the classic growth pattern (93). Fibronectin staining is preserved in basement membranes around the LCIS associated with invasive lobular carcinoma. Because fibronectins have properties that contribute to cell adhesiveness (95), the paucity of this glycoprotein in the stroma of invasive lobular carcinoma may contribute to its linear and dispersed growth pattern.

E-cadherin is an epithelium-specific molecule involved in cell-to-cell adhesion that acts as a tumor invasion-suppressor gene. Compared with invasive duct carcinoma, E-cadherin expression was markedly reduced or absent in invasive lobular carcinomas (96–99a), and there was also loss of reactivity for α-, β-, and γ-catenins (97). In patients with invasive lobular carcinomas, staining for E-cadherin was also absent from LCIS, whereas intraductal carcinoma tended to display strong immunoreactivity for E-cadherin (99) (see figures in front of book). Mutations have been reported in the E-cadherin gene in invasive lobular carcinomas (100,101). In one study, a molecular abnormality was detected in 2 of 20 examples (10%) of invasive lobular carcinoma that were examined. Because only exons 5 through 8 were studied, these investigators could not exclude the possibility of different point mutations in other cases (100). They also found a protein-truncating mutation in an E-cadherin exon in 21 of 32 (66%) invasive lobular carcinomas with loss of immunoreactivity for E-cadherin (102). Loss of heterozygosity (LOH) at 16q22.1, the location coding for the E-cadherin gene, was found with greater frequency in invasive lobular carcinoma than in invasive ductal carcinoma (103).

Immunohistochemical study revealed expression of cyclin D1 in 80% of invasive lobular carcinomas but extremely infrequent immunoreactivity in LCIS (104). Most cells immunoreactive for cyclin-D1 did not stain for Ki67, a protein expressed in proliferating cells. There was no correlation between cyclin-D1 and p27 expression in invasive lobular carcinoma. These observations suggested that cyclin-D1 does not act to accelerate the rate of cell cycling in invasive lobular carcinomas.

## FLOW CYTOMETRY AND MOLECULAR GENETICS

When studied by flow cytometry, classic invasive lobular carcinomas were typically diploid and with a low S-phase fraction, and these factors played a minor role as predictors of prognosis (105,106).

Nayar et al. studied LOH on chromosome 11q13 in invasive lobular carcinomas using the microsatellite markers INT-2 and PYGM (107). LOH was found in 9 of 22 (41%) informative cases. It has been postulated that LOH at the 11q13 region is associated with the loss of one or more tumor suppressor genes, an alteration that could contribute to mammary carcinogenesis.

Nishizaki et al. compared the frequency of genetic alterations in invasive ductal and lobular carcinomas (108). Gains in DNA copy number were significantly lower in lobular carcinomas; however, 79% (15 of 19) of invasive lobular carcinomas had increased copy numbers of 1q; 12 (63%) exhibited loss of 16q. These genetic alterations were not significantly correlated with nodal status or classification as classic or pleomorphic subtype. The frequency of 16q loss was higher in lobular than in ductal carcinomas, but a lower frequency of 8q and 20q gains was found in invasive lobular carcinomas.

The fragile histidine triad (FHIT) gene, a candidate tumor suppressor gene, encodes the FHIT protein (108a). LOH in FHIT was detected more often in invasive ductal carcinomas (59%) than in invasive lobular carcinomas (19%) (108a). Genetic alterations in FHIT were significantly associated with reduced immunohistochemical expression of FHIT in ductal and lobular carcinomas.

## ELECTRON MICROSCOPY

Electron microscopy has yielded variable ultrastructural findings in invasive lobular carcinoma (76,109–111). In some cases, the cells of *in situ* and invasive lobular carcinoma have pale or clear, organelle-poor cytoplasm. Intracytoplasmic lumina are often but not always present. Cells with darker, irregular nuclei and organelle-rich cytoplasm correspond to examples of "myoid" invasive lobular carcinoma. It has been found that neoplastic cells in the alveolar form of invasive lobular carcinoma have organelle-poor cytoplasm with oval, pale nuclei and inconspicuous nucleoli (76,111).

## CYTOLOGY

The diagnosis of invasive lobular carcinoma may be suggested by a fine needle aspirate (FNA) (112,113). The sample is often sparsely cellular, a circumstance that can lead to false-negative reports (114). In one series of 56 patients, only 29 FNAs (52%) from invasive lobular carcinomas yielded diagnostic cytology specimens (115). Ten of the 27 patients with nondiagnostic aspirations were subsequently diagnosed by needle-core biopsy. Similar results were reported by Mitnick et al. in a series of 66 patients with invasive lobular carcinoma who had FNAs performed (32). The cytologic specimens were diagnostic of carcinoma in 27 (41%) and suspicious or atypical in 20 (30%). Negative aspirates were obtained from 19 (28%) patients. The cytologic results were not significantly influenced by tumor size. The same series included 15 patients who had a needle core biopsy that proved to be diagnostic of carcinoma in 13 (87%) and suspicious in another case.

Small cells with scanty, inconspicuous cytoplasm are dispersed singly or in small groups on the slide in a FNA from invasive lobular carcinoma (116). Signet-ring cell forms may be found, but they are conspicuous in a minority of cases. In one study, intracytoplasmic lumina were found in 58% of aspirates from invasive lobular carcinomas (116). Some cytoplasmic lumina contain a central globule of condensed secretion which, if present, helps to distinguish true lumina from nonspecific vacuoles (Fig.34.21) (117). Linear arrays of tumor cells are a characteristic feature in the aspirate from classic invasive lobular carcinoma. The FNA specimen obtained from invasive pleomorphic lobular carcinoma is a "hybrid" between the appearances of lobular and ductal carcinoma (118,118a). The specimens are more cellular than aspirates from classic lobular carcinoma, the cells are larger, and the nuclei are more pleomorphic. A "rosette-like" pattern may be found in the aspirate from the alveolar variant of lobular carcinoma (118). Intranuclear vacuoles are reported to be less frequent in variant forms than in classic invasive lobular carcinoma (119).

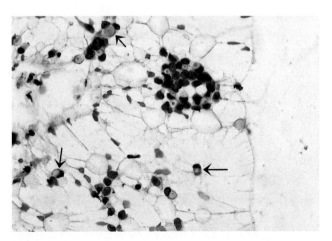

**FIG. 34.21.** *Invasive lobular carcinoma, cytology.* Signet-ring cells with cytoplasmic vacuoles which contain secretion (*arrows*) are shown in this fine needle aspiration specimen from a classic invasive lobular carcinoma.

## PATTERNS OF METASTASES

Invasive lobular carcinoma can metastasize via lymphatics or by hematogenous dissemination. Metastatic deposits of lobular carcinoma tend to duplicate the cytologic features of the primary tumor (Fig. 34.22). On occasion, signet-ring cell formation is more or less conspicuous in metastases than in the primary lesion (120). Axillary lymph node metastases derived from invasive lobular carcinoma of the classic type may be distributed largely in sinusoids, or they may involve sinusoids and lymphoid areas (Fig. 34.23). When lymph node involvement is sparse, the distinction between tumor cells and histiocytes can be difficult. Problems also may be encountered when there are extensive nodal metastases that are limited to sinusoids because the appearance resembles severe sinus histiocytosis. This pattern of metastatic spread has been described as *sinus catarrh*. In this setting, tumor cells are sometimes also distributed individually or in small groups in the lymphoid areas. On occasion, one may encounter lymph nodes in which metastatic lobular carcinoma is concentrated in sinusoids of the hilum.

Reactive changes in histiocytes in the sinusoids of lymph nodes may resemble metastatic lobular carcinoma. Vacuolated histiocytes associated with silicone mastitis resemble signet-ring cells, but ordinarily they are not limited to the sinusoids, and a giant cell reaction is typically present. Signet-ring cell sinus histiocytosis, a rare nonneoplastic reactive change of unknown cause, is especially difficult to distinguish from metastatic lobular carcinoma (Fig. 34.24) (121,122). Signet-ring histiocytes resemble metastatic lobular carcinoma in routine hematoxylin and eosin (H&E) sections, necessitating the use of histochemical and immunohistochemical procedures. Cytoplasmic staining with periodic acid-Schiff that is abolished with diastase and a weakly to moderately positive mucicarmine reaction can be found in signet-ring cell histiocytes. These cells are not immunoreactive with markers associated with epithelial cells such as cytokeratin or GCDFP-15, and they are reactive for histiocytic markers, including lysozyme, CD68, and $\alpha_1$-antitrypsin (121). Electron microscopic examination reveals an open cytoplasmic vacuole or amorphous, electron-dense lipid in signet-ring histiocytes (121). The etiology of signet-ring his-

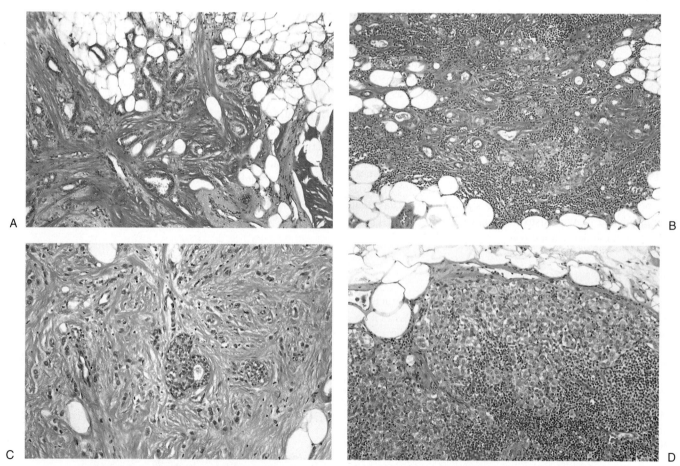

**FIG. 34.22.** *Invasive lobular carcinoma with lymph node metastases.* This patient had separate primary invasive duct and lobular carcinomas in the same breast. **A:** Invasive duct carcinoma, well-differentiated tubular type in the breast. **B:** Metastatic tubular carcinoma in an axillary lymph node and in perinodal fat. **C:** Invasive lobular carcinoma, classic type in the breast. **D:** Metastatic lobular carcinoma fills the subcapsular sinuses in an axillary lymph node.

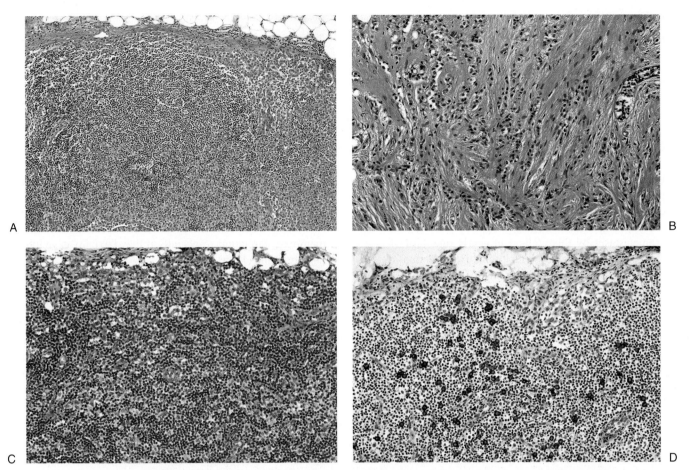

**FIG. 34.23.** *Invasive lobular carcinoma, axillary lymph node metastasis.* **A:** Metastatic carcinoma cells are present in the subcapsular sinuses and in lymphoid tissue. **B–D** are from another patient. **B:** Invasive lobular carcinoma in the breast. **C:** A sentinel lymph node with no apparent metastatic carcinoma. **D:** The same region of the sentinel lymph node in **C** prepared with the CAM5.2 cytokeratin immunostain displays isolated metastatic carcinoma cells (avidin-biotin).

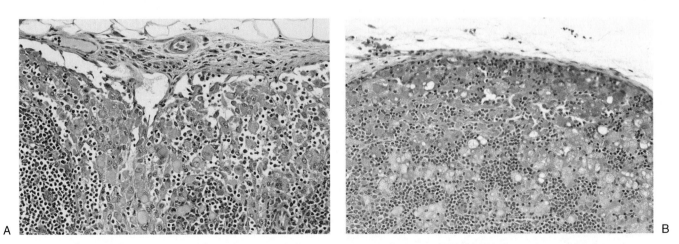

**FIG. 34.24.** *Signet-ring cell histiocytes.* **A:** The subcapsular sinuses are filled with signet-ring cell histiocytes. **B:** The cytoplasm of the histiocytes is tinted pink with the mucicarmine stain, but the cytoplasmic vacuoles are not mucicarminophilic.

tiocytes is uncertain, but most reported patients have had prior surgery involving the chest wall for breast carcinoma or coronary artery disease (121–123). The lipid present in these cells may derive from injury to fat caused by prior operations.

When the presence of metastatic lobular carcinoma in lymph nodes cannot be determined with confidence in routine histologic sections, immunohistochemical studies for cytokeratin can be used to detect inapparent micrometastases. Presently, there is no consensus on the utility of routine immunohistochemical study of lymph nodes from patients with invasive lobular carcinoma for detecting micrometastases, but published data suggest that this is a useful procedure. Some investigators reported finding occult micrometastases by this method in nearly one-third of cases (124,125). Cote et al. used additional H&E sections as well as cytokeratin immunohistochemistry to detect metastatic carcinoma in axillary lymph nodes previously reported as negative in women with invasive lobular carcinoma or mixed invasive lobular and duct carcinoma (126). Occult metastases were found in 39% of 64 cases by immunohistochemistry and in 3% with H&E sections. Presently, cytokeratin immunohistochemistry should be used in the diagnosis of all sentinel lymph nodes and is advisable for all other lymph nodes from patients with invasive lobular carcinoma.

Difficulty in distinguishing metastatic lobular carcinoma

from histiocytes has been described at sites other than lymph nodes (54). Orbital metastases can be mistaken for malinant lymphoma or melanoma (Fig. 34.25). In the eyelid, the lesion may resemble a chalazion (69,127). Isolated tumor cells in the bone marrow can resemble hematopoietic elements (128,128a). A retrospective review of bone marrow core biopsies, all proven to harbor metastatic breast carcinoma by cytokeratin immunohistochemistry, revealed that metastatic lobular carcinoma was correctly identified in routine sections from 39% of these cases (129). In the same study, carcinoma was detected in 58% of bone marrow core biopsies from patients with ductal carcinoma. It is recommended that immunohistochemical cytokeratin studies be included in the routine workup of bone marrow biopsies from patients with mammary carcinoma, especially if they have invasive lobular carcinoma (128a).

Distinctive patterns of systemic metastases also are associated with invasive lobular carcinoma. Investigators have compared the metastatic patterns of duct and lobular carcinoma at autopsy (130) or from clinical records (131). Both approaches revealed statistically significant greater frequencies of metastatic lobular carcinoma in the peritoneum and retroperitoneum, leptomeninges, gastrointestinal tract, and gynecologic organs and a lower frequency of pulmonary or pleural metastases. Bone is a common site of metastases from invasive lobular carcinoma (129,132). In one study,

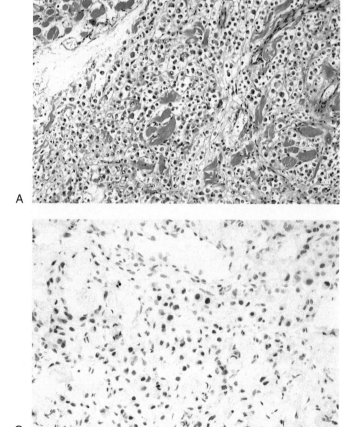

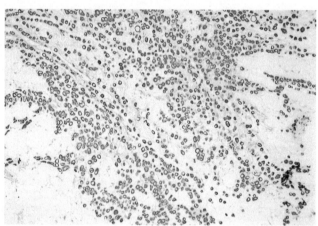

**FIG. 34.25.** *Invasive lobular carcinoma, metastatic.* **A:** Metastatic lobular carcinoma in the muscles of the orbit resembles a histiocytic infiltrate. **B:** The tumor cells are immunoreactive for cytokeratin CK7. **C:** Nuclear immunoreactivity for estrogen receptor is shown (avidin-biotin).

parenchymal metastases in the liver, lungs, and brain were detected less often clinically or at autopsy in patients with invasive lobular carcinoma than in those with invasive duct carcinoma (132). Others reported that hepatic metastases were significantly more frequent with invasive lobular than with invasive duct carcinoma (133), or that there was no significant difference in the frequency of liver metastases (130,131). No significant differences have been found in the distribution of metastases between patients with the classic and variant patterns of invasive lobular carcinoma (10).

Central nervous system involvement usually takes the form of carcinomatous meningitis and consists of diffuse leptomeningeal infiltration (130,132,134,135). Occult carcinoma presenting with symptoms attributable to leptomeningeal metastases has been described (136). Jayson et al. found that 67% of patients with carcinomatous meningitis had lobular or mixed lobular and duct carcinomas (137). The disease had a rapidly progressive course with the median interval of 10.9 months from primary diagnosis to meningeal recurrence. Cerebral infarcts were ascribed to mucin emboli in a patient with invasive lobular carcinoma that had prominent signet-ring cell features (138). Signet-ring cells are typically present in the cerebrospinal fluid when there are meningeal metastases (136).

Intraabdominal metastases tend to involve the serosal surfaces and retroperitoneum (64,130,132,133,139) or ovaries (130,140) (Fig. 34.26). At surgery, exploration sometimes reveals thickening of serosal, mesenteric, and retroperitoneal tissues with no discrete mass. Ureteral obstruction can develop as a consequence of retroperitoneal metastases (135). In other cases, there is diffuse spread to the uterus and ovaries with ovarian enlargement creating the features of Krukenberg's tumor. Computed tomography (CT) scanning has proven especially useful for the detection of abdominal metastases of invasive lobular carcinoma (141,141a).

Metastatic lobular carcinoma in the uterus also can present a challenging diagnostic problem (142). The carcinoma cells

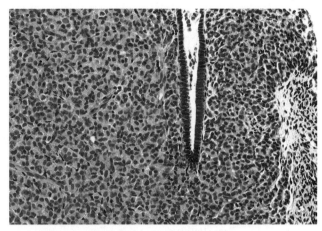

**FIG. 34.27.** *Metastatic lobular carcinoma in the endometrium.* Metastatic lobular carcinoma in the endometrium resembles stromal cells.

blend with normal endometrial stromal cells and may be overlooked in endometrial curettings obtained from a patient with vaginal bleeding (Fig. 34.27). The cells of metastatic lobular carcinoma in the endometrium may be detectable in a cervicovaginal smear (143,144). Liebmann et al. described a patient with a previously unrecognized invasive lobular carcinoma in the breast who had metastatic lobular carcinoma discovered in a uterine leiomyoma (145).

Invasive lobular carcinoma can result in serosal and mural metastases involving the stomach (Fig. 34.28). The clinical and pathologic findings may be indistinguishable from those of a primary gastric carcinoma (120,132,146–148). An immunohistochemical stain for estrogen receptor can be employed in this situation, but a weakly positive result does not rule out gastric carcinoma. Estrogen receptor has been detected in gastric adenocarcinoma by biochemical (149,150) and immunohistochemical (151,152) procedures, largely in Oriental patients. In one study, estrogen receptor was detected significantly more often in poorly differentiated than

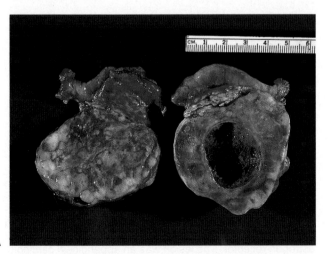

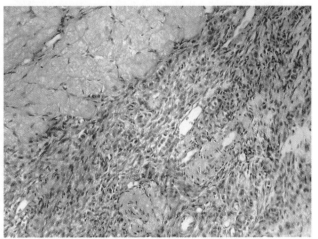

**FIG. 34.26.** *Metastatic lobular carcinoma in the ovary.* **A:** The bisected ovary is diffusely involved by metastatic lobular carcinoma around a cyst. **B:** Carcinoma cells are difficult to recognize in the ovarian stroma next to a corpus albicans.

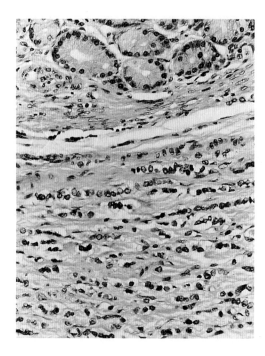

**FIG. 34.28.** *Metastatic lobular carcinoma in the stomach.* Carcinoma in the submucosa has the growth pattern of classic lobular carcinoma.

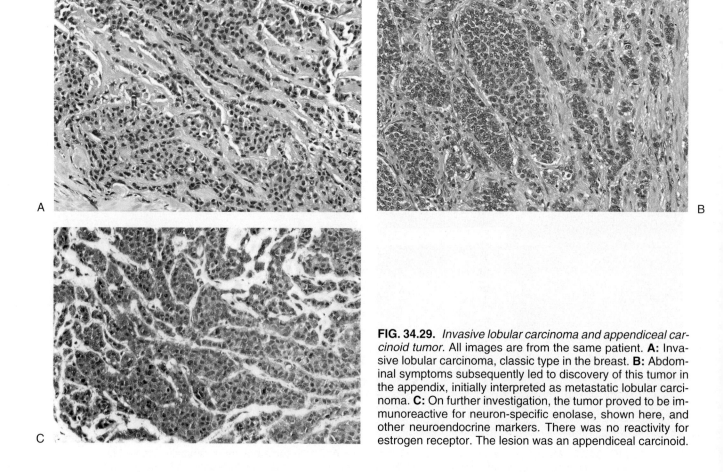

A

B

C

**FIG. 34.29.** *Invasive lobular carcinoma and appendiceal carcinoid tumor.* All images are from the same patient. **A:** Invasive lobular carcinoma, classic type in the breast. **B:** Abdominal symptoms subsequently led to discovery of this tumor in the appendix, initially interpreted as metastatic lobular carcinoma. **C:** On further investigation, the tumor proved to be immunoreactive for neuron-specific enolase, shown here, and other neuroendocrine markers. There was no reactivity for estrogen receptor. The lesion was an appendiceal carcinoid.

in well-differentiated gastric carcinomas, and immunoreactivity was not sex related (152). Chaubert et al. reported that immunoreactivity was absent from gastric carcinoma in European patients (153). Metastatic mammary signet-ring cell carcinoma involving the stomach and other sites is likely to be positive with the antibody to GCDFP-15, whereas primary gastric carcinoma is rarely immunoreactive. Loss of E-cadherin expression has been found in gastric carcinomas, and familial gastric carcinoma has been associated with germ-line mutations of the E-cadherin gene (154). Metastatic lobular carcinoma in the colon may mimic a primary colonic carcinoma (155). The distinction between metastatic lobular carcinoma and some carcinoid tumors can present a challenging diagnostic problem (Fig. 34.29).

## PROGNOSIS AND TREATMENT

Numerous studies reported on the prognosis of patients with invasive lobular carcinoma. Newman's article that described 72 patients with classic invasive lobular carcinoma was the first to provide substantial prognostic data (2). He found that 5 of 36 stage I (14%) and 17 of 37 stage II (46%) patients died of disease, with follow-up averaging nearly 8 years. Ashikari et al. reported 5- and 10-year survivals of 86% and 74%, respectively, for stage I patients with invasive lobular carcinoma not further stratified on the basis of tumor size (9). No significant differences in survival were found when the patients were compared with women treated for invasive ductal carcinoma with similar nodal status.

A few series included enough patients to compare the prognosis of patients with classic and variant types of invasive lobular carcinoma. Dixon et al. studied 103 women with invasive lobular carcinoma (6). Overall, the combined group had a significantly more favorable prognosis than women with invasive duct carcinomas; however, the groups of lobular and ductal carcinoma patients were not matched specifically for stage and treatment and hence may not have been comparable. Dixon et al. also found that patients with classic invasive lobular carcinoma had a more favorable prognosis than those with variant forms of invasive lobular carcinoma (6). Because the patients with classic and variant forms of invasive lobular carcinoma were not stratified by stage, these results may also be misleading. For example, the frequency of stage I cases varied from 33% among those with a mixed histologic pattern to 74% in the group with alveolar variant tumors. Most patients included in the study did not have an axillary dissection.

Analysis of 171 patients with invasive lobular carcinoma by du Toit et al. revealed that women with the classic subtype had a slightly better prognosis than those with alveolar and solid variants (43). The best prognosis, a 12-year actuarial survival of 100%, was observed in patients with tubulolobular carcinoma. Systemic recurrences were found in 44% of patients with classic invasive lobular carcinoma and in 40% to 57% of patients with variant forms. Unfortunately, the results in this study are difficult to assess because patients were not stratified by stage, and they were not treated in a consistent manner. Primary surgery consisted of "simple mastectomy, subcutaneous mastectomy or a lumpectomy followed by whole breast irradiation" and "lymph node status was determined by a triple node biopsy technique" rather than by conventional axillary dissection.

Frost et al. reviewed 92 patients with invasive lobular carcinoma subclassified by histologic growth pattern (156). There was no statistically significant relationship between the type of invasive lobular carcinoma (classic, alveolar, solid, mixed) and prognosis. Variant lesions were similar in regard to age distribution, tumor size, nodal status, and hormone receptor expression.

DiCostanzo et al. studied 230 patients with stage I and II invasive lobular carcinoma treated by mastectomy and axillary dissection (10). They compared 176 women with classic invasive lobular carcinoma with 54 women with variant histologic patterns (10 solid, 14 alveolar, 30 mixed). The classic group was significantly younger at diagnosis (52 vs. 57 years). The groups did not differ significantly in tumor size, nodal status, or TNM stage. Overall survival and recurrence-free survival were similar in the two groups (Fig. 34.30). Although not statistically significant, the survival of stage I and level I node-positive stage II patients with classic invasive lobular carcinoma was better than that of patients with variant tumors of similar stage (Fig. 34.31). Compared with patients with classic invasive lobular carcinoma, each of the variant subsets showed a trend to more frequent recurrence and death from disease, but none of the differences was statistically significant (Fig. 34.32).

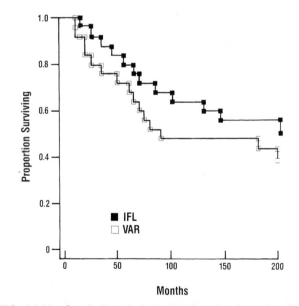

**FIG. 34.30.** *Survival analysis comparing classic and variant forms of invasive lobular carcinoma.* The difference in survival between patients with classic *(IFL)* and variant *(VAR)* forms of carcinoma was not statistically significant. (From DiCostanzo D, Rosen PP, Gareen I, et al. Prognosis in infiltrating lobular carcinoma: an analysis of "classical" and variant tumors. *Am J Surg Pathol* 1990;14:12–23, with permission.)

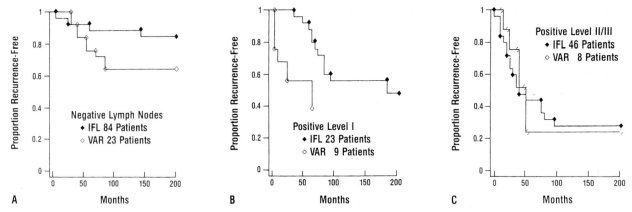

**FIG. 34.31.** *Survival analysis comparing classic invasive lobular carcinoma* (IFL) *with variant forms* (VAR) *stratified by stage.* **A–C:** Although patients with variant forms tend to have a lower recurrence-free survival in each subset, the differences are not statistically significant. (From DiCostanzo D, Rosen PP, Gareen I, et al. Prognosis in infiltrating lobular carcinoma: an analysis of "classical" and variant tumors. *Am J Surg Pathol* 1990;14:12–23, with permission.)

In a further analysis, women with classic invasive lobular carcinoma were compared with a series of patients treated for invasive duct carcinoma, matched for age, tumor size, and nodal status (10) (Fig. 34.33). When stratified by stage, stage I patients with lesions of the classic lobular type had a significantly better recurrence-free survival (Fig. 34.34). No significant difference in survival was found when stage II patients were compared.

Two studies compared patients with pure invasive lobular, mixed duct and lobular, and nonlobular carcinomas. Sastre-Garau et al. reported that patients with invasive lobular carcinoma tended to have larger tumors, but they also had the lowest frequency of nodal metastases (157). The three groups did not differ significantly with respect to overall survival, locoregional control, or distant metastases. Patients with invasive lobular carcinoma had a significantly lower frequency of lung metastases and a higher frequency of bone

metastases. A comparison of the prognosis of patients with invasive lobular and ductal carcinoma by Silverstein et al. revealed a significantly more favorable overall outcome in the lobular carcinoma group (158).

Weidner and Semple found that patients who had the pleomorphic variant of invasive lobular carcinoma had a significantly worse recurrence-free survival than those with classic invasive lobular carcinoma (72). The comparison was based on groups similar with respect to tumor size and nodal status. Analysis of relative risk for recurrence was carried out by comparison with patients with classic invasive lobular carcinoma and negative lymph nodes. The relative risks for recurrence were 4.13 for node-negative pleomorphic carcinoma, 7.35 for node positive classic carcinoma, and 30.4 for node-positive pleomorphic lobular carcinoma. A subsequent comparative study from the same institution revealed a shorter relapse-free survival for patients with pleomorphic

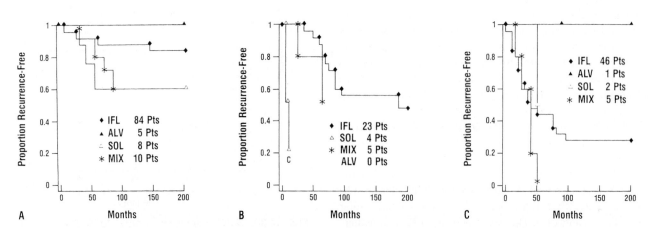

**FIG. 34.32.** *Survival analysis comparing classic invasive lobular carcinoma* (IFL) *with subtypes of variant forms.* The differences are not statistically significant in each stage grouping. **A:** Negative node patients. **B:** Patients with lymph nodes metastases at level I. **C:** Patients with lymph node metastases at levels II/III. *ALV,* alveolar; *SOL,* solid; *MIX,* mixed. (From DiCostanzo D, Rosen PP, Gareen I, et al. Prognosis in infiltrating lobular carcinoma: an analysis of "classical" and variant tumors. *Am J Surg Pathol* 1990;14:12–23, with permission.)

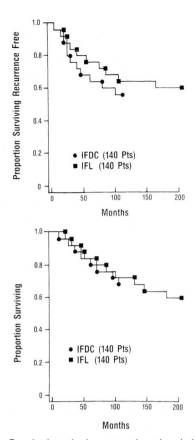

**FIG. 34.33.** *Survival analysis comparing classic invasive lobular carcinoma* (IFL) *and invasive duct carcinoma* (IFDC). Survival and recurrence-free survival were virtually the same for the two groups of patients matched for age and primary tumor stage. (From DiCostanzo D, Rosen PP, Gareen I, et al. Prognosis in infiltrating lobular carcinoma: an analysis of "classical" and variant tumors. *Am J Surg Pathol* 1990; 14:12–23, with permission.)

lobular carcinoma, but no significant difference was found compared with overall survival of patients with classic lobular carcinoma (159). Bentz et al. reported a fatal outcome in 9 of 12 (75%) patients with pleomorphic lobular carcinoma with a median survival of 2.1 years after diagnosis (74). This outcome was significantly worse than for comparison groups of patients with invasive ductal and classic invasive lobular carcinoma.

Compared with classic invasive lobular carcinoma, pleomorphic lobular carcinoma was more often aneuploid with a higher S-phase (160), and the cells had larger nuclear diameters (160), a higher mitotic rate (159), and a higher Ki67 labeling index (159). The two types of lobular carcinoma did not differ significantly with respect to intratumoral vascular density (159).

In summary, various studies of prognosis in patients with invasive lobular carcinoma have not shown a consistent difference from patients with invasive duct carcinoma treated by mastectomy when stage at diagnosis is taken into consideration. Most studies indicated that patients with classic invasive lobular carcinoma had a better prognosis than those

with variant forms as a group, but the differences have not been statistically significant. No reproducible differences in prognosis have been demonstrated among patients with non-pleomorphic variant lesions, and it is evident that large numbers of cases are needed to document significant differences, if they exist.

The most important determinants of prognosis for patients with invasive lobular carcinoma are primary tumor size and nodal status (161). Analysis of more than 15,000 patients in the Colorado Tumor Registry demonstrated that tumor size was the most significant indicator of axillary lymph node status (162). The frequency of axillary lymph node metastases was nearly identical for patients with invasive ductal and lobular carcinomas when stratified by tumor size. Among women with tumors 2 cm or smaller, axillary lymph nodes were positive in 25% with lobular and 27% with ductal carcinomas, and for tumors 0.5 cm or smaller, the frequencies of axillary metastasis were 13% and 12%, respectively (162).

Yeatman et al. reported that mastectomy rather than lumpectomy with breast conservation was performed

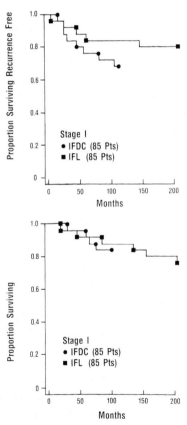

**FIG. 34.34.** *Survival analysis comparing stage I patients with classic invasive lobular carcinoma* (IFL) *and invasive duct carcinoma* (IFDC). The difference between the two groups was statistically significant for recurrence-free survival rate (*p* = 0.02) but not for overall survival rate. (From DiCostanzo D, Rosen PP, Gareen I, et al. Prognosis in infiltrating lobular carcinoma: an analysis of "classical" and variant tumors. *Am J Surg Pathol* 1990;14:12–23, with permission.)

significantly more often in patients with invasive lobular carcinoma than with invasive duct carcinoma (25). Conversion from lumpectomy to mastectomy because of positive margins after reexcision occurred more frequently among patients treated for invasive lobular carcinoma. If a mastectomy is performed, it should be a total mastectomy to minimize the chance of leaving breast tissue at the surgical site. Subcutaneous mastectomy is not appropriate for these patients.

Several reports of treatment by breast conservation with radiotherapy have appeared (33,157,163–168). The data, obtained from nonrandomized studies, indicated that local control and survival for patients with invasive lobular carcinoma treated by breast conservation are similar to the results obtained for duct carcinoma at 5 years of follow-up (169). Most of the available reports do not have comprehensive data for 10 years of follow-up, an important consideration because of the observed trend to later local recurrence of invasive lobular carcinoma in the breast described by some investigators (41).

Warneke et al. analyzed 111 patients treated for stage I–II invasive lobular carcinoma over a 10-year period at the University of Arizona (170). Among 34 (37%) who had lumpectomy with radiotherapy, one (3%) local recurrence occurred, with a mean overall survival of 83.6 months. The remaining 59 patients (63%) underwent modified radical mastectomy, after which there were two (30%) local recurrences. Compared with the lumpectomy and radiotherapy patients, the mastectomy group was characterized by larger clinical tumor size (3.0 cm vs. 1.6 cm), larger pathologic tumor size (2.6 cm vs. 2.1 cm), and more frequent axillary lymph node metastases (44% vs. 27%).

Kurtz et al. found that local failure in the breast after 5 years was more frequent in patients with invasive lobular carcinoma (13.5%) than after treatment of invasive duct carcinoma (8.8%), but the difference was not statistically significant (163). Virtually all recurrences in the breast were at some distance from the primary tumor or were multifocal. The 5-year actuarial survival rates were 100% and 77% for node-negative and node-positive patients, respectively. Schnitt et al. reported that the 5-year actuarial risk for local recurrence was nearly identical for patients with invasive lobular (12%) and ductal carcinomas (11%) (166). The local recurrence rate for invasive lobular carcinoma was greater than the recurrence rate for patients with invasive ductal carcinoma that lacked an extensive intraductal component (5%), but the rate was lower than the 23% recurrence rate encountered for ductal carcinoma with extensive intraductal carcinoma. In this series, all recurrences of invasive lobular carcinoma were in the vicinity of the initial primary tumor. Features of invasive lobular carcinoma associated with higher frequencies of local treatment failure were multifocal invasion in the primary tumor, signet-ring cell cytology, and variant histologic pattern. Because of the high incidence of positive margins in the initial excision for invasive lobular carcinoma, these patients are more likely than those with ductal carcinoma to require a reexcision as part of breast conservation therapy (170a).

Poen et al. studied 60 patients with invasive lobular carcinoma with follow-up of 2.5 to 10 years (mean, 5.5 yrs) after lumpectomy and radiation therapy (165). Two patients had recurrences in local nodal regions, and one developed recurrent carcinoma in the affected breast. The 5-year actuarial locoregional control rate was 95%. During the same interval, 11 patients were found to have distant metastases, leading to death in six cases. White et al. reported 5-year local recurrence rates of 3.3% and 4.2%, respectively, for infiltrating lobular and infiltrating duct carcinoma (33).

Analysis of data from the state of Rhode Island tumor registry for the years 1984 to 1994 included 4,886 women diagnosed and treated for invasive ductal and lobular carcinoma (169). Women with invasive lobular carcinoma had a significantly older mean age at diagnosis (lobular, 64.5 years vs. ductal, 61.6 years) and larger tumor size (lobular, 28.6 mm vs. ductal, 23.9 mm) with a nearly identical frequencies of axillary nodal metastases (lobular, 33.4% vs. ductal, 33.1%). There were no significant differences in 5-year survival (lobular, 68% vs. ductal, 71%), in 5-year local recurrence after breast conservation (lobular, 2.8% vs. ductal, 2.5%), or in the incidence of contralateral carcinoma (lobular, 6.6% vs. ductal, 6.5%).

Routine biopsy of the contralateral breast is not indicated by currently available data for patients with invasive lobular carcinoma (44,48,167). When LCIS is excluded, the overall yield of significant findings from this procedure is not greater than for patients with invasive ductal carcinoma. Contralateral biopsy is appropriate when indicated by mammographic or clinical findings and possibly in patients with a strong family history or other evidence of a genetic predisposition to breast carcinoma. The issue of differences in the long-term risk of bilateral breast carcinoma (metachronous as well as synchronous) between patients with invasive ductal and lobular carcinoma in one breast is unresolved. Data based on patients treated before the use of tamoxifen and other treatments that inhibit the development of contralateral carcinoma may not be directly applicable after the introduction of this and other selective estrogen receptor-modulating drugs.

## REFERENCES

1. Foote Jr FW, Stewart FW. Lobular carcinoma *in situ:* a rare form of mammary cancer. *Am J Pathol* 1941;17:491–496.
2. Newman W. Lobular carcinoma of the female breast: report of 73 cases. *Ann Surg* 1966;164:305–314.
3. Richter GO, Dockerty MB, Clagett OT. Diffuse infiltrating scirrhous carcinoma of the breast: special consideration of the single filing phenomenon. *Cancer* 1967;20:363–370.
4. Henson D, Tarone R. A study of lobular carcinoma of the breast based on the Third National Cancer Survey in the United States of America. *Tumori* 1979;65:133–142.
5. Fu L, Tsuchiya S, Matsuyama I, et al. Clinicopathologic features and incidence of invasive lobular carcinoma in Japanese women. *Pathol Int* 1998;48:348–354.
6. Dixon JM, Anderson TJ, Page DL, et al. Infiltrating lobular carcinoma of the breast. *Histopathology* 1982;6:149–161.
7. Martinez V, Azzopardi JG. Invasive lobular carcinoma of the breast: incidence and variants. *Histopathology* 1979;3:467–488.

8. Steinbrecher JS, Silverberg SG. Signet ring cell carcinoma of the breast. The mucinous variant of infiltrating lobular carcinoma. *Cancer* 1976;37:828–840.

8a.Li CI, Anderson BO, Porter P, et al. Changing incidence rate of invasive lobular breast carcinoma among older women. *Cancer* 2000;88:2561–2568.

9. Ashikari R, Huvos AG, Urban JA, et al. Infiltrating lobular carcinoma of the breast. *Cancer* 1973;31:110–116.

10. DiCostanzo D, Rosen PP, Gareen I, et al. Prognosis in infiltrating lobular carcinoma: an analysis of "classical" and variant tumors. *Am J Surg Pathol* 1990;14:12–23.

11. Fechner RE. Infiltrating lobular carcinoma without lobular carcinoma in situ. *Cancer* 1972;29:1539–1545.

12. Fechner RE. Histologic variants of infiltrating lobular carcinoma of the breast. *Hum Pathol* 1975;6:373–378.

13. Rosen PP, Lesser ML, Kinne DW. Breast carcinoma at the extremes of age: a comparison of patients younger than 35 years and older than 75 years. *J Surg Oncol* 1985;28:90–96.

14. Rosen PP, Lesser ML, Senie RT, et al. Epidemiology of breast carcinoma. IV. Age and histologic tumor type. *J Surg Oncol* 1982;19:44–47.

15. Monti F, Ravaioli A, Tassinari D, et al. Infiltrating lobular breast carcinoma in a woman with HIV infection. *Eur J Cancer* 1998;34:591.

16. Cuvier C, Espie M, Extra JM, et al. Breast cancer and HIV infection: two case reports. *Eur J Cancer* 1997;33:507–508.

17. Mayer AP, Greenberg ML. FNB diagnosis of breast carcinoma associated with HIV infection: a case report and review of HIV associated malignancy. *Pathology* 1996;28:90–95.

18. Spina M, Nasti G, Simonelli C, et al. Breast cancer in a woman with HIV infection: a case report. *Ann Oncol* 1994;5:661–662.

19. Mendelson EB, Harris KM, Doshi N, et al. Infiltrating lobular carcinoma: mammographic patterns with pathologic correlation. *Am J Radiol* 1989;153:265–271.

20. Helvie MA, Paramagul C, Oberman HA, et al. Invasive lobular carcinoma imaging features and clinical detection. *Invest Radiol* 1993;28:202–207.

21. Krecke KN, Gisvold JJ. Invasive lobular carcinoma of the breast: mammographic findings and extent of disease at diagnosis in 184 patients. *AJR Am J Roentgenol* 1993;161:957–960.

22. Le Gal M, Ollivier L, Asselain B, et al. Mammographic features of 455 invasive lobular carcinomas. *Radiology* 1992;185:705–708.

23. Newstead GM, Bante PB, Toth HK. Invasive lobular and ductal carcinoma: mammographic findings and stage at diagnosis. *Radiology* 1992;184:623–627.

24. Porter PL, El-Bastawissi AY, Mendelson MT, et al. Breast tumor characteristics as predictors of mammographic detection: comparison of interval- and screen-detected cancers. *J Natl Cancer Inst* 1999;91:2020–2028.

25. Yeatman TJ, Cantor AB, Smith TJ, et al. Tumor biology of infiltrating lobular carcinoma. Implications for management. *Ann Surg* 1995;222:549–561.

26. Esserman L, Hylton N, Yassa L, et al. Utility of magnetic resonance imaging in the management of breast cancer: evidence for improved preoperative staging. *J Clin Oncol* 1999;17:110–119.

27. Rodenko GN, Harms SE, Pruneda JM, et al. MR imaging in the management before surgery of lobular carcinoma of the breast: correlation with pathology. *AJR Am J Roentgenol* 1996;167:1415–1419.

28. Harvey JA, Fechner RE, Moore MM. Apparent ipsilateral decrease in breast size at mammography: a sign of infiltrating lobular carcinoma. *Radiology* 2000;214:883–889.

29. Butler RS, Venta LA, Wiley EL, et al. Sonographic evaluation of infiltrating lobular carcinoma. *AJR Am J Roentgenol* 1999;172:325–330.

30. Berg WA, Gilbreath PL. Multicentric and multifocal cancer: whole-breast US in preoperative evaluation. *Radiology* 2000;214:59–66.

31. Skaane P, Skjorten F. Ultrasonographic evaluation of invasive lobular carcinoma. *Acta Radiol* 1999;40:369–375.

32. Mitnick JS, Gianutsos R, Pollack AH, et al. Comparative value of mammography, fine-needle aspiration biopsy, and core biopsy in the diagnosis of invasive lobular carcinoma. *Breast J* 1998;4:75–83.

33. White JR, Gustafson GS, Wimbish K, et al. Conservative surgery and radiation therapy for infiltrating lobular carcinoma of the breast: the role of preoperative mammograms in guiding treatment. *Cancer* 1994;74:640–647.

34. Peeters PHM, Verbeek ALM, Hendriks JHCL, et al. The occurrence of interval cancers in the Nijmegen screening programme. *Br J Cancer* 1989;59:929–932.

35. Broët P, de la Rochefordière A, Scholl SM, et al. Contralateral breast cancer: annual incidence and risk parameters. *J Clin Oncol* 1995;13:1578–1583.

36. Bernstein JL, Thompson WD, Risch N, et al. Risk factors predicting the incidence of second primary breast cancer among women diagnosed with a first primary breast cancer. *Am J Epidemiol* 1992;136:925–936.

37. Horn PL, Thompson WD. Risk of contralateral breast cancer: associations with factors related to initial breast cancer. *Am J Epidemiol* 1988;128:309–323.

38. Kollias J, Ellis IO, Elston CW, et al. Clinical and histologic predictors of contralateral breast cancer. *Eur J Surg Oncol* 1999;25:584–589.

39. Dixon JM, Anderson TJ, Page DL, et al. Infiltrating lobular carcinoma of the breast: an evaluation of the incidence and consequence of bilateral disease. *Br J Surg* 1983;70:513–516.

40. Lesser ML, Rosen PP, Kinne DW. Multicentricity and bilaterality in invasive breast carcinoma. *Surgery* 1982;1:234–240.

41. Bouvet M, Ollila DW, Hunt KK, et al. Role of conservation therapy for invasive lobular carcinoma of the breast. *Ann Surg Oncol* 1997;4:650–654.

42. Hislop TG, Ng V, McBride ML, et al. Incidence and risk factors for second breast primaries in women with lobular breast cancer. *Breast Dis* 1990;3:95–105.

43. du Toit RS, Locker AP, Ellis IO, et al. Invasive lobular carcinomas of the breast—the prognosis of histopathological subtypes. *Br J Cancer* 1989;60:605–609.

44. Yeatman TJ, Lyman GH, Smith SK, et al. Bilaterality and recurrence rates for lobular breast cancer: considerations for treatment. *Ann Surg Oncol* 1997;4:198–202.

45. Lee JS, Grant CS, Donohue JH, et al. Arguments against routine contralateral mastectomy or undirected biopsy for invasive lobular breast cancer. *Surgery* 1995;118:640–647.

46. Babiera GV, Lowy AM, Davidson BS, et al. The role of contralateral prophylactic mastectomy in invasive lobular carcinoma. *Breast J* 1997;3:2–6.

47. Simkovich AH, Sclafani LM, Masri M, et al. Role of contralateral breast biopsy in infiltrating lobular cancer. *Surgery* 1993;114:555–557.

48. Cody HS. Routine contralateral breast biopsy: helpful or irrelevant? Experience in 871 patients, 1979–1993. *Ann Surg* 1997;225:370–376.

49. Rosen PP, Menendez-Botet CJ, Senie RT, et al. Estrogen receptor protein (ERP) and the histopathology of human mammary carcinoma. In: McGuire WL, ed. *Hormones, receptors and breast cancer.* New York: Raven Press, 1978:71–83.

50. Lesser ML, Rosen PP, Senie RT, et al. Estrogen and progesterone receptors in breast carcinoma: correlations with epidemiology and pathology. *Cancer* 1981;48:299–309.

51. Shousha S, Backhous CM, Alaghband-Zadeh J, et al. Alveolar variant of invasive lobular carcinoma of the breast. *Am J Clin Pathol* 1986;85:1–5.

52. Radhi JM. Immunohistochemical analysis of pleomorphic lobular carcinoma: higher expression of p53 and chromogranin and lower expression of ER and PgR. *Histopathology* 2000;36:156–160.

53. Foote Jr FW, Stewart FW. A histologic classification of carcinoma of the breast. *Surgery* 1946;19:74–99.

54. Underwood JCE, Parsons MA, Harris SC, et al. Frozen section appearances simulating invasive lobular carcinoma in breast tissue adjacent to inflammatory lesions and biopsy sites. *Histopathology* 1988;13:232–234.

55. Chetty R, Butler AE. Lymphocytic mastopathy associated with infiltrating lobular breast carcinoma. *J Clin Pathol* 1993;46:376–377.

55a.Cristina S, Boldorini R, Brustia F, et al. Lymphoepithelioma-like carcinoma of the breast. An unusual pattern of infiltrating lobular carcinoma. *Virchows Arch* 2000;437:198–202.

56. Cserni G. Reproducibility of a diagnosis of invasive lobular carcinoma. *J Surg Oncol* 1999;70:217–221.

57. Kiaer H, Andersen JA, Rank F, et al. Quality control of patho-anatomical diagnosis of carcinoma of the breast. *Acta Oncol* 1988;27:745–747.

58. Van Bogaert L-J, Maldaque P. Infiltrating lobular carcinoma of the female breast: deviations from the usual histopathologic appearance. *Cancer* 1980;45:979–984.

59. Fisher ER, Gregorio RM, Redmond C, et al. Tubulolobular invasive

breast carcinoma: a variant of lobular invasive cancer. *Hum Pathol* 1977;8:679–683.

60. Davis RP, Nora PF, Kooy RG, et al. Experience with lobular carcinoma of the breast: emphasis on recent aspects of management. *Arch Surg* 1979;114:485–488.

61. Breslow A, Brancaccio ME. Intracellular mucin production by lobular breast carcinoma cells. *Arch Pathol Lab Med* 1976;100:620–621.

62. Gad A, Azzopardi JG. Lobular carcinoma of the breast: a special variant of mucin secreting carcinoma. *J Clin Pathol* 1975;28:711–716.

63. Frost AR, Terahata S, Yeh I-T, et al. The significance of signet ring cells in infiltrating lobular carcinoma of the breast. *Arch Pathol Lab Med* 1995;119:64–68.

64. Merino MJ, LiVolsi VA. Signet ring carcinoma of the female breast: a clinicopathologic analysis of 24 cases. *Cancer* 1981;48:1830–1837.

65. Battifora H. Intracytoplasmic lumina in breast carcinoma. *Arch Pathol* 1975;99:614–617.

66. Erlandson RA, Carstens PHB. Ultrastructure of tubular carcinoma of the breast. *Cancer* 1972;29:987–995.

67. Hull MT, Seo IS, Battersby JS, et al. Signet-ring cell carcinoma of the breast: a clinicopathologic study of 24 cases. *Am J Clin Pathol* 1980;73:31–35.

68. Allenby PL, Chowdhury LN. Histiocytic appearance of metastatic lobular breast carcinoma. *Arch Pathol Lab Med* 1986;110:759–760.

69. Hood CI, Font RI, Zimmerman LE. Metastatic mammary carcinoma in the eyelid with histiocytoid appearance. *Cancer* 1973;31:793–800.

70. Shimizu S, Kitamura H, Ito T, et al. Histiocytoid breast carcinoma: histological, immunohistochemical, ultrastructural, cytological and clinicopathological studies. *Pathol Int* 1998;48:549–556.

71. Eusebi V, Magalhaes F, Azzopardi JG. Pleomorphic lobular carcinoma of the breast: an aggressive tumor showing apocrine differentiation. *Hum Pathol* 1992;23:655–662.

72. Weidner N, Semple JP. Pleomorphic variant of invasive lobular carcinoma of the breast. *Hum Pathol* 1992;23:1167–1171.

73. Walford N, Ten Velden J. Histiocytoid breast carcinoma: an apocrine variant of lobular carcinoma. *Histopathology* 1989;14:515–522.

74. Bentz JS, Yassa N, Clayton F. Pleomorphic lobular carcinoma of the breast: clinicopathologic features of 12 cases. *Mod Pathol* 1998;11:814–822.

74a.Middleton LP, Palacios DM, Bryant BR, et al. Pleomorphic lobular carcinoma: morphology, immunohistochemistry, and molecular analysis. *Am J Surg Pathol* 2000;24:1650–1656.

75. Morphopoulos G, Pearson M, Ryder WDJ, et al. Tumour angiogenesis as a prognostic marker in infiltrating lobular carcinoma of the breast. *J Pathol* 1996;180:44–49.

76. Nesland JM, Holm R, Johannessen JV. Ultrastructural and immunohistochemical features of lobular carcinoma of the breast. *J Pathol* 1985;145:39–52.

77. Lee AK, Rosen PP, DeLellis RA, et al. Tumor marker expression in breast carcinomas and relationship to prognosis: an immunohistochemical study. *Am J Clin Pathol* 1985;84:687–696.

78. Kuhajda FP, Offutt LE, Mendelsohn G. The distribution of carcinoembryonic antigen in breast carcinoma: diagnostic and prognostic implications. *Cancer* 1983;52:1257–1264.

79. Lee AK, DeLellis RA, Rosen PP, et al. Alphalactalbumin as an immunohistochemical marker for metastatic breast carcinomas. *Am J Surg Pathol* 1984;8:93–100.

80. Mazoujian G, Pincus GS, Davis S, et al. Immunohistochemistry of a breast gross cystic disease fluid protein (GCDFP-15): a marker of apocrine epithelium and breast carcinomas with apocrine features. *Am J Pathol* 1983;110:105–111.

81. Mazoujian G, Bodian C, Haagensen Jr DE, et al. Expression of GCDFP-15 in breast carcinomas: relationship to pathologic and clinical factors. *Cancer* 1989;63:2156–2161.

82. Eusebi V, Betts C, Haagensen DE Jr, et al. Apocrine differentiation in lobular carcinoma of the breast: a morphologic, immunologic, and ultrastructural study. *Hum Pathol* 1984;15:134–140.

83. Porter PL, Garcia R, Moe R, et al. C-*erb*B-2 oncogene protein in *in situ* and invasive lobular breast neoplasia. *Cancer* 1991;68:331–334.

84. Domagala W, Markiewski M, Kubiak R, et al. Immunohistochemical profile of invasive lobular carcinoma of the breast: predominantly vimentin and p53 protein negative cathepsin D and oestrogen receptor positive. *Virchows Arch* 1993;423:497–502.

85. Martinazzi M, Crivelli F, Zampatti C, et al. Epidermal growth factor receptor immunohistochemistry in different histological types of infiltrating breast carcinoma. *J Clin Pathol* 1993;46:1009–1010.

86. Sainsbury JRC, Nicholson S, Angus B, et al. Epidermal growth factor receptor status of histological sub-types of breast cancer. *Br J Cancer* 1988;58:458–460.

87. Charpin C, Devictor B, Bonnier P, et al. Epidermal growth factor receptor in breast cancer: correlation of quantitative immunocytochemical assays to prognostic factors. *Breast Cancer Res Treat* 1993;25:203–210.

88. Gould VE, Chejfec G. Lobular carcinoma of the breast with secretory features. *Ultrastruct Pathol* 1980;1:151–156.

89. Jundt G, Schulz A, Heitz PU, et al. Small cell neuroendocrine (oat cell) carcinoma of the male breast. *Virchows Arch* 1984;404:213–221.

90. Wade PM, Mills SE, Read M, et al. Small cell neuroendocrine (oat cell) carcinoma of the breast. *Cancer* 1983;52:121–125.

91. d'Ardenne AJ, Burns J, Sykes BC, et al. Fibronectin and type III collagen in epithelial neoplasms of gastrointestinal tract and salivary gland. *J Clin Pathol* 1983;36:756–763.

92. Stenman S, Vaheri A. Fibronectin in human solid tumours. *Int J Cancer* 1981;27:427–435.

93. d'Ardenne AJ, Barnard NJ. Paucity of fibronectin in invasive lobular carcinoma of breast. *J Pathol* 1989;157:219–224.

94. Gusterson BA, Warburton MJ, Mitchell D, et al. Distribution of myoepithelial cells and basement membrane protein in the normal breast and in benign and malignant breast diseases. *Cancer Res* 1982;42:4763–4770.

95. Yamada KM, Olden K. Fibronectins-adhesive glycoproteins of cell surface and blood. *Nature* 1978;275:179–184.

96. Moll R, Mitze M, Frixen UH, et al. Differential loss of E-cadherin expression in infiltrating ductal and lobular breast carcinomas. *Am J Pathol* 1993;143:1731–1742.

97. De Leeuw WJ, Berx G, Vos CB, et al. Simultaneous loss of E-cadherin and catenins in invasive lobular breast cancer and lobular carcinoma in situ. *J Pathol* 1997;183:404–411.

98. Ioffe O, Silverberg SG, Simsir A. Lobular lesions of the breast: immunohistochemical profile and comparison with ductal proliferations. *Mod Pathol* 2000;13:23A.

99. Acs G, Lawton TJ, Livolsi VA, et al. Differential expression of E-cadherin in ductal and lobular carcinoma of the breast. *Mod Pathol* 2000;13:17A.

99a.Lehr HA, Folpe A, Yaziji H, et al. Cytokeratin 8 immunostaining pattern and E-cadherin expression distinguish lobular from ductal breast carcinoma. *Am J Clin Pathol* 2000;114:190–196.

100. Kanai Y, Oda T, Tsuda H, et al. Point mutation of the E-cadherin gene in invasive lobular carcinoma of the breast. *Jpn J Cancer Res* 1994;85:1035–1039.

101. Berx G, Cleton-Jansen AM, Nollet F, et al. E-cadherin is a tumour/invasion suppressor gene mutated in human lobular breast cancers. *EMBO J* 1995;14:6107–6115.

102. Berx G, Cleton-Jansen AM, Strumane K, et al. E-cadherin is inactivated in a majority of invasive human lobular breast cancers by truncation mutations throughout its extracellular domain. *Oncogene* 1996;13:1919–1925.

103. Huiping C, Sigurgeirsdottir JR, Jonasson JG, et al. Chromosome alterations and E-cadherin gene mutations in human lobular breast cancer. *Br J Cancer* 1999;81:1103–1110.

104. Oyama T, Kashiwabara K, Yoshimoto K, et al. Frequent overexpression of the cyclin D1 oncogene in invasive lobular carcinoma of the breast. *Cancer Res* 1998;58:2876–2880.

105. Pandis N, Idvall I, Bardi G, et al. Correlation between karyotypic pattern and clinicopathologic features in 125 breast cancer cases. *Int J Cancer* 1996;66:191–196.

106. Frost AR, Karcher DS, Terahata S, et al. DNA analysis and S-phase fraction determination by flow cytometric analysis of infiltrating lobular carcinoma of the breast. *Mod Pathol* 1996;9:930–937.

107. Nayar R, Zhuang Z, Merino MJ, et al. Loss of heterozygosity on chromosome 11q13 in lobular lesions of the breast using tissue microdissection and polymerase chain reaction. *Hum Pathol* 1996;28:277–282.

108. Nishizaki T, Chew K, Chu L, et al. Genetic alterations in lobular breast cancer by comparative genomic hybridization. *Int J Cancer* 1997;74:513–517.

108a.Huiping C, Jonasson JG, Agnarsson BA, et al. Analysis of the fragile histidine triad (FHIT) gene in lobular breast cancer. *Eur J Cancer* 2000;36:1552–1557.

109. Eusebi V, Pich A, Macchiorlatti E, et al. Morphofunctional differentiation in lobular carcinoma of the breast. *Histopathology* 1977;1:301–314.

110. Shousha S, Bull TB, Burn I. Alveolar variant of invasive lobular carcinoma of the breast. *Ultrastruct Pathol* 1986;10:311–319.

111. Nesland JM, Holm R, Lunde S, et al. Diagnostic problems in breast pathology: the benefit of ultrastructural and immunocytochemical analysis. *Ultrastruct Pathol* 1987;11:293–311.

112. Kline TS, Kannan V, Kline IK. Appraisal and cytomorphologic analysis of common carcinomas of the breast. *Diagn Cytopathol* 1985;1:188–193.

113. Oertel YC. *Fine needle aspiration of the breast*. Stoneham: M.A. Butterworth, 1987:145–149.

114. Lerma E, Furmanal V, Carreras A, et al. Undetected invasive lobular breast cancer: review of false negative smears. *Diagn Cytopathol* 2000;23:303–307.

115. Sadler GP, McGee S, Dallimore NS, et al. Role of fine-needle aspiration cytology and needle-core biopsy in the diagnosis of lobular carcinoma of the breast. *Br J Surg* 1994;81:1315–1317.

116. Jayaram G, Swain M, Chew MT, et al. Cytologic appearances in invasive lobular carcinoma of the breast. A study of 21 cases. *Acta Cytol* 2000;44:169–174.

117. Robinson IA, McKee G, Jackson PA, et al. Lobular carcinoma of the breast: cytological features supporting the diagnosis of lobular cancer. *Diagn Cytopathol* 1995;13:196–201.

118. Auger M, Huttner I. Fine-needle aspiration cytology of pleomorphic lobular carcinoma of the breast: comparison with the classic type. *Cancer (Cancer Cytopathol)* 1997;81:29–32.

118a.Abdulla M, Hombal S, Juwaiser A, et al. Cytomorphologic features of classic and variant lobular carcinoma: a comparative study. *Diagn Cytopathol* 2000;22:370–375.

119. Greeley CF, Frost AR. Cytologic features of ductal and lobular carcinoma in fine needle aspirates of the breast. *Acta Cytol* 1997;41:333–340.

120. Raju UR, Ma CK, Shaw A. Signet ring variant of lobular carcinoma of the breast: a clinicopathologic and immunohistochemical study. *Mod Pathol* 1993;6:516–520.

121. Frost AR, Shek YH, Lack EE. "Signet ring" sinus histiocytosis mimicking metastatic adenocarcinoma: report of two cases with immunohistochemical and ultrastructural study. *Mod Pathol* 1992;5:497–500.

122. Gould E, Perez J, Albores-Saavedra J, et al. Signet ring cell sinus histiocytosis: a previously unrecognized histologic condition mimicking metastatic adenocarcinoma in lymph nodes. *Am J Clin Pathol* 1989;92:509–512.

123. Cappellari J, Islander S, Woodruff R. Signet ring cell sinus histiocytosis. *Am J Clin Pathol* 1990;94:800–801.

124. Trojani M, de Mascarel I, Bonichon F, et al. Micrometastases to axillary lymph nodes from carcinoma of breast: detection by immunohistochemistry and prognostic significance. *Br J Cancer* 1987;55:303–306.

125. Wells CA, Heryet A, Brochier HJ, et al. The immunocytochemical detection of axillary micrometastases in breast cancer. *Br J Cancer* 1984;50:193–197.

126. Cote RJ, Peterson HF, Chaiwun B, et al. Role of immunohistochemical detection of lymph-node metastases in management of breast cancer. International Breast Cancer Study Group. *Lancet* 1999;354:896–900.

127. Weinstein GW, Goldman JN. Metastatic adenocarcinoma of the breast masquerading as chalazion. *Am J Opthamol* 1970;69:259–264.

128. Bitter MA, Fiorito D, Corkell ME, et al. Bone marrow involvement by lobular carcinoma of the breast cannot be identified reliably by routine histological examination alone. *Hum Pathol* 1994;25:781–788.

128a.Lyda MH, Tetef M, Carter NH, et al. Keratin immunohistochemistry detects clinically significant metastases in bone marrow biopsy specimens in women with lobular breast carcinoma. *Am J Surg Pathol* 2000;24:1593–1599.

129. Dearnaley DP, Sloane JP, Ormerod MG, et al. Increased detection of mammary carcinoma cells in marrow smears using antisera to epithelial membrane antigen. *Br J Cancer* 1981;44:85–90.

130. Lamovec J, Bracko M. Metastatic pattern of infiltrating lobular carcinoma of the breast: an autopsy study. *J Surg Oncol* 1991;48:28–31.

131. Borst MJ, Ingold JA. Metastatic patterns of invasive lobular versus invasive ductal carcinoma of the breast. *Surgery* 1993;114:637–642.

132. Harris M, Howell A, Chrissohou M, et al. A comparison of the metastatic pattern of infiltrating lobular carcinoma and infiltrating duct carcinoma of the breast. *Br J Cancer* 1984;50:23–30.

133. Dixon AR, Ellis IO, Elston CW, et al. A comparison of the clinical metastatic patterns of invasive lobular and ductal carcinomas of the breast. *Br J Cancer* 1991;63:634–635.

134. Olsen ME, Chernik NL, Posner JB. Infiltration of the leptomeninges by systemic cancer: a clinical and pathologic study. *Arch Neurol* 1974;30:122–137.

135. Smith DB, Howell A, Harris M, et al. Carcinomatous meningitis associated with infiltrating lobular carcinoma of the breast. *Eur J Surg Oncol* 1985;11:33–36.

136. Heimann A, Merino MJ. Carcinomatous meningitis as the initial manifestation of breast cancer. *Acta Cytol* 1986;30:25–28.

137. Jayson GC, Howell A, Harris M, et al. Carcinomatous meningitis in patients with breast cancer: an aggressive disease variant. *Cancer* 1994;74:3135–3141.

138. Deck JHN, Lee MA. Mucin embolism to cerebral arteries: a fatal complication of carcinoma of the breast. *Can J Neurol Sci* 1978;5:327–330.

139. Feun L, Drelichman A, Singhakowinta A, et al. Ureteral obstruction secondary to metastatic breast carcinoma. *Cancer* 1979;44:1164–1171.

140. Gagnon Y, Tetu B. Ovarian metastases of breast carcinoma. A clinicopathologic study of 59 cases. *Cancer* 1989;64:892–898.

141. Kidney DD, Cohen AJ, Butler J. Abdominal metastases of infiltrating lobular breast carcinoma: CT and fluoroscopic imaging findings. *Abdom Imaging* 1997;22:156–159.

141a.Winston CB, Hadar O, Teicher JB, et al. Metastatic lobular carcinoma of the breast: patterns of spread in the chest, abdomen, and pelvis on CT. *AJR Am J Roentgenol* 2000;175:795–800.

142. Kumar NB, Hart WR. Metastases to the uterine corpus from extragenital cancers: a clinicopathologic study of 63 cases. *Cancer* 1982;50:2163–2169.

143. Mallow DW, Humphrey PA, Soper JT, et al. Metastatic lobular carcinoma of the breast diagnosed in cervicovaginal samples: a case report. *Acta Cytol* 1997;41:549–555.

144. Vadmal M, Brones C, Hajdu SI. Metastatic lobular carcinoma of the breast in a cervical-vaginal smear [letter]. *Acta Cytol* 1997;41:1236–1237.

145. Liebmann RD, Jones KD, Hamid R, et aal. Fortuitous diagnosis in a uterine leiomyoma of metastatic lobular carcinoma of the breast [Letter]. *Histopathology* 1998;32:577–578.

146. Cormier WJ, Gaffey TA, Welch JM, et al. Linitis plastica caused by metastatic carcinoma of the breast. *Mayo Clin Proc* 1980;55:747–753.

147. Hartmann, WH, Sherlock P. Gastroduodenal metastases from carcinoma of the breast. An adrenal steroid induced phenomenon. *Cancer* 1961;14:426–431.

148. Yoshida Y. Metastases and primary neoplasms of the stomach in patients with breast cancer. *Surgery* 1973;125:738–743.

149. Matsui M, Kokima O, Uehara Y, et al. Characterization of estrogen receptor in human gastric cancer. *Cancer* 1991;68:305–308.

150. Tokunaga A, Nishi K, Matsukura N, et al. Estrogen and progesterone receptors in gastric cancer. *Cancer* 1986;57:1376–1379.

151. Harrison JD, Morris DL, Ellis IO, et al. The effect of tamoxifen and estrogen receptor status on survival in gastric carcinoma. *Cancer* 1989;64:1007–1010.

152. Yokozaki H, Takemura N, Takanashi A, et al. Estrogen receptors in gastric adenocarcinoma: a retrospective immunohistochemical analysis. *Virchows Arch* 1988;413:297–302.

153. Chaubert P, Bouzourene H, Saraga E. Estrogen and progesterone receptors and pS2 and ERD5 antigens in gastric carcinomas from the European population. *Mod Pathol* 1996;9:189–193.

154. Keller G, Vogelsang H, Becker I, et al. Diffuse type gastric and lobular breast carcinoma in a familial gastric cancer patient with an E-cadherin germline mutation. *Am J Pathol* 1999;155:337–342.

155. Voravud N, El-Naggar AK, Balch CM, et al. Metastatic lobular breast carcinoma simulating primary colon cancer. *Am J Clin Oncol* 1992;15:365–369.

156. Frost AR, Terahata S, Siegel RS, et al. An analysis of prognostic features in infiltrating lobular carcinoma of the breast. *Mod Pathol* 1995;8:830–836.

157. Sastre-Garau X, Jouve M, Asselain B, et al. Infiltrating lobular carcinoma of the breast. Clinicopathologic analysis of 975 cases with reference to data on conservative therapy and metastatic patterns. *Cancer* 1996;77:113–120.

158. Silverstein MJ, Lewinsky BS, Waisman JR, et al. Infiltrating lobular carcinoma. Is it different from infiltrating duct carcinoma? *Cancer* 1994;73:1673–1677.

159. Cha I, Weidner N. Correlation of prognostic factors and survival with classical and pleomorphic variants of invasive lobular carcinoma. *Breast J* 1996;2:385–393.

160. Weidner N, Bennington J. Correlation of DNA ploidy, DNA S-phase and nuclear diameter with classical and pleomorphic variants of invasive lobular carcinoma. *Lab Invest* 1994;70:24A.

161. Moreno-Elola A, Aguilar A, Roman JM, et al. Prognostic factors in invasive lobular carcinoma of the breast: a multivariate analysis. A multicentre study after seventeen years of follow-up. *Ann Chir Gynaecol* 1999;88:252–258.

162. Leonard CE, Philpott P, Shapiro H, et al. Clinical observations of axillary involvement for tubular, lobular, and ductal carcinomas of the breast. *J Surg Oncol* 1999;70:13–20.

163. Kurtz JM, Jacquemier J, Torhorst J, et al. Conservation therapy for breast cancers other than infiltrating ductal carcinoma. *Cancer* 1989;63:1630–1635.

164. Mate TP, Carter D, Fischer DB, et al. A clinical and histopathologic analysis of the results of conservation surgery and radiation therapy in stage I and II breast carcinoma. *Cancer* 1986;58:1995–2002.

165. Poen JC, Tran L, Juillard G, et al. Conservation therapy for invasive lobular carcinoma of the breast. *Cancer* 1992;69:2789–2795.

166. Schnitt SJ, Connolly JL, Recht A, et al. Influence of lobular histology on local tumor control in breast cancer patients treated with conservative surgery and radiotherapy. *Cancer* 1989;64:448–454.

167. Haffty BG, Perrotta PL, Ward B, et al. Conservatively treated breast cancer: outcome by histologic subtype. *Breast J* 1997;3:7–14.

168. Francis M, Cakir B, Bilous M, et al. Conservative surgery and radiation therapy for invasive lobular carcinoma of the breast. *Aust N Z J Surg* 1999;69:450–454.

169. Chung MA, Cole B, Wanebo HJ, et al. Optimal surgical treatment of invasive lobular carcinoma of the breast. *Ann Surg Oncol* 1997;4:545–550.

170. Warneke J, Berger R, Johnson C, et al. Lumpectomy and radiation treatment for invasive lobular carcinoma of the breast. *Am J Surg* 1996;172:496–500.

170a. Moore MM, Borossa G, Imbrie JZ, et al. Association of infiltrating lobular carcinoma with positive surgical margins after breast-conservation therapy. *Ann Surg* 2000;231:877–882.

# CHAPTER 35

# Unusual Clinical Presentations of Carcinoma

## CARCINOMA IN PREGNANCY AND LACTATION

The reported frequency of coincident pregnancy in women with breast carcinoma is 1% to 3% (1). The average age of women who have breast cancer in pregnancy is in the mid to late 30s (1). About 6% of women with breast carcinoma diagnosed by age 35 years are pregnant when the tumor is detected (2). With the trend for women in some ethnic and social groups to delay pregnancy to their late 30s and 40s, it is likely that more instances of coincident pregnancy and breast carcinoma will be encountered. Breast carcinoma has been reported in pregnant teenage girls (3,4). Data from one study suggest that women from BRCA1-positive families may be at increased risk to develop breast carcinoma during and after pregnancy (5).

### Clinical Presentation

The usual presenting symptom is a painless mass that may be obscured by surrounding physiologic hyperplasia. These factors can contribute to delay on the part of the patient in seeking medical attention, as well as physician delay in obtaining a biopsy. In one study, more than 50% of patients with breast carcinoma diagnosed postpartum had a palpable mass detected and followed during pregnancy (6). Because of concern about exposing the fetus to radiation, mammography may not be obtained early in pregnancy. The effectiveness of mammography is reduced during pregnancy by increased parenchymal density. In one study, the sensitivity of mammography for detecting carcinoma during pregnancy or within 1 year postpartum was 78% (7). Ultrasound was 100% sensitive as a method for detecting solid tumors in this series of pregnant women and is the preferred initial diagnostic procedure (8). A case-control study of BRCA1 and BRCA2 mutation carriers found that parous carriers were significantly more likely to develop breast cancer before age 40 than nulliparous carriers, and that early first pregnancy was not protective (8a).

### Pathology

A diagnosis of carcinoma during pregnancy and lactation can be made by fine needle aspiration (FNA) biopsy (9).

However, caution should be exercised when interpreting cytology specimens in this setting, because hyperplastic and lactating parenchyma can appear atypical in cytologic preparations and the material often consists of abundant discohesive cells (10). Incisional or excisional biopsy is preferable.

The histologic spectrum of pregnancy-associated breast carcinoma is not significantly different from breast carcinoma unrelated to pregnancy in women of a comparable age (6,11,12). In one case-control study, intraductal carcinoma was present in 4.8% of control patients and in 1.6% of women with pregnancy-related carcinoma (11). Invasive duct carcinoma was present in about 90% of both groups. There were small numbers of patients with mucinous, medullary, and other types of carcinoma. Tumors were significantly larger, vascular invasion was more frequent in the pregnancy group, and these women had axillary nodal metastases significantly more often. Infiltrating lobular carcinoma has been described in pregnancy (13). Axillary lymph node metastases were present in 60% to 70% of women with pregnancy-related breast carcinoma (6,11,14).

Biochemically measured estrogen and progesterone receptors are significantly more often negative in carcinomas from pregnant and lactating women than in tumors from nonpregnant age-matched controls (11). Similar results have been obtained with tissues studied by immunohistochemistry.

### Treatment and Prognosis

Primary treatment generally is surgical. The role of adjuvant chemotherapy and breast conservation with primary radiotherapy depend on the circumstances in individual cases. Mastectomy has been performed in most cases because of a desire to avoid radiation of the fetus in breast conservation therapy. In some instances, radiation has been delayed until after delivery of the child. Kuerer et al. (15) reported results in nine patients treated by breast conservation in pregnancy. The patients were all stage I and II, with a median fetal gestational age of 7 months. After a median follow-up of 24 months, there were no recurrences in the breast, although three women had distant recurrences.

The overall prognosis of women with breast carcinoma diagnosed in pregnancy and lactation is relatively poor due to the high proportion of patients with nodal metastases. In one study, axillary nodal metastases were present in 74% of patients under 40 years of age with breast cancer diagnosed during pregnancy, whereas 37% of nonpregnant patients in the same age group had positive nodes (16). When stratified by stage, some investigators reported no significant difference in outcome between pregnancy-related and nonpregnancy-related patients of comparable age (6,12,14). In a number of reports, 75% to 80% of node-negative patients remained alive or recurrence-free with follow-up of 5 to 10 years. In one case-control study, node-negative women in the pregnancy and lactation group had a poorer survival (85%) at 10 years than women with nonpregnancy-associated breast carcinoma (93%), but the outcome for both groups was exceptionally favorable (11). The same series reported a much greater discrepancy in node-positive cases, with survival of 62% and 37% in the nonpregnant and pregnant groups, respectively. Others also found the prognosis of pregnancy-associated breast carcinoma to be relatively unfavorable after adjustment for tumor size and nodal status (17).

The impact of pregnancy and childbearing on prognosis in women previously treated for breast carcinoma remains uncertain (18). Most studies of this subject conducted retrospectively appear to indicate that the prognosis for such patients is the same as, or better than, patients who do not become pregnant (19,20). One case-control study compared 53 women who became pregnant after treatment of breast carcinoma with a cohort without subsequent pregnancy matched for stage of disease at diagnosis and a disease-free survival that was at least as long as the interval to pregnancy in the study individual (21). There were five deaths due to breast carcinoma among 53 women (9.6%), with subsequent pregnancies and 34 deaths among 265 controls (13%). The relative risk for death due to breast carcinoma in the subsequent pregnancy group was 0.8 (95% confidence interval, 0.3 to 2.3), a result indicative of no increase in risk associated with subsequent pregnancy. Many biases could explain these results, and a prospective study is necessary to fully evaluate this issue, especially in the context of current breast conservation and systemic adjuvant therapy.

An unusual complication of pregnancy concurrent with, or subsequent to, the diagnosis of breast carcinoma is the development of placental metastases. This is most likely to occur in women who have disseminated metastatic tumors (22,23). Gross evidence of metastatic carcinoma usually is apparent on the placental surface. Microscopic examination discloses tumor cells in the intervillous spaces, rarely with villous invasion.

## PATHOLOGY OF BREAST CARCINOMA AT THE EXTREMES OF AGE

The average age at diagnosis of patients with breast carcinoma is in the mid 50s. The ages of the great majority of af-

fected women are within two decades above or below this midpoint. Within this framework, the extremes of age among adults may be considered younger than 35 years and older than 75 years.

Breast carcinoma is widely thought to have a relatively poor prognosis in women less than 35 years of age, whereas it has been described as an indolent disease in those older than 75 years. Many published studies of this issue are not easily compared because of differences in defining age extremes or in the treatment that patients received. These are important considerations, especially when comparing data from the era when therapy consisted of surgery alone to more recent data including adjuvant chemotherapy, breast conservation, and radiation therapy. Data obtained from a statewide tumor registry for patients treated between 1985 and 1992 suggest that age-related differences in prognosis may be influenced by the stage at diagnosis (24). Among stage I patients, women older than 80 years had the poorest 5-year disease-free survival when compared to younger women stratified by decade. In stages II and III, the groups of patients 40 years or younger and women older than 80 years had significantly lower 5-year disease-free survival than those whose ages were in the intervening decades.

Feldman and Welch (25) studied 29 women who were younger than 30 years when they were diagnosed and treated for breast carcinoma. The patients were identified between 1953 and 1983 in the records of an urban teaching hospital. Age at diagnosis ranged from 20 to 29 years. Seven (26%) were pregnant at the time of diagnosis. Stage at diagnosis, determined in 27 cases, was II or higher in 26; only one patient was stage I. Twenty-two patients (76%) died of breast carcinoma, including three who developed recurrences 12.7, 14.6, and 19.9 years after diagnosis. Virtually all patients were treated by mastectomy, and none received systemic adjuvant therapy.

Further evidence of the relatively unfavorable prognosis of breast carcinoma in youthful patients was obtained from a review of records in the Laboratory of Pathology at the National Cancer Institute (NCI) (26). As a referral center, the NCI may receive a disproportionate sampling of patients with more advanced disease and this might introduce a bias, but the data are consistent with reports from other sources. The investigators identified 191 women younger than 40 years of age when treated at the NCI between 1980 and 1992. Axillary lymph node metastases were present in 65% of documented cases. Among women assessed for clinical stage, 19% were classified as stage 0 or I, and 81% were stage II to IV. Twelve percent had a history of breast carcinoma in a first-degree relative, and 5% had pregnancy-associated carcinoma. Histologic classification of tumors was as follows: ductal, 83%; lobular, 11%; and special types (tubular, mucinous, metaplastic, etc.), 6%. The majority of 11 patients with intraductal carcinoma alone had a comedo growth pattern. Poorly differentiated nuclear and histologic grade and vascular invasion were present in 68%, 60%, and 67% of cases, respectively. Estrogen receptors were positive in 57% of evaluable cases, and the same percentage of carcinomas were progesterone receptor–positive. Recurrences were documented in 102 patients (54%), with approximately half of the recurrences detected within 2 years of initial diagnosis. The 5-year disease-free survival for the entire group was 29.6%, with an overall 5-year survival rate of 72.3%. Factors associated with poorer outcome were pregnancy-associated carcinoma, axillary nodal metastases, and negative hormone receptor status.

Most studies of clinical issues in the diagnosis of breast carcinoma in younger women focused on the relatively large group of patients 40 to 49 years of age. A study of 809 consecutive patients biopsied for nonpalpable, mammographically detected lesions revealed carcinoma in 5% of biopsies prior to age 40 years, in 15% of biopsies in the 40- to 50-year age group, and in 34% of biopsies from women over 50 years (27). Twenty-five percent of carcinomas in women 40 to 49 years old and 16% in women 50 years or older were noninvasive. Mean tumor size was the same in both groups (1.5 cm), but nodal metastases were present more often in the 40- to 49-year age group (25%) than in the group 50 years or older (17%).

McPherson et al. (28) investigated the relationship of method of tumor detection to prognosis in women 40 to 49 years of age using a database of patients diagnosed in North Dakota, South Dakota, and Minnesota. When compared to the risk of dying from carcinomas detected by mammography, the relative risks for dying from carcinomas detected by breast self-examination (BSE) (2.5), by clinical breast examination (CE) (2.7), or by the patient incidentally (2.8) were significantly greater. The mean size of mammographically detected tumors (1.9 cm) was significantly smaller than those in the CE (2.3 cm), BSE (2.8 cm), and incidental (2.9 cm) groups. After adjusting for stage (tumor size and nodal status), the relative risks for dying of breast cancers detected by BSE (1.5), CE (1.9), or incidentally (1.6), when compared to tumors detected by mammography, were greater. These results suggest that mammography makes a contribution to breast cancer diagnosis in women 40 to 49 years of age. The implication of these observations for mammographic screening in this age group and in women younger than 40 years has been controversial.

Clinical problems encountered in the diagnosis of breast carcinoma in women 49 years and younger were detailed in a report by Lannin et al. (29). The authors analyzed the results of mammography and physical examination in a consecutive series of patients evaluated in a university hospital clinic in order to compare women 20 to 49 years of age with those 50 years and older. The positive predictive value (PPV) of mammography was 28% for women younger than 50 years and 53% in those older than 50 years. The PPV of an abnormal physical examination resulting in biopsy was 11% and 57% in women younger and older than 50 years, respectively. There also was a significant difference in the sensitivity of mammography between patients younger than and older than 50 years (68% and 91%, respectively).

The sensitivity of physical examination did not differ significantly between the two groups. Nonpalpable tumors were smaller (mean size, 1.0 cm) than palpable tumors in women older than 50 (mean size, 1.0 and 4.1 cm, respectively). This discrepancy was not observed between nonpalpable and palpable tumors in women younger than 50 years (mean size, 4.0 and 3.4 cm, respectively). These results led the authors to conclude that physical examination and mammography were less sensitive in women 20 to 49 years old when compared to women 50 years or older and that this phenomenon resulted from "biologic factors of the disease." They suggested that "tumors in young women are nonpalpable, not because they are small, but because of background density of the mammary tissue or because of the more diffuse growth pattern of tumors at this age. These are exactly the same reasons mammography is less sensitive in young women." The addition of FNA or needle core biopsy to mammography and clinical examination constitutes the "triple test" approach to the diagnosis of breast tumors. This combination has been advocated as a method for improving diagnostic accuracy, especially in younger women (30).

A number of pathologic features of breast carcinoma do not differ appreciably at the extremes of age (31–34). The distribution of primary size is not significantly different when young and elderly patients are compared (33). Approximately 50% of patients have tumors 2 cm or smaller, 40% have tumors in the range from 2.1 to 5.0 cm, and the remainder have tumors larger than 5 cm. The left breast is affected more often than the right in both age extremes. The position in the breast of the primary tumor (lateral vs. medial-central), overall frequency of bilaterality, and concurrent bilaterality are not significantly different at the extremes of the age distribution.

Several differences with respect to tumor type exist at the extremes of age. Patients younger than 35 years have a higher proportion of medullary carcinoma (10% vs. 1.0%) but lower proportions of infiltrating lobular (2.0% vs. 11.0%) and colloid carcinoma (1.0% vs. 7.0%) in comparison to patients older than 75 years. A marked lymphocytic reaction occurs in a higher proportion of women younger than 35 years than in the elderly group (34% vs. 12%).

Studies of growth rate and tumor cell kinetics suggest an inverse relationship between patient age and the proliferative activity in the carcinoma (35,36). Growth rate tends to be reduced in breast carcinomas that arise in elderly women (36). Others have reported that the presence of axillary lymph node metastases in breast carcinoma patients 34 years or younger is significantly related to p53 positivity and high proliferative index (37). Walker et al. (38) found an inverse relationship between p53 immunopositivity and age, with positive staining in 67% and 37% of tumors from women 25 to 29 and 50 to 67 years of age, respectively. Proliferative rate, assessed by Ki67 immunostaining, also was inversely related to age, with 72% of tumors in patients 25 to 29 years old classified as "high" compared to 40% in the group 50 to 67 years of age.

The proportion of estrogen receptor-positive tumors is increased in postmenopausal women, and there is evidence indicating that the growth rate and estrogen receptor status of breast carcinomas are directly related (36,39). The proportion of estrogen and progesterone receptor-positive tumors does not increase significantly with advancing age in postmenopausal women 65 years or older (40). Although these observations appear to support the perception that breast carcinoma tends to have less aggressive biologic features and a more favorable clinical course in the elderly, when patients younger than 35 years and older than 75 years were matched on the basis of tumor stage, no significant differences in prognosis were observed (32).

Limited data are available regarding the effect of other markers on prognosis in young women. Bertheau et al. (41) compared marker expression in women 35 years or younger and in women 36 to 50 years old. The presence of HER2/*neu* expression was associated with a significantly poorer outcome in the younger group, whereas p53 was a significant prognostic marker for women 36 to 50 years old when assessed by multivariate analysis.

Women 35 to 40 years of age or younger are more likely to develop breast recurrences after conservation surgery and radiotherapy than older patients (42–46). This phenomenon has been attributed to more frequent poorly differentiated carcinomas in this age group, difficulty in determining the extent of the carcinoma intraoperatively, and a high prevalence of carcinomas with an extensive intraductal component or lymphatic emboli in the surrounding tissue (43). The addition of adjuvant systemic chemotherapy appears to lower the risk of breast recurrence in women younger than 35 years who are treated by breast conservation (44,47,48). Chest wall irradiation has been recommended if carcinoma is present at, or close to (<5 mm), the deep margin of a mastectomy (49). The risk of breast recurrence after breast conservation does not appear to be affected by a family history of breast cancer (50).

The necessity of performing an axillary dissection in elderly women with invasive carcinoma is controversial (51,52). Existing data suggest that the procedure is appropriate in some instances and that no overall recommendation can be made. As additional data from sentinel lymph node mapping become available, this may prove to be an alternative to axillary dissection for many elderly patients. Lacking a randomized prospective trial, the question has been addressed through retrospective studies (34). In one study of women 70 years of age or older with T1 tumors, none of the 78 patients studied received adjuvant chemotherapy, regardless of nodal status (51). The 10 patients in this series who did not have an axillary dissection had an outcome similar to that of women subjected to axillary lymphadenectomy with or without nodal metastases. Adjuvant tamoxifen was given more often to women whose axillary status was not determined surgically in this study. Others concluded that axillary

dissection should be performed in women 75 years or older only if they are candidates for adjuvant chemotherapy or for local control if there are clinically evident axillary nodal metastases (52). Al-Hilaly et al. (53) analyzed 159 women 70 years or older treated for breast carcinoma who did not undergo axillary dissection. The regional recurrence rate, including the axilla, after a median follow-up of 54 months was 14%, largely in patients with high-grade tumors.

## CARCINOMA ARISING IN FIBROADENOMAS AND PHYLLODES TUMORS

Fibroepithelial neoplasms consist of proliferating epithelial and stromal mammary tissues. Fibroadenomas arise from the stroma and epithelium of lobular–terminal duct units, whereas phyllodes tumors are composed predominantly of periductal stroma and duct epithelium.

In 1931, Cheatle and Cutler (54) described carcinoma arising in a fibroadenoma, and similar lesions were reported in 1940 by Harrington and Miller (55). The first series consisting of 26 patients was published in 1967 (56). More than 200 patients (27–35) were subsequently reported (57–61). Carcinoma occurs in less than 0.5% of fibroadenomas (59,62), and concurrence of the lesions probably is coincidental. Carcinoma occurs in 1% to 2% of phyllodes tumors (59,60).

### Clinical Presentation

The age of patients with carcinoma arising in a fibroadenoma ranged from 15 to 70 years (mean, 42 to 44 years) (59,62). The mean age of women with *in situ* carcinoma was 42 to 45 years, and the mean age of patients with invasion in the fibroadenoma was 47 to 52 years (57). Because patients who have carcinoma in a fibroadenoma tend to be somewhat older than those with fibroadenomas that lack carcinoma, the possibility of encountering carcinoma should be anticipated when a fibroadenoma is excised from a patient older than 35 years. The age distribution of women with carcinoma in, or associated with, a phyllodes tumor is not appreciably different from women with phyllodes tumors generally.

There are no specific clinical or radiologic clues to indicate the presence of *in situ* carcinoma within a fibroadenoma. Invasive carcinoma in, or associated with, a fibroadenoma may distort or blur the margin of the tumor in a mammogram. Rarely, the pattern of calcifications in a fibroadenoma can suggest intraductal carcinoma (63). Carcinoma is more likely to be detected in a fine needle aspirate from a fibroadenoma if the carcinomatous component is extensive. The diagnosis depends on recognizing neoplastic cells in the customary background of benign epithelium and stromal cells obtained from a typical fibroadenoma (64,65). If the lesion consists of *in situ* carcinoma limited to a small part of the tumor, the FNA specimen is unlikely to contain sufficient material to be diagnostic. Because there are no good clinical indicators of the presence of carcinoma in a fibroadenoma, the diagnosis generally is not suspected unless a needle core biopsy is obtained or the excised tumor has been studied pathologically. There also are no clinical signs to indicate that a phyllodes tumor harbors carcinoma.

### Gross Pathology

When *in situ* carcinoma is present in a fibroadenoma or phyllodes tumor, it usually will not be apparent on gross inspection (57). Fibroepithelial tumors that harbor carcinoma are not especially large, and many do not exceed 2 cm. Areas of unusual firmness may develop at the site of intraductal carcinoma, particularly the comedo type with calcifications. Invasive carcinoma confined to a fibroadenoma is generally inconspicuous and may not be appreciated, but invasion into the adjacent breast can distort the tumor enough to be evident grossly.

### Microscopic Pathology

The distinction between hyperplasia and *in situ* carcinoma in a fibroadenoma or phyllodes tumor is based on the same criteria that are used to assess epithelial proliferation in the mammary parenchyma. The presence and character of ep-

ithelial abnormalities within a fibroadenoma or phyllodes tumor does not necessarily reflect the proliferative status of the surrounding breast. Atypical epithelial lesions in fibroadenomas are prone to have a conspicuous myoepithelial component, and they often are characterized by a variety of proliferative abnormalities, including sclerosing adenosis, cysts, and apocrine metaplasia that constitute the so-called complex fibroadenoma.

### *Fibroadenoma*

The morphology of carcinomas that arise in fibroadenomas is not peculiar to this setting, but the relative frequency of the types of carcinoma differs from that of carcinomas found in the breast parenchyma. In published reports, more than 50% of the affected fibroadenomas had lobular carcinoma *in situ* (Figs. 35.1 and 35.2) (57,58). Among patients who were treated by mastectomy, lobular carcinoma *in situ* was found in the surrounding breast in about half of the cases. Nearly 20% of fibroadenomas with carcinoma had intraductal carcinoma (Figs. 35.3 and 35.4). Invasive duct carcinoma accounted for 20% of the cases (Fig. 35.5), and about 10% had invasive lobular carcinoma (Fig. 35.6). The invasive duct carcinomas have been well- to moderately differentiated lesions. It is exceedingly unusual for special

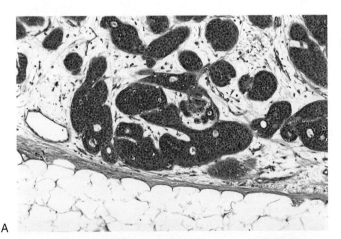

A

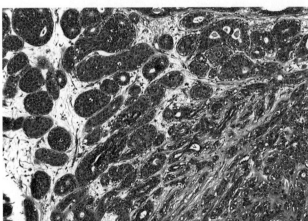

B

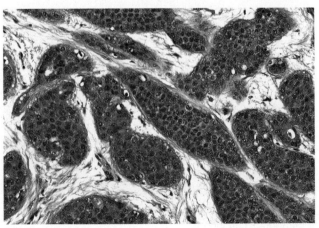

C

**FIG. 35.1.** *Fibroadenoma, lobular carcinoma* in situ. All images are from the same tumor. **A:** Epithelial component of the lesion is expanded by *in situ* lobular carcinoma. Lobular carcinoma *in situ* does not extend beyond the border of the fibroadenoma with edematous stroma. **B,C:** Lobular carcinoma *in situ* replaces part of the benign epithelium in this complex fibroadenoma in which there is sclerosing adenosis.

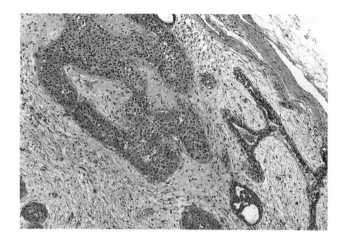

**FIG. 35.2.** *Fibroadenoma, lobular carcinoma* in situ. Much of the epithelial element is greatly expanded by lobular carcinoma *in situ*.

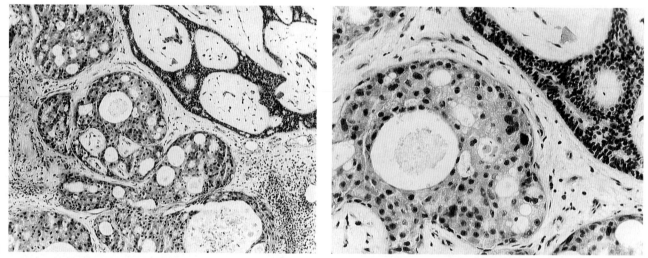

A                                                                                                B

**FIG. 35.3.** *Fibroadenoma, intraductal carcinoma.* **A:** Cribriform growth pattern. **B:** Apocrine cytology.

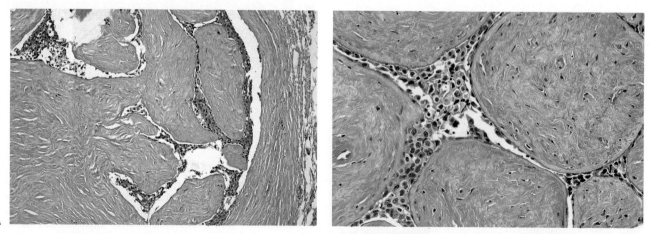

A                                                                                                B

**FIG. 35.4.** *Fibroadenoma, intraductal carcinoma.* **A,B:** The usual epithelium in these two different sclerotic fibroadenomas has been replaced by high-grade intraductal carcinoma.

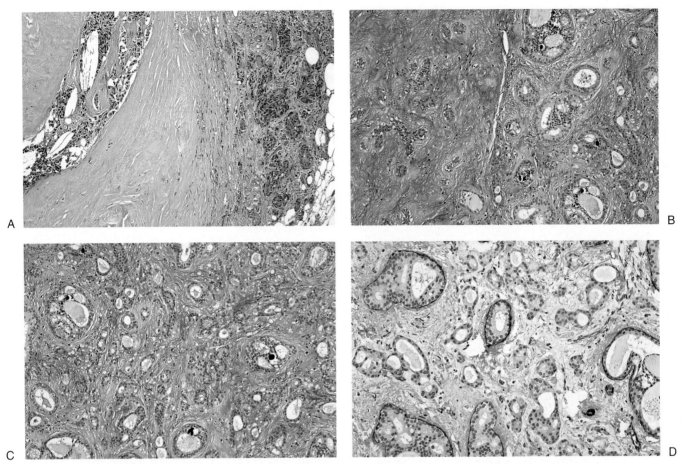

**FIG. 35.5.** *Fibroadenoma, invasive duct carcinoma.* **A:** Invasive duct carcinoma involving the periphery of a sclerotic fibroadenoma. Intraductal carcinoma is shown on the *left* (same tumor as shown in Fig. 35.4A). **B:** Cribriform intraductal carcinoma with calcifications in a myxoid fibroadenoma from a 30-year-old woman. Noncarcinomatous epithelium is on the *left* and invasive carcinoma is on the *far right.* **C:** Several ducts with cribriform intraductal carcinoma and calcifications in the midst of invasive well-differentiated duct carcinoma. **D:** Immunoreactivity for smooth muscle myosin heavy chain is shown around intraductal carcinoma. Staining is absent around invasive carcinoma (avidin-biotin). Images **B–D** are from the same tumor.

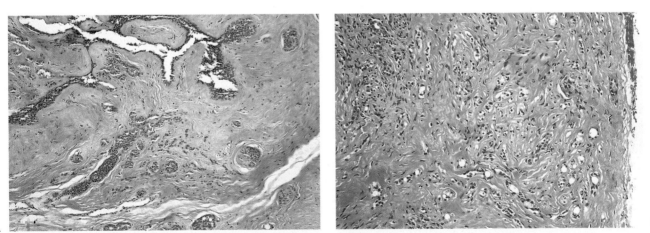

**FIG. 35.6.** *Fibroadenoma, invasive lobular carcinoma.* **A:** Small focus of *in situ* and invasive lobular carcinoma (*lower center*) in a fibroadenoma. **B:** Severe sclerosing adenosis in a complex fibroadenoma. This pattern simulates invasive lobular carcinoma.

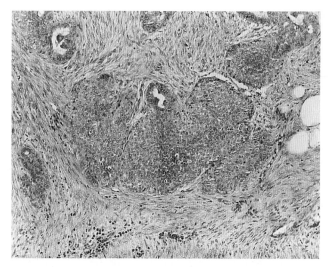

**FIG. 35.7.** *Phyllodes tumor, benign, with lobular carcinoma* in situ.

types of duct carcinoma (e.g., mucinous or papillary) to arise in fibroadenomas or phyllodes tumors.

The probability of finding carcinoma in the breast outside the fibroadenoma has been difficult to determine on the basis of published reports, because many patients have been treated only by excisional biopsy. A literature review of 62 published cases found extraadenomatous carcinoma in 42% of patients (62). Diaz et al. (57) reported that the type and amount of carcinoma in the fibroadenoma and the age at diagnosis were not significant predictors of the likelihood of finding carcinoma in the surrounding breast. Among women treated by mastectomy, carcinoma was limited to the fibroadenoma in a third to a half of cases that had *in situ* lobular carcinoma, intraductal carcinoma, or invasive lobular carcinoma (59,62). Invasive duct carcinoma that arose in a fibroadenoma involved the surrounding breast in at least 50% of cases. With rare exceptions, the same type of carcinoma has been found in the fibroadenoma and in the breast. Lobular carcinoma *in situ* may be detected in multiple fi-

broadenomas in one breast or in bilateral fibroadenomas (58). Axillary lymph node metastases have arisen from invasive carcinoma within a fibroadenoma in two cases (55,66). These exceptional situations must be distinguished from the more common circumstance in which a fibroadenoma that contained *in situ* carcinoma was present coincidentally with a separate invasive carcinoma that gave rise to axillary metastases. Ten to fifteen percent of patients had contralateral carcinomas concurrently or previously treated (56,58,59). The opposite breast contained invasive duct carcinoma in the majority of these cases. Subsequent contralateral carcinoma has been described in about 6% of cases (57).

### Phyllodes Tumor

Very florid hyperplasia involving epithelial and myoepithelial cells often is encountered in phyllodes tumors. The intensity and degree of atypia in the epithelial hyperplasia parallels that of the stromal component in some but not all cases. Mitoses may be seen in hyperplastic epithelial and myoepithelial cells.

Carcinomas arising in phyllodes tumors are similar histologically to carcinomas developing in fibroadenomas. Most have been *in situ* lobular carcinoma (Fig. 35.7), but intraductal (Fig. 35.8) and infiltrating duct carcinoma (Fig. 35.9) also have been described (59,60,67,68), and invasive lobular carcinoma also can be found in this setting. Phyllodes tumors that harbor carcinoma are usually benign or low-grade malignant tumors (68). A high-grade malignant phyllodes tumor that contains carcinoma is a form of carcinosarcoma, because these lesions are, by definition, neoplasms that contain carcinomatous and sarcomatous elements derived independently from the mammary epithelium and stroma. Carcinoma has been found in the surrounding breast tissue concurrently, or subsequent to, excision of a phyllodes tumor that contained carcinoma (60). Well-differentiated infiltrating duct carcinoma (69) and tubular carcinoma (70) have been described in phyllodes tumors. The latter case was un-

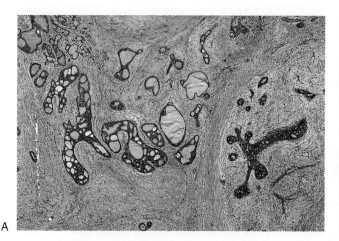

A

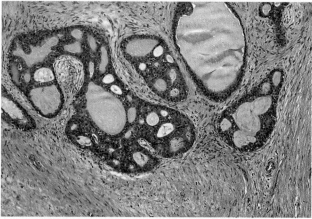

B

**FIG. 35.8.** *Phyllodes tumor, benign, with intraductal carcinoma.* **A,B:** Cribriform intraductal carcinoma has replaced most of the epithelium.

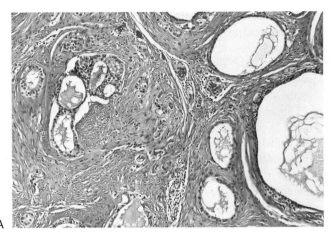 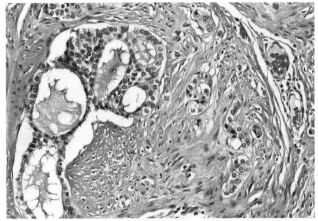

**FIG. 35.9.** *Phyllodes tumor, benign, with intraductal and invasive duct carcinoma.* **A,B:** Cribriform intraductal carcinoma is next to invasive duct carcinoma.

usual in that tubular carcinoma was found in the second recurrence of a benign phyllodes tumor. The first recurrence contained lobular carcinoma *in situ*. Other unusual pathologic presentations have been coexistent intraductal and *in situ* lobular carcinoma in a benign phyllodes tumor (71), as well as separate infiltrating duct carcinoma coincidental with benign (60) and malignant (72) phyllodes tumors and lobular carcinoma *in situ* in a phyllodes tumor with liposarcomatous stroma (73).

### Prognosis and Treatment

There have been very few deaths due to carcinoma arising in a fibroadenoma, and these have been attributable to invasive duct carcinomas (59,62). Recurrence in the breast following excisional biopsy of *in situ* lobular or intraductal carcinoma has been uncommon and appears to be less frequent than when the same lesions occurring outside of fibroadenomas have been treated only by excisional surgery (57). Some clinical series have reported recurrence rates in the breast greater than 10% following excisional biopsy of intraductal carcinoma with or without radiation, after follow-up of 10 years or less (74,75). There are virtually no published data on breast conservation therapy that used radiation in addition to excisional surgery. The overall lower frequency of subsequent carcinomas may reflect to some extent the relatively short follow-up, averaging less than 10 years in most series of patients with carcinoma arising in a fibroadenoma.

### OCCULT CARCINOMA PRESENTING WITH AXILLARY LYMPH NODE METASTASES

Fewer than 1% of patients who have mammary carcinoma present with an axillary lymph node metastasis as the first clinical manifestation of the disease (76,77). Among 10,014 primary operable breast carcinoma patients treated at one institution, 35 (0.35%) had occult carcinoma presenting with axillary metastases.

### Clinical Presentation

This condition occurs throughout virtually the entire age distribution of breast carcinoma from 30 to 83 years (76–82), with the mean and median age around 57 years. The right axilla and breast were affected slightly more often (54%) than the left in one series (80), but others reported left predominance (83,84). A positive family history of breast carcinoma has been reported in nearly 50% of patients (80,82), with about 25% having a maternal first-degree relative affected (76).

The initial clinical abnormality is enlargement of one or more axillary lymph nodes. An abnormality may be reported on clinical examination of the ipsilateral breast in 25% of patients, but often it is not regarded as suspicious, or on later follow-up it may not correlate with the location in the breast where carcinoma is detected (78,80,85). This observation is consistent with data complied by Rosen et al. (86), who studied nearly 3,500 patients with palpable lesions who had undergone mammography. Carcinoma was diagnosed in 64 women. The palpable lesion was carcinoma in 54 of these cases, but in 10 women the palpable tumor was benign and carcinoma was a nonpalpable lesion detected by mammography alone. In this series, none of the patients was initially examined because of axillary nodal involvement, but the study demonstrated the capacity of mammography to detect clinically occult carcinoma in the presence of a benign, palpable mass.

To rule out an extramammary tumor or other metastases, most women have been studied by at least one of a variety of techniques that include chest x-ray, bone scan, abdominal sonogram, scans of the liver and spleen, computed tomographic scans, gastrointestinal contrast studies, and intravenous pyelogram (78,80,81). Marcantonio and Libshitz (87) demonstrated axillary lymph node enlargement by computed tomography in patients with pulmonary carcinoma and proved the presence of metastatic carcinoma by biopsy in six cases, confirming the lung as one of the alternate primary sites for an occult carcinoma that presents with axillary metastases.

Mammography has revealed abnormalities in 12% (78), 25% (82), 26.5% (76), 31% (84), and 35% (80,85) of patients examined. The majority of these patients can therefore be classified as having false-negative mammograms. Tartter et al. (88) compared women with false-negative and positive mammography. The two groups were similar with respect to tumor differentiation, tumor size, mean S-phase fraction, and estrogen receptor status. However, women with false-negative mammography had a lower frequency of intraductal carcinoma and significantly more frequent metastases in axillary lymph nodes. Some investigators excluded patients with significant mammographic abnormalities from the syndrome of subclinical carcinoma presenting with axillary metastases (79,89), but others found no consistent correlation between the location of the radiologic abnormality and the site at which a carcinoma ultimately was located (80). If mastectomy is delayed, repeat mammograms of patients who initially had negative studies may reveal new findings suggestive of carcinoma (85). In one study, the interval until the detection of a breast abnormality clinically or by mammography was 6 to 39 months, with a mean of 15 months in women who did not undergo a mastectomy (90). The presence of mammographically detectable calcifications in metastatic carcinoma in axillary lymph nodes may be a clue to the diagnosis of a subclinical mammary carcinoma (91,92).

Magnetic resonance imaging (MRI) has proven to be an effective method for detecting occult carcinomas that are not evident mammographically. In one study, enhancement on magnetic resonance images led to the diagnosis of a clinically occult primary carcinoma in 9 of 12 women who presented with axillary nodal metastases (93). No tumor was found at the site of magnetic resonance enhancement in a tenth patient, and two women had no tumor found in the breast after a negative magnetic resonance study. Other investigators reported finding a tumor by magnetic resonance in each of four patients, including one woman with two lesions (94). Stomper et al. (95) used magnetic resonance to examine eight women who had negative mammograms when they presented with axillary nodal metastases (95). Sites of enhancement found in two (25%) cases proved to be invasive duct carcinoma. Henry-Tillman et al. located occult primary breast carcinomas in 8 of 10 women with negative mammography using 3D RODEO MRI (95a).

Occasionally, nodal enlargement occurs in the contralateral axilla of a patient treated previously for mammary carcinoma (96). This phenomenon was observed in 52 (3.6%) of 1,440 patients in one series (97). Most of these patients were judged to have systemic disease. Six (0.04%) of the 52 patients were treated by mastectomy, and two had a primary tumor in the contralateral breast. Breslow (98) reported that six (0.39%) of 1,543 patients with unilateral breast carcinoma subsequently developed carcinoma in contralateral axillary lymph nodes, and that a primary tumor was detected in four of the opposite breasts. In a series of patients presenting with axillary metastases from subclinical breast carcinoma, about 8% were previously treated for contralateral breast carcinoma (76,78) or developed subsequent

carcinoma in the contralateral breast (76,79). One patient had an augmentation prosthesis in the breast that harbored a subclinical carcinoma (76). It is very unlikely that the prior contralateral carcinoma is the source of axillary metastases in these situations and, in most instances, an occult primary gives rise to the newly apparent nodal metastases.

Clonal analysis may be used to evaluate metastatic carcinoma in contralateral axillary lymph nodes if material from the ipsilateral tumor is available for comparison. In the majority of cases, clonal analysis of the carcinomas in both breasts of patients with bilateral tumors has demonstrated cytogenetic differences indicative of independent origin of the lesions (99,100). Rarely, the pattern of clonal abnormalities in both tumors suggests metastatic spread from one breast to the other (100). A similar conclusion would be supported by finding that a primary carcinoma and metastatic tumor at another site, such as the chest wall or contralateral axillary lymph nodes, shared the same karyotypic abnormalities (99).

Occult breast carcinoma presenting as an axillary lymph node metastasis is exceedingly unusual in men (101–103). In some cases, axillary metastases from a nonmammary primary, such as carcinoma of the lung, have been documented in men generally after treatment of the pulmonary primary (90,104,105). There is insufficient experience with this presentation of male breast carcinoma to compare with female patients.

## Gross Pathology

The frequency with which a primary tumor was detected pathologically in the ipsilateral breast varies from 55% (81) to 82% (77,84). In most series, the proportion with a documented primary was about 75% (76,78,80,82,85). Although not clinically palpable, the majority of carcinomas were found upon gross examination of a mastectomy or excisional biopsy specimen (Fig. 35.10). Rarely, the breast contained

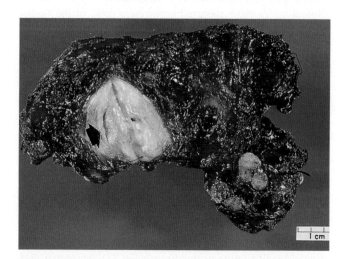

**FIG. 35.10.** *Occult carcinoma, mastectomy.* The *arrow* indicates a small invasive duct carcinoma that was not palpable clinically. A bisected axillary lymph node with metastatic carcinoma is shown in the lower right portion of the specimen.

two separate, grossly evident invasive primary carcinomas, each accompanied by an *in situ* component (82). The lesions have measured up to 6.5 cm (77,81,82), but most were 1 to 2 cm or less in diameter. In one series, the median size was 1.9 cm and the mean size was 1.5 cm, with 82% classified at T1, 14% as T2, and 4% as T3 (82). Smaller tumors often were discrete, with a stellate or circumscribed contour, but those larger than 2 cm more often had ill-defined margins and tended to blend grossly with the surrounding breast. The majority of the primary lesions occurred in the upper outer quadrant and less often in other quadrants (78,80–82,84). The occult primary tumor has been detected in the central or subareolar regions or in the axillary tail.

About 30% of the clinically occult primary carcinomas were not grossly evident. These lesions were found by taking multiple random sections of breast. They usually were located in tissue that appeared grossly normal. Consequently, sampling should not be limited to grossly abnormal parenchyma. Radiography of breast biopsies and mastectomies has not been helpful for locating the primary and cannot be relied on for guidance in the selection of tissue for histologic study. This is not unexpected in view of the lack of success with clinical mammography in these patients.

The likelihood of finding a primary lesion in the breast is related to the thoroughness with which the available tissue has been studied. In some cases, the primary tumor remains undetected because a breast biopsy and/or mastectomy were not performed. Despite the most careful and extensive gross and microscopic examination of a mastectomy, there are rare instances in which no primary is found. Patients not proven to have a primary breast carcinoma or a primary tumor at another site have a similar age distribution, similar lymph node findings, and comparable survival results as those with a pathologically demonstrated clinically occult breast carcinoma. In one series, none of the 12 patients without a documented primary lesion in the breast was later shown to have an extramammary primary (80).

Among patients subjected to axillary dissection, the number of lymph nodes found to be involved histologically varies from one to as many as 65 (77,78,82,85). When numerous lymph nodes are involved, they may form a matted mass with extranodal extension, but in most instances metastatic tumor is limited to discrete lymph nodes. In one series, half of the 40 patients had no more than three involved lymph nodes (one to three positive), including 13 patients whose only positive node was the one removed for diagnosis (Fig. 35.11). Among 15 women with carcinoma in four or more lymph nodes, the median number involved was 11.

## Microscopic Pathology

Metastatic adenocarcinoma in the axillary lymph nodes derived from an occult breast carcinoma usually has one of three patterns (Table 35.1). About 65% of the lymph nodes contain extensive infiltrates of large cells, often with apo-

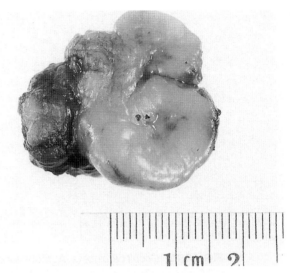

**FIG. 35.11.** *Occult carcinoma.* This lymph node containing metastatic carcinoma is more than 2 cm in diameter. No primary tumor was detected in the breast by clinical palpation, mammography, or gross examination of a mastectomy specimen.

crine features, diffusely distributed in the lymphoid tissue as well as in sinusoids (Figs. 35.12 and 35.13). Some of these lymph nodes contain predominantly sinusoidal metastases. Apocrine features include substantial cytoplasmic eosinophilia in most cases, but in some metastases, there is prominent cytoplasmic clearing (Fig. 35.14). Little or no gland formation is evident in this type of metastasis, but mucicarmine-positive secretion can be demonstrated in at least a few cells in most cases. Nuclei tend to be large, round, or oval and to be vacuolated with prominent, frequently eosinophilic nucleoli. This cell type and pattern sometimes are suggestive of metastatic malignant melanoma (Fig. 35.15), and metastatic renal cell carcinoma may be considered if cytoplasmic clearing is prominent. When the tumor cells are dispersed singly or in small groups throughout a lymph node, the resulting pattern might be confused with diffuse malignant lymphoma (Fig. 35.16). Small well-differentiated glandular metastases in an otherwise hyperplastic lymph node may be the presenting manifestation of an occult

**TABLE 35.1.** *Lymph node pathology in patients with and without primary breast carcinoma*

|  | With primary (N = 31) | Without primary (N = 12) |
|---|---|---|
|  | No. (%) | No. (%) |
| Large apocrine cells | 20 (65) | 8 (67) |
| Mammary carcinoma pattern | 7 (23) | 1 (8) |
| Mixed pattern | 4 (13) | 3 (25) |

Adapted from Haupt HM, Rosen PP, Kinne DW. Breast carcinoma presenting with axillary lymph node metastases. An analysis of specific histopathologic features. *Am J Surg Pathol* 1985;9:165–175.

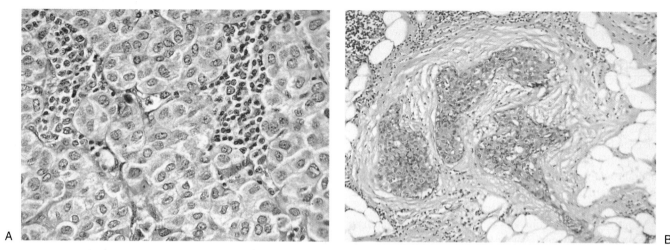

**FIG. 35.12.** *Occult carcinoma.* **A:** Metastatic adenocarcinoma in an axillary lymph node. The tumor cells have apocrine features consisting of abundant, finely granular eosinophilic cytoplasm, large open nuclei, and prominent nucleoli. **B:** This microscopic focus of intraductal carcinoma with periductal fibrosis and lymphocytic reaction was the only parenchymal lesion in the mastectomy.

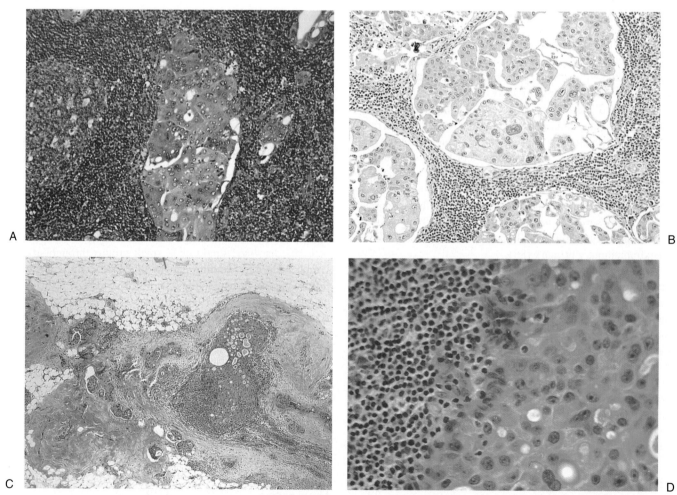

**FIG. 35.13.** *Occult carcinoma, apocrine.* **A:** Metastatic carcinoma, apocrine type, in a sinusoidal space of an axillary lymph node. **B:** Intracytoplasmic mucin is demonstrated with mucicarmine stain. **C:** Non-palpable intraductal and infiltrating primary carcinoma in the breast has focal lymphocytic infiltrates. **D:** Apocrine differentiation in the primary carcinoma. *(continued)*

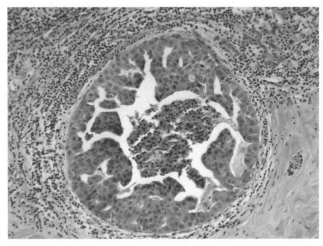

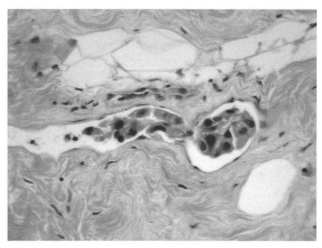

E F

**FIG. 35.13.** *Continued.* **E:** Intraductal carcinoma, papillary, with necrosis. **F:** Lymphatic tumor emboli in the primary carcinoma. All images are from one case.

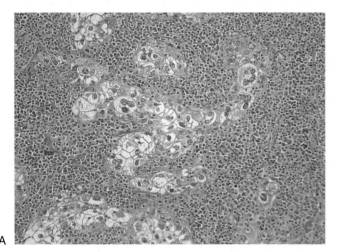

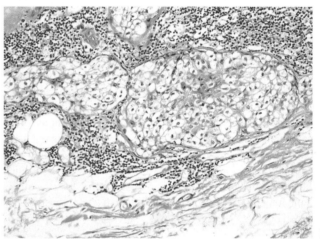

A B

**FIG. 35.14.** *Occult carcinoma, clear cell.* **A:** This metastatic carcinoma in an axillary lymph node was the initial manifestation of breast carcinoma in this patient. **B:** Clinically unapparent focus of intraductal carcinoma, clear cell type, with a surrounding lymphocytic reaction was found in the breast.

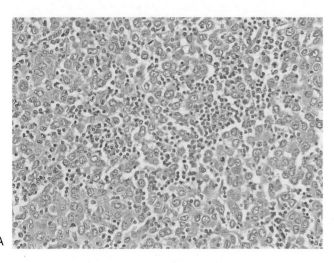

A

**FIG. 35.15.** *Occult carcinoma, diffuse.* **A:** The patient presented with an enlarged axillary lymph node found to contain malignant cells diffusely infiltrating the lymphoid tissue. *(continued)*

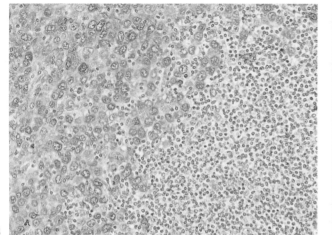

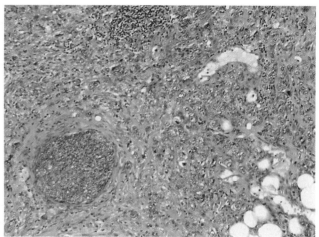

**FIG. 35.15.** *Continued.* **B:** The tumor cells are immunoreactive for S-100 protein (shown here) and for cytokeratin (avidin-biotin). **C:** Poorly differentiated infiltrating duct carcinoma found in the breast.

tubular carcinoma (Fig. 35.17). In these cases, the lymph node is enlarged by lymphoid hyperplasia, possibly in response to the metastatic carcinoma. These metastases should not be misinterpreted as benign glandular inclusions.

About 20% of axillary lymph node metastases consist of adenocarcinoma with growth patterns similar to those more commonly encountered in primary carcinomas in the breast. These include cribriform, papillary, glandular, and comedo forms of invasive carcinoma (Fig. 35.18). A scirrhous stromal reaction is rarely present in these nodal metastases. The remaining 15% of the lymph nodes contain mixtures of tumor with the conventional patterns and diffuse apocrine cells. Metastatic carcinoma from a nonmammary site, such as the lung, may be difficult to distinguish from breast carcinoma (Fig. 35.19).

Approximately 50% of the lymph nodes in each of the three patterns of metastases had some mucicarmine-positive cells (80). Among cases in which paraffin blocks were available to cut fresh sections for the mucicarmine stain, 75% gave a positive reaction. A lower proportion of positivity (30%) was found when the mucicarmine stain was done after decolorization of hematoxylin and eosin sections. A positive result with this simple procedure narrows the differential diagnosis substantially. Because mucin production often is inconspicuous and focal in these cases, the tumor should not be regarded as mucin negative unless several different blocks have been studied, whenever possible from different lymph nodes. It is not unusual to find mucin-positive cells limited to one of several lymph nodes.

If a diagnosis of adenocarcinoma is not apparent from the

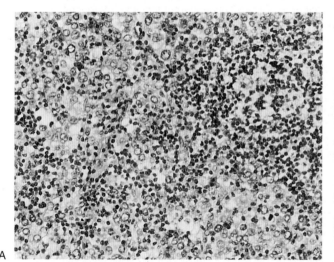

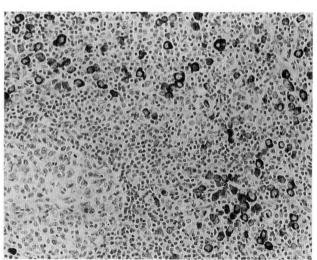

**FIG. 35.16.** *Occult carcinoma, diffuse.* **A:** Enlarged axillary lymph node in which poorly differentiated malignant cells, most prominent in the *upper left corner*, mingle with lymphocytes. The differential diagnosis for this pattern includes malignant lymphoma, metastatic carcinoma, and metastatic melanoma. **B:** Tumor cells were immunoreactive for cytokeratin (anti-CAM5.2, avidin-biotin).

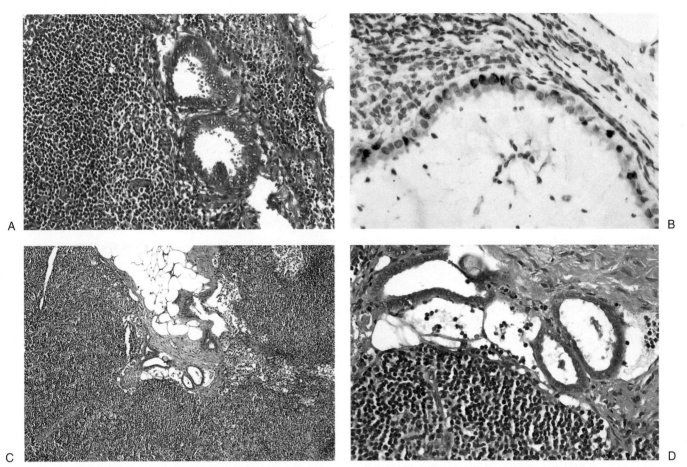

**FIG. 35.17.** *Occult carcinoma, tubular type.* **A:** Two glands of metastatic tubular carcinoma in the superficial lymph node tissue. **B:** Nuclear immunoreactivity for estrogen receptor is shown in one of the glands from **A** (avidin-biotin). **C,D:** Metastatic tubular carcinoma in subcapsular sinusoids of a hyperplastic lymph node.

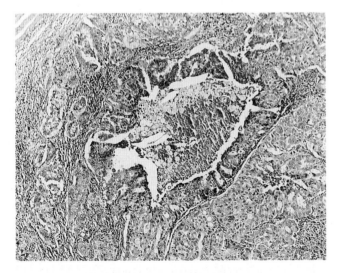

**FIG. 35.18.** *Occult carcinoma, cribriform.* Focal necrosis in metastatic cribriform carcinoma in an axillary lymph node.

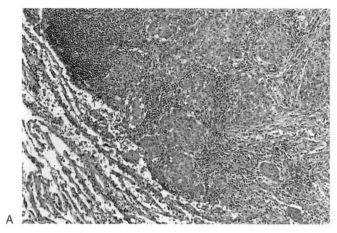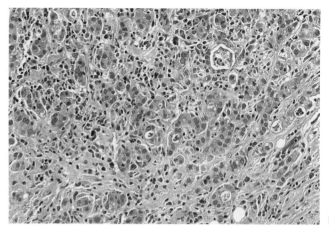

**FIG. 35.19.** Metastatic nonmammary carcinoma. **A:** Poorly differentiated adenocarcinoma of the lung. **B:** Metastatic pulmonary carcinoma in an axillary lymph node.

growth pattern and mucin stain, other studies may be helpful. Immunohistochemical procedures for cytokeratins, especially CK7 and CK20, epithelial membrane antigen, S-100 protein, carcinoembryonic antigen, lymphoid markers, and other cellular constituents usually resolve the differential diagnosis. Mammary carcinoma typically is immunoreactive for CK7 but not for CK20. It is rarely necessary to use electron microscopy (106).

When adenocarcinoma has been diagnosed in tissue removed from an axillary mass, there may be uncertainty as to whether this represents a metastasis or a primary axillary tumor. Because this distinction cannot be made on the basis of a needle biopsy, excisional biopsy is essential. Variation in the characteristics of tumor among affected lymph nodes can be helpful for diagnosis. It may require several sections of a mass of matted nodes to find a portion of uninvolved lymph node. The distinction between medullary carcinoma and metastatic carcinoma in a lymph node can be a particularly vexing problem. A reticulin stain is useful in this situation to reveal the underlying architecture of ducts that may be present in a primary carcinoma or the structure of a lymph node obscured by metastatic tumor. Tissue around the lymph node should be studied for evidence of axillary breast tissue. If found, this is presumptive evidence in support of an axillary primary, but it is necessary to find *in situ* carcinoma in conjunction with an invasive axillary lesion to establish a diagnosis of carcinoma arising in axillary breast tissue.

An unusual, largely hypothetical, source for mammary carcinoma arising in the axilla is heterotopic breast tissue in an axillary lymph node (107,108). This phenomenon is not likely to be recognized in a case presenting with an enlarged lymph node, because the heterotopic tissue probably will have been overgrown by the carcinoma. Because normal-appearing heterotopic mammary tissue is an extreme rarity in routine axillary dissections, transformation of these glands to carcinoma could account for only a very small proportion of breast carcinomas presenting as nodal metastases. Benign lesions that may be associated with axillary lymph nodes, such

as nevus cell aggregates and heterotopic glands, should not be misinterpreted as metastatic carcinoma (109).

Estrogen and progesterone receptors have been examined biochemically and immunohistochemically in axillary nodal metastases from patients with occult carcinoma (76,82, 106,110,111). The two largest series thus far reported presented similar results, with 32% to 35% positive for estrogen and progesterone receptors, 24% to 27% positive for estrogen and negative for progesterone receptors, and 38% to 44% negative for both receptors (76,82). Others also reported that estrogen and progesterone receptors were negative in the majority of axillary lymph nodes analyzed (83). The presence of one or both receptors in amounts regarded as positive is highly suggestive of, but not specific for, mammary carcinoma.

In most cases, the histologic characteristics of the primary tumor and nodal metastases were similar (Fig. 35.12). Nearly two-thirds of the primary tumors were invasive duct carcinomas. A striking characteristic of many of the primary lesions, particularly tumors too small to be palpable, was a prominent lymphocytic reaction in and around the lesion (Figs. 35.13, 35.14, and 35.20) (80,84). This was especially conspicuous when the primary lesion appeared to be largely or entirely *in situ*.

An exceptionally high proportion of the primary duct carcinomas had apocrine cytology, and there was a tendency to cytoplasmic clearing in the primary lesions as well as in metastases (Figs. 35.12–35.13). The invasive carcinomas tended to be poorly differentiated histologically and cytologically. The data presented in Table 35.2 show some cases in which the only carcinoma detected in the breast appeared to be noninvasive. This has been described in several studies (78,85,110,112). It is thought that metastases in these cases arose from invasive carcinoma that was inapparent with the light microscope in the *in situ* lesion (77,78,84,111,112), from foci of "healed" invasive carcinoma (Fig. 35.18), or from undetected invasive foci. The occurrence of axillary nodal metastases in women with intraductal carcinoma has also been documented by sentinel lymph node mapping

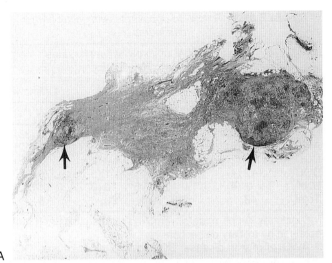

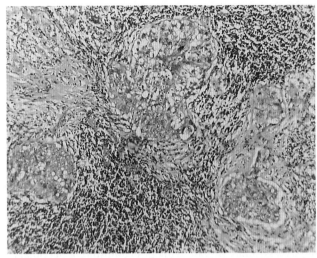

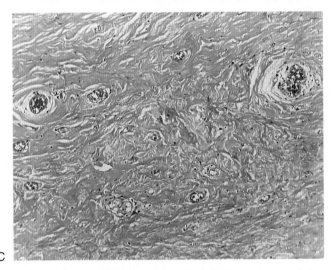

**FIG. 35.20.** *Occult carcinoma.* **A:** The entire occult carcinoma represented in this section consists of two nodular foci of intraductal carcinoma with lymphocytic reaction *(arrows)* and an intervening zone of fibrosis. **B:** Focus of intraductal carcinoma in the right-hand nodule. **C:** Dense collagenous tissue in the center of the lesion could be the site of "healed" invasive carcinoma.

(see Chapter 46). Infrequent examples of infiltrating lobular (77,78), medullary (84,98,106,113), mucinous (77), tubular (84), and papillary (77) carcinoma have been described. Analysis of hormone receptors in one series of primary tumors revealed positive levels of estrogen receptors in four (46%) of 11 and progesterone receptors in four (44%) of 9 (84).

**TABLE 35.2.** *Primary carcinomas found in breast*

|  | No. (%) |
| --- | --- |
| Invasive | 22 (79) |
|   Invasive duct | (65) |
|   Invasive lobular | (6) |
|   Medullary | (6) |
|   Colloid | (3) |
| Noninvasive | 7 (21) |
|   Intraductal | (12) |
|   *In situ* lobular | (6) |
|   Intraductal and *in situ* lobular | (3) |

Adapted from Rosen PP, Kimmel M. Occult breast carcinoma presenting with axillary lymph node metastases; a follow-up study of 48 patients. *Hum Pathol* 1990;21:518–523.

## Treatment

After it has been determined that an excised lymph node contains metastatic adenocarcinoma consistent with mammary origin in the absence of clinical evidence of a nonmammary tumor, treatment should be based on the assumption that there is an invasive primary carcinoma in the ipsilateral breast. A random biopsy of the breast may be obtained before initiating therapy, but without localizing clinical or radiologic signs this procedure is unlikely to detect the primary lesion. The majority of patients described in reports published in the past three decades were treated by mastectomy, often supplemented by local irradiation or chemotherapy. Mastectomy offers an opportunity to characterize and stage the primary tumor. Axillary dissection is performed to minimize the risk of recurrence in the axilla, and it provides prognostic information about the number of affected lymph nodes.

Breast-conserving surgery coupled with axillary dissection usually has been followed by breast irradiation (76,89). In some reports, radiation was given to the breast and axilla after the diagnosis of carcinoma was established by excisional or needle biopsy of an enlarged axillary lymph node (79,89,113). The 5-year disease-free survival reported with this approach varied from 66% to 76% (79,113–116). A primary tumor was detected clinically during follow-up in the ipsilateral breast of 7% to 33% of these patients.

Another approach to managing these patients has been to observe the ipsilateral breast, which remained unbiopsied and not irradiated. In 1907, Halsted (117) reported that up to 2 years might elapse before a primary tumor became clinically apparent in the breast if the patient did not undergo a biopsy or mastectomy. A more recent series included 17 patients with an untreated ipsilateral breast and a negative mammogram (84). Nine (52%) developed a clinically apparent primary tumor within 2 to 34 months (mean, 13 months). Two of the remaining eight patients died of progressive systemic disease without manifesting a mammary primary and six remained disease free, with an average follow-up of 6 years. Another report included 13 patients who did not have breast surgery or radiotherapy (83). Seven women (54%) developed a clinically evident primary tumor in the ipsilateral breast 11 to 47 months after diagnosis of the axillary metastasis (average, 27 months). Three of the carcinomas were in the upper outer and two in the upper inner quadrant. One lesion was subareolar, and diffuse involvement was observed in the seventh woman. Others observed a subsequent breast primary in two (13%) of 15 (116), one (20%) of five (118), and seven (88%) of eight (119) patients after average follow-up of 7.7, 2.2, and 3.5 years, respectively.

## Prognosis

The first large series with follow-up from a single institution, the Mayo Clinic, was published in 1954 (120). The article included the first reported example of this condition in a man. Follow-up of 25 patients revealed that nine (36%) died of breast carcinoma, three (12%) died of other causes, and 13 (52%) remained well. The authors concluded that these patients had "a better prognosis than is observed for the average carcinoma of the breast with nodal metastasis."

Several later studies also described a relatively favorable clinical course for patients treated by mastectomy and axillary dissection. Patel et al. (81) reported that 29% of patients died of disease, suggesting that the "prognosis is as good or better than it is for palpable breast cancer with axillary metastases." Two follow-up studies from Memorial Hospital in New York reported that 23% (76) and 25% (82) of patients died of breast carcinoma. In reports based on smaller series, 9% (78) and 12% (80) of patients had recurrent carcinoma and/or died of breast carcinoma.

Survival results for a series of 48 patients are shown in Table 35.3 (82). Follow-up ranged from 5 to 267 months (mean, 71 months; median, 60 months). Among patients alive and disease free, follow-up ranged from 33 to 367 months (median, 64 months; mean, 73 months). The intervals between diagnosis of breast carcinoma and the deaths of

**TABLE 35.3.** *Follow-up of patients with occult breast carcinoma*

| Status | Total patients | Number of involved lymph nodes[a] | | |
|---|---|---|---|---|
| | | 1–3 | ≥4 | Unknown |
| | No. (%) | No. (%) | No. (%) | No. (%) |
| NED | 29 (60) | 12 (60) | 14 (70) | 3 (38) |
| AWD | 3 (6) | 1 (5) | 1 (5) | 1 (12) |
| DOD | 12 (25) | 5 (25) | 4 (20) | 3 (38) |
| DOC | 2 (4) | 1 (5) | 1 (5) | 0 (0) |
| UNK | 2 (4) | 1 (5) | 0 (0) | 1 (12) |
| Total | 48 | 20 | 20 | 8 |

[a] Includes lymph node(s) removed for diagnosis and those obtained by axillary dissection.

AWD, alive with disease; DOC, died of other causes; DOD, died of disease; NED, alive, no evidence of disease; UNK, unknown.

Based on Rosen PP, Kimmel M. Occult breast carcinoma presenting with axillary lymph node metastases; a follow-up study of 48 patients. *Hum Pathol* 1990;21:518–523.

two patients from causes other than mammary carcinoma were 91 and 204 months. Two other patients surviving with recurrent carcinoma were alive 53 to 166 months after the original excision of carcinoma in an axillary lymph node. Patients who died of metastatic carcinoma survived 5 to 68 months (median, 26 months; mean, 31 months). Overall, 29 (60%) of the 48 patients remained alive and disease free. Two (4%) women died of causes other than mammary carcinoma, and the status of two (4%) patients was unknown. Recurrences occurred in 15 (31%) cases, including 12 (25%) patients who died of metastatic breast carcinoma. There was not a significant difference in the frequency of recurrence or of death due to disease between patients with one to three positive lymph nodes and those with four or more affected nodes, although the recurrence rate was higher in the latter group.

Twenty-two of the patients found to have a measurable primary tumor at mastectomy were chosen for a case-control analysis of survival (82). Matching was based on tumor size (±0.5 cm in T category), total number of involved lymph nodes (one to three vs. four or more, selected for closest total count), tumor type, and age at diagnosis. All patients were treated by mastectomy, and almost all patients received systemic adjuvant chemotherapy in both groups. The distributions of primary tumor size and axillary nodal involvement in the two groups were very similar. A comparison of follow-up results revealed a lower frequency of recurrence and death due to disease among patients who presented with axillary metastases and an occult primary tumor (Table 35.4). Survival curve analysis for the two groups is shown in Fig. 35.21. Although patients with occult lesions exhibited a more favorable prognosis overall, as well as when stratified by tumor size and nodal status, the differences were not statistically significant (Figs. 35.22 and 35.23). Patients who presented with palpable breast tumors had a less favorable

**TABLE 35.4.** *Follow-up of matched patients with occult and palpable breast carcinomas*

| Patient status | Total | | 1–3 | | ≥4 | |
| --- | --- | --- | --- | --- | --- | --- |
| | Occult (%) | Palpable (%) | Occult (%) | Palpable (%) | Occult (%) | Palpable (%) |
| NED | 16 (73) | 15 (36) | 9 (75) | 9 (38) | 7 (70) | 6 (33) |
| AWD | 1 (5) | 4 (10) | 1 (8) | 3 (13) | 0 (0) | 1 (6) |
| DOD | 5 (23) | 18 (43) | 2 (17) | 7 (29) | 3 (30) | 11 (61) |
| DOC | 0 (0) | 5 (12) | 0 (0) | 5 (21) | 0 (0) | 0 (0) |
| Total | 22 | 42 | 12 | 24 | 10 | 18 |

AWD, alive with disease; DOC, died of other causes; DOD, died of disease; NED, alive, no evidence of disease.

From Rosen PP, Kimmel M. Occult breast carcinoma presenting with axillary lymph node metastases: a follow-up study of 48 patients. *Hum Pathol* 1990;21:518–523, with permission.

outcome despite similar treatment that included chemotherapy for both groups.

Four other studies also described survival curve analysis of patients with occult stage II carcinoma (76,81,83,84). In a series of 29 women, the 5- and 10-year disease-free survival rates were 28% and 17%, respectively (81). These authors reported similar results for a comparison group of 127 patients who presented with palpable mammary primary tumors, but they gave no indication as to how patients with "known" breast carcinoma were chosen. Their patients with occult carcinoma did not have substantially larger primary tumors or more numerous involved lymph nodes than have been reported in other recent series, and the data provide no other obvious explanation for the unusually poor survival rate of stage II patients in both groups. Baron et al. (76) carried out a survival analysis of 35 patients and found that 63% were alive and disease free. Their study did not include a matched series of women who presented with palpable breast tumors.

Ellerbroek et al. (83) reported an overall survival rate of 71.8% at 5 years and 65% at 10 years. This study included two features found to be significantly associated with 5-year survival: axillary dissection (performed, 88.9% survival; not performed, 46.7% survival) and gross residual tumor in axilla after surgery (absent, 79.9% survival; present, 20% survival). In this study, there was not a significant difference in survival between patients treated by mastectomy and those treated by breast conservation. Although patients who received adjuvant chemotherapy had a better 5-year survival (92.9%) than those who did not receive systemic treatment (63.5%), the difference was not statistically significant.

Merson et al. (84) reported survival rates at 5 and 10 years of 76.6% and 58.3%, respectively. There was a trend to more favorable prognosis if metastases involved not more than three axillary lymph nodes when compared to women with four or more nodal metastases, but the difference was not statistically significant. Prognosis also appeared to be better in the group of patients who underwent mastectomy or breast irradiation when compared to patients who had no treatment of the breast (*p* = 0.06). Adjuvant systemic therapy did not significantly influence survival. Read et al. (113) also reported a lower frequency of local breast recurrence and a lower systemic recurrence rate in women with three or fewer nodal metastases after breast irradiation and axillary dissection. In this latter series, disease-free survival was higher in the group of patients who received systemic adjuvant therapy, but the difference from untreated patients was not statistically significant.

Several studies compared the outcome of patients with occult breast carcinoma treated by mastectomy with those who had breast preservation and radiation (76,83,84). Survival rates did not differ significantly for the two treatment groups.

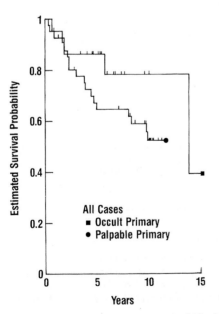

**FIG. 35.21.** *Occult carcinoma, overall survival.* Kaplan-Meier survival rate comparison of patients with clinically occult primary tumors to stage-matched patients who presented with a palpable breast tumor. Patients with clinically unapparent (occult) primary tumors had a more favorable survival, but the difference was not statistically significant. (From Rosen PP, Kimmel M. Occult breast carcinoma presenting with axillary lymph node metastases: a follow-up study of 48 patients. *Hum Pathol* 1990;21:518–523, with permission.)

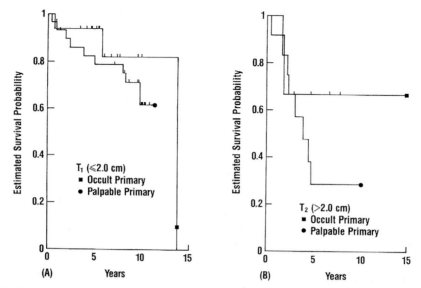

**FIG. 35.22.** *Occult carcinoma, tumor size and survival.* Kaplan-Meier survival rate comparison of matched patients stratified by primary tumor size. Differences are not statistically significant. *Left,* T1 tumors; *right,* T2 tumors. (From Rosen PP, Kimmel M. Occult breast carcinoma presenting with axillary lymph node metastases: a follow-up study of 48 patients. *Hum Pathol* 1990;21:518–523, with permission.)

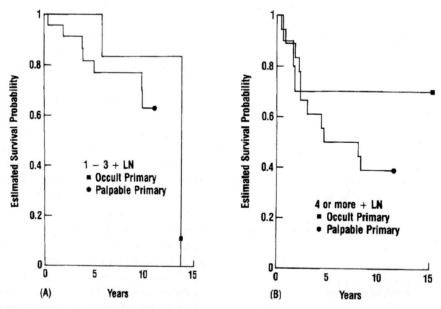

**FIG. 35.23.** *Occult carcinoma, lymph node status and survival.* Kaplan-Meier survival rate comparison of patients stratified for the number of involved lymph nodes (*LN*). Differences are not statistically significant. *Left,* one to three positive nodes; *right,* four or more positive nodes. (From Rosen PP, Kimmel M. Occult breast carcinoma presenting with axillary lymph node metastases: a follow-up study of 48 patients. *Hum Pathol* 1990;21:518–523, with permission.)

Breast recurrences have been reported in 19% and 23% of patients treated with mammary radiation (79,83). In one of these reports, the intervals between diagnosis of the axillary metastasis and detection of the primary breast carcinoma were 8, 44, and 106 months (83).

In conclusion, available data indicate that stage II patients who present with an axillary nodal metastasis and an inapparent breast primary have a prognosis similar to, and possibly better than, that of stage II patients who present with a palpable breast carcinoma. This probably reflects the fact that the majority of the stage II patients with clinically and, in most cases, radiographically occult carcinomas prove to have relatively small, grossly measurable invasive tumors detected in their breast on pathologic examination of the mastectomy specimen. The actual pathologically determined TNM stage is probably a more important determinant of prognosis than the apparent clinical stage when the patient is first examined. Magnetic resonance imaging is a very useful procedure for detecting an occult primary when none is evident on mammography.

## CARCINOMA IN ECTOPIC BREAST TISSUE

Supernumerary breast tissue is subject to proliferative conditions that affect the normal mammary gland, including cysts, papilloma with apocrine metaplasia (121), and other common hyperplastic changes (122). Adenomas have been described in supernumerary breast tissue, most commonly in the axilla (123) and vulva (124,125). These develop for the most part during pregnancy or lactation, and they represent nodules of lactational hyperplasia that persist in an adenomatous form (126). The tumors measured from 1.0 to 6.0 cm. Bilateral vulvar fibroadenomas have been reported (125). Patients with vulvar fibroadenomas generally have been between 20 and 50 years of age. A benign phyllodes tumor that originated in vulvar mammary tissue has been described in a 20-year-old woman (127). Breast tissue surrounding the tumor showed fibrocystic changes, including apocrine metaplasia and papillomatosis. The lesion recurred locally 8 months after excisional biopsy.

Carcinoma has been described arising in axillary (122,128,129) and vulvar (129–134) breast tissue. The most frequent site is in the axilla, but origin from parasternal, subclavicular, and inframammary ectopic breast has been reported (135). Histologically, most adenocarcinomas arising in supernumerary breast tissue had a ductal growth pattern (135). Infrequent examples of medullary, papillary, and infiltrating lobular carcinoma have been reported (Fig. 35.24) (135). Separate primary carcinomas arising concurrently in ectopic axillary breast tissue and in the ipsilateral breast are an extremely unusual coincidence (135). Ectopic breast tissue, especially when located in the axilla, may be distributed

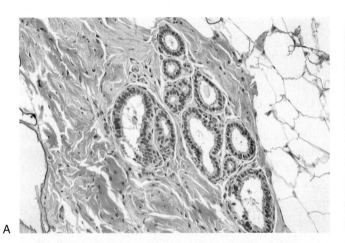

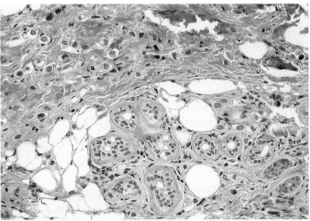

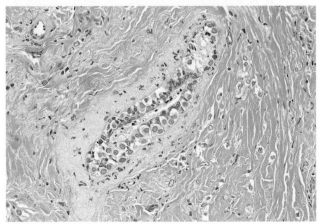

**FIG. 35.24.** *Ectopic breast in axilla with invasive lobular carcinoma.* **A:** Normal lobule in axillary breast tissue. **B:** Invasive lobular carcinoma in axillary tissue above a lobule. **C:** Pagetoid lobular carcinoma *in situ* in a duct and invasive lobular carcinoma. All images are from a single axillary tumor.

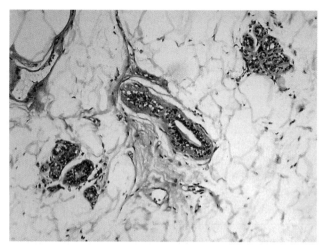

**FIG. 35.25.** *Ectopic breast in axilla.* Mammary duct and lobular glands found in the fat of an axillary lymph node dissection.

in subcutaneous tissue (Fig. 35.25) and the deep dermis of the skin. The breast tissue may mingle with normal skin appendage glands rather than forming a discrete, independent structure. In this circumstance, it can be difficult to distinguish between carcinoma of mammary and skin appendage gland origin. As discussed in Chapter 44, biologic markers such as hormone receptors can be helpful but are not always definitive for resolving this issue.

Residual breast tissue, not necessarily ectopic in its distribution, is a potential source for a new primary carcinoma on the chest wall after mastectomy (136,137). The presence of noncancerous breast tissue and/or an *in situ* component will distinguish such a new primary from a conventional local recurrence. It is essential that a lesion labeled clinically as a "local recurrence" at the site of a prior mastectomy be examined carefully for evidence of residual breast tissue and *in situ* carcinoma (Fig. 35.26). The presence of the latter features establish the tumor as a new primary carcinoma, with a clinical course determined by its specific histologic and bio-

logic properties. Rarely, there may be substantial differences in histology between the initial carcinoma and the new primary tumor that arises in residual breast tissue (Fig. 35.27).

Inflammatory carcinoma arising in the vulva was described in one patient (133). Another woman had asynchronous bilateral mammary carcinomas and a separate mammary type adenocarcinoma that arose in supernumerary vulvar breast tissue (132). Metastatic mammary carcinoma in the vulva that arose from a breast primary could mimic carcinoma arising in ectopic breast tissue (138).

Adenocarcinoma metastatic from carcinoma that arose in supernumerary breast tissue has been reported in ipsilateral axillary (128,129) and groin lymph nodes (131,134). In one case, analysis of metastatic tumor in a lymph node revealed estrogen and progesterone receptor levels of 297 and 27 fmol per milligram of cytosol protein, respectively (134). Another patient also had positive levels of estrogen (280 fmol per milligram protein) and progesterone receptors (51 fmol per milligram protein) in an inguinal lymph node metastasis (131). Immunoreactivity for estrogen and progesterone receptors and for gross cystic disease fluid protein has been reported in patients who had positive groin lymph nodes (130).

Treatment for ectopic invasive mammary carcinomas is wide local excision and regional lymphadenectomy. Lesions arising in the axilla are treated by axillary dissection, possibly including the tail of Spence. Mastectomy is not indicated if origin in supernumerary axillary breast tissue can be documented and there is no evidence of a separate primary tumor in the breast. Vulvar lesions are managed by partial vulvectomy and ipsilateral groin dissection. Many of these tumors had an aggressive clinical course with systemic metastases reported after axillary (128) and vulvar lesions (134). Adjuvant treatment with tamoxifen has been reported (130,131). Two patients died of metastatic carcinoma (132,134).

Breast tissue in a teratoma is a potential site for occult mammary carcinoma (Fig. 35.28). Extramammary Paget's disease has been described in ovarian and retroperitoneal

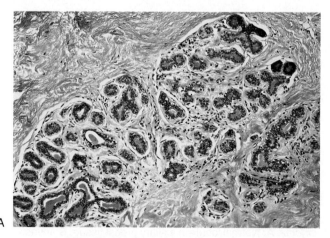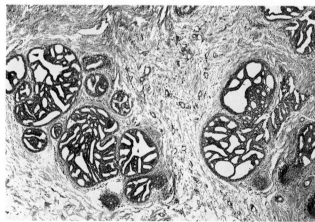

A  B

**FIG. 35.26.** *Residual breast tissue with carcinoma after mastectomy.* **A:** Residual breast tissue in the chest wall 8 years after a mastectomy. **B:** Mass at this site contained intraductal cribriform carcinoma and invasive well-differentiated duct carcinoma.

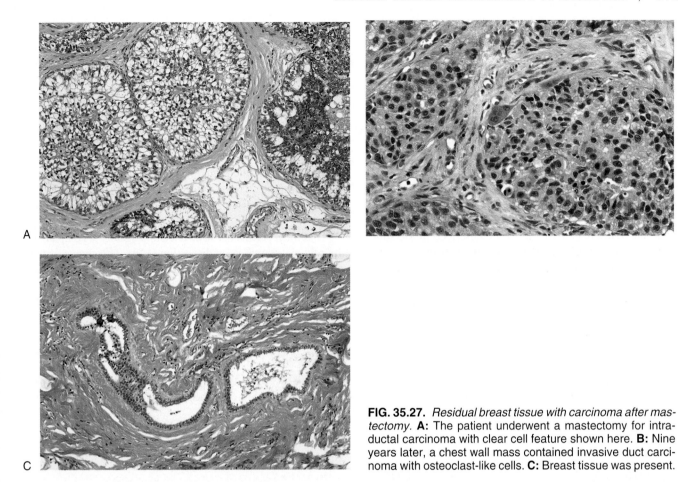

**FIG. 35.27.** *Residual breast tissue with carcinoma after mastectomy.* **A:** The patient underwent a mastectomy for intraductal carcinoma with clear cell feature shown here. **B:** Nine years later, a chest wall mass contained invasive duct carcinoma with osteoclast-like cells. **C:** Breast tissue was present.

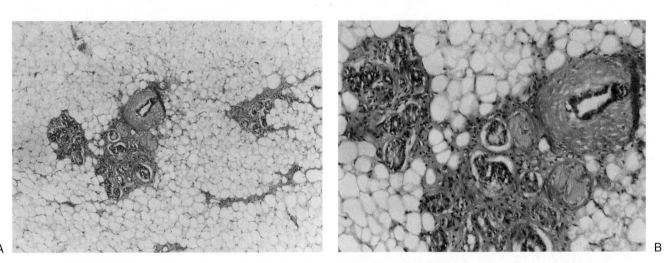

**FIG. 35.28.** *Breast tissue in a mediastinal teratoma.* **A:** Duct and atrophic lobular glands in fat. **B:** Magnified view of **A**.

teratomas (139–141), including one with invasive carcinoma (142).

A diagnosis of carcinoma arising in aberrant breast tissue (beyond the usual anatomic extent of the breast) can be made if intraductal and/or invasive carcinoma is found in subcutaneous mammary glandular parenchyma beyond the normal extent of the breast (Fig. 35.29). The distinction between breast tissue remaining after mastectomy and aberrant breast tissue largely depends on location, and the lesions arising in the two settings are indistinguishable. In the absence of *in situ* changes and glandular parenchyma, the histologic appearance of the invasive carcinoma often is indistinguishable from carcinoma of sweat gland origin. Carcinoma originating in aberrant breast tissue has been described in the subclavicular and anterior axillary regions, over the sternum (138), and in the upper abdominal skin (143–145) outside the distribution of the milk lines (146). The tumors have been infiltrating ductal adenocarcinomas in most cases. One patient had cystic papillary carcinoma in the inframammary upper abdominal region (144). One carcinoma was positive for estrogen receptors (99 fmol per milligram protein) and negative for progesterone receptors (143).

Diagnosis by FNA of carcinoma arising in aberrant breast tissue has been reported (143,147,148). In addition to carcinoma arising in ectopic breast tissue, the differential diagnosis of an FNA specimen containing atypical epithelial cells obtained from an axillary mass includes a proliferative lesion in ectopic breast and metastatic carcinoma in a lymph node. Proliferative epithelium is most likely to be encountered when ectopic breast tissue enlarges during pregnancy or, in rare instances, of fibroepithelial neoplasms arising from such tissue (149). One unusual case in which the diagnosis was made by aspiration biopsy involved a 45-year-old woman with a 3.0-cm subcutaneous lesion on the submammary chest wall (150). Excisional biopsy confirmed the presence of infiltrating duct carcinoma that arose in ectopic breast tissue.

Treatment consists of wide excision, usually accompanied by regional lymph node dissection (143). The choice of the lymph node group most likely to be involved by metastases may be difficult if, for example, the lesion is located over the sternum or the upper abdomen (146). Sentinel lymph node mapping may be helpful in this situation.

## INFLAMMATORY CARCINOMA

In 1807, Charles Bell (151) reported that "when a purple color is on the skin over the tumor it is a very unpropitious

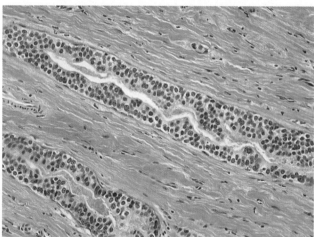

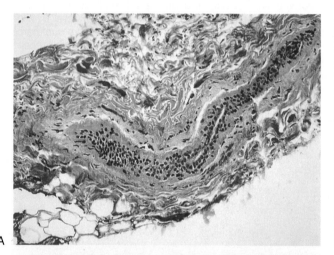

**FIG. 35.29.** *Aberrant breast.* **A:** Mammary duct in the subcutaneous tissue around a carcinoma excised from the upper abdominal wall below the inframammary fold. **B:** Intraductal carcinoma in the same specimen. **C:** Infiltrating duct carcinoma.

beginning." This is said to be the first clinical reference to inflammatory carcinoma. Reviewing the subject in 1916, Learmonth (152) commented that the many synonyms were "verily a distressful commentary on the 'chaotic condition' of the present-day terminology of diseases of the breast." Lee and Tannenbaum (153) proposed the currently used term *inflammatory carcinoma* in 1924.

Inflammatory carcinoma refers to the clinical appearance of patients with this condition. It is not a specific histologic subtype of mammary carcinoma. However, some investigators included histopathologic findings among their diagnostic criteria. An assessment of the frequency of this uncommon condition largely depends on clinical reporting. In population-based studies of over 50,000 patients, inflammatory carcinoma constituted 10.1% and 6.2% (154,155) of carcinomas in blacks and whites, respectively, when the diagnosis was made on clinical and/or pathologic criteria (156). If the diagnosis was entirely based on pathologic features, the reported frequencies were 0.7% for blacks and 0.5% for whites. Clinically diagnosed inflammatory carcinoma was said to be present in 9% of blacks and 5.8% of whites. Information provided by the Surveillance, Epidemiology, and End Results (SEER) Program of the National Cancer Institute revealed an increased incidence among whites (0.3 to 0.7 cases per 100,000 person-years) and African-Americans (0.6 to 1.1 cases per 100,000 person-years) in the periods 1975 to 1977 and 1990 to 1992 (157). In institutional series, the frequency of inflammatory carcinoma reportedly varies from 1% to 10% depending on diagnostic criteria and the nature of the institution. Patients with this condition often are referred to tertiary treatment centers, where they constitute a relatively higher proportion of patients than would be encountered in general clinical practice.

The age distribution of primary inflammatory carcinoma is not significantly different from common infiltrating duct carcinoma, averaging about 55 years (152,158,159). It is only rarely encountered in children (160,161) and men (162). Pregnancy and lactation do not predispose to the clinical presentation of inflammatory carcinoma, although breast carcinomas that arise in this setting are prone to have lymphatic tumor emboli in the breast parenchyma (158,163).

## Clinical Features

*Primary inflammatory carcinoma* was classified as stage IIIb by the American Joint Committee on Cancer in 1988 (164), but more recently it has been categorized as a T4d tumor (165). The latter staging system does not require that dermal lymphatic tumor emboli be demonstrated. Carcinoma that develops inflammatory features in a recurrence, but with no inflammatory changes seen initially, is referred to as *secondary inflammatory carcinoma*.

*Primary inflammatory carcinoma* is characterized by erythema of the mammary skin (Fig. 35.30). Typically, the skin is thickened, especially at the edge of the erysipeloid area, with *peau d'orange* changes usually conspicuous over dependent portions of the breast (159,166,167). When the condition is advanced, these changes may extend to the skin of the chest wall (Fig. 35.31). In most patients, the breast is diffusely indurated or a mass can be palpated centrally, but at an early stage some patients do not have a palpable lesion when cutaneous changes are initially evident (168). Skin thickening is invariably seen on mammography, whereas

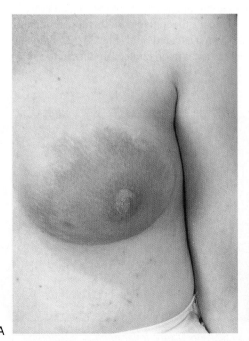
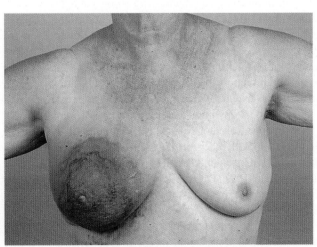

**FIG. 35.30.** *Primary inflammatory carcinoma.* **A:** Cutaneous erythema predominantly over the dependent part of the breast. **B:** Most of the swollen breast is involved, and there is desquamation of the skin.

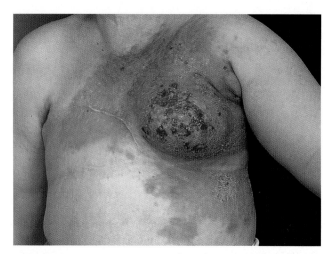

**FIG. 35.31.** *Primary inflammatory carcinoma.* Spread to the chest wall is evident.

within the breast, there may be a mass, stromal coarsening, or diffusely increased parenchymal density (169–171). Thickening of the skin due to edema is not a specific radiologic feature of inflammatory carcinoma, because it can be found in patients with lesions that lack inflammatory features (167,172). Calcifications may be present with or without a mammographically detectable mass (169). Magnetic resonance imaging cannot be relied on to distinguish between mastitis and inflammatory carcinoma, but patients with inflammatory carcinoma are more likely to have greater than 100% enhancement of their lesion in the first minute after contrast administration (173).

Focal cutaneous erythema sometimes is localized to the region overlying a palpable tumor. Detection of a mass may precede the appearance of the skin change. Haagensen (158) observed that the diagnosis of inflammatory carcinoma requires that at least one-third of the mammary skin be affected. However, it has been noted that the prognosis of patients with less extensive cutaneous changes is as grave as that of women with classic inflammatory carcinoma (174). Patients with inflammatory carcinoma tend to be younger than women with locally advanced carcinoma that does not have an inflammatory component, and their tumors are more likely to be estrogen receptor negative (174,175).

Inflammatory carcinoma may be mistaken at first for a nonneoplastic inflammatory condition because of the rapid onset and pain described by the patient (153). Diffuse leukemic or lymphomatous involvement of the breast may simulate inflammatory carcinoma. A substantial number of these patients present with other features of locally advanced carcinoma manifested by enlarged axillary and/or supraclavicular lymph nodes (159). Patients with the clinical syndrome of rapidly progressing breast carcinoma described in Tunisia usually have inflammatory carcinoma (176).

The primary tumor of inflammatory carcinoma has been negative for estrogen and progesterone receptors in about 60% of cases (175,177–179). Lymphatic tumor emboli and dermal deposits of carcinoma in a skin biopsy from a patient with in-

flammatory carcinoma constitute only a small part of the specimen. The availability of immunohistochemical procedures makes it possible to selectively examine the tumor in such samples. Most have proven to be receptor negative by this method, but occasionally the tumor cells have been found to have estrogen receptors demonstrable by immunohistochemistry.

Amplified expression of HER2/*neu* has been found in inflammatory breast carcinomas (178). There was a trend toward more frequent amplified expression in cases with negative estrogen receptors or with positive lymph nodes. In another study, all 22 samples of inflammatory carcinoma were immunoreactive for HER2/*neu* and cathepsin D (177). A transplantable xenograft model of human inflammatory carcinoma displayed the same absence of estrogen and progesterone receptors, and p53 and epidermal growth factor receptor as the primary tumor used to develop the xenograft (180). However, the xenograft exhibited amplification of HER2/*neu* that was not present in the primary tumor, as well as 10- to 20-fold overexpression of E-cadherin. Molecular characteristics of inflammatory carcinoma also have been investigated (181).

*Secondary inflammatory carcinoma* usually occurs at metastatic foci in the skin of patients who had axillary lymph node metastases when initially treated. Clinically, the inflammatory form of recurrent carcinoma is characterized by the same discoloration and edema of the skin as primary inflammatory lesions. These changes tend to develop on the chest wall at the site of prior mastectomy, but they also can be found associated with distant cutaneous recurrences (182). Inflammatory changes at distant sites are not specific for mammary carcinoma, because they have been reported in metastases from carcinoma of the pancreas, stomach, lung, and other sites (183,184). Occasionally, secondary inflammatory carcinoma is limited to the treated region in patients who receive postoperative radiotherapy, or it may occur only outside of an irradiated field (Fig. 35.32). Palpable tumor infiltrates are a common clinical finding in the skin (159).

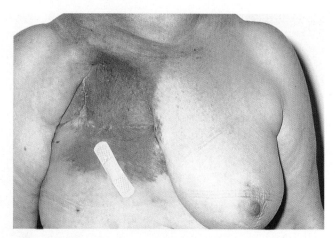

**FIG. 35.32.** *Recurrent inflammatory carcinoma.* Inflammatory carcinoma appears clinically to be restricted to the area of radiation on the chest wall and supraclavicular region.

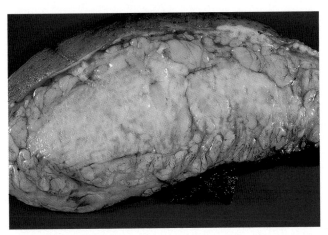

**FIG. 35.33.** *Inflammatory carcinoma, mastectomy.* Invasive carcinoma is present throughout the breast without forming a discrete tumor. Note *peau d'orange* change in the skin surface.

## Gross Pathology

Patients with primary inflammatory carcinoma have an underlying invasive mammary carcinoma. The primary tumor typically is indistinct clinically, radiologically, and pathologically. If a mastectomy is performed, the size of the tumor may not be recorded because the gross margins cannot be defined (Fig. 35.33). Frequently, the breast is said to be diffusely involved, or a large tumor is described (185). As a consequence, accurate data about the size distribution of the primary tumors are unavailable. In one series, localized tumors measured 2 to 12 cm, averaging 6 cm in greatest diameter (185). The majority of the carcinomas were central, or they were large enough to occupy virtually the entire breast. Diffuse induration of the mammary parenchyma was palpable and the skin was visibly thickened. The skin was 2 to 8 mm thick (average, 4 mm). This is substantially more than the normal thickness that varies from $1 \pm 0.2$ mm over the upper outer quadrant to $1.5 \pm 0.4$ mm over the areola (186). Despite diffuse dermal involvement by tumor emboli or direct invasion into the skin, cutaneous ulceration is found only in very advanced cases. Paget's disease of the nipple is uncommon, although the nipple often is retracted (186). When present, Paget's disease typically is accompanied by intraductal carcinoma of major lactiferous ducts.

## Microscopic Pathology

*Primary inflammatory carcinoma* usually is a manifestation of infiltrating duct carcinoma that almost always is poorly differentiated (Fig. 35.34) (185,186). Tumor emboli usually

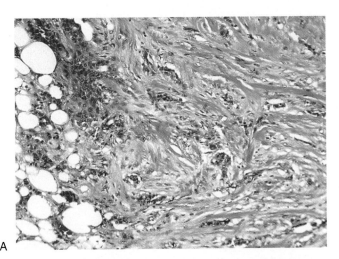

A

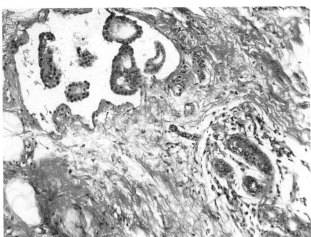

B

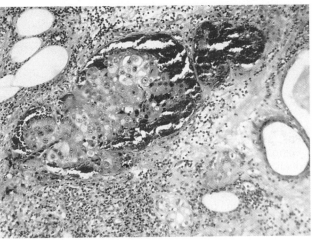

C

**FIG. 35.34.** *Primary Inflammatory carcinoma.* **A:** The primary tumor is an infiltrating, poorly differentiated duct carcinoma. **B:** Clusters of carcinoma cells in a dilated lymphatic channel. **C:** Carcinomatous emboli in a vascular channel with red blood cells.

are encountered throughout the breast, but in a few cases this has been an inconspicuous feature. Many of the vascular spaces that contain tumor, devoid of red blood cells, are considered to be lymphatics. However, channels of similar structure and caliber containing erythrocytes and tumor emboli also are encountered, especially in patients with extensive vascular and lymph node involvement. Hence, a distinction between blood vessel and lymphatic emboli often is difficult.

A lymphoplasmacytic reaction may be encountered in the tumor or in the surrounding breast, but it does not differ in intensity, pattern, or frequency from the findings in patients with noninflammatory carcinoma (159,185,186). The intensity of the reaction in the breast and skin usually are similar, but these reactive components have not been found to correlate with the severity and distribution of the clinical cutaneous manifestations of the disease. That is, patients with the most marked lymphoplasmacytic reaction do not necessarily

have the most intense cutaneous erythema or the most severe edema (176). There also is no direct relationship between the number of lymphatic tumor emboli or the extent of vascular distension and the clinical findings. Neutrophils, eosinophils, or numerous mast cells are not a common feature of inflammatory carcinoma.

Because the cutaneous manifestations of inflammatory carcinoma are so striking clinically, there has been a great deal of interest in the microscopic pathology of the skin. Often, a biopsy of the skin is performed for diagnostic purposes, but the diagnosis of carcinoma can be made easily by needle biopsy of the breast if there is an underlying palpable mass. It is not necessary to obtain a skin biopsy to establish the diagnosis of inflammatory carcinoma when a patient presents with characteristic clinical findings.

The skin often displays a variety of histologic alterations associated with inflammatory carcinoma (Fig. 35.35). The

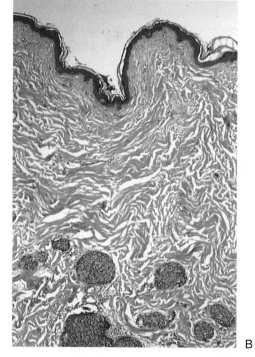

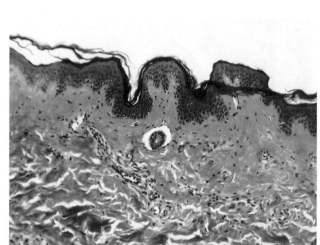

**FIG. 35.35.** *Primary inflammatory carcinoma, cutaneous pathology.* **A:** Cluster of carcinoma cells is present in a lymphatic space in the reticular dermis. **B:** Numerous groups of carcinoma cells distend vascular channels in the deep dermis. The reticular dermis is thickened and composed of coarse collagen bundles. **C:** Carcinomatous emboli in small lymphatic spaces are accompanied by a perivascular lymphocytic reaction in the reticular dermis.

collagenous reticular dermal layer is broader than normal due to increased amounts of collagen and edema. Dilation of lymphatics tends to be prominent in the papillary and reticular dermis, and intralymphatic tumor emboli can be found at either level of the dermis. When present, a lymphoplasmacytic reaction is localized around dilated lymphatic and vascular channels.

The microscopic pathology of the skin varies greatly among patients with inflammatory carcinoma. Histologic features of the skin are not necessarily correlated with the clinical findings. Samples of skin from within and outside the zone of erythema and edema may appear histologically identical, with lymphatic tumor emboli detectable in areas that appear clinically uninvolved. When carcinoma is found in the skin of a patient with primary inflammatory carcinoma, it usually is limited to lymphatic emboli. Nodular or plaquelike extralymphatic dermal tumor infiltrates are uncommon.

In some patients with the classic clinical appearance of inflammatory carcinoma, tumor may not be found in biopsies of the skin, even if serial sections of the specimen have been prepared (114,166–168,186). The skin biopsy was reportedly negative in 50% of patients (167). As a consequence, no pattern of histologic findings is specifically associated with the clinical diagnosis of primary inflammatory carcinoma.

*Inflammatory recurrent carcinoma* usually is accompanied by nodules and plaques of invasive carcinoma in the dermis of the skin, as well as intralymphatic tumor emboli (Fig. 35.36). In some of these cases, lymphatic tumor emboli are inconspicuous or not detectable. Clinically, erythema and edema occur equally in the skin over and around palpable dermal tumor infiltrates, regardless of the presence of dermal lymphatic tumor emboli.

A review of the primary lesions in patients who developed inflammatory recurrence suggested some predisposing features (159). All patients had infiltrating duct carcinomas, including a disproportionately high number with apocrine cytology. Inflammatory recurrence was rarely found following treatment of papillary, medullary, and mucinous carcinomas. Although these patients did not exhibit the clinical signs of inflammatory carcinoma when initially treated, parenchymal intralymphatic tumor emboli were seen in many of the mastectomy specimens. A number of these patients also had lymphatic tumor emboli in the nipple and/or the skin of the breast (Fig. 35.37). The majority of patients with an inflammatory recurrence initially had metastases involving many enlarged axillary lymph nodes, but this type of recurrence can develop in a patient who did not have axillary lymph node metastases.

The term *occult inflammatory carcinoma* describes a group of patients who have cutaneous and parenchymal lymphatic tumor emboli associated with their primary tumor in the absence of cutaneous erythema and other clinical changes that typify inflammatory carcinoma (155,186). Occult inflammatory carcinoma occurs in 1% to 2% of patients with invasive carcinomas that are not clinically inflammatory (186). The primary tumors tend to be central, larger than 4 cm, and often multicentric. The pathologic findings are not appreciably different from those in women with primary inflammatory carcinoma. These patients are predisposed to develop inflammatory recurrences (159). When compared to women with primary inflammatory carcinoma, patients with occult inflammatory carcinoma may have a relatively better prognosis (186a).

### Prognosis and Treatment

Until the introduction of combined modality treatment including intensive chemotherapy, less than 5% of patients with inflammatory carcinoma reportedly survived 5 years (159,187). Although one group of investigators suggested

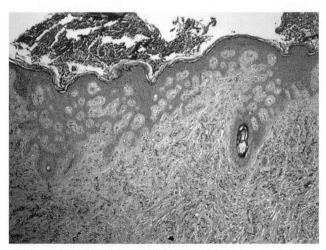

**FIG. 35.36.** *Inflammatory recurrent carcinoma.* Diffuse dermal infiltration of poorly differentiated duct carcinoma in a patient with recurrent carcinoma on the chest wall and the clinical manifestations of inflammatory carcinoma.

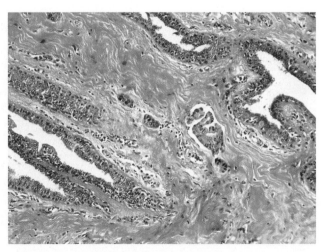

**FIG. 35.37.** *Lymphatic tumor emboli in the nipple.* Carcinoma cells in lymphatic channels in the stroma of the nipple in a patient who did not have clinical manifestations of inflammatory carcinoma. Recurrent carcinoma in such a patient is likely to have inflammatory features clinically.

that inflammatory carcinoma patients with no detectable dermal lymphatic tumor emboli had a more favorable prognosis (154), others did not find this to be the case (168,186,188). Patients with occult inflammatory carcinoma may have a slightly less acute clinical course, but ultimately not a better survival, than women with classic primary inflammatory carcinoma.

Reports in the 1980s and early 1990s described a substantial improvement in prognosis, with 5-year survival rates ranging from 25% to 48% (188,189–191) and a 10-year survival rate of 32% (191). One series had a projected 5-year relapse-free survival rate of 31% (188). Clinical stage at the time of diagnosis had an important influence on prognosis with a better 5-year survival rate observed in those with localized than with regional disease (189,191). Clinical features at the time of presentation that were associated with a less favorable prognosis were diffuse erythema, axillary lymph node metastases, and chest wall adhesion. Mastectomy alone was shown in the past to be ineffective and rarely indicated for inflammatory carcinoma (159), but it now is considered an integral part of the multimodality treatment program. Mastectomy has been more effective for obtaining local control of the primary tumor when preceded by combination chemotherapy followed by radiation (179,192–196). Treatment with anthracycline-based neoadjuvant chemotherapy followed by surgery and/or radiotherapy and additional radiotherapy can result in local control in at least 80% of patients and 5-year survival rates greater than 50% (197).

Radiation and chemotherapy often cause a diminution in the clinical manifestations of inflammatory carcinoma prior to a mastectomy. The effects of treatment include some or all of the following: decrease or elimination of erythema, reduction in breast size, loss of cutaneous edema, and decrease in the size of a palpable tumor if present. Enlarged axillary lymph nodes in the radiation treatment field may become smaller. In a few patients, clinical signs disappeared entirely, but residual carcinoma was found microscopically at mastectomy in virtually all cases (179,190,193,195–198). Clinical complete response has been reported in 12% to 52% of

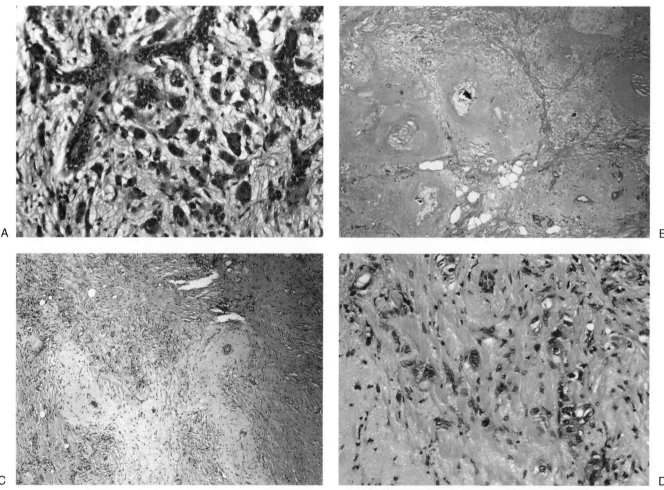

**FIG. 35.38.** *Chemotherapy effect in inflammatory carcinoma.* **A:** Invasive, poorly differentiated carcinoma surrounds mammary ductules. **B:** Three months after treatment with combination chemotherapy, broad areas of hypocellular, loose stroma with scattered calcifications remain in areas where the carcinoma was destroyed by treatment and resorbed. **C:** Fibrosis and mild chronic inflammation beginning to occupy an area of resorbed carcinoma. **D:** Microscopic foci of carcinoma remaining in the treated breast.

patients, with pathologic complete response in 4% to 33% (197). Various sequences of treatment have been shown to reliably improve local control and disease-free survival. Amelioration of edema, erythema, breast enlargement, and tumor mass was associated with a relatively longer disease-free survival than was achieved in patients who did not respond to treatment (188,193,199).

The clinical description of response to treatment does not always correlate well with the pathologic findings in the mastectomy specimen. Considerable residual tumor, often with substantial lymphatic tumor emboli, may persist despite a "complete" clinical response. Alternatively, women reported to have partial or minimal response may prove to have little or no microscopically demonstrable tumor. In the latter situation, one typically finds substantial alterations in the mammary parenchyma where the tumor has been destroyed (Fig. 35.38). These changes, which vary from simple fibrosis to chronic granulomatous inflammation, are described in detail in Chapter 43. A similar effect was observed in axillary lymph nodes that were pathologically devoid of tumor after treatment, although there appeared to be little response clinically. It has been suggested that pathologic findings in the mastectomy specimen predict prognosis more accurately than the clinical assessment of response to treatment (199,200). In one study, "therapeutic response parameters" associated with the most favorable outcome were complete regression after induction therapy within 8 months of diagnosis and complete regression of inflammatory symptoms within 3 months of neoadjuvant therapy (191). Patients who exhibit a good response clinically and pathologically appear to have the best prognosis. The number of involved lymph nodes may be a particularly important prognostic factor, and for this reason surgical staging has been advocated (200). However, pretreatment with chemotherapy may result in downstaging of axillary involvement in patients who have a response that destroys axillary metastases without leaving residual fibrosis in the nodes. Cytokeratin immunohistochemistry can be used to detect microscopic residual carcinoma in axillary lymph nodes or in the breast after chemotherapy and radiation therapy. There is no precedent for attributing focal nodal scarring to metastatic carcinoma in the absence of demonstrable neoplastic cells in these lesions.

# REFERENCES

## Carcinoma in Pregnancy and Lactation

1. Wallack MK, Wolf JA Jr, Bedwenek J, et al. Gestational carcinoma of the female breast. *Curr Probl Cancer* 1983;7:1–58.
2. Rosen PP, Lesser ML, Kinne DW, et al. Breast carcinoma in women 35 years of age or younger. *Ann Surg* 1984;199:133–142.
3. Birks DM, Crawford GM, Ellison LG, et al. Carcinoma of the breast in women 30 years of age or less. *Surg Gynecol Obstet* 1973;137:21–25.
4. Richards SR, Chang F, Moynihan V, et al. Metastatic breast cancer complicating pregnancy. *J Reprod Med* 1984;29:211–213.
5. Johannsson O, Loman N, Borg A, et al. Pregnancy-associated breast cancer in BRCA1 and BRCA2 germline mutation carriers. *Lancet* 1998;352:1359–1360.
6. Petrek JA, Dukoff R, Rogatko A. Prognosis of pregnancy-associated breast cancer. *Cancer* 1991;67:869–872.
7. Liberman L, Geiss CS, Dershaw DD, et al. Imaging of pregnancy-associated breast cancer. *Radiology* 1994;191:245–248.
8. Hogge JP, Shaw de Paredes E, Magnant DM, et al. Imaging and management of breast masses during pregnancy and lactation. *Breast J* 1999;5:272–283.
8a. Jernström H, Lerman C, Ghadirian P, et al. Pregnancy and risk of early breast cancer in carriers of BRCA1 and BRCA2. *Lancet* 1999;364:1846–1850.
9. Bottles K, Taylor RN. Diagnosis of breast masses in pregnant and lactating women by aspiration cytology. *Obstet Gynecol* 1985;66:76S–78S.
10. Novotny DB, Maygarden SJ, Shermer RW, et al. Fine needle aspiration of benign and malignant breast masses associated with pregnancy. *Acta Cytol* 1991;35:676–686.
11. Ishida T, Yokoe T, Kasumi F, et al. Clinicopathologic characteristics and prognosis of breast cancer patients associated with pregnancy and lactation: analysis of case-control study in Japan. *Jpn J Cancer Res* 1992;83:1143–1149.
12. Tobon H, Horowitz LF. Breast cancer during pregnancy. *Breast Dis* 1993;6:127–134.
13. King RM, Welch JS, Martin JK Jr, et al. Carcinoma of the breast associated with pregnancy. *Surg Gynecol Obstet* 1985;160:228–232.
14. Ribeiro G, Jones DA, Jones M. Carcinoma of the breast associated with pregnancy. *Br J Surg* 1980;73:607–609.
15. Kuerer HM, Cunningham JD, Bleiweiss IJ, et al. Conservative surgery for breast carcinoma associated with pregnancy. *Breast J* 1999;4:171–176.
16. Nugent P, O'Connell TX. Breast cancer in pregnancy. *Arch Surg* 1985;120:1221–1224.
17. Guinee VF, Olsson H, Möller T, et al. Effect of pregnancy on prognosis for young women with breast cancer. *Lancet* 1994;343:1587–1589.
18. Surbone A, Petrek JA. Childbearing issues in breast carcinoma survivors. *Cancer* 1997;79:1271–1278.
19. Danforth DN. How subsequent pregnancy affects outcome in women with a prior breast cancer. *Oncology* 1991;11:23–29.
20. Petrek JA. Pregnancy safety after breast cancer. *Cancer* 1994;74:528–531.
21. Velentgas P, Daling JR, Malone KE, et al. Pregnancy after breast carcinoma: outcomes and influence on mortality. *Cancer* 1999;85:2424–2432.
22. Salamon MA, Sherer DM, Saller DNJ, et al. Placental metastases in a patient with recurrent breast carcinoma. *Am J Obstet Gynecol* 1994;171:573–574.
23. Eltorky M, Khare VK, Osborne P, et al. Placental metastasis from maternal carcinoma. A report of three cases. *J Reprod Med* 1995;40:399–403.

## Pathology of Breast Carcinoma at the Extremes of Age

24. Chung M, Chang HR, Bland KI, et al. Younger women with breast carcinoma have a poorer prognosis than older women. *Cancer* 1996;77:97–103.
25. Feldman AL, Welch JP. Long-term outcome in women less than 30 years of age with breast cancer. *J Surg Oncol* 1998;68:193–198.
26. Bertheau P, Steinberg SM, Cowan K, et al. Breast cancer in young women: clinicopathologic correlation. *Semin Diagn Pathol* 1999;16:248–256.
27. Lein BC, Alex WR, Zebley M, et al. Results of needle localized breast biopsy in women under age 50. *Am J Surg* 1996;171:356–359.
28. McPherson CP, Swenson KK, Jolitz G, et al. Survival of women ages 40–49 years with breast carcinoma according to method of detection. *Cancer* 1997;79:1923–1932.
29. Lannin DR, Harris RP, Swanson FH, et al. Difficulties in diagnosis of carcinoma of the breast in patients less than fifty years of age. *Surg Gynecol Obstet* 1993;177:457–462.
30. Vetto JT, Pommier RF, Schmidt WA, et al. Diagnosis of palpable breast lesions in younger women by the modified triple test is accurate and cost-effective. *Arch Surg* 1996;131:967–974.
31. Rosen PP, Lesser ML, Kinne DW, et al. Breast carcinoma in women 35 years of age or younger. *Ann Surg* 1984;199:133–142.
32. Rosen PP, Lesser ML, Kinne DW. Breast carcinoma at the extremes of age: a comparison of patients younger than 35 years and older than 75 years. *J Surg Oncol* 1985;28:90–96.

33. Schaefer G, Rosen PP, Lesser ML, et al. Breast carcinoma in elderly women: pathology, prognosis, and survival. *Pathol Annu* 1984;19[Pt 1]:195–219.

34. Ashkanani F, Eremin O, Heys SD. The management of cancer of the breast in the elderly. *Eur J Surg Oncol* 1998:24:396–402.

35. Meyer JS, Bauer WC, Rao BR. Subpopulations of breast carcinoma defined by S-phase fraction, morphology and estrogen receptor content. *Lab Invest* 1978;39:225–235.

36. Silvestrini R, Daidore MG, Gentili C. Biologic characteristics of breast cancer and their clinical relevance. *Commun Res Breast Dis* 1981;2:1–40.

37. Gattuso P, Bloom K, Yaremko L, et al. Prognostic predictors of lymph node metastasis in young patients with breast carcinoma. *Mod Pathol* 1997;10:19A.

38. Walker RA, Lees E, Webb MB, et al. Breast carcinomas occurring in young women (<35 years) are different. *Br J Cancer* 1996;74: 1796–1800.

39. Olszewski W, Darzynkiewicz D, Rosen PP, et al. Flow cytometry of breast carcinoma. II. Relations of tumor cell cycle distribution to histology and estrogen receptor. *Cancer* 1981;48:985–988.

40. Dhodapkar MV, Ingle JN, Cha SS, et al. Prognostic factors in elderly women with metastatic breast cancer treated with tamoxifen. An analysis of patients entered on four prospective clinical trials. *Cancer* 1996;77:683–690.

41. Bertheau P, Steinberg SM, Merino MJ. C-erbB-2, p53, and nm23 gene product expression in breast cancer in young women: immunohistochemical analysis and clinicopathologic correlation. *Hum Pathol* 1998;29:323–329.

42. Recht A, Connolly JL, Schnitt SJ, et al. The effect of young age on tumor recurrence in the treated breast after conservative surgery and radiotherapy. *Int J Radiat Oncol Biol Phys* 1998;14:3–10.

43. Kurtz JM, Jacquemier J, Amalric R, et al. Why are local recurrences after breast-conserving therapy more frequent in younger patients? *J Clin Oncol* 1990;8:591–598.

44. Fowble BL, Schultz DJ, Overmoyer B, et al. The influence of young age on outcome and early stage breast cancer. *Int J Radiat Oncol Biol Phys* 1994;30:23–33.

45. Matthews RH, McNeese MD, Montague ED, et al. Prognostic implications of age in breast cancer patients treated with tumorectomy and irradiation or with mastectomy. *Int J Radiat Oncol Biol Phys* 1988;14:659–663.

46. Fourquet A, Campana F, Zafrani B, et al. Prognostic factors of breast recurrence in the conservative management of early breast cancer: a 25-year follow-up. *Int J Radiat Oncol Biol Phys* 1989;17:719–725.

47. Rose MA, Henderson IC, Gelman R, et al. Premenopausal breast cancer patients treated with conservative surgery, radiotherapy and adjuvant chemotherapy have a low risk of local failure. *Int J Radiat Oncol Biol Phys* 1989;17:711–717.

48. Haffty BG, Fischer D, Rose M, et al. Prognostic factors for local recurrence in the conservatively treated breast cancer patient: a cautious interpretation of the data. *J Clin Oncol* 1991;9:997–1003.

49. Freedman GM, Fowble BL, Hanlon AL, et al. A close or positive margin after mastectomy is not an indication for chest wall irradiation except in women aged fifty or younger. *Int J Radiat Oncol Biol Phys* 1998;41:599–605.

50. Chabner E, Nixon A, Gelman R, et al. Family history and treatment outcome in young women after breast-conserving surgery and radiation therapy for early-stage breast cancer. *J Clin Oncol* 1998;16:2045–2051.

51. Feigelson BJ, Acosta JA, Feigelson HS, et al. T1 breast carcinoma in women 70 years of age and older may not require axillary lymph node dissection. *Am J Surg* 1996;172:487–490.

52. Naslund E, Fernstad R, Ekman S, et al. Breast cancer in women over 75 years: is axillary dissection always necessary? *Eur J Surg* 1996;162:867–871.

53. Al-Hilaly M, Willsher PC, Robertson JFR, et al. Audit of a conservative management policy of the axilla in elderly patients with operable breast cancer. *Eur J Surg Oncol* 1997;23:339–340.

## Carcinoma Arising in Fibroadenomas and Phyllodes Tumors

54. Cheatle GL, Cutler M. *Tumours of the breast. Their pathology, symptoms, diagnosis and treatment.* London: Edward Arnold & Co., 1931:483–484.

55. Harrington SW, Miller JM. Malignant changes in fibro-adenoma of the mammary gland. *Surg Gynecol Obstet* 1940;70:615–619.

56. McDivitt RW, Stewart FW, Farrow JH. Breast carcinoma arising in solitary fibroadenomas. *Surg Gynecol Obstet* 1967;125:572–576.

57. Diaz NM, Palmer JO, McDivitt RW. Carcinoma arising within fibroadenomas of the breast. A clinicopathologic study of 105 patients. *Am J Clin Pathol* 1991;95:614–622.

58. Fondo EY, Rosen PP, Fracchia AA, et al. The problem of carcinoma developing in a fibroadenoma. Recent experience at Memorial Hospital. *Cancer* 1979;43:563–567.

59. Ozzello L, Gump FE. The management of patients with carcinomas in fibroadenomatous tumors of the breast. *Surg Gynecol Obstet* 1985;160:99–103.

60. Rosen PP, Urban JA. Coexistent mammary carcinoma and cystosarcoma phyllodes. *Breast* 1975;1:9–15.

61. Yoshida Y, Takaoka M, Fukumoto M. Carcinoma arising in fibroadenoma. Case report and review of the world literature. *J Surg Oncol* 1985;29:132–140.

62. Pick PW, Iossifides IA. Occurrence of breast carcinoma within a fibroadenoma. A review. *Arch Pathol Lab Med* 1984;108:590–594.

63. Baker KS, Monsees BS, Diaz NM, et al. Carcinoma within fibroadenomas: mammographic features. *Radiology* 1990;176:371–374.

64. Gupta RK. Fine needle aspiration (FNA) cytology of concurrent breast carcinoma in fibroadenoma. *Cytopathology* 1995;6:201–203.

65. Psarianos T, Kench JG, Ung OA, et al. Breast carcinoma in a fibroadenoma: diagnosis by fine needle aspiration cytology. *Pathology* 1998;30:419–421.

66. Goldman RL, Friedman NB. Carcinoma of the breast arising in fibroadenomas, with emphasis on lobular carcinoma. *Cancer* 1969;23:544–550.

67. Gittleman MA, Horstmann JP. Cystosarcoma phyllodes with concurrent infiltrating ductal carcinoma. *Breast* 1983;9:15–17.

68. Grimes MM. Cystosarcoma phyllodes of the breast: histologic features, flow cytometry analysis, and clinical correlations. *Mod Pathol* 1992;5:232–239.

69. Klausner JM, Lelcuk S, Ilia B, et al. Breast carcinoma originating in cystosarcoma phyllodes. *Clin Oncol* 1983;9:71–74.

70. Leon AS-Y, Meredith DJ. Tubular carcinoma developing within a recurring cystosarcoma phyllodes of the breast. *Cancer* 1980;46: 1863–1867.

71. Knudsen PJ, Ostergaard J. Cystosarcoma phyllodes with lobular and ductal carcinoma *in situ. Arch Pathol Lab Med* 1987;111:873–875.

72. Huntrakoon M. Malignant cystosarcoma phyllodes with simultaneous carcinoma in the ipsilateral breast. *South Med J* 1984;77:1176–1178.

73. Padmanabhan V, Dahlstrom JE, Chong GC, et al. Phyllodes tumor with lobular carcinoma in situ and liposarcomatous stroma. *Pathology* 1997;29:224–226.

74. Gallagher WJ, Koerner FC, Wood WC. Treatment of intraductal carcinoma with limited surgery: long term follow-up. *J Clin Oncol* 1989;7:376–380.

75. Page DL, DuPont WD, Rogers LW, et al. Intraductal carcinoma of the breast: follow-up after biopsy only. *Cancer* 1982;49:751–758.

## Occult Carcinoma Presenting with Axillary Lymph Node Metastases

76. Baron PL, Moore MP, Kinne DW, et al. Occult breast cancer presenting with axillary metastases: updated management. *Arch Surg* 1990;125:210–215.

77. Fitts WT Jr, Steiner GC, Enterline HT. Prognosis of occult carcinoma of the breast. *Am J Surg* 1963;106:460–463.

78. Ashikari R, Rosen PP, Urban JA, et al. Breast cancer presenting as an axillary mass. *Ann Surg* 1976;183:415–417.

79. Campana F, Fourquet A, Ashby MA, et al. Presentation of axillary lymphadenopathy without detectable breast primary (T0N1b breast cancer): experience at Institut Curie. *Radiother Oncol* 1989;15: 321–325.

80. Haupt HM, Rosen PP, Kinne DW. Breast carcinoma presenting with axillary lymph node metastases. An analysis of specific histopathologic features. *Am J Surg Pathol* 1985;9:165–175.

81. Patel J, Nemoto T, Rosner D, et al. Axillary lymph node metastasis from an occult breast cancer. *Cancer* 1981;47:2923–2927.

82. Rosen PP, Kimmel M. Occult breast carcinoma presenting with axillary lymph node metastases: a follow-up study of 48 patients. *Hum Pathol* 1990;21:518–523.

83. Ellerbroek N, Holmes F, Singletary E, et al. Treatment of patients with isolated axillary nodal metastases from an occult primary carcinoma consistent with breast origin. *Cancer* 1990;66:1461–1467.

84. Merson M, Andreola S, Galimberti V, et al. Breast carcinoma presenting as axillary metastases without evidence of a primary tumor. *Cancer* 1992;70:504–508.

85. Westbrook KC, Gallager HS. Breast carcinoma presenting as an axillary mass. *Am J Surg* 1971;122:607–611.

86. Rosen EL, Sickles E, Keating D. Ability of mammography to reveal nonpalpable breast cancer in women with palpable breast masses. *AJR Am J Roentgenol* 1999;172:309–312.

87. Marcantonio DR, Libshitz HI. Axillary lymph node metastases of bronchogenic carcinoma. *Cancer* 1995;76:803–806.

88. Tartter PI, Weiss S, Ahmed S, et al. Mammographically occult breast cancers. *Breast J* 1999;5:22–35.

89. Vilcoq JR, Calle R, Ferme F, et al. Conservative treatment of axillary adenopathy due to probable subclinical breast cancer. *Arch Surg* 1982;117:1136–1138.

90. Jackson B, Scott-Conner C, Moulder J. Axillary metastasis from occult breast carcinoma: diagnosis and management. *Am Surg* 1995;61:431–434.

91. Dunnington GL, Pearce J, Sherrod A, et al. Breast carcinoma presenting as mammographic microcalcifications in axillary lymph nodes. *Breast Dis* 1995;8:193–198.

92. Helvie MA, Rebner M, Sickles EA, et al. Calcifications in metastatic breast carcinoma in axillary lymph nodes. *Am J Radiol* 1988;151:921–922.

93. Morris EA, Schwartz LH, Dershaw DD, et al. MR imaging of the breast in patients with occult primary breast carcinoma. *Radiology* 1997;205:437–440.

94. Tilanus-Linthorst MMA, Obdeijn AIM, Bontenbal M, et al. MRI in patients with axillary metastases of occult breast carcinoma. *Breast Cancer Res Treat* 1997;44:179–182.

95. Stomper PC, Waddell BE, Edge SB, et al. Breast MRI in the evaluation of patients with occult primary breast carcinoma. *Breast J* 1999;5:230–234.

95a. Henry-Tillman RS, Harms SE, Westbrook KC, et al. Role of breast magnetic resonance imaging in determining breast as a source of unknown metastatic lymphadenopathy. *Am J Surg* 1999;178:496–500.

96. Jaffer S, Goldfarb AB, Gold JE, et al. Contralateral axillary lymph node metastasis as the first evidence of locally recurrent breast carcinoma. *Cancer* 1995;75:2875–2878.

97. Devitt JE, Michalchuk AW. Significance of contralateral axillary metastases in carcinoma of the breast. *Can J Surg* 1969;12:178–180.

98. Breslow A. Occult carcinoma of second breast following mastectomy. *JAMA* 1973;226:1000–1001.

99. Noguchi S, Motomura K, Inaji H, et al. Differentiation of primary and secondary breast cancer with clonal analysis. *Surgery* 1994;115:458–462.

100. Pandis N, Teixeira MR, Gerdes A-M, et al. Chromosome abnormalities in bilateral breast carcinomas. Cytogenetic evaluation of the clonal origin of multiple primary tumors. *Cancer* 1995;76:250–258.

101. Axelsson J, Andersson A. Cancer of the male breast. *World J Surg* 1983;7:281–287.

102. Balish SM, Khandekhar JD, Sener SF. Cancer of the male breast presenting as an axillary mass. *J Surg Oncol* 1993;53:68–70.

103. Yap HY, Tashima CK, Blumenschein GR, et al. Male breast carcinoma—a natural history study. *Cancer* 1979;44:748–754.

104. Kemeny MM, Rivera DE, Terz JJ, et al. Occult primary adenocarcinoma with axillary metastases. *Am J Surg* 1986;152:43–47.

105. Riquet M, Le Pimpec-Barthes F, Danel C. Axillary lymph node metastases from bronchogenic carcinoma. *Ann Thorac Surg* 1998;66:920–922.

106. Inglehart JD, Ferguson BJ, Shingleton WW, et al. An ultrastructural analysis of breast carcinoma presenting as isolated axillary adenopathy. *Ann Surg* 1982;196:8–13.

107. Walker AN, Fechner RE. Papillary carcinoma arising from ectopic breast tissue in an axillary lymph node. *Diagn Gynecol Obstet* 1982;4:141–145.

108. Layfield LJ, Mooney E. Heterotopic epithelium in an intramammary lymph node. *Breast J* 2000;6:63–67.

109. Ridolfi R, Rosen PP, Thaler H. Nevus cell aggregates associated with lymph nodes: estimated frequency and clinical significance. *Cancer* 1977;39:164–171.

110. Bhatia SK, Saclarides TJ, Witt TR, et al. Hormone receptor studies in axillary metastases from occult breast cancers. *Cancer* 1987;59:1170–1172.

111. Grundfest S, Steiger E, Sebek B. Metastatic axillary adenopathy. Use of estrogen receptor protein as an aid in diagnosis. *Arch Surg* 1978;113:1108–1109.

112. Rosen PP. Axillary lymph node metastases in patients with occult noninvasive breast carcinoma. *Cancer* 1980;46:1298–1306.

113. Read NE, Strom EA, McNeese MD. Carcinoma in axillary nodes in women with unknown primary site—results of breast-conserving therapy. *Breast J* 1996;2:403–409.

114. Whillis D, Brown PW, Rodger A. Adenocarcinoma from an unknown primary presenting in women with an axillary mass. *Clin Oncol (R Coll Radiol)* 1990;2:189–192.

115. Merson M, Andreola S, Galimberti V, et al. Breast carcinoma presenting as axillary metastases without evidence of a primary tumor. *Cancer* 1992;70:504–508.

116. van Ooijen B, Bontenbal M, Henzen-Logmans SC, et al. Axillary nodal metastases from an occult primary consistent with breast carcinoma. *Br J Surg* 1993;80:1299–1300.

117. Halsted WS. Results of radical operation for the cure of carcinoma of breast. *Ann Surg* 1907;46:1–9.

118. Jackson B, Scott-Conner C, Moulder J. Axillary metastasis from occult breast carcinoma: diagnosis and management. *Am Surg* 1995;61:431–434.

119. van de Weijer GH, van Ooijen B, Hesp WL, et al. Expectant management concerning the breast in five patients with occult breast carcinoma. *Ned Tijdschr Geneeskd* 1995;139:1648–1650.

120. Owen HW, Dockerty MB, Gray HK. Occult carcinoma of the breast. *Surg Gynecol Obstet* 1954;98:302–308.

## Carcinoma in Ectopic Breast Tissue

121. Rickert RR. Intraductal papilloma arising in supernumerary vulvar breast tissue. *Obstet Gynecol* 1980;55:84S–87S.

122. DeCholnoky T. Accessory breast tissue in the axilla. *N Y State J Med* 1951;5:2245–2248.

123. O'Hara MF, Page DL. Adenomas of the breast and ectopic breast under lactational influences. *Hum Pathol* 1985;16:707–712.

124. Foushee JHS, Pruitt AB. Vulvar fibroadenoma from aberrant breast tissue—report of two cases. *Obstet Gynecol* 1967;29:819–823.

125. Hassim AM. Bilateral fibroadenoma in supernumerary breasts of the vulva. *Br J Obstet Gynecol* 1969;76:275–277.

126. Garcia JJ, Verkauf BS, Hochberg CJ, et al. Aberrant breast tissue of the vulva. A case report and review of the literature. *Obstet Gynecol* 1978;52:225–228.

127. Tabakhi A, Cowan DF, Kumor D, et al. Recurring phyllodes tumor in aberrant breast tissue of the vulva. *Am J Surg Pathol* 1993;17:946–950.

128. Cogswell HD, Czerny EW. Carcinoma of aberrant breast of axilla. *Am Surg* 1961;27:388–390.

129. Smith GMR, Greening WP. Carcinoma of aberrant breast tissue. A report of 3 cases. *Br J Surg* 1972;59:89–90.

130. Bailey CL, Sankey HZ, Donovan JT, et al. Case report. Primary breast cancer of the vulva. *Gynecol Oncol* 1993;50:379–383.

131. Cho D, Buscema J, Rosenshein NB, et al. Primary breast cancer of the vulva. *Obstet Gynecol* 1985;66:79–81.

132. Guerry RL, Pratt-Thomas HR. Carcinoma of supernumerary breast of vulva with bilateral mammary cancer. *Cancer* 1976;38:2570–2574.

133. Hoogerland DL, Buchler DA. Inflammatory carcinoma of the vulva. *Gynecol Oncol* 1979;8:240–245.

134. Simon KE, Dutcher JP, Runowicz CD, et al. Adenocarcinoma arising in vulvar breast tissue. *Cancer* 1988;62:2234–2238.

135. Marshall MB, Moynihan JJ, Frost A, et al. Ectopic breast cancer: case report and literature review. *Surg Oncol* 1994;3:295–304.

136. Miller LA, Khan SA. Second ipsilateral breast cancer after modified radical mastectomy: a case report and review of the literature. *Surgery* 1997;121:109–111.

137. Willemsen HW, Kaas R, Peterse JH, et al. Breast carcinoma in residual breast tissue after prophylactic bilateral subcutaneous mastectomy. *Eur J Surg Oncol* 1998;24:331–332.

138. Falk VS. Carcinoma in aberrant breast tissue. *Wis Med J* 1950;49:1007.

139. Shimizu S, Kobayashi H, Suchi T, et al. Extramammary Paget's disease arising in mature cystic teratoma of the ovary. *Am J Surg Pathol* 1991;15:1002–1006.

140. Zaino RJ. Paget's disease in a retroperitonial teratoma. *Hum Pathol* 1991;15:622–624.

141. Monteagudo C, Torres J-V, Llombart-Bosch A. Extramammary Paget's disease arising in a mature cystic teratoma of the ovary. *Histopathology* 1999;35:579–585.

142. Randall BJ, Hutchinson RC. Paget's disease and invasive undifferentiated carcinoma occurring in a mature cystic teratoma of the ovary. *Histopathology* 1991;18:469–470.

143. Dyes DL, Tucker JA, Ferrara JJ. Carcinoma in a supernumerary nipple/breast complex: case report and review of the literature. *Breast Dis* 1995;8:77–84.

144. Finical S, Pennanen MF, Magnant CM, et al. Intracystic papillary carcinoma of aberrant breast tissue. Report of a case and review of the literature. *Breast Dis* 1993;6:295–301.

145. Kao GF, Graham JG, Helwig EB. Paget's disease of the ectopic breast with an underlying intraductal carcinoma. *J Cutan Pathol* 1986;13:59–66.

146. Petrek J, Rosen PP, Robbins GF. Carcinoma of aberrant breast tissue. *Clin Bull* 1980;10:13–15.

147. Bhambhani S, Rajwanshi A, Pant L, et al. Fine needle aspiration cytology of supernumerary breasts. Report of three cases. *Acta Cytol* 1987;31:311–312.

148. Youn SN, Kim YK, Park YL. A case report of infiltrating ductal carcinoma originating from aberrant breast tissue. *J Dermatol* 1994;21:960–964.

149. Velanovich V. Fine needle aspiration cytology in the diagnosis and management of ectopic breast tissue. *Am Surg* 1995;61:277–278.

150. Vargas J, Nevado M, Rodríguez-Peralto J, et al. Fine needle aspiration diagnosis of carcinoma arising in an ectopic breast. A case report. *Acta Cytol* 1995;39:941–944.

## Inflammatory Carcinoma

151. Bell C. *A system of operative surgery*. Longman, Herst, Rees, Arne, Cadell, and Davies 1807;1:180.

152. Learmonth GE. Acute mammary carcinoma (Volkmann's mastitis carcinomatosa). *Can Med Assoc J* 1916;6:499–511.

153. Lee BJ, Tannenbaum E. Inflammatory carcinoma of the breast: a report of twenty-eight cases from the breast clinic of the Memorial Hospital. *Surg Gynecol Obstet* 1924;39:580–595.

154. Ellis DL, Teitelbaum SL. Inflammatory carcinoma of the breast. A pathologic definition. *Cancer* 1974;33:1045–1047.

155. Saltzstein SL. Clinically occult inflammatory carcinoma of the breast. *Cancer* 1974;34:382–388.

156. Levine PH, Steinhorn SC, Ries LG, et al. Inflammatory breast cancer: the experience of the Surveillance, Epidemiology, and End Results (SEER) Program. *J Natl Cancer Inst* 1985;74:291–297.

157. Chang S, Parker SL, Pham T, et al. Inflammatory breast carcinoma incidence and survival: the Surveillance, Epidemiology, and End Results program of the National Cancer Institute, 1975–1992. *Cancer* 1998;82:2366–2372.

158. Haagensen CD. Inflammatory carcinoma. In: *Diseases of the breast*, 2nd ed. Philadelphia: WB Saunders, 1971:576–584.

159. Robbins GF, Shah J, Rosen P, et al. Inflammatory carcinoma of the breast. *Surg Clin North Am* 1974;54:801–810.

160. Chamadol W, Pesie M, Puapairoj A. Inflammatory carcinoma of the breast in a 12 year old Thai girl. *J Med Assoc Thai* 1987;70:543–547.

161. Nichini F, Holdman L, Lapayowker M, et al. Inflammatory carcinoma of the breast in a 12–year-old girl. *Arch Surg* 1972;105:505–508.

162. Treves N. Inflammatory carcinoma of the breast in a male patient. *Surgery* 1953;34:810–820.

163. Stocks L, Patterson S. Inflammatory carcinoma of the breast. *Surg Gynecol Obstet* 1976;143:885–889.

164. Beahrs O, Henson D, Huffer RVP, et al., eds. *Manual for staging of cancer,* 3rd ed. Philadelphia: JB Lippincott, 1988;145–150.

165. UICC International Union Against Cancer. In: Sobin LH, Wittekind C, eds. *TNM classification of malignant tumours.* New York: Wiley-Liss, 1997:123–130.

166. Barker JL, Nelson AJ III, Montague ED. Inflammatory carcinoma of the breast. *Radiology* 1976;121:173–176.

167. Droulias CA, Sewell CW, McSweeney MB, et al. Inflammatory carcinoma of the breast. A correlation of clinical radiologic and pathologic findings. *Ann Surg* 1976;184:217–222.

168. Nussbaum H, Kagan AR, Gilbert H, et al. Management of inflammatory breast carcinoma. *Breast* 1977;3:25–28.

169. Dershaw DD, Moore MP, Liberman L, et al. Inflammatory breast carcinoma: mammographic findings. *Radiology* 1994;190:831–834.

170. Tardivon AA, Viala J, Rudelli AC, et al. Mammographic patterns of inflammatory breast carcinoma: a retrospective study of 92 cases. *Eur J Radiol* 1997;24:124–130.

171. Kushwaha AC, Whitman GJ, Stelling CB, et al. Primary inflammatory carcinoma of the breast: retrospective review of mammographic findings. *AJR Am J Roentgenol* 2000;174:535–538.

172. Shukla HS, Hughes LE, Gravelle IH, et al. The significance of mammary skin edema in noninflammatory breast cancer. *Ann Surg* 1979;89:53–57.

173. Rieber A, Tomczak RJ, Mergo PJ, et al. MRI of the breast in the differential diagnosis of mastitis versus inflammatory carcinoma and follow-up. *J Comp Assist Tomogr* 1997;21:128–132.

174. Piera JM, Alonso MC, Ojeda MB, et al. Locally advanced breast cancer with inflammatory component: a clinical entity with a poor prognosis. *Radiother Oncol* 1986;7:199–204.

175. Kokal WA, Hill RL, Porudominsky D, et al. Inflammatory breast carcinoma: a distinct entity? *J Surg Oncol* 1985;30:152–155.

176. Mourali N, Muenz LR, Tabbane F, et al. Epidemiologic features of rapidly progressing breast cancer in Tunisia. *Cancer* 1980;46:2741–2746.

177. Charpin C, Bounier P, Khouzami A, et al. Inflammatory breast carcinoma: an immunohistochemical study using monoclonal anti-pHER-2/neu, pS2, cathepsin, ER and PR. *Anticancer Res* 1992;12:591–598.

178. Guerin M, Gabillot M, Mathieu M-C, et al. Structure and expression of c-erbB-2 and EGF receptor genes in inflammatory and non-inflammatory breast cancer: prognostic significance. *Int J Cancer* 1989;43:201–208.

179. Schäfer P, Alberto P, Forni M, et al. Surgery as part of a combined modality approach for inflammatory breast carcinoma. *Cancer* 1987;59:1063–1067.

180. Alpaugh ML, Tomlinson JS, Shao ZM, et al. A novel human xenograft model of inflammatory breast cancer. *Cancer Res* 1999;59:5079–5084.

181. van Golen KL, Davies S, Wu ZF, et al. A novel putative low-affinity insulin-like growth factor-binding protein, LIBC (lost in inflammatory breast cancer), and RhoC GTPase correlate with the inflammatory breast cancer phenotype. *Clin Cancer Res* 1999;5:2511–2519.

182. Tschen EH, Apisarnthanarax P. Inflammatory metastatic carcinoma of the breast. *Arch Dermatol* 1981;177:120–121.

183. Brownstein MH, Helwig EB. Spread of tumors to the skin. *Arch Dermatol* 1973;107:80–86.

184. Hazelrigg DC, Rudolph AH. Inflammatory metastatic carcinoma. *Arch Dermatol* 1977;113:69–70.

185. Meyer AC, Dockerty MB, Harrington SW. Inflammatory carcinoma of the breast. *Surg Gynecol Obstet* 1948;87:417–424.

186. Lucas FV, Perez-Mesa C. Inflammatory carcinoma of the breast. *Cancer* 1978;41:1595–1605.

186a. Ruizs A, Climent-Duran MA, Lluch-Hernandez A, et al. Inflammatory breast carcinoma: pathological or clinical entity? *Breast Cancer Res Treat* 2000;64:269–273.

187. Gradishar WJ. Inflammatory breast cancer: the evolution of multimodality treatment strategies. *Semin Surg Oncol* 1996;12:352–363.

188. Fastenberg NA, Buzdar AV, Montague ED, et al. Management of inflammatory carcinoma of the breast. A combined modality approach. *Am J Clin Oncol* 1985;8:134–141.

189. McBride CM, Hortobagyi GN. Primary inflammatory carcinoma of the female breast: staging and treatment possibilities. *Surgery* 1985;98:792–798.

190. Moore MP, Ihde JK, Crowe JP Jr, et al. Inflammatory breast cancer. *Arch Surg* 1991;126:304–306.

191. Palangie T, Mosseri V, Mihura J, et al. Prognostic factors in inflammatory breast cancer and therapeutic implications. *Eur J Cancer* 1994;30A:921–927.

192. Brun B, Otmezguine Y, Feuilhade F, et al. Treatment of inflammatory breast cancer with combination chemotherapy and mastectomy versus breast conservation. *Cancer* 1988;61:1096–1103.

193. Chevallier B, Asselain B, Kunlin A, et al. Inflammatory breast cancer. Determination of prognostic factors by univariate and multivariate analysis. *Cancer* 1987;60:897–902.

194. Jaiyesimi IA, Buzdar AU, Hortobagyi G. Inflammatory breast cancer: a review. *J Clin Oncol* 1992;10:1014–1024.

195. Knight CD Jr, Martin JK Jr, Welch JS, et al. Surgical considerations

after radiation therapy for inflammatory breast cancer. *Surgery* 1986;99:385–391.

196. Picciocchi A, Masetti R, Terribile D, et al. Inflammatory breast carcinoma: contribution of surgery as part of a combined modality approach. *Breast Dis* 1994;7:143–149.

197. Carlson RW, Favret AM. Multidisciplinary management of locally advanced breast cancer. *Breast J* 1999;5:303–307.

198. Crowe J, Hakes T, Rosen PP, et al. Changing trends in the management of inflammatory breast cancer: a clinical-pathological review of 69 patients. *Am J Clin Oncol* 1985;8:21.

199. Feldman LD, Hortobagyi GN, Buzdar AW, et al. Pathological assessment of response to induction chemotherapy in breast cancer. *Cancer Res* 1986;46:2578–2581.

200. McCready DR, Hortobagyi GN, Kau SW, et al. The prognostic significance of lymph node metastases after preoperative chemotherapy for locally advanced breast cancer. *Arch Surg* 1989;124:21–25.

# CHAPTER 36

# Metastases in the Breast from Nonmammary Malignant Neoplasms

In 1936, Dawson (1) described a 25-year-old woman who had diffuse lymphatic metastases in both breasts from signet-ring cell gastric adenocarcinoma. Her review of the literature revealed four patients with breast metastases from gastric carcinoma as well as two with metastatic ovarian carcinoma. All of these patients had generalized metastases, as did three women with breast metastases from uterine cervical carcinoma reported in 1947 (2) and 1948 (3). The first patient with metastatic intestinal carcinoid in the breast documented in 1952 was a 43-year-old woman who presented with carcinoid syndrome, an enlarged liver, and multiple metastatic nodules in both breasts (4). Autopsy disclosed a malignant ileal carcinoid.

Ten more patients with metastases in the breast were described by Charache (5) in 1953. This series included two men with malignant melanoma and individual men with carcinomas of the prostate gland and kidney. The man with prostatic carcinoma presented with a breast mass, and the primary site was not detected until autopsy. This is probably the first reported case of an occult neoplasm presenting as a metastatic tumor in the breast in the absence of coincidental systemic metastases. Included in the article were two women who had metastatic ovarian carcinoma in the breast, and there were single instances of malignant melanoma, as well as individuals with metastases from carcinoma of a kidney, the thyroid gland, and the endometrium. One of the patients with ovarian carcinoma developed a solitary breast mass 4 years after treatment of the ovarian primary.

A series of patients reported by Sandison (6) in 1959 included four women whose breast tumors were the initial manifestation of occult nonmammary neoplasms. The primary lesions were chloroma, oat cell carcinoma of the lung, and carcinomas of the stomach and kidney. Subsequent systemic metastases and a rapidly fatal course were described in the four cases. Also included in Sandison's report were patients who had breast involvement as part of systemic spread of the following neoplasms: malignant melanoma, lymphoma, leiomyosarcoma, and cutaneous squamous carcinoma.

## CLINICAL PRESENTATION

A lesion in the breast is the initial manifestation of a nonmammary malignant neoplasm in about 25% of patients who have metastatic tumor in the breast. The primary tumor is usually a carcinoma. Reported primary sites are the lung, including small cell (oat cell) carcinoma (7–9), the kidney (6,10,11), stomach (1,6,12), intestinal carcinoid tumor (13–15), ovarian carcinoma (16–19), uterine cervix (20), and thyroid gland (21). Occult alveolar soft part sarcoma also has presented as a breast metastasis (22). In an exceptional case, metastatic carcinoma in the breast was the first evidence of an occult renal primary in a woman who previously had mammary carcinoma in the same breast treated by lumpectomy (11).

Previously diagnosed tumors that have given rise to metastases in the breast, sometimes rather late in the clinical course of the patient, include melanoma (9,23,24) and sarcomas (6,9,24–26), in addition to various carcinomas such as transitional cell carcinoma of the urinary bladder (27) and carcinoma of the lung (24,28). An uncommon cause of metastatic tumor in the postpartum breast is choriocarcinoma (29).

Several types of malignant lymphoma have been included under the heading of metastases in the breast. However, these neoplasms in the breast are best regarded as primary breast tumors or as part of a systemic disease affecting the lymphoid system. The inclusion or exclusion of lymphomas from this category influences statistics on the frequency of metastases in the breast. Malignant lymphoma in the breast is discussed in Chapter 42.

Two reviews listing primary tumors that gave rise to mammary metastases reported through 1981 are available (9,30). Subsequent articles on the subject generally describe similar patterns in small groups of cases or in case reports. One series included two patients with metastatic mucoepidermoid carcinoma of the parotid gland, a lesion not often considered a source of metastatic tumor in the breast (31). Metastatic carcinoma that originated from mucoepidermoid carcinoma of the minor salivary glands in the floor of the mouth also has been reported (Fig. 36.1) (32). The primary tumor and the mammary metastasis were discovered coincidentally. In another patient, metastatic epidermoid carcinoma involved one breast and bone at the time that a primary tumor in the pharynx was identified (33). The author also had the opportunity to examine an example of metastatic acinic cell carcinoma of salivary gland origin in the breast (Fig. 36.2).

Adenocarcinomas of the gastrointestinal tract, especially the colon and rectum, are rarely the source of metastatic carcinoma in the breast despite their relative frequency in the population at large (34). Metastatic gastrointestinal muci-nous carcinoma is histologically indistinguishable from primary mucinous carcinoma of the breast (Figs. 36.3 and 36.4). Carcinoid tumors of the small bowel are a surprisingly frequent source of breast metastases. In some of these cases, the breast metastasis was the first clinical finding (15,35,36). In other instances, the breast metastasis occurred in patients who had a known carcinoid tumor and/or carcinoid syndrome (4,15,37). The cytologic diagnosis of metastatic carcinoid in the breast by fine needle aspiration has been reported in a woman previously treated for an ileal carcinoid (38). Without knowledge of an extramammary primary, metastatic carcinoid tumor in the breast is easily mistaken for a primary mammary tumor with neuroendocrine differentiation (Fig. 36.5). Radionuclide imaging has been used to detect metastatic carcinoid tumors in the breast (39). Merkel's cell carcinoma of the skin is also a source of metastatic carcinoma with neuroendocrine features (40).

One woman developed metastatic bronchial carcinoid in

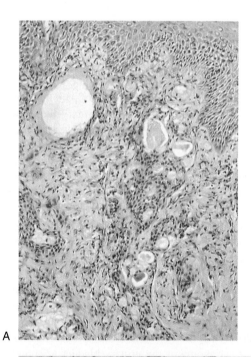

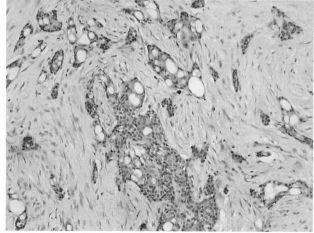

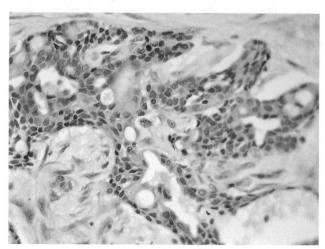

**FIG. 36.1.** *Metastatic minor salivary gland mucoepidermoid carcinoma.* **A:** Primary tumor in the base of the tongue. **B,C:** Metastatic tumor in the breast.

A

B

C

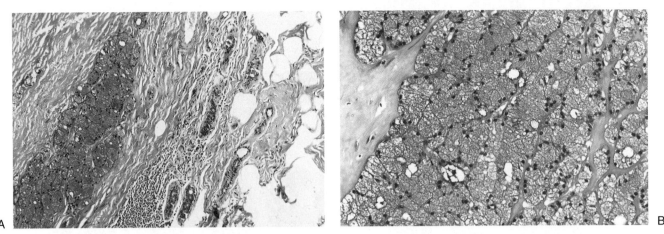

**FIG. 36.2.** *Metastatic salivary gland acinic cell carcinoma.* **A:** Metastatic acinic cell carcinoma in the breast. **B:** Typical vacuolated basophilic tumor cells.

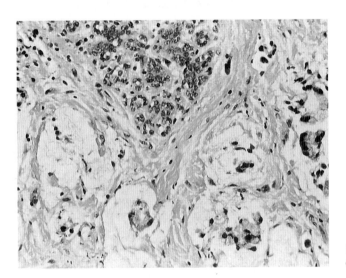

**FIG. 36.3.** *Metastatic gastric carcinoma.* The metastatic focus next to a lobule has mucinous differentiation.

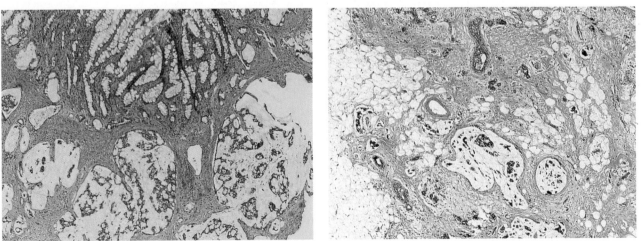

**FIG. 36.4.** *Metastatic colonic carcinoma.* **A:** Primary mucinous adenocarcinoma in the sigmoid colon of a 28-year-old woman. **B:** Two years later, this metastatic mucinous carcinoma was detected in one breast.

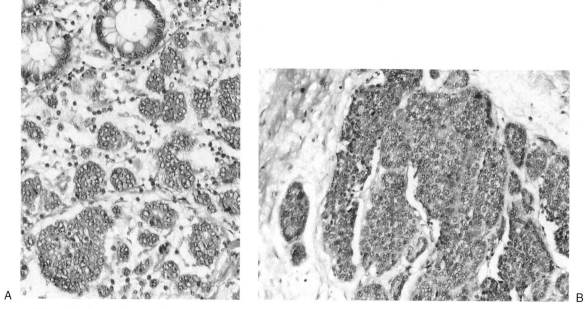

**FIG. 36.5.** *Metastatic colonic carcinoid tumor.* **A:** Primary tumor in the colonic mucosa. **B:** Metastasis in the breast from the tumor shown in **A**.

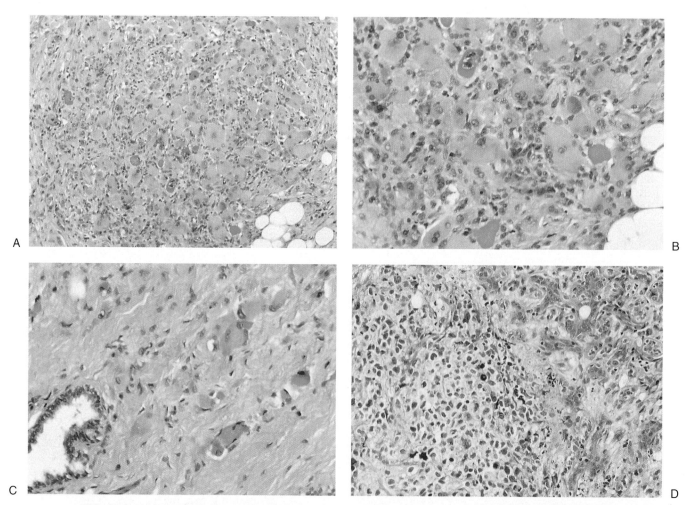

**FIG. 36.6.** *Metastatic embryonal rhabdomyosarcoma.* **A,B:** Metastatic tumor exhibiting maturation in a breast from a 15-year-old girl. **C:** Tumor cells in the mammary stroma are characterized by peripheral nuclei and cytoplasmic eosinophilia. **D:** Undifferentiated metastasis in the breast from a retroperitoneal primary in a 27-year-old patient.

the breast from a bronchial primary (15). The case report suggests that the lung tumor may have been present for 19 years prior to appearance of the breast metastasis, but resection of the lung tumor was performed only 4 years before the breast biopsy. In another case, a breast metastasis was detected 13 months after diagnosis of a primary bronchial carcinoid (41).

Mammary metastases from medulloblastoma (42,43), rhabdomyosarcoma (Fig. 36.6) (44–46), and neuroblastoma (23) have been reported in children and adults. The distinction between metastatic small cell pulmonary carcinoma and lymphoma can present a difficult diagnostic problem (23,28). Metastatic melanoma presenting clinically as a breast tumor may be difficult to recognize if the primary lesion is occult, if the pathologist is not informed that the patient received prior treatment for such a lesion, or if the primary site is clinically occult (Figs. 36.7–36.10) (47). Metastases in the breast have been found at autopsy rela-

tively often from malignant melanoma and from carcinomas of the lung, prostate gland, cervix, ovary, and urinary bladder (48). Malignant melanoma arising in the breast is usually a form of metaplastic carcinoma, and these tumors display focal reactivity for cytokeratin (see Chapter 44).

In men, involvement of the breast by metastatic prostatic adenocarcinoma has been a relatively frequent finding at autopsy. Microscopic breast involvement was found in 11 (26%) of the 46 men with breast tissue available in one series of 222 autopsied patients with prostatic carcinoma, although none had clinically apparent metastases (49). With two exceptions, the men had gynecomastia, and all had been treated with estrogens. Several authors described patients with bilateral breast metastases from prostatic carcinoma (50–52). It has been suggested that estrogen treatment for prostatic carcinoma predisposes patients to develop metastases in the breast. However, this remains speculative, because estrogens were widely used to treat prostatic

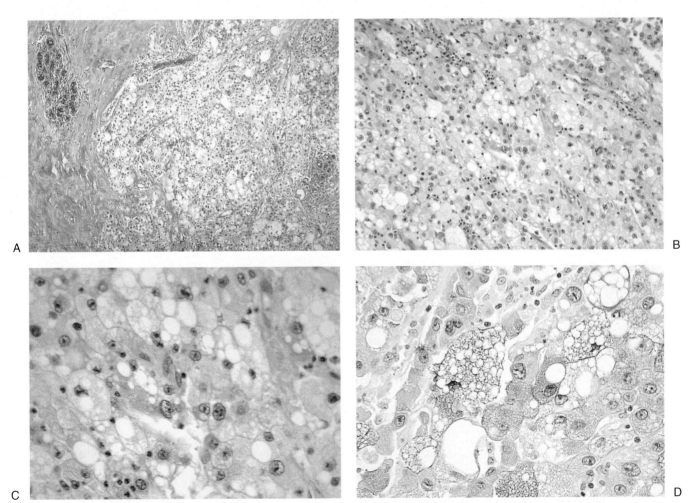

**FIG. 36.7.** *Metastatic malignant melanoma, clear cell type.* **A,B:** Metastatic tumor in the breast composed of epithelioid cells with pale-to-clear cytoplasm. **C:** Cytoplasmic features and prominent nucleoli suggest apocrine carcinoma. **D:** Melanin pigment was not seen in routine histologic sections. Melanosomes were demonstrated by electron microscopy. The tumor cells were immunoreactive for S-100 protein, but not for keratin, gross cystic disease fluid protein, or epithelial membrane antigen. The only cutaneous lesion found was suggestive of a regressed melanoma (anti–S-100 protein, avidin-biotin).

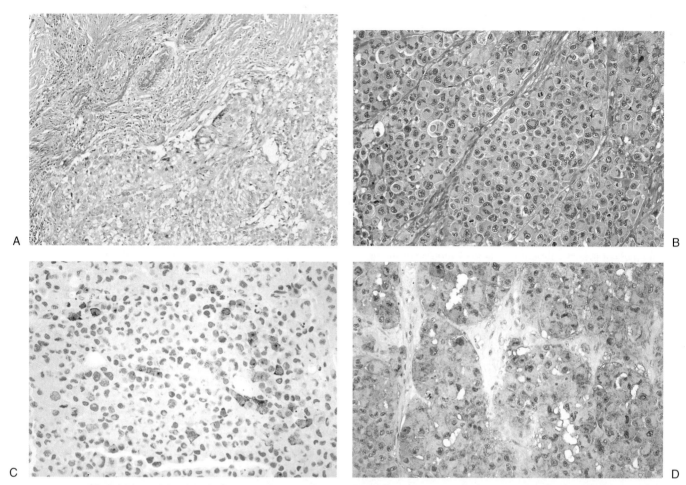

**FIG. 36.8.** *Metastatic malignant melanoma, epithelioid.* **A:** Sharp juxtaposition of the metastatic tumor and breast tissue is evident. **B:** Numerous intranuclear inclusions typically seen in malignant melanoma. **C:** Immunoreactivity for HMB45 in the cytoplasm of tumor cells (avidin-biotin). **D:** Nuclear and cytoplasmic reactivity for S-100 protein (avidin-biotin).

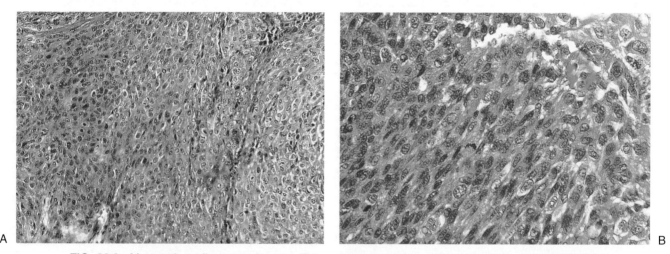

**FIG. 36.9.** *Metastatic malignant melanoma.* This metastasis had a mixture of spindle and epithelioid cells. **A:** Predominantly round cell component of the tumor. **B:** Spindle cell area in the tumor. *(continued)*

**FIG. 36.10.** *Metastatic malignant melanoma, epithelioid.* **A,B:** Metastatic tumor in the breast that was mistaken for alveolar lobular carcinoma. Subsequent metastases in the opposite breast led to further studies that established the diagnosis of metastatic melanoma, including reactivity for vimentin **(C)**, S-100 **(D)**, and MEL-A **(E). F:** The tumor was not reactive for any cytokeratin reagent tested (CK7 shown). All immunostains used avidin-biotin method.

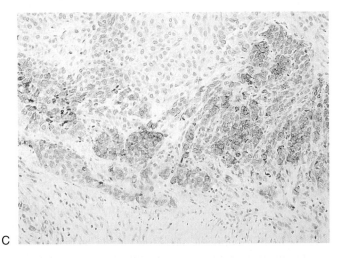

C

**FIG. 36.9.** *Continued.* **C:** Immunoreactivity for HMB45 (avidin-biotin).

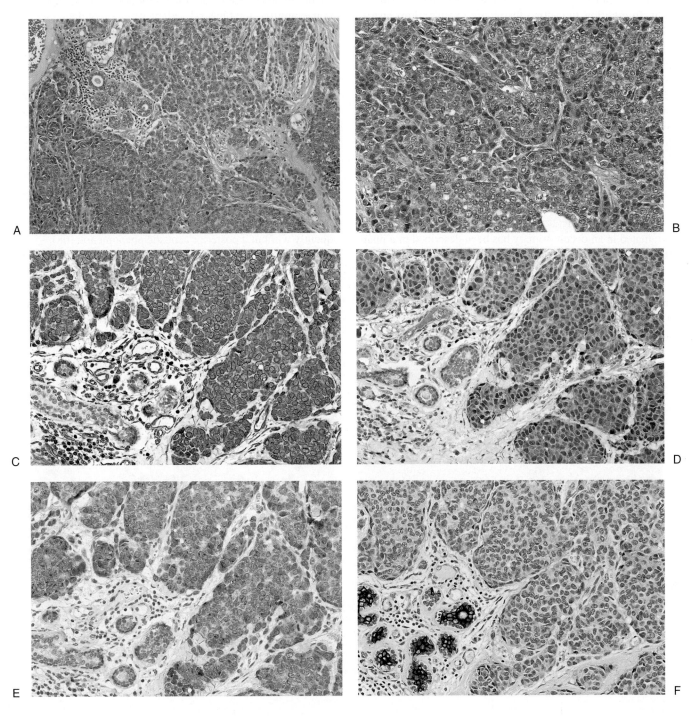

A

B

C

D

E

F

carcinoma, but breast metastases were relatively infrequent and some patients with breast metastases did not receive estrogens. Although a breast mass in a patient with prostatic carcinoma often proves to be metastatic from the prostatic tumor, there have been a few patients described who had independent synchronous or metachronous primary carcinomas of the prostate and breast (53,54). On review, some other purported examples of male mammary carcinoma that arose after estrogen therapy appear to be instances of metastatic prostatic carcinoma (55).

When a breast mass is discovered in a man known to have prostatic carcinoma, excisional biopsy is preferable to needle biopsy or fine needle aspiration, although the latter procedures sometimes may provide samples adequate for evaluation. In addition to routine histologic examination, histochemical studies for mucin and immunostains should be obtained for prostate-specific antigen, prostatic acid phosphatase (56,57), estrogen receptor (ER), progesterone receptor (PR), androgen receptor, gross cystic disease fluid protein 15 (GCDFP-15), CK7, and CK20. Prostate-specific antigen has been detected in breast carcinomas from men and women; therefore, a positive immunostain is not specific for prostatic carcinoma (58–60). The typical immunoprofile for prostatic carcinoma is as follows: ER and PR(−) or variably(+); CK7(−); GCDFP-15(−) (Fig. 36.11). Mammary carcinoma in men typically has the following immunophenotype: ER(+); PR variably(+); CK7(+); GCDFP(+) (see Chapter 38). Metastatic clear cell renal carcinoma that originated in an occult primary has been described in a man (61).

It is important to consider metastatic tumor in the differential diagnosis when faced with any breast lesion that has unusual clinical, radiologic, gross, or microscopic features. This concern applies to routine biopsy and cytology specimens (23) and to mammography (9,31). The pathologist, cytologist, or radiologist does not always have information about previously treated malignant tumors. Or, the primary lesion may be a new, occult neoplasm. The preoperative clinical workup of an apparently healthy patient with a breast mass often is perfunctory and unlikely to exclude an occult extramammary primary.

Radiographically, metastatic lesions tend to be discrete, round shadows without spiculation (9,31). They usually are not distinguishable from circumscribed primary breast carcinomas, which may be of the papillary, medullary, or colloid type (Fig. 36.12). Microcalcifications are uncommon but have been described in metastatic ovarian carcinoma (62–64) and in metastatic medullary thyroid carcinoma (65). Metastatic foci usually are solitary initially, but they may become multiple and bilateral with progression of the patient's clinical course. In one case, metastatic renal carcinoma was detected as a solitary nodule in the breast 15 years after treatment of the primary tumor (66). Metastatic squamous carcinoma of the uterine cervix studied by ultrasound appeared to be a solid tumor with hypoechoic areas (20). In adolescent girls, metastatic rhabdomyosarcoma appeared as "heterogeneous nodules which were quite different from the usual benign lesions," although no consistent sonographic pattern was observed (67). A study of various tumors in the breast, including metastatic lesions and lymphoma, led the authors to conclude that the "gray-scale" sonographic features of nonmammary malignancies of the breast are a hypoechoic mass with indistinct and occasionally irregular margins, frequently without a posterior acoustic phenomenon (68).

Some clinical features are helpful in recognizing that a neoplasm in the breast is a metastatic tumor. The average interval to the development of a mammary metastasis is approximately 2 years for patients with previously treated cancer. Usually, there have already been metastases at other sites, or they are detected coincidentally. Isolated initial metastases

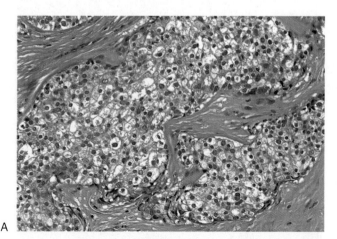
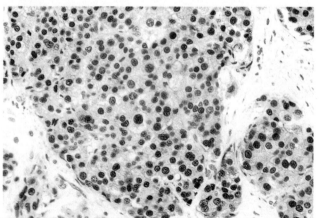

A      B

**FIG. 36.11.** *Metastatic prostatic carcinoma.* The primary tumor was diagnosed 1 year earlier. The patient presented with an elevated serum prostate-specific antigen, bone metastases, and a breast tumor shown here. **A:** The carcinoma had prominent clear cell features that were present focally in the primary prostatic tumor. **B:** Strong diffuse nuclear immunoreactivity for androgen receptors. The carcinoma displayed cytoplasmic reactivity for prostate-specific antigen (not shown). There was no nuclear reactivity for estrogen and progesterone receptors. Immunostains for CK7 and CK20 were negative (avidin-biotin).

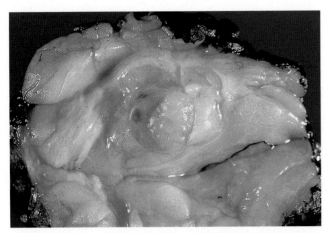

**FIG. 36.12.** *Metastatic ovarian carcinoma, gross.* This bulging, circumscribed mucoid-appearing tumor is grossly indistinguishable from a primary breast tumor.

limited to the breast are uncommon. However, when it occurs, metastatic tumor in the breast is at first a single lesion in about 85% of cases (9). A minority of patients have multiple (10%) or diffuse (5%) involvement initially. With progression, multiple breast metastases may become evident, and bilateral breast metastases eventually are found in about 25% of patients. Metastases have been described in ipsilateral axillary lymph nodes in 25% to 48% of patients (9). The frequency of axillary lymph node involvement tends to be higher in series that include malignant lymphomas. In patients with metastatic carcinoma or melanoma in the breast, involvement of the ipsilateral axillary lymph nodes is generally a manifestation of systemic spread, and it is not unusual to also find metastatic tumor in the supraclavicular lymph nodes and at other sites, including the contralateral axilla.

## MICROSCOPIC PATHOLOGY

An unusual histologic pattern and clinical information about a prior neoplasm are the best clues for identifying a metastatic tumor in the breast. It is important to be sensitive to morphologic patterns that are not typical for breast carcinoma. Certain histologic patterns present especially difficult problems because tumors of similar or identical appearance arise in the breast as well as in other organs. Included in this group are squamous, mucinous (colloid), mucoepidermoid, and clear cell carcinomas, as well as spindle cell lesions such as malignant melanoma, renal carcinoma, and sarcomas. Metastatic ovarian carcinomas generally have been serous rather than mucinous or clear cell, and in the absence of a known ovarian primary may be mistaken for papillary mammary carcinoma (Fig. 36.13) (16,69). Metastatic endometrial carcinoma with a solid growth pattern may mimic poorly differentiated mammary carcinoma (Fig. 36.14). Among sarcomas metastatic to the breast, hemangiopericytoma (25,70), leiomyosarcoma, and malignant fibrous histiocytomas may be difficult to distinguish from primary mammary sarcomas, sarcomatoid renal carcinoma, and some metaplastic mammary carcinomas (Figs. 36.15 and 36.16). Metastatic medullary carcinoma of the thyroid gland has been described growing in the breast with the pattern of infiltrating lobular carcinoma (71,72). Metastatic clear cell renal carcinoma resembles mammary carcinoma of the clear cell type (Fig. 36.17). Papillary and follicular carcinoma of the thyroid may rarely metastasize to the breast (73) (Fig. 36.18).

A search should be made for *in situ* carcinoma to confirm origin in the breast, but because this cannot be found in all primary mammary lesions, the absence of *in situ* carcinoma is not conclusive evidence that one is dealing with a metastasis. Metastatic tumor often surrounds and displaces normal-appearing breast parenchyma, which typically shows little or no hyperplasia. A peripheral symmetrically distributed lymphocytic infiltrate and stromal reaction are not unusual at the site of metastatic tumor in the breast. The finding of more than two grossly evident tumor nodules should lead one to consider metastatic tumor, especially if the histologic pattern is unusual. Lymphatic tumor emboli may result from metastases in the breast, as well as from primary breast

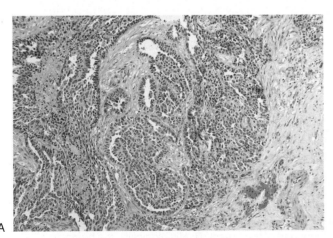

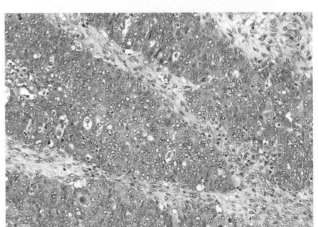

**FIG. 36.13.** *Metastatic ovarian carcinoma.* **A:** Papillary growth. **B:** Solid growth, poorly differentiated.

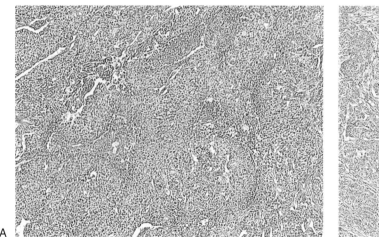
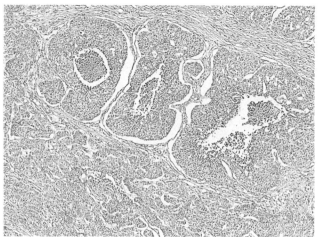

**FIG. 36.14.** *Metastatic endometrial carcinoma.* **A:** Solid, infiltrating, poorly differentiated carcinoma of the endometrium in the uterus. Note focal comedonecrosis in this primary tumor. **B:** Metastatic endometrial carcinoma in the breast with areas of comedonecrosis.

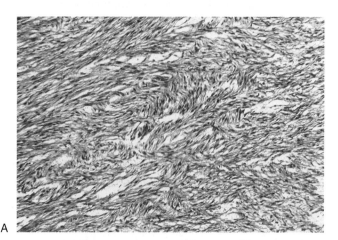
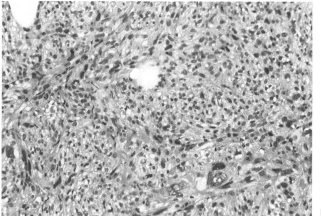

**FIG. 36.15.** *Metastatic leiomyosarcoma.* **A:** Primary tumor in the thigh. **B:** Metastatic lesion in the breast 1 year later showing spindle cells and pleomorphic giant cells.

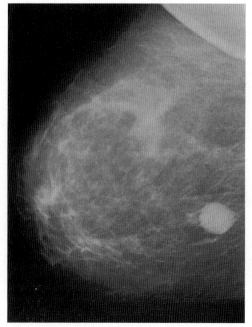
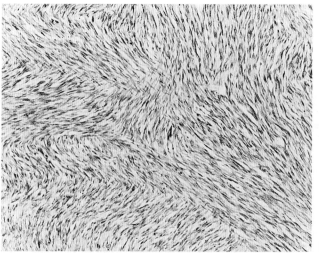

**FIG. 36.16.** *Metastatic sarcomatoid renal carcinoma.* **A:** Mammogram shows a dense, well-circumscribed tumor in the inferior part of the breast. **B:** Histologically, the breast tumor was composed of spindle cells arranged in a storiform pattern. *(continued)*

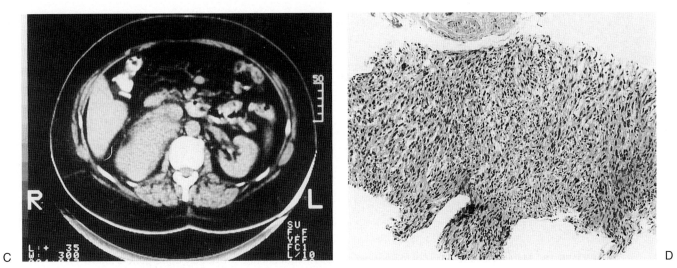

**FIG. 36.16.** *Continued.* **C:** Computed tomographic scan demonstrated a tumor of the right kidney. **D:** Needle biopsy of the right renal mass revealed sarcomatoid carcinoma.

carcinomas. Diffuse lymphatic spread within the breast can occur, rarely producing the clinical appearance of inflammatory carcinoma (69). Electron microscopy, lymphocyte markers, and ER analysis may be helpful in the differential diagnosis of a neoplasm suspected to be metastatic in the breast. Nuclear immunoreactivity for estrogen receptors has been found in nonsmall cell pulmonary adenocarcinomas by some investigators. A series of 248 consecutive lung tumors studied by DiNunno et al. had no detectable nuclear reactivity for estrogen or progesterone receptors (74).

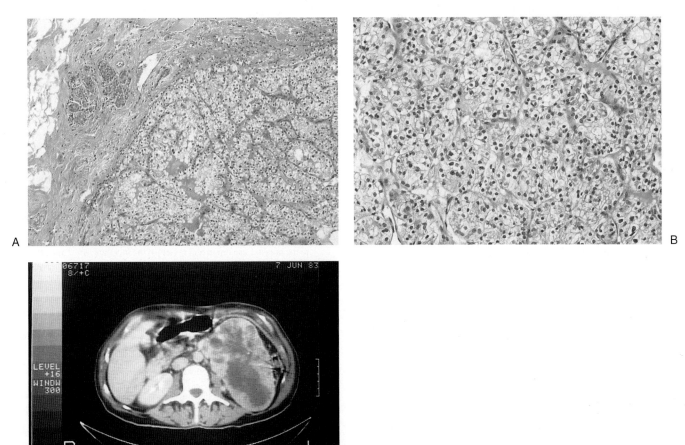

**FIG. 36.17.** *Metastatic clear cell renal carcinoma.* **A,B:** Metastatic tumor in the breast. **C:** Scan demonstrating the primary tumor in the left kidney.

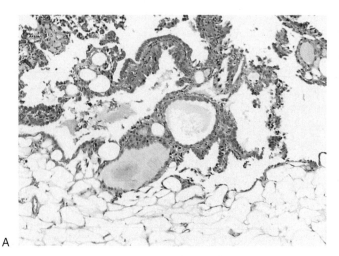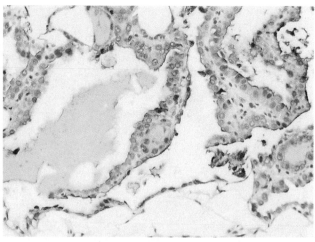

A                                  B

**FIG. 36.18.** *Metastatic carcinoma of the thyroid gland.* The patient had previously undergone a total thyroidectomy for "diffuse nodular hyperplasia." **A:** Metastatic, well-differentiated thyroid carcinoma with papillary and follicular features. **B:** Breast lesion was immunoreactive for thyroglobulin (avidin-biotin).

## PROGNOSIS AND TREATMENT

The distinction between a primary breast tumor and a metastasis in the breast is critical for treatment. Some types of metastatic tumor in the breast can be accurately diagnosed by needle aspiration cytology if the patient has a previously diagnosed nonmammary malignant neoplasm (24,57,75). However, excisional biopsy generally is recommended to ensure accurate identification of the lesion, because, in many cases, immunohistochemical studies, electron microscopy, or other procedures may be necessary. When an occult extramammary neoplasm presents with a breast metastasis, workup of the patient will be influenced by morphologic features of the tumor that may suggest one of more particular primary sites. Mastectomy is not appropriate for metastatic tumor in the breast in most cases, but it may be performed to obtain local control of bulky, ulcerated, necrotic, or otherwise symptomatic lesions. Wide excision can be supplemented by radiotherapy to the breast for radiosensitive neoplasms, and axillary dissection may be performed, especially if the lymph nodes seem grossly involved. Emphasis should necessarily be placed on systemic treatment appropriate to the primary lesion. Metastatic involvement of the breast is a manifestation of generalized metastases in virtually all cases. The prognosis depends on the clinical characteristics of the specific neoplasm.

## REFERENCES

1. Dawson EK. Metastatic tumour of the breast, with report of a case. *J Pathol Bacteriol* 1936;43:53–60.
2. de Alvarez PP, Russell P. Causes of death in cancer of the cervix uteri. *Am J Obstet Gynecol* 1947;54:91–96.
3. Speert H, Greeley AV. Cervical cancer with metastasis to breast. *Am J Obstet Gynecol* 1948;55:894–895.
4. Zetzel L, Scully RE. Case records of the Massachusetts General Hospital. *N Engl J Med* 1957;256:703–707.
5. Charache H. Metastatic tumors in the breast with a report of ten cases. *Surgery* 1953;33:385–390.
6. Sandison AT. Metastatic tumours in the breast. *Br J Surg* 1959;47:54–58.
7. Hajdu SI, Urban JA. Cancers metastatic to the breast. *Cancer* 1972;29:1691–1696.
8. Kelly C, Henderson D, Corris P. Breast lumps: rare presentation of oat cell carcinoma of lung. *J Clin Pathol* 1988;41:171–172.
9. Toombs BD, Kalisher L. Metastatic disease in the breast: clinical, pathologic and radiographic features. *AJR Am J Roentgenol* 1977;129:673–676.
10. Chica GA, Johnson DE, Ayala AG. Renal cell carcinoma presenting as breast carcinoma. *J Urol* 1980;15:389–390.
11. Kannan V. Fine-needle aspiration of metastatic renal-cell carcinoma masquerading as primary breast carcinoma. *Diagn Cytopathol* 1998;18:343–345.
12. Silverman EM, Oberman HA. Metastatic neoplasms in the breast. *Surg Gynecol Obstet* 1974;138:26–28.
13. Harrist TJ, Kalisher L. Breast metastasis: an unusual manifestation of a malignant carcinoid tumor. *Cancer* 1977;40:3102–3106.
14. Hawley PP. A case of secondary carcinoid tumors in both breasts following excision of primary carcinoid of the duodenum. *Br J Surg* 1966;53:818–820.
15. Kashlan RB, Powell RW, Nolting SF. Carcinoid and other tumors metastatic to the breast. *J Surg Oncol* 1982;20:25–30.
16. Elit LM, Cunnane MF. Breast metastasis from ovarian carcinoma: report of two cases and literature review. *J Surg Pathol* 1995;1:69–74.
17. Frauenhoffer EE, Ro JY, Silva EG, et al. Well differentiated serous ovarian carcinoma presenting as a breast mass: a case report and flow cytometric DNA study. *Int J Gynecol Pathol* 1991;10:79–87.
18. Ron I-G, Inbar M, Halpern M, et al. Endometrioid carcinoma of the ovary presenting as primary carcinoma of the breast. A case report and review of the literature. *Acta Obstet Gynecol Scand* 1992;71:81–83.
19. Yamasaki H, Saw D, Zdanowitz J, et al. Ovarian carcinoma metastasis to the breast. Case report and review of the literature. *Am J Surg Pathol* 1993;17:193–197.
20. Kelkar PS, Helbich TH, Becherer A, et al. Solitary breast metastasis as the first sign of a squamous cell carcinoma of the cervix: imaging findings. *Eur J Radiol* 1997;24:159–162.
21. Ascani S, Nati S, Liberati F, et al. Breast metastasis of thyroid follicular carcinoma. *Acta Oncol* 1994;33:71–73.
22. Hanna NN, O'Donnell K, Wolfe GRZ. Alveolar soft part sarcoma metastatic to the breast. *J Surg Oncol* 1996;61:159–162.
23. Silverman JF, Feldman PS, Covell JL, et al. Fine needle aspiration cytology of neoplasms metastatic to the breast. *Acta Cytol* 1987;31:291–300.
24. Sneige N, Zachariah S, Fanning TV, et al. Fine needle aspiration cytology of metastatic neoplasms in the breast. *Am J Clin Pathol* 1989;92:27–35.
25. Breitbart AS, Harris MN, Vazquez M, et al. Metastatic hemangiopericytoma of the breast. *N Y State J Med* 1992;92:158–160.
26. Tulasi NR, Kurian S, Mathew G, et al. Breast metastases from primary leiomyosarcoma. *Aust N Z J Surg* 1997;67:71–72.

27. Belton AL, Stull MA, Grant T, et al. Mammographic and sonographic findings in metastatic transitional cell carcinoma of the breast. *AJR Am J Roentgenol* 1997;168:511–512.

28. Domanski HA. Metastases to the breast from extramammary neoplasms. A report of six cases with diagnosis by fine needle aspiration cytology. *Acta Cytol* 1996;40:1293–1300.

29. Fowler CA, Nicholson S, Lott M, et al. Choriocarcinoma presenting as a breast lump. *Eur J Surg Oncol* 1995;21:576–578.

30. Nielsen M, Andersen JA, Henriksen FW, et al. Metastases to the breast from extramammary carcinomas. *Acta Pathol Microbiol Scand (A)* 1981;89:251–256.

31. Bohman L, Bassett LW, Gold RH, et al. Breast metastases from extramammary malignancies. *Radiology* 1982;144:309–312.

32. Kirsch RLA, Rosen PP. An unusual well-circumscribed breast tumor. *Mem Hosp Bull* 1976;6:60–61.

33. Nunez DA, Sutherland CGC, Sood RK. Breast metastasis from a pharyngeal carcinoma. *J Laryngol Otol* 1989;103:227–228.

34. Alexander HR, Turnbull AD, Rosen PP. Isolated breast metastases from gastrointestinal carcinomas. *J Surg Oncol* 1989;42:264–266.

35. Schurch W, Lamoureux E, Lefebre R, et al. Solitary breast metastasis: first manifestation of an occult carcinoid of the ileum. *Virchows Arch [A]* 1980;386:117–124.

36. Turner M, Gallager HS. Occult appendiceal carcinoid. Report of a case with fatal metastases. *Arch Pathol* 1959;88:188–190.

37. Chodoff RJ. Solitary breast metastasis from carcinoid of the ileum. *Am J Surg* 1965;109:814–815.

38. Lozowski MS, Faegenberg D, Mishriki Y, et al. Carcinoid tumor metastatic to breast diagnosed by fine needle aspiration. Case report and literature review. *Acta Cytol* 1989;33:191–194.

39. Kaltsas GA, Putignano P, Mukherjee JJ, et al. Carcinoid tumours presenting as breast cancer: the utility of radionuclide imaging with $^{123}$I-MIBG and $^{111}$In-DTPA pentetreotide. *Clin Endocrinol* 1998;49:685–689.

40. Schnabel T, Glag M. Breast metastases of Merkel cell carcinoma. *Eur J Cancer* 1996;32A:1617–1618.

41. Helvie MA, Frank TS. Enhancing breast metastases from bronchial neuroendocrine carcinoid carcinoma. *Breast Dis* 1993;6:233–236.

42. Baliga M, Holmquist ND, Espinoza CG. Medulloblastoma metastatic to breast diagnosed by fine-needle aspiration biopsy. *Diagn Cytopathol* 1994;10:33–36.

43. Kapila K, Sarkar C, Verma K. Detection of metastatic medulloblastoma in a fine needle breast aspirate. *Acta Cytol* 1996;40:384–385.

44. Howarth GB, Caces JN, Pratt CB. Breast metastases in children with rhabdomyosarcoma. *Cancer* 1980;46:2520–2524.

45. Hogge JP, Magnant CM, Lage JM, et al. Rhabdomyosarcoma metastatic to the breast. *Breast J* 1996;2:270–274.

46. Kwan WH, Choi PHK, Li CK, et al. Breast metastasis in adolescents with alveolar rhabdomyosarcoma of the extremities: report of two cases. *Pediatr Hematol Oncol* 1996;13:277–285.

47. Cangiarella J, Symmans WF, Cohen JM, et al. Malignant melanoma metastatic to the breast. A report of seven cases diagnosed by fine-needle aspiration cytology. *Cancer (Cancer Cytopathol)* 1998;84:160–162.

48. Abrams HL, Spiro R, Goldstein M. Metastases in carcinoma: analysis of 1000 autopsied cases. *Cancer* 1950;3:74–85.

49. Salyer WR, Salyer DC. Metastases of prostatic carcinoma to the breast. *J Urol* 1973;109:671–675.

50. Hartley LCJ, Little JH. Bilateral mammary metastases from carcinoma of the prostate during oestrogen therapy. *Med J Aust* 1971;1:434–436.

51. Malek GA, Madsen PO. Carcinoma of the prostate with unusual metastases. *Cancer* 1969;24:194–197.

52. Scott J, Robb-Smith AHT, Burns I. Bilateral breast metastases from carcinoma of the prostate. *Br J Urol* 1974;46:209–214.

53. Moldwin RM, Orihuela E. Breast masses associated with adenocarcinoma of the prostate. *Cancer* 1989;63:2229–2233.

54. Wilson SE, Hutchinson WB. Breast masses in males with carcinoma of the prostate. *J Surg Oncol* 1976;8:105–112.

55. Jakobsen AHI. Bilateral mammary carcinoma in the male following stilboestrol therapy. *Acta Pathol Microbiol Scand* 1952;31:61–66.

56. Choudhury M, DeRosas J, Papsidero L, et al. Metastatic prostatic carcinoma to the breast or primary breast carcinoma. *J Urol* 1982;19:297–299.

57. Green LK, Klima M. The use of immunohistochemistry in metastatic prostatic adenocarcinoma to the breast. *Hum Pathol* 1991;22:242–246.

58. Gupta RK. Immunoreactivity of prostate-specific antigen in male breast carcinoma: two examples of a diagnostic pitfall in discriminating a primary breast cancer from metastatic prostatic carcinoma. *Diagn Cytopathol* 1999:21:167–169.

59. Bodey B, Bodey B Jr, Kaiser HE. Immunocytochemical detection of prostate specific antigen expression in human breast carcinoma cells. *Anticancer Res* 1997;17:2577–2581.

60. Yu H, Levesque MA, Clark GM, et al. Enhanced prediction of breast cancer prognosis by evaluating expression of p53 and prostate-specific antigen in combination. *Br J Cancer* 1999;81:490–495.

61. Gibbons CER, Lewi HJE, Kashif KM. Breast lump—an unusual presentation of renal cell carcinoma. *Br J Urol* 1995;76:131.

62. Duda RB, August CZ, Schink JC. Ovarian carcinoma metastatic to the breast and axillary node. *Surgery* 1991;110:552–556.

63. Raptis S, Kanbour AI, Dusenbery D, et al. Fine-needle aspiration cytology of metastatic ovarian carcinoma to the breast. *Diagn Cytopathol* 1996;15:1–6.

64. Moncada R, Cooper RA, Garces M, et al. Calcified metastases from malignant ovarian neoplasm. *Radiology* 1974;113:31–35.

65. Soo MS, Williford ME, Elenberger CD. Medullary thyroid carcinoma metastatic to the breast: mammographic appearance. *AJR Am J Roentgenol* 1995;165:65–66.

66. Bowditch MG, Peck R, Shorthouse AJ. Metastatic renal adenocarcinoma presenting in a breast screening programme. *Eur J Surg Oncol* 1996;22:641–643.

67. Chateil JF, Arboucalot F, Pérel Y, et al. Breast metastases in adolescent girls: US findings. *Pediatr Radiol* 1998;28:832–835.

68. Yang WT, Metreweli C. Sonography of nonmammary malignancies of the breast. *AJR Am J Roentgenol* 1999;172:343–348.

69. Moore DH, Wilson DK, Hurteau JA, et al. Gynecologic cancers metastatic to the breast. *J Am Coll Surg* 1998;187:178–181.

70. Kindblom L-G, Ullman A. Malignant hemangiopericytoma with admixed glandular structures in breast and lung metastases. *Appl Pathol* 1983;1:50–59.

71. Kiely N, Willimas N, Wilson G, et al. Medullary carcinoma of the thyroid metastatic to breast. *Postgrad Med* J 1995;71:744–754.

72. Ali SD, Teichberg S, Attie JN, et al. Medullary thyroid carcinoma metastatic to breast masquerading as infiltrating lobular carcinoma. *Ann Clin Lab Sci* 1994;24:441–447.

73. Loureiro MM, Leite VH, Boavida JM, et al. An unusual case of papillary carcinoma of the thyroid with cutaneous and breast metastases only. *Eur J Endocrinol* 1997;137:267–269.

74. DiNunno L, Larsson LG, Rinehart JJ, et al. Estrogen and progesterone receptors in non-small cell lung cancer in 248 consecutive patients who underwent surgical resection. *Arch Pathol Lab Med* 2000;124:1467–1470.

75. Vazquez MF, Mitnick JS, Roses DF. Diagnosis of metastatic melanoma to the breast by aspiration biopsy. *Breast Dis* 1995;8:387–390.

# CHAPTER 37

# Benign Proliferative Lesions of the Male Breast

## PAPILLOMA

Several examples of intraductal papilloma arising in the male breast have been reported (Figs. 37.1 and 37.2) (1–4). Patients have ranged in age from 3 months to 82 years. The usual presenting symptom is nipple discharge that is bloody or blood tinged. Cystic lesions may be palpable. The ultrasound appearance of a benign cystic papillary tumor of the male breast has been documented (5). One patient treated with phenothiazines for more than 10 years had a multiloculated cystic tumor measuring $7 \times 6 \times 3$ cm that recurred as a $1 \times 1$ cm cystic lesion 6 months after initial excision (3). Microscopic examination revealed an orderly benign papillary tumor composed of cells with apocrine features and prominent secretory activity. Syringocystadenoma papilliform is an extremely unusual benign papillary tumor of the male breast (6).

Local recurrence of a multiloculated cystic papilloma in an 82-year-old man was described by David (7). Because of the relatively high proportion of papillary carcinomas of the male breast, all male papillary tumors should be carefully evaluated pathologically (Fig. 37.2).

## FLORID PAPILLOMATOSIS OF THE NIPPLE

Less than 5% of the reported examples of florid papillomatosis of the nipple have been in men (8–10). Some of these lesions contained carcinoma (8,10). The histologic features are identical to those of florid papillomatosis in women (see Chapter 5).

## FIBROEPITHELIAL TUMORS

Phyllodes tumors described in the male breast usually have arisen in patients with gynecomastia (11–15). A number of these patients have been treated with estrogens, resulting in gynecomastia with lobular differentiation (13–15). Most phyllodes tumors in men have been histologically and clinically benign. In one case, the stromal component of a 12-cm tumor was described as malignant, but the histologic appearance of the lesion was not illustrated.

Fibroadenomas occur in the male breast, but in retrospect, many of the lesions described in case reports were poorly documented or appear to have been nodular foci of gynecomastia (Fig. 37.3). Tumors measuring up to 5 cm have been described (16). Four male patients with fibroadenomas have been reported from the Armed Forces Institute of Pathology (12). Age at diagnosis in this series ranged from 37 to 71 years. One patient had been treated with estrogens, and another had received methyldopa and chlordiazepoxide. Gynecomastia with lobular differentiation was present microscopically in each case. A particularly unusual patient was a 15-year-old boy with a 7-cm benign fibroepithelial tumor that arose in unilateral gynecomastia (17). He had not received any medications. Gynecomastia was found histologically in the surrounding breast tissue, but there was no evidence of lobular differentiation.

Nielsen documented a 16-cm fibroadenomatoid tumor that arose in one breast of a 69-year-old man with bilateral gynecomastia (18). The patient had chronic heart disease treated with digoxin and furosemide for 23 years, during which time his breasts appeared clinically normal. Breast enlargement and the appearance of the unilateral tumor began after spironolactone was added to his medications, suggesting that this drug contributed to the mammary lesion. Gynecomastia has been associated with digitalis (19) and spironolactone (20).

## DUCT ECTASIA

Duct dilation or ectasia and periductal mastitis, a relatively common condition in the female breast, also has been described in men (1,21,22). Andersen and Gram (21) found duct ectasia in nine (26%) of 35 "normal" breasts and in 19 (35%) of 55 breasts with gynecomastia examined at autopsy. The histologic appearance is similar in men and women, there being less inflammation and fibrosis in lesions that are clinically asymptomatic.

## BENIGN PROLIFERATIVE CHANGES

Proliferative changes ("fibrocystic changes") resembling those of the female are only rarely encountered in the male

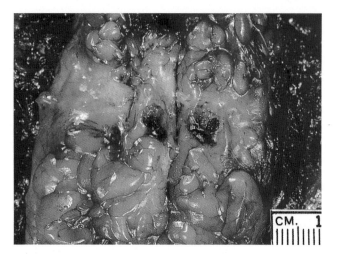

**FIG. 37.1.** *Papilloma.* Intracystic papilloma in the male breast.

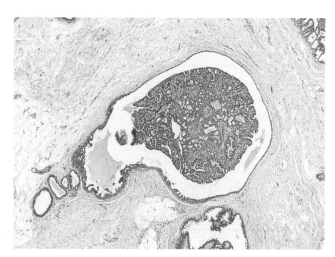

**FIG. 37.2.** *Papilloma.* Papilloma in a cystically dilated duct.

breast. Three case reports document men 28, 33, and 41 years of age (23–25). Two of the men were described as karyotypically and phenotypically normal (23,24). One patient reported having swelling of the affected breast for 17 years, which doubled in size during the year prior to biopsy (25). Grossly, each patient had a circumscribed multicystic tumor. The lesions include cysts with apocrine metaplasia, papillary apocrine metaplasia, duct hyperplasia, and duct stasis with mastitis. Gynecomastia was evident histologically in two cases. The gross and microscopic features in these lesions resemble juvenile papillomatosis (25).

Sclerosing adenosis arising in lobules was described as an incidental finding in the postmortem examination of a 41-year-old man with disseminated pulmonary oat cell carcinoma (26). Grossly, the lesion was a unilateral firm white 1.8 × 1.5 × 1.0-cm nodule. Ectopic hormone production was not documented in this case.

An unusual retroareolar mass in a 38-year-old man proved to be a 2.5-cm cyst lined by benign squamous epithelium (27). There were no skin appendage glands in the cyst wall, and surrounding tissue contained mammary gland ducts.

## GYNECOMASTIA

Gynecomastia is the most common clinical and pathologic abnormality of the male breast. Mammary enlargement may be due to a discrete, nodular increase in subareolar tissue or a diffuse accumulation of tissue. Gynecomastia is extremely common in newborn male infants, reflecting exposure to maternal estrogens. Gynecomastia in prepubertal boys is relatively infrequent (28), but it has been reported in 30% to 40% of adolescent (29) and adult males (30–32). Both breasts are affected in the majority of gynecomastic patients at all ages. Among those with unilateral gynecomastia, the left breast is

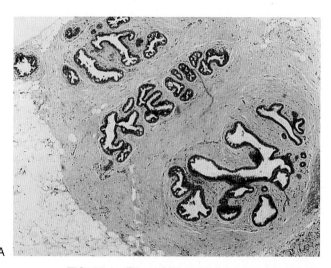

A

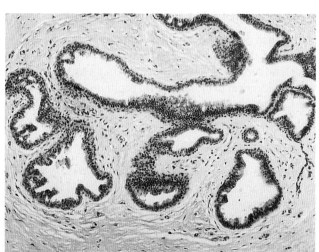

B

**FIG. 37.3.** *Fibroadenomatoid gynecomastia.* **A,B:** Nodular gynecomastia with early lobular differentiation. The patient was being treated with estrogen for prostatic carcinoma.

involved more often than the right (33). Bilateral involvement usually is synchronous, but it may be asynchronous.

Numerous conditions have been associated with gynecomastia. Systemic diseases include hyperthyroidism, cirrhosis of the liver, chronic renal failure, chronic pulmonary disease, and hypogonadism. Gynecomastia has been related to the use of hormones, such as estrogens and androgens, and many commonly used drugs, including digitalis, cimetidine, spironolactone, marijuana, and tricyclic antidepressants. Androgen administrated to develop muscular strength in athletes can cause gynecomastic breast enlargement and rarely has been associated with the development of male breast carcinoma. Gynecomastia is the most frequent adverse side effect of finasteride administration to treat prostatic hyperplasia (34). Neoplasms that are most likely to cause gynecomastia as a result of hormone production by the tumor are pulmonary carcinoma and testicular germ cell tumors.

Clinically invasive carcinoma arising in gynecomastia usually can be detected as a localized, asymmetric area of firmness. Mammography is helpful for distinguishing between gynecomastia and carcinoma and may identify carcinoma developing in gynecomastia (35). Two mammographic patterns associated with gynecomastia are a dendritic configuration featuring retroareolar density with prominent radial extensions into the breast and a triangular subareolar density lacking radiating extensions. The triangular pattern is more common in gynecomastia of recent onset, whereas gynecomastia present for six months or longer tends to have the dendritic configuration. High-frequency ultrasound also has proved useful for distinguishing between these patterns (36).

The initial clinical signs of gynecomastia are breast enlargement and a palpable mass that may be accompanied by pain or tenderness. Enlargement of the nipple and areola occur in a minority of patients. Nipple retraction and discharge are rarely encountered. The palpable mass is located in the central subareolar region in all but a very small number of patients who have eccentric or peripherally located lesions. Patients with bilateral involvement tend to have diffuse lesions, whereas unilateral gynecomastia is more likely to produce a discrete tumor. On clinical examination, the tumor may measure 10 cm or larger, but in most cases the mass is 2 to 6 cm in diameter.

Gynecomastic breast tissue contains receptors for estradiol (37–40), dihydrotestosterone (38), androgen (39), progesterone (37–39), and glucocorticoids (38,39). In one series, estradiol and dihydrotestosterone receptors were detected in about 75% of gynecomastia samples (38). Overall, approximately 35% of gynecomastia samples studied by the dextran charcoal method have been reported to be estrogen receptor-positive. Using an immunohistochemical procedure, Andersen et al. (41) demonstrated nuclear reactivity for estrogen receptor in 89% of gynecomastia specimens examined. Positive staining was limited to the nuclei of epithelial cells in the proliferating ducts. In this series, 18 of 22 specimens with negative biochemical levels of estrogen receptor were immunohistochemically positive. Strong, focal immunoreactivity for prostate-specific antigen (PSA) has been detected in nonhyperplastic and hyperplastic duct epithelium in gynecomastia (42). The epithelium was not immunoreactive for prostatic acid phosphatase.

Gross examination reveals soft rubbery or firm, gray or white tissue that forms a discrete mass or an ill-defined area of induration. Rarely, fat is dispersed in the fibrous tissue.

Histopathologic studies show similar microscopic alterations regardless of etiologic factors (28,32,33,43–45). Three phases of proliferative change have been described. Florid gynecomastia, ordinarily seen within 1 year of onset, is characterized by prominent epithelial proliferation in ducts that may have papillary and cribriform-like patterns (Fig. 37.4). There usually is concomitant myoepithelial hyperplasia (Fig. 37.5). Duct ectasia is not conspicuous during this phase. Increased amount and cellularity of periductal stroma are accompanied by prominent vascularity, edema, and a round cell infiltrate.

*Gynecomastia-like hyperplasia,* a proliferative lesion of the female breast that is indistinguishable histologically

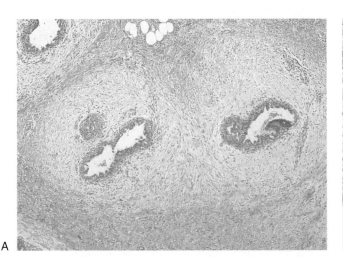
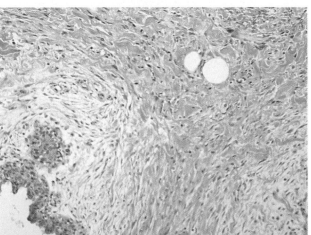

A                                          B

**FIG. 37.4.** *Gynecomastia, florid.* **A:** Periductal edema and cellular stroma with epithelial hyperplasia. **B:** Gynecomastic tissue with pseudoangiomatous stromal hyperplasia.

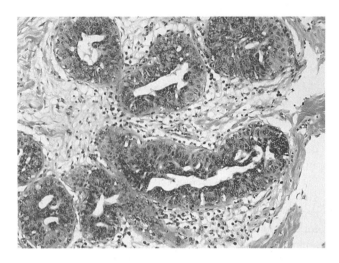

**FIG. 37.5.** *Gynecomastia, florid.* Epithelial hyperplasia with periductal edema and a slight lymphocytic infiltrate. The hyperplastic epithelium is composed of epithelial and myoepithelial cells.

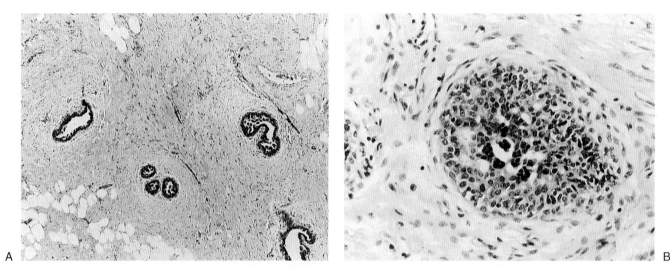

**FIG. 37.6.** *Gynecomastia-like hyperplasia in the female breast.* **A:** Periductal stromal proliferation with a mild lymphocytic infiltrate and epithelial hyperplasia. **B:** Micropapillary hyperplasia.

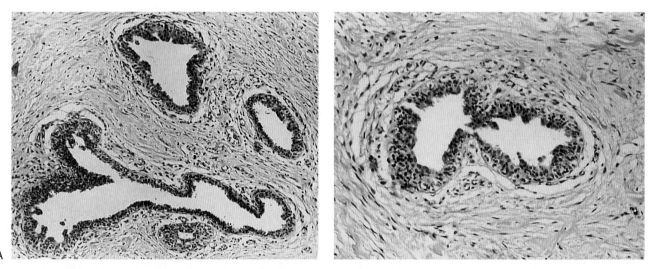

**FIG. 37.7.** *Gynecomastia, inactive.* **A:** Periductal edema is considerably reduced and collagenized stroma surrounds the ducts. **B:** Minimal epithelial hyperplasia is present.

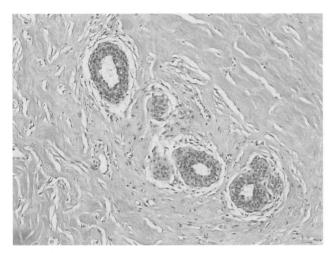

**FIG. 37.8.** *Gynecomastia, pseudoangiomatous stromal hyperplasia.*

from florid gynecomastia, is rarely encountered (Fig. 37.6). Umlas described gynecomastia-like tumors in four women 34 to 60 years old (46). Two tumors were palpable and 2 were detected by mammography. Ultrasounds performed in 3 cases were "negative." The excised tumors measured 1 to

3 cm. In another series, the female patients ranged in age from 33 to 54 years (47). The lesion may appear on mammography as an asymmetric density or as a nodule, but the radiographic features are nonspecific.

Fibrous or inactive gynecomastia typically occurs after the lesion has been present for 6 months or longer. The epithelial proliferation is much less conspicuous than in the florid phase, the stroma is more collagenous, with less edema, and there is reduced vascularity (Fig. 37.7). Intermediate gynecomastia that has florid and fibrous components tends to be present for 12 months or less. It constitutes a transitional phase in maturation of the lesion. Pseudoangiomatous hyperplasia of the stroma may be found in any phase of gynecomastia, but it is more pronounced in the active and intermediate stages (Fig. 37.8).

A variety of other proliferative epithelial changes have been found in gynecomastia. Lobule formation, initially attributed to exogenous estrogen administration (48), has been associated with diverse etiologies, including prepubertal gynecomastia (49), spironolactone treatment (Fig. 37.9), and androgen administration (Fig. 37.10). Pseudolactational hyperplasia occurs rarely in lobules formed in gynecomastia (Fig. 37.11). Apocrine metaplasia occurs in all three phases (Fig. 37.12). Focal squamous metaplasia is most common in

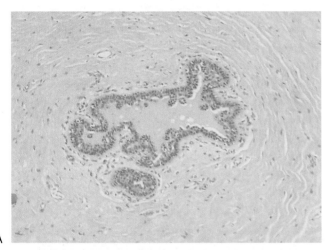

A

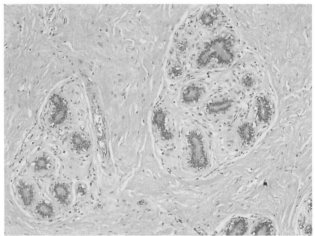

B

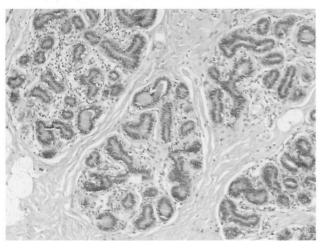

C

**FIG. 37.9.** *Gynecomastia, lobular differentiation.* The patient had cirrhosis of the liver and was being treated with spironolactone. **A:** Duct with micropapillary hyperplasia. **B:** Lobules with distinct epithelial and myoepithelial components. **C:** Lobules with secretory hyperplasia.

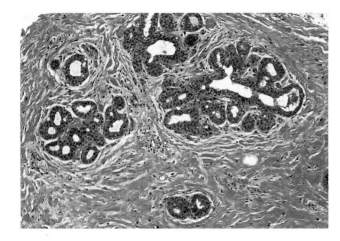

**FIG. 37.10.** *Gynecomastia, lobular differentiation.* Lobules were present in this biopsy of gynecomastia from a 27-year-old man who was using "over-the-counter" androgen supplements for body-building.

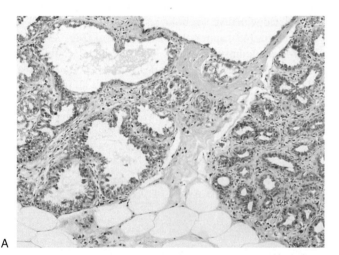

A

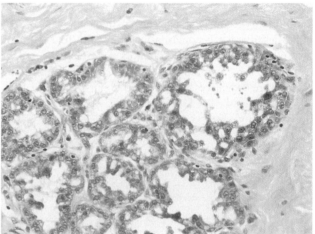

B

**FIG. 37.11.** *Gynecomastia.* **A,B:** Pseudolactational hyperplasia.

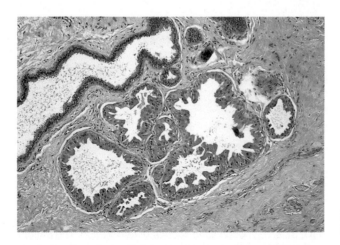

**FIG. 37.12.** *Gynecomastia, apocrine metaplasia.* Apocrine metaplasia is present in a duct and adjacent cysts.

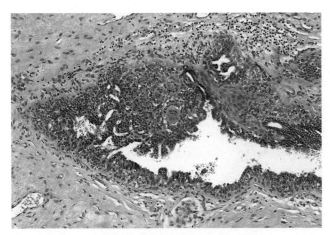

**FIG. 37.13.** *Gynecomastia, squamous metaplasia.* Squamous metaplasia is present in the partly papillary epithelial hyperplasia.

the florid stage (Fig. 37.13). Extensive squamous metaplasia is present in rare cases (50).

The cytologic features and growth pattern of the epithelial proliferation in ducts may be atypical. This occurs most often in the florid phase. Atypical features are the development of fenestrated and solid growth patterns, and papillary proliferation in which a cytologically atypical cell type appears to overgrow the usual dimorphic cell population that characterizes florid gynecomastia (Figs. 37.14–37.16). Mitotic activity usually is sparse, but it may be more abundant in ducts exhibiting severely atypical hyperplasia. Cytologic atypia in gynecomastia also has been associated with flutamide therapy for prostatic carcinoma (Fig. 37.17) (51). Marked cytologic atypia has also been observed in ductal hyperplasia in gynecomastia associated with finasteride treatment for alopecia (52).

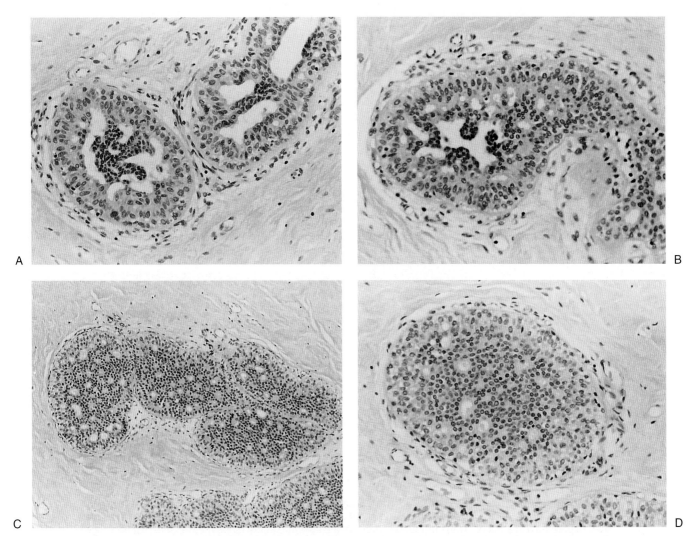

**FIG. 37.14.** *Gynecomastia, atypical duct hyperplasia.* All illustrations are from one biopsy specimen. **A:** Micropapillary hyperplasia. **B:** Micropapillary hyperplasia with peripheral fenestration. **C:** Atypical duct hyperplasia with a fenestrated (cribriform) growth pattern and a dimorphic cellular composition. **D:** Magnified view of the atypical duct hyperplasia.

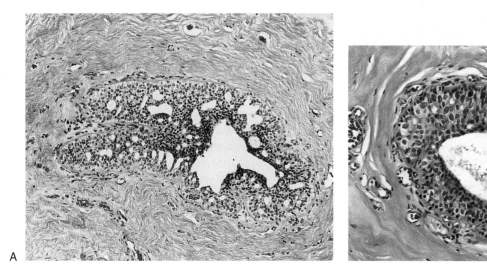

**FIG. 37.15.** *Gynecomastia, atypical duct hyperplasia.* **A:** Fenestrated epithelial hyperplasia with predominantly peripheral microlumens that have irregular shapes. **B:** Solid atypical duct hyperplasia.

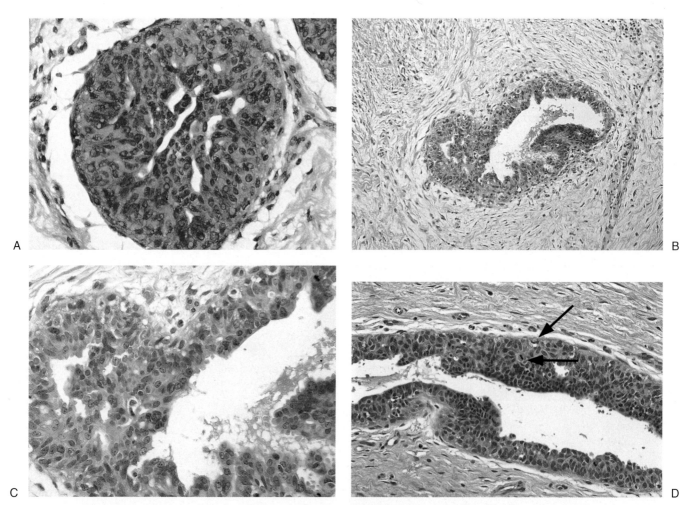

**FIG. 37.16.** *Gynecomastia, atypical duct hyperplasia.* **A:** Disorderly proliferation of epithelial cells nearly fills the duct. Some cellular heterogeneity and slight streaming are evident. **B,C:** Focal atypical papillary duct hyperplasia in a patient with intraductal carcinoma elsewhere in the biopsy. Extensive histologic examination of the specimen should be done when this is the most extreme finding in a biopsy. A mitotic figure can be seen in the *upper right corner* of **C. D:** Atypical hyperplasia lines this duct. The cells have a disorderly distribution. Note that nuclei become smaller and hyperchromatic near the lumen. Two mitotic figures are shown *(arrows).*

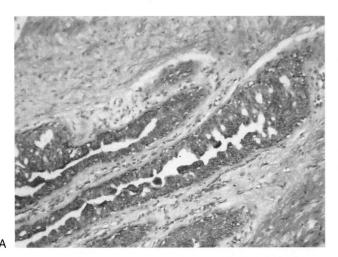
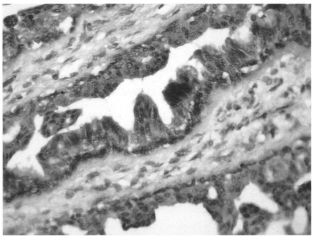

A

B

**FIG. 37.17.** *Gynecomastia, atypical duct hyperplasia.* The patient was treated for prostatic carcinoma with flutamide. **A,B:** Atypical micropapillary hyperplasia.

Fine needle aspiration cytology is useful for confirming a clinical diagnosis of gynecomastia (53). The character of the specimen depends on the phase of the process, but samples tend to have sparse cellularity. Apocrine cells are rarely present in the aspiration cytology specimen from gynecomastia (54).

Electron microscopy confirms the presence in gynecomastia of proliferating myoepithelial and epithelial cells (55). Splitting and duplication of the basement membrane, which may be interrupted by gaps formed by protruding epithelial cells, is seen frequently. The stroma contains fibroblasts and myofibroblasts. The ultrastructural features are similar to those encountered in duct hyperplasia of the female breast.

Regression of gynecomastia has been described in patients with hyperthyroidism (44) and alcoholic liver disease (56) when the underlying conditions were treated; however, breast enlargement usually persists. Radiation has been effective in preventing gynecomastia in patients receiving exogenous estrogens to treat prostatic carcinoma (57,58). Regression of gynecomastia has been reported after treatment with antiestrogens, such as tamoxifen and danazol. Excisional biopsy is indicated to exclude primary or metastatic carcinoma. Although carcinoma may arise in conjunction with gynecomastia, there is no evidence based on long-term follow-up studies that atypical proliferative changes in gynecomastia are associated with an increased risk for the subsequent development of carcinoma.

## REFERENCES

1. Detraux P, Benmussa M, Tristant H, et al. Breast disease in the male: galactographic evaluation. *Radiology* 1985;154:605–606.
2. Giltman LI. Solitary intraductal papilloma of the male breast. *South Med J* 1976;74:774.
3. Sara, AS, Gottfried MR. Benign papilloma of the male breast following chronic phenothiazine therapy. *Am J Clin Pathol* 1987;87:649–650.
4. Simpson JS, Barson AJ. Breast tumors in infants and children. *Can Med Assoc J* 1969;101:100–102.
5. Navas MDM, Povedano JLR, Mendivil EA, et al. Intracystic papilloma

in male breast: ultrasonography and pneumocystography diagnosis. *J Clin Ultrasound* 1993;21:38–40.
6. Nowak M, Pathan A, Fatteh S, et al. Syringocystadenoma papilliferum of the male breast. *Am J Dermatopathol* 1998;20:422–424.
7. David VC. Papillary cystadenoma of the male breast. *Ann Surg* 1922;75:652–657.
8. Burdick C, Reinhart RM, Matsumoto T, et al. Nipple adenoma and Paget's disease in a man. *Arch Surg* 1965;91:835–838.
9. Shapiro L, Karpas CM. Florid papillomatosis of the nipple. First reported case in a male. *Am J Clin Pathol* 1965;44:155–159.
10. Waldo ED, Sidhu GS, Hu AW. Florid papillomatosis of male nipple after diethylstilbestrol therapy. *Arch Pathol* 1975;99:364–366.
11. Nielsen VT, Andreasen C. Phyllodes tumour of the male breast. *Histopathology* 1987;11:761–765.
12. Ansah-Boateng Y, Tavassoli FA. Fibroadenoma and cystosarcoma phyllodes of the male breast. *Mod Pathol* 1992;5:114–116.
13. Bartoli C, Zurrida SM, Clemente C. Phyllodes tumor in a male patient with bilateral gynecomastia induced by oestrogen therapy for prostatic carcinoma. *Eur J Surg Oncol* 1991;17:215–217.
14. Panotoja E, Llobert RE, Lopez E. Gigantic cystosarcoma phyllodes in a man with gynecomastia. *Arch Surg* 1976;111:611.
15. Reingold IM, Ascher GS. Cystosarcoma phyllodes in a man with gynecomastia. *Am J Clin Pathol* 1970;53:852–856.
16. Uchida T, Ishii M, Motomiya Y. Fibroadenoma associated with gynaecomastia in an adult man. Case report. *Scand J Plast Reconstr Hand Surg* 1993;27:327–329.
17. Hilton DA, Jameson JS, Furness PN. Acellular fibroadenoma resembling a benign phyllodes tumour in a young male with gynecomastia. *Histopathology* 1991;18:476–477.
18. Nielsen BB. Fibroadenomatoid hyperplasia of the male breast. *Am J Surg Pathol* 1990;14:774–777.
19. Lewinn EB. Gynecomastia during digitalis therapy. *N Engl J Med* 1953;248:316–319.
20. Mann NM. Gynecomastia during therapy with spironolactone. *JAMA* 1963;184:778–780.
21. Andersen JA, Gram JB. Male breast at autopsy. *Acta Microbiol Immunol Scand (A)* 1982;90:191–197.
22. Tedeschi LG, McCarthy PE. Involutional mammary duct ectasia and periductal mastitis in a male. *Hum Pathol* 1974;5:232–236.
23. Banik S, Hale R. Fibrocystic disease in the male breast. *Histopathology* 1988;12:214–216.
24. McClure J, Banerjee SS, Sandilands DGD. Female type cystic hyperplasia in a male breast. *Postgrad Med J* 1985;61:441–443.
25. Sund BS, Topstad TK, Nesland JM. A case of juvenile papillomatosis of the male breast. *Cancer* 1992;70:126–128.
26. Bigotti G, Kasznica J. Sclerosing adenosis in the breast of a man with pulmonary oat cell carcinoma: report of a case. *Hum Pathol* 1986;17:861–863.
27. Newcomer TA, Green AE Jr, Sutton J, et al. Epithelial inclusion cyst in a male breast. *Breast Dis* 1995;8:91–95.

28. August GP, Chandra R, Hung W. Prepubertal male gynecomastia. *J Pediatr* 1972;80:259–263.

29. Nydick M, Bustos J, Dale JH Jr, et al. Gynecomastia in adolescent boys. *JAMA* 1961;178:449–454.

30. Carlson HE. Gynecomastia. *N Engl J Med* 1980;303:795–799.

31. Nuttall FQ. Gynecomastia as a physical finding in normal men. *J Clin Endocrinol Metab* 1979;48:338–340.

32. Williams MJ. Gynecomastia. Its incidence, recognition and host characterization in 447 autopsy cases. *Am J Med* 1963;34:103–112.

33. Bannayan GA, Hajdu SI. Gynecomastia: clinicopathologic study of 351 cases. *Am J Clin Pathol* 1972;57:431–437.

34. Green L, Wysowski DK, Fourcroy JL. Gynecomastia and breast cancer during finasteride therapy. *N Engl J Med* 1996;335:823.

35. Michels LG, Gold RH, Arndt RD. Radiography of gynecomastia and other disorders of the male breast. *Radiology* 1977;122:117–122.

36. Cilotti A, Campassi C, Bagnolesi P, et al. Gynecomastia: diagnostic value of high-frequencies ultrasound (10–13 MHz). *Breast Dis* 1996;9:61–69.

37. Contesso G, Delarue JC, Guerinot F, et al. Recepteurs aux estrogenes et aux progestogenes en pathologie mammaire chez l'homme. *Nouv Presse Med* 1977;6:1951–1953.

38. Grilli S, DeGiovanni C, Galli MC, et al. The simultaneous occurrence of cytoplasmic receptors for various steroid hormones in male breast carcinoma and gynecomastia. *J Steroid Biochem* 1980;13:813–820.

39. Pacheco MM, Oshima CF, Lopes MP, et al. Steroid hormone receptors in male breast diseases. *Anticancer Res* 1986;6:1013–1018.

40. Rosen PP, Menendez-Botet CJ, Nisselbaum JS, et al. Estrogen receptor in lesions of the male breast. *Cancer* 1976;37:1866–1868.

41. Andersen J, Orntoft TF, Andersen JA, et al. Gynecomastia. *Acta Pathol Microbiol Immunol Scand* 1987;95:263–267.

42. Gatalica Z, Norris BA, Kovatich AJ. Immunohistochemical localization of prostate-specific antigen in ductal epithelium of male breast. Potential diagnostic pitfall in patients with gynecomastia. *Appl Immunohistochem Molecul Morphol* 2000;8:158–161.

43. Andersen JA, Gram JB. Gynecomasty. Histological aspects in a surgical material. *Acta Pathol Microbiol Immunol Scand* 1982;90:185–190.

44. Becker KL, Matthews MJ, Higgins GA Jr, et al. Histologic evidence of gynecomastia in hyperthyroidism. *Arch Pathol* 1974;98:257–260.

45. Nicolis GL, Modlinger RS, Gabrilove JL. A study of the histopathology of human gynecomastia. *J Clin Endocrinol Metab* 1971;32:173–178.

46. Umlas J. Gynecomastia-like lesions in the female breast. *Arch Pathol Lab Med* 2000;124:844–847.

47. Selland D-LG, Korbin CD, Lester SC, et al. Gynecomastoid hyperplasia: imaging findings in six patients. *Radiology* 2000;214:553–555.

48. Schwartz IS, Wilens SL. The formation of acinar tissue in gynecomastia. *Am J Pathol* 1963;43:797–807.

49. Haibach H, Rosenholtz MJ. Prepubertal gynecomastia with lobules and acini: a case report and review of the literature. *Am J Clin Pathol* 1983;80:252–255.

50. Gottfried MR. Extensive squamous metaplasia in gynecomastia. *Arch Pathol Lab Med* 1986;110:971–973.

51. Pinedo F, Vargas J, deAgustín P, et al. Epithelial atypia in gynecomastia induced by chemotherapeutic drugs. A possible pitfall in fine needle aspiration biopsy. *Acta Cytol* 1991;35:229–233.

52. Zimmerman RL, Fogt F, Cronin D, et al. Cytologic atypia in a 53-year-old man with finasteride-induced gynecomastia. *Arch Pathol Lab Med* 2000;124:625–627.

53. Gupta RK, Naran S, Simpson J. The role of fine needle aspiration cytology (FNAC) in the diagnosis of breast masses in males. *Eur J Surg Oncol* 1988;14:317–320.

54. Gupta RK, Naran S, Lallu S, et al. Incidence of apocrine cells in fine-needle aspirates of gynecomastia: a study of 100 cases. *Diag Cytopathol* 2000;22:286–287.

55. Hassan MO, Olaizola MY. Ultrastructural observations in gynecomastia. *Arch Pathol Lab Med* 1979;103:624–630.

56. Becker KL, Matthews MJ, Winnacker J, et al. Sequential histological study of the regression of gynecomastia in a patient with alcoholic liver disease. *Am J Med Sci* 1967;254:685–691.

57. Waterfall NB, Glaser MG. A study of the effects of radiation on prevention of gynecomastia due to oestrogen therapy. *Clin Oncol* 1979;5:257–260.

58. Wolf H, Madsen PO, Vermundn H. Prevention of estrogen-induced gynecomastia by external irradiation. *J Urol* 1969;102:607–609.

# CHAPTER 38

# Carcinoma of the Male Breast

## EPIDEMIOLOGY

Breast carcinoma is an uncommon neoplastic condition among men, accounting for not more than 1% of all breast carcinomas and less than 0.1% of male cancer deaths (1–4). Worldwide, the incidence is generally less than one case per 100,000 men per year. Racial variations have been described, with the incidence reportedly lower among Japanese (5) and higher among blacks in West Africa (6) and the United States (7) when compared with whites. The average annual age-adjusted breast carcinoma death rate is higher among nonwhite men in the United States (4) and lower among Japanese men in Japan (5) than among white men in the United States, Canada, Europe, or Scandinavia. A higher incidence of breast carcinoma has been found among Jewish men when compared with other white ethnic subgroups (2,4,8,9). The incidence and age-specific death rate for male breast carcinoma increase in a linear fashion with advancing age among different racial and ethnic groups (1,4,5,8). This straight-line relationship between incidence and age among men differs from female breast carcinoma, which is characterized by a less steep slope after age 50 years among postmenopausal women (10).

Several risk factors for the development of male breast carcinoma have been identified. Some investigators found increased levels of estradiol and other estrogenic hormones in men with breast carcinoma (11,12), but others did not detect increased or abnormal estrogen concentrations (13–15). Case-control studies by Schottenfeld et al. (4) and Mabuchi et al. (2) found a relatively high frequency of antecedent mumps orchitis among men with breast carcinoma. It was suggested that testicular atrophy after orchitis causes relative hyperestrogenism. A follow-up study of 132 men who had mumps orchitis in one community revealed that the median age of patients with mumps was 8 years, and for those with mumps orchitis the median age was 29 years (16). Follow-up of 20 years or more was obtained for 36% of the patients, revealing testicular neoplasms in two. The absence of subsequent male mammary carcinoma in this cohort may reflect the relative youth of the patients at follow-up and the lack of

information about most of the men. Nicolis et al. (17) described a patient who developed breast carcinoma 30 years after mumps orchitis that resulted in testicular atrophy. Casagrande et al. (18) found no relationship between mumps in adulthood and male breast carcinoma, but they did not evaluate orchitis as a specific factor. An association with antecedent testicular trauma was observed by Mabuchi et al. (2), who found no relationship with prior orchiectomy, the presence of an undescended testis, or prostatic disease. A case-control study that compared men with breast and lung carcinoma, and lymphoma found that testicular trauma was reported more often by the breast carcinoma patients and that there was a significant association with hernia surgery (19). Further evidence that testicular dysfunction contributes to male breast carcinoma risk was reported by Thomas et al. (20), who studied 227 patients and 300 controls. The strongest association was detected for undescended testes, but orchitis, injury, late puberty, and infertility also were relevant factors.

An international comparison of age standardized incidence rates for prostatic and male breast carcinoma revealed a direct relationship between the two diseases (21). On the other hand, the actual reported frequency of both diseases in individual patients is quite low, occurring in less than 1% of 397 men in one study (22). There is limited evidence that the administration of exogenous estrogens to treat prostatic carcinoma contributes to the development of male breast carcinoma. Epidemiologic studies have failed to demonstrate an excess frequency of breast carcinoma among men with prostatic carcinoma (23). This is somewhat surprising, because most patients treated with estrogens for this disease develop gynecomastia. However, the duration of treatment rarely exceeds 10 years; therefore, the exposure may not be sufficient for mammary carcinogenesis to become apparent. Schlappack et al. (24) described two men who had breast carcinoma diagnosed after 12 years of estrogen therapy for prostatic carcinoma. Wilson and Hutchinson (25) described another man with a 7-year interval. Carlsson et al. (26) reported four patients who developed carcinoma after estrogen therapy. Case reports of breast carcinoma that developed in men with prostatic carcinoma are difficult to evaluate because of the well-known predilection of the latter to metastasize to the breast. The sporadic occurrence of primary concurrent prostatic and mammary carcinoma has been reported (27). Breast carcinoma has been described in transsexuals after castration and prolonged estrogen treatment (28–30). Benign histologic changes in the breast associated with this therapy include fully formed lobules, apocrine metaplasia, and pseudolactational hyperplasia.

Traumatic injury of the breast has been cited in some studies as a possible predisposing event (4). That most patients who related their carcinoma to trauma reported a single incident, rather than sustained or repeated injury, has led most investigators to discount this as a significant factor. In many instances, documentation that the carcinoma arose at the site of injury is not available. Occupational exposure has not been explored in most studies. An association with employment in steel works, blast furnaces, and rolling mills was noted by Mabuchi et al. (2). Other occupations reportedly associated with excess risk were work as a butcher and employment associated with exposure to high environmental temperatures (31,32). Cocco et al. (33) carried out a case-control study that compared 178 male breast carcinoma patients with 1,041 controls. There was a significantly increased risk of breast carcinoma among men employed in occupations with exposure to blast furnaces, steel works, and rolling mills (odds ratio [OR], 3.4; 95% confidence interval [CI], 1.1 to 10.1) and in motor vehicle manufacturing (OR, 3.1; 95% CI, 1.2 to 8.2). Breast cancer risk was not significantly related to exposure to electromagnetic fields, herbicides, pesticides, high temperatures, and organic solvents.

Radiation exposure has been implicated as a risk factor. In some instances, radiation was administered to the breast to treat gynecomastia or other local conditions or for intrathoracic diseases (10,34–37). Male breast carcinoma has been associated with one source of radiation linked to increased breast carcinoma risk among women, multiple fluoroscopic examinations (38), but not to atomic bomb explosions (39). Although not statistically significant, Casagrande et al. (18) found a trend to more frequent breast carcinoma in men who had the greatest thoracic radiation exposure by fluoroscopy or during therapy (18). One patient received radiotherapy for chondrosarcoma of a rib prior to developing breast carcinoma (22).

A potential role for lesions of the pituitary gland was suggested by a case-control study that found a greater frequency of head injuries that caused concussions or fractures among men with breast carcinoma (19). It was suggested that traumatic injuries of the hypothalamus or hypophyseal stalk could interfere with normal hypothalamic control of prolactin secretion. Further evidence for prolactin as a possible etiologic agent was the finding in the same study that drug treatment associated with prolactin elevation was more frequent in the male breast carcinoma cohort. Others also have reported excess risk of breast carcinoma among men treated with medications that cause hyperprolactinemia (31). Bilat-

eral breast carcinoma has been described in a man treated for a prolactin-secreting pituitary adenoma (40). Olsson et al. (14) found that plasma prolactin levels in 15 male breast carcinoma patients were elevated when compared to controls with other neoplasms. Concurrent breast carcinoma and pituitary prolactinoma were described in a 68-year old male who did not have gynecomastia (41). Lactational change was not evident in the carcinoma.

Klinefelter's syndrome, a genetic abnormality that usually becomes evident during or after puberty, has been associated with an increased risk for development of male breast carcinoma. Prominent clinical manifestations are gynecomastia and testicular atrophy. Microscopic examination of the testes reveals hyalinization of spermatic tubules with disappearance of germ cells and Sertoli cells. Hyperplasia with pleomorphism of interstitial cells develop concurrently (42). Dodge et al. (43) described coexistent mammary carcinoma and interstitial cell tumor in a patient with Klinefelter's syndrome. The majority of patients with Klinefelter's syndrome have at least two X chromosomes and a Y chromosome. The extra X, or 47th, chromosome is identified cytologically as the nuclear Barr body. Abnormal hormonal findings include reduced testosterone production, low plasma testosterone, and a high estradiol-to-testosterone ratio at least partially augmented by increased testicular estrogen secretion.

Most papers relating male breast carcinoma to Klinefelter's syndrome have been individual case reports in which the chromosomal abnormality was documented by genetic studies (43–46). The reported incidence of breast carcinoma among patients with Klinefelter's syndrome varies from 1% to 3% (47,48). Breast carcinoma also has been described in a phenotypic male with an XX genotype (49).

It has been estimated that 1% to 3% of male breast carcinoma patients have Klinefelter's syndrome (50,51). Using fluorescence *in situ* hybridization (FISH) to examine tissues from men with breast carcinoma, Hultborn et al. (52) found the prevalence of Klinefelter's syndrome to be 7.5% in this patient group. The authors concluded that individuals with Klinefelter's syndrome had a 50-fold increased risk for developing breast carcinoma when compared to normal males. Klinefelter's syndrome did not have a significant effect on the median age at diagnosis or on survival after diagnosis.

Cutuli et al. (22) found a positive family history of breast carcinoma in 5.6% of 397 men with breast carcinoma. A twofold increased risk of breast carcinoma among first-degree relatives of male breast carcinoma patients, largely due to an excess of carcinoma in sisters, was reported by Casagrande et al. (18). Rosenblatt et al. (53) reported that the increased risk associated with sisters having breast carcinoma was significantly greater among men with carcinoma diagnosed before age 60 years. The relative risk of male breast carcinoma among men with an affected sister was 3.93. The relative risk in men whose mothers had breast carcinoma also was increased (2.33). Gough et al. (54) found a positive family history of breast carcinomas associated with 27% of male breast carcinomas treated at the Mayo Clinic.

Uterine carcinoma among female relatives also was associated with an increased OR (2.66), whereas the OR for prostatic carcinoma among male relatives was low (0.90). Others also reported a lower incidence of prostatic carcinoma among male relatives of men with breast carcinoma (55).

Several instances of the familial occurrence of male breast carcinoma have been described, in which father and son (53,56–58), brothers (53,59,60), and other groups of male relatives (53,61–64) were affected. Multiple female and male relatives have been affected in some kindreds (61). One family included an individual with Klinefelter's syndrome (56). Genetic analysis of two brothers who developed breast carcinoma at age 55 and 75 years, respectively, revealed a mutation consisting of a G-to-A substitution in exon 3 of the androgen receptor gene (65). Both men were born with penoscrotal hypospadias and undescended testes. A study of deoxyribonucleic acid (DNA) extracted from the tumor tissue of 12 male breast cancer patients who did not have clinical features of androgen insensitivity failed to reveal comparable mutations of the androgen receptor gene (66).

Analysis of 22 families with at least one male and multiple female breast carcinomas revealed no linkage to the BRCA1 locus (67). Other investigators reported that approximately 16% of families with multiple females and one or more males affected are attributable to BRCA1 mutation (68). In the same study, analysis of 26 families with one or more male breast carcinomas revealed that 76% were associated with BRCA2 mutations. Male carriers of BRCA2 mutations were found to have a cumulative risk of 6.3% to develop breast carcinoma by age 70 years (69). Analysis of 111 families with BRCA2 mutations revealed that 11% of breast carcinomas diagnosed in these families occurred in men (70). Among 18 Hungarian males with breast carcinoma, six (33%) had truncating mutations in the BRCA2 gene (71). None of the six patients with BRCA2 mutations reported a family history of breast/ovarian carcinoma, but four other men without BRCA2 mutations had such a history. A study of Icelandic men with breast carcinoma revealed that 40% had a BRCA2 mutation (72). These results are of interest in view of a study of 30 men with "sporadic" breast carcinoma reported by Prechtel et al. (73). None of the men belonged to a "breast cancer family," defined as "3 or more cases of breast cancer in a first- and second-degree relative with at least one patient younger than 50 years of age." Loss of heterozygosity was detected on chromosome 13q12–13 in 16 (67%) of 24 evaluable cases. Data from a Danish cancer registry revealed that the relative risk for developing breast carcinoma in daughters of affected men was 16.4 (95% CI, 3.3 to 47.7) (74). Linkage to mutations in the BRCA2 region on chromosome 13q has been demonstrated in one family with multiple cases of male breast carcinoma (75). Others have reported finding loss of heterozygosity on chromosome 11q13 in 13 (68.4%) of 19 male breast carcinomas (76) and on chromosome 8 in 19 (83%) of 23 cases studied (77).

Increased urinary estrogen excretion has been reported among male relatives of male patients with breast carcinoma (57,59). Many of these families had relatives with other malignant neoplasms (56,57,59,60,63,78). The incidence of breast carcinoma and other malignant neoplasms in wives of men with breast carcinoma is similar to that in the general population (55).

The relationship between gynecomastia and the development of male breast carcinoma is not clear. A major factor that has contributed to the problem is differing definitions of gynecomastia, including the distinction between clinical and pathologic manifestations of the condition. Gynecomastia has florid or proliferative and quiescent phases, but the histologic diagnosis sometimes is limited to the former pattern, although clinical manifestations may be as prominent when the process is inactive. Evidence linking gynecomastia to the pathogenesis of male breast carcinoma includes epithelial atypia in gynecomastia, relatively lower mean age at diagnosis of breast carcinoma when associated with gynecomastia, association of gynecomastia and carcinoma with Klinefelter's syndrome, and the finding of microscopic gynecomastia associated with 5% to 40% of carcinomas (79,80). Histologic transitions from epithelial hyperplasia in gynecomastia to intraductal carcinoma have very rarely been described (80,81).

Finasteride, a medication used since 1992 to treat prostatic hyperplasia, blocks the conversion of testosterone to dihydrotesterone, thereby causing an increase in the ratio of estrogen to androgen. Gynecomastia has been the most frequent adverse side effect of finasteride (82). Two of 214 men reported to the United States Food and Drug Administration as having gynecomastia related to finasteride also had intraductal carcinoma. Long-term follow-up studies will be necessary to determine if this is more than a coincidental association.

It seems likely that the coexistence of male breast carcinoma and gynecomastia is due to the fact that both conditions sometimes are related to one or more common predisposing factors. However, evidence suggests that gynecomastia rarely serves as a precancerous condition or as an intermediate step in the development of carcinoma.

Other factors that have been associated with the development of male breast carcinoma in various studies include liver disease, obesity, tuberculosis, and therapeutic use of digitalis, although the relationship has not been statistically significant in all instances (18,31,42).

Several authors have commented on the development of nonmammary malignant neoplasms (NMMN) among men with mammary carcinoma (10,22,80,83–85). The frequency of NMMN ranges from 3.5% (22) to 13% (85,86). The more common sites of NMMN include the colon and rectum, stomach, and prostate gland. A study of 229 male patients with breast carcinoma diagnosed over a 40-year period in Canada revealed prior or subsequent NMMN in 24.5%, including tumors of the skin and undocumented sites (87). In view of the relatively advanced age of men with mammary carcinoma, the frequency of NMMN in this population does not appear to be excessive, especially if one includes NMMN diagnosed before and after the breast lesion.

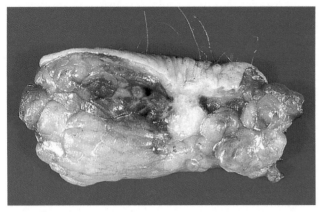

**FIG. 38.1.** *Male breast carcinoma.* In this gross specimen, a carcinoma in the central part of the breast has caused retraction of the nipple.

## CLINICAL PRESENTATION

The majority of male breast carcinomas are located centrally in a retroareolar position (Fig. 38.1), but eccentric lesions, particularly in the upper outer quadrant, have been described (3,88). Rarely, the tumor may arise in the nipple and invade the underlying breast (Fig. 38.2). Synchronous, clinically evident bilateral carcinoma is exceedingly unusual (85,89,90). It has been estimated that the cumulative risk for bilaterality is 3% or less (34,83).

About 75% of patients present with a painless mass. When a mass is absent, the lesion invariably is detected because of nipple ulceration, retraction, or discharge. Carcinoma is found in about 75% of male patients with a mass and bloody discharge. Approximately half of the patients with serous discharge and a mass prove to have carcinoma (91). Serous

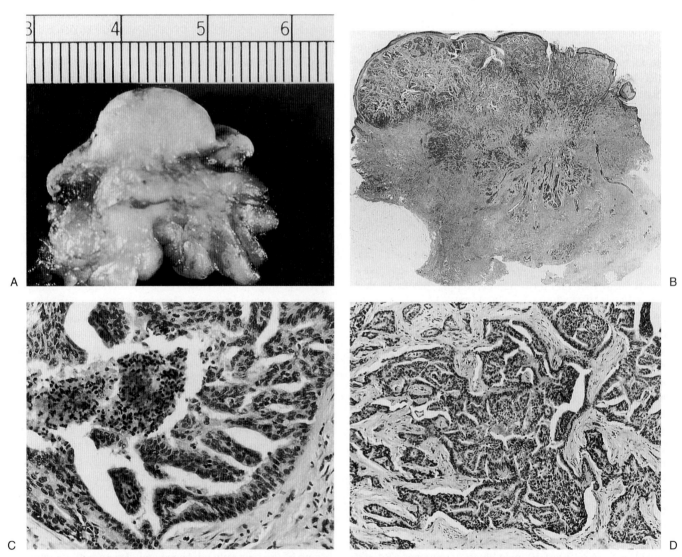

**FIG. 38.2.** *Male breast carcinoma in the nipple.* **A:** Gross hemisection of the nipple and underlying tissue with carcinoma in the nipple. **B:** Whole-mount histologic section of invasive carcinoma in the nipple. **C:** Papillary intraductal carcinoma in the tumor. **D:** Infiltrating papillary carcinoma in the nipple tumor.

discharge alone may indicate intraductal carcinoma (92,93). The mean duration of symptoms prior to clinical consultation has been reported to be between 6 months (94) and nearly 1 year (84). Age at diagnosis averages about 60 years, approximately 5 years older than women. However, breast carcinoma has been diagnosed in males at virtually all ages, including children and young adults less than 30 years of age (86,95). Among men with intraductal carcinoma, six of 31 patients were younger than 40 years and the median age at diagnosis was 58 years (22). Hittmair et al. (96) reported an age range from 25 to 94 years and a median age of 65 years in 84 men with intraductal carcinoma.

Mammograms of men with breast carcinoma typically reveal distinct lesions with invasive margins that contrast sharply with the surrounding fatty tissue (97,98), but carcinoma may be obscured by concurrent gynecomastia (99,100). Cystic papillary carcinoma produces a discrete round mass that may contain calcifications. The cystic character of such a lesion and the presence of an internal papillary component can be demonstrated by ultrasonography (101,102). An irregular border around a cystic lesion may be evidence of invasion (103). Mammograms of gynecomastia typically reveal accentuated glandular tissue and ducts extending from the nipple. Ultrasonography is useful for distinguishing between gynecomastia and carcinoma (62). The mammographic density associated with gynecomastia usually is symmetric. It often has a triangular configuration at an early stage but may develop a dendritic pattern in established lesions (97,104).

Microcalcifications are found in 9% to 30% of male breast carcinomas studied mammographically (88,99,100). Mammographic detection of occult carcinoma in the contralateral breast of a man previously treated for breast carcinoma was reported by Dershaw (97). Inflammatory carcinoma of the male breast produces diffuse enlargement of the affected breast and skin thickening (105). Invasion of the skin and enlarged lymph nodes may be evident radiographically (106).

Fine needle aspiration cytology has been used to evaluate tumors of the male breast (107). Joshi et al. (108) reviewed breast aspirates from 507 men. Satisfactory specimens were obtained from 393 (78%), of which 70 (13.8%) revealed carcinoma.

Cellular aspirates may be obtained from carcinomas or gynecomastia, but the specimens exhibit qualitative differences (109). The specimen from florid gynecomastia contains abundant epithelial cells, largely arranged in sheets and cohesive clusters, with only scattered isolated cells (107,109). Dispersed epithelial cells are a prominent feature of most male carcinomas, but epithelioid cell clusters may be encountered in specimens from papillary tumors (110,111). Considerable cytologic atypia that can occur in the epithelial hyperplasia of gynecomastia may present a diagnostic problem in a fine needle aspiration specimen (107,112). Mitotic figures may be found in aspirates from gynecomastia, but they are more frequent in carcinoma (109). Myoepithelial cells, which feature small dark nuclei, are seen in almost all

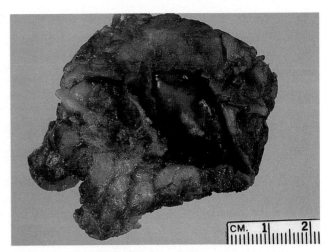

**FIG. 38.3.** *Cystic papillary carcinoma.* Specimen from the right breast of a 72-year-old man. The cyst, shown here opened, measured 5.5 cm. On the *left*, there is an intracystic papillary tumor with an underlying nodule of invasive carcinoma. On the *right*, the inner surface of the cyst is smooth.

aspirates from gynecomastia (112). They are more numerous in material from florid lesions, and such specimens also may have a scattering of lymphocytes. The aspirate from mature, stable gynecomastia ordinarily is sparsely cellular, consisting of scanty epithelial elements largely in loosely cohesive sheets and connective tissue.

A high frequency of estrogen receptor–positive male breast carcinomas was noted in 1976 (113). Subsequent reports confirmed this observation, revealing that approximately 85% of the lesions had positive levels of estradiol receptor (114–117). The expression of estrogen receptor in male breast carcinoma does not appear to be age related (118). When tested biochemically, many male breast carcinomas also had substantial levels of receptors for progesterone (114,119), dihydrotestosterone (119), androgen (114,120), and glucocorticoid (114,120). Positive levels of estrogen receptor corresponding to the primary tumor have been reported in liver metastases (117). Gynecomastic breast tissue also contains receptors for estradiol (113,120,121), dihydrotestosterone (112), androgen (120), progesterone (112,120), and glucocorticoid (112,120).

## GROSS PATHOLOGY

Carcinoma of the male breast appears identical grossly to carcinoma arising in the female breast. Cystic papillary carcinomas may present as striking tumors grossly (Fig. 38.3).

## MICROSCOPIC PATHOLOGY

Approximately 85% of male mammary carcinomas are of the infiltrating duct variety (Fig. 38.4). An intraductal component is found in 35% to 50% of male and 75% of female infiltrating duct carcinomas (79). Extensive intraductal carcinoma constituting more than 25% of the tumor and

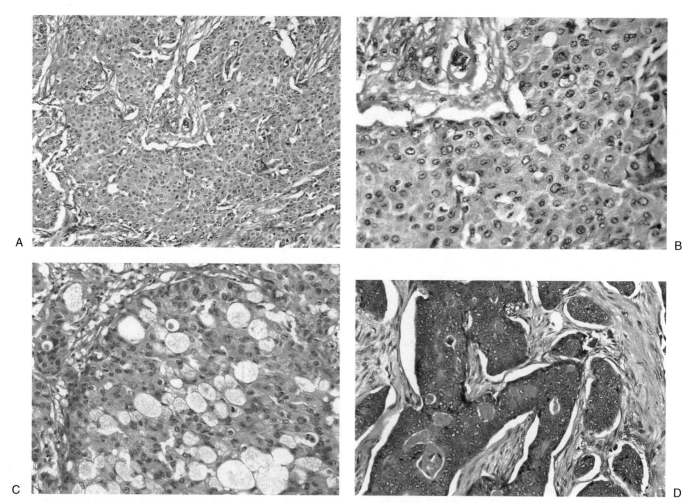

**FIG. 38.4.** *Male breast carcinoma, infiltrating duct type.* **A,B:** Solid infiltrating duct carcinoma. Carcinoma has apocrine cytologic features. **C:** Marked cytoplasmic clearing and vacuolization. **D:** High-grade invasive duct carcinoma. This histologic appearance resembles a pattern seen in prostatic carcinoma.

involving surrounding breast is uncommon (93). The pattern of associated intraductal carcinoma usually resembles the invasive tumor, often growing as solid or comedocarcinoma (96). The majority of the invasive tumors are moderately or poorly differentiated (122), but low-grade and tubular carcinomas have been described (Fig. 38.5) (79,122–124). The growth patterns seen in male infiltrating duct carcinomas duplicate those encountered in the female breast, including cribriform, comedo, papillary, solid, or gland-forming components (Fig. 38.6).

Periductal elastosis is found in some invasive duct carcinomas (125). Apocrine differentiation, which has rarely been described, may be present in intraductal as well as invasive lesions (126,127). Approximately 2% of male breast carcinomas are complicated by Paget's disease of the nipple, nearly the same frequency as Paget's disease in women (45,86,128,129). Bilateral Paget's disease was reported in a patient with Klinefelter's syndrome and multiple other malignant neoplasms (130). Secondary Paget's disease occurs when an underlying invasive tumor extends into the epidermis of the nipple or adjacent skin.

Papillary carcinomas, often with a prominent cystic com-

ponent, are relatively more common among men than women, constituting 3% to 5% of male carcinomas (7,79,80,122,123) but only 1% to 2% of carcinomas in women. The majority of male papillary carcinomas are

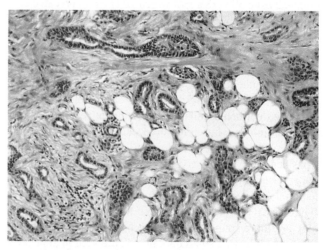

**FIG. 38.5.** *Male breast carcinoma, tubular type.*

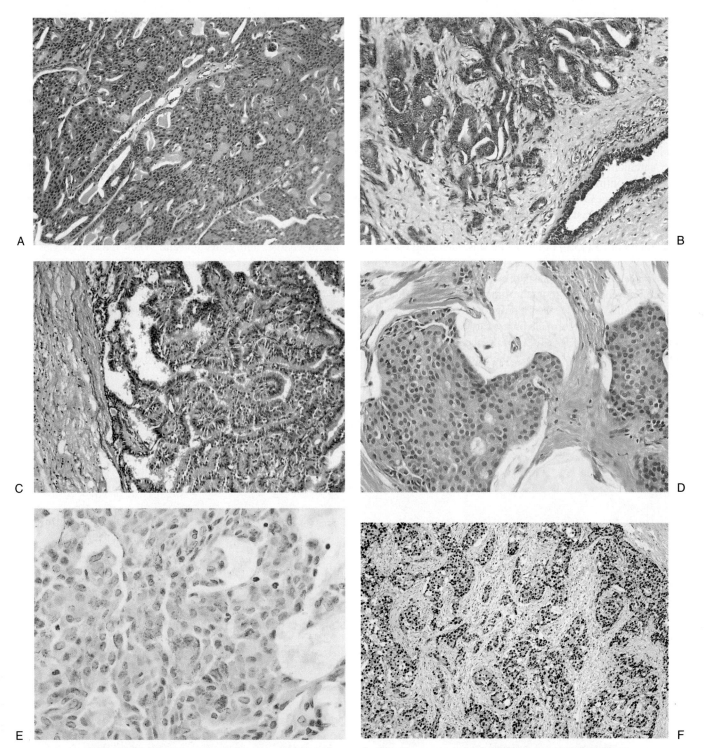

**FIG. 38.6.** *Male breast carcinoma, growth patterns.* **A:** Cribriform carcinoma. **B:** Moderately differentiated infiltrating duct carcinoma. **C:** Papillary carcinoma. **D:** Mucinous carcinoma. **E:** Positive Grimelius stain in the carcinoma shown in **D**. **F:** Diffuse, strong nuclear immunoreactivity for estrogen receptor in an invasive duct carcinoma (avidin-biotin).

intracystic and noninvasive. A very orderly papillary carcinoma may be mistaken for papillary hyperplasia (Fig. 38.7). Neurosecretory-type, electron-dense, membrane-bound cytoplasmic granules were found by electron microscopy in one male papillary carcinoma (131). The granules proved to be argyrophilic, and they were not reactive immunohistochemically for S-100 protein, lactalbumin, or a variety of endocrine substances, including calcitonin, bombesin, corticotropin, and vasoactive intestinal peptide. Melanin in another papillary carcinoma of the male breast was evident in routine sections and confirmed by histochemical stains (132).

Alm et al. (133) studied 51 consecutively treated examples of male breast carcinoma for evidence of neuroendocrine differentiation. Chromogranin immunoreactivity was found in 23 (45%) of the neoplasms, including one example of intraductal carcinoma. "Endocrine-like" granules were detected in the cytoplasm of six tumors studied by electron microscopy. Chromogranin immunoreactivity did not have a significant influence on prognosis.

About 5% to 10% of male breast carcinomas are entirely intraductal lesions (7,79,81,82,86). In one series, 26% of the lesions were intraductal (80). Others found 12% (93) and 17% (134) to be noninvasive. A review of 282 cases identified in 10 United States population-based cancer registries revealed 10.4% to be intraductal (118). The histologic appearance duplicates that of intraductal carcinoma in women, including comedo, cribriform, solid micropapillary, and papillary patterns (Fig. 38.8). Myoepithelial cells may persist and become hyperplastic in intraductal carcinoma of the male breast (Figs. 38.8 and 38.9). Male intraductal carcinoma without invasion is papillary, cribriform, or micropapillary in about 75% of patients and infrequently solid and comedo (96).

Associated clinically apparent abnormalities that may be responsible for the detection of intraductal carcinoma include nipple erosion caused by Paget's disease, bloody nipple discharge, and gynecomastia. When intraductal carcinoma arises in gynecomastia, it is rarely possible to find transitions from atypical hyperplasia in gynecomastic ducts to carcinoma (48). Comedonecrosis and epithelial clear cell change are features more strongly associated with intraductal carcinoma than with hyperplasia in gynecomastia. In one case, comedo intraductal carcinoma treated only by excisional biopsy was followed 4 years later by the

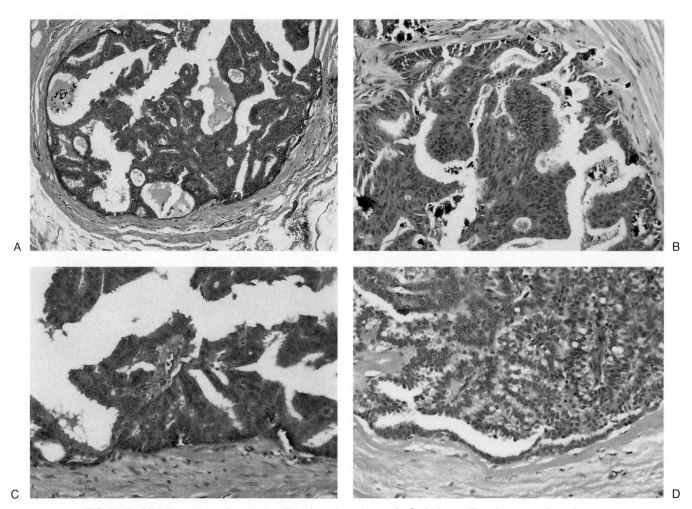

**FIG. 38.7.** *Male breast carcinoma, papillary intraductal type.* **A:** Orderly papillary intraductal carcinoma. **B,C:** Carcinoma has apocrine features and microcalcifications. **D:** Columnar epithelium and clear cells.

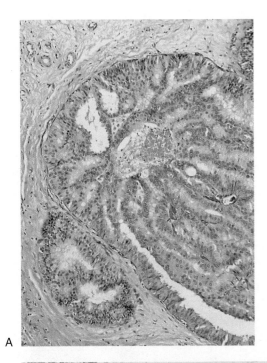

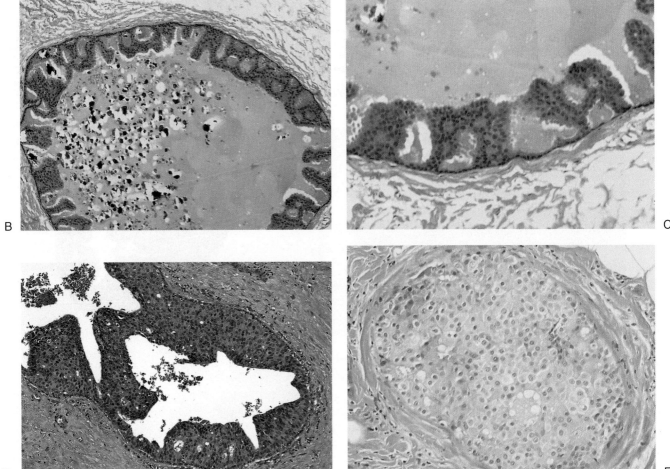

**FIG. 38.8.** *Male breast carcinoma, intraductal.* **A:** Papillary carcinoma with focal necrosis. **B,C:** Micropapillary carcinoma with calcifications. **D:** Solid type distributed at the periphery of a duct. Note the prominent myoepithelial cell layer. **E:** Solid apocrine type. *(continued)*

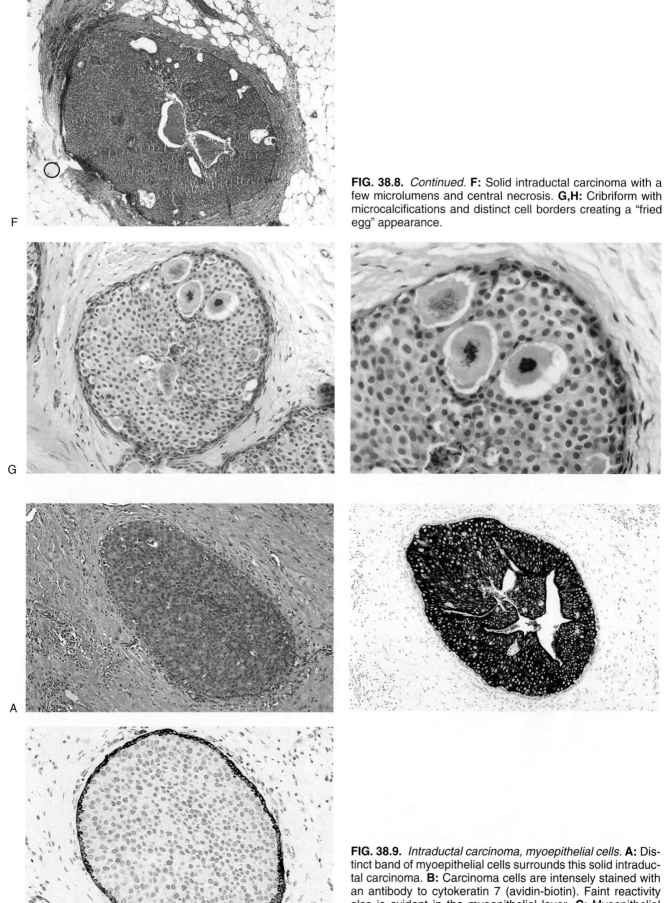

**FIG. 38.8.** *Continued.* **F:** Solid intraductal carcinoma with a few microlumens and central necrosis. **G,H:** Cribriform with microcalcifications and distinct cell borders creating a "fried egg" appearance.

**FIG. 38.9.** *Intraductal carcinoma, myoepithelial cells.* **A:** Distinct band of myoepithelial cells surrounds this solid intraductal carcinoma. **B:** Carcinoma cells are intensely stained with an antibody to cytokeratin 7 (avidin-biotin). Faint reactivity also is evident in the myoepithelial layer. **C:** Myoepithelial cells are highlighted with the antibody to smooth muscle myosin heavy chain (avidin-biotin).

development of invasive duct carcinoma in the same breast, leading to osseous metastases (81). Replacement of most of the intraductal carcinoma by granulation tissue was observed in one remarkable specimen (Fig. 38.10). This finding suggests that the phenomenon of "healing" can occur in male as well as in female intraductal carcinoma (see Chapter 13).

Because lobular differentiation is so rarely seen in the male breast, the existence of lobular carcinoma has been questioned in this setting. Isolated examples of "small cell carcinoma" or lobular carcinoma have been described (31,80,123,135–138), but there were none in several larger series (10,79,86,122). The microscopic appearance of the lesions depicted in several of the papers is consistent with invasive lobular carcinoma (136–138). *In situ* lobular carcinoma has reportedly been found in two cases (136,137). Michaels et al. (139) described a 59-year-old man with infiltrating lobular carcinoma, no *in situ* lobular carcinoma, and a normal male karyotype. None of these tumors were studied immunohistochemically for E-cadherin.

Other uncommon types of invasive carcinoma encountered in the male breast include medullary (3,7,80,122,123) mucinous (79,80,122,123,135), and adenoid cystic (140,141) tumors. The ultrastructural features of carcinoma of the male breast appear to be similar to those in the female breast (142).

Metastatic prostatic adenocarcinoma involving one or both breasts has been well documented (25,143–145). On occasion, the distinction between a primary carcinoma of the breast and metastatic prostatic carcinoma may be difficult. Both types of carcinoma may express estrogen receptors. Patients with prostatic adenocarcinoma treated with estrogens invariably have gynecomastia, which may exhibit markedly atypical papillary epithelial hyperplasia. Such proliferative changes should not be misinterpreted as intraductal carcinoma. In men with known prostatic carcinoma, the diagnosis of mammary carcinoma is relatively easy in the presence of convincing evidence of intraductal carcinoma, usually cribriform or comedo type, or the finding of specific growth

patterns such as tubular, medullary, mucinous, or cystic papillary carcinoma. Greater difficulty is encountered with poorly differentiated carcinomas that lack an intraductal component (Fig. 38.4). The immunohistochemical demonstration of prostate-specific antigen (PSA) favors a diagnosis of metastatic prostatic carcinoma, whereas finding intracellular mucin supports a diagnosis of mammary carcinoma. However, aberrant expression of PSA detected by immunohistochemistry has been reported in breast carcinomas from men (146) and women (147). The tissue concentration of PSA in breast carcinomas may be prognostically significant (148). Strong nuclear reactivity for androgen receptor typically is associated with prostatic carcinoma (see Chapter 36).

Several markers reported to be prognostically significant in female breast carcinoma have been studied in men. Cathepsin D immunoreactivity was found in 62% of 21 tumors, 86% of which were estrogen receptor positive (149). Cathepsin D reactivity did not appear to influence prognosis. Another series reported cathepsin D reactivity in 47% of male carcinomas (150).

Fox et al. (151) reported detecting membrane immunoreactivity for epidermal growth factor receptor (EGFR) in 76% of 21 male breast carcinomas, of which 86% were estrogen receptor positive. Others found EGFR expression in only 13.8% of carcinomas (152).

Membrane immunoreactivity for HER2/*neu* has been found in 17% (152,153), 29% (154), 35% (155), 39% (156), 41% (157), and 81% (150) of male breast carcinomas. In one series, HER2/*neu* reactivity was present in three (17%) of 18 invasive ductal carcinomas (153). It was absent from three examples of intraductal carcinoma and 12 specimens of gynecomastia. These authors also detected immunoreactivity for the pregnancy-specific B-1 glycoprotein in 27% of invasive duct carcinomas in the male breast. Nuclear immunoreactivity for p53 protein has been detected in 2% (158), 6% (150), 14% (159), 21% (154), 25% (160), 29% (157), 31% (152), 53% (161), and 62% (162) of male breast carcinomas.

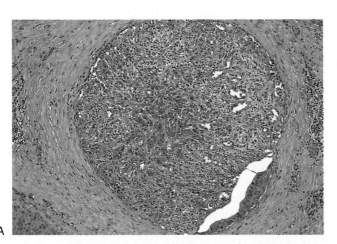
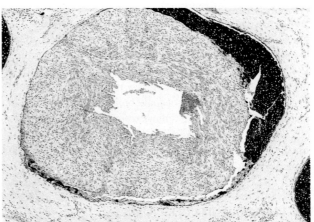

**FIG. 38.10.** *Intraductal carcinoma with granulation tissue.* **A:** Most of the duct lumen is filled with granulation tissue. Persisting carcinoma is evident in the *lower right corner.* **B:** Residual carcinoma displays reactivity with the antibody to cytokeratin 7 (avidin-biotin).

Most authors have not found the expression of HER2/*neu* and p53 to be prognostically significant in men (150, 152,154), but Joshi et al. (157) reported that HER2/*neu* immunoreactivity was prognostically unfavorable, and Pich et al. (162) reported that p53 positivity was significantly associated with a poor prognosis in a multivariate analysis. Co-expression of p53 and HER2/*neu* was prognostically significant in one report that found no five-year survivors among men whose tumors were immunoreactive for both oncogenes, whereas all patients with nonreactive tumors survived nearly five years (162a).

Rayson et al. (154) detected androgen receptor by immunohistochemistry in 95% of male breast carcinomas and *bcl*-2 in 94%. Cyclin D1 was positive in 58% and MIB1 in 38%. Tumors classified as cyclin D1 positive had a significantly better disease-free survival, whereas MIB1-positive tumors had a decreased disease-free survival.

Expression of *bcl*-2 was evident in 28 (82%) of 34 male breast carcinomas studied by Pich et al. (163). The *bcl*-2 was not significantly related to prognosis, p53 expression, or proliferative activity in the tumor.

Expression of the estrogen inducible gene pS2 was detected in 71% of 38 male breast carcinomas studied by immunohistochemistry (164). The presence or absence of detectable pS2 was not significantly related to survival or tumor grade.

A report on the distribution of type IV collagen in the male breast described the immunohistochemical localization of this protein in the basement membrane region in proliferative lesions at the epithelial–stromal junction (165). A fibrillary network of type IV collagen was found in the stroma of invasive carcinomas. These observations led the authors to suggest that type IV collagen could be "an important mediator of epithelial–stromal interactions" (165).

Molecular analysis of DNA extracted from paraffin-embedded male breast carcinomas revealed p53 mutations in 12 (41.4%) of 29 tumors analyzed (166). Only one of these tumors gave a positive reaction for the p53 protein by immunohistochemistry. The presence or absence of p53 mutations was not significantly related to prognosis, although it was observed that patients with altered p53 had a shorter median disease-free and overall survival (166). Nayak et al. (167) reported that p53 mutations occurred in exons 5 or 6 of the p53 gene in 33% of female breast carcinomas studied with positive immunohistochemistry in all cases. Mutations in p53 were found in 90% of male breast carcinomas (all in exon 6), and 86% of these tumors were immunohistochemically positive for p53. Anelli et al. (168) found p53 mutations in 41% of male breast carcinoma, with alterations distributed among exons 5 to 8.

## TREATMENT AND PROGNOSIS

Most patients have been treated by total mastectomy and axillary dissection. Total mastectomy alone has occasionally been used for patients with intraductal carcinoma. Lumpec-

tomy and radiation therapy have only rarely been recommended, but may be used in elderly patients (84). Two patients who underwent partial mastectomies without radiotherapy for intraductal carcinoma developed recurrent intraductal carcinoma in the conserved breasts 30 and 108 months after primary surgery (134). Mastectomy may be followed by radiation of the chest wall in patients with large tumors for whom the risk of local recurrence is relatively high (169,170), but it has not been demonstrated that this improves overall prognosis (171–173).

Numerous studies described the prognosis of male breast carcinoma after treatment by mastectomy and axillary dissection. Prognosis was significantly related to stage at diagnosis as determined by tumor size and nodal status (3,79,85,171,173–177). The presence of lymphatic tumor emboli negatively influences prognosis (157). Breast carcinoma is very uncommon in men younger than 45 years, but it may have a relatively unfavorable prognosis in this age group (178). Hill et al. (179) reported that a family history of breast carcinoma did not have a significant effect on the age and stage at diagnosis or on the prognosis of men with breast carcinoma.

Several investigators concluded that male and female patients with the same stage of disease have a similar prognosis (83,85,172,176,180), but others reported a less favorable outcome among men when compared with women by stage (175). Heller et al. (79) reported that node-negative male and female patients had nearly identical survivals when compared 5 and 10 years after treatment. In the same study, node-positive male and female patients did not differ in survival at 5 years, but there were substantially fewer survivors among the men 10 years after treatment. Survival at 5 and 10 years in pathologically node-negative patients was 70% to 84% (79,85,171,172,175–177). Among node-positive patients, the 5-year survival rate has been reported to be $59\% \pm 18\%$ (79), 57% (175), and 37% (171). The 10-year survival rate has been reported as $25\% \pm 14\%$ (177) and $11\% \pm 13\%$ (79). When stratified by the number of lymph nodes with metastases, survival was 73% at 5 years and 44% at 10 years for one to three positive nodes, and 55% at 5 years and 14% at 10 years for four or more nodal metastases (176). Many reports present data in terms of clinical rather than pathologic stage and are difficult to interpret because of the acknowledged inaccuracy of clinical staging. Unfavorable prognostic factors regardless of nodal status are tumor size larger than 2 cm (85,177) and poor histologic differentiation (172,177).

Attempts to correlate DNA ploidy with prognosis in male breast carcinoma have produced inconsistent results. In one study, DNA ploidy measured in 32 paraffin-embedded male breast carcinomas was not a significant predictor of survival (181). In another series, analysis of DNA ploidy and S-phase fraction (SPF) by flow cytometry using paraffin-embedded tissue revealed that 57.6% of male carcinomas were aneuploid (182). The median SPF was 8.9% for all tumors with a significantly higher median for aneuploid (14.3%) than for diploid/tetraploid tumors (6.6%). In this series, ploidy was significantly related to tumor size but not to grade or nodal status. Ploidy and SPF were not predictive of prognosis. Pich et al. reported that ploidy was a significant prognostic factor in univariate, but not in multivariate, analysis (162). Mani et al. found DNA ploidy to be prognostically significant for disease-free survival in univariate and multivariate analyses (183). SPF was not a significant prognostic indicator in this series.

There have been few studies of systemic adjuvant therapy in male breast carcinoma. Treves et al. (184) observed that bilateral orchiectomy could cause regression of the unresected primary tumor when performed in men who presented with systemic metastases. Estradiol and, to a lesser degree, estrone levels are reduced following orchiectomy (185), and the procedure has proven effective in producing symptomatic relief as well as objective responses in metastatic disease, especially in bone (186). Orchiectomy has not been adopted as an adjuvant measure in men with potentially curable tumors.

Adjuvant chemotherapy trials in a limited number of patients suggest this may be effective, but none of the studies included a randomized control group for comparison (84,173,187). Ribeiro (84) reported a 5-year survival rate of 55% among 23 stage II to III men given adjuvant tamoxifen. The 5-year survival rate in a prior period for men with equivalent stages was 28% without adjuvant tamoxifen. Patel et al. (187) described 11 men with stage II to III carcinoma treated with 5-fluorouracil and cyclophosphamide combined with either doxorubicin or methotrexate. After a median follow-up of 52 months, seven were recurrence free, and their estimated 5-year survival rate was greater than 85%. Spence et al. (173) were unable to detect benefit from adjuvant hormone therapy in seven patients or from adjuvant chemotherapy in another seven men. Donegan et al. (188) were not able to demonstrate an overall beneficial effect of adjuvant chemotherapy or hormonal therapy in a multiinstitutional database. Subset analysis demonstrated a beneficial effect among node-positive patients from both types of adjuvant treatment.

Hormonal treatments have been used with variable success to treat metastatic breast carcinoma in men. Ribeiro (189) reported a 38% response rate to diethylstilbestrol. Others described patients treated with dimethyltestosterone (190); buserelin, an analogue of luteinizing hormone–releasing hormone that inhibits the pituitary gonadal axis (191); aminoglutethimide (192); tamoxifen (193,194); adrenalectomy (193); and other endocrine agents (116,195,196).

# REFERENCES

1. Ewertz M, Holmberg L, Karjalainen S, et al. Incidence of male breast cancer in Scandinavia 1943–1982. *Int J Cancer* 1989;43:27–31.
2. Mabuchi K, Bross DS, Kessler II. Risk factors for male breast cancer. *J Natl Cancer Inst* 1985;74:371–375.
3. Ouriel K, Lotze MT, Hinshaw JR. Prognostic factors of carcinoma of the male breast. *Surg Gynecol Obstet* 1984;159:373–376.
4. Schottenfeld D, Lilienfeld AM, Diamond H. Some observations on the epidemiology of breast cancer among males. *Am J Public Health* 1963;53:890–897.
5. Moolgavkar SH, Lee JAH, Hade RD. Comparison of age-specific mortality from breast cancer in males in the United States and Japan. *J Natl Cancer Inst* 1978;60:1223–1225.
6. Ajayi DOS, Osegbe DN, Ademiluyi SA. Carcinoma of the male breast in West Africans and a review of world literature. *Cancer* 1982;50:1664–1667.
7. Simon MS, McKnight E, Schwartz A, et al. Racial differences in cancer of the male breast—15 years experience in the Detroit metropolitan area. *Breast Cancer Res Treat* 1992;21:55–62.
8. Steinitz R, Katz L, Ben-Hur M. Male breast cancer in Israel: selected epidemiological aspects. *Isr J Med Sci* 1981;17:816–821.
9. Newill VA. Distribution of cancer mortality among ethnic subgroups of the white population of New York City 1953–1958. *J Natl Cancer Inst* 1961;26:405–417.
10. Hultborn R, Friberg S, Hultborn KA. Male breast carcinoma. I. A study of the total material reported to the Swedish Cancer Registry 1958–1967 with respect to clinical and histopathologic parameters. *Acta Oncol* 1987;26:241–256.
11. Dao TL, Morreal C, Nemoto T. Urinary estrogen excretion in men with breast cancer. *N Engl J Med* 1973;289:138–140.
12. Nirmul D, Pegoraro RJ, Jialal I, et al. The sex hormone profile of male patients with breast cancer. *Br J Cancer* 1982;48:423–427.
13. Ballerini P, Recchione C, Cavalleri A, et al. Hormones in male breast cancer. *Tumori* 1990;76:26–28.
14. Olsson H, Alm P, Aspegren K, et al. Increased plasma prolactin levels in a group of men with breast cancer—a preliminary study. *Anticancer Res* 1990;10:59–62.
15. Ribeiro GG, Phillips HV, Skinner IG. Serum oestradiol-17 beta testosterone luteinizing hormones in males with breast cancer. *Br J Cancer* 1980;41:474–477.
16. Beard C, Benson RC Jr, Kelalis PP, et al. The incidence and outcome of mumps orchitis in Rochester, Minnesota, 1935 to 1974. *Mayo Clin Proc* 1977;52:3–7.
17. Nicolis GL, Sabetghadam R, Hsu CCS, et al. Breast cancer after mumps orchitis. *JAMA* 1973;223:1032–1033.
18. Casagrande JT, Hanisch R, Pike MC, et al. A case-control study of male breast cancer. *Cancer Res* 1988;48:1326–1330.
19. Olsson H, Ranstam J. Head trauma and exposure to prolactin-elevating drugs as risk factors for male breast cancer. *J Natl Cancer Inst* 1988;80:679–683.
20. Thomas DB, Jimenez LM, McTiernan A, et al. Breast cancer in men: risk factors with hormonal implications. *Am J Epidemiol* 1992;135:734–748.
21. Sobin LH, Sherif M. Relation between male breast cancer and prostate cancer. *Br J Cancer* 1980;42:787–790.
22. Cutuli B, Lacroze M, Dilhuydy JM, et al. Male breast cancer: results of the treatments and prognostic factors in 397 cases. *Eur J Cancer* 1995;31A:1960–1964.
23. McClure JA, Higgins CC. Bilateral carcinoma of the male breast after estrogen therapy. *JAMA* 1951;146:7–9.
24. Schlappack OK, Braun O, Maier V. Report of two cases of male breast cancer after prolonged estrogen treatment for prostatic carcinoma. *Cancer Detect Prevent* 1986;9:319–322.
25. Wilson SE, Hutchinson WB. Breast masses in males with carcinoma of the prostate. *J Surg Oncol* 1976;8:105–112.
26. Carlsson G, Hafstrom L, Jonsson P-E. Male breast cancer. *Clin Oncol* 1981;7:149–155.
27. Tajika M, Tuchiya T, Yasuda M, et al. A male case of synchronous double cancers of the breast and prostate. *Int Med* 1994;33:31–35.
28. Pritchard TJ, Pankowsky DA, Crowe JP, et al. Breast cancer in a male-to-female transsexual. A case report. *JAMA* 1988;259:2278–2280.
29. Symmers WStC. Carcinoma of breast in trans-sexual individuals after surgical and hormonal interference with the primary and secondary sex characteristics. *Br Med J* 1968;2:83–85.
30. Ganly I, Taylor EW. Breast cancer in a trans-sexual man receiving hormone replacement therapy. *Br J Surg* 1995;82:341.
31. Lenfant-Pejovic M-H, Mlika-Cabanne N, Bouchardy C, et al. Risk factors for male breast cancer: a Franco-Swiss case-control study. *Int J Cancer* 1990;45:661–665.
32. Rosenblaum PF, Vena JE, Zielezny MA, et al. Occupational exposures associated with male breast cancer. *Am J Epidemiol* 1994;139:30–36.
33. Cocco P, Figgs L, Dosemeci M, et al. Case-control study of occupational exposures and male breast cancer. *Occup Environ Med* 1998;55:599–604.

34. Crichlow RW. Carcinoma of the male breast. *Surg Gynecol Obstet* 1972;134:1011–1019.
35. Eldar S, Nash E, Abrahamson J. Radiation carcinogenesis in the male breast. *Eur J Surg Oncol* 1989;15:274–278.
36. Lowell DM, Martineau RG, Luria SB. Carcinoma of the male breast following radiation: report of a case occurring 35 years after radiation therapy for unilateral prepubertal gynecomastia. *Cancer* 1968;22:581–586.
37. Young GS, Wong JYC, Pezner RD. Bilateral breast cancer in a male after radiation therapy for Hodgkin's disease: a case report and review of the literature. *Breast Dis* 1995;8:185–191.
38. Boice JD Jr, Monson RA. Breast cancer in women after repeated fluoroscopic examinations of the chest. *J Natl Cancer Inst* 1977;59:823–832.
39. Tokunaga M, Norman JE Jr, Asano M, et al. Malignant breast cancers among atomic bomb survivors, Hiroshima and Nagasaki, 1950–1974. *J Natl Cancer Inst* 1979;62:1347–1359.
40. Olsson H, Alm P, Kristofferson V, et al. Hypophyseal tumor and gynecomastia preceding bilateral breast cancer development in a man. *Cancer* 1984;53:1974–1977.
41. Haga H, Watanabe O, Shimizu T, et al. Breast cancer in a male patient with prolactinoma. *Jpn J Surg* 1993;23:251–255.
42. El-Gazayerli MM, Abdel-Aziz A-S. On bilharziasis and male breast cancer in Egypt: a preliminary report and review of the literature. *Br J Cancer* 1963;17:566–571.
43. Dodge OG, Jackson AW, Muldal S. Breast cancer and interstitial tumor in a patient with Klinefelter's syndrome. *Cancer* 1969;24:1027–1032.
44. Brown PW, Terz JJ. Breast carcinoma associated with Klinefelter syndrome: a case report. *J Surg Oncol* 1978;10:413–415.
45. Coley GM, Otis RD, Clark WE II. Multiple primary tumors including bilateral breast cancers in a man with Klinefelter's syndrome. *Cancer* 1971;27:1476–1481.
46. Nadel M, Koss LG. Klinefelter's syndrome and male breast cancer. *Lancet* 1967;2:366.
47. Evans DB, Crichlow RW. Carcinoma of the male breast and Klinefelter's syndrome: is there an association? *Cancer* 1987;37:246–251.
48. Scheike O, Visfeldt J. Male breast cancer. 4. Gynecomastia in patients with breast cancer. *Acta Pathol Microbiol Scand (A)* 1973;81:359–365.
49. Giammarini A, Rocchi M, Zennaro W, et al. XX male with breast cancer. *Clin Genet* 1980;18:103–108.
50. Harnden DG, Maclean N, Langlands AO. Carcinoma of the breast and Klinefelter's syndrome. *J Med Genet* 1971;8:460–461.
51. Scheike O, Visfeldt J, Peterson B. Male breast cancer. 3. Breast carcinoma in association with the Klinefelter syndrome. *Acta Pathol Microbiol Scand (A)* 1973;81:351–358.
52. Hultborn R, Hanson C, Köpf I, et al. Prevalence of Klinefelter's syndrome in male breast cancer patients. *Anticancer Res* 1997;17:4293–4297.
53. Rosenblatt KA, Thomas DB, McTiernan A, et al. Breast cancer in men: aspects of familial aggregation. *J Natl Cancer Inst* 1991;83:849–854.
54. Gough DB, Donohue JH, Evans MM, et al. A 50-year experience of male breast cancer: is outcome changing? *Surg Oncol* 1993;2:325–333.
55. Olsson H, Andersson H, Johansson O, et al. Population-based cohort investigations of the risk for malignant tumors in first-degree relatives and wives of men with breast cancer. *Cancer* 1993;71:1273–1278.
56. Lynch HT, Kaplan AR, Lynch JF. Klinefelter syndrome and cancer. A family study. *JAMA* 1974;229:809–811.
57. Manheimer LH. Breast cancer in a father and son. *Breast* 1977;3:21–23.
58. Schwartz RM, Newell RB, Hauch JF, et al. A study of familial male breast carcinoma and a second report. *Cancer* 1980;46:2697–2701.
59. Everson RB, Fraumeni JF Jr, Wilson RE, et al. Familial male breast cancer. *Lancet* 1976;1:9–12.
60. Marger D, Urdaneta N, Fischer JJ. Breast cancer in brothers. Case reports and a review of 30 cases of male breast cancer. *Cancer* 1975;36:458–461.
61. Hauser AR, Lerner IJ, King RA. Familial male breast cancer [Letter]. *Am J Med Genet* 1992;44:839–840.
62. Jackson VP, Gilmor RL. Male breast carcinoma and gynecomastia. Comparison of mammography with sonography. *Radiology* 1983;149:533–536.

63. Kozak FK, Hall JG, Baird PA. Familial breast cancer in males. A case report and review of the literature. *Cancer* 1986;58:2736–2739.
64. Siddiqui T, Weiner R, Moreb J, et al. Cancer of the male breast with prolonged survival. *Cancer* 1988;62:1632–1636.
65. Wooster R, Mangion J, Eeles R, et al. A germline mutation in the androgen receptor gene in two brothers with breast cancer and Reifenstein syndrome. *Nat Genet* 1992;2:132–134.
66. Hiort O, Naber SP, Lehners A, et al. The role of androgen receptor gene mutations in male breast carcinomas. *J Clin Endocrinol Metab* 1996;81:3404–3407.
67. Stratton MR, Ford D, Neuhasen S, et al. Familial male breast cancer is not linked to the BRCA1 locus on chromosome 17q. *Nat Genet* 1994;7:103–107.
68. Ford D, Easton DF, Stratton M, et al. Genetic heterogeneity and penetrance analysis of the BRCA1 and BRCA2 genes in breast cancer families. The Breast Cancer Linkage Consortium. *Am J Hum Genet* 1998;62:676–689.
69. Easton DF, Steele L, Fields P, et al. Cancer risks in two large breast cancer families linked to BRCA2 on chromosome 13q-12–13. *Am J Hum Genet* 1987;61:120–128.
70. Neuhausen SL, Godwin AK, Gershoni-Baruch R, et al. Haplotype and phenotype analysis of nine recurrent BRCA2 mutations in 111 families: results of an international study. *Am J Hum Genet* 1998;62:1381–1388.
71. Csokay B, Udvarhelyi N, Sulyok Z, et al. High frequency of germ-line BRCA2 mutations among Hungarian male breast cancer patients without family history. *Cancer Res* 1999;59:995–998.
72. Thorlacius S, Sigurdsson S, Bjarnadottir H, et al. Study of a single BRCA2 mutation with high carrier frequency in a small population. *Am J Hum Genet* 1997;60:1079–1084.
73. Prechtel D, Werenskiold AK, Prechtel K, et al. Frequent loss of heterozygosity at chromosome 13q12–13 with BRCA2 markers in sporadic male breast cancer. *Diagn Mol Pathol* 1998;7:57–62.
74. Storm HH, Olsen J. Risk of breast cancer in offspring of male breast-cancer patients. *Lancet* 1999;353:209.
75. Thorlacius S, Tryggvadottir L, Oladsdottir GH, et al. Linkage to BRCA2 region in hereditary male breast cancer. *Lancet* 1995;346:544–545.
76. Sanz-Ortega J, Chuaqui R, Zhuang Z, et al. Loss of heterozygosity on chromosome 11q13 in microdissected human male breast carcinomas. *J Natl Cancer Inst* 1995;87:1408–1410.
77. Chuaqui RF, Sanz-Ortega J, Vocke C, et al. Loss of heterozygosity on the short arm of chromosome 8 in male breast carcinomas. *Cancer Res* 1995;55:4995–4998.
78. Reinbach D, McGregor JR, O'Dwyer PJ, et al. Synchronous male breast carcinoma and soft tissue sarcoma occurring within a cancer family. *Eur J Surg Oncol* 1992;18:624–626.
79. Heller KS, Rosen PP, Schottenfeld D, et al. Male breast cancer. A clinicopathologic study of 97 cases. *Ann Surg* 1978;188:60–65.
80. Wolff M, Reinis MS. Breast cancer in the male: clinicopathologic study of 40 patients and review of the literature. In: Fenoglio M, Wolff M, eds. *Progress in Surgical Pathology, volume III.* New York: Masson Publishers, USA, 1981:77–109.
81. Cole FM, Qizilbash AH. Carcinoma in situ of the male breast. *J Clin Pathol* 1979;32:1128–1134.
82. Green L, Wysowski DK, Fourcroy JL. Gynecomastia and breast cancer during finasteride therapy. *N Engl J Med* 1996;335:823.
83. Langlands AO, Maclean N, Kerr GR. Carcinoma of the male breast: report of a series of 88 cases. *Clin Radiol* 1976;27:21–25.
84. Ribeiro G. Male breast carcinoma—a review of 301 cases from the Christie Hospital & Holt Radium Institute, Manchester. *Br J Cancer* 1985;51:115–119.
85. Yap HY, Tashima CK, Blumenschein GR, et al. Male breast cancer: a natural history study. *Cancer* 1979;44:748–754.
86. Gadenne C, Contesso G, Travagli JP, et al. Tumeurs du sein chez l'homme. Etude anatomoclinique. 73 observations. *Nouv Presse Med* 1982;11:2331–2334.
87. Goss PE, Reid C, Pintilie M, et al. Male breast carcinoma: a review of 229 patients who presented to the Princess Margaret Hospital during 40 years: 1955–1996. *Cancer* 1999;85:629–639.
88. Ouimet-Oliva D, Hebert G, Ladouceur J. Radiographic characteristics of male breast cancer. *Radiology* 1978;129:37–40.
89. Brodie EM, King ER. Histologically different synchronous bilateral carcinoma of the male breast (a case report). *Cancer* 1974;34:1276–1277.

90. Wolloch Y, Zer M, Dintsman M, et al. Simultaneous bilateral primary breast carcinoma in the male. *Isr J Med Sci* 1972;8:158–162.

91. Treves N, Robbins GF, Amoroso WL. Serous and serosanguinous discharge from the male nipple. *Arch Surg* 1956;73:319–329.

92. Ranier E, D'Andrea MR, D'Alessio A, et al. Male breast carcinoma in situ. Report of a case diagnosed by nipple discharge cytology alone. *Anticancer Res* 1995;15:1589–1592.

93. Wang Y, Abreau M, Hoda S. Mammary duct carcinoma in situ in males: pathological findings and clinical considerations. *Mod Pathol* 1997;10:27A.

94. Scheike O. Male breast cancer. 5. Clinical manifestations in 257 cases in Denmark. *Br J Cancer* 1973;28:552–561.

95. Saltzstein EC, Tavaf AM, Latorraca R. Breast carcinoma in a young man. *Arch Surg* 1978;113:880–881.

96. Hittmair AP, Lininger RA, Tavassoli FA. Ductal carcinoma in situ (DCIS) in the male breast: a morphologic study of 84 cases of pure DCIS and 30 cases of DCIS associated with invasive carcinoma—a preliminary report. *Cancer* 1998;83:2139–2149.

97. Dershaw DD. Male mammography. *AJR Am J Roentgenol* 1986;146:127–131.

98. Chantra PK, So GJ, Wollman JS, et al. Mammography of the male breast. *AJR Am J Roentgenol* 1995;164:853–858.

99. Tükel S, Özcan H. Mammography in men with breast cancer: review of the mammographic findings in five cases. *Australas Radiol* 1996;40:387–390.

100. Dershaw DD, Borgen PI, Deutch BM, et al. Mammographic findings in men with breast cancer. *AJR Am J Roentgenol* 1993;160:267–270.

101. Fallentin E, Rothman L. Intracystic carcinoma of the male breast. *J Clin Ultrasound* 1994;22:118–120.

102. Sonksen CJ, Michell M, Sundaresan M. Case report: intracystic papillary carcinoma of the breast in a male patient. *Clin Radiol* 1996;51:438–439.

103. Chinn C, Kalisher L, Rickert RR. Intracystic papillary breast carcinoma in a 55-year-old man: radiologic and pathologic correlation. *J Can Assoc Radiol* 1989;40:40–42.

104. Michels LG, Gold RH, Arndt RD. Radiography of gynecomastia and other disorders of the male breast. *Radiology* 1977;122:117–122.

105. Weiss LM, Durhan LS, Esposito MJ, et al. Mammographic appearance of inflammatory carcinoma in the male breast. *Breast Dis* 1987;1:33–36.

106. Kalisher L, Peyster RG. Xerographic manifestations of male breast cancer. *AJR Am J Roentgenol* 1975;125:656–661.

107. Lilleng R, Paksoy N, Vural G, et al. Assessment of fine needle aspiration cytology and histopathology for diagnosing male breast masses. *Acta Cytol* 1995;39:877–881.

108. Joshi A, Kapila K, Verma K. Fine needle aspiration cytology in the management of male breast masses. Nineteen years of experience. *Acta Cytol* 1999;43:334–338.

109. Das DK, Junaid TA, Mathews SB, et al. Fine needle aspiration cytology diagnosis of male breast lesions. A study of 185 cases. *Acta Cytol* 1995;39:870–876.

110. Bhagat P, Kline TS. The male breast and malignant neoplasms. Diagnosis by aspiration biopsy cytology. *Cancer* 1989;65:2338–2341.

111. Russin T, Lachowicz C, Kline TS. Male breast lesions: gynecomastia and its distinction from carcinoma by ABC. *Diagn Cytopathol* 1989;5:243–247.

112. Gupta RK, Naran S, Simpson J. The role of fine needle aspiration cytology (FNAC) in the diagnosis of breast masses in males. *Eur J Surg Oncol* 1988;14:317–320.

113. Rosen PP, Menendez-Botet CJ, Nisselbaum JS, et al. Estrogen receptor in lesions of the male breast. *Cancer* 1976;37:1866–1868.

114. Everson RB, Lippman ME, Thompson EB, et al. Clinical correlations of steroid receptors and male breast cancer. *Cancer Res* 1980;40:991–997.

115. Friedman MA, Hoffman PG Jr, Dandolos EM, et al. Estrogen receptors in male breast cancer: clinical and pathologic correlations. *Cancer* 1981;47:134–137.

116. Lopez M, DiLauro L, Lazzaro B, et al. Hormonal treatment of disseminated male breast cancer. *Oncology* 1985;42:345–349.

117. Nomura Y, Kondo H, Yamagata J, et al. Detection of the estrogen receptor and response to endocrine therapy in male breast cancer patients. *Gann* 1977;68:333–336.

118. Stalsberg H, Thomas DB, Rosenblatt KA, et al. Histologic types and hormone receptors in breast cancer in men: a population-based study in 282 United States men. *Cancer Causes Control* 1993;4:143–151.

119. Thompson EB, Perlin E, Tormey D. Steroid-binding proteins in carcinoma of the human male breast. *Am J Clin Pathol* 1976;65:360–363.

120. Pacheco MM, Oshima CF, Lopes MP, et al. Steroid hormone receptors in male breast diseases. *Anticancer Res* 1986;6:1013–1018.

121. Rajendran KG, Shah PN, Bagli NP, et al. Oestradiol receptors in non-neoplastic gynaecomastic tissue of phenotypic males. *Horm Res* 1976;7:193–200.

122. Visfeldt J, Sheike O. Male breast cancer. I. Histologic typing and grading of 187 Danish cases. *Cancer* 1973;32:985–990.

123. Norris HJ, Taylor HB. Carcinoma of the male breast. *Cancer* 1969;23:1428–1435.

124. Taxy JB. Tubular carcinoma of the male breast. Report of a case. *Cancer* 1975;36:462–465.

125. Raju GC, Lee Y-S. Elastosis in the male breast. *Histopathology* 1988;12:203–209.

126. Bryant J. Male breast carcinoma: a case of apocrine carcinoma with psammoma bodies. *Hum Pathol* 1981;12:751–753.

127. Costa MJ, Silverberg SG. Oncocytic carcinoma of the male breast. *Arch Pathol Lab Med* 1989;113:1396–1399.

128. Crichlow RW, Czernobilsky B. Paget's disease of the male breast. *Cancer* 1969;24:1033–1040.

129. Serour F, Birkenfeld S, Amsterdam E, et al. Paget's disease of the male breast. *Cancer* 1988;62:601–605.

130. Coley GM, Kuehn PG. Paget's disease of the male breast. *Am J Surg* 1972;123:444–450.

131. Ramos CV, Boeshart C, Restrepo GL. Intracystic papillary carcinoma of the male breast. *Arch Pathol Lab Med* 1985;109:858–861.

132. Romanelli R, Toncini C. Pigmented papillary carcinoma of the male breast. *Tumori* 1986;72:105–108.

133. Alm P, Alumets J, Bak-Jensen E, et al. Neuroendocrine differentiation in male breast carcinomas. *APMIS* 1992;100:720–726.

134. Camus MG, Joshi MG, Mackarem G, et al. Ductal carcinoma in situ of the male breast. *Cancer* 1994;74:1289–1293.

135. Giffler RF, Kay S. Small cell carcinoma of the male mammary gland. A tumor resembling infiltrating lobular carcinoma. *Am J Clin Pathol* 1976;66:715–722.

136. Nance KVA, Reddick RL. In situ and infiltrating lobular carcinoma of the male breast. *Hum Pathol* 1989;20:1220–1222.

137. Sanchez AG, Villaneuva AG, Redondo C. Lobular carcinoma of the breast in a patient with Klinefelter's syndrome: a case with bilateral synchronous histologically different breast tumors. *Cancer* 1986;57:1181–1183.

138. Yogore MG III, Sahgal S. Small cell carcinoma of the male breast. Report of a case. *Cancer* 1977;39:1748–1751.

139. Michaels BM, Nunn CR, Roses DF. Lobular carcinoma of the male breast. *Surgery* 1994;115:402–405.

140. Hjorth S, Magnusson PH, Blomquist P. Adenoid cystic carcinoma of the breast. Report of a case in a male and review of the literature. *Acta Chir Scand* 1977;143:156–158.

141. Verani RR, Van der Bel-Kahn J. Mammary adenoid cystic carcinoma with unusual features. *Am J Clin Pathol* 1973;59:653–658.

142. Hassan MO, Olaizola MY. Male breast carcinoma. An ultrastructural study. *Arch Pathol Lab Med* 1979;103:191–195.

143. Berge T. Metastases to the male breast. *Acta Pathol Microbiol Scand (A)* 1971;79:491–496.

144. Campbell JH, Cummins SD. Metastases simulating mammary cancer in prostatic carcinoma under estrogenic therapy. *Cancer* 1951;4:303–311.

145. Hartley LCJ, Little JH. Bilateral mammary metastases from carcinoma of the prostate during oestrogen therapy. *Med J Aust* 1971;1:434–436.

146. Gupta RK. Immunoreactivity of prostate-specific antigen in male breast carcinomas: two examples of a diagnostic pitfall in discriminating a primary breast cancer from metastatic prostate carcinoma. *Diagn Cytopathol* 1999;21:167–169.

147. Bodey B, Bodey B Jr, Kaiser HE. Immunohistochemical detection of prostate specific antigen expression in human breast carcinoma cells. *Anticancer Res* 1997;17:2577–2581.

148. Yu H, Levesque MA, Clark GM, et al. Enhanced prediction of breast cancer prognosis by evaluating expression of p53 and prostate-specific antigen in combination. *Br J Cancer* 1999;81:490–495.

149. Rogers S, Day CA, Fox SB. Expression of cathepsin D and estrogen receptor in male breast carcinoma. *Hum Pathol* 1993;24:148–151.

150. Youngson BJ, Borgen P, Senie R, et al. Prognostic markers in male breast carcinoma (MBC): an immunohistochemical study. *Lab Invest* 1994;70:25A.

151. Fox SB, Rogers S, Day CA, et al. Oestrogen receptor and epidermal growth factor receptor expression in male breast carcinoma. *J Pathol* 1992;166:13–18.

152. Moore J, Friedman MI, Gramlich TL, et al. Prognostic indicators in male breast cancer. *Lab Invest* 1994;70:19A.

153. Dawson PJ, Paine TM, Wolman SR. Immunocytochemical characterization of male breast cancer. *Mod Pathol* 1992;5:621–625.

154. Rayson D, Erlichman C, Suman VJ, et al. Molecular markers in male breast carcinoma. *Cancer* 1998;83:1947–1955.

155. Gattuso P, Reddy V, Green L, et al. "New" prognostic factors in invasive breast cancer in men. *Mod Pathol* 1992;5:13A.

156. Leach IH, Ellis IO, Elston CW. C-erbB-2 expression in male breast carcinoma. *J Clin Pathol* 1992;45:942.

157. Joshi MG, Lee AKC, Loda M, et al. Male breast carcinoma: an evaluation of prognostic factors contributing to a poorer outcome. *Cancer* 1996;77:490–498.

158. Hecht JR, Wong JT, Ramos L, et al. Male breast cancers rarely overexpress p53 protein. *Lab Invest* 1994;35:214.

159. Weber-Chappuis K, Bieri-Burger S, Hurlimann J. Comparison of prognostic markers detected by immunohistochemistry in male and female breast carcinomas. *Eur J Cancer* 1996;32A:1686–1692.

160. Dawson PJ, Schroer KR, Wolman SR. ras and p53 genes in male breast cancer. *Mod Pathol* 1996;9:367–370.

161. Wieczorek R, Heller P, Feiner H, et al. p53 protein overexpression in male breast cancer: clinicopathologic (CPC) correlation. *Lab Invest* 1994;70:24A.

162. Pich A, Margaria E, Chiusa L, et al. DNA ploidy and p53 expression correlate with survival and cell proliferative activity in male breast carcinoma. *Hum Pathol* 1996;27:676–682.

162a.Pich A, Margaria E, Chiusa L. Oncogenes and male breast carcinoma: c-erbB-2 and p53 expression predicts a poor survival. *J Clin Oncol* 2000;18:2948–2956.

163. Pich A, Margaria E, Chiusa L. Bcl-2 expression in male breast carcinoma. *Virchows Arch* 1998;433:229–235.

164. Kardas I, Seitz G, Limon J, et al. Retrospective analysis of prognostic significance of the estrogen-inducible pS2 gene in male breast carcinoma. *Cancer* 1993;72:1652–1656.

165. Magro G, Lanzafame S, Colombatti A. Immunohistochemical staining patterns of type VI collagen in the normal, hyperplastic, and neoplastic adult male breast. *Pathologica* 1994;86:142–145.

166. Anelli A, Anelli TFM, Youngson B, et al. Mutations of the p53 gene in male breast cancer. *Cancer* 1995;75:2233–2238.

167. Nayak BK, Baral RN, Das BR. p53 gene mutation in relation to p53 protein accumulation in male and female breast cancer. *Neoplasia* 1996;43:305–310.

168. Anelli A, Anelli TFM, Youngson B, et al. Mutations of the p53 gene in male breast cancer. *Cancer* 1995;75:2233–2238.

169. Robison R, Montague ED. Treatment results in males with breast cancer. *Cancer* 1982;49:403–406.

170. Schuchardt U, Seegenschmiedt MH, Kirschner M, et al. Adjuvant radiotherapy for breast carcinoma in men: a 20-year clinical experience. *Int J Clin Oncol* 1996;19:330–336.

171. Erlichman C, Murphy KC, Elhakim T. Male breast cancer: a 13-year review of 89 patients. *J Clin Oncol* 1984;2:903–909.

172. Scheike O. Male breast cancer. 6. Factors influencing prognosis. *Br J Cancer* 1974;30:261–271.

173. Spence RAJ, Mackenzie G, Anderson JR, et al. Long-term survival following cancer of the male breast in Northern Ireland. A report of 81 cases. *Cancer* 1985;55:648–652.

174. Adami H-O, Hakulinen T, Ewertz M, et al. The survival pattern in male breast cancer. An analysis of 1429 patients from the Nordic countries. *Cancer* 1989;64:1177–1182.

175. Ciatto S, Iossa A, Bonardi R, et al. Male breast carcinoma: review of a multicenter series of 150 cases. *Tumori* 1990;76:555–558.

176. Guinee VF, Olsson H, Moller T, et al. The prognosis of breast cancer in males. A report of 335 cases. *Cancer* 1993;71:154–161.

177. Hultborn R, Friberg S, Hultborn KA, et al. Male breast carcinoma. II. A study of the total material reported to the Swedish Cancer Registry 1958–1967 with respect to treatment prognostic factors and survival. *Acta Oncol* 1987;26:327–341.

178. Mejias A, Sittler S, Mies C. Poor prognostic features are prevalent in young men with breast carcinoma. *Lab Invest* 1994;70:18A.

179. Hill A, Yagmur Y, Tran KN, et al. Localized male breast carcinoma and family history. An analysis of 142 patients. *Cancer* 1999;86: 821–825.

180. Borgen P, Senie RT, McKinnon WMP, et al. Carcinoma of the male breast. Analysis of prognosis compared with matched female patients. *Ann Surg Oncol* 1997;5:385–388.

181. Gattuso P, Reddy VB, Green L, et al. Prognostic significance of DNA ploidy in male breast carcinoma. A retrospective analysis of 32 cases. *Cancer* 1992;70:777–780.

182. Hatschek T, Wingren S, Carstensen J, et al. DNA content and S-phase fraction in male breast carcinomas. *Acta Oncol* 1994;33: 609–613.

183. Mani S, Haffty BG, Sinard J, et al. DNA ploidy as a significant predictor of recurrence-free survival in male patients with breast cancer. *Breast J* 1995;1:356–361.

184. Treves N, Abels JC, Woodard HQ, et al. The effects of orchiectomy on primary and metastatic carcinoma of the breast. *Surg Gynecol Obstet* 1944;79:589–605.

185. Hellman L, Fishman J. Oestradiol production rates in men before and after orchiectomy for cancer. *J Endocrinol* 1970;46:113–114.

186. Kraybill WG, Kaufman R, Kinne D. Treatment of advanced male breast cancer. *Cancer* 1981;47:2183–2189.

187. Patel HZ II, Buzdar AV, Hortobagyi GN. Role of adjuvant chemotherapy in male breast cancer. *Cancer* 1989;64:1583–1585.

188. Donegan WL, Redlich PN, Lang PJ, et al. Carcinoma of the breast in males: a multiinstitutional survey. *Cancer* 1998;83:498–509.

189. Ribeiro GG. The results of diethylstilbestrol therapy for recurrent and metastatic carcinoma of the male breast. *Br J Cancer* 1976;33: 465–467.

190. Horn Y, Roof B. Male breast cancer: two cases with objective regressions from calusterone (7-alpha-17-beta-dimethyltestosterone) after failure of orchiectomy. *Oncology* 1976;33:188–191.

191. Vorobiof DA, Falkson G. Nasally administered buserelin inducing complete remission of lung metastases in male breast cancer. *Cancer* 1987;59:688–689.

192. Harris AL, Dowsett M, Stuart-Harris R, et al. Role of aminoglutethimide in male breast cancer. *Br J Cancer* 1986;54:657–660.

193. Patel JK, Nemoto T, Dao TL. Metastatic breast cancer in males. Assessment of endocrine therapy. *Cancer* 1984;53:1344–1346.

194. Patterson JS, Battersby LA, Bach BK. Use of tamoxifen in advanced male breast cancer. *Cancer Treat Rep* 1980;64:801–804.

195. Kantarjian H, Yay HY, Hortobagyi G, et al. Hormonal therapy for metastatic male breast cancer. *Arch Intern Med* 1983;143:237–240.

196. Lopez M. Cyproterone acetate in the treatment of metastatic cancer of the male breast. *Cancer* 1985;55:2334–2336.

# CHAPTER 39

# Breast Tumors in Children

## JUVENILE PAPILLOMATOSIS

### Clinical Presentation

The localized benign proliferative lesion known as juvenile papillomatosis (JP) usually occurs in women less than 30 years of age. At the time of diagnosis, two-thirds of the patients are younger than 25 years (Fig. 39.1). JP is uncommon prior to puberty and after the age of 40 years (1,2). No clinical data on the prevalence of JP are available. However, JP was found in one of 519 forensic autopsies of females 14 years or older performed by a state medical examiner over a 5-year interval (3). Because JP was not formally characterized prior to 1980, it was not recognized as a specific lesion in earlier reports that, in retrospect, described this condition (4).

The typical clinical finding is a solitary, firm, discrete unilateral tumor that suggests a fibroadenoma. Bilateral JP may be synchronous or metachronous. Very rare instances of multifocal tumors in one breast have been reported. Separate coexistent fibroadenomas are common.

Few descriptions of the mammographic findings in JP are available, because mammography usually is not performed preoperatively in these young women. The films reveal a localized area of increased density with a border that generally is not as well defined as that of a fibroadenoma (Fig. 39.2) (2,5). The sonographic appearance of JP is that of an inhomogeneous, ill-defined mass with hypoechoic areas largely at the periphery (5,6).

At the time of diagnosis, patients with JP report a frequency of positive family history for breast carcinoma that is similar to that of patients who have mammary carcinoma (7,8). With further follow-up, the frequency of positive family history exceeds 50% (9). Because of the youth of JP patients, the high frequency of breast carcinoma in these families is particularly remarkable, because it may be assumed that female relatives of patients with JP tend to be younger than comparable relatives of breast carcinoma patients.

The female relatives of JP patients most likely to be affected by breast carcinoma are their mothers and maternal aunts. Breast carcinoma and other benign breast tumors, including JP, have only rarely been seen in the sisters of JP patients. JP is not associated with an increased frequency of breast carcinoma in paternal female relatives, and there is no association with any type of nonmammary neoplasm. A variety of chromosomal copy number changes have been detected in JP, most commonly involving chromosome 16 but also in 3p and 18p (10). No studies that analyzed JP patients or their relatives for BRCA1 or BRCA2 mutations have been published.

### Gross Pathology

The excised tumor is a firm discrete mass that appears to be distinct from the surrounding breast on the cut surface but lacks the sharply circumscribed border typical of a fibroadenoma. The lesions measure 1 to 8 cm (average, 4 cm) in diameter (Fig. 39.3). The most prominent gross feature is multiple cysts ranging from 1 mm to 2 cm. The intervening tissue often has white or yellow flecks that resemble comedonecrosis (Fig. 39.4).

### Microscopic Pathology

Histologic examination reveals a spectrum of benign proliferative changes that are present in varying proportions in individual cases. Cysts and duct hyperplasia are constant features (Figs. 39.5–39.7). The epithelium of cysts and proliferative foci frequently exhibits apocrine metaplasia (Fig. 39.8). Stasis of secretion in cysts and ducts manifested by collections of lipid-laden histiocytes is seen in most specimens (Fig. 39.9). These inflammatory changes correspond to the yellow and white flecks observed grossly. Sclerosing adenosis, lobular hyperplasia, and fibroadenomatoid hyperplasia are variably present.

In most cases, the ductal proliferative changes consist of ordinary hyperplasia. Apocrine metaplasia, largely in cysts, may be flat or papillary. Sometimes ductal hyperplasia is accompanied by sclerosis that produces a radial scar pattern.

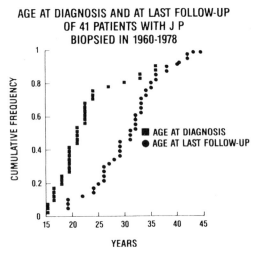

FIG. 39.1. *Juvenile papillomatosis, age distribution.* In this series of patients with relatively long-term follow-up, the mean and median ages at diagnosis were 19 and 21 years, respectively. (From Rosen PP, Kimmel M. Juvenile papillomatosis of the breast: a follow-up study of 41 patients having biopsies before 1979. *Am J Clin Pathol* 1990;93:599–603, with permission.)

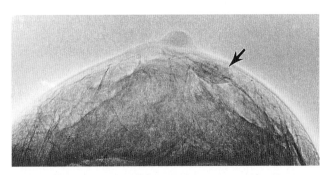

FIG. 39.2. *Juvenile papillomatosis, mammography.* The lesion forms the oval mass indicated by the *arrow* in this xeromammogram.

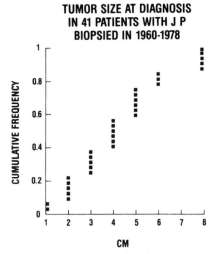

FIG. 39.3. *Juvenile papillomatosis, tumor size.* Median size was 4 cm (range 1 to 8 cm). (From Rosen PP, Kimmel M. Juvenile papillomatosis of the breast: a follow-up study of 41 patients having biopsies before 1979. *Am J Clin Pathol* 1990;93:599–603, with permission.)

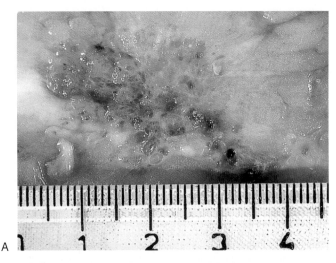

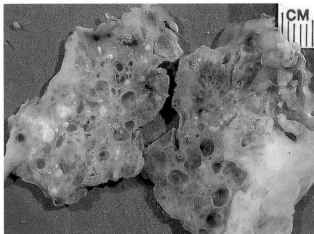

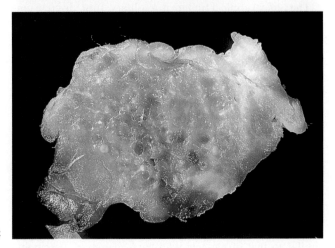

FIG. 39.4. *Juvenile papillomatosis, gross appearance.* **A–C:** Three different specimens showing localized lesions with multiple small cysts and white or yellow flecks.

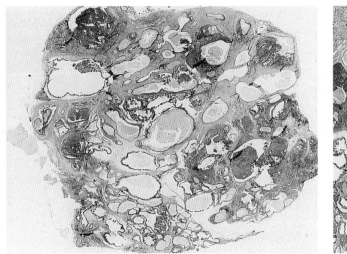
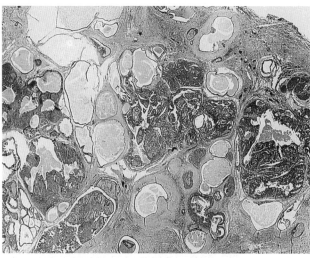

A

B

**FIG. 39.5.** *Juvenile papillomatosis.* **A,B:** Whole-mount histologic sections of two lesions. Papillary duct hyperplasia is more pronounced in **B**.

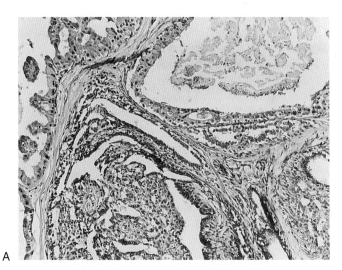
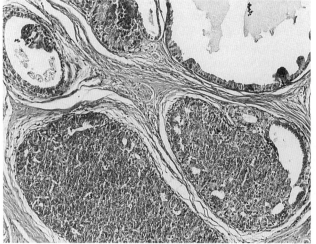

A

B

**FIG. 39.6.** *Juvenile papillomatosis, cysts and duct hyperplasia.* **A,B:** Two microscopic fields showing patterns of duct hyperplasia characteristic of juvenile papillomatosis.

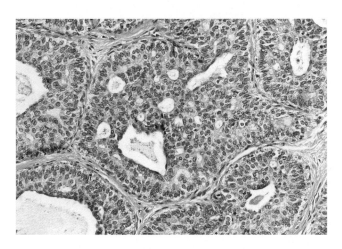

**FIG. 39.7.** *Juvenile papillomatosis, duct hyperplasia.* This cribriform pattern is often present.

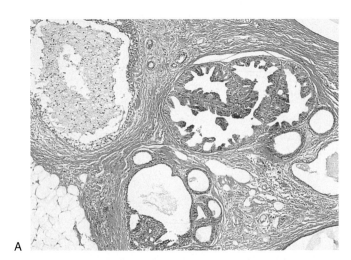
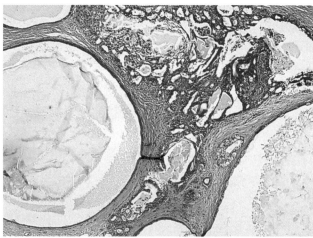

**FIG. 39.8.** *Juvenile papillomatosis, apocrine metaplasia.* **A:** Papillary apocrine metaplasia. **B:** Apocrine metaplasia of cyst epithelium and in papillary duct hyperplasia.

Atypical changes in ductal hyperplasia include cribriform or micropapillary growth patterns and intraductal necrosis (Fig. 39.10). In one series, there was significant atypia in 40% and intraductal necrosis in 15% of JP cases (9).

The diagnosis of JP should not be used for lesions that consist only of cysts, cystic papillomas, or papillomas. For example, illustrations of the lesion reported as "juvenile papillomatosis" by Talisman et al. (11) show cysts and intracystic papillomas rather than the typical features of JP. Specimens showing only solitary papilloma, multiple dispersed papillomas, and sclerosing papillomas with a radial scar configuration, included in the group of lesions termed *papillary duct hyperplasia,* are not part of the spectrum of JP (12–15).

It is not unusual for patients with JP to have had one or more biopsies of the ipsilateral or contralateral breast prior to the diagnosis of JP. Concurrent contralateral biopsies and subsequent biopsies of either breast have been reported (9). Most prior biopsies have been for fibroadenomas or benign proliferative lesions other than JP. Similar findings have been reported in most concurrent contralateral biopsies, but rare patients had carcinoma in the opposite breast.

Subsequent biopsies of one or both breasts are not unusual. About one-third of subsequent ipsilateral biopsies reveal JP. Other lesions encountered subsequently include benign proliferative changes without the configuration of typical JP, fibroadenoma, scar, and rarely carcinoma.

### Juvenile Papillomatosis and Carcinoma

From 10% to 15% of patients with JP also have breast carcinoma (2,8,9). Virtually all of these women had a positive family history for breast carcinoma, usually affecting their

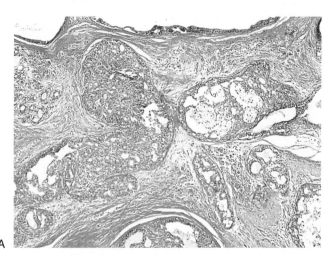
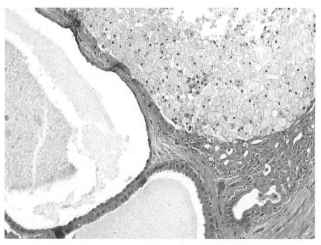

**FIG. 39.9.** *Juvenile papillomatosis, histiocytes.* **A:** Histiocytes in a focus of duct hyperplasia. **B:** One of three cysts lined by apocrine epithelium is filled with lipid histiocytes. Cysts like this are seen grossly as yellow flecks.

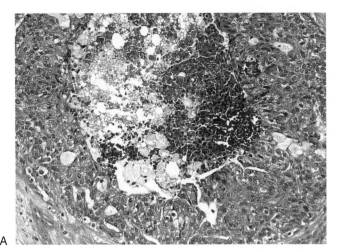
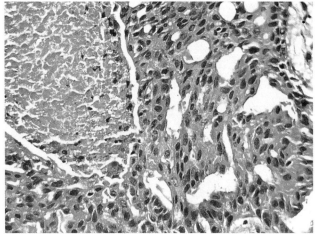

A     B

**FIG. 39.10.** *Juvenile papillomatosis, epithelial necrosis.* **A:** Necrosis, hemorrhage, and histiocytes in duct hyperplasia. **B:** Comedo-type necrosis in a focus of sclerosing papillary hyperplasia.

mother or a maternal aunt (8,9). Women with JP and coexistent carcinoma usually are in the upper quartile of the age distribution of JP.

The types of breast carcinoma that have been encountered include intraductal carcinoma, infiltrating lobular carcinoma, lobular carcinoma *in situ,* infiltrating duct carcinoma, and secretory (juvenile) carcinoma. Carcinoma and JP were diagnosed concurrently in most of these patients (Figs. 39.11 and 39.12) (8,9). With few exceptions, the carcinoma was within, and appeared to arise from, the JP. One exceptional patient had JP in one breast and concurrent contralateral secretory carcinoma not associated with JP.

Sufficient follow-up data are accumulating to begin assessing the risk for subsequent carcinoma in patients who had JP excised previously. A review of 41 patients with at least 10 years of follow-up after the diagnosis of JP (median

14 years) found that four (10%) patients subsequently developed breast carcinoma after an interval of 5 to 15 years (Fig. 39.13) (9). These patients were 25 to 42 years old when JP was diagnosed; thus, all were older than the mean age for JP. Three of the patients had multifocal or bilateral JP. Intraductal carcinoma was diagnosed in two of these women, and a third had intraductal carcinoma with microinvasion. The fourth patient had unilateral JP at the age of 29 years. Thirteen years later, recurrent ipsilateral JP was found and concurrent biopsy of the contralateral breast revealed intraductal carcinoma not associated with JP.

## Treatment and Prognosis

JP is rarely considered as the preoperative diagnosis. In most instances, the clinical findings suggest a fibroadenoma.

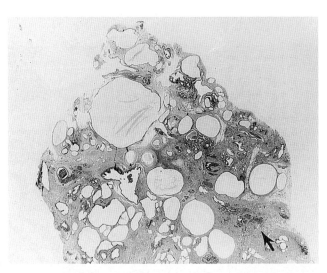
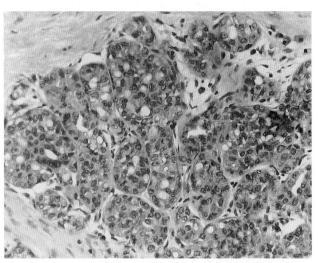

A     B

**FIG. 39.11.** *Juvenile papillomatosis with lobular carcinoma* in situ. **A:** *Arrow* indicates a focus of *in situ* lobular carcinoma in this histologic section of juvenile papillomatosis. **B:** Lobular carcinoma *in situ* shown in **A**.

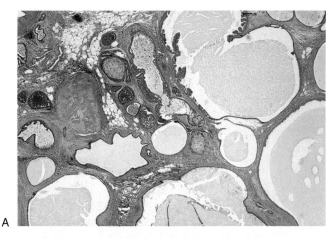

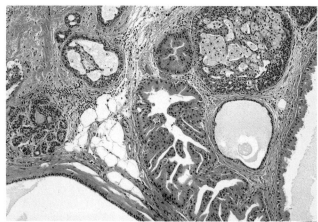

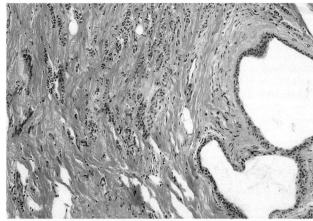

**FIG. 39.12.** *Invasive lobular carcinoma.* The specimen is from a 46-year-old woman. **A,B:** Cysts, duct hyperplasia, and apocrine metaplasia in juvenile papillomatosis. **C:** Invasive carcinoma adjacent to cysts in the tumor shown in **A** and **B**.

Consequently, excisional biopsy often is performed with little margin. Incomplete excision probably predisposes to local recurrence, but this may occur even when the margins appear to be adequate histologically. Reexcision of the biopsy site is recommended if the lesion has not been grossly excised, especially if there is atypia.

Unless carcinoma is found in the tumor, no treatment is necessary after excisional biopsy. Follow-up examinations

should be scheduled annually or more frequently for patients who have multifocal, bilateral, or recurrent JP and if there are other risk factors such as a positive family history. Mammography should be used judiciously during follow-up, especially for patients under 35 years of age. Ultrasonography is a useful alternative to mammography. Female relatives of JP patients, especially on the maternal side, are advised to have regular breast surveillance. No data are currently avail-

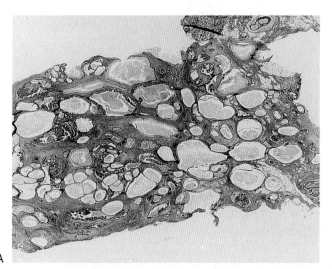

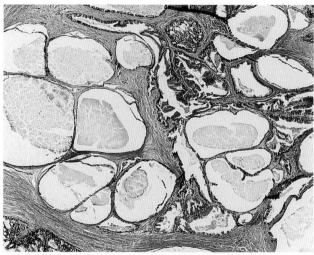

**FIG. 39.13.** *Juvenile papillomatosis with subsequent carcinoma.* **A:** Juvenile papillomatosis of the right breast at age 20 years. **B:** Juvenile papillomatosis of the left breast at age 24 years. *(continued)*

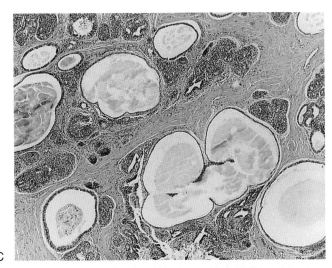

C

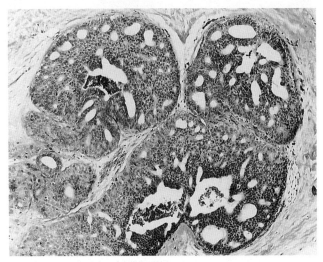

D

FIG. 39.13. *Continued.* **C:** Recurrent juvenile papillomatosis of the left breast at age 32 years. **D:** Intraductal carcinoma in the left breast in recurrent juvenile papillomatosis. **(A,B,D:** From Rosen PP, Holmes G, Lesser ML, et al. Juvenile papillomatosis and breast carcinoma. *Cancer* 1985;55:1345–1352, with permission.)

able regarding the presence of BRCA mutations in JP patients or their relatives. However, a variety of genetic alterations have been detected in JP lesions (10).

Presently, the frequency of carcinoma in JP patients does not warrant considering this to be a precancerous condition. Care should be taken *not* to exaggerate the near-term risk for developing breast carcinoma in JP patients. The importance of risk factors such as positive family history of breast carcinoma and pathologic atypia remains to be determined.

## PAPILLOMA AND PAPILLARY DUCT HYPERPLASIA IN CHILDREN AND YOUNG WOMEN

### Clinical Presentation

Papillary duct hyperplasia and papillomas are infrequent breast lesions in patients less than 30 years old (16). With few exceptional male cases (17), the patients are female with a median age of 17 years (18). The majority (70%) are 15 to 25 years of age, but a sizable group (24%) is younger, including rare neonatal patients.

The most frequent presenting symptom is a mass. Less than 20% of patients have nipple discharge, which may be bloody or clear. There is no predilection for either breast. Any part of the breast may be affected, but periareolar or subareolar lesions are most common. Very few patients had mammography, and the results are nonspecific (18). Microcalcifications have been found in a few cases. These patients have a moderate frequency (13%) of breast carcinoma among family members most often affecting maternal female relatives.

### Gross Pathology

Lesions measuring up to 5 cm have been reported. The tumors have been well circumscribed or ill defined. Numerous 1- to 3-mm cysts that contain papillary excrescences may be present in papillomatosis. The author has seen in consultation an 11-cm complex, partly cystic papillary tumor from a 3-year-old girl (Fig. 39.14).

### Microscopic Pathology

Three microscopic growth patterns have been described. *Sclerosing papilloma* has been found in nearly 50% of cases (Figs. 39.15 and 39.16). This radial scar-like lesion is fundamentally a papilloma distorted and disrupted by a desmoplastic proliferation of myoepithelial and stromal cells. Small clusters of epithelial cells and lobules incorporated into the stromal proliferation may be mistaken for invasive carcinoma.

About one-third of the lesions are *papillomas* with little or no sclerosis, limited to a single focus. Papillomas consist of one or more contiguous dilated ducts that contain papillary fronds of epithelial cells in single or multiple layers, supported by fibrovascular stroma (Figs. 39.14, 39.17, and 39.18). Infrequent mitoses may be encountered in the epithelium. Myoepithelial cell hyperplasia is variably present (Fig. 39.19).

Papillary hyperplasia involving multiple ducts, *papillomatosis*, is encountered in about 25% of cases. Papillary fronds supported by fibrovascular stroma are seen in some foci, but the hyperplasia often has a solid or micropapillary pattern lacking stroma (Figs. 39.20 and 39.21). In micropapillary areas, the nuclei of hyperplastic epithelial cells tend to become smaller and more hyperchromatic at the tips of

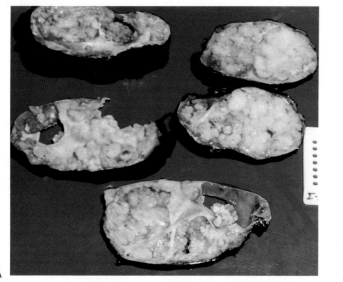
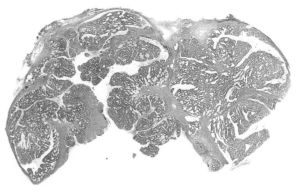

**FIG. 39.14.** *Papilloma.* **A,B:** An 11-cm tumor from a 3-year-old child.

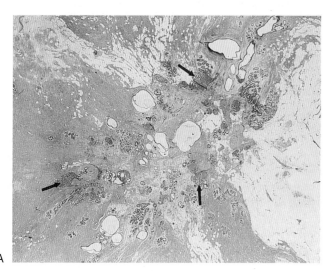
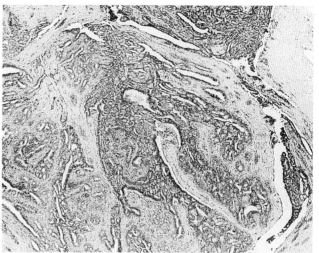

**FIG. 39.15.** *Papillary duct hyperplasia, sclerosing type.* The patient was a 15-year-old girl with a palpable tumor. **A:** The lesion has a radial scar configuration. Some papillary foci are indicated by *arrows.* **B:** Part of a sclerosing papilloma in the tumor.

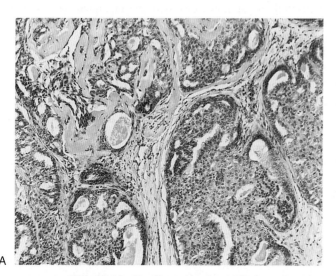
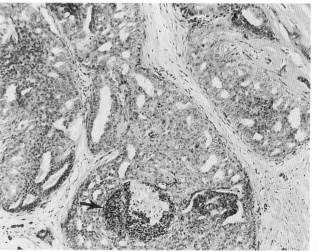

**FIG. 39.16.** *Papillary duct hyperplasia, sclerosing type.* The lesion was a palpable tumor in a 14-year-old girl. **A:** Sclerosing papilloma. **B:** Focal necrosis in the hyperplastic epithelium *(arrow).*

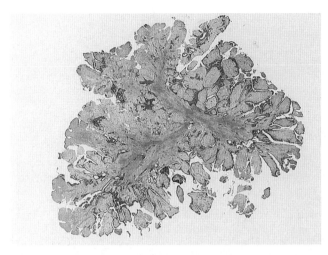

**FIG. 39.17.** *Papilloma.* Papilloma removed from the subareolar tissue of a 14-year-old girl who had bloody nipple discharge.

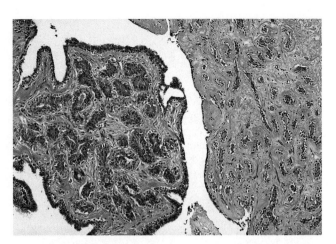

**FIG. 39.19.** *Papilloma, myoepithelial hyperplasia.* Myoepithelial hyperplasia is evident around glands in proliferative *(left)* and sclerotic *(right)* portions of this papilloma from a 14-year-old girl.

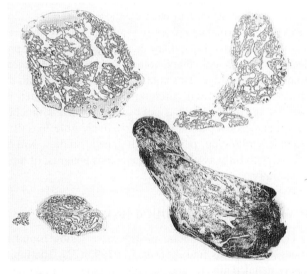

A

**FIG. 39.18.** *Papilloma.* The patient was a 13-year-old girl with a subareolar tumor. **A:** Multiple fragments of the papilloma in one histologic section. The darkened tissue in the *lower right* is hemorrhagic as a result of infarction. **B:** Magnified view of the papilloma demonstrating diffuse, epithelial hyperplasia. **C:** Micropapillary hyperplasia.

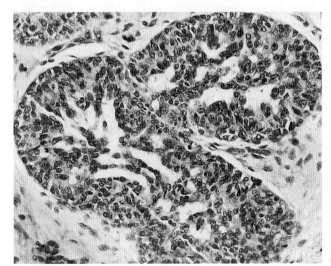

B

C

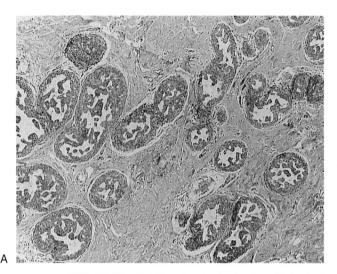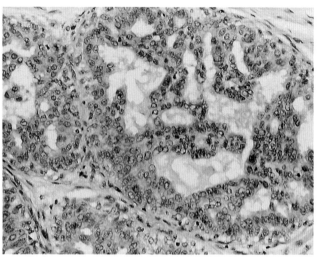

**FIG. 39.20.** *Papillary hyperplasia of multiple ducts.* Biopsy was obtained from a 16-year-old girl with a palpable tumor. **A:** Papillary hyperplasia involves multiple ducts. **B:** Proliferation has a micropapillary pattern.

individual papillae. Myoepithelial cell hyperplasia may be present. Some lesions exhibit cytologic atypia that may be severe.

Prominent cyst formation, extensive apocrine metaplasia, stasis, mastitis, and other benign proliferative changes that characterize JP are largely absent from these forms of papillary duct hyperplasia (19).

### Treatment and Prognosis

Most patients can be managed by excisional biopsy. Large lesions may require quadrantectomy.

In one series, breast recurrences were detected in 16% of patients after a median interval of 3 years (18). Recurrence was more frequent in patients with sclerosing papilloma and solitary papilloma than in those with papillomatosis.

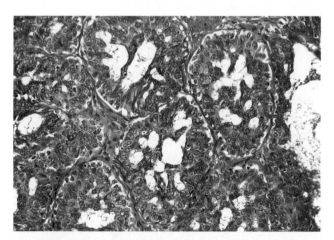

**FIG. 39.21.** *Papillary hyperplasia of multiple ducts.* This magnified view of a lesion from an 11-year-old girl shows cytologic atypia with small nucleoli. Note streaming pattern of growth centrally in the hyperplastic ducts.

Follow-up rarely has exceeded 10 years. A single patient developed invasive carcinoma in one breast 27 years after bilateral papillomatosis had been diagnosed at the age of 11 years (20). Information presently available supports the view that these patterns of papillary duct hyperplasia do not predispose children and young women to develop breast carcinoma at an early age. This conclusion is consistent with the observation that breast carcinoma detected in women 35 years of age or younger has not been associated with a history of antecedent papillary proliferative breast lesions (21). Extended follow-up, perhaps with genetic studies, will be necessary to fully assess the precancerous potential of these proliferative conditions.

### JUVENILE ATYPICAL DUCT HYPERPLASIA

This microscopic ductal proliferative lesion found in young women was first described in 1992 (22). The initial report included nine female patients who were 18 to 26 years old (mean, 21 years) at diagnosis. The ductal hyperplasia was found in biopsies of breast "thickening" (four cases) or in specimens from patients who underwent reduction mammoplasty for "mammary hypertrophy" (five cases). A family history of breast carcinoma was reported in three (33%) of the patients. Follow-up at the time of the report averaged 39 months (range, 5 to 68 months), during which time rebiopsy in two cases revealed persistent atypical hyperplasia. Long-term follow-up will be necessary to assess the precancerous significant of this lesion.

There are no specific gross features indicative of juvenile atypical duct hyperplasia. The specimens generally are described as fibrous breast tissue with variable amounts of fat. No discrete lesion is produced by the ductal proliferation.

Histologic examination reveals widely separated, isolated ducts with epithelial hyperplasia that has micropapillary or cribriform features. In the typical specimen, the area between

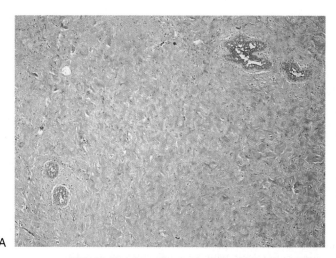
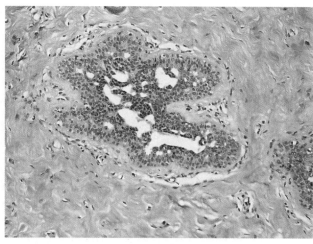

**FIG. 39.22.** *Juvenile atypical duct hyperplasia.* The patient was 18 years old. **A:** Ducts with hyperplastic epithelium in the *upper right* and *lower left* corners are separated by dense collagenized stroma. **B:** Hyperplastic epithelium has micropapillary features. Myoepithelial cells form a continuous layer around the duct.

the hyperplastic ducts is occupied by dense, collagenous stroma in which there are also widely spaced ducts without hyperplasia and lobules (Fig. 39.22). The hyperplastic changes tend to develop focally in the epithelium of an affected duct (Fig. 39.23). In some ducts, the hyperplastic epithelium forms a laciform network in the lumen (Fig. 39.24). Myoepithelial cells are present in a continuous or discontinuous fashion (Fig. 39.25). Juxtaposition of duct cross sections showing juvenile atypical duct hyperplasia with ducts lacking hyperplasia is a characteristic feature (Figs. 39.26 and 39.27).

## FIBROEPITHELIAL TUMORS IN CHILDREN AND ADOLESCENTS

### Fibroadenoma

Fibroadenomas account for at least 75% of breast tumors in this age group (23–25). Most of these fibroadenomas are similar histologically to comparable tumors in young adult women (26). Pericanalicular and intracanalicular growth patterns are encountered. Focal stromal hyalinization as well as epithelial hyperplasia can be found in childhood fibroadenomas (Fig. 39.28) (27). Between 5% and 10% of fibroadenomas in adolescent girls attain a substantial size to qualify for the term *giant fibroadenoma*. Despite their rapid growth, sometimes with stromal cellularity that rarely contains mitotic figures, giant fibroadenomas have a benign clinical course (28). A more complete discussion of fibroadenomas can be found in Chapter 8.

Fibroadenomas with multiple cysts may suggest JP grossly (Figs. 39.29 and 39.30). In some instances, histologic examination reveals the complex proliferative pattern of JP in fibroadenomatous stroma. The precise relationship of these infrequent lesions to the conventional presentation or JP remains to be determined. Fibroadenomas containing

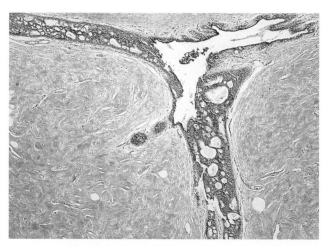
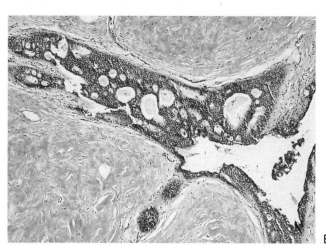

**FIG. 39.23.** *Juvenile atypical duct hyperplasia.* The specimens shown in **A–C** were obtained from a 20-year-old woman who had a reduction mammoplasty for mammary "hypertrophy." **A:** Epithelial hyperplasia is present focally in two of three branches of this duct system. *(continued)*

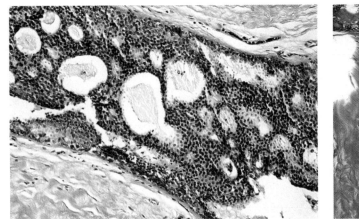
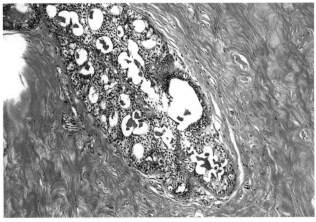

C

D

**FIG. 39.23.** *Continued.* **B,C:** Hyperplastic epithelium has a cribriform pattern. **D:** Reduction mammoplasty for macromastia revealed this pattern of cribriform hyperplasia with clear cell cytology in a 17-year-old girl.

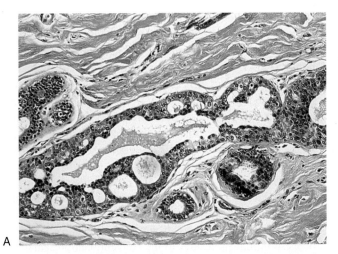
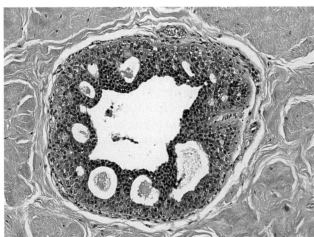

A

B

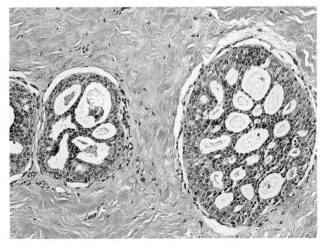

C

**FIG. 39.24.** *Juvenile atypical duct hyperplasia.* This 23-year-old patient had a breast biopsy for an area of "thickening." **A:** A terminal duct cut longitudinally as it enters an undeveloped lobule. The hyperplastic epithelium forms a peripheral arcade. **B:** Transverse section of a duct similar to **A**, in which the hyperplastic epithelium forms a circumferential arcade. **C:** Adjacent duct cross sections with laciform (cribriform) hyperplasia.

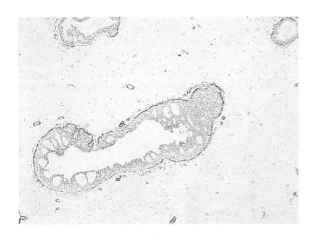

**FIG. 39.25.** *Juvenile atypical duct hyperplasia.* The specimen is from the same patient as shown in Fig. 39.23. The peripheral myoepithelial layer is highlighted by the immunostain for smooth muscle actin (avidin-biotin).

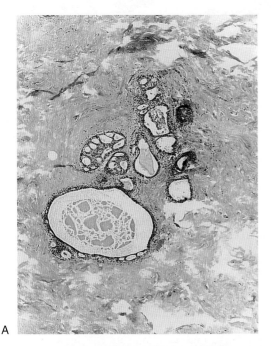

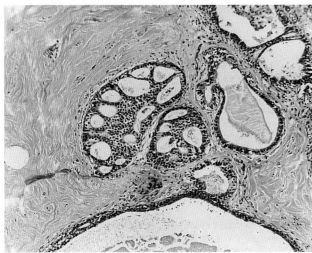

**FIG. 39.26.** *Juvenile atypical duct hyperplasia.* The specimen is from a 21-year-old woman. **A,B:** Two duct cross sections with cribriform hyperplasia are shown in close proximity to dilated ducts without hyperplasia.

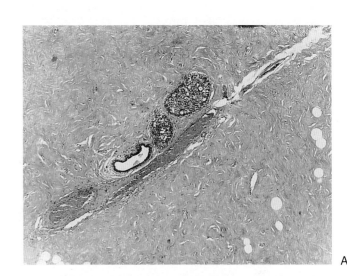

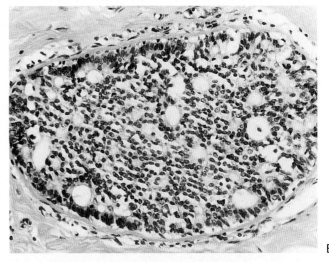

**FIG. 39.27.** *Juvenile atypical duct hyperplasia.* The same patient as shown in Fig. 39.25. **A:** Three duct cross sections, probably representing a single duct passing in and out of the plane of section, next to a small blood vessel. **B:** Duct lumen is filled by cribriform hyperplasia. Persisting columnar duct epithelium is present predominantly on the left perimeter.

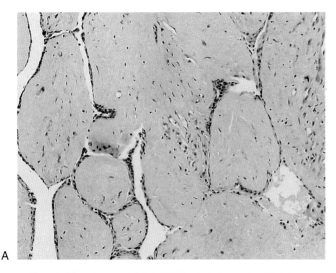

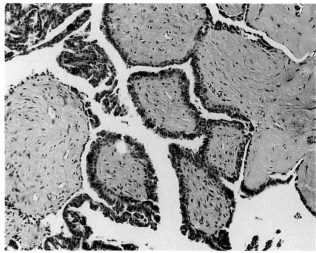

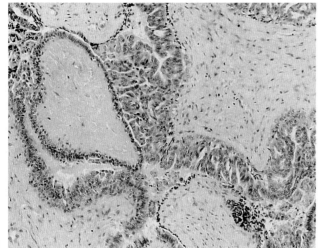

**FIG. 39.28.** *Fibroadenoma with stromal and epithelial heterogeneity.* The tumor was obtained from a 15-year-old girl. **A:** Part of the lesion with hyalinized stroma and flat epithelium. **B:** Mild epithelial hyperplasia. **C:** Moderate epithelial hyperplasia with some detached epithelial fragments.

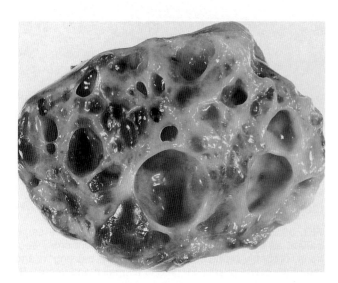

**FIG. 39.29.** *Fibroadenoma with cysts.* This tumor from a 20-year-old woman exhibits striking cyst formation reminiscent of juvenile papillomatosis, but histologically the lesion lacked the characteristic proliferative components.

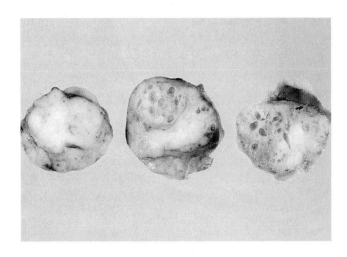

**FIG. 39.30.** *Fibroadenoma with juvenile papillomatosis-like hyperplasia.* Proliferative changes similar to juvenile papillomatosis were present in the localized cystic area within this fibroadenoma.

only cysts lined by flat or cuboidal epithelium are not considered to be part of JP.

### Phyllodes Tumor

Some of the neoplasms described as phyllodes tumors in children or adolescents are probably juvenile fibroadenomas with cellular stroma. Phyllodes tumors in this age group have the same histologic characteristics as comparable tumors in adults (29). Important features that distinguish phyllodes tumors from giant or juvenile fibroadenomas include marked stromal overgrowth relative to the epithelium, a tendency for cellularity to be greatest in the subepithelial stroma, the presence of mitoses, especially in the subepithelial zone, and an invasive border. Uncommon stromal differentiation includes adipose, leiomyomatous, and rhabdomyoid elements, as well as myofibroblastic proliferation that resembles myofibroblastoma (Fig. 39.31). Cystic papillary phyllodes tumors,

which may be benign or malignant, can occur in children (Fig. 39.32). Tagaya et al. (30) described a benign cystic and papillary phyllodes tumor in an 11-year-old child who presented with nipple bleeding. Although most phyllodes tumors in children follow a benign clinical course after excision, rare instances of local recurrence (Fig. 39.33) and malignant tumors with systemic metastases have been reported (Fig. 39.34) (29,31–34). Additional discussion of phyllodes tumors can be found in Chapter 8.

### CARCINOMA IN CHILDREN AND ADOLESCENTS

The most frequent breast tumors in female infants and children are fibroadenomas and juvenile macromastia (35–38). Carcinoma of the breast is extremely unusual in this age group. A literature review published in 1977 listed 74 cases reported between 1888 and 1972 (39). A few case reports subsequently have documented infiltrating duct carcinomas (40–43).

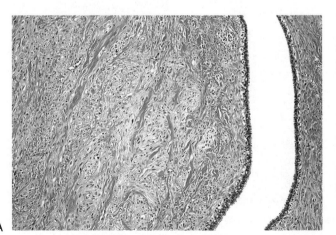
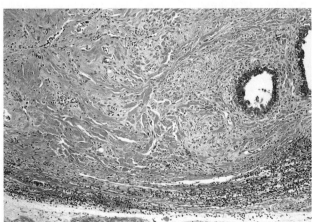

A    B

**FIG. 39.31.** *Phyllodes tumor with myofibroblastoma-like stroma.* **A:** The stroma in this benign tumor from a 12-year-old girl shows myofibroblastic hyperplasia and collagen bands. Note the phyllodes epithelial structure. **B:** The tumor has a circumscribed border. Traces of pseudoangiomatous structure are present.

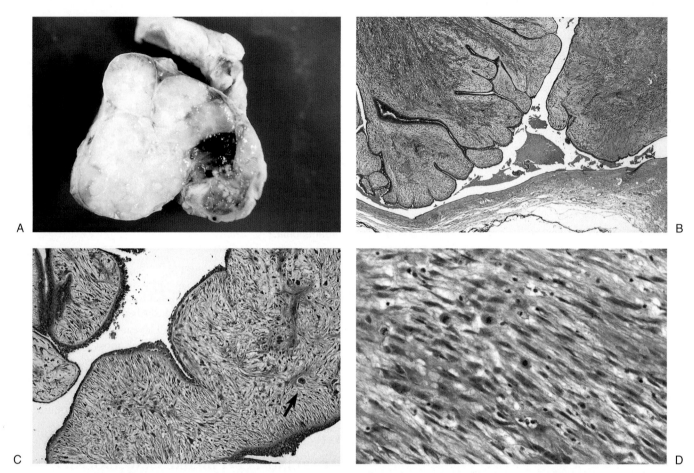

**FIG. 39.32.** *Cystic papillary phyllodes tumor.* **A:** Part of the cystic portion of this benign tumor from a 12-year-old girl contains clotted blood *(lower right)*. **B:** Cystic papillary low-grade malignant phyllodes tumor from a 13-year-old girl. **C:** Moderate stromal cellularity and one atypical mitosis *(arrow)* in the same lesion as shown in **B**. **D:** Focus with multiple mitoses from the tumor shown in **B**.

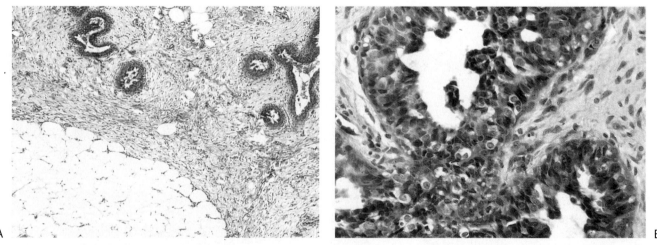

**FIG. 39.33.** *Phyllodes tumor.* **A,B:** This female patient was 11 years old when a benign phyllodes tumor with invasive margins was excised. *(continued)*

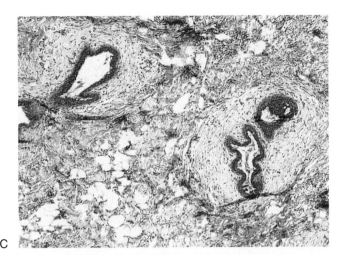

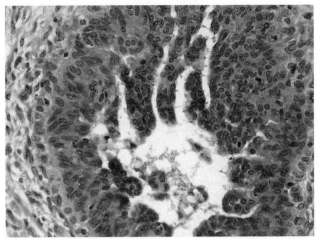

**FIG. 39.33.** *Continued.* **C,D:** Locally recurrent phyllodes tumor with histologic features similar to the primary tumor.

Prior irradiation appears to be a predisposing factor in some instances. Close and Maximov (44) described a poorly differentiated carcinoma in the left breast of a 17-year-old patient who had received mediastinal radiation for an enlarged thymus gland at 3 months of age. Carcinoma in the breast of an 18-year-old boy has been reported after thymic radiation during childhood (45). Radiation in the region of the breast in children and young adults has been associated with breast carcinoma diagnosed in adulthood (46–49).

Most of the patients have been female with an average age of about 13 years. With few exceptions, the presenting sign has been a mass. Nipple discharge and diffuse breast enlargement are uncommon. The carcinomas have ranged in size from 1 to 9 cm.

Histologically, a substantial number of the tumors have been of the secretory (juvenile) type (Figs. 39.35 and 39.36), an entity discussed in Chapter 26. Other types of carcinoma commonly found in adults have been described (39,50).

Small cell carcinoma of the breast in children is a highly malignant neoplasm that is difficult to distinguish from lymphoma and embryonal rhabdomyosarcoma in routine sections (Fig. 39.37) (43,44,51,52). *In situ* carcinoma may not be found, and the tumor cells do not have the cytologic features of typical infiltrating lobular carcinoma such as mucin secretion. Immunoreactivity for cytokeratin usually is detectable, and the cells are not reactive with markers for lymphoma or myosarcoma. Cystic papillary carcinoma is extremely rare in girls (Fig. 39.38). Breast carcinoma in boys is usually the secretory type, but other types are rarely encountered (Fig. 39.39).

## Other Tumors

The juvenile breast may be involved by systemic diseases such as lymphoma or leukemia. Metastases from primary tumors arising at other sites, such as rhabdomyosarcoma and

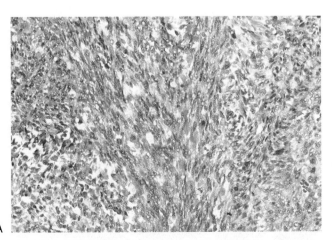

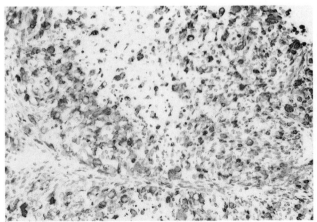

**FIG. 39.34.** *Myosarcoma in malignant phyllodes tumor.* **A:** Cells with eosinophilic cytoplasm (round on *lower left* and strap-shaped *centrally*) are indicative of rhabdomyosarcoma in this malignant phyllodes tumor from a 13-year-old girl. **B:** Tumor cells are immunoreactive for desmin (avidin-biotin).

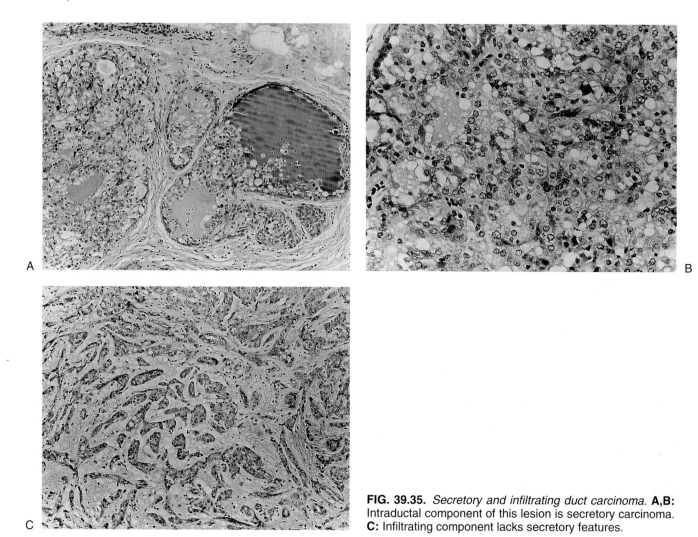

A

B

C

**FIG. 39.35.** *Secretory and infiltrating duct carcinoma.* **A,B:** Intraductal component of this lesion is secretory carcinoma. **C:** Infiltrating component lacks secretory features.

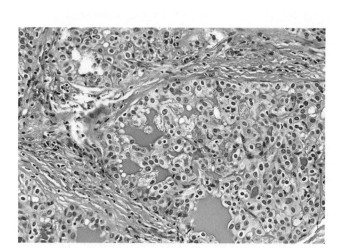

**FIG. 39.36.** *Secretory carcinoma.* This tumor is from a 5-year-old girl.

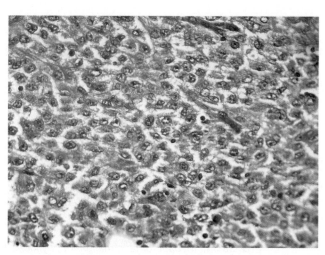

**FIG. 39.37.** *Small cell carcinoma.* The patient was a 17-year-old girl.

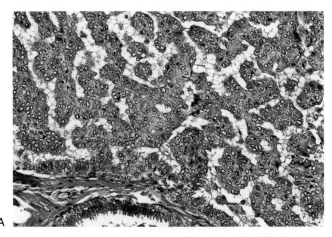 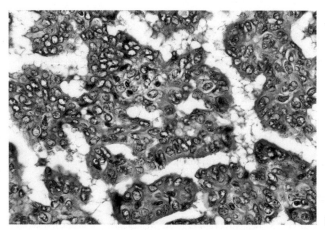

A                                                            B

**FIG. 39.38.** *Papillary carcinoma.* **A:** Cystic papillary carcinoma in a 12-year-old girl. **B:** Epithelial proliferation lacks stroma and myoepithelial cells.

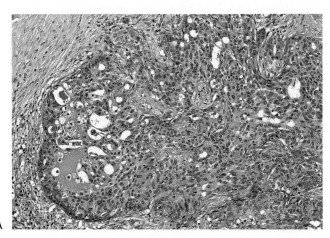 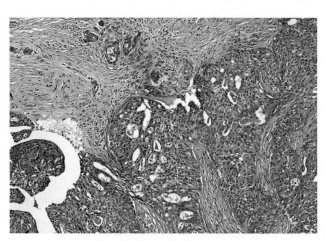

A                                                            B

**FIG. 39.39.** *Solid papillary carcinoma.* This tumor is from a 16-year-old boy. Metastatic tumor was found in an axillary lymph node. **A:** Solid papillary growth with apocrine and secretory features. **B:** Focal invasion is shown at the upper border of the tumor.

medulloblastoma, have been reported. Primary mammary sarcoma is exceedingly uncommon in this age group. For further discussion of these topics, see relevant sections elsewhere in this volume.

## REFERENCES

### Juvenile Papillomatosis

1. Rosen PP, Cantrell B, Mullen DL, et al. Juvenile papillomatosis (Swiss cheese disease) of the breast. *Am J Surg Pathol* 1980;4:3–12.
2. Rosen PP, Holmes G, Lesser ML, et al. Juvenile papillomatosis and breast carcinoma. *Cancer* 1985;55:1345–1352.
3. Bartow SA, Pathak DR, Black WC, et al. Prevalence of benign, atypical and malignant breast lesions in populations at different risk for breast cancer. A forensic autopsy study. *Cancer* 1987;60:2751–2760.
4. Uriburu JV, Mosta AM, Gomez MA. Displasia proliferative juvenil focalizada. *Pren Med Argentina* 1975;62:172–176.
5. Kersschot EAJ, Hermans M-E, Pauwels C, et al. Juvenile papillomatosis of the breast: sonographic appearance. *Radiology* 1988; 169:631–633.
6. Hidalgo F, Llano JM, Marhuenda A. Juvenile papillomatosis of the breast (Swiss cheese disease). *AJR Am J Roentgenol* 1997;169:912.
7. Rosen PP, Lyngholm B, Kinne DW, et al. Juvenile papillomatosis of the breast and family history of breast carcinoma. *Cancer* 1982;49: 2591–2595.
8. Bazzocchi F, Santini D, Martinelli G, et al. Juvenile papillomatosis (epitheliosis) of the breast. *Am J Clin Pathol* 1986;86:745–748.
9. Rosen PP, Kimmel M. Juvenile papillomatosis of the breast: a follow-up study of 41 patients having biopsies before 1979. *Am J Clin Pathol* 1990;93:599–603.
10. Osin P, Lu Y-J, Shipley J, et al. Comparative genomic hybridisation of juvenile papillomatosis—changes in chromosome 16 suggest its neoplastic nature. *Mod Pathol* 2000;13:44A.
11. Talisman R, Nissim F, Rothstein H, et al. Juvenile papillomatosis of the breast. *Eur J Surg* 1993;159:317–319.
12. Batchelor JS, Farah G, Fisher C. Multiple breast papillomas in adolescence. *J Surg Oncol* 1993;54:64–66.
13. Kiaer HW, Kiaer WW, Linell F, et al. Extreme duct papillomatosis of the juvenile breast. *Acta Pathol Microbiol Immunol Scand (A)* 1979;87A:353–359.
14. Rosen PP. Papillary duct hyperplasia of the breast in children and young adults. *Cancer* 1985;56:1611–1617.
15. Wilson M, Cranor ML, Rosen PP. Papillary duct hyperplasia of the breast in children and young women. *Mod Pathol* 1993;6:570–574.

### Papilloma and Papillary Duct Hyperplasia in Children and Young Women

16. Rosen PP. Papillary duct hyperplasia of the breast in children and young adults. *Cancer* 1985;56:1611–1617.
17. Hughes DE, Orr JD, Smith NM. Intraduct papillomatosis of the breast in a peripubertal male. *Pediatr Pathol* 1994;14:561–565.

18. Wilson M, Cranor ML, Rosen PP. Papillary duct hyperplasia of the breast in children and young women. *Mod Pathol* 1993;6:570–574.
19. Rosen PP, Cantrell B, Mullen DL, et al. Juvenile papillomatosis (Swiss cheese disease) of the breast. *Am J Surg Pathol* 1980;4:3–12.
20. Kiaer HW, Kiaer WW, Linell F, et al. Extreme duct papillomatosis of the juvenile breast. *Acta Pathol Microbiol Immunol Scand (A)* 1979; 87A:353–359.
21. Rosen PP, Lesser ML, Kinne DW, et al. Breast carcinoma in women 35 years of age or younger. *Ann Surg* 1984;199:133–142.

## Juvenile Atypical Duct Hyperplasia

22. Eliasen CA, Cranor ML, Rosen PP. Atypical duct hyperplasia of the breast in young females. *Am J Surg Pathol* 1992;16:246–251.

## Fibroepithelial Tumors in Children and Adolescents

23. Bower R, Bell ML, Ternbergh JL. Management of breast lesions in children and adolescents. *J Pediatr Surg* 1976;11:337–346.
24. Diehl T, Kaplan DW. Breast masses in adolescent females. *J Adolesc Health Care* 1985;6:353–357.
25. Stone AM, Shenker IR, McCarthy K. Adolescent breast masses. *Am J Surg* 1977;134:275–277.
26. Ashikari R, Farrow JH, O'Hara J. Fibroadenomas in the breast of juveniles. *Surg Gynecol Obstet* 1971;32:259–262.
27. Kern WH, Clark RW. Retrogression of fibroadenomas of the breast. *Am J Surg* 1973;126:59–62.
28. Raganoonan C, Fairbairn JK, Williams S, et al. Giant breast tumours of adolescence. *Aust N Z J Surg* 1987;57:243–247.
29. Rajan PB, Cranor ML, Rosen PP. Cystosarcoma phyllodes in adolescent girls and young women: a study of 45 patients. *Am J Surg Pathol* 1998;22:64–69.
30. Tagaya N, Kodaira H, Kagure H, et al. A case of phyllodes tumor with bloody nipple discharge in juvenile patient. *Breast Cancer* 1999;6: 207–210.
31. Gibbs BF, Roe RD, Thomas DF. Malignant cystosarcoma in a pre-pubertal female. *Ann Surg* 1968;167:229–231.
32. Hoover HC, Trestioreanu A, Ketcham AS. Metastatic cystosarcoma phylloides in an adolescent girl: an unusually malignant tumor. *Ann Surg* 1975;181:279–282.
33. Levéque J, Meunier B, Wattier E, et al. Malignant cystosarcomas phyllodes of the breast in adolescent females. *Eur J Obstet Gynecol Reprod Biol* 1994;54:197–203.
34. Roisman I, Barak V, Okon E, et al. Benign cystosarcoma phyllodes of breast in an adolescent female. *Breast Dis* 1991;4:299–305.

## Carcinoma in Children and Adolescents

35. Bower R, Bell ML, Ternbergh JL. Management of breast lesions in children and adolescents. *J Pediatr Surg* 1976;11:337–346.
36. Pettinato G, Manivel JC, Kelly DR, et al. Lesions of the breast in children exclusive of typical fibroadenoma and gynecomastia. A clinicopathologic study of 113 cases. *Pathol Annu* 1989;24[Pt 2]: 295–326.
37. Simpson JS, Barson AJ. Breast tumours in infants and children: a 40-year review of cases at a Children's Hospital. *Can Med Assoc J* 1969;101:100–102.
38. Stone AM, Shenker IR, McCarthy K. Adolescent breast masses. *Am J Surg* 1977;134:275–277.
39. Ashikari H, Jun MY, Farrow JH, et al. Breast carcinoma in children and adolescents. *Clin Bull* 1977;7:55–62.
40. Bauer BS, Jones KM, Talbot CW. Mammary masses in the adolescent female. *Surg Gynecol Obstet* 1987;165:63–65.
41. Hammer B. Childhood breast carcinoma: a report of a case. *J Pediatr Surg* 1981;16:77–78.
42. Munoz FS, Fernandez EAY, Varela De Ugarte A. Cancer de mama en una nina de 6 anos. *Rev Clin Esp* 1980;159:289–290.
43. Roisman I, Barak V, Robinson E, et al. Breast malignancies in adolescents in Israel (1967–1989). *Breast Dis* 1992;5:149–168.
44. Close MB, Maximov NG. Carcinoma of breast in young girls. *Arch Surg* 1965;91:386–389.
45. Deutsch M, Altomare F, Mastrian AS, et al. Carcinoma of male breast following thymic irradiation. *Radiology* 1975;116:413–414.
46. Lowell DM, Martineau RG, Luria SB. Carcinoma of the male breast following radiation; report of a case occurring 35 years after radiation therapy for unilateral prepubertal gynecomastia. *Cancer* 1968;22: 581–586.
47. Rogers DA, Lobe TE, Rao BN, et al. Breast malignancy in children. *J Pediatr Surg* 1994;29:48–51.
48. Tefft M, Vawter GE, Mitus A. Second primary neoplasms in children. *AJR Am J Roentgenol* 1968;103:814–821.
49. Yahalom J, Petrek JA, Biddinger P, et al. Breast cancer in patients irradiated for Hodgkin's disease: a clinical and pathological analysis of 45 events in 37 patients. *J Clin Oncol* 1992;10:1674–1681.
50. Corpron CA, Black CT, Singletary SE, et al. Breast cancer in adolescent females. *J Pediatr Surg* 1995;30:322–324.
51. Nichini F, Goldman L, Lapayowker M, et al. Inflammatory carcinoma of the breast in a 12-year-old girl. *Arch Surg* 1972;105:505–508.
52. Ramirez G, Ansfield FJ. Carcinoma of the breast in children. *Arch Surg* 1968;96:222–225.

# CHAPTER 40

# Benign Mesenchymal Neoplasms

## FIBROMATOSIS

Fibromatosis is an infiltrating, histologically low-grade spindle cell proliferation composed of fibroblastic cells with variable amounts of collagen. Relatively few instances of fibromatosis originating in the breast have been reported. With the exception of three series totaling 67 patients (1–3), the literature on this subject consists of anecdotal case reports (4–11). Alternative diagnoses used for these lesions include extraabdominal desmoid, low-grade or grade I fibrosarcoma, and aggressive fibromatosis.

Adair and Herrmann (12) referred to a 2-cm mammary "desmoid" in the breast and pectoral muscle of a recently parturient 32-year-old woman in 1946. More than two decades later, Norris and Taylor (13) mentioned two tumors with "a desmoid pattern" in a review of mammary sarcomas. One woman was pregnant, and both "appeared to involve the deep dermis secondarily" (13). Three instances of mammary involvement by fibromatosis were listed by DasGupta et al. (14) in a review of extraabdominal desmoids. A patient with Gardner's syndrome and fibromatosis of the breast was reported in 1964 (15), and 6 years later a case of bilateral mammary fibromatosis associated with this genetic syndrome was described (7). Most authors have preferred the term *fibromatosis* for extraabdominal desmoid tumors of the breast.

### Clinical Presentation

Patients with mammary fibromatosis range in age from 13 to 80 years at diagnosis, averaging 37 (2), 43 (3), and 48.7 (1) years in three reported series. The median age at diagnosis was 25 years in one series (2). The lesions usually are painless, but pain and tenderness have been described (10). Patients with mammary fibromatosis almost always present with a palpable, firm or hard tumor in the breast that may suggest carcinoma on clinical examination. When present, dimpling or retraction of the overlying skin is likely to reinforce the clinical impression of carcinoma. The tumor typically is found in one of the quadrants and infrequently in the

subareolar area. Origin in axillary breast tissue has been reported (8,16). A case of multiple pedunculated lesions described as "fibromatosis of the breast" appears on review to be an example of dermatofibrosarcoma protuberans (17).

Mammography reveals a stellate tumor that may be indistinguishable from carcinoma (1,3,5,6,8). Calcifications are rarely formed in mammary fibromatosis, but they may be present in a benign proliferative lesion such as sclerosing adenosis that has been engulfed by the tumor. Rarely, the tumor may be nonpalpable and initially detected by mammography (6,18).

Antecedent injury or trauma has been reported at the site of fibromatosis in some patients, but this has been described infrequently for mammary lesions. One patient developed fibromatosis in a breast struck by falling concrete (19), and in another the tumor arose at an operative site 3 years after surgical drainage of postpartum mastitis (5). Also reported are one patient who had prior surgery for a fibroadenoma and another who had trauma in the area where fibromatosis developed (2). Inadvertent minor injury may occur more often, but it appears unlikely that trauma is responsible for the development of mammary fibromatosis in most patients.

An association with breast augmentation implants has been reported in several cases (Fig. 40.1). Three women each developed unilateral fibromatosis 2 years after having bilateral silicone implants placed for reconstruction after subcutaneous mastectomies for fibrocystic disease (9,20,21). One implant was filled with saline (9) and two with silicone gel (20,21). In the latter case, the "desmoid appeared to arise from the capsule of the implant." In another instance, mammary fibromatosis developed in one breast "several years" after bilateral placement of saline-filled silicone implants (2). A fourth patient with a silicone implant developed a dumbbell-shaped mass, one lobe of which infiltrated the chest wall and protruded into the thorax (22).

Very few cases have been associated with Gardner's syndrome (7,15,23). Other possible predisposing genetic conditions are not known. The positive family history of breast carcinoma mentioned in a few case reports (6,10) probably

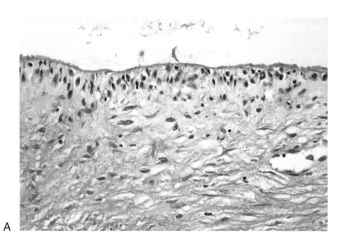
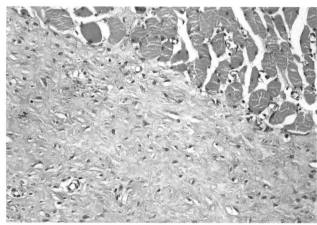

A

B

**FIG. 40.1.** *Fibromatosis and breast implant.* The images are from a 19-year-old woman who had undergone silicone implant breast augmentation. **A:** Synovial metaplasia lined the implant pocket. The wall of the implant capsule consisted of fibromatosis *(below).* **B:** Fibromatosis invaded the pectoral muscle.

is coincidental. Two patients had invasive duct carcinoma of the contralateral breast (2). One other woman was 22 years old when she developed unilateral mammary fibromatosis 5 years after treatment of Hodgkin's disease by chemotherapy alone (2).

The idea that hormonal disturbances contribute to the development of fibromatosis has been suggested by a number of observations. When assayed in nonmammary extraabdominal fibromatosis, estrogen and progesterone receptor levels have been negative (24,25). Negative hormone receptor results were obtained in one mammary tumor from a 54-year-old woman who was receiving exogenous estrogens to treat menopausal symptoms (2). In another report, positive levels of estrogen and progesterone receptors were found in mammary fibromatosis from a 44-year-old woman who had received exogenous estrogens for 5 years following bilateral oophorectomy for an ovarian cyst (1). Estrogen and progesterone receptors were not detected in six examples of mammary fibromatosis studied by immunohistochemistry, and the tumors also were not immunoreactive for the estrogen-inducible protein pS2 (26). Despite the association of abdominal desmoid tumors with pregnancy, the fact that very few of the breast lesions have been pregnancy related suggests that the occasional coexistence of the two conditions is most likely coincidental, probably a consequence of the broad age range of the women, including a substantial number younger than 40 years (1,3,5,13).

Four patients with bilateral fibromatosis were included among 67 cases (6%) summarized in the three large published series (1–3). There are two other reported examples of bilateral mammary fibromatosis. Only one of these patients had Gardner's syndrome (7). The bilateral lesions appear to have been independent processes, because extension across the midline was not reported. With the exception of one woman with asynchronous tumors separated by a 2-year in-

terval, bilateral lesions have been simultaneous. Among patients with unilateral lesions, the left and right breast are affected with approximately equal frequency.

**Gross Pathology**

Tumor size varied from 1 to 10 cm (average, 2.5 to 3.0 cm) (2,3). The lesion typically is described as a poorly circumscribed or ill-defined firm area of white, tan, or gray fibrous tissue (Fig. 40.2). Some examples of fibromatosis have a distinct stellate configuration. Others are described as circumscribed or "well demarcated" nodules (Fig. 40.3). Occasionally, the cut surface is said to have a whorled or trabecular appearance.

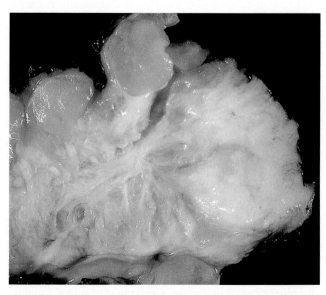

**FIG. 40.2.** *Fibromatosis, gross appearance.* The lesion forms a stellate mass composed of white tissue.

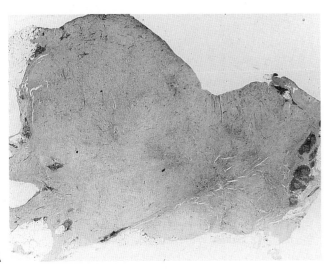 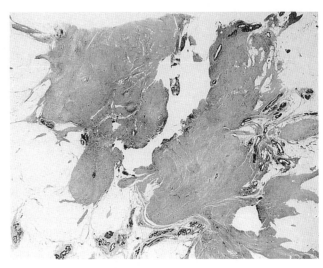

**FIG. 40.3.** *Fibromatosis.* **A:** Whole-mount histologic section of a tumor with a circumscribed and invasive border. Dark nodules along the right margin are lymphoid aggregates. **B:** Whole-mount histologic section of a stellate tumor.

## Microscopic Pathology

The histologic features of mammary fibromatosis are identical to those of the lesion when it develops in other anatomic sites. It is not unusual to discover varied growth patterns in a single lesion. The microscopic components of the tumor are spindle cells and collagen. Areas in which the collagenous element is accentuated have a keloidal appearance (Fig. 40.4). More commonly, the lesion features a moderately cellular, spindle cell proliferation in which there is modest collagen deposition (Fig. 40.5). Mitotic figures are inconspicuous or undetectable in most cases, although a rate of three mitotic figures per 10 high power fields (hpf) has been reported (2). In most tumors, the cells have a small pale oval or spindly nuclei with little pleomorphism (Fig. 40.6). Cells with nuclear atypia or pleomorphism are very uncommon (Fig. 40.7).

Cytoplasmic inclusion bodies identical to those seen in infantile digital fibromatosis were described in three mammary lesions (27,28). Two of these tumors appear to have been fibromatosis (28), whereas the third had an epithelial component suggestive of a phyllodes tumor (27). Round eosinophilic cytoplasmic inclusions measuring 3 to 10 μm were observed in the cytoplasm of tumor cells, often in a juxtanuclear location. The inclusions stained red with Masson's trichrome but were negative for periodic acid-Schiff (PAS), cytokeratin, desmin, and S-100. A ring of immunoreactivity for muscle-specific actin was apparent around the inclusion bodies. Ultrastructurally, loosely granular material formed the core of inclusion bodies, while at the periphery there was a "microfibrillary structure" that merged with cytoplasmic microfilaments. These findings suggest that myofibroblasts play a significant role in this form of mammary fibromatosis.

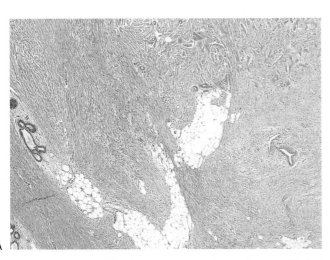 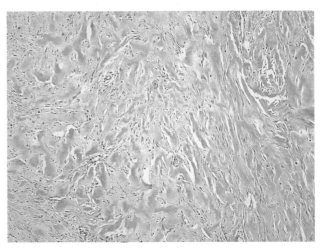

**FIG. 40.4.** *Fibromatosis, keloidal.* **A:** Broad keloidal bands of collagen are present in the tumor near the *upper border.* **B:** Keloidal area. *(continued)*

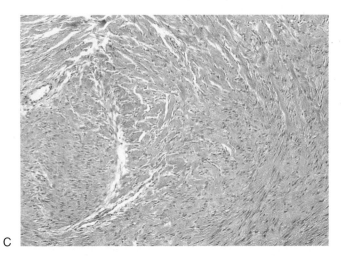

**FIG. 40.4.** *Continued.* **C:** Bands of collagen are blue when the tissue is stained with Masson's trichrome.

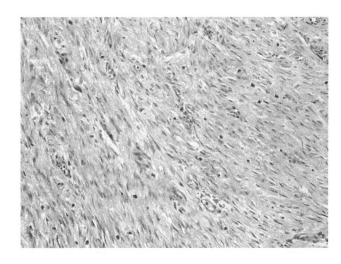

**FIG. 40.5.** *Uniform spindle cells with mild nuclear pleomorphism and hyperchromasia in a typical moderately cellular tumor.*

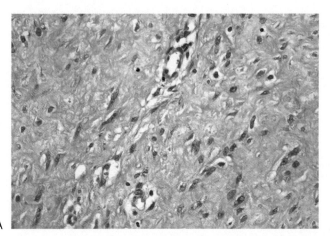
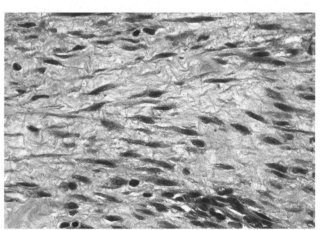

**FIG. 40.6.** *Fibromatosis.* Two examples of fibromatosis composed of uniform spindle cells without nuclear atypia. **A:** Hypocellular, nonkeloidal lesion. **B:** Moderately cellular tumor.

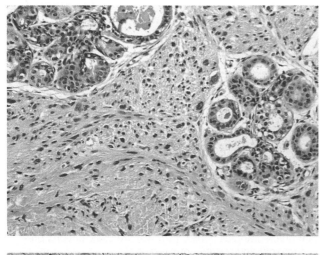

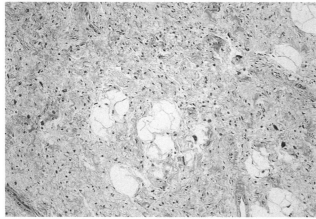

**FIG. 40.7.** *Fibromatosis.* **A:** In this tumor, a few cells infiltrating between lobules have large, hyperchromatic nuclei. **B:** Another tumor with multinucleated stromal giant cells.

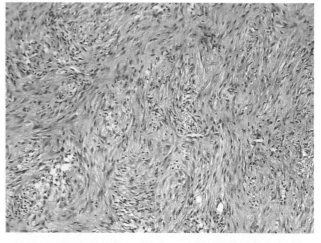

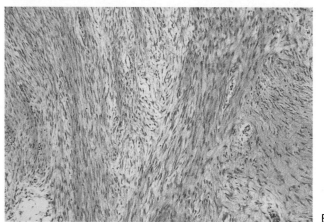

**FIG. 40.8.** *Fibromatosis.* **A:** Storiform pattern. **B:** Interlacing bundles of cells and collagen in a herringbone pattern.

The tumor cells usually are distributed in broad sheets, sometimes in a storiform configuration or in the form of interlacing bundles with a herringbone pattern (Fig. 40.8). In addition to varied amounts of collagenization, the stroma sometimes has focal myxoid areas (Fig. 40.9) and calcification is rarely seen histologically (Fig. 40.10).

Many tumors are relatively more cellular at the periphery, and there is a tendency to collagenization centrally. Focal lymphocytic infiltrates are found in nearly half of the tumors. These are more prominent at the periphery. Some lymphoid nodules have germinal centers (Fig. 40.11). Regardless of how well demarcated the lesions seem to be grossly, all have some stellate extensions into the surrounding fat and glandular parenchyma (Fig. 40.12). It usually is possible to identify ducts and lobules engulfed by these extensions at the periphery of the tumor (Fig. 40.13). The appearance created in these infiltrative areas at the margin may mimic the growth pattern of a phyllodes tumor (Fig. 40.14). Glandular parenchymal elements are less conspicuous or absent toward the center of fibromatosis.

The surrounding breast parenchyma is generally quiescent. Mild epithelial hyperplasia sometimes is present in ducts trapped by infiltrating extensions of some tumors.

Several lesions must be considered in the differential diagnosis of mammary fibromatosis. Some examples of spindle cell and squamous metaplastic carcinoma have readily identified metaplastic or carcinomatous components. Rarely the distinction between duct hyperplasia in fibromatosis and

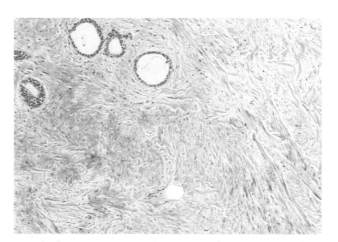

**FIG. 40.9.** *Fibromatosis, myxoid.* Basophilic stromal ground substance is prominent in this example of fibromatosis that surrounds cystic lobular glands.

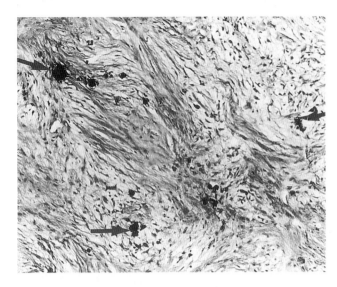

**FIG. 40.10.** *Fibromatosis, myxoid with calcifications.* The irregular black granular bodies *(arrows)* are calcifications present in myxoid and collagenous regions.

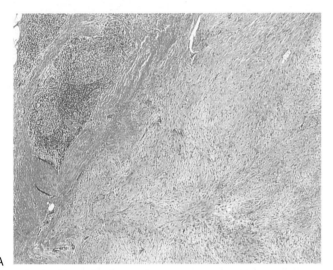

A

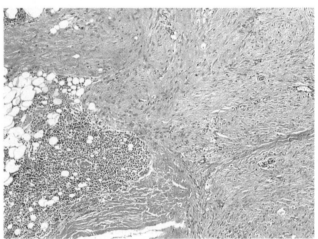

B

**FIG. 40.11.** *Fibromatosis, lymphocytic aggregates.* **A:** Lymphocytic nodule with germinal center formation is present at the edge of the tumor. **B:** Ill-defined lymphocytic infiltrate.

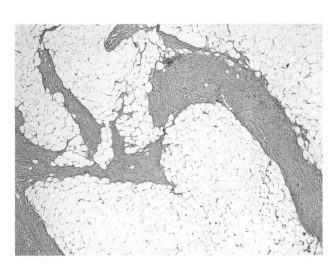

**FIG. 40.12.** *Fibromatosis, invasive border.* Slender tentacles of tumor extending into mammary fat.

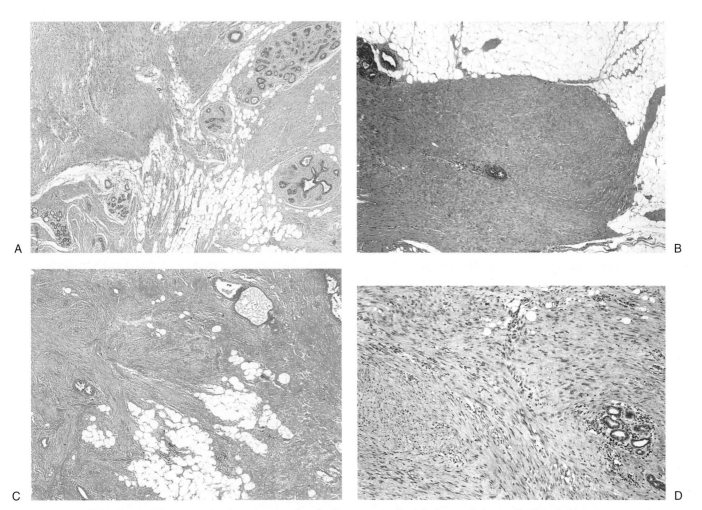

**FIG. 40.13.** *Fibromatosis, invasive border.* **A:** Tumor engulfs lobules and ducts. **B:** Small duct surrounded by fibromatosis. **C:** Tumor *(left)* blends with fibrous mammary stroma *(right)*. There is no clear demarcation between the tumor and normal stroma. **D:** Atrophic lobule *(lower right)* is surrounded by fibromatosis.

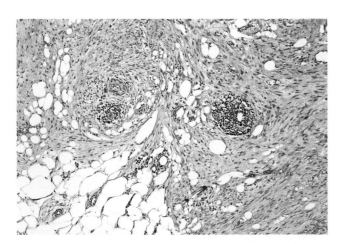

**FIG. 40.14.** *Fibromatosis.* Presence of focal lymphocytic infiltrates favors a diagnosis of fibromatosis over benign phyllodes tumor.

intraductal carcinoma may be difficult. One feature favoring metaplastic carcinoma is a highly cellular and pleomorphic spindle cell component, whereas desmoid-like foci and lymphoid aggregates suggest fibromatosis. An inflammatory reaction that may be predominantly lymphocytic occurs in and around most metaplastic carcinomas. The distinction between fibromatosis and high-grade fibrosarcoma or undifferentiated "stromal sarcoma" is determined on the basis of cellularity, cytologic pleomorphism, and especially mitotic activity. Although a mitotic rate of 3/10 hpf has been described in fibromatosis, this is exceptional. Typically the mitotic rate does not exceed 1/10 hpf, and usually no mitoses can be found.

A lesion said to be "the first described case of ossifying fibromatosis" in the breast was not well characterized and lacks follow-up (29). The histologic appearance illustrated would be compatible with metaplastic carcinoma containing an osseous heterologous component.

Another neoplasm included in the differential diagnosis is fibrous histiocytoma. Although mammary fibromatosis may have storiform areas, this is rarely a prominent pattern. Epithelioid, histiocytic, and multinucleated cells often found in fibrous histiocytoma are not a feature of fibromatosis.

Scars from healed fat necrosis, remote trauma, and surgery must be distinguished from fibromatosis. Calcifications are more likely to be associated with fat necrosis, but rarely they can occur in fibromatosis. Foreign body granulomas, sometimes with partly absorbed suture material, are an indication of prior surgery. If the patient has recurrent fibromatosis, reparative changes caused by an earlier operation may mingle with recurrent tumor, further complicating the diagnosis. Lymphoid infiltrates that commonly occur in fibromatosis should not lead to the erroneous diagnosis of an inflammatory condition such as nodular fasciitis. The inflammatory component of fibromatosis typically is limited to isolated separate lymphoid aggregates at the periphery of the lesion. In fasciitis, inflammatory cells are dispersed more diffusely at the periphery and within the lesion, although localized areas of inflammation also occur. "Myoid" and multinucleated cells characteristically found in nodular fasciitis are not a feature of fibromatosis (30).

Because the clinical presentation of mammary fibromatosis may mimic that of carcinoma, it is not surprising that a few examples have been subjected to needle aspiration or core biopsy for diagnosis (5,6,11,31,32). The diagnosis of fibromatosis may be suspected on the basis of findings in a fine needle aspiration biopsy usually described as "limited in cellularity" or "scanty." The specimen consists of small uniform spindle cells dispersed singly or in groups that may be clusters or relatively flat sheets. The spindle cells, largely devoid of cytoplasm, are represented by nuclei. Epithelial cells in groups and sheets and lymphocytes may be found in the background. The differential diagnosis of such a fine needle aspiration specimen includes fibroadenoma and benign phyllodes tumor. A feature favoring the diagnosis of fibromatosis is a sparse epithelial component relative to the number of stromal cells and the virtual absence of flat sheets of epithelium commonly found in a fibroepithelial tumor. The findings in a needle core biopsy may suggest fibromatosis, but in most instances, immunohistochemistry and excisional biopsy are necessary to exclude other lesions such as metaplastic carcinoma (31).

Electron microscopic studies of mammary fibromatosis have been reported (6,28,32). The spindle cells are predominantly fibroblasts with lesser numbers of myofibroblasts. Only a few cells in these tumors prove to be immunoreactive with antibodies for actin.

## Treatment and Prognosis

Recommended treatment is wide local excision. Because of the ill-defined character of most lesions, it is difficult to judge the adequacy of margins intraoperatively by inspec-

tion or frozen section. The excisional biopsy specimen should be inked and the margins sampled generously. When a tumor is adherent to fascia, muscle, or skin, the excision should be extended to include the affected area, and it may be necessary to perform a mastectomy to achieve adequate margins of resection. In many cases, the nature of the tumor has not been established prior to surgery and the surgeon does not anticipate the need for a particularly generous margin. Although the risk of recurrence is higher in patients with documented positive margins (3), recurrences have been observed in cases with apparently negative margins. Not all patients with positive margins develop recurrences, and there have been unusual instances in which locally advanced lesions stabilized or regressed after incomplete excision (1). The frequency of local recurrence ranges from 21% to 27% (1–3). Most recurrences occur within 3 years of diagnosis, but in a few instances they were not detected for nearly a decade. Histologic features such as cellularity, mitotic activity, and cellular pleomorphism are not helpful for predicting recurrence.

Immediate reexcision of the biopsy site should be considered when the initial biopsy is small and margins are positive, especially for lesions located deep in the breast or peripherally near the chest wall. Recurrences at these sites may be difficult to control and are best avoided (Fig. 40.15). On the other hand, follow-up is preferable to reexcision of relatively superficial lesions or subareolar fibromatosis, which might require excision of the nipple. There is no evidence that postoperative radiotherapy or chemotherapy are reliable as adjuncts to surgery for primary treatment or to control large or extensive recurrences.

There are several reports of attempts to use hormonal treatment for fibromatosis. Administration of antiestrogens or hormones has resulted in remission in some patients with nonmammary fibromatosis given this treatment (33–36). One review found a response rate of 51% in 35 cases in the

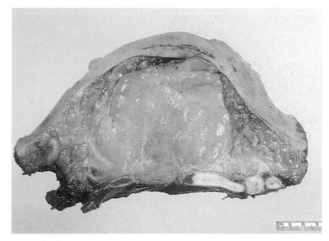

FIG. 40.15. *Fibromatosis, chest wall invasion.* Recurrent fibromatosis forming a distinct tumor that occupies most of the breast and invades the chest wall between the ribs.

literature (37). The effect of these medications on mammary fibromatosis has not been determined.

## FIBROUS TUMOR

This condition presents as a discrete breast mass composed of collagenized mammary stroma. It was first characterized by Haagensen (38) as fibrous disease. Other names that have been given to this entity include fibrous mastopathy (39), fibrosis of the breast (40), and focal fibrous disease (41). Because of the clinical presentation as a distinct mass, the term *fibrous tumor* is preferable to distinguish it from more frequent nonspecific and involutional stromal changes (42). Some tumors illustrated and described as focal fibrous disease (41) and fibrous tumor (42) appear to be examples of pseudoangiomatous stromal hyperplasia (PASH). Other lesions sampled by needle core biopsy that are diagnosed as "focal fibrous" probably represent examples of fibrous tumor (43).

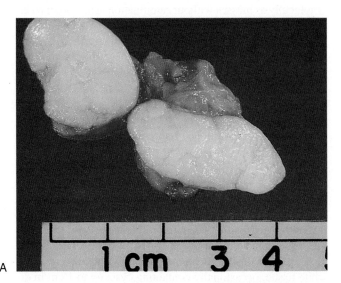

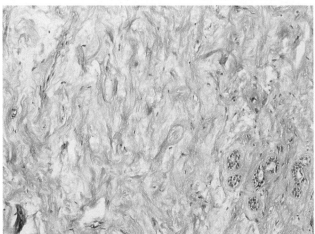

**FIG. 40.16.** *Fibrous tumor.* **A:** Circumscribed white tumor. **B:** Atrophic lobule is present in the collagenous stroma that contains scattered fibroblasts.

## Clinical Presentation

Fibrous tumor is a disease of premenopausal women. On palpation it is a firm-to-hard, distinct tumor measuring 2 to 5 cm. Skin retraction and dimpling are not evident. Mammography reveals an area of density with borders varying from irregular to smooth. Calcifications are not a feature of fibrous tumor (44).

Cytogenetic analysis of a lesion reported to be a fibrous tumor in a 26-year-old woman revealed a clonal translocation in mesenchymal cells that was characterized as t(4;14)(q24–25;q24.3) (45). The histologic features illustrated in this report are best interpreted as PASH.

## Gross Pathology

Fibrous tumor forms a firm-to-hard mass (Fig. 40.16). The extent of the lesion can be appreciated on palpation by the operating surgeon. The excised specimen typically has the appearance of a discrete tumor. The cut surface of the bisected tumor reveals white, homogeneous rubbery tissue.

## Microscopic Pathology

Histologically, fibrous tumor consists of collagenous stroma that contains markedly decreased or absent atrophic ductal and lobular elements (Fig. 40.16). Capillaries, other vascular structures, and nerves are very sparse; perivascular and perilobular inflammatory infiltrates are absent. Cysts with apocrine metaplasia, sclerosing adenosis, and duct hyperplasia are not features of fibrous tumor. The diagnosis of fibrous tumor may be suggested if a needle core biopsy sample from a nonpalpable relatively discrete mammographically detected lesion consists of hypocellular collagenous tissue devoid of glandular structures.

## Treatment and Prognosis

Fibrous tumor is a benign, self-limited stromal proliferation adequately treated by local excision.

## PSEUDOANGIOMATOUS HYPERPLASIA OF MAMMARY STROMA

PASH can be mistaken for angiosarcoma. The term *pseudoangiomatous* was proposed to emphasize the fact that the histologic pattern mimics, but does not actually constitute, a vasoformative proliferation. The presence of myoid differentiation in examples of PASH led some authors to classify the lesions as hamartomas (46). This is an inappropriate use of the term *hamartoma,* defined as "a benign tumor or tumor-like lesion composed of one or more tissues, normal to the organ but abnormally mixed and overgrown" (47). PASH is a lesion formed by myofibroblasts with variable

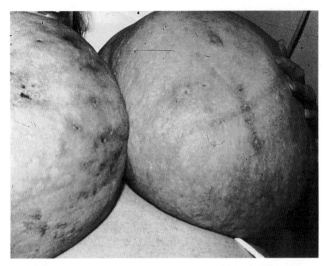

**FIG. 40.17.** *Pseudoangiomatous stromal hyperplasia.* This patient developed massive breast enlargement during pregnancy. A biopsy revealed diffuse pseudoangiomatous stromal hyperplasia.

expression of myoid and fibroblastic features. Glandular hyperplasia is sometimes also present.

### Clinical Presentation

With one exception, reported examples of tumor-forming PASH have been in women. The exceptional case report described the finding of PASH in rapidly growing gynecomastia in axillary breast tissue of a 39-year-old man (48). PASH is a frequent incidental component of gynecomastia, having been found in 44 (47.4%) of 93 consecutive male breast biopsies, of which 43 of the 44 specimens with PASH exhibited gynecomastia (49). Milanezi et al. (50) found PASH in 21 (23.8%) of 88 cases of gynecomastia (50). Gynecomastia-like hyperplasia of the breast has been described in a renal transplant patient during cyclosporine treatment (51).

The published images suggest florid PASH and the breast lesion regressed after cyclosporin was discontinued (51). Baildam et al. (52) described a series of patients who developed multiple, often bilateral breast tumors while being treated with cyclosporine after renal transplantation. The lesions were described clinically as "fibroadenomas" but not biopsied, and these might represent other examples of gynecomastia-like hyperplasia in this setting.

Age at diagnosis in females ranges from the teens to the mid 50s, with a median age in the mid to late 30s (53–56). Almost all patients have been premenopausal. Most women have a palpable painless unilateral mass that is firm or rubbery. One patient presented with unilateral mildly painful breast enlargement with *peau d'orange* change of the skin suggesting inflammatory carcinoma (54). *Peau d'orange* and skin necrosis has been observed in patients who have massive breast enlargement due to PASH during pregnancy (Fig. 40.17).

Although most women present with a clinically palpable mass, PASH has been detected by mammography in patients who were asymptomatic (57,58). The lesions appear radiographically as masses without calcification. The borders usually are smooth, but a minority of the tumors are spiculated or have ill-defined margins sometimes obscured by surrounding tissue. Ultrasound reveals a well-defined hypoechoic mass (58). Clinically asymptomatic PASH detected by mammography may occur in postmenopausal patients, whereas palpable lesions are almost always found in premenopausal women or in postmenopausal women who have been treated with hormone replacement therapy.

### Gross Pathology

In patients with localized PASH, the excised tumors are well demarcated and the smooth external surface sometimes resembles a capsule. The tumors measure 2 to 15 cm in greatest dimension (average, 5 cm) (Fig. 40.18). The cut surface usually consists of homogeneous fibrous tan, gray, or white tissue, occasionally containing cysts up to 1 cm in di-

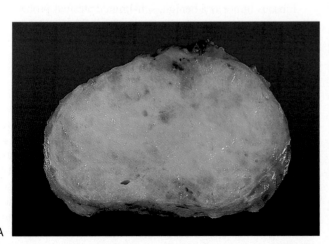
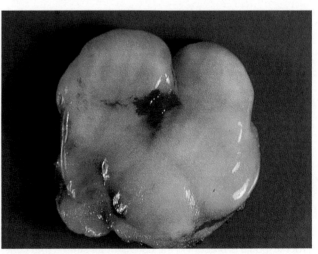

A               B

**FIG. 40.18.** *Pseudoangiomatous stromal hyperplasia, gross appearance.* **A,B:** Circumscribed oval tumor measured 5 cm in the long axis. The tumor is circumscribed and lobulated.

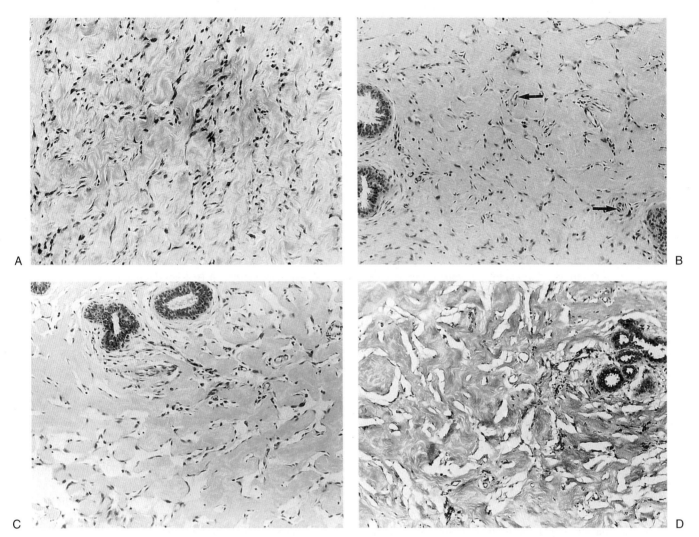

**FIG. 40.19.** *Pseudoangiomatous stromal hyperplasia.* Various histologic appearances. **A:** Slender cords of myofibroblasts with almost no spaces between them. **B:** Inconspicuous spaces and true capillaries *(arrows).* **C:** Well-formed anastomosing spaces. **D:** Dilated spaces.

ameter. A minority of the tumors are grossly nodular (Fig. 40.18). No areas of hemorrhage or necrosis are seen except in tumors subjected to needle biopsy or aspiration.

## Microscopic Pathology

In hematoxylin and eosin-stained sections of paraffin-embedded tissue, the tumors are composed of intermixed stromal and epithelial elements. The lobular and duct structures of the breast parenchyma usually are separated by an increased amount of stroma. Collagenization of intralobular stroma and duct attenuation producing fibroadenoma-like features are common. Nonspecific proliferative epithelial changes include mild hyperplasia of duct and lobular epithelium, often with some accentuation of myoepithelial cells, and apocrine metaplasia with or without cyst formation.

The most striking histologic finding is a complex pattern of largely empty, often anastomosing spaces in the dense collagenous stroma (Figs. 40.19 and 40.20). These slits,

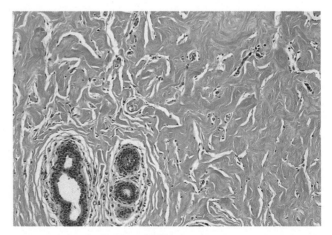

**FIG. 40.20.** *Pseudoangiomatous stromal hyperplasia.* A diffuse complex network of spaces is evident at low magnification.

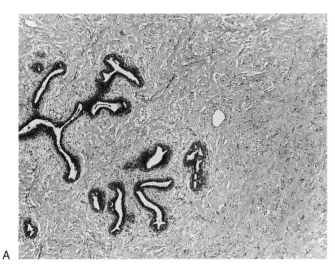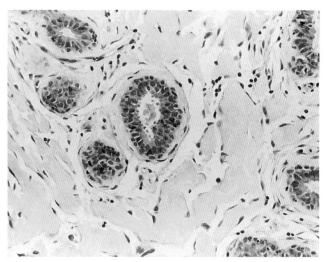

A
B

**FIG. 40.21.** *Pseudoangiomatous stromal hyperplasia, lobular involvement.* **A,B:** Pseudoangiomatous spaces involve perilobular and intralobular stroma.

sufficiently large to be identified at low magnification, often are present in intralobular as well as interlobular stroma (Fig. 40.21). The spaces rarely contain a few red blood cells. Collagen fibrils may traverse the space. Myofibroblasts, present singly and intermittently at the margins of the spaces, resemble endothelial cells (Fig. 40.22). The nuclei of the myofibroblasts usually are attenuated, lack atypia, and do not show mitotic activity, but some of these cells are enlarged and have noticeably hyperchromatic nuclei (Fig. 40.22). Also present in the stroma are round or oval blood-containing true capillaries lined by endothelial cells. Myofibroblasts in PASH usually are CD34 immunoreactive (Fig. 40.23).

The myofibroblasts may accumulate in distinct fascicles in a background of conventional PASH, forming fascicular PASH (Figs. 40.24 and 40.25). These groups of cells are ev-

idence of a more pronounced proliferation of myofibroblasts that retain immunoreactivity for CD34 (Fig. 40.26). The most extreme examples of this cellular form of PASH have a growth pattern reminiscent of a myofibroblastoma (Figs. 40.25 and 40.27). This is especially the case when the myofibroblasts have abundant cytoplasm and PASH occurs as a localized tumor rather than as a diffuse process (Fig. 40.28). Myofibroblastoma and PASH are related conditions, representing the spectrum of lesions, sharing a common histogenesis in the myofibroblast.

Stromal pseudoangiomatous spaces can be seen in frozen sections, indicating that they are not simply an artifact of formalin-fixed, paraffin-embedded tissue. Basement membrane material is not demonstrable around the slit-like spaces. Alcian blue staining, demonstrable in the spaces, is removed by

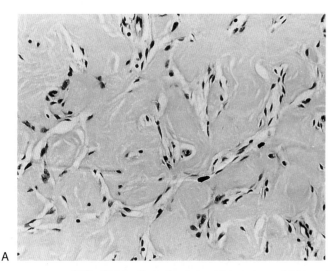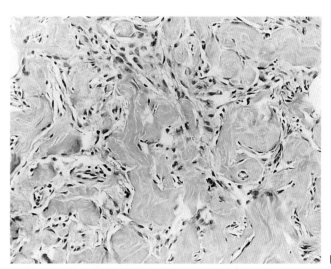

A
B

**FIG. 40.22.** *Pseudoangiomatous stromal hyperplasia.* **A:** Connected slits outlined by myofibroblasts with uniform, small flat nuclei are shown. Strands of collagen traverse some spaces. **B:** Focal myofibroblastic hyperplasia in which some cells have enlarged, hyperchromatic nuclei.

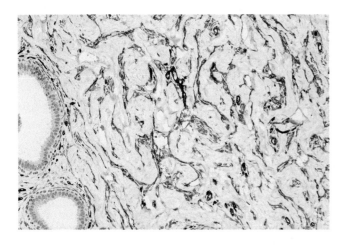

**FIG. 40.23.** *Pseudoangiomatous stromal hyperplasia, CD34.* The myofibroblasts are strongly CD34 immunoreactive (avidin-biotin).

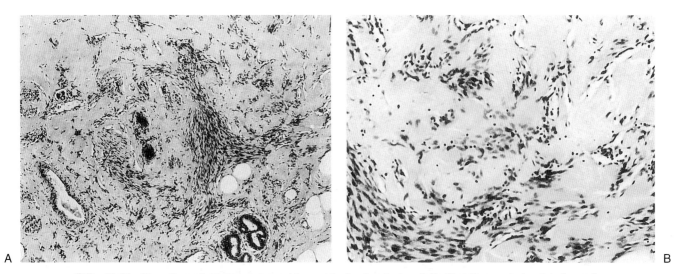

A

B

**FIG. 40.24.** *Pseudoangiomatous stromal hyperplasia, fascicular.* **A,B:** Bundles and sheets of myofibroblasts in a background of conventional pseudoangiomatous stroma hyperplasia.

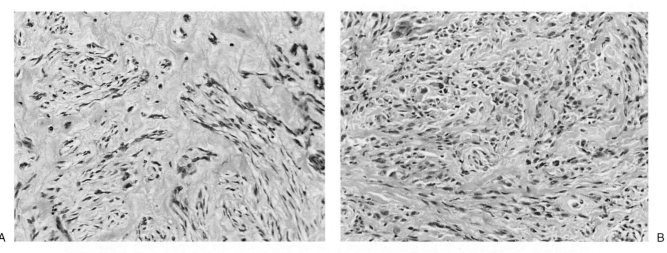

A

B

**FIG. 40.25.** *Pseudoangiomatous stromal hyperplasia, fascicular.* Bundles of myofibroblasts sectioned longitudinally **(A)** and transversely **(B)**. Areas such as those shown here can occur in myofibroblastoma.

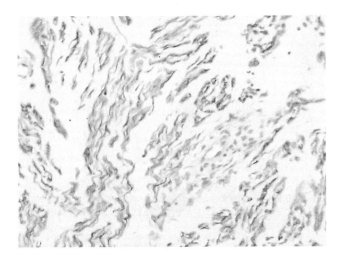

**FIG. 40.26.** *Pseudoangiomatous stromal hyperplasia, fascicular.* These fascicles of myofibroblasts are immunoreactive for CD34 (avidin-biotin).

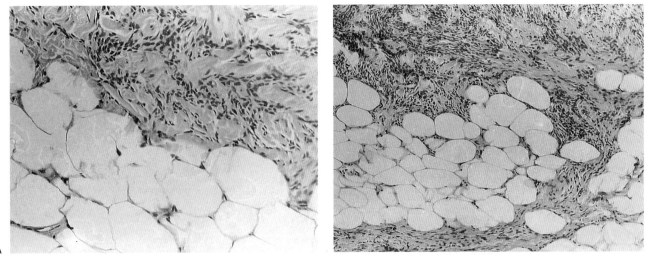

**FIG. 40.27.** *Pseudoangiomatous stromal hyperplasia, fascicular.* **A,B:** Pronounced fascicular growth that resembles a myofibroblastoma.

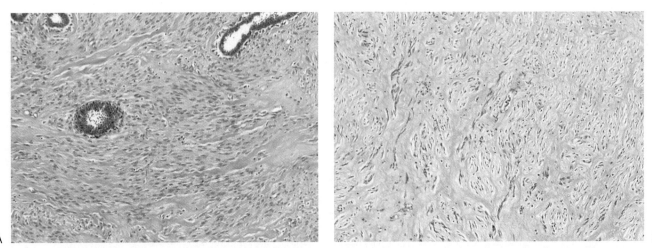

**FIG. 40.28.** *Pseudoangiomatous stromal hyperplasia, fascicular.* **A,B:** The collagen bands and fascicles of myofibroblasts with abundant cytoplasm separated by collagen bands resemble a classic myofibroblastoma.

hyaluronidase treatment. Myofibroblasts lining pseudoangiomatous spaces exhibit strong immunoreactivity for vimentin, variable immunoreactivity for actin, and no immunoreactivity for cytokeratin or factor VIII-related antigen (Fig. 40.29). The nuclei of myofibroblasts in PASH sometimes are immunoreactive for progesterone receptor (53,59), and progesterone receptor has been detected in PASH by biochemical analysis (46). Estrogen receptor has not been detected biochemically (46,53) and is absent or only weakly present when the tissues are studied by immunohistochemistry (46,50,59,60).

CD34 reactivity can be demonstrated in the majority of lesions (Fig. 40.23) (50,59,60). The presence of CD34 reactivity in cells staining for vimentin, desmin, and smooth muscle actin in PASH suggests that it is a marker for myofibroblastic differentiation. An extremely unusual variant of PASH has cytoplasmic inclusion bodies of the type found in digital fibromas. The inclusions are immunoreactive for actin and desmin (Fig. 40.30). Isolated foci of smooth muscle differentiation can be encountered in PASH (Fig. 40.31).

Cytologic alterations of myofibroblasts sometimes are encountered in PASH. Myoid differentiation to smooth muscle phenotype can occur in isolated cells, and rarely this is a diffuse process that resembles multiple ill-defined leiomyomas (Fig. 40.31). Pleomorphic nuclei are infrequent. They can be found in conventional and in fascicular PASH, sometimes accompanied by mitotic activity (Fig. 40.32). The author has encountered two instances of tumor-forming PASH in teenage girls, characterized by marked cytologic atypia, multinucleated cells, and mitotic activity (Fig. 40.33). These appear to be instances of myofibroblastic sarcoma arising in PASH. Insufficient information is available to characterize the clinical course of these tumors.

Samples from two tumors examined by electron microscopy revealed similar findings (54,55). Well-formed vascular structures, usually capillaries, were readily distinguished from pseudoangiomatous spaces at the ultrastructural level. True vessels lined by endothelial cells joined by

tight junctions were surrounded by a basement membrane and pericytes. Pinocytotic vesicles, intermediate filaments, and Weibel-Palade bodies were evident in endothelial cells. On the other hand, pseudoangiomatous spaces were lined by an incomplete layer of spindle cells that featured a fairly well-developed endoplasmic reticulum and prominent Golgi apparatus. Slender cytoplasmic processes extended along and around the spaces, sometimes joined by small rudimentary cell junctions, or they terminated in the collagenous stroma.

At the ultrastructural level, the intervening stroma consisted of collagen fibrils and slender cells with longitudinally arranged highly attenuated cytoplasmic processes joined by occasional tight or rudimentary cell junctions. The cytoplasmic processes of these cells, thought to be modified pericytes, retained fragments of basement membrane on both surfaces, pinocytotic vesicles, and occasional small clusters of intermediate filaments.

The diagnosis of PASH by fine needle aspiration has been reported (56). The specimens are likely to be hypocellular with bipolar spindle cells and benign epithelial clusters. The distinction between PASH and a benign fibroepithelial tumor would be difficult in such a specimen.

### Prognosis and Treatment

PASH that forms a clinically palpable tumorous mass appears to be a highly exaggerated manifestation of physiologic changes commonly encountered microscopically. In this setting, PASH seems to be part of the proliferative process rather than a separate lesion. This form of PASH often contributes to the clinical impression of a mass when the histologic findings are described as fibrocystic changes (60). Vogel et al. (61) described distinct alterations in mammary epithelium and stroma at various phases of the menstrual cycle. They found "loose, broken" stroma in the luteal phase (days 15 to 20) and a "loose, edematous" stroma in the secretory phase (days 21 to 27). The open clefts of PASH

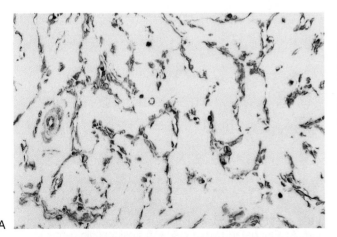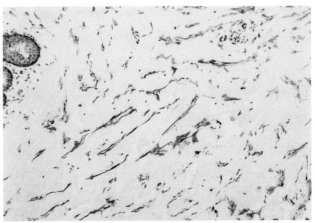

A B

**FIG. 40.29.** *Pseudoangiomatous stromal hyperplasia, vimentin and actin.* **A:** Immunoreactivity for vimentin highlights the pseudoangiomatous structure. **B:** Immunoreactivity for smooth muscle actin (both avidin-biotin).

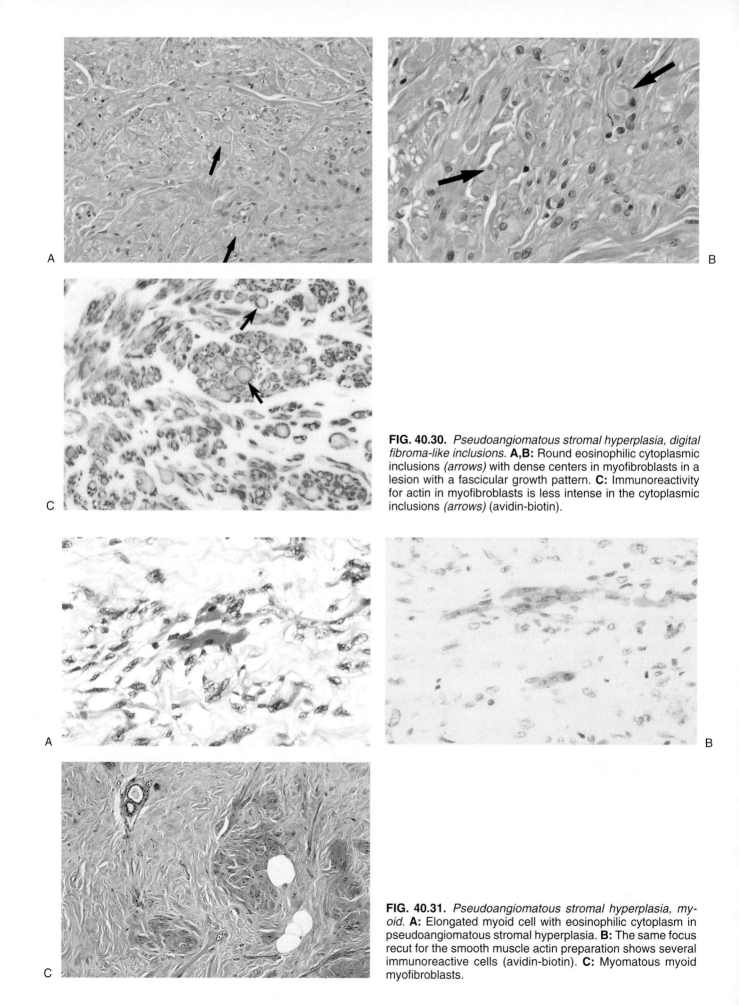

**FIG. 40.30.** *Pseudoangiomatous stromal hyperplasia, digital fibroma-like inclusions.* **A,B:** Round eosinophilic cytoplasmic inclusions *(arrows)* with dense centers in myofibroblasts in a lesion with a fascicular growth pattern. **C:** Immunoreactivity for actin in myofibroblasts is less intense in the cytoplasmic inclusions *(arrows)* (avidin-biotin).

**FIG. 40.31.** *Pseudoangiomatous stromal hyperplasia, myoid.* **A:** Elongated myoid cell with eosinophilic cytoplasm in pseudoangiomatous stromal hyperplasia. **B:** The same focus recut for the smooth muscle actin preparation shows several immunoreactive cells (avidin-biotin). **C:** Myomatous myoid myofibroblasts.

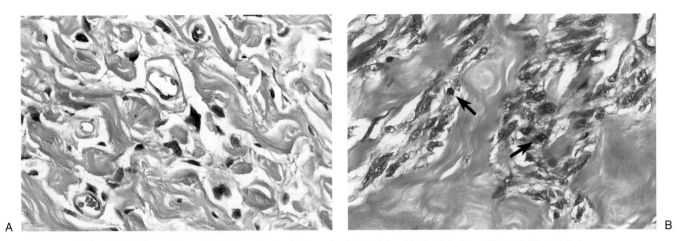

**FIG. 40.32.** *Pseudoangiomatous stromal hyperplasia, atypia.* **A:** Nuclei of myofibroblasts are hyperchromatic and pleomorphic. **B:** Nuclear pleomorphism and two mitoses *(arrows)* in fascicular pseudoangiomatous stromal hyperplasia.

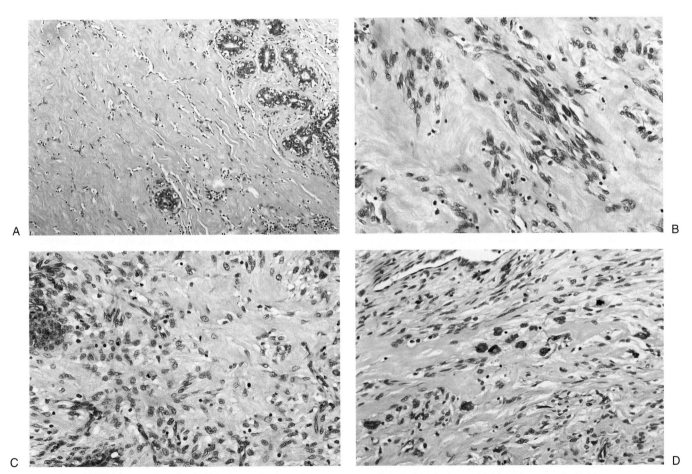

**FIG. 40.33.** *Pseudoangiomatous stromal hyperplasia, giant cells and atypia.* All images are from a specimen obtained from an 18-year-old nonpregnant girl with a breast mass. **A:** Region showing conventional pseudoangiomatous stromal hyperplasia (PASH). The scattered lymphocytic reaction is unusual. **B:** Fascicular growth. **C:** Cellular overgrowth obscures the PASH architecture in this region. **D:** Atypical multinucleated stromal cells. Note the mitotic figure *(upper right)*.

contain hyaluronidase-sensitive mucopolysaccharide and resemble physiologic changes depicted in figures 4 and 5 of the report by Vogel et al. (61).

Ibrahim et al. (54) found microscopic foci of PASH in 23% of 200 consecutive breast specimens obtained for benign or malignant conditions. Eighty-nine percent of the patients were younger than 50 years. The majority of these specimens exhibited epithelial hyperplasia, sometimes including secretory changes in lobules. It appears that under as-yet-undefined conditions, microscopic and clinically inapparent pseudoangiomatous hyperplasia becomes capable of autonomous growth. That almost all patients with tumorous pseudoangiomatous stroma have been premenopausal underscores the probable importance of hormonal factors in the development of this lesion. Hormonal influence is further suggested by the frequent presence of PASH in gynecomastia and fibroepithelial neoplasms (60). Traces of PASH can be found in breast tissue from a postmenopausal woman, but well-developed PASH in this age group almost always is associated with hormone-replacement therapy.

In several instances, biopsies of PASH have been misinterpreted as low-grade angiosarcoma, and this has led to treatment by mastectomy. Most patients have remained well after excisional biopsy of PASH, but ipsilateral recurrences have occurred in some cases. Rarely, patients had asynchronous or concurrent bilateral PASH. Incomplete excision probably predisposes to local recurrence, but it also is possible that residual breast stroma may become susceptible to the same unknown stimuli even after apparently complete removal of the tumor. Lesions followed by recurrence are histologically indistinguishable from PASH in women who did not have recurrences. Recurrent lesions ordinarily exhibit no change in cellularity or other atypical features.

The recommended treatment is wide local excision. Mastectomy rarely becomes necessary to control multiple recurrent tumors. No information presently is available about the effectiveness of radiation or antiestrogen treatment in patients with recurrent lesions. The administration of estrogenic hormone-replacement therapy to a perimenopausal woman with a prior history of PASH, but no recently active lesions, resulted in the development of breast tumors consistent with PASH.

## MYOFIBROBLASTOMA

Myofibroblasts are spindle-shaped or fusiform mesenchymal cells probably derived from fibroblasts (62). They are present in small numbers in virtually all tissues outside the central nervous system. Proliferation of myofibroblasts triggered by cytokines is conspicuous in various inflammatory conditions such as healing wounds (63). They are a component of various benign mesenchymal tumors (64) and some sarcomas (65,66). Soft tissue neoplasms of the breast thought to be composed of myofibroblasts have been classified as myofibroblastomas (67). The structural and immunohistochemical characteristics of these tumors are similar to those of a solitary fibrous tumor (68,69). Some investigators suggested that myofibroblastomas of the breast should be regarded as solitary fibrous tumors and diagnosed by this name (69). Others attempted to distinguish between the two entities on the basis of structural, cytologic, and immunohistochemical features (70). The latter authors reserved the diagnosis of myofibroblastoma for lesions expressing actin and CD34 reactivity and classified actin-negative, CD34-positive lesions as solitary fibrous tumors. These hair-splitting distinctions seem totally unwarranted in view of the "plasticity" of myofibroblastic phenotypic expression (71). It is appropriate to use the term *myofibroblastoma* for these tumors in the breast. If so-called *solitary fibrous tumors* at other sites take origin from myofibroblasts, perhaps they also should be designated as myofibroblastomas.

Myofibroblastic proliferation occurs in many mammary carcinomas, being most prominent in scirrhous, desmoplastic tumors (72,73). The presence of myofibroblasts in scirrhous breast carcinomas has been confirmed by electron microscopy (72–74) and immunohistochemistry (73,75). It has been possible to characterize myofibroblasts, isolated *in vitro* from scirrhous carcinomas, by electron microscopy and immunohistochemistry (76).

Myofibroblasts are distinguished from spindled myoepithelial cells largely on the basis of their distribution as well as their immunohistochemical and electron microscopic characteristics (74). Ultrastructurally, both types of cells have cytoplasmic actin-like microfilaments measuring 5 to 7 nm in diameter, with focal dense bodies and pinocytotic vesicles (more numerous in myoepithelial cells). In contrast to myoepithelial cells, myofibroblasts lack prekeratin tonofilaments. Desmosomes are readily found between myoepithelial cells, whereas they are absent or poorly formed between myofibroblasts. Depending on their phenotypic state, both types of cells may be reactive with antiactin antibodies. Myoepithelial cells are immunoreactive for smooth muscle myosin heavy chain, which stains myofibroblasts weakly or not at all. Myoepithelial cells are variably positive for S-100 protein and cytokeratin, such as 34BE12, in their epithelial phenotype, but myofibroblasts are negative with both antibodies.

### Clinical Presentation

Mammary neoplasms derived largely or entirely from myofibroblasts are uncommon. Two of the lesions described by Toker et al. (77) as "benign spindle cell breast tumors" probably were myofibroblastomas. Ultrastructural study of one right breast tumor revealed prominent myofibroblasts as well as smooth muscle cells. Both patients were men 55 and 66 years of age. The latter patient had two identical separate tumors in his left breast treated by simple mastectomy. Seventeen years later, he underwent a right mastectomy with the finding of six foci of the same neoplastic process in that breast. Synchronous bilaterality and unilateral multicentricity also have been reported, respectively, in two men (78).

Wargotz et al. (79) described 16 patients ranging in age from 41 to 85 years (median, 64 years). Eleven (69%) were men. Each patient presented with a solitary unilateral mass in the breast. In a case reported by Bégin (80), the 77-year-old patient experienced progressive breast enlargement for 7 years resulting in a 6.5 × 6.0 × 4.5-cm tumor. Although the majority of patients reported to have myofibroblastoma have been men, the lesion occurs in women as well (78). One woman developed a myofibroblastoma in a breast 4 years after ipsilateral lumpectomy and radiotherapy for intraductal carcinoma (81). Concurrent gynecomastia was present in one male patient (69). The author has seen the specimen from a 76-year-old woman in whom moderately differentiated invasive duct carcinoma coexisted with and invaded a mammary myofibroblastoma. Two men with myofibroblastoma of the breast and coincidental primary carcinomas of the pancreas and kidney, respectively, also have been seen in consultation.

Radiographically, the tumors are homogeneous, lobulated, and well circumscribed, and they lack microcalcifications (82,83). Nonpalpable myofibroblastomas have been detected by mammography (84). Ultrasonography suggests a fibroadenoma (84). Magnetic resonance imaging of a myofibroblastoma in the male breast revealed homogeneous enhancement with internal septations (85). There is no attachment to the skin.

## Gross Pathology

The average diameter of the tumors is about 2 cm, with most smaller than 4 cm. Size extremes include one lesion that measured 0.9 cm (78) and one tumor that was 10 cm (86). The excised mass is firm and rubbery, with a lobulated external surface. The cut surface consists of homogeneous, bulging gray-to-pink whorled or lobulated tissue that, in one case, had myxoid gelatinous areas (Fig. 40.34) (80). Cystic degeneration, necrosis, and hemorrhage have not been reported.

## Microscopic Pathology

Microscopically, the classic type of myofibroblastoma is devoid of mammary ducts and lobules, but compressed breast parenchyma forms a pseudocapsule. Two distinctive histologic features are bundles of slender, bipolar uniform spindle-shaped cells typically arranged in clusters and broad bands of hyalinized collagen distributed throughout the tumor (Fig. 40.35). Multinucleated giant cells are uncommon, and mitotic figures are sparse or undetectable. In a minority of lesions fat cells are present, reflecting invasion of surrounding tissue, and cartilaginous differentiation has been described in two lesions (79,87). A perivascular lymphoplasmacytic infiltrate sometimes is identified. The border of

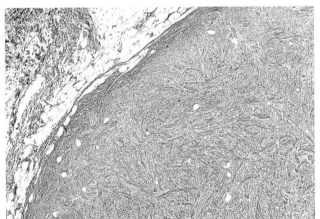

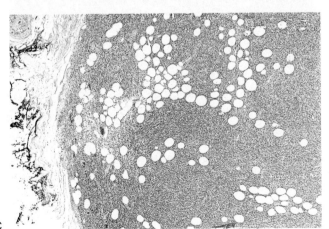

**FIG. 40.34.** *Myofibroblastoma, gross appearance.* **A,B:** Tumor is grossly well circumscribed, fleshy, and nodular. **B:** Whole-mount histologic section showing the circumscribed border and solid growth. **C:** This well-circumscribed tumor contains abundant fat.

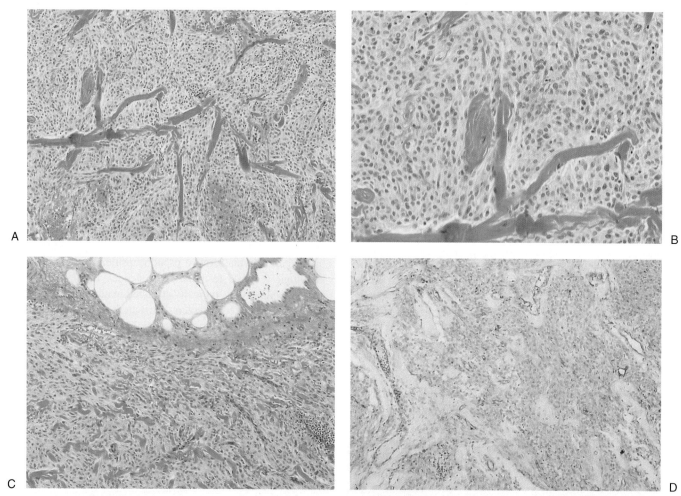

**FIG. 40.35.** *Myofibroblastoma, classic type.* **A,B:** Tumor is composed of a homogeneous population of predominately spindle-shaped cells with ovoid nuclei and pale cytoplasm. **C:** Circumscribed border. A small cluster of lymphocytes can be seen in the tumor on the *right*. **D:** Immunoreactivity for CD34 is present in the tumor cells (avidin-biotin).

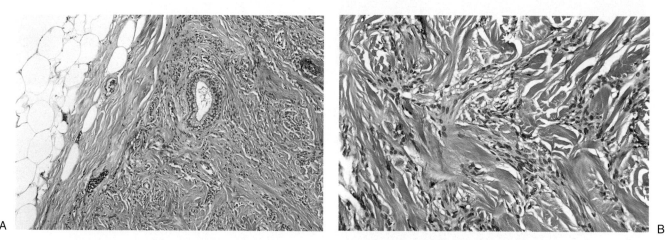

**FIG. 40.36.** *Myofibroblastoma, collagenized or fibrous variant.* **A,B:** Spindle-shaped tumor cells are embedded in collagenous stroma. The structure resembles fascicular pseudoangiomatous stromal hyperplasia. The circumscribed border with one duct incorporated in the tumor is shown in **A**.

the tumor usually is circumscribed microscopically, but in a minority of cases, the tumor has an invasive margin. Small amounts of mammary glandular tissue may be incorporated into the lesion, but the pattern differs from that of infiltrative myofibroblastoma described later (78).

Variant forms of myofibroblastoma have received little attention. These tumors exhibit a spectrum of histologic appearances between classic myofibroblastoma and PASH, a myofibroblastic lesion that was described in detail earlier in this chapter. The variant forms of myofibroblastoma have not been well characterized pathologically or clinically (87).

In a *collagenized* or *fibrous myofibroblastoma,* the spindle cells are distributed in collagenous stroma (Fig. 40.36). The broad, deeply eosinophilic fibrous bands, which are so prominent in a classic myofibroblastoma, are absent or greatly reduced in number. Irregular slit-like spaces formed between tumor cells and the stroma are reminiscent of PASH, and some of these tumors have a fascicular structure.

The *epithelioid variant* of myofibroblastoma features polygonal or epithelioid cells arranged in alveolar groups (Fig. 40.37). Epithelioid areas may be mixed with more classic elements, or they can constitute the predominant growth pattern. The term *epithelioid variant* is used arbitrarily for

tumors in which more than 50% of the lesion has this histologic pattern. Epithelioid cells in these tumors are immunoreactive for desmin and sometimes for CD34. Epithelioid myofibroblastoma with sclerotic stroma can have a linear growth pattern that resembles invasive lobular carcinoma. There is no reactivity for cytokeratin in epithelioid myofibroblastoma. The epithelioid cells were not immunoreactive for actin and had little or no CD34 reactivity in a small group of tumors available to study.

A *cellular variant* of myofibroblastoma features a dense proliferation of spindle-shaped neoplastic myofibroblasts (Fig. 40.38). Collagenous bands may be absent in some parts of the lesion. These tumors tend to have infiltrative borders microscopically. The tumor cells are immunoreactive for actin and desmin. Rarely, cellular and collagenous or fibrous growth patterns are combined in a single tumor (Fig. 40.39). The existence of these hybrid tumors supports the conclusion that breast tumors with the appearance of solitary fibrous tumor are myofibroblastomas.

The *infiltrative variant* of myofibroblastoma is characterized by entirely invasive growth. These lesions form a tumor grossly that consists not only of the lesional tissue but also fat, mammary stroma, ducts, and lobules (Fig. 40.40). This pattern differs from that of the classic and other foregoing

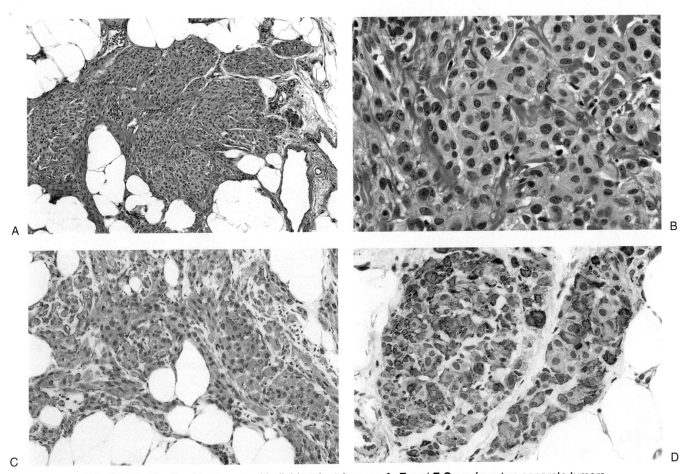

**FIG. 40.37.** *Myofibroblastoma, epithelioid variant.* Images **A–E** and **F,G** are from two separate tumors. **A:** Tumor has a stellate border. **B:** Tumor cells are arranged in alveolar groups. **C:** Desmin immunoreactivity. **D:** Immunoreactivity for smooth muscle actin is present in epithelioid cells. *(continued)*

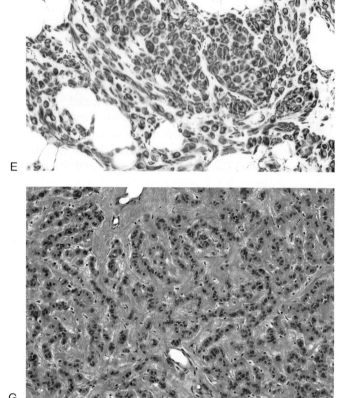

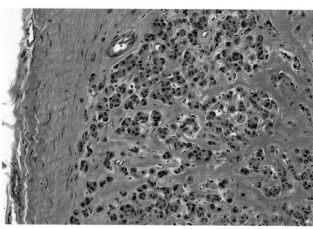

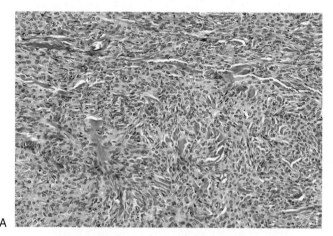

**FIG. 40.37.** *Continued.* **E:** Vimentin immunoreactivity. Tumor cells were not immunoreactive for S-100 and cytokeratin. **F:** This tumor was from a 60-year-old woman. Note the circumscribed border and alveolar clustering of the tumor cells.**G:** Epithelioid myofibroblastic tumor cells have a linear growth pattern in this part of the tumor. It is not surprising that a needle core biopsy sample of this tumor, obtained prior to excision, was interpreted as invasive lobular carcinoma. The tumor was immunoreactive for smooth muscle actin and CD34 but not for cytokeratin.

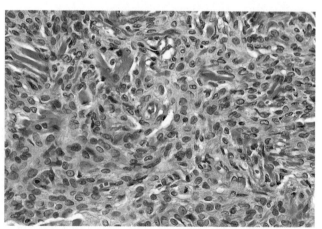

**FIG. 40.38.** *Myofibroblastoma, cellular variant.* **A,B:** Interlacing plump spindle cells and scant deeply eosinophilic collagen fibers. *(continued)*

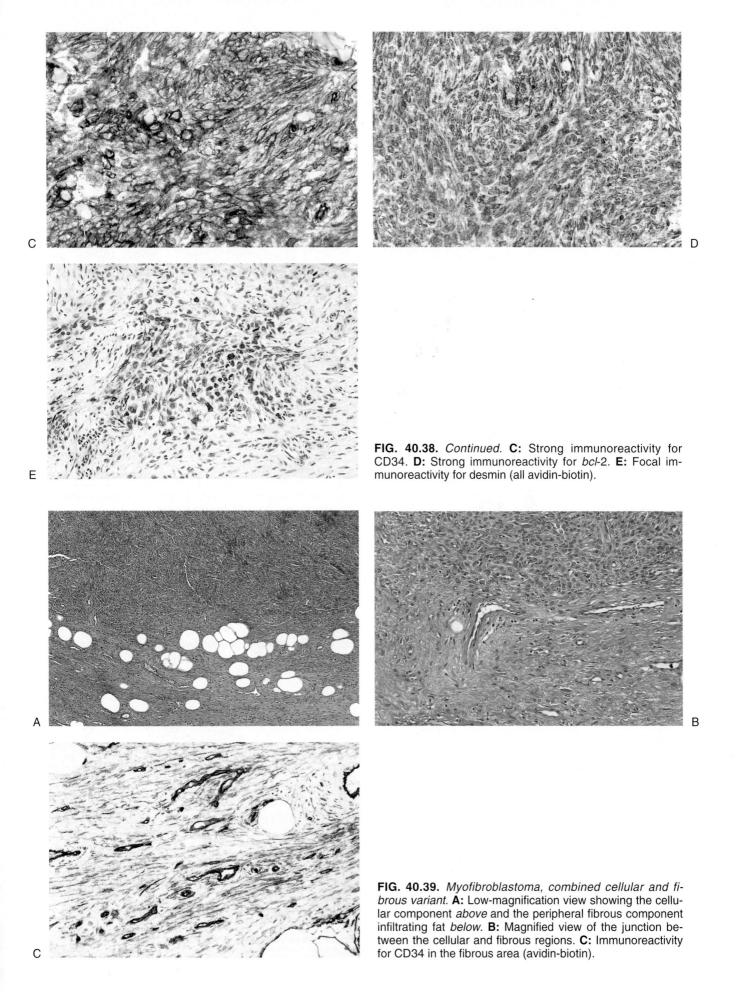

**FIG. 40.38.** *Continued.* **C:** Strong immunoreactivity for CD34. **D:** Strong immunoreactivity for *bcl*-2. **E:** Focal immunoreactivity for desmin (all avidin-biotin).

**FIG. 40.39.** *Myofibroblastoma, combined cellular and fibrous variant.* **A:** Low-magnification view showing the cellular component *above* and the peripheral fibrous component infiltrating fat *below*. **B:** Magnified view of the junction between the cellular and fibrous regions. **C:** Immunoreactivity for CD34 in the fibrous area (avidin-biotin).

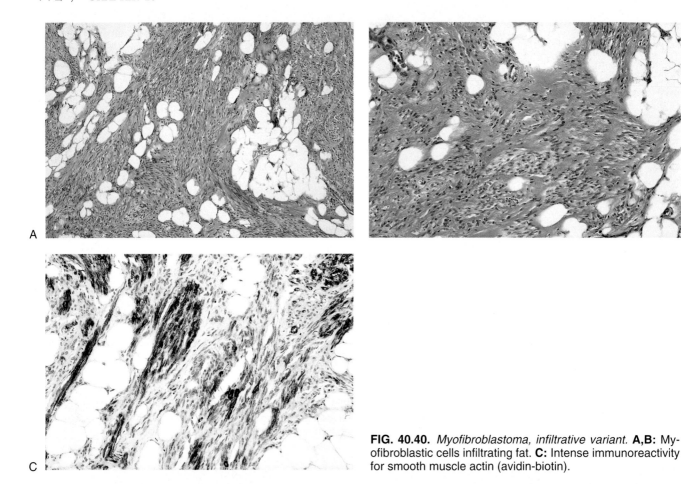

A

B

C

**FIG. 40.40.** *Myofibroblastoma, infiltrative variant.* **A,B:** Myofibroblastic cells infiltrating fat. **C:** Intense immunoreactivity for smooth muscle actin (avidin-biotin).

variants of myofibroblastoma, which incorporate fat, glandular tissue, or both into what is essentially a discrete tumor composed in large measure of the lesional tissue. The infiltrative variant of myofibroblastoma consists of bundles of relatively evenly dispersed spindle, ovoid, and epithelioid cells embedded in collagenous stroma. Some of these lesions exhibit a peculiar tendency for the neoplastic myofibroblasts to be oriented around blood vessels.

Rarely, the cells in a myofibroblastoma may have a histo-

logic appearance that resembles well-differentiated smooth muscle cells, and cartilage may be formed (Fig. 40.41). The myoid myofibroblasts are strongly immunoreactive for actin and desmin, but not for CD34 (88). The author has encountered a tumor that appeared to be a *myxoid myofibroblastoma* (Fig. 40.42).

The fine needle aspiration cytology specimen from a myofibroblastoma consists of cells distributed singly or in clusters (Fig. 40.43) (82,89–92). A fascicular arrangement may

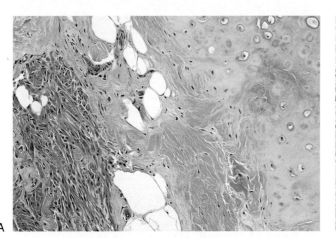

A

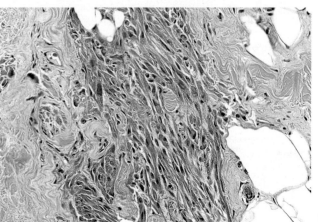

B

**FIG. 40.41.** *Myofibroblastoma with myoid and cartilaginous differentiation.* **A:** Myoid cells *(left)* and cartilage *(right).* **B:** Magnified view of the myoid focus.

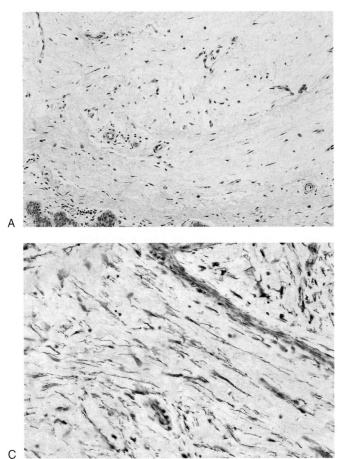

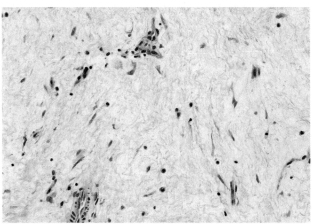

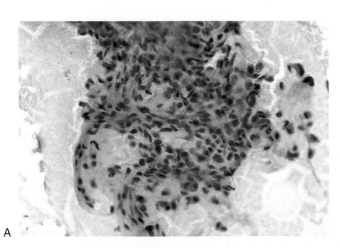

**FIG. 40.42.** *Myofibroblastoma with myxoid variant.* The tumor presented as a palpable, discrete soft mass. **A,B:** Excised lesion consisted of dispersed stellate and spindle cells in myxoid stroma. **C:** Actin-positive cells had long slender cytoplasmic processes (avidin-biotin).

be evident in cell clusters (90). The oval nuclei have fine granular chromatin that may be divided by a "nuclear groove." Nucleoli are small and inconspicuous.

The majority of myofibroblastomas typically are immunoreactive for desmin, vimentin, actin, and CD34. The pattern of reactivity is demonstrable in fine needle aspiration specimens (92). The tumors are not immunoreactive for cy-

tokeratin or factor VIII, and only rarely are they weakly reactive for S-100 protein. Nuclear immunoreactivity for androgen receptor was detected in each of five myofibroblastomas studied by Morgan and Pitha (93). Others have reported strong nuclear reactivity for progesterone and estrogen receptors in a myofibroblastoma (91).

Myofibroblastoma must be considered in the differential

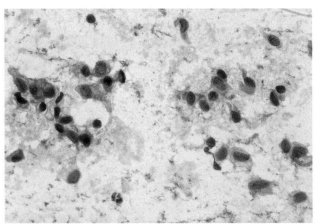

**FIG. 40.43.** *Myofibroblastoma, cytology.* **A:** Cohesive spindle cells with a few discohesive epithelioid cells *(right)*. **B:** Discohesive epithelioid cells from a myofibroblastoma. This sample could suggest carcinoma. Note the presence of some oval nuclei and spindle cells.

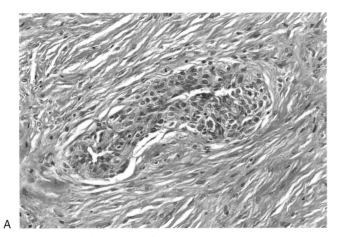
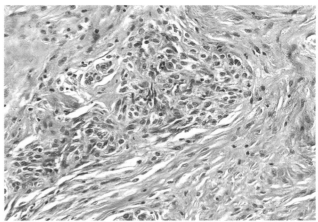

A
B

**FIG. 40.44.** *Perivascular myocytic neoplasm.* **A:** Epithelioid myocytic cells surround a slit-shaped vascular space. **B:** Nodular focus that contains inconspicuous vascular channels.

diagnosis of spindle cell mammary tumors. Malignant neoplasms, such as sarcoma and metaplastic carcinoma, are typically more cellular than myofibroblastomas with frequent mitoses, and many have distinguishing histologic features (e.g., squamous metaplasia). Fibromatosis tends to be a stellate invasive lesion. Plump myoid cells and the inflammatory reaction of fasciitis are not seen in myofibroblastoma. Fibromatosis exhibits abundant collagen and spindle cells arranged in broad bands rather than short fascicular clusters. Spindle cell lipomas also have a male predominance and sometimes may be well circumscribed. They have more abundant adipose tissue than myofibroblastomas. However, the distinction between spindle cell lipoma and myofibroblastoma by light microscopy sometimes can be difficult (77).

### Treatment and Prognosis

No recurrences have been reported after follow-up of 3 to 126 months. Two patients have been treated by mastectomy after an erroneous diagnosis of sarcoma (79), and in one instance mastectomy was necessary for a 10-cm tumor in a man (86). Virtually all patients were managed by excisional biopsy (79,80,82).

## TUMORS WITH PERIVASCULAR MYOID DIFFERENTIATION

Tumors with perivascular myoid differentiation have been described under various names. Most involve the skin and subcutaneous tissue, commonly in the extremities. Breast involvement has rarely been cited in published reports, but the author has encountered several mammary tumors with this appearance. A striking feature of these lesions is nodular fibrohistiocytic growth, predominantly with a perivascular localization (Fig. 40.44). Osteoclast-like giant cells are variably present (Fig. 40.45). Immunoreactivity of actin is present in the spindle cells, whereas the histiocytic elements are KP1 positive (94).

The terms *myofibromatosis-type perivascular myoma* and *myopericytoma* have been applied to an unusual and histologically distinctive group of neoplasms characterized by

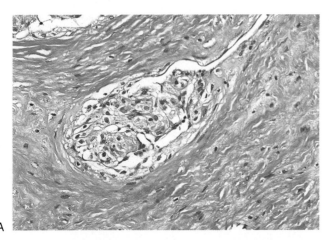
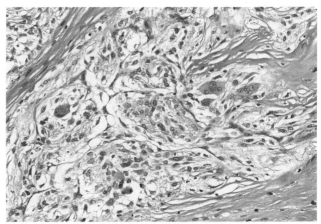

A
B

**FIG. 40.45.** *Perivascular myocytic neoplasm.* **A:** Small vascular channel extends from the upper right to the center of the image where it is distorted by the perivascular myocytic proliferation. **B:** More complex nodular focus from the same case with osteoclast-like giant cells. *(continued)*

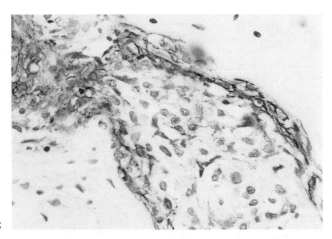
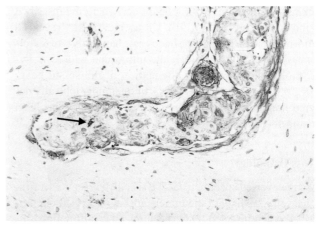

C

D

**FIG. 40.45.** *Continued.* **C:** Reactivity for factor VIII is localized to endothelial cells. **D:** Immunoreactivity for smooth muscle actin is shown. Note the mitotic figure *(arrow).*

spindle cell perivascular proliferation (95). Areas with a hemangiopericytoma-like and glomangiopericytoma patterns may be encountered in these tumors. The spindle cells are consistently immunoreactive for actin.

Local recurrence in soft tissues at the primary extramammary site has been described in several reports of the various lesions in this group of tumors. Occasional patients had repeated recurrences over two or more decades, and metastases have rarely been reported (96). No systematic study of these lesions in the breast has been published, but the author has observed instances of local recurrence. Angioblastic sarcoma is discussed in Chapter 41.

## GIANT CELL FIBROBLASTOMA

This uncommon soft tissue tumor of children has only rarely been encountered in the breast (97). The lesion presents as a lobulated, circumscribed, firm, superficial mass that is composed of grossly homogeneous pale tissue. Microscopic examination reveals spindle and multinucleated giant cells that often lie at the borders of clefts in the collagenous stroma. This pattern bears a close resemblance to PASH, although the latter usually lacks multinucleated stromal cells. Some giant cell fibroblastomas are immunoreactive for CD34. Electron microscopy reveals multisegmented nuclei and some cells with multiple nuclei. Numerous cytoplasmic microfilaments have been described (97), and the ultrastructural findings suggest that the spindle cells are of fibroblastic or myofibroblastic origin. Local recurrence may occur after incomplete excision.

## GRANULAR CELL TUMOR

The first report of this tumor is attributed to Abrikossof (98), who described a granular cell tumor of the tongue. He proposed origin from striated muscle cells; consequently, the lesion was termed a myoblastoma (98). Tissue culture studies of three granular cells tumors, including two from the breast, appeared to support this interpretation (99). Subse-

quently, accumulated evidence has cast doubt on the myogenous histogenesis of granular cell neoplasms, and it has been shown that the tumors are derived from the Schwann cells of peripheral nerves. Granular cell tumors occur throughout the body, with about 5% of them originating in the breast (100).

### Clinical Presentation

The first description of a mammary granular cell tumor was published by Abrikossof (101) in 1931. In 1946, Haagensen and Stout (102) described five patients 24 to 74 years of age and emphasized the importance of distinguishing this benign tumor from carcinoma.

Granular cell tumor of the breast (GCTB) is encountered most often in women 30 to 50 years old, but it has been described in adolescents and elderly women with an overall age range of 17 to 74 years (100,103–105). About 10% of GCTB occur in the male breast (103–106).

In most cases, the patient presents with a firm or hard, painless mass. The left and right breast are affected with equal frequency. GCTB may arise in any part of the breast parenchyma, including the axillary tail, or in a subcutaneous location. The lesions tend to develop more often in the upper and medial quadrants. Superficial lesions may cause skin retraction, and nipple inversion has been reported when the tumor is in a subareolar location. Large tumors or those that arise deep in the breast may be adherent to the pectoral fascia. GCTB usually occurs as a solitary unilateral lesion, but rare instances of multiple and bilateral tumors have been reported. Patients who have multiple granular cell tumors at various sites may have one or more lesions in the breast (107,108). Unusual clinical presentations include nonpalpable GCTB detected by mammography (109,110), coincidental GCTB and intraductal carcinoma (110), or infiltrating duct carcinoma (111) in the same breast and GCTB in the contralateral breast of a patient with previously treated ductal carcinoma of the other breast (109).

On mammography, GCTB is difficult to distinguish from carcinoma (112–114). It typically forms a stellate mass lacking calcifications with a dense core, but circumscribed lesions occur rarely (115,116). Ultrasound usually reveals a solid mass with posterior shadowing suggestive of carcinoma (109,115–117); rarely, the ultrasound pattern is hypoechoic with or without attenuation of the sound beam (106,109,118,119). The diagnosis of mammographically detected nonpalpable GCTB by needle core biopsy has been described (120).

## Gross Pathology

In the excised specimen, GCTB usually presents as a firm or hard mass. Many of the tumors appear to be well circumscribed when bisected. Other examples have ill-defined infiltrative borders. The cut surface is white or gray, or it may have a yellow-to-tan color (Fig. 40.46). Lesions measuring up to 6 cm have been reported, but the tumors generally are 3 cm or smaller.

## Microscopic Pathology

With very rare exceptions, GCTB is a benign neoplasm. The histologic, histochemical, and ultrastructural features of GCTB are indistinguishable from those of granular cell tumors arising at other sites. The tumor is composed of compact nests or sheets of cells that contain eosinophilic cytoplasmic granules. The granules usually are prominent and fill the cytoplasm, but in some lesions, there is a tendency to cytoplasmic vacuolization and clearing (Fig. 40.47). The cytoplasmic granules are diastase resistant and PAS positive. Cell borders typically are well defined, and the cells vary in shape from polygonal to spindle. Variable amounts of collagenous stroma are present (Fig. 40.48). One group of investigators reported a direct correlation between the amount of stromal fibrosis and the presence of elastosis in the lesion (121). Nuclei are round to slightly oval, with an open chromatin pattern. Nucleoli tend to be prominent. In some cases, a modest amount of nuclear pleomorphism, occasional multinucleated cells, and rare mitoses may be found, but these features should not be interpreted as evidence of a malignant neoplasm. Small nerve bundles sometimes are seen in the tu-

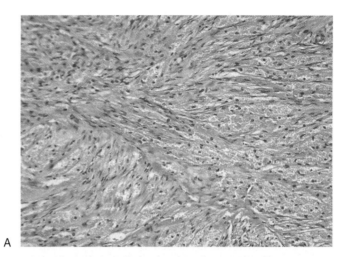

A

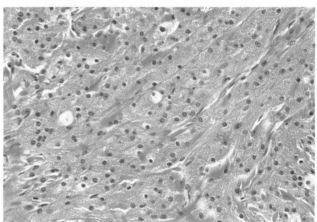

B

**FIG. 40.47.** *Granular cell tumor.* **A:** Tumor cells are arranged in a fascicular pattern. **B:** Tumor cells with small round nuclei and granular eosinophilic cytoplasm.

mor or in close association with stellate extensions of the lesion peripherally (Fig. 40.48). Cells that resemble those of granular cell tumor have been observed in nerves close to, but not directly involved by, granular cell tumors (122).

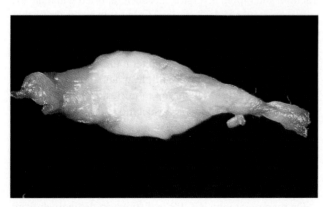

**FIG. 40.46.** *Granular cell tumor, gross appearance.* Pale yellow homogeneous tumor that blends with the fibrous parenchyma.

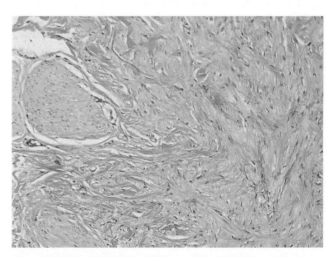

**FIG. 40.48.** *Granular cell tumor, collagenous stroma.* Tumor cells are distributed between wavy bands of collagen. A nerve is associated with the tumor *(left).*

Although many of the tumors appear grossly circumscribed, microscopic examination usually reveals an infiltrating growth pattern at the margins of the lesion. Ducts and lobules typically are surrounded by the invasive tumor cells and incorporated into the lesion. Granular cell tumor cells may infiltrate into lobules and superficially into the dermis of the skin.

Histologically, GCTB must be distinguished from mammary carcinoma, histiocytic lesions, and metastatic neoplasms. The infiltrative character of GCTB composed of cells with prominent nucleoli, especially when the lesion has collagenous stroma, results in a close resemblance to scirrhous carcinoma, particularly in frozen sections. The similarity between apocrine carcinoma and GCTB sometimes is striking. The presence of intraductal carcinoma, often with lobular extension, as well as cytologic pleomorphism, usually serve to identify apocrine carcinoma. In some instances, the lesions can only be distinguished with confidence by histochemical studies, especially if *in situ* carcinoma is not evident. Apocrine carcinomas are immunoreactive for cytokeratin and usually for epithelial membrane antigen. GCTB is not reactive for these epithelial markers and does not contain mucin. Strong, diffuse immunoreactivity for S-100 protein and carcinoembryonic antigen, which characterizes granular cell tumors, does not by itself distinguish these lesions from mammary carcinoma, because some carcinomas are also S-100 positive (Fig. 40.49) (114,123–126). A high proportion of granular cell tumors are reactive for vimentin, which is detectable in relatively few carcinomas (123). GCTB is negative for estrogen and progesterone receptors.

The distinction between GCTB and mammary carcinoma, especially apocrine carcinoma, is particularly difficult in fine needle aspiration cytology specimens (124,126–128). This difficulty can result in a false-positive diagnosis of carcinoma on fine needle aspiration (129,130). The aspirate usually is cellular, and the cells, which are dispersed separately or in irregular clusters, have mildly pleomorphic nuclei that may contain nucleoli (106). Numerous granules distributed throughout the background, as well as in the cells, stain blue with Romanovsky stains or red with the Papanicolaou and hematoxylin and eosin stains.

A superficial resemblance between the cells of GCTB and histiocytes can lead to confusion with a granulomatous inflammatory reaction or a histiocytic tumor. GCTB is immunohistochemically negative for histiocyte-associated antigens, such as α₁-antitrypsin, α₁-antichymotrypsin, and muramidase (114,123), but reactivity for CD68 (KP1) has been described in GCTB (131). Histiocytes and GCTB are immunoreactive for S-100.

GCTB must be distinguished from metastatic neoplasms in the breast that have oncocytic or clear cell features, such as renal carcinoma and malignant melanoma. The differential diagnosis also includes alveolar soft part sarcoma. Granular cell tumors are not immunoreactive for myoglobin (125). The cytoplasmic granules in these tumors are Luxol fast blue positive, an observation that suggests they contain myelin (132).

Electron microscopy reveals myelin figures as well as numerous lysosomes in granular cell tumors (105,114, 123,125). Observations in one electron microscopic study suggested that the granules are formed by infolding of the cell membrane, resulting in myelin figures that are phagocytosed by lysosomes (132). The process appeared to be analogous to the mechanism by which myelin is formed around axons in nerves. Some cells also have angulate bodies, which are rounded triangular membrane-bound structures that contain microtubules and microfibrils.

## Prognosis and Treatment

Benign GCTB is treated by wide excision. Local recurrence may occur after incomplete excision, but sometimes it is difficult to distinguish between recurrence and asynchronous multifocal lesions. Direct invasion of an axillary lymph node by a GCTB that arose in the axillary tail has been reported (119). No recurrence was evident after 47 months of follow-up.

Less than 1% of all granular cell tumors, including mammary lesions, are malignant (Fig. 40.50). Systemic metastases have been described in patients with nonmammary malignant granular cell tumors (133). One woman presented with a 4-cm breast tumor and multiple pulmonary metastases that were confirmed histologically to be metastatic granular cell tumor (134). Another patient was found to have axillary metastases when a tumor initially excised from the upper anterior chest wall recurred in her right breast (135). The microscopic features of this tumor were not exceptional. There were no detectable mitotic figures, the cells exhibited no anaplasia, and there was minimal nuclear pleomorphism. In some instances, it may not be possible to distinguish between the clinical presentation of multifocal benign granular cell tumors, including breast lesions, and metastatic malignant granular cell tumor.

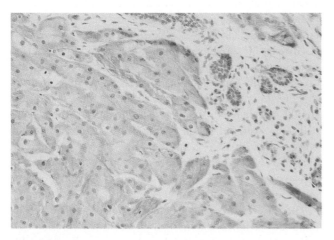

**FIG. 40.49.** *Granular cell tumor, S-100 protein.* Tumor cells invading a lobule are immunoreactive for S-100 protein (avidin-biotin).

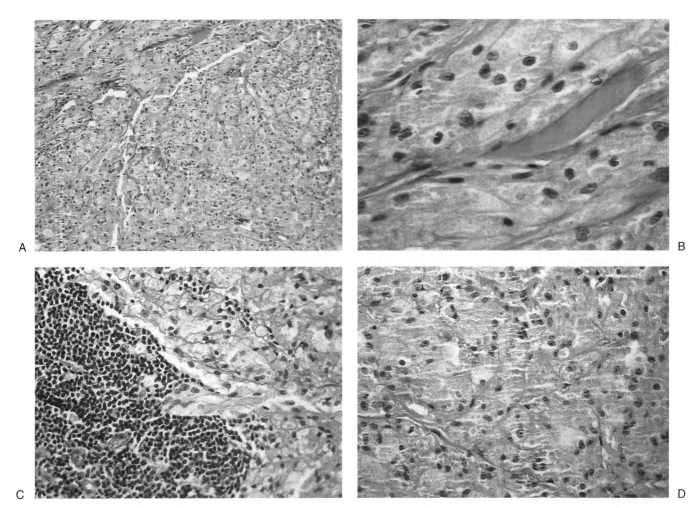

**FIG. 40.50.** *Granular cell tumor, malignant.* **A,B:** The histologic appearance of the cells in the primary tumor is not exceptional. **C,D:** Metastatic granular cell tumor in an axillary lymph node that arose from the tumor shown in **A** and **B**.

## TUMORS OF NERVE AND NERVE SHEATH ORIGIN

Benign neural neoplasms commonly found in the soft tissues at various sites occur rarely in the breast. Benign nerve sheath tumors of the breast have been reported, usually diagnosed as "neurilemomas" or as schwannomas (136–139). Many of these tumors arose in the mammary subcutaneous tissue, but parenchymal lesions also were described. Patients with von Recklinghausen's disease develop neurofibromas in the subcutaneous tissues and the breast, but massive neurofibromatosis of the breast is uncommon (140,141). A patient with two schwannomas of one breast has been reported (142). The age range at diagnosis is 15 to 81 years, with most patients in their 30s to 50s. Although most patients have been female, benign neural neoplasms of the male breast have been described (143,144). A patient with von Recklinghausen's disease can develop mammary carcinoma; therefore, the appearance of a new breast tumor should prompt appropriate diagnostic evaluation (145).

The lesion presents as a painless, well-defined mass that is clinically indistinguishable from a fibroadenoma. Either breast may be involved, and there is no predilection for a specific site in the breast. One tumor measured 14 cm in greatest diameter (146), but most are smaller and one schwannoma was an asymptomatic 7-mm lesion detected by mammography (147).

Grossly, the circumscribed tumor consists of dense, firm gray or white tissue that may have soft mucoid regions (Fig. 40.51). Microscopic examination reveals the typical histologic features of a benign nerve sheath tumor, consisting of spindle cells in bundles, sometimes with nuclei arranged in a palisading pattern (Antoni type A). Less cellular areas with thick-walled blood vessels, the Antoni B pattern, may be present as well. Vascular thrombi, hyalinized blood vessels, cells with atypical nuclei, and xanthomatous areas are found in sclerotic schwannomas.

The differential diagnosis includes other spindle cell tumors such as fibroadenomas, phyllodes tumor, fibromatosis, and metaplastic carcinoma. These lesions usually are readily distinguished in histologic sections, but difficulty may be encountered in material obtained by fine needle aspiration

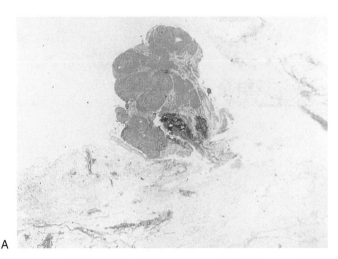

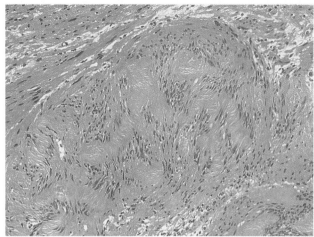

A

B

**FIG. 40.51.** *Schwannoma.* **A:** Whole-mount histologic section of a circumscribed, nodular tumor that presented as a nonpalpable lesion detected by mammography. Hemorrhage in the lesion is the result of a needle core biopsy. **B:** Palisading of tumor cells. (Courtesy of Dr. S. Hoda.)

(142,144,148,149). The nuclei of cells seen in the aspirate typically are spindly or oval with homogeneous fine chromatin. Pleomorphic irregular, hyperchromatic nuclei may be encountered, particularly in the lesions termed "ancient" nerve sheath tumors (150). The diagnosis of a benign peripheral nerve sheath tumor is supported by a positive immunohistochemical stain for S-100 protein, a negative immunostain for actin, and the absence of mitotic activity. Palisaded cells may be evident in an fine needle aspiration specimen (136). Complete excision provides adequate therapy.

## HAMARTOMA

*Stedman's Medical Dictionary* defines hamartoma as "a focal malformation that resembles a neoplasm, grossly and even microscopically, but results from faulty development in an organ; it is composed of an abnormal mixture of tissue elements, or an abnormal proportion of a single element normally present at that site . . ." (151).

This term was applied to lesions of the breast in 1971 by Arrigoni et al. (152), who described 10 patients with encapsulated breast tumors that clinically and grossly resembled fibroadenomas. Microscopic examination revealed "mammary glandular tissue with a prominent lobular arrangement, fibrous stroma, and fat in variable proportions." Cystic and papillary apocrine metaplasia were evident in some lesions.

There has been a tendency among some authors to use the diagnosis of mammary hamartoma broadly and to apply it to a variety of benign circumscribed lesions, such as PASH (153,154). That the radiologic appearances of these lesions are quite similar has reinforced this misconception, which obscures the definition of hamartoma by lumping together several pathologically distinct lesions. This is exemplified by one lesion diagnosed as mammary hamartoma, which was reported twice with identical illustrations, but is an ex-

ample of PASH (155,156). Two tumors reported to be "multiple hamartomas" in the breast of a 20-year-old woman had a radiologic appearance consistent with this diagnosis but appear grossly and histologically to be fibroadenomas (157). In another case report, a 14-cm mass with the radiologic appearance of a hamartoma proved to be "juvenile hypertrophy" histologically (158).

Tumors that best qualify as hamartoma of the breast occur most often in premenopausal women, but they have been described in teenagers and in women in their 60s. Association with pregnancy has been noted in a minority of cases (159). Some patients report slow enlargement, whereas others describe rapid growth. The tumors have been as large as 17 cm, often resulting in substantial asymmetry. In some cases, large tumors responsible for macromastia may not be palpable as distinct lesions, although they are clearly evident in a mammogram. Mammography reveals a well-circumscribed, dense, round or oval mass surrounded by a narrow lucent zone (159–161). Hamartomas of the breast were diagnosed in 16 of 10,000 mammography examinations reviewed by Hessler et al. (161). The ultrasound appearance of mammary hamartoma is reported to be variable and not specific, an observation that reflects intrinsic differences in the lesions and probably inclusion of assorted entities in this diagnostic category (162). The two common variants of mammary hamartoma are *adenolipoma* and *chondrolipoma*.

*Adenolipoma* has a broad age distribution, having been reported in women in their 20s and 80s (163). The mean age at diagnosis in the largest series was 45 years (161). Several patients were pregnant. The presenting symptom is a painless mass that measures up to 13 cm in diameter. On clinical examination, the tumor forms a dominant mass that may be well defined and mobile or indistinct. In some cases, the lesion is difficult to appreciate on palpation, although it is readily apparent by mammography. Radiologic exam demonstrates a sharply defined round or oval tumor that appears to be encapsulated and surrounded by a radiolucent

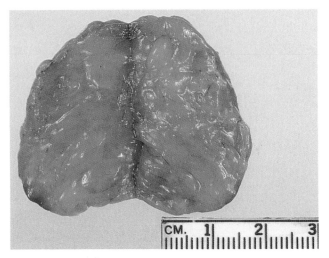

**FIG. 40.52.** *Hamartoma, gross appearance.*

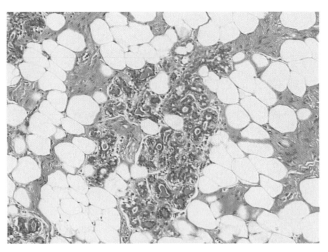

**FIG. 40.54.** *Hamartoma, adenolipoma type.* Lobular aggregates lack distinctive stroma and tend to blend with the fat.

ring. Predominantly fatty tumors may have the lucent appearance of lipomas, whereas those with abundant glandular tissue appear dense (161,163,164). Ultrasonography reveals a mixed pattern of echogenic and sonolucent regions (165).

Gross examination discloses a soft, circumscribed, sometimes lobulated mass bordered by a thin fibrous pseudocapsule (Fig. 40.52). The cut surface has a variegated pattern of fat and fibrous breast parenchyma. Lesions with the most abundant fat resemble lipomas. Small cysts may be seen.

Microscopically, the tissue consists of mature fat and mammary parenchyma mixed in varying proportions, delimited by a pseudocapsule of compressed breast tissue (Fig. 40.53). Lobules and ducts present in the lesion appear structurally normal, with little or no proliferative change. The most significant abnormality is the unusual tissue distribution (Fig. 40.54). In this setting, the term *dysplastic* has been used to describe the structural composition of the lesion, rather than proliferative and cytologic abnormalities (161).

Adenolipoma differs structurally from other mammary lesions that contain fat. It lacks the adenomatous component seen in fibroadenomas with adipose metaplasia and does not exhibit the cytologic atypia seen in phyllodes tumors with adipose stroma (166).

Adenolipoma should be treated by excisional biopsy. Good cosmetic results have been reported, even when tumors larger than a quadrant were treated by excision (161).

*Chondrolipomas* are composed of mature adipose tissue and hyaline cartilage (149,167–169). The patients have been adult women 37 to 79 years of age who presented with palpable tumors. One tumor was present for several years, but most were noted no more than 2 months before diagnosis. Several chondrolipomas measured 2 cm in diameter, and one lesion was 6 cm. Mammography revealed a well-circumscribed mass without calcification resembling a fibroadenoma. In one case, the radiographic findings were described as "probably mammary dysplasia" (169).

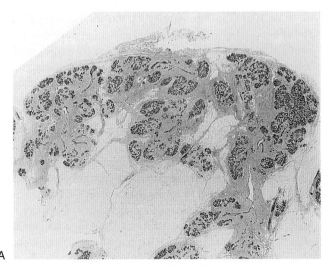

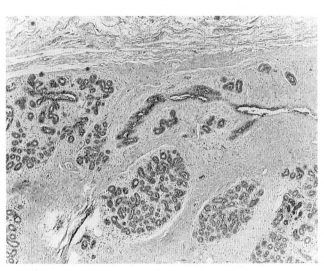

**FIG. 40.53.** *Hamartoma, adenolipoma type.* **A:** Nodular aggregates of lobular breast parenchyma in a circumscribed lipomatous tumor. **B:** Lobular structure is normal. Note circumscribed tumor border above.

The excised tumor is a soft or rubbery, circumscribed, lobulated mass composed of gray or pink-white tissue that is not obviously fat. Plate-like foci of cartilage and gritty areas may be evident grossly (167). Microscopic examination reveals sharply defined islands of hyaline cartilage distributed in mature fat and fibrofatty glandular mammary parenchyma. Smooth muscle was been noted rarely, and these lesions probably are myofibroblastomas with chondroid and myoid differentiation (170). The margin of the tumor is demarcated by compressed mammary tissue resulting in an encapsulated appearance (169). Glandular elements were absent from the main tumor in two lesions (169,171,172). The cytologic specimen obtained by fine needle aspiration reveals benign hyaline cartilage and fat (172).

Chondrolipoma is treated by excisional biopsy. No recurrences have been reported.

## LEIOMYOMA

Most *leiomyomas* of the breast arise from smooth muscle in the nipple and areola (173). Parenchymal leiomyomas

probably arise as a result of smooth muscle metaplasia of myoepithelial or myofibroblastic cells or from blood vessels (Fig. 40.55). Myoid differentiation of myofibroblastic cells was discussed and illustrated earlier in this chapter. The diagnosis of leiomyoma should be restricted to lesions composed entirely of smooth muscle. Fibroadenomas (174) and sclerosing adenosis (175) with myomatous metaplasia should be excluded from this category. The so-called *adenoleiomyoma* described by Haagensen (176) is an example of adenosis with leiomyomatous hyperplasia of myoepithelial cells.

### Clinical Presentation

Leiomyoma of the breast presents as a palpable, solitary mass. Pain or discomfort has been reported with parenchymal and nipple lesions. There is no predilection as to the location of parenchymal lesions. Patients tend to be middle aged, ranging in age from 34 to 69 years. Radiologic examination of a parenchymal leiomyoma revealed a circumscribed 3-cm tumor without calcification (177). A

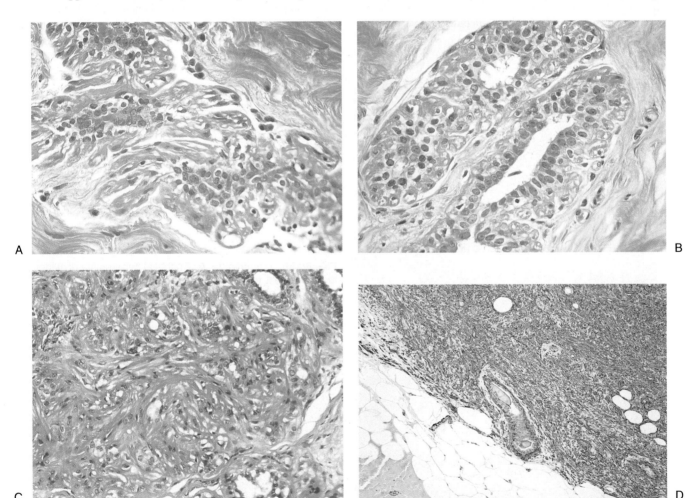

**FIG. 40.55.** *Myoid metaplasia of myoepithelial cells.* **A:** Myoepithelial cells with a myoid phenotype are cut longitudinally in this section of a terminal duct–lobular complex. **B:** Myoid myoepithelial cells are cut transversely in this section of a duct. **C:** Nodular myoid metaplasia in sclerosing adenosis. **D:** Actin immunostain of a lesion similar to **C** showing abundant myoepithelial cells with a myoid phenotype (avidin-biotin).

nonpalpable leiomyoma was detected in the course of routine follow-up mammography of a 50-year-old woman receiving adjuvant tamoxifen for a prior contralateral invasive carcinoma (178). The tumor was a distinct, slightly lobulated oval nodule 9 mm in largest dimension. Leiomyoma of the male breast has been reported (179). The mammographic appearance of a subareolar leiomyoma of the male breast was described by Velasco et al. (180).

### Pathology

Grossly, the tumor forms a firm, circumscribed mass with a whorled cut surface. Tumors as large as 13 cm have been reported, but most are smaller than 5 cm.

Microscopically, circumscription also is evident. The growth pattern features interlacing fascicles of spindle cells with eosinophilic cytoplasm (Fig. 40.56). Cytologic atypia, mitoses, and necrosis, which characterize leiomyosarcoma, are absent. An epithelioid variant of mammary parenchymal leiomyoma was described by Roncaroli et al. (181). The tumor cells had fine granular cytoplasm and were immunoreactive for desmin and actin, but not for S-100 protein. Similar staining results are obtained in nonepithelioid variants of mammary leiomyoma.

### Treatment and Prognosis

Complete excision is recommended. This may necessitate removing the nipple if the lesion is in the subareolar region or nipple. Local recurrence has rarely been reported (173,182). Two of the recurrences were treated by reexcision. A third recurrence growing as leiomyosarcoma with mitoses and necrosis was treated by mastectomy (182).

## MYOID "HAMARTOMA"

This tumor, also termed *muscular hamartoma,* is a benign proliferative lesion composed of ducts, lobules, stroma, and bands of smooth muscle cells. Most examples of this neoplasm are adenosis tumors with leiomyomatous myoid metaplasia of the myoepithelial cell component. Regrettably, the designation of these tumors as hamartomas is now well entrenched in the literature.

### Clinical Presentation

Myoid "hamartoma" forms a circumscribed palpable tumor ranging from 2 to 11 cm in diameter (183–185). A duration of 5 years or longer sometimes is reported (186,187). The tumor is located most often in the upper outer quadrant.

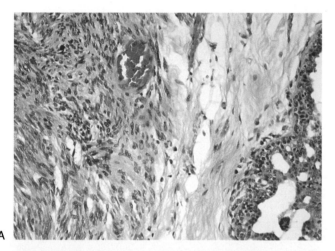

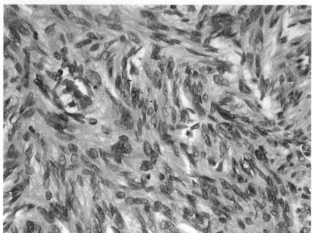

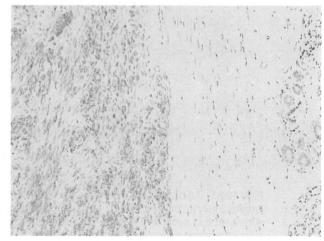

**FIG. 40.56.** *Leiomyoma.* **A:** Epithelial hyperplasia is evident in a duct next to the tumor. **B:** Interlacing spindle cells that have oval nuclei. **C:** Cytoplasm is immunoreactive for desmin (avidin-biotin).

Mammography reveals a well-demarcated lesion of variable density, often with a radiolucent halo (184,185,187,188). Cystic areas may be suggested by the radiographic appearance or by sonography (184–186).

### Gross Pathology

The tumor is a grossly well-circumscribed, bosselated, firm mass appearing fibrous on the cut surface. Adipose tissue usually is not evident grossly in the lesion. Cysts of varying size containing brown fluid have been described in a minority of cases (184,186,187).

### Microscopic Pathology

The histologic composition of myoid "hamartomas" is variable, depending on the relative proportions of glandular, cystic, myomatous, and fibrous elements. In most lesions, interlacing bundles of smooth muscle constitute focal leiomyoma formation. In a minority of tumors, the myoid component mingles more diffusely with adipose and fibrous tissue. Epithelioid

differentiation of myoepithelial cells can result in a pattern resembling infiltrating lobular carcinoma, especially in the limited sample of a needle core biopsy (185). Adequate sampling reveals foci of sclerosing adenosis in virtually all examples of myoid "hamartoma." At these sites, origin of the myoid element can be traced to myoepithelial cells (Figs. 40.55 and 40.57) (189). Associated "fibrocystic changes" include cystic apocrine metaplasia and duct hyperplasia. The histologic features of myoid "hamartoma" have been found in a fibroadenoma, a not unexpected observation because sclerosing adenosis develops occasionally in fibroadenomas (187).

Electron microscopy and immunohistochemistry confirm the myoid character of the spindle cell component of the lesion and support origin from myoepithelial cells (183,186,187).

### Treatment and Prognosis

Myoid "hamartoma" is adequately treated by excisional biopsy performed by "shelling out" the tumor. There is no tendency to local recurrence, multifocality, or bilaterality.

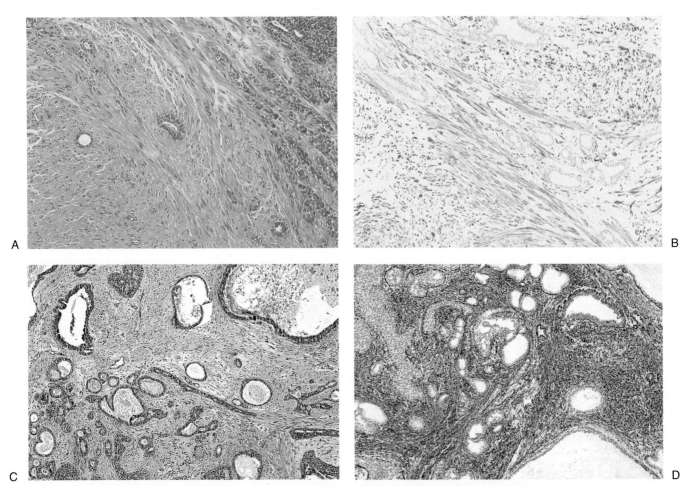

**FIG. 40.57.** *Myoid "hamartoma."* **A:** Myomatous nodule *(lower left)* in the tumor adjacent to sclerosing adenosis. A few glands remain in the myomatous area. **B:** Desmin reactivity in the myomatous tissue around sclerosing adenosis (avidin-biotin). **C:** Another lesion in which cystic adenosis glands are surrounded by myomatous stroma. **D:** Smooth muscle actin immunoreactivity in the stroma (avidin-biotin).

## MYELOID METAPLASIA

Tumorous extramedullary hematopoiesis (myeloid meta-plasia) may involve virtually any organ. The breast is one of the least frequent sites of this condition (190–192). In most instances, tumorous myeloid metaplasia occurs late in the course of myelosclerosis or myelofibrosis, and multiple sites are involved. Lesions limited to the breast (190) or breast and axillary lymph nodes (192) are unusual. The circumscribed firm tumor may suggest carcinoma clinically (192).

Histologic examination reveals fibrosis of the breast parenchyma, with a diffuse infiltrate of mature hematopoietic cells. Megakaryocytes with large, hyperchromatic nuclei are conspicuous. Association of the infiltrate with vascular structures has been reported (192). Axillary lymph nodes may harbor the same infiltrate. To the unwary, the infiltrative pattern and fibrosis may suggest an infiltrating carcinoma, especially if the tissue is not well fixed. The presence of myeloid cells can be confirmed with the Leder stain for myeloperoxidase.

## MYXOMA

A myxoma presented as a slowly enlarging tumor of the left breast in a 19-year-old woman (193). The lesion measured 6.5 cm in the subareolar region. An ultrasound study was interpreted as a "mucinous cyst." The patient remained well 1 year after radical mastectomy. Grossly, the tumor was a well-defined multinodular mass involving subcutaneous tissue and the breast parenchyma. Microscopic examination revealed hypocellular myxoid neoplastic tissue containing stellate and spindle-shaped undifferentiated mesenchymal cells (Fig. 40.58). Chondroid and lipoblastic differentiation were absent. The myxoid material was positive with Alcian blue at pH 2.5, which did not stain the neoplastic cells. A few

tumor cells were weakly immunoreactive for S-100 and $\alpha_1$-antichymotrypsin. There was no reactivity for $\alpha_1$-antitrypsin, vimentin, epithelial membrane antigen, cytokeratin, or estrogen and progesterone receptors. Electron microscopy of the cells revealed abundant dilated rough endoplasmic reticulum, scant secondary lysosomes, and no junctional complexes or basal lamina. Another example of mammary myxoma was described in a 64-year-old woman (194). The tumor measured 8 cm and lacked electron microscopic features of a myxoid neurofibroma. Although these appear to have been benign lesions, the reported follow-up was brief at best. In a case examined by the author, local recurrence and progression to high-grade sarcoma with features of malignant fibrous histiocytoma were observed.

The differential diagnosis of myxoma includes myxoid neurofibroma, myxoid sarcoma, myxoid fibroadenoma, and myxoid stromal change (myxomatosis). The latter two lesions, reported to occur in the breast of patients with Carney's syndrome, are the result of a specific genetic defect that results in excessive production of proteoglycans by stromal cells (195). The presence of epithelial elements and multiple myxoid nodules distinguishes these conditions from myxoma. Strong immunoreactivity with markers of neural differentiation, such as S-100, serves to identify myxoid neurofibroma (196).

## MUCINOSIS

The histogenesis of this extremely rare stromal tumor has not been determined. Michal et al. (197) described three patients, one man 40 years old and two women 28 and 29 years old. They did not have evidence of Carney's syndrome. Mucinosis has been described in the nipple (197,198), but it may occur at other sites in the breast. The lesion consists of myxoid material in fibrocollagenous stroma (Fig. 40.59). Epithelial elements are not evident in routine sections, and

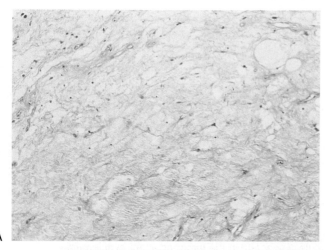
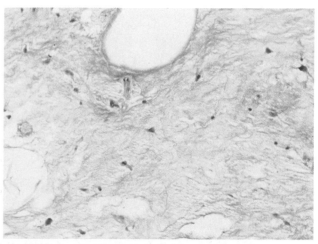

A                                                                                                 B

**FIG. 40.58.** *Myxoma.* **A,B:** The tumor is hypocellular and consists of cytologically benign, widely scattered cells with ill-defined cytoplasm suspended in myxoid stromal matrix.

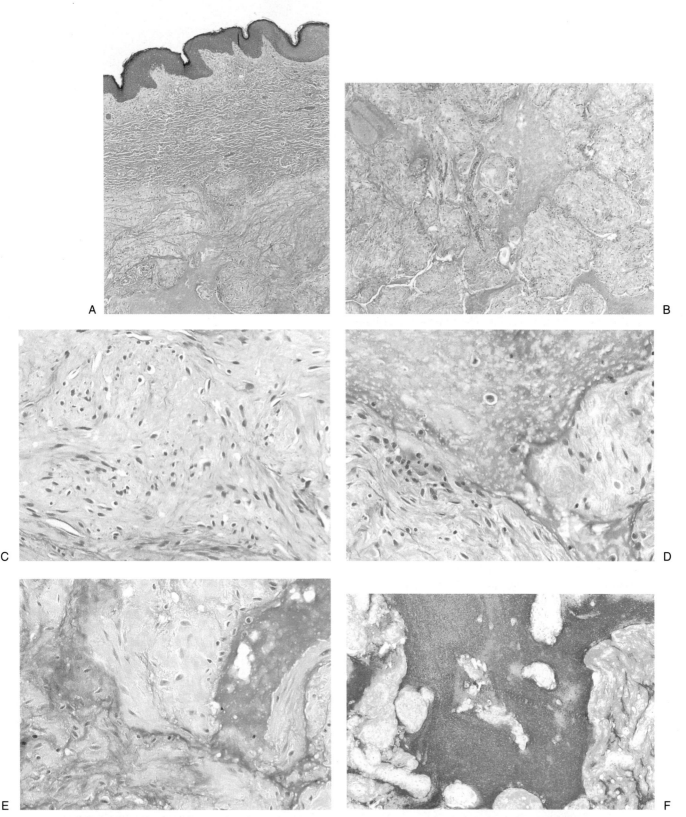

**FIG. 40.59.** *Mucinosis.* **A:** This lesion occurred in the nipple of a 16-year-old girl. No duct structures are evident in the basophilic myxoid stromal tumor. **B:** Serpiginous myxoid deposits in the vascularized stroma. A few histiocytes are evident at this magnification. **C:** Basophilic material is present in the stroma. **D:** A few histiocytes scattered in the myxoid substance and at its interface with the collagenous stroma should not be mistaken for epithelial cells. **E:** Myxoid material stains with the mucicarmine stain in the stroma and in isolated deposits. **F:** Intense staining with colloidal iron.

they are not demonstrated with immunostains for cytokeratin. The basophilic myxoid substance forms distinct, irregular pools that contain scattered histiocytes, and it also is dispersed in the fibrocollagenous matrix from which it appears to arise. This stromal myxoid material stains intensely with the Alcian blue and colloidal iron stains (197). Alcian blue and colloidal iron staining are diastase resistant and are eliminated by hyaluronidase treatment. It is imperative that a diagnosis of mucinous carcinoma or mucocele-like tumor be ruled out by carefully searching for epithelial elements. Further investigation will be needed to determine if mucinosis is related to pathologic changes in the breast that have been associated with Carney's syndrome (199).

## LIPOMA

Lipomas of the breast usually are solitary tumors, but multiple lipomas may be encountered. Many of these lesions are located in the subcutaneous fat. The tumors are circumscribed, well-defined masses of mature adipose tissue. In some instances, a clinically palpable lesion proves to be mature fat without the characteristic circumscription of lipoma. Fat necrosis within a lipoma may present as a spiculated lesion on mammography (200).

*Hibernomas* are tumors composed of brown fat. In the mammary region, hibernomas occur in the axillary tail of the breast or in the axilla (Fig. 40.60).

*Fibrolipomas* are grossly well-circumscribed tumors composed of mature adipose tissue and collagenous stroma that contain prominent fibroblasts (Fig. 40.61). Microscopically, the lesion may blend with glandular parenchyma. The stromal cells do not manifest myoid features of myofibroblasts.

*Spindle cell lipomas* rarely occur in the breast (201–203). One lesion presented as an asymptomatic, 2.1-cm, well-circumscribed mass on mammography that was hyperechoic on ultrasonography (203). Biopsy reveals lipomatous tissue

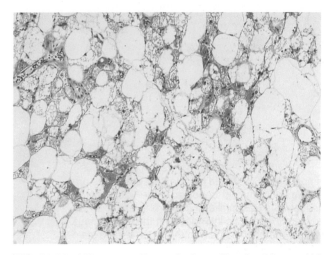

**FIG. 40.60.** *Hibernoma.* Tumor in the axilla of a 24-year-old woman.

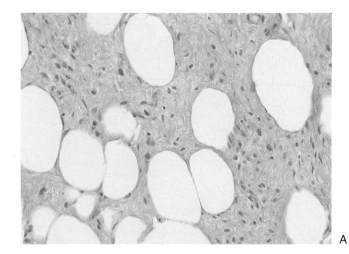

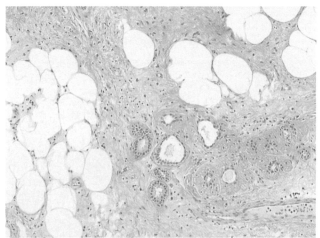

**FIG. 40.61.** *Fibrolipoma.* **A:** Cellular collagenous stroma and fat cells. **B:** Lobular glands present in the lesion.

mixed with spindly myofibroblasts and variably collagenous stroma (Fig. 40.62). CD34 immunoreactivity can be demonstrated in the myofibroblastic component (204).

## ANGIOMAS AND OTHER BENIGN VASCULAR LESIONS OF THE BREAST

The majority of the vascular lesions of the breast described in published reports have been angiosarcomas. Major textbooks of breast or surgical pathology emphasize the need for extreme caution in the interpretation of grossly evident vascular tumors, because portions of angiosarcomas may appear deceptively bland histologically. Azzopardi (205) indicated that "a benign angioma has never to date constituted a palpable or symptom-producing breast tumor." McDivitt et al. (206) stated that "after the perilobular angiomas have been eliminated, it must be inferred that all the capillary tumors . . . [of the breast] . . . are malignant."

Pathologic analysis of more than 400 mammary vascular tumors studied by the author has revealed diverse grossly ev-

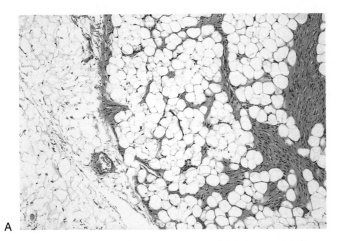

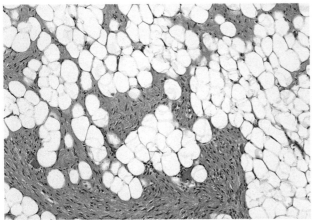

**FIG. 40.62.** *Spindle cell lipoma.* **A:** Tumor has a distinct border *(left).* **B:** Spindle cells in collagenous stroma course through the lipomatous fat.

ident angiomas and other nonmalignant vascular lesions of the breast, as well as nonparenchymal hemangiomas of the mammary subcutaneous fat (Table 40.1).

## PERILOBULAR HEMANGIOMAS

### Clinical Presentation

The perilobular hemangioma is a microscopic benign vascular lesion detected in sections of breast tissue taken to

**TABLE 40.1.** *Benign vascular lesions of the breast*

Perilobular hemangioma
Hemangioma (cavernous, capillary, or complex)
Angiomatosis (lymphangiomatosis)
Venous hemangioma
Subcutaneous nonparenchymal hemangiomas
   Angiolipoma
   Cavernous
   Capillary
   Juvenile
   Venous
   Papillary endothelial hyperplasia
Aneurysm

**TABLE 40.2.** *Perilobular hemangiomas*

| Feature evaluated | Authors of study | |
| --- | --- | --- |
| | Rosen and Ridolfi (209) | Lesueur et al. (208) |
| Type of specimen | Surgical mastectomy | Forensic autopsy |
| Laterality | 519 unilateral, 18 bilateral | 210 bilateral |
| Number of patients | 537 | 210 |
| Number of breasts | 555 | 420 |
| Number of patients with hemangioma | 7 | 23 |
| Percentage of patients with hemangioma | 1.3 | 11 |

evaluate various unrelated benign and malignant lesions (207). Although a few have reportedly measured between 2 and 4 mm on histologic section, none were grossly apparent (208,209). The presence of these vascular lesions is not appreciated until the tissue has been examined microscopically.

Two studies (Table 40.2) evaluated the frequency and clinicopathologic features of perilobular hemangiomas (208,209). They were found in 1.3% of mastectomies performed for carcinoma (209), 4.5% of biopsies for benign breast lesions, and in 11% of women whose breast tissue was sampled in forensic autopsies (208). The age distribution apparently reflects the ages of patients studied. Patients with perilobular hemangiomas found at autopsy ranged in age from 29 to 82 years (mean, 51.5 years) (208).

### Microscopic Pathology

Multiple perilobular hemangiomas may be found in one breast, and a number of patients had these lesions in both breasts (208–210). Microscopically, perilobular hemangiomas are not limited to a perilobular distribution (Fig. 40.63). Many are partially or completely within the lobular stroma (208,209,211), whereas others are located in extralobular stroma, sometimes in proximity to ducts, or apparently in no particular relationship to a duct or lobule (209) (Fig. 40.64). In a series studied by Lesueur et al. (208), only two of 32 microscopic hemangiomas had a perilobular position. Although the term *perilobular* does not accurately describe the microanatomic distribution of many of these lesions, it is widely used and there is no compelling reason to propose an alternative name.

Perilobular hemangiomas often can be identified at low magnification because they usually contain many red blood cells. In some instances, the contents lack erythrocytes and consist of fluid that may be lymph. The lesion typically is a sharply defined collection of small, distinct vascular channels arranged in a meshwork fashion. Rarely it may have ill-defined borders with vessels that extend into the adjacent fatty and fibrous stroma. The vessels vary in caliber from capillary size to ectatic miniature cavernous channels. Anas-

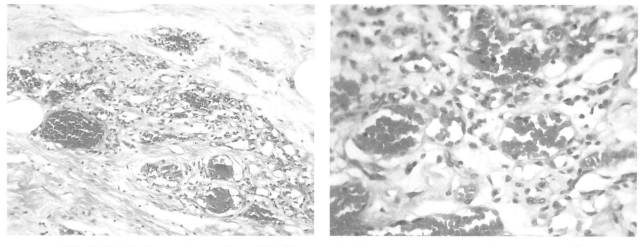

**FIG. 40.63.** *Perilobular hemangioma.* **A,B:** Circumscribed hemangioma composed of congested capillaries is located in the extralobular stroma.

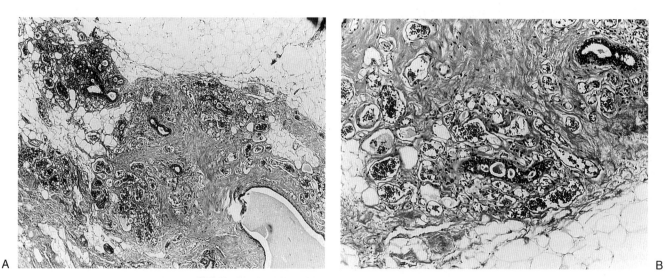

**FIG. 40.64.** *Perilobular hemangioma.* **A,B:** Capillary proliferation mingles with lobules and surrounds small ducts. (**A:** From Jozefczyk MA, Rosen PP. Vascular tumors of the breast. II. Perilobular hemangiomas and hemangioma. *Am J Surg Pathol* 1985;9:491–503, with permssion.)

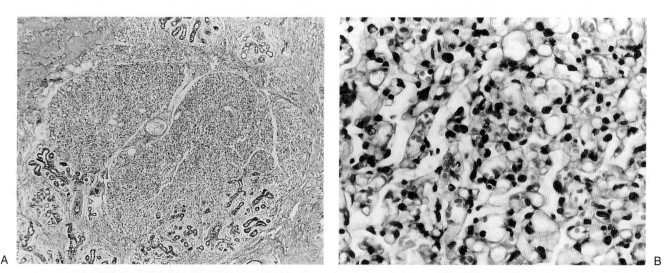

**FIG. 40.65.** *Perilobular hemangioma.* This 2-mm lesion has previously been referred to as an "atypical" hemangioma. **A:** The compact circumscribed lesion involving intralobular and perilobular stroma is subdivided by fibrous septae. The well-formed central vessel is probably a branch of the feeding vessel. **B:** Capillary channels, some anastomosing, with prominent hyperchromatic nuclei are present. (From Jozefczyk MA, Rosen PP. Vascular tumors of the breast. II. Perilobular hemangiomas and hemangioma. *Am J Surg Pathol* 1985;9:491–503, with permssion.)

tomosing channels may be seen. The thin, delicate vessels consist of endothelial cells encased in inconspicuous stroma without a supporting smooth muscle coat. It is not unusual to find varying numbers of lymphocytes in the stroma regardless of the presence or absence of erythrocytes within the vascular spaces.

Some microscopic vascular lesions with the general features of perilobular hemangiomas have endothelial cells that appear cytologically atypical because they have prominent, hyperchromatic nuclei (207). Interconnected channels often are present, but endothelial papillary proliferation, mitotic activity, and extensive vascular anastomoses are not seen in these so-called *atypical perilobular hemangiomas*. Most atypical perilobular hemangiomas have rounded, circumscribed contours and are separated into aggregates of vessels or vascular lobules by slender fibrous septa (Fig. 40.65). A few lesions with irregular margins have been noted (Fig. 40.66).

### Prognosis and Treatment

Perilobular hemangiomas, whether unifocal, multiple, or bilateral, require no treatment. There is no evidence that angiosarcoma arises from these lesions, although the existence of cytologically atypical variants leaves this issue open to speculation. Given the rarity of mammary angiosarcoma and the relatively frequent detection of perilobular hemangiomas in "normal" breast tissue or in specimens examined for various unrelated conditions, malignant transformation of perilobular hemangiomas must be exceedingly uncommon, if it does occur it all.

Whether treated by mastectomy or local excision, no patient with an atypical perilobular hemangioma is known to

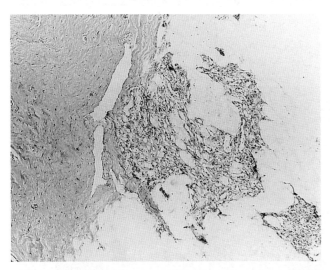

**FIG. 40.66.** *Perilobular hemangioma.* Irregularly shaped capillary proliferation in extralobular fibrofatty tissue previously characterized as atypical. A dilated feeder vessel is present at the left border of the lesion. (From Jozefczyk MA, Rosen PP. Vascular tumors of the breast. II. Perilobular hemangiomas and hemangioma. *Am J Surg Pathol* 1985;9: 491–503, with permssion.)

have experienced recurrence of the lesion or progression to angiosarcoma. No treatment other than local excision is recommended for atypical perilobular hemangiomas.

## HEMANGIOMAS

### Clinical Presentation

Hemangiomas are benign vascular tumors large enough to be clinically palpable or detected by mammography (207). The lesions measure between 0.3 and 2.5 cm, and they occur in patients ranging in age from 18 months to 82 years (207,212,213). Magnetic resonance imaging was used to assess the relationship of the hemangioma to the breast bud in the infantile and immature breasts of patients 5 months to 7 years old (214). Multiple mammary hemangiomas were demonstrated by magnetic resonance imaging in the breast of a 41-year-old woman with Kasabach-Merritt syndrome (215).

A substantial number of hemangiomas currently are detected by mammography, with no clinically palpable tumor (Fig. 40.67), or by ultrasonography (Fig. 40.68). Nonpalpable hemangiomas range in size from 0.4 to 2.0 cm, with a mean diameter of 0.9 cm. The majority of patients have been women 19 to 82 years of age (mean, 60 years). The mammographic appearance usually is that of a well-defined, lobulated mass that may have fine or coarse calcifications (216,217). Almost all palpable vascular tumors of the male breast have been hemangiomas.

### Gross Pathology

Grossly, hemangiomas tend to be well circumscribed. There is no predilection for any particular location in the breast. Palpable lesions are described as firm.

### Microscopic Pathology

Most hemangiomas have well-circumscribed borders grossly, but microscopically the vascular channels may blend with the surrounding breast parenchyma. As part of this process, the vessels are infrequently seen within lobules, although they much more often grow around and displace glandular structures.

*Cavernous hemangiomas* are the most common form of mammary hemangioma. The lesion typically is described as a dark-red or brown circumscribed mass that may grossly appear spongy (207,212,218). Microscopic examination reveals dilated vessels congested with red blood cells (Fig. 40.69). Small vessels of capillary dimension may be seen in portions of a cavernous hemangioma. The individual channels appear to be independent, with few if any anastomosing vessels (Fig. 40.70). Endothelial nuclei are inconspicuous and flat. The vessels are supported by fibrous stroma that tends to be more prominent toward the central part of the tumor. Calcification may occur in the stroma (207,212). Thrombosis within cavernous channels sometimes elicits a

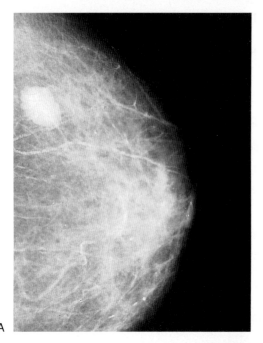

A

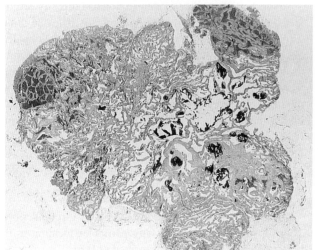

B

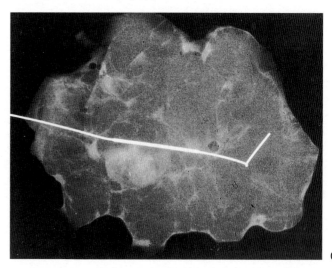

C

**FIG. 40.67.** *Hemangioma, mammography.* **A:** The lesion is a well-circumscribed lobulated oval mass in this mammogram. **B:** Whole-mount histologic section of the hemangioma shown in **A**. **C:** Radiographic appearance of a different hemangioma in a biopsy specimen with a localization wire.

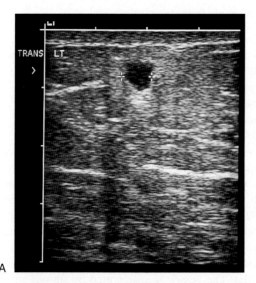

A

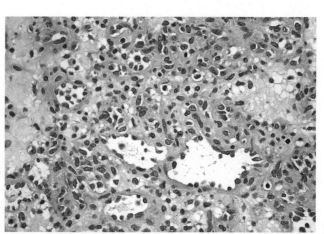

B

**FIG. 40.68.** *Hemangioma, ultrasonography.* **A:** The dark circumscribed nodule between the markers in this ultrasound image was a hemangioma. **B:** The lesion was a compact capillary hemangioma shown here.

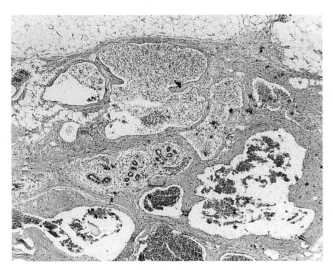

**FIG. 40.69.** *Cavernous hemangioma.* Dilated, congested vascular spaces surround a lobule.

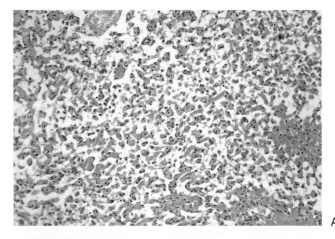

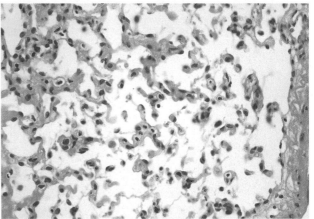

**FIG. 40.71.** *Papillary endothelial hyperplasia in cavernous hemangioma.* **A,B:** Vascular space is filled with a complex network of fibrous stroma lined by endothelial cells with conspicuous, hyperchromatic nuclei.

lymphocytic reaction, and endothelial proliferation may be seen within the organizing clot. These alterations can result in papillary endothelial hyperplasia that should not be mistaken for angiosarcoma (Fig. 40.71).

There is considerable variability in the degree of circumscription seen microscopically. In many cavernous hemangiomas, vascular channels drift into the fatty parenchyma, becoming smaller at the periphery. This pattern duplicates the histologic appearance of peripheral parts of some well-differentiated angiosarcomas (Fig. 40.72).

Other types of hemangioma comprise a heterogeneous group of lesions. Because of their dimensions, atypical cytologic features in some instances, and concern that they might be precursors of angiosarcoma, many were initially characterized as "atypical" hemangiomas (207). Additional follow-up has demonstrated that so-called *atypical* angiomas are not borderline or low-grade variants of angiosarcoma and provides no evidence that they predispose to the development of

angiosarcoma (212). Consequently, they should simply be classified as types of *noncavernous hemangiomas* for which the designation "atypical" is no longer warranted in most cases.

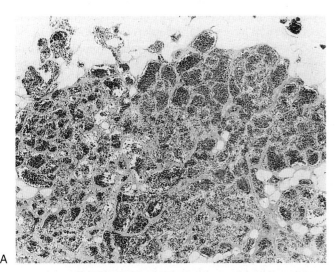

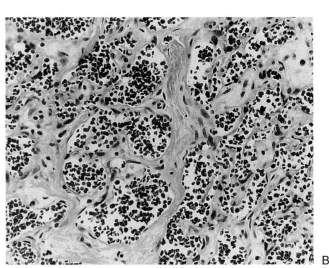

**FIG. 40.70.** *Cavernous hemangioma.* **A:** The core of the lesion is a compact mass of separate distended, congested vascular channels. **B:** Fibrous septae extend between the vascular spaces lined by inconspicuous endothelium.

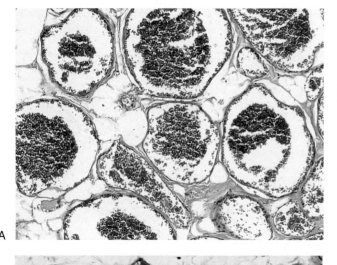

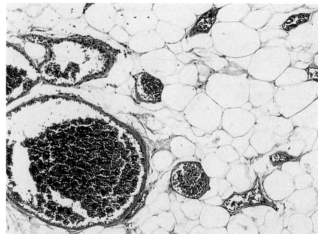

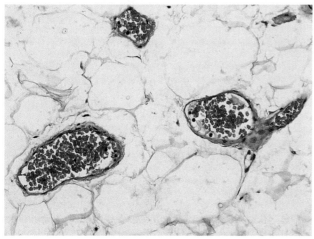

**FIG. 40.72.** *Cavernous hemangioma.* **A:** Cavernous vascular channels are present in the *center* of the lesion. **B,C:** Smaller vessels extend into the fat at the periphery.

Microscopically, slender fibrous septa frequently divide noncavernous hemangiomas into segments resulting in a lobulated structure. Some of the tumors have prominent anastomosing vascular channels. Papillary endothelial hyperplasia may be present, usually at sites of organizing thrombosis. Florid papillary endothelial hyperplasia can obscure the basic angiomatous character of the lesion or even suggest a well-differentiated angiosarcoma (219). When present in the breast, papillary endothelial hyperplasia invariably arises in a hemangioma, and it does not represent a specific category of breast tumor. Mast cells frequently are present individually or in small clusters.

*Capillary hemangiomas* tend to be cellular and to superficially resemble pyogenic granulomas. The mean gross size of these hemangiomas is 1.0 cm. Many of these lesions have been detected by mammography. Microscopically, capillary hemangiomas are composed of small, vascular channels lined by endothelial cells that may have hyperchromatic nuclei (Fig. 40.73). Fibrous bands are variably present subdividing the lesion. Larger, muscular vessels may be found within and at the periphery of the tumor, apparently constituting branches of a *feeding vessel* or vessels (Fig. 40.74).

These are nonneoplastic muscular vessels with features of arteries and/or veins. Often, the muscular component of these vessels seems malformed or incomplete, and the vessels have a sinuous character. The resultant configuration suggests that the hemangioma arose from the feeding vessel. Capillary hemangiomas usually are well circumscribed, but some lesions have irregular borders (Fig. 40.75).

Some hemangiomas have a more complex vascular pattern consisting of dilated vascular channels of varying size as well as compact, dense aggregates of capillary structures (Fig. 40.76). Many of these *complex hemangiomas,* which measure 1.0 cm or less (average, 0.7 cm), have been detected by mammography. A feeding vessel may be evident at the periphery of the tumor. Some complex hemangiomas have conspicuous anastomosing vascular channels (Fig. 40.77).

Hemorrhage and infarction can occur in hemangiomas, especially lesions detected radiologically and subjected to needle core biopsy or needle localization excision (Fig. 40.78). This should not be confused with the pattern of hemorrhagic necrosis that results in the formation of "blood lakes" characteristically found in high grade angiosarcomas. Calcification may occur in organized thrombi, sometimes associated

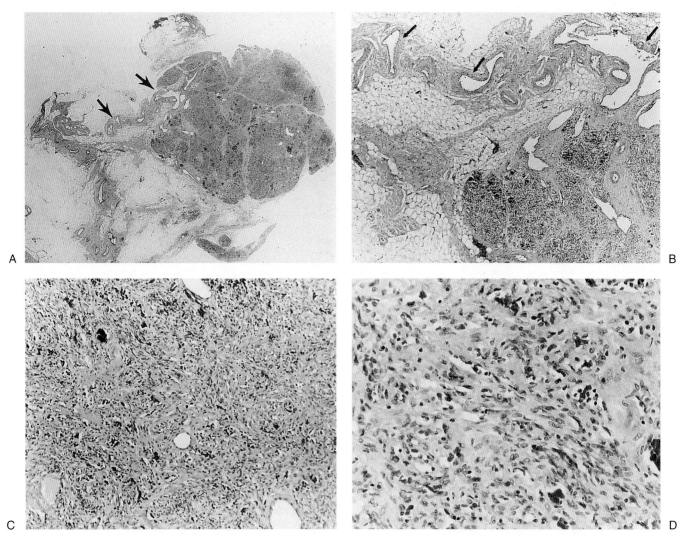

**FIG. 40.73.** *Capillary hemangioma.* **A,B:** Sinuous, branching feeding vessel is shown at the border of the lobulated tumor *(arrows).* **C,D:** Tumor is composed of small, compressed capillaries with prominent intervening spindle cells. (From Jozefczyk MA, Rosen PP. Vascular tumors of the breast. II. Perilobular hemangiomas and hemangioma. *Am J Surg Pathol* 1985;9:491–503, with permssion.)

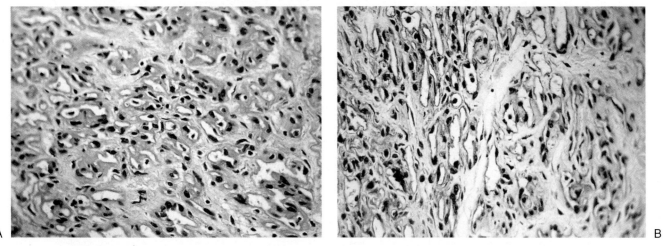

**FIG. 40.74.** *Capillary hemangioma.* **A:** Delicate clusters of capillaries that have prominent hyperchromatic nuclei are shown. **B:** Collagen between the capillaries is stained green with a trichrome stain. *(continued)*

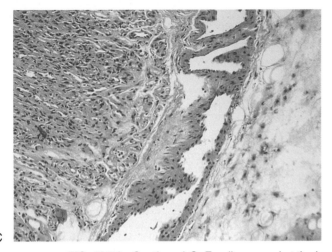

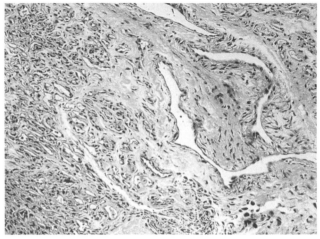

**FIG. 40.74.** *Continued.* **C:** Feeding vessel at the border of the tumor. **D:** Branches of the feeding vessel within a fibrous septum are highlighted by the trichrome stain.

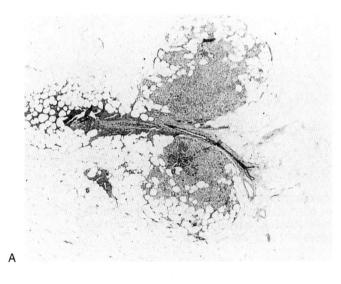

**FIG. 40.75.** *Capillary hemangioma.* **A:** Whole-mount histologic section showing a central feeding vessel. The lesion has the shape of a butterfly. **B,C:** Hemangiomatous capillaries blending with fat are illustrated. (**A:** From Hoda SA, Cranor ML, Rosen PP. Hemangiomas of the breast with atypical histological features. Further analysis of histological subtypes confirming their benign character. *Am J Surg Pathol* 1992;16:553–560, with permission.)

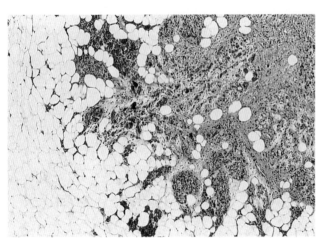

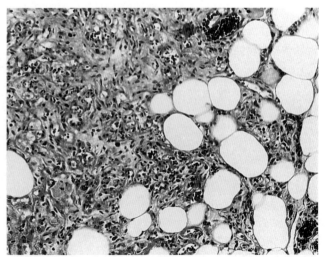

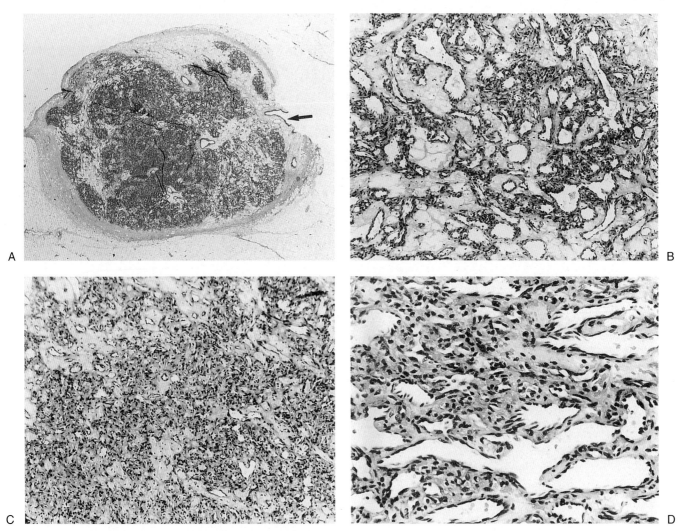

**FIG. 40.76.** *Complex hemangioma.* **A:** Whole-mount histologic section of a circumscribed, seemingly encapsulated tumor. Part of the feeding vessel is shown at the right border *(arrow)*, and several branches of this vessel are present in fibrous septae within the hemangioma. **B:** Compressed capillaries. **C:** Dilated, irregular, sometimes anastomosing vascular channels. **D:** Anastomosing vascular channels with an avian shape. (From Jozefczyk MA, Rosen PP. Vascular tumors of the breast. II. Perilobular hemangiomas and hemangioma. *Am J Surg Pathol* 1985;9:491–503, with permssion.)

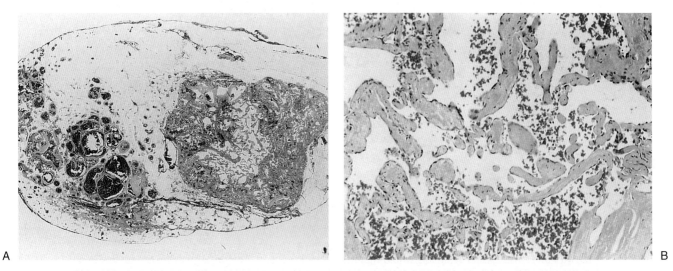

**FIG. 40.77.** *Complex hemangioma.* **A:** In this whole-mount histologic section, the area on the *left* has the diffuse pattern of a conventional cavernous hemangioma, whereas the circumscribed component on the *right* has numerous anastomosing vascular channels. **B:** The endothelium is flat and inconspicuous. Red blood cells are present. (From Rosen PP, Oberman HA. Tumors of the mammary gland. In: *Atlas of tumor pathology.* Washington, DC: Armed Forces Institute of Pathology, 1993, with permission.)

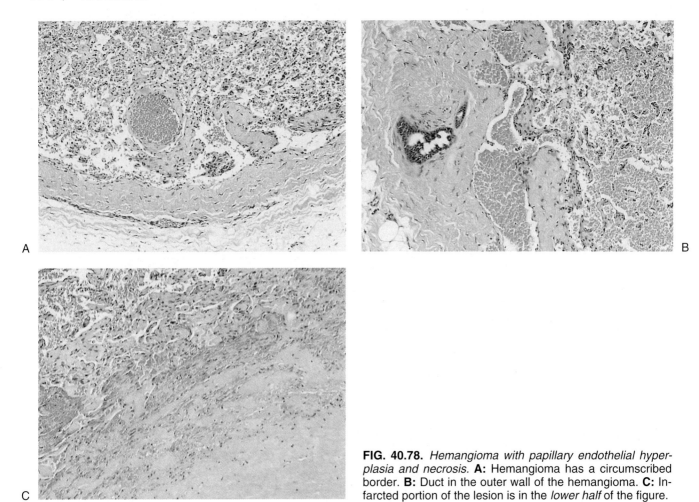

**FIG. 40.78.** *Hemangioma with papillary endothelial hyperplasia and necrosis.* **A:** Hemangioma has a circumscribed border. **B:** Duct in the outer wall of the hemangioma. **C:** Infarcted portion of the lesion is in the *lower half* of the figure.

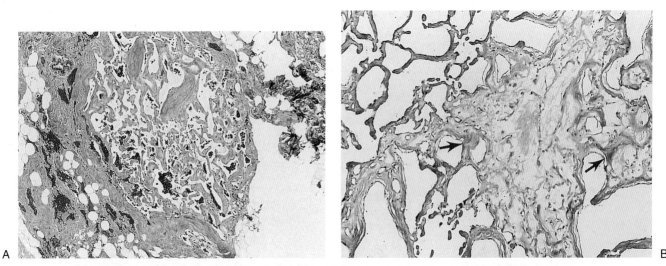

**FIG. 40.79.** *Hemangioma.* **A:** In this whole-mount histologic section, hemorrhage in the breast tissue on the *left* around the hemangioma was caused by needle localization of the mammographically detected lesion. Fibrosis of septae between anastomosing vascular channels is apparent. **B:** Dark zones within the fibrous septae represent delicate bands of calcification *(arrows)*.

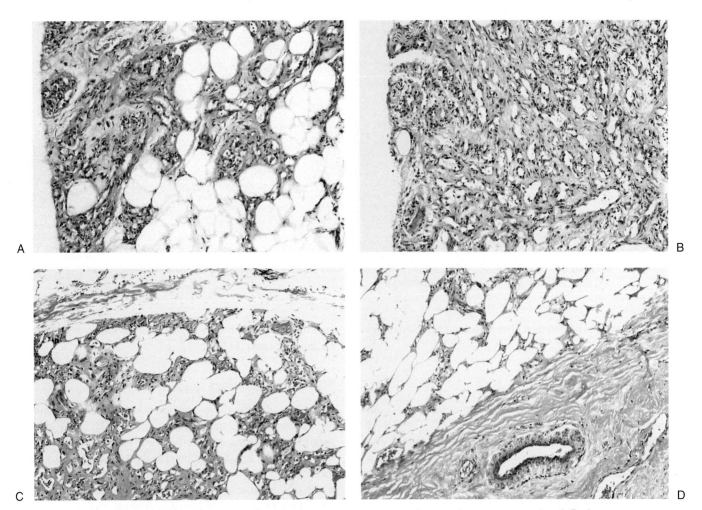

**FIG. 40.80.** *Hemangioma, needle core biopsy.* The lesion was detected by mammography. **A,B:** Areas in the needle core samples showing varying cellularity and spread into the fat. **C,D:** The excised tumor was a capillary hemangioma.

with endothelial hyperplasia, or in fibrous septa between vascular spaces. Marked septal fibrosis sometimes is found in hemangiomas (Fig. 40.79).

### Treatment and Prognosis

Reexcision of the biopsy site may be indicated if it appears that a substantial portion of the lesion has not been extirpated. Further surgery is not necessary if only a few peripheral capillaries extend to the margin of excision. It often is not possible to recognize residual hemangioma in the granulation tissue of a healing biopsy site.

Complete excision of a hemangioma is necessary for accurate diagnosis. The material obtained with a needle core biopsy is not sufficient for this purpose (Fig. 40.80). Peripheral portions of a cavernous hemangioma may be indistinguishable from low-grade angiosarcoma in a small sample. Hemangiomas rarely exceed 2.0 cm in diameter, whereas few angiosarcomas are smaller than 3.0 cm.

Most hemangiomas have been treated by excision. Mastectomy is not indicated but has been performed in a few in-

stances when the lesion was diagnosed incorrectly as angiosarcoma. No patient with any of the foregoing types of hemangiomas has had a recurrence with follow-up averaging 44 months but extending as long as 140 months.

### ANGIOMATOSIS

The name *angiomatosis* is a descriptive compromise when applied to these tumors that often are composed of hemangiomatous and lymphangiomatous channels. An example of angiomatosis in a 49-year-old woman with prominent lymphangiomatous features has been described as a "cystic hygroma of the breast" (220). This condition should be distinguished from "hemangiomatosis," the diagnosis recommended by Hamperl (221) for patients with several perilobular hemangiomas. It is preferable to refer to this latter condition as multiple perilobular hemangiomas, although rarely perilobular hemangiomas may be so numerous as to suggest a diffuse vascular proliferation. Multiple perilobular hemangiomas retain the localized capillary structure that typifies these lesions and thus are easily distinguished from

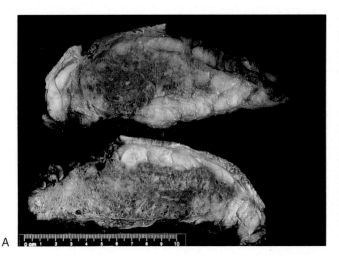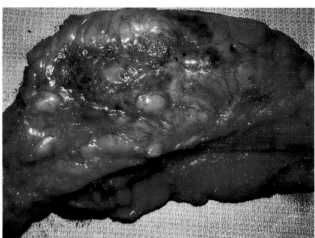

**FIG. 40.81.** *Angiomatosis, gross appearance.* **A,B:** Two bisected mastectomy specimens demonstrating diffuse cystic hemorrhagic angiomatosis.

the larger, irregularly shaped channels that characterize angiomatosis.

### Clinical Presentation

This is a diffuse benign vascular lesion of the breast. Four female patients have been described (222,223). Three were adults 19 to 40 years old when the lesion was diagnosed, and the fourth had a congenital tumor. Each presented with a mass in the breast. In excisional biopsies, the lesions from the adult women measured 11.0, 9.3, and 9.0 cm in largest diameter, respectively.

### Gross Pathology

The lesions are grossly cystic and spongy. One tumor had a 15-cm blood-filled cyst (222). When the vascular spaces contain blood, the tumor appears hemorrhagic, resembling an angiosarcoma (Fig. 40.81).

### Microscopic Pathology

Microscopically, the tumors are composed of anastomosing, large vascular channels extending diffusely in the breast parenchyma. They surround ducts and lobules but do not to invade into the lobular stroma. The vessels are lined by flat inconspicuous endothelium with sparse supporting mural tissue that is virtually devoid of smooth muscle. The lesions consist predominantly of hemangiomatous erythrocyte-containing channels or lymphangiomatous, empty, channels accompanied by lymphoid aggregates, or a mixture of the two vascular patterns (Fig. 40.82). Angiomatosis may occur in breast tissue involved by other conditions such as a fibroadenoma (Fig. 40.83). An extremely unusual capillary

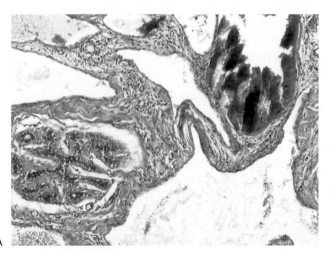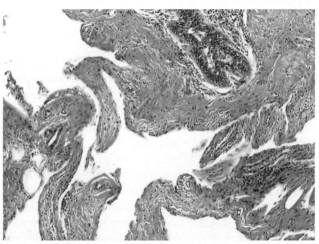

**FIG. 40.82.** *Angiomatosis.* **A:** Blood-filled and empty dilated vascular channels that surround a lobule. The stroma contains sparse smooth muscle cells and lymphocytes. **B:** The flat endothelium is very inconspicuous.

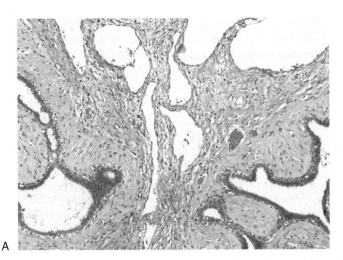
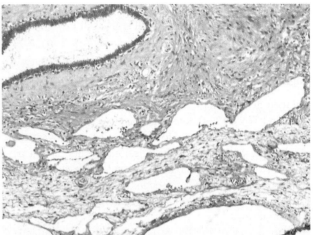

**FIG. 40.83.** *Angiomatosis in a fibroadenoma.* **A,B:** Lymphangiomatous vascular proliferation is present in a fibroadenoma and in the surrounding breast.

variant of angiomatosis presents as a breast mass. The specimen consists of numerous clusters of histologically benign-appearing capillaries throughout fibrous and fatty breast tissue (Fig. 40.84). Association with renal failure and dialysis in one case may be coincidental.

Although angiomatosis forms a mass clinically and on gross pathologic examination, it does not have the microscopically circumscribed structure that typifies mammary hemangiomas. The bulk of the tumor is composed of normal breast parenchyma distributed among the vascular channels. This configuration is similar to that of somatic angiomatosis as described by Enzinger and Weiss (224):

> A proliferation of small to medium-sized vessels of irregular shape that diffusely infiltrate skin, subcutis, muscle and even bone in a given area. The vessels are usually thin walled or at best contain a few poorly formed fascicles of smooth muscle. They may be blood filled or empty and are sometimes surrounded by foci of lymphocytes, features that raise the question of focal lymphangiomatosis differentiation.

The microscopic distinction between low-grade angiosarcoma and angiomatosis may be difficult, especially in a small biopsy sample. Anastomosing channels that are "empty" or contain erythrocytes occur in both lesions. When multiple areas are sampled, significant differences are apparent. The vascular channels in angiomatosis are distributed uniformly throughout the tumor with very little variation. On the other hand, even the most well-differentiated angiosarcoma has a heterogeneous pattern of vessels that are numerous in some regions and more widely separated elsewhere. At the periphery of low-grade angiosarcomas, neoplastic vessels of capillary size merge with the surrounding tissue, whereas those of angiomatosis do not become smaller peripherally. In angiosarcomas, the vascular channels grow into lobules that consequently are destroyed, whereas lobules are spared in angiomatosis as the vascular proliferation surrounds but does not invade them. Finally, endothelial nuclei are histologically normal in angiomatosis, or they may be so attenuated that they may be difficult to find. More

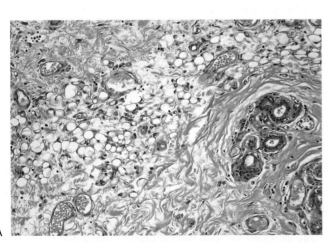
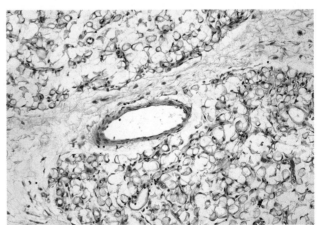

**FIG. 40.84.** *Angiomatosis, capillary type.* **A:** Small, uniform capillaries are distributed in the fat. **B:** Two discrete adjacent foci of capillary proliferation in fat.

prominent, hyperchromatic endothelial nuclei are found in angiosarcomas except in peripheral regions of low grade tumors.

### Prognosis and Treatment

In their discussion of angiomatosis of the soft tissues, Enzinger and Weiss (224) noted that the "lesions are capable of repeated local recurrence. However, we are not aware that malignant degeneration of these lesions occurs or that acceptable cases have given rise to metastatic disease . . . a conservative surgical approach seems advisable initially, and more extensive surgery should be reserved for persistently recurring lesions."

Angiomatosis of the breast is comparable to similar lesions that arise at other anatomic sites. The large size attained in the breast without the development of a histologically or clinically malignant component indicates that these are benign tumors. It may be necessary to perform a mastectomy to control a bulky lesion, but less extensive surgery is preferable whenever possible. Recurrence may occur, sometimes after a long interval, indicating that the lesion is a chronic condition in some patients (223). Radiation therapy used for many years to treat cutaneous hemangiomas in infants is likely to be complicated by mammary hypoplasia when applied prior to full breast development (225,226). No data are available about the effectiveness of radiotherapy in the treatment of angiomatosis of the adult breast.

The clinical course of one patient with a congenital tumor is of particular interest. At birth she had a cavernous hemangioma of the right anterior chest. It measured "3 × 4 inches" and was described as "not smooth but rolling as if enlarged vessels lie underneath." At surgery a tumor was found "extending from beneath the right nipple upward . . . to the level of the clavicle and outward . . . to the anterior axillary fold." The specimen, resected when the patient was 11 weeks old, consisted of many empty channels of varying size lined by

flat endothelium. Although no breast tissue was described histologically, the breast did not develop fully at puberty, presumably because part of the breast bud was removed. Twenty-eight years later, the patient underwent bilateral mammoplasty with insertion of a right breast prosthesis. Six years after this operation, when the patient was 34 years old, a mass was resected from the right superior lateral chest wall and proved to be angiomatosis in fat and skeletal muscle. Many of the vascular space were congested with red blood cells. At 39 years of age, the patient presented with two soft masses near the areola involving the upper and lower inner quadrants overlying the breast implant. Microscopic examination revealed angiomatosis in the mammary parenchyma (Fig. 40.85).

### VENOUS HEMANGIOMAS

The microscopic appearance of these vascular tumors of the breast corresponds most closely to that of soft tissue (227) and bone (228) lesions that have been termed *venous hemangiomas* or *vascular anomalies*. It is not known whether these are true neoplasms, but progressive enlargement of extramammary venous hemangiomas has been observed as a result of growth in fat, skeletal muscle, and bone. It is unlikely that trauma contributes to the development of venous hemangiomas, although antecedent injury was reported by one patient with a mammary venous hemangioma. Fat necrosis and hemosiderin-laden macrophages, which would be expected in a trauma-associated vascular lesion, have been largely absent from venous hemangiomas.

### Clinical Presentation

Five cases have been reported (229). The patients ranged in age from 24 to 59 years (average, 40 years). Each presented with a palpable tumor. One patient reported that the mass had been present for 13 years. Another patient became aware of the lesion after trauma to the breast.

### Gross Pathology

The tumors have measured from 1.0 to 5.3 cm in greatest diameter (average, 3.2 cm). They were well circumscribed, firm, and darkly colored. Hemorrhagic cysts 0.5 to 1.3 cm in diameter were noted in one lesion.

### Microscopic Pathology

The lesions are characterized by some histologic diversity. All have dilated venous channels with smooth muscle walls of varying structural completeness (Fig. 40.86). Red blood cells are present in the lumens of some vascular spaces. Others are empty or contain lymph. Thick-walled arterial channels and capillaries are not conspicuous, except for one of the larger tumors that had capillary-forming areas. A large, well-formed muscular artery was found at the margin of one tumor (Fig. 40.87). A few lobules and ducts sometimes are

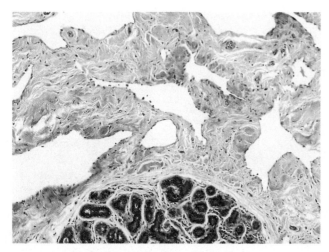

**FIG. 40.85.** *Angiomatosis.* Recurrent lymphangioma in the breast growing as angiomatosis.

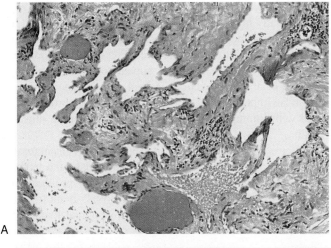
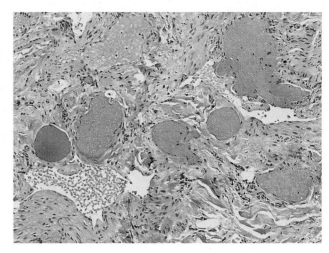
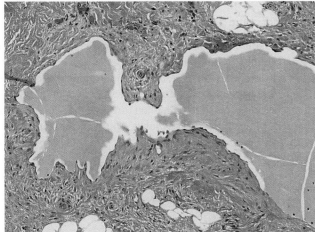

**FIG. 40.86.** *Venous hemangioma.* **A:** Vascular spaces contain variable amounts of blood. **B:** Many congested vessels are present in this region. **C:** The vessel contains homogeneous pink fluid.

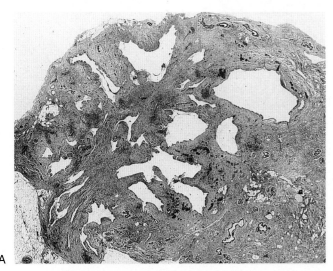
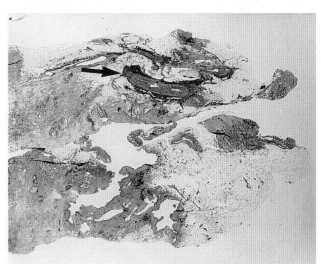

**FIG. 40.87.** *Venous hemangioma.* **A:** This whole-mount histologic section reveals a circumscribed group of irregular dilated vascular channels. **B:** Large feeding artery is present in the upper piece of tissue from the periphery of the tumor (*arrow*). The lower sample contains less well-formed, thin-walled vascular channels characteristic of the venous hemangioma. (**B:** From Rosen PP, Jozefczyk MA, Boram LH. Vascular tumors of the breast. IV. The venous hemangioma. *Am J Surg Pathol* 1985;9:659–665, with permission.)

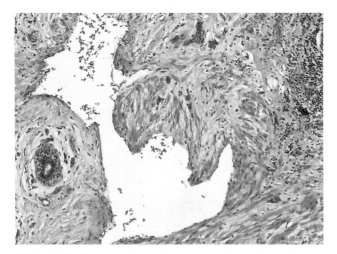

**FIG. 40.88.** *Venous hemangioma.* A small duct is shown on the *left* and a perivascular lymphocytic infiltrate on the *right*.

distributed in the mammary stroma between vascular channels that form the lesion (Fig. 40.88). Focal perivascular lymphocytic infiltrates also are present in the stroma, often accompanied by congested capillaries. Lobular carcinoma *in situ* was present in breast tissue outside the venous hemangioma in one case (229).

The dilated vascular channels are irregularly shaped and vary greatly in caliber. A smooth muscle layer is evident in the wall of some of the tumor vessels, but often it does not encompass the entire circumference (Fig. 40.89). In some areas, smooth muscle elements appear to be incompletely formed or absent in sections stained with hematoxylin and eosin, an impression that is confirmed with a trichrome stain and with immunohistochemical stains for smooth muscle actin.

Microscopic features most often associated with angiosarcoma are absent. These include pleomorphism and hyperchromasia of endothelial cell nuclei, papillary proliferation of endothelium, endothelial cell mitoses, hemorrhagic necrosis, and destructive invasion into glandular mammary parenchyma.

### Prognosis and Treatment

One patient underwent a mastectomy because the lesion was thought to be adherent to the pectoral muscle at the time of surgery. However, the vascular tumor was confined to the breast. Another patient who had coincidental lobular carcinoma *in situ* had no residual tumor in the specimen obtained when the original biopsy site was reexcised. The other three patients were treated by excisional biopsy. With

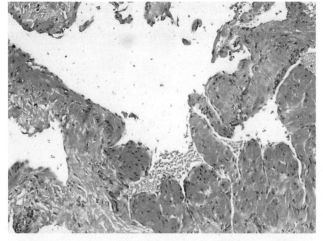

A

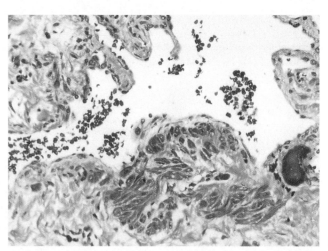

B

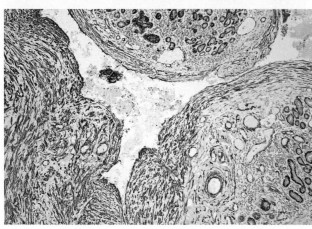

C

**FIG. 40.89.** *Venous hemangioma.* **A:** Bundles of smooth muscle cells are present around part of the vascular channel. **B:** The smooth muscle is red in this section stained with Masson's trichrome. **C:** Vascular channel between lobules with abundant actin-positive mural smooth muscle (avidin-biotin).

follow-up ranging from 6 months to 11 years, there have been no recurrences of the venous hemangiomas. Excisional biopsy is the recommended treatment for this benign vascular lesion.

## NONPARENCHYMAL HEMANGIOMAS OF THE MAMMARY REGION

For many years, considerable emphasis was placed on the distinction between subcutaneous and intraparenchymal vascular lesions of the breast. Virtually all of the former proved to be benign, whereas the majority of the latter were interpreted as angiosarcomas. However, location alone is not sufficient to determine the diagnosis, because the existence of intraparenchymal hemangiomas is now well documented and angiosarcoma may involve the mammary skin and subcutaneous tissue.

Little attention has been paid to the clinical and pathologic characteristics of nonparenchymal hemangiomas of the breast. In 1933, Menville and Bloodgood (230) reported several patients with mammary subcutaneous cavernous and capillary hemangiomas. They emphasized the difference between hemangiomas of the skin and subcutaneous tissue, noting that "subcutaneous lesions have no connection with the epidermis." The distinction was important because "the recognition of angiomas has been difficult . . . in regards to the diagnosis of malignancy and benignancy." Two of the seven hemangiomas in their series were misdiagnosed as angiosarcomas and treated by mastectomy. Madding and Hershberger (231) described a 23-year-old patient with a "birthmark" of her right breast that was treated with radiation. Subsequent ulceration and persistent bleeding led to a mastectomy, which revealed an 8 × 7 × 6 cm vascular tumor of the subcutaneous tissue. Microscopically, "no breast ducts were observed admixed with the tumor," and the authors described the vessels as "for the most part dilated capillaries." They noted that "few of the larger vessels showed scattered muscle fibers but no elastic tissue. These latter vessels were interpreted to be small venules." The figures that accompany the paper illustrate vascular channels typically associated with venous hemangiomas.

### Clinical Presentation

A variety of nonparenchymal mammary hemangiomas occur in the mammary region (232). Dermal or cutaneous hemangiomas, the majority of which are capillary hemangiomas that present no diagnostic problem, are excluded from this category. Almost all patients are women ranging in age from 20 to 76 years (average, 53 years). Nonparenchymal subcutaneous hemangiomas of the male breast also have been encountered. The right and left breast are involved with nearly equal frequency. Some lesions occur in the inframammary region, but the majority are distributed in various quadrants. The presenting symptom is a mass. A cavernous hemangioma of the pectoralis muscle presented as a 2.5-cm

tumor deep in the breast on mammography (233). At surgery, the lesion proved to be intramuscular.

Benign angiomatous lesions that occur in the skin after radiation therapy are discussed in Chapter 41.

### Pathology

Tumor size ranges from 0.8 to 3.2 cm (average, 1.8 cm). Breast parenchyma may be included in the biopsy specimen. The lesion is classified as nonparenchymal if the neoplastic vessels are not present in glandular tissue.

The diagnosis of nonparenchymal vascular tumors is based on the descriptions and the classification of soft tissue vascular tumors provided by Enzinger and Weiss (227). Several types of hemangiomas have been identified: angiolipoma (Figs. 40.90 and 40.91), cavernous hemangioma (Fig. 40.92), hemangioma with papillary endothelial hyperplasia (Fig. 40.93), capillary hemangioma (Fig. 40.94), and venous hemangioma. The frequency of these types of hemangioma corresponds roughly to their relative frequency in the soft tissues generally. This suggests that there is not a strong predilection for a particular type of hemangioma to occur in the mammary subcutaneous tissue.

It is possible that selected regions of the breast are prone to develop certain types of hemangiomas. In one study, two angiolipomas were located in the upper inner quadrant, and two cavernous hemangiomas were excised from the inframammary region (232). Yu et al. (234) described a 2-cm "cellular" angiolipoma that was excised from the left upper inner quadrant of a 64-year-old woman. A study of angiolipomas noted that "many of the lesions were removed from sites subject to repeated pressure and irritation" (235). About 8% of the angiolipomas occurred on the anterior chest, but the frequency of the lesions in the female breast was not stated.

The histologic appearances of various types of hemangiomas in the mammary subcutaneous tissue does not differ from comparable lesions in other subcutaneous locations.

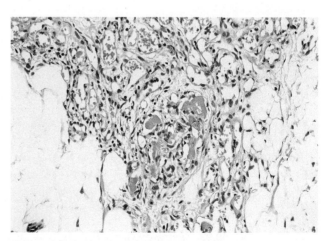

**FIG. 40.90.** *Nonparenchymal angiolipoma.* Capillaries meshed in delicate fibrous stroma. Fibrin thrombi are present.

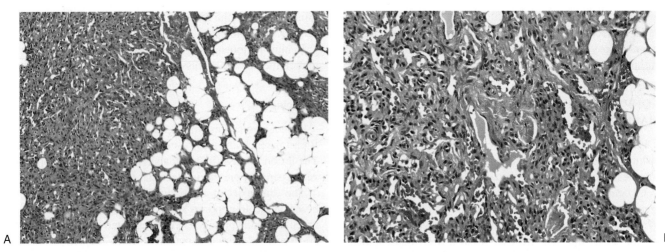

**FIG. 40.91.** *Nonparenchymal angiolipoma.* **A:** The capillary component of this tumor has a relatively solid growth pattern. **B:** The capillaries form a network of small anastomosing channels.

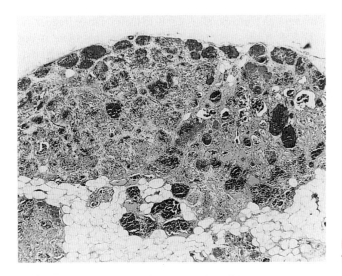

**FIG. 40.92.** *Nonparenchymal cavernous hemangioma.* The tumor is well circumscribed along one border.

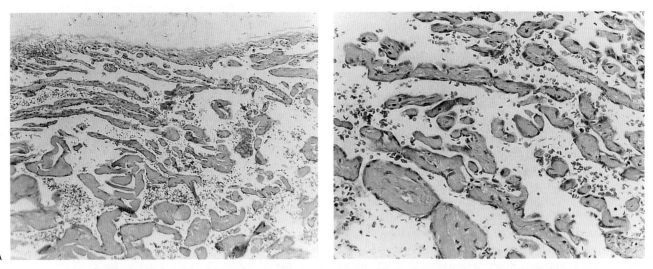

**FIG. 40.93.** *Nonparenchymal hemangioma, papillary endothelial hyperplasia.* **A:** The tumor has a well-circumscribed border. **B:** Widely anastomosing vascular spaces are distributed among branching, disrupted papillary fronds of collagenous stroma. (**B:** From Rosen PP. Vascular tumors of the breast. V. Non-parenchymal hemangiomas of mammary subcutaneous tissue. *Am J Surg Pathol* 1985;9:723–729, with permission.)

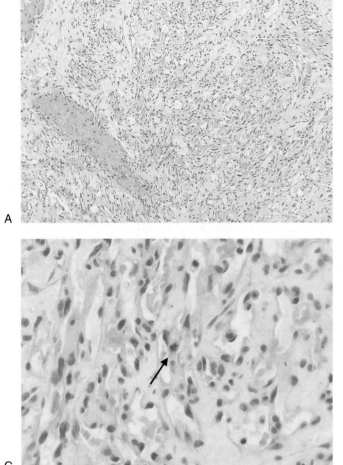

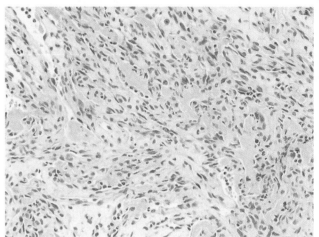

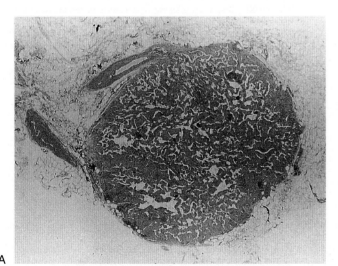

C

**FIG. 40.94.** *Nonparenchymal capillary hemangioma.* **A:** A few distended vascular spaces contain fibrin thrombi. Most of the tumor is compact and the vascular spaces are compressed slits. **B:** Region with conspicuous stromal spindle cells. **C:** A mitotic figure *(arrow)* is present in the center between the capillaries.

Some hemangiomas found in mammary subcutaneous tissue feature interconnected vascular channels (Fig. 40.95). Areas in which these septa are disrupted have a pseudopapillary pattern (Fig. 40.93). The vascular spaces can be larger to-ward the center than at the periphery, where they tend to spread into the subcutaneous fat producing an ill-defined margin. Encapsulation of angiolipomas often is difficult to determine after the lesions have been dissected. Concern

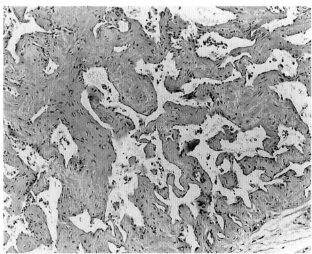

**FIG. 40.95.** *Nonparenchymal hemangioma.* **A:** This whole-mount histologic section shows a circumscribed vascular tumor in fat. Two segments of feeding vessel were captured on the *left* in this fortuitous section. The appearance suggests that they may be afferent and efferent portions, respectively, of a single artery that gives rise to the hemangioma. **B:** Complex network of anastomosing vascular channels with intervening fibrous septae. *(continued)*

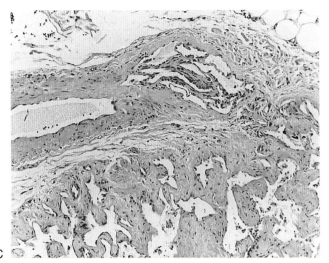

C

**FIG. 40.95.** *Continued.* **C:** Magnified view of the upper feeding vessel shown in **A**. The vascular proliferation extends into the lumen of the artery.

about the diagnosis often arises because of uncertainty about whether the lesion is truly extraparenchymal and the abundant closely opposed vascular spaces with intervening spindle cell stroma (234).

### Prognosis and Treatment

Nonparenchymal subcutaneous hemangiomas of the breast are benign vascular tumors adequately treated by local excision. Reexcision of the biopsy site may be indicated when the location of the lesion (subcutaneous versus parenchymal) is in doubt or if there is uncertainty about the adequacy of the margins. Complete removal of the tumor also helps to exclude the possibility that the benign-appearing vascular lesion in a small biopsy is a subcutaneous extension from an underlying low-grade angiosarcoma.

### ANEURYSM

Aneurysms occurring in and around the breast are very uncommon nonneoplastic vascular tumors. Two aneurysms apparently arose at the sites of stereotactic needle core biopsies and were detected on follow-up mammograms 6 and 9 months, respectively, after the needle biopsy procedures (236,237). Two reports described hypertensive patients. One was a 57-year-old woman with a 3-cm smooth mobile tumor in the upper outer quadrant of the right breast (238). The lesion was brought to clinical attention because of sudden severe pain and ecchymosis in the area. Angiography revealed an aneurysmal arteriovenous fistula arising from the underlying intercostal artery. The excised specimen was described as "a false aneurysm filled with blood clot in continuity with the feeding artery" with no evidence of atherosclerotic, traumatic, or inflammatory etiology or of medial degeneration. The other hypertensive patient was a 55-year-old woman with a painful, pulsatile 1 × 1.5-cm tumor accompanied by

ecchymosis involving the left medial breast and chest wall (239). A diagnosis of pseudoaneurysm was made radiologically and successfully treated by percutaneous insertion of an occluding wire embolus. The specific artery affected was not identified.

In a fifth instance, mammography demonstrated a bilobed 3.5-cm mass adjacent to arterial calcifications in the breast of a 57-year-old woman (240). It was predominantly cystic on ultrasonography and appeared to be pulsatile. The patient had systemic lupus in remission and was receiving anticoagulant therapy after a heart valve replacement. Histologic examination revealed a false aneurysm arising in the wall of a medium-sized artery with medial calcification. No arteritis was evident.

Davies and Kulka (241) reviewed histologic sections of 107 surgically excised radial sclerosing lesions and reported finding false aneurysms in five cases. All of the radial sclerosing lesions that had an aneurysm were 10 mm or larger. Fine needle aspiration had been performed in four cases 18 to 22 days previously. The interval was 121 days in one case.

### REFERENCES

#### Fibromatosis

1. Gump FE, Sternschein MJ, Wolff M. Fibromatosis of the breast. *Surg Gynecol Obstet* 1981;15:57–60.
2. Rosen PP, Ernsberger D. Mammary fibromatosis. A benign spindle cell tumor with significant risk for local recurrence. *Cancer* 1989;63:1363–1369.
3. Wargotz ES, Norris HJ, Austin RM, et al. Fibromatosis of the breast. A clinical and pathological study of 28 cases. *Am J Surg Pathol* 1987;11:38–45.
4. Ali M, Fayemi AO, Braun EV, et al. Fibromatosis of the breast. *Am J Surg Pathol* 1979;3:501–505.
5. Cederlund CG, Gustavsson S, Linell F, et al. Fibromatosis of the breast mimicking carcinoma at mammography. *Br J Radiol* 1984;57:98–101.
6. El-Naggar A, Abdul-Karim FW, Marshalleck JJ, et al. Fine needle aspiration of fibromatosis of the breast. *Diagn Cytopathol* 1987; 3:320–322.
7. Haggitt RC, Booth JF. Bilateral fibromatosis of the breast in Gardner's syndrome. *Cancer* 1970;25:161–166.
8. Kalisher L, Long JA, Peyster RG. Extra-abdominal desmoid of the axillary tail mimicking breast carcinoma. *AJR Am J Roentgenol* 1976;126:903–906.
9. Jewett ST Jr, Mead JH. Extra-abdominal desmoid arising from a capsule around a silicone breast implant. *Plast Reconstr Surg* 1979;63:577–579.
10. Pierce VE Jr, Rives DA, Sisley JF, et al. Estradiol and progesterone receptors in a case of fibromatosis of the breast. *Arch Pathol Lab Med* 1987;111:870–872.
11. Tani EM, Stanley MW, Skoog L. Fine needle aspiration cytology presentation of bilateral mammary fibromatosis. Report of a case. *Acta Cytol* 1988;32:555–558.
12. Adair FE, Herrmann JB. Sarcoma of the breast with a report of thirty cases. *Surgery* 1946;19:55–73.
13. Norris HJ, Taylor HB. Sarcomas and other mesenchymal tumors of the breast. *Cancer* 1968;22:22–28.
14. DasGupta TK, Brasfield RD, O'Hara J. Extra-abdominal desmoids. *Ann Surg* 1969;170:109–121.
15. Simpson RD, Harrison EG. Mesenteric fibromatosis in familial polyposis: a variant of Gardner's syndrome. *Cancer* 1964;17:526–534.
16. Needelman P, Leibman J, Capasse J. Fibromatosis of the axillary breast in a young patient. *Breast Dis* 1996;9:171–175.
17. Gupta AK, Atri SC, Naithani YP. Multiple pedunculated fibromatosis of the breast. *J Indian Med Assoc* 1978;10:228–229.

18. Kalbhen CL, Cooper RA, Candel AG. Mammographic and stereotactic core biopsy findings in fibromatosis of the breast: case report. Can Assoc Radiol J 1998;49:229–231.
19. Bogomoletz WV, Boulenger E, Simatos A. Infiltrating fibromatosis of the breast. J Clin Pathol 1981;34:30–34.
20. Schuh ME, Radford DM. Desmoid tumor of the breast following augmentation mammaplasty. Plast Reconstr Surg 1994;93:603–605.
21. Aaron AD, O'Mara JW, Legendre KE, et al. Chest wall fibromatosis associated with silicone breast implants. Surg Oncol 1996;5:93–99.
22. Schiller VL, Arndt RD, Brenner RJ. Aggressive fibromatosis of the chest associated with a silicone breast implant. Chest 1995;108:1466–1468.
23. Zayid I, Dihmic C. Familial multicentric fibromatosis-desmoids. Cancer 1969;24:786–795.
24. Chaudhuri PK, Walker MJ, Beattie CW, et al. Presence of steroid receptors in human soft tissue sarcomas of diverse histological origin. Cancer Res 1980;40:861–865.
25. Hayry P, Reitamo JJ, Vihko R, et al. The desmoid tumor. III. A biochemical and genetic analysis. Am J Clin Pathol 1982;77:681–685.
26. Rasbridge SA, Gillert CE, Millis RR. Oestrogen and progesterone receptor expression in mammary fibromatosis. J Clin Pathol 1993;46:349–351.
27. Bittesini L, Dei Tos AP, Doglioni C, et al. Fibroepithelial tumor of the breast with digital fibroma-like inclusions in the stromal component. Case report with immunocytochemical and ultrastructural analysis. Am J Surg Pathol 1994;18:296–301.
28. Pettinato G, Manivel JC, Gould EW, et al. Inclusion body fibromatosis of the breast. Two cases with immunohistochemical and ultrastructural findings. Am J Clin Pathol 1994;101:714–718.
29. Mayers MM, Evans P, MacVicar D. Case report: ossifying fibromatosis of the breast. Clin Radiol 1994;49:211–212.
30. Fritsches HG, Muller EA. Pseudosarcomatous fasciitis of the breast. Cytologic and histologic features. Acta Cytol 1983;27:73–75.
31. Shuler FJ, Cronin EB, Ricci A Jr, et al. Fibromatosis of the breast diagnosed by stereotaxic core biopsy. AJR Am J Roentgenol 1997;168:846–847.
32. Pettinato G, Manivel JC, Petrella G, et al. Fine needle aspiration cytology, immunocytochemistry and electron microscopy of fibromatosis of the breast. Report of two cases. Acta Cytol 1991;35:403–408.
33. Kinzbrunner B, Ritter S, Domingo J, et al. Remission of rapidly growing desmoid tumors after tamoxifen therapy. Cancer 1983;52:2201–2204.
34. Klein WA, Miller HH, Anderson M, et al. The use of indomethacin, sulindac, and tamoxifen for the treatment of desmoid tumors associated with familial polyposis. Cancer 1987;60:2863–2868.
35. Procter H, Singh L, Baum M, et al. Response of multicentric desmoid tumors to tamoxifen. Br J Surg 1987;74:401.
36. Sportiello DJ, Hoogerland DL. A recurrent pelvic desmoid tumor successfully treated with tamoxifen. Cancer 1991;67:1443–1446.
37. Wilcken N, Tattersall MHN. Endocrine therapy for desmoid tumors. Cancer 1991;68:1384–1388.

## Fibrous Tumor

38. Haagensen CD. Fibrous disease of the breast. In: Haagensen CD. Diseases of the breast, 2nd ed. Philadelphia: WB Saunders, 1971:185–190.
39. Minkowitz S, Hedayati H, Miller S, et al. Fibrous mastopathy: a clinical histopathologic study. Cancer 1973;32:913–916.
40. Vassar PS, Culling CF. Fibrosis of the breast. Arch Pathol 1959;67:128–133.
41. Rivera-Pomar JM, Vilanova JR, Burgos-Bretones JJ, et al. Focal fibrous disease of breast. A common entity in young women. Virchows Arch [A] 1980;386:59–64.
42. Puente JL, Potel J. Fibrous tumor of the breast. Arch Surg 1974;109:391–394.
43. Rosen EL, Soo MS, Bentley RC. Focal fibrosis: a common breast lesion diagnosed at imaging-guided core biopsy. AJR Am J Roentgenol 1999;173:1657–1662.
44. Venta LA, Wiley EL, Gabriel H, et al. Imaging features of focal breast fibrosis: mammographic-pathologic correlation of noncalcified breast lesions. AJR Am J Roentgenol 1999;173:309–316.
45. Belda F, Lester SC, Pinkus JL, et al. Lineage-restricted chromosome translocation in a benign fibrous tumor of the breast. Hum Pathol 1993;24:923–927.

## Pseudoangiomatous Hyperplasia of Mammary Stroma

46. Fisher CJ, Hanby AM, Robinson L, et al. Mammary hamartoma—a review of 35 cases. Histopathology 1992;20:99–106.
47. Churchill's illustrated medical dictionary. New York:Churchill-Livingstone, 1989.
48. Seidman JD, Borkowski A, Aisner SC, et al. Rapid growth of pseudoangiomatous hyperplasia of mammary stroma in axillary gynecomastia in an immunosuppressed patient. Arch Pathol Lab Med 1993;117:736–738.
49. Badve S, Sloane JP. Pseudoangiomatous hyperplasia of male breast. Histopathology 1995;26:463–466.
50. Milanezi MF, Saggioro FP, Zanati SG, et al. Pseudoangiomatous hyperplasia of mammary stroma associated with gynaecomastia. J Clin Pathol 1998;51:204–206.
51. Kollias J, Gill PG, Leong AS, et al. Gynaecomastia presenting as fibroadenomatoid tumours of the breast in a renal transplant recipient associated with cyclosporin treatment. Aust N Z J Surg 1998;68:679–681.
52. Baildam AD, Higgins RM, Hurley E, et al. Cyclosporin A and multiple fibroadenomas of the breast. Br J Surg 1996;83:1755–1757.
53. Anderson C, Ricci A Jr, Pedersen CA, et al. Immunocytochemical analysis of estrogen and progesterone receptors in benign stromal lesions of the breast. Evidence for hormonal etiology in pseudoangiomatous hyperplasia of mammary stroma. Am J Surg Pathol 1991;15:145–149.
54. Ibrahim RE, Sciotto CG, Weidner N. Pseudoangiomatous hyperplasia of mammary stroma. Some observations regarding its clinicopathologic spectrum. Cancer 1989;63:1154–1160.
55. Vuitch MF, Rosen PP, Erlandson RA. Pseudoangiomatous hyperplasia of mammary stroma. Hum Pathol 1986;17:185–191.
56. McCluggage WG, Allen M, Anderson NH. Fine needle aspiration cytology of mammary pseudoangiomatous stromal hyperplasia. A case report. Acta Cytol 1999;43:1147–1149.
57. Polger MR, Denison CM, Lester S, et al. Pseudoangiomatous stromal hyperplasia: mammographic and sonographic appearances. AJR Am J Roentgenol 1996;166:349–352.
58. Cohen MA, Morris EA, Rosen PP, et al. Pseudoangiomatous stromal hyperplasia: mammographic, sonographic and clinical patterns. Radiology 1996;198:117–120.
59. Powell CM, Cranor ML, Rosen PP. Pseudoangiomatous stromal hyperplasia (PASH): a mammary stromal tumor with myofibroblastic differentiation. Am J Surg Pathol 1995;19:270–277.
60. Zanella M, Falconieri G, Lamovec J, et al. Pseudoangiomatous hyperplasia of the mammary stroma: true entity or phenotype? Pathol Res Pract 1998;194:535–540.
61. Vogel PM, Georgiade NG, Fetter BF, et al. The correlation of histologic changes in the human breast with the menstrual cycle. Am J Pathol 1981;104:23–34.

## Myofibroblastoma

62. Schurch W, Seemayer TA, Gabbiani G. The myofibroblast. A quarter century after its discovery. Am J Surg Pathol 1998;22:141–147.
63. Majno G. The story of the myofibroblasts. Am J Surg Pathol 1979;3:535–542.
64. Nakanishi I, Kajikawa K, Okada Y, et al. Myofibroblasts in fibrous tumors and fibrosis in various organs. Acta Pathol Jpn 1981;31:423–437.
65. Lagacé R, Schürch W, Seemayer TA. Myofibroblasts in soft tissue sarcomas. Virchows Arch [A] 1980;389:1–11.
66. Vasudev KS, Harris M. A sarcoma of myofibroblasts. An ultrastructural study. Arch Pathol Lab Med 1987;102:185–188.
67. Herrera GA, Johnson WW, Lockard VG, et al. Soft tissue myofibroblastomas. Mod Pathol 1991;4:571–577.
68. Lee AHS, Sworn MJ, Theaker JM, et al. Myofibroblastoma of the breast: an immunohistochemical study. Histopathology 1993;22:75–78.
69. Damiani S, Miettinen M, Peterse JL, et al. Solitary fibrous tumour (myofibroblastoma) of the breast. Virchows Arch [A] 1994;425:89–92.
70. Salomao DR, Crotty TB, Nascimento AG. Myofibroblastoma and solitary fibrous tumor of the breast: histopathological and immunohistochemical comparative study. Mod Pathol 1997;10:25A.

71. Schmitt-Graff A, Desmouliere A, Gabbiani G. Heterogeneity of my-ofibroblast phenotypic features: an example of fibroblastic cell plasticity. *Virchows Arch* 1994;425:3–24.

72. Seemayer TA, Schurch W, Lagacé R, et al. Myofibroblasts in the stroma of invasive and metaplastic carcinoma. A possible host response to neoplasia. *Am J Surg Pathol* 1979;3:525–533.

73. Schürch W, Lagacé R, Seemayer TA. Myofibroblastic stromal reaction in retracted scirrhous carcinoma of the breast. *Surg Gynecol Obstet* 1982;154:351–358.

74. Ohtani H, Sansano N. Myofibroblasts and myoepithelial cells in human breast carcinoma. An ultrastructural study. *Virchows Arch [A]* 1980;385:247–261.

75. Bussolati G, Alfani V, Weber K, et al. Immunocytochemical detection of actin on fixed and embedded tissues. Its potential use in routine pathology. *J Histochem Cytochem* 1980;28:169–173.

76. Barsky SH, Green WR, Grotendorst GR, et al. Desmoplastic breast carcinoma as a source of human myofibroblasts. *Am J Pathol* 1984;115:329–333.

77. Toker C, Tang C-K, Whitely JF, et al. Benign spindle cell breast tumor. *Cancer* 1981;48:1615–1622.

78. Hamele-Bena D, Cranor ML, Sciotto C, et al. Uncommon presentation of mammary myofibroblastoma. *Hum Pathol* 1996;9:786–790.

79. Wargotz ES, Weiss SW, Norris HJ. Myofibroblastoma of the breast. Sixteen cases of a distinctive benign mesenchymal tumor. *Am J Surg Pathol* 1987;11:493–502.

80. Bégin LR. Myogenic stromal tumor of the male breast (so-called myofibroblastoma). *Ultrastruct Pathol* 1991;15:613–622.

81. Yagmur Y, Prasad MJ, Osborne MP. Myofibroblastoma in the irradiated breast. *Breast J* 1999;5:136–140.

82. Ordi J, Riverola A, Solé M, et al. Fine needle aspiration of myofibroblastoma of the breast in a man: a report of two cases. *Acta Cytol* 1992;36:194–198.

83. Rebner M, Raju U. Myofibroblastoma of the male breast. *Breast Dis* 1993;6:157–160.

84. Greenberg JS, Kaplan SS, Grady C. Myofibroblastoma of the breast in women: imaging appearances. *AJR Am J Roentgenol* 1998;171:71–72.

85. Vourtsi A, Kehagias D, Antoniou A, et al. Male breast myofibroblastoma and MR findings. *J Comput Assist Tomogr* 1999;23:414–416.

86. Ali S, Teichberg S, Derisi DC, et al. Giant myofibroblastoma of the male breast. A case report. *Am J Surg Pathol* 1994;18:1170–1176.

87. Fukunaga M, Ushigome S. Myofibroblastoma of the breast with diverse differentiations. *Arch Pathol Lab Med* 1997;121:599–603.

88. Thomas TMM, Mying A, Mak CKL, et al. Mammary myofibroblastoma with leiomyomatous differentiation. *Am J Clin Pathol* 1997;107:52–55.

89. Amin MB, Gottlieb CA, Fitzmaurice M, et al. Fine needle aspiration cytologic study of myofibroblastoma of the breast: immunohistochemical and ultrastructural findings. *Am J Clin Pathol* 1993;99:593–597.

90. Negri S, Bonzanini M, Togni R, et al. Fine needle aspiration of myofibroblastoma of the breast. Case report. *Pathologica* 1995;87:719–722.

91. Deligeorgi-Politi H, Kontozoglou T, Joseph M, et al. Myofibroblastoma of the breast: cytologic, histologic, immunohistochemical, and ultrastructural findings in two cases with differing cellularity. *Breast J* 1997;3:365–371.

92. Schmitt FC, de La Cruz Mera A. Fine needle aspiration cytology presentation of a cellular variant of breast myofibroblastoma. Report of a case with immunohistochemical studies. *Acta Cytol* 1998;42:721–724.

93. Morgan MB, Pitha JV. Myofibroblastoma of the breast revisited: an etiologic association with androgens? *Hum Pathol* 1998;29:347–351.

## Tumors with Perivascular Myoid Differentiation

94. Hollowood K, Holley MP, Fletcher CDM. Plexiform fibrohistiocytic tumour: clinicopathological, immunohistochemical and ultrastructural analysis in favour of a myofibroblastic lesion. *Histopathology* 1991;19:503–513.

95. Granter SR, Badizadegan K, Fletcher CD. Myofibromatosis in adults, glomangiopericytoma, and myopericytoma. A spectrum of tumors showing perivascular myoid differentiation. *Am J Surg Pathol* 1998;22:513–525.

96. Dictor M, Alner Å, Andersson T, et al. Myofibromatosis-like hemangiopericytoma metastasizing as differentiated vascular smooth-muscle and myosarcoma. Myopericytes as a subset of "myofibroblasts." *Am J Surg Pathol* 1992;16:1239–1247.

## Giant Cell Fibroblastoma

97. Pinto A, Hwang W-S, Wong AL, et al. Giant cell fibroblastoma in childhood: immunohistochemical and ultrastructural study. *Mod Pathol* 1992;5:639–642.

## Granular Cell Tumor

98. Abrikossof AI. Über myome, ausgehend von der quergestreifter willkür licher Muskulatur. *Virchows Arch [A]* 1926;260:215–233.

99. Murray MR. Cultural characteristics of three granular-cell myoblastomas. *Cancer* 1951;4:857–865.

100. Turnbull AD, Huvos AG, Ashikari R, et al. Granular-cell myoblastoma of the breast. *N Y State J Med* 1971;71:436–438.

101. Abrikossof AI. Weitere untersuchungen über Myoblastenmyome. *Virchows Arch [A]* 1931;280:723–740.

102. Haagensen CD, Stout AP. Granular cell myoblastoma of the mammary gland. *Ann Surg* 1946;124:218–227.

103. Weitzner S, Nascimento AG, Scanlon LJ. Intramammary granular cell myoblastoma. *Am J Surg* 1979;45:34–37.

104. Boulat J, Mathoulin M-P, Vacheret H, et al. Tumeurs à cellules granuleuses du sein. *Ann Pathol* 1994;14:93–100.

105. DeMay RM, Kay S. Granular cell tumor of the breast. *Pathol Ann* 1984;19[Pt 2]:121–148.

106. Placidi A, Aversa A, Foggi CM, et al. Granular cell tumour of breast in a young man preoperatively diagnosed by fine needle aspiration (FNA) cytology. *Cytopathology* 1995;6:343–348.

107. Moscovic EA, Azar HA. Multiple granular cell tumors ("myoblastomas"). *Cancer* 1967;20:2032–2047.

108. Murray DE, Seaman E, Utzinger W. Granular cell myoblastomas in successive generations. *J Surg Oncol* 1969;1:193–197.

109. Loyer E, Sahin A, David C. Granular cell tumor of the breast: sonographic and histologic patterns. *Breast Dis* 1996;9:101–106.

110. Tai G, D, Costa H, Lee D, et al. Case report: coincident granular cell tumour of the breast with invasive ductal carcinoma. *Br J Radiol* 1995;68:1034–1036.

111. Tran TA, Kallakury BVS, Carter J, et al. Coexistence of granular cell tumor and ipsilateral infiltrating ductal carcinoma of the breast. *South Med J* 1997;90:1149–1151.

112. Bassett LW, Cove HC. Myoblastoma of the breast. *AJR Am J Roentgenol* 1979;132:122–123.

113. D'Orsi CJ, Felhaus L, Sonnenfeld M. Unusual lesions of the breast. *Radiol Clin North Am* 1983;21:67–80.

114. Willen R, Willen H, Balldin G, et al. Granular cell tumor of the mammary gland simulating malignancy. *Virchows Arch [A]* 1984;403:391–400.

115. Green DH, Clark AH. Case report: granular cell myoblastoma of the breast: a rare benign tumour mimicking breast carcinoma. *Clin Radiol* 1995;50:799.

116. Vos LD, Tjon A Tham RT, Vroegindweij D, et al. Granular cell tumor of the breast: mammographic and histologic correlation. *Eur J Radiol* 1994;19:56–59.

117. Scatarige JC, Hsiu JG, de la Torre R, et al. Acoustic shadowing in benign granular cell tumor (myoblastoma) of the breast. *J Ultrasound Med* 1987;6:545–547.

118. Baum JK, Robins JR, Schnitt S, et al. The ultrasound appearance of granular cell tumor of the breast: a case report. *Breast Dis* 1994;7:281–285.

119. Gibbons D, Leitch M, Coscia J, et al. Fine needle aspiration cytology and histologic findings of granular cell tumor of the breast: review of 19 cases with clinical/radiologic correlation. *Breast J* 2000;6:27–30.

120. Horiguchi J, Iino Y, Takei H, et al. Granular cell tumor of the breast diagnosed by core needle biopsy: a case report. *Breast Cancer* 1999;6:69–71.

121. McMahon JN, Rigby HS, Davies JD. Elastosis in granular cell tumours: prevalence and distribution. *Histopathology* 1990;16:37–41.

122. Fust JA, Custer RP. On the neurogenesis of so-called granular cell myoblastoma. *Am J Clin Pathol* 1949;19:522–535.

123. Buley ID, Gatter KC, Kelly PMA, et al. Granular cell tumours revisited. An immunohistochemical and ultrastructural study. *Histopathology* 1988;12:263–274.

124. Hahn HJ, Iglesias J, Flenker H, et al. Granular cell tumor in differential diagnosis of tumors of the breast. *Pathol Res Pract* 1992;188:1091–1094.

125. Ingram DL, Mossler JA, Snowhite J, et al. Granular cell tumors of the breast. Steroid receptor analysis and localization of carcinoembryonic antigen, myoglobin and S-100 protein. *Arch Pathol Lab Med* 1984;108:897–901.

126. Shousha S, Lyssiotis T. Granular cell myoblastoma: positive staining for carcino-embryonic antigen. *J Clin Pathol* 1979;32:219–244.

127. Franzen S, Steinkvist B. Diagnosis of granular cell myoblastoma by fine-needle aspiration biopsy. *Acta Pathol Microbiol Scand* 1968;72:391–395.

128. Löwhagen T, Rubio CA. The cytology of the granular cell myoblastoma of the breast. *Acta Cytol* 1977;21:314–315.

129. Mitnick JS, Vazquez MF, Pressman PI, et al. Stereotactic fine-needle aspiration biopsy for the evaluation of nonpalpable breast lesions: report of an experience based on 2,988 cases. *Ann Surg Oncol* 1996;3:185–191.

130. Chhieng DC, Cangiarella JF, Waisman J, et al. Fine-needle aspiration cytology of spindle cell lesions of the breast. *Cancer* 1999; 87:359–371.

131. Sirgi KE, Sneige N, Fanning TV, et al. Fine-needle aspirates of granular cell lesions of the breast: report of three cases, with emphasis on differential diagnosis and utility of immunostaining for CD68 (KP1). *Diagn Cytopathol* 1996;15:403–408.

132. Mittal KR, True LD. Origin of granules in granular cell tumor. Intracellular myelin formation with autodigestion. *Arch Pathol Lab Med* 1988;112:302–303.

133. Gamboa LG. Malignant granular cell myoblastoma. *Arch Pathol* 1955;60:663–668.

134. Crawford ES, DeBakey ME. Granular cell myoblastoma: two unusual cases. *Cancer* 1953;6:786–789.

135. Uzoaru I, Firfer B, Ray V, et al. Malignant granular cell tumor. *Arch Pathol Lab Med* 1992;116:206–208.

## Tumors of Nerve and Nerve Sheath Origin

136. Bernardello F, Caneva A, Bresaola E, et al. Breast solitary schwannoma: fine-needle aspiration biopsy and immunocytochemical analysis. *Diagn Cytopathol* 1994;10:221–223.

137. DasGupta TK, Brasfield RD, Strong EW, et al. Benign solitary schwannomas (neurilemomas). *Cancer* 1969;24:355–366.

138. Fisher PE, Estabrook A, Cohen MB. Fine needle aspiration biopsy of intramammary neurilemoma. *Acta Cytol* 1990;34:36–37.

139. van der Walt JD, Reid HA, Shaw JHF. Neurilemoma appearing as a lump in the breast. *Arch Pathol Lab Med* 1982;106:539–540.

140. Lipper S, Wilson CF, Copeland KC. Pseudogynecomastia due to neurofibromatosis: a light and ultrastructural study. *Hum Pathol* 1981;12:755–759.

141. Sherman JE, Smith JW. Neurofibromas of the breast and nipple-areolar area. *Am Plast Surg* 1981;7:302–307.

142. Galant C, Mazy S, Berlier M, et al. Two schwannomas presenting as lumps in the same breast. *Diagn Cytopathol* 1997;16:281–284.

143. Hock YL, Mohamid W. Myxoid neurofibroma of the male breast: fine needle aspiration cytodiagnosis. *Cytopathology* 1995;6:44–47.

144. Martinez-Onsurbe P, Fuentes-Vaamonde E, Gonzalez-Estecha A, et al. Neurilemoma of the breast in a man. A case report. *Acta Cytol* 1992;36:511–513.

145. Murayama Y, Yamamoto Y, Shimojima N, et al. T1 breast cancer associated with von Recklinghausen's neurofibromatosis. *Breast Cancer* 1999;6:227–230.

146. Cohen MB, Fisher PE. Schwann cell tumours of the breast and mammary region. *Surg Pathol* 1991;4:47–56.

147. Gultekin SH, Cody HS III, Hoda SA. Schwannoma of the breast. *South Med J* 1996;89:238–239.

148. Hood IC, Qizilbash AH, Young JEM, et al. Needle aspiration cytology of a benign and a malignant schwannoma. *Acta Cytol* 1984; 28:157–164.

149. Silverman JF, Geisinger KR, Frable WJ. Fine-needle aspiration cytology of mesenchymal tumors of the breast. *Diagn Cytopathol* 1988;4:50–58.

150. Ryd W, Mugal S, Ayyash K. Ancient neurilemoma. A pitfall in the cytologic diagnosis of soft-tissue tumors. *Diagn Cytopathol* 1986; 2:244–247.

## Hamartoma

151. *Stedman's medical dictionary,* 24th ed. Baltimore: Williams & Wilkins, 1982:619.

152. Arrigoni MG, Dockerty MB, Judd ES. The identification and treatment of mammary hamartoma. *Surg Gynecol Obstet* 1971;133: 577–582.

153. Daya D, Trus T, D'Souza TJ, et al. Hamartoma of the breast, an underrecognized breast lesion. A clinicopathologic and radiographic study of 25 cases. *Am J Clin Pathol* 1995;103:685–689.

154. Oberman HA. Hamartomas and hamartoma variants of the breast. *Semin Diagn Pathol* 1989;6:135–145.

155. Andersson I, Hildell J, Linell F, et al. Mammary hamartomas. *Acta Radiol [Diagn]* 1979;20:712–720.

156. Ljungqvist U, Andersson I, Hildell J, et al. Mammary hamartoma, a benign breast lesion. *Acta Chir Scand* 1979;145:227–230.

157. Altermatt HJ, Gebbers J-O, Laissue J-A. Multiple hamartomas of the breast. *Appl Pathol* 1989;7:145–148.

158. Cooper RA, Johnson MS. Juvenile hypertrophy presenting as a discrete breast mass. *Can Assoc Radiol J* 1992;43:218–220.

159. Linell F, Ostberg G, Soderstrom J, et al. Breast hamartomas. An important entity in mammary pathology. *Virchows Arch [A]* 1979; 383:253–264.

160. Evers K, Yeh I-T, Troupin RH, et al. Mammary hamartomas. The importance of radiologic-pathologic correlation. *Breast Dis* 1992;5: 35–43.

161. Hessler C, Schnyder P, Ozzello L. Hamartoma of the breast: diagnostic observation of 16 cases. *Radiology* 1978;126:95–98.

162. Adler DD, Jeffries DO, Helvie MA. Sonographic features of breast hamartomas. *J Ultrasound Med* 1990;9:85–90.

163. Borochovitz D. Adenolipoma of the breast: a variant of adenofibroma. *Breast* 1982;8:32–33.

164. Crothers JG, Butler NF, Fortt RW, et al. Fibroadenolipoma of the breast. *Br J Radiol* 1985;58:191–202.

165. Yasuda S, Kubota M, Noto T, et al. Two cases of adenolipoma of the breast. *Tokai J Exp Clin Med* 1992;17:139–144.

166. Oberman HA, Nozanchuk JS, Frazer JE. Periductal stromal tumors of breast with adipose metaplasia. *Arch Surg* 1969;98:384–387.

167. Kaplan L, Walts AE. Benign chondrolipomatous tumor of the human female breast. *Arch Pathol Lab Med* 1977;101:149–151.

168. Lugo M, Reyes JM, Putony PB. Benign chondrolipomatous tumor of the human female breast. *Arch Pathol Lab Med* 1982;106:691–692.

169. Marsh WL Jr, Lucas JG, Olsen J. Chondrolipoma of the breast. *Arch Pathol Lab Med* 1989;113:369–371.

170. Metcalf JS, Ellis B. Choristoma of the breast. *Hum Pathol* 1985;16:739–740.

171. Peison B, Benisch B, Tonzola A. Case report: benign chondrolipoma of the female breast. *N J Med* 1994;91:401–402.

172. Fushimi H, Kotoh K, Nishihara K, et al. Chondrolipoma of the breast: a case report with cytological and histological examination. *Histopathology* 1999;35:478–479.

## Leiomyoma

173. Nasciemento AG, Rosen PP, Karas M. Leiomyoma of the nipple. *Am J Surg Pathol* 1979;3:151–154.

174. Eusebi V, Cunsolo A, Fedeli F, et al. Benign smooth muscle cell metaplasia in breast. *Tumori* 1980;66:643–653.

175. Davies JD, Riddell RH. Muscular hamartomas of the breast. *J Pathol* 1973;111:209–211.

176. Haagensen CD. Non-epithelial neoplasms of the breast. In: Haagensen CD. *Diseases of the breast,* 2nd ed. Philadelphia: WB Saunders, 1971:292–325.

177. Diaz-Arias AA, Hurt MA, Loy TS, et al. Leiomyoma of the breast. *Hum Pathol* 1989;20:396–399.

178. Son EJ, Oh KK, Kim EK, et al. Leiomyoma of the breast in a 50-year-old woman receiving tamoxifen. *AJR Am J Roentgenol* 1998; 171:1684–1686.

179. Allison JG, Dodds HM. Leiomyoma of the male nipple. A case report and literature review. *Am Surg* 1989;55:501–502.

180. Velasco M, Ubeda B, Autonel F, et al. Leiomyoma of the male areola infiltrating the breast tissue. *AJR Am J Roentgenol* 1995;164:511–512.

181. Roncaroli F, Rossi R, Severi B, et al. Epithelioid leiomyoma of the breast with granular cell change: a case report. *Hum Pathol* 1993; 24:1260–1263.

182. Boscaino A, Ferrara G, Orabona P, et al. Smooth muscle tumors of the breast: clinicopathologic features of two cases. *Tumori* 1994;80: 241–245.

## Myoid "Hamartoma"

183. Daroca PJ Jr, Reed RJ, Love GL, et al. Myoid hamartomas of the breast. *Hum Pathol* 1985;16:212–219.
184. Huntrakoon M, Lin F. Muscular hamartoma of the breast. *Virchows Arch [A]* 1984;403:307–312.
185. Garfein CF, Aulicino MR, Leytin A, et al. Epithelioid cells in myoid hamartoma of the breast. *Arch Pathol Lab Med* 1996;120:676–680.
186. Shepstone BJ, Wells CA, Berry AR, et al. Mammographic appearance and histopathological description of a muscular hamartoma of the breast. *Br J Radiol* 1985;58:459–461.
187. Eusebi V, Cunsolo A, Fedeli F, et al. Benign smooth muscle cell metaplasia in breast. *Tumori* 1980;66:643–653.
188. Fiirgaard B, Kristensen S. Muscular hamartomas of the breast. A case report. *Acta Radiol* 1992;33:115–116.
189. Davies JD, Riddell RH. Muscular hamartomas of the breast. *J Pathol* 1973;111:209–211.

## Myeloid Metaplasia

190. Brooks JJ, Krugman DT, Damjanov I. Myeloid metaplasia presenting as a breast mass. *Am J Surg Pathol* 1980;4:281–285.
191. Glew RH, Haese WM, McIntyre PA. Myeloid metaplasia with myelofibrosis. The clinical spectrum of extramedullary hematopoiesis and tumor formation. *Johns Hopkins Med J* 1973;132:253–265.
192. Martinelli G, Santini D, Bazzocchi F, et al. Myeloid metaplasia of the breast. A lesion which clinically mimics carcinoma. *Virchows Arch [A]* 1983;401:203–207.

## Myxoma

193. Arihiro K, Inai K, Kurihara K, et al. Myxoma of the breast: report of a case with unique histological and immunohistochemical appearances. *Acta Pathol Jpn* 1993;43:340–346.
194. Chan YF, Yeung HY, Ma L. Myxoma of the breast: report of a case and ultrastructural study. *Pathology* 1986;18:153–157.
195. Carney JA, Toorkey BC. Myxoid fibroadenoma and allied conditions (myxomatosis) of the breast. A heritable disorder with special associations including cardiac and cutaneous myxomas. *Am J Surg Pathol* 1991;15:713–721.
196. Wee A, Tan CEL, Raju GC. Nerve sheath myxoma of the breast. A light and electron microscopic, histochemical and immunohistochemical study. *Virchows Arch [A]* 1989;416:163–167.

## Mucinosis

197. Michal M, Ludvíková M, Zámecník M. Nodular mucinosis of the breast: report of three cases. *Pathol Int* 1998;48:542–544.
198. Tavasolli FA. Diseases of the nipple. In: Tavasolli FA. *Pathology of the breast.* Norwalk, CT: Appleton & Lange, 1992:589.
199. Carney JA, Toorkey BC. Myxoid fibroadenoma and allied conditions (myxomatosis) of the breast. A heritable disorder with special associations including cardiac and cutaneous myxomas. *Am J Surg Pathol* 1991;18:713–721.

## Lipoma

200. Hansen PE, Williamson EO. Lipoma with central fat necrosis: is core biopsy a good way to diagnose fat necrosis of the breast? *Breast J* 1999;5:202–203.
201. Chan KW, Ghadially FN, Alagaratnam TT. Benign spindle cell tumour of breast—a variant of spindle cell lipoma or fibroma of breast? *Pathology* 1984;16:331–336.
202. Lew WY. Spindle cell lipoma of the breast. A case report and literature review. *Diagn Cytopathol* 1993;9:434–437.
203. Smith DN, Denison CM, Lester SC. Spindle cell lipoma of the breast. A case report. *Acta Radiol* 1996;37:893–895.

204. Magro G, Bisceglia M, Pasquinelli G. Benign spindle cell tumor of the breast with prominent adipocytic component. *Ann Diagn Pathol* 1998;2:306–311.

## Angiomas and Other Benign Vascular Lesions of the Breast

205. Azzopardi JG. *Major problems in pathology, vol. 11, problems in breast pathology.* Philadelphia: WB Saunders, 1979:371.
206. McDivitt RW, Stewart FW, Berg JW. *Tumors of the breast. Atlas of tumor pathology, 2nd series, fascicle 2.* Washington, DC: Armed Forces Institute of Pathology, 1968:128.

## Perilobular Hemangiomas

207. Jozefczyk MA, Rosen PP. Vascular tumors of the breast. II. Perilobular hemangiomas and hemangiomas. *Am J Surg Pathol* 1985;9: 491–503.
208. Lesueur GC, Brown RW, Bhathal PS. Incidence of perilobular hemangioma in the female breast. *Arch Pathol Lab Med* 1983;107: 308–310.
209. Rosen PP, Ridolfi RL. The perilobular hemangioma. A benign vascular lesion of the breast. *Am J Clin Pathol* 1977;68:21–23.
210. Hamperl H. Hämangiome der menschlichen Mamma. *Geburtsh Frauenheilk* 1973;33:13–17.
211. Nielsen B. Haemangiomas of the breast. *Pathol Res Pract* 1983; 176:253–257.

## Hemangiomas

212. Hoda SA, Cranor ML, Rosen PP. Hemangiomas of the breast with atypical histological features. Further analysis of histological subtypes confirming their benign character. *Am J Surg Pathol* 1992;16: 553–560.
213. Nagar H, Marmor S, Hammar B. Haemangiomas of the breast in children. Case report. *Eur J Surg* 1992;158:503–505.
214. Miaux Y, Lemarcharnd-Venencie F, Cyna-Gorse F. MR imaging of breast hemangioma in female infants. *Pediatr Radiol* 1992;22: 463–464.
215. Courcoutsakis NA, Hill SC, Chow CK, Breast hemangiomas in a patient with Kasabach-Merritt syndrome: imaging findings. *AJR Am J Roentgenol* 1997;169:1397–1399.
216. Webb LA, Young JR. Case report: haemangioma of the breast—appearances on mammography and ultrasound. *Clin Radiol* 1996;51: 523–524.
217. Tabar L, Dean PB. In: *Teaching atlas of mammography,* 2nd ed. New York: George Thieme Verlag Stuttgart, 1985:45, 209.
218. Sebek BA. Cavernous hemangioma of the female breast. *Cleve Clin Q* 1984;51:471–474.
219. Branton PR, Ashton MA, Tavassoli FA. The great impostor for angiosarcoma: papillary endothelial hyperplasia of the breast. *Mod Pathol* 1997;10:16A.

## Angiomatosis

220. Sieber PR, Sharkey FE. Cystic hygroma of the breast. *Arch Pathol Lab Med* 1986;110:353.
221. Hamperl H. Hämangiome der menschlichen Mamma. *Geburtsh Frauenheilk* 1973;33:13–17.
222. Morrow M, Berger D, Thelmo W. Diffuse cystic angiomatosis of the breast. *Cancer* 1988;62:2392–2396.
223. Rosen PP. Vascular tumors of the breast. III. Angiomatosis. *Am J Surg Pathol* 1985;9:652–655.
224. Enzinger FM, Weiss SW. *Soft tissue tumors.* St. Louis: CV Mosby, 1983:407–409.
225. Kolar J, Bek V, Vrabec R. Hypoplasia of the growing breast after contact X-ray therapy for cutaneous angiomas. *Arch Dermatol* 1967;96:427–430.
226. Weidman AI, Zimany A, Kopf AW. Underdevelopment of the human breast after radiotherapy. *Arch Dermatol* 1966;93:708–710.

## Venous Hemangiomas

227. Enzinger FM, Weiss SW. *Soft tissue tumors.* St. Louis: CV Mosby, 1983:387–391.
228. Wold LE, Swee RG, Sim FH. Vascular lesions of bone. *Pathol Annu* 1985;20[Pt 2]:101–138.
229. Rosen PP, Jozefczyk MA, Boram LH. Vascular tumors of the breast. IV. The venous hemangioma. *Am J Surg Pathol* 1985;9:659–665.

## Nonparenchymal Hemangiomas of the Mammary Region

230. Menville JG, Bloodgood JC. Subcutaneous angiomas of the breast. *Ann Surg* 1933;97:401–413.
231. Madding GF, Hershberger LR. Hemangioma of the breast. *Surgery* 1949;26:685–687.
232. Rosen PP. Vascular tumors of the breast V. Non-parenchymal hemangiomas of mammary subcutaneous tissue. *Am J Surg Pathol* 1985;9:723–729.
233. Perugini G, Bonini G, Giardina C. Cavernous hemangioma of the pectoralis muscle mimicking a breast tumor. *AJR Am J Roentgenol* 1994;162:1321–1322.

234. Yu GH, Fishman SJ, Brooks JSJ. Cellular angiolipoma of the breast. *Mod Pathol* 1993;6:497–499.
235. Howard WR, Helwig EB. Angiolipoma. *Arch Dermatol* 1960;82:924–931.

## Aneurysm

236. Beres RA, Harrington DG, Wenzel MS. Percutaneous repair of breast pseudoaneurysm: sonographically guided embolization. *AJR Am J Roentgenol* 1997;169:425–427.
237. Smith SM. Breast pseudoaneurysm after core biopsy. *AJR Am J Roentgenol* 1996;167:817.
238. Dehn TCB, Lee ECG. Aneurysm presenting as a breast mass. *Br Med J* 1986;292:240.
239. Pettinger TW, Dublin AB, Lindfors KK. Percutaneous embolotherapy of an arterial pseudoaneurysm of the breast: a case report. *Breast Dis* 1995;87:97–101.
240. Daunt N. An intramammary pseudoaneurysm presenting as a breast mass. *Austral Radiol* 1995;39:71–72.
241. Davies JD, Kulka J. Traumatic arterial damage after fine-needle aspirational cytology in mammary complex sclerosing lesions. *Histopathology* 1996;28:65–70.

# CHAPTER 41

# Sarcoma

Mammary sarcomas are a heterogeneous group of malignant neoplasms that arise from the mammary stroma. Excluded from this presentation are malignant lymphomas and malignant phyllodes tumor, which are covered in other chapters. Neoplasms included in the category of mammary sarcoma or stromal "sarcoma" are thought to arise from interlobular mesenchymal elements that constitute the supporting mammary stroma.

The diagnosis of mammary sarcomas should be reported in the same histogenetic terms as are used for soft-part sarcomas, which occur throughout the body. The relative frequency of different types of breast sarcomas is difficult to determine from the literature because these lesions sometimes have been referred to by the general term *stromal sarcoma*. Some differences in frequency do appear to exist, however. For example, one of the most common forms of mammary sarcoma, angiosarcoma, is proportionately less common among somatic sarcomas. Other distinct mammary sarcomas include liposarcoma, fibrosarcoma, leiomyosarcoma, sarcomas with bone and cartilage, and malignant fibrous histiocytoma.

As a group, mammary sarcomas vary greatly in size, ranging from 1 cm or smaller to 30 cm or larger. In most studies, the mean and median size is 3 to 4 cm. The gross appearance of the tumors is influenced in part by the specific histologic characteristics of the lesion, but the specimens typically consist of fleshy, moderately firm, pale tissue with varying amounts of hemorrhage and necrosis (Fig. 41.1). Most sarcomas appear to be well circumscribed grossly, even if the border is histologically invasive.

Grading of mammary sarcomas is prognostically important, as has been demonstrated in the case of angiosarcoma. Lesions at the low-grade end of the spectrum of fibrosarcoma constitute the group of neoplasms discussed elsewhere under the heading of *fibromatosis*. Although mammary fibromatosis does not metastasize, it can pursue an inexorable course of local recurrence, resulting in extensive local destruction and even death as a consequence of visceral invasion.

A diagnosis of mammary sarcoma can be established only after metaplastic carcinoma is excluded. The distinction is important for treatment as well as for prognosis. The lesion should be sampled extensively for evidence of *in situ* or invasive carcinoma. Perhaps the most difficult distinction lies between fibrosarcoma and a metaplastic spindle cell squamous carcinoma. Immunohistochemical studies for epithelial markers are useful for detecting evidence of epithelial origin or inconspicuous foci of epithelial cells in a carcinoma that has undergone virtually complete conversion into a spindle cell neoplasm.

A review of the reported incidence of local recurrence in relation to primary treatment suggests that total mastectomy should be recommended for most sarcomas of the breast. Axillary lymph node metastases are exceedingly uncommon at the time of primary therapy, and therefore axillary dissection ordinarily is not indicated (1,2). When a total mastectomy or a more extensive operation was the initial treatment, 8% of patients had local failures, whereas recurrence in the breast was reported in 53% of patients treated by excisional surgery. Excisional surgery is more likely to be successful if performed for low-grade lesions and for tumors smaller than 5 cm, and mastectomy is indicated for larger or high-grade sarcomas (1). Contemporary multimodal approaches, including radiation and chemotherapy, may reduce the frequency of local and systemic recurrence of somatic sarcomas, but results to date are inconclusive in patients with mammary sarcoma (1,3,4).

## STROMAL SARCOMA

This term was introduced in 1962 to describe 25 primary mammary sarcomas that did not qualify for a diagnosis of malignant phyllodes tumor or angiosarcoma (5). The histologic appearance included "fibrous, myxoid and fatty patterns." A liposarcomatous component was identified in six tumors, and others had elements that resembled leiomyosarcoma or "neurosarcoma." None of the tumors exhibited osseous or rhabdomyosarcomatous differentiation. These researchers concluded that the neoplasms had a common "basic stromal-like structure" composed of elongated cells with an "off center" nucleus, and on this basis chose the term *stromal*

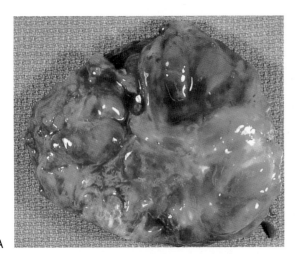

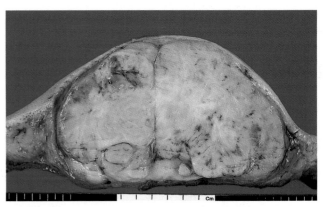

**FIG. 41.1.** *Sarcoma, gross appearance.* **A:** This tumor had areas of osteogenic and liposarcoma. **B:** Fibrosarcoma in a 42-year-old woman replaces much of the breast parenchyma in this mastectomy specimen. Necrosis imparts a pale yellow color centrally. Viable tumor forms a beige rim to the mass and deep secondary nodules (Courtesy of Hyunee Kim, M.D.).

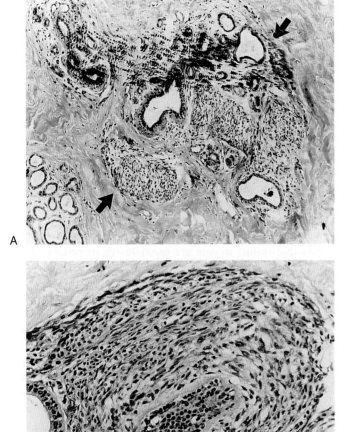

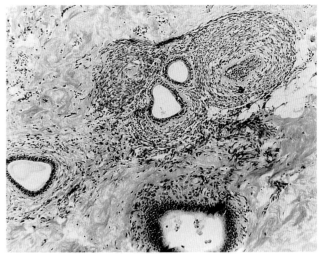

**FIG. 41.2.** *True stromal sarcoma.* **A:** Sarcoma limited to the intralobular stroma between the *arrows*. The interlobular stroma is normal. **B,C:** Sarcoma limited to periductal stroma in the same tumor as **A**. (**A,B:** From Callery CD, Rosen PP, Kinne DW. Sarcoma of the breast: a study of 32 patients with reappraisal of classification and therapy. *Ann Surg* 1985;201: 527–532, with permission.)

*sarcoma.* The 25 patients ranged in age from 25 to 64 years, averaging 48 years. All but one were women. Among 15 patients treated by local excision, nine developed local recurrences within 5 years, and five of these patients died of disease. A sixth patient treated by local excision died of sarcoma without local recurrence. Local recurrence occurred in one patient treated by mastectomy whose tumor initially invaded the chest wall. No patient had axillary lymph node metastases. The actuarial 5-year survival rate was 60%.

In retrospect, the illustrations and microscopic descriptions suggest that most of the tumors included in the report would be classified currently as liposarcoma, malignant fibrous histiocytoma, or fibrosarcoma. Despite the apparent lack of specificity, the diagnosis of stromal sarcoma is still sometimes used, although it is now considered preferable to subclassify mammary sarcomas according to their growth patterns (6,7).

The breast is composed of specialized hormone-responsive stroma localized in lobules and around ducts as well as fibrous, adipose, and other mesenchymal tissues. If the term *stromal sarcoma* were selected to designate any of the mesenchymal neoplasms of the breast, it should be applied to those derived from the hormonally responsive specialized stroma. Most of these neoplasms, phyllodes tumors, also have a proliferative epithelial component. Purely sarcomatous tumors of this specialized stroma, which are exceptionally rare, can be classified as true stromal sarcomas of the breast (8) (Fig. 41.2). Most nonphyllodes mesenchymal neoplasms are best classified with the same terminology as sarcomas at other anatomic sites.

## LEIOMYOSARCOMA

This form of sarcoma probably originates from blood vessels or the smooth muscle of the nipple–areolar complex in some cases. A predisposition of smooth muscle in the nipple to give rise to neoplasms is evidenced by reports of leiomyomata (9–11) and leiomyosarcomas (12,13) at this site. One leiomyosarcoma may have arisen in an ectopic areola (14).

Myoid transformation of myoepithelial cells and myofibroblasts are other histogenetic mechanisms (15,16).

### Clinical Presentation

Most cases have been in female patients, but origin in the male breast has been reported (12,17,18). The age at diagnosis is typically in the fifth decade, with an age range from 24 to 86 years. The presenting symptom is a mass measuring 1.5 to 9 cm, averaging about 4 cm. Nearly half the tumors are in or near the nipple–areola complex, but any quadrant may be affected. The tumors are circumscribed and firm. Pain is rarely reported. Mammography reveals a dense, lobulated lesion with a defined border.

### Pathology

Gross examination reveals a circumscribed, firm, lobulated pale tumor. Areas of necrosis may be grossly apparent.

Microscopically, the neoplasm consists of interlacing bundles of fusiform cells characteristic of a smooth-muscle tumor with typical blunt-end nuclei (Figs. 41.3 and 41.4). Cells with an epithelioid phenotype are variably present. Malignant cytologic features reported in most cases have been nuclear hyperchromasia, pleomorphism (sometimes with multinucleated giant cells), and readily identified mitoses ranging from 2 to 29 per 10 high-power fields (hpf), with an average of 18 mitoses/10 hpf. Focal areas of degeneration are characterized by nuclear pyknosis, necrosis, and lymphocytic infiltration. Areas of hyalinized stromal fibrosis with a pattern that resembles pseudoangiomatous stromal hyperplasia may be present (Fig. 41.5). Mammary ducts and lobules, sometimes with proliferative changes, can be incorporated into the neoplasm, particularly at the periphery, a feature that may lead to considering alternative diagnoses, such as metaplastic carcinoma and phyllodes tumor. One tumor classified as leiomyosarcoma contained areas of "benign" metaplastic bone and cartilage (19) and another tumor had focal rhabdomyoblastic dif-

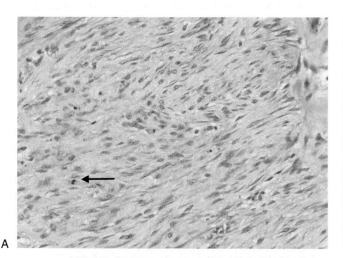
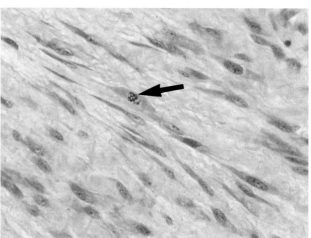

A                            B

**FIG. 41.3.** *Leiomyosarcoma.* **A:** A moderately cellular tumor composed of fusiform tumor cells with blunt-end nuclei. One mitosis is evident *(arrow).* **B:** A mitotic figure is shown *(arrow).*

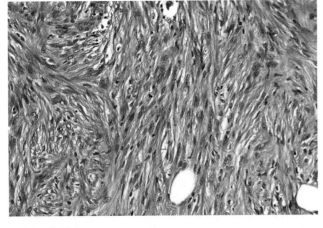

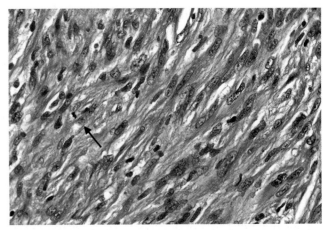

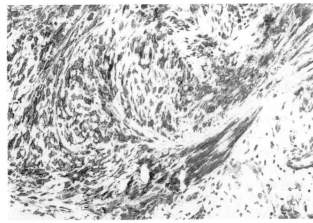

**FIG. 41.4.** *Leiomyosarcoma.* **A:** A highly cellular tumor composed of interlacing fascicles of spindle cells. **B:** A mitotic figure is shown *(arrow).* **C:** Immunoreactivity for actin (anti–smooth-muscle actin; avidin-biotin).

ferentiation (20). Leiomyosarcoma with osteoclast-like giant cells can occur in the breast (Fig. 41.6).

Immunohistochemical stains are usually at least focally positive for desmin, smooth-muscle actin, and vimentin (Figs. 41.4 and 41.6). Some tumors classified as leiomyosarcoma were weakly positive for cytokeratin (13) and S-100 (13,21,22) and focally positive for epithelial membrane antigen (21), and a few were negative for actin or desmin (22,23). Weak reactivity for vimentin has been described

(13,24). The precise classification of these tumors with aberrant cytokeratin immunoreactivity remains uncertain.

Electron microscopy revealed myofilaments in three cases (12,21,25), whereas in another report electron microscopy was described as "unhelpful showing undifferentiated polygonal and spindle cells" (13).

The fine needle aspiration (FNA) specimen consists of clustered and dissociated spindle or polygonal cells. The extent of pleomorphism, hyperchromasia, and mitotic activity in the FNA specimen reflects the histologic appearance of the neoplasm (13,25).

### Treatment and Prognosis

With the exception of a few instances of local excision alone (21,26), primary treatment consisted of total mastectomy. Local recurrence in the breast has been reported when primary treatment was limited to excision (21,26) and on the chest wall after mastectomy (27). No instance of axillary nodal metastases has been reported.

About 25% of patients with mammary leiomyosarcoma with reported follow-up died of metastatic sarcoma (13,21,23,28–30). Outcome has not correlated well with the mitotic rate in the primary tumor because fatalities occurred in cases with 2 or 3 mitoses/10 hpf as well as higher rates. Late recurrences and death from disease 16 and 20 years after initial diagnoses have been reported (26,27,31).

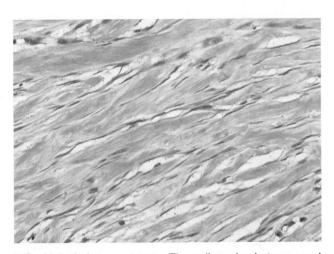

**FIG. 41.5.** *Leiomyosarcoma.* The collagenized stroma and clefts resemble pseudoangiomatous stromal hyperplasia.

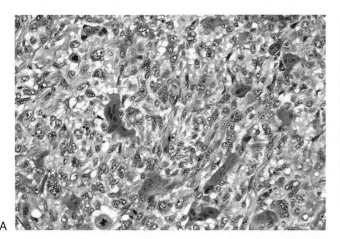
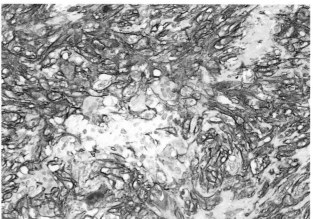

A

B

**FIG. 41.6.** *Leiomyosarcoma, osteoclast-like giant cells.* **A:** Osteoclast-like giant cells mingle with epithelioid myosarcoma cells. Mitoses are present in sarcoma cells. **B:** Strong actin immunoreactivity is limited to the sarcoma cells. The giant cells were immunoreactive for CD68, a histiocytic marker (not shown) and no reactivity for cytokeratin was present (anti–smooth-muscle actin; avidin-biotin).

## LIPOSARCOMA

This malignant neoplasm may arise from periductal–perilobular stroma in the form of a malignant phyllodes tumor (32,33) or from interlobular stroma to present as a primary stromal sarcoma (32). Liposarcoma arising in a phyllodes tumor is discussed in Chapter 8.

### Clinical Presentation

Patients range in age from 26 to 76 years at the time of diagnosis, with an average age of 49 years. The presenting symptom is a mass of variable duration occasionally with pain (32,34). Two instances of bilateral low-grade liposarcoma have been reported (34,35). Two male patients have been described (32). Radiation-related pleomorphic liposarcoma of the chest wall has been reported 10 years after mastectomy (36).

On clinical examination, the tumor is typically firm and well circumscribed, but ill-defined lesions have been reported. Mammography in a patient with bilateral involvement revealed "a bizarre pattern of widespread density in the posterior and axillary region of each breast" (34).

### Pathology

Grossly, the tumors have measured 2 to 40 cm, averaging about 8 cm. Some tumors were described as well circumscribed or encapsulated, whereas others were multinodular or infiltrative. The cut surface was yellow to tan. Gelatinous areas were evident if there was a myxoid liposarcoma component.

The histologic features of liposarcoma in the breast are identical to those of liposarcoma arising in the extremities or trunk. Among current published reports, including 25 mammary tumors classified in these terms, 12 (48%) were myxoid (Fig. 41.7), 6 (24%) were well differentiated, 4 (16%) were pleomorphic, and 3 (12%) were poorly differentiated (32,34,37–43). No apparent consistent relationship between tumor type, size, and age at diagnosis was found.

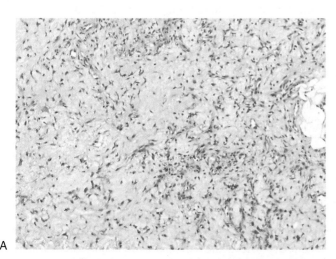
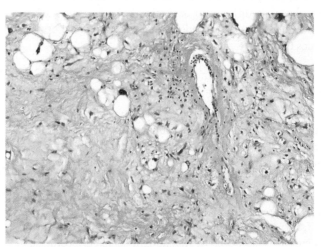

A

B

**FIG. 41.7.** *Liposarcoma, myxoid type.* **A:** The characteristic myxoid stroma and vascular pattern are shown. **B:** An occasional tumor cell with an enlarged, hyperchromatic nucleus. *(continued)*

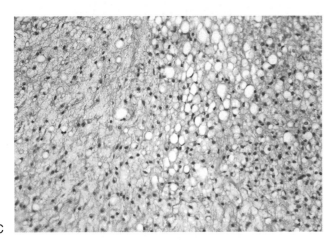

C

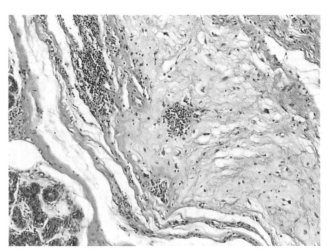

D

**FIG. 41.7.** *Continued.* **C:** Most tumor cells have small, round nuclei. **D:** Myxoliposarcoma invading breast parenchyma.

## Treatment and Prognosis

With rare exceptions, treatment has consisted of simple or radical mastectomy (32). Axillary lymph node metastases have not been reported. With follow-up ranging from less than a year to 20 years, about 70% of patients have remained recurrence free, 6% were alive with systemic recurrence, and 24% died of metastatic liposarcoma (32,34,37–44). Systemic recurrences and deaths from disease usually occurred within 2 years of diagnosis and were limited to patients with pleomorphic or high-grade tumors. Tumor size by itself was not predictive of outcome.

## OSTEOGENIC SARCOMA AND CHONDROSARCOMA

Most mammary neoplasms with malignant osseous and cartilaginous differentiation are variants of heterologous metaplastic carcinoma or malignant phyllodes tumor. Pure osteogenic sarcomas and chondrosarcomas of the mammary stroma are uncommon, but the precise frequency of these neoplasms is difficult to determine because some case reports do not clearly exclude metaplastic carcinoma or phyllodes tumor.

## Clinical Presentation

The presenting symptom is a mass, typically described as circumscribed and freely movable. A minority of the tumors are irregular or multinodular. Mammography reveals a dense mass that may exhibit calcifications (45,46); by ultrasound, one tumor had heterogeneous echogenicity with an anterior halo and posterior shadowing and enhancement (46). The tumor may be positive in a technetium-99 diphosphonate scan (47,48). Age at diagnosis ranges from 23 to 84 years, averaging 55 years (49–59). Radiation-associated, postmastectomy osteogenic sarcoma and chondrosarcoma of the chest wall has been reported (60).

## Pathology

The excised tumors have measured 5 to 25 cm in diameter, with an average size of 10 cm. A well-defined border is described in most cases. The cut surface usually has a somewhat variegated appearance, with areas of softening or gelatinous degeneration and foci of necrosis distributed in firm gray or white tissue. A gritty sensation is encountered when cutting the tumor in areas of ossification. Gross calcification also may be visible and palpable (54).

Histologic examination reveals a spectrum of microscopic patterns (Fig. 41.8). The tumors have in common a prominent component of high-grade spindle cell sarcoma with a variable mitotic rate. Tumors with chondroid differentiation alone are less frequent than those with osseous differentiation in which there may be a chondroid element (50,55). Multinucleated osteoclastic giant cells are usually present in areas of bone formation. Rarely, giant cells constitute a conspicuous element and may be associated with hemorrhagic cysts with a telangiectatic appearance (57).

Special stains, including immunohistochemistry for cytokeratin, are helpful in ruling out an epithelial component. Areas with cartilaginous differentiation can be immunoreactive for epithelial membrane antigen (58), and staining for S-100 sometimes is found in spindle cell portions of the lesion (55,58). An unusual form of metaplastic carcinoma with osseous and chondroid differentiation features infrequent squamoid cell clusters in the midst of otherwise sarcomatous tumor tissue. In one case report, osteoclastic giant cells within the tumor were immunoreactive for KP-1 (CD68), a marker of histiocytic differentiation (45). The findings in a FNA specimen depend on the composition of the lesion (46,51,54,57). If the predominant elements are spindle and giant cells, the distinction between a primary sarcoma, a malignant phyllodes tumor, and a metaplastic carcinoma cannot be made with certainty. The electron microscopic features of mammary osteogenic sarcoma and chondrosarcoma have been reported (54,55,61). Desmosomes have been observed linking undifferentiated cells in osteogenic sarcoma (61).

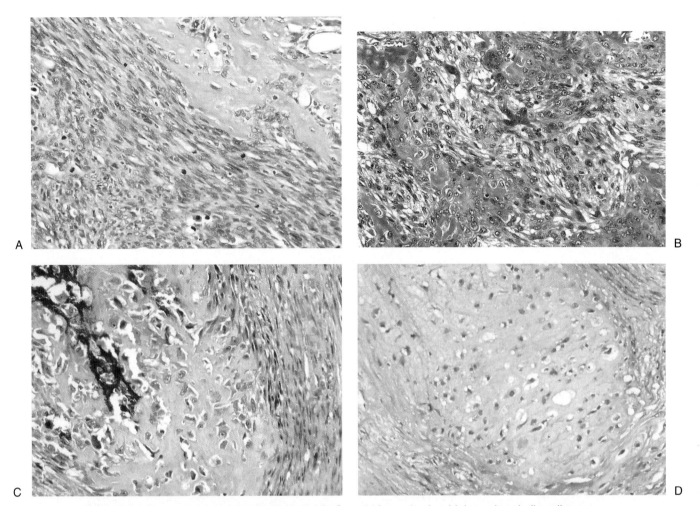

**FIG. 41.8.** *Osteogenic and chondrosarcoma.* **A:** Osteoid formation in a high-grade spindle cell sarcoma. **B:** Patches of osteoid formation in the midst of high-grade spindle cell sarcoma. **C:** Ossification in osteogenic sarcoma. **D:** Chondrosarcoma.

### Treatment and Prognosis

A minority of patients have been treated by local excision, and they remained disease free 2 to 3 years after treatment (51,55). Most patients had a simple, modified, or radical mastectomy. Lymph node metastases have not been reported. One patient treated by mastectomy died of an unrelated cause within 1 year, four died of metastatic sarcoma in less than a year, one died of lung metastases 9 years after diagnosis (62), and three were alive with recurrent sarcoma at last follow-up.

### MALIGNANT FIBROUS HISTIOCYTOMA

Histologic descriptions of spindle cell sarcomas of the breast have not always clearly distinguished between fibrosarcoma and malignant fibrous histiocytoma. As noted by Jones et al., "these two tumors have many features in common; thus, classification of some into one or the other group can be arbitrary" (63). In this chapter, a breast tumor was accepted as malignant fibrous histiocytoma if this was the reported diagnosis and the growth pattern was predominantly storiform (63–70).

### Clinical Presentation

Most patients have been women, but low-grade (63) and high-grade (71,72) malignant fibrous histiocytoma of the male breast has been described. The initial symptom is a mass, which may be located in any portion of the breast. The tumors are usually solitary, but patients with multiple tumors have been described. Ulceration of the overlying skin can occur (67,68). Antecedent trauma occasionally is reported. Numerous case reports suggested an association between prior irradiation for breast carcinoma and the development of malignant fibrous histiocytoma (73,74). In most of these instances, the sarcoma arose in the chest wall after mastectomy (75–78) or in sites of nodal irradiation, such as the axilla (76,79,80). In one patient, the sarcoma appeared in the conserved breast 2 years after excisional surgery and radiotherapy for mammary carcinoma (81). The interval between radiation and the diagnosis of sarcoma in the breast has been 2 to 7 years.

Age at diagnosis of primary malignant fibrous histiocytoma of the breast ranges from 24 to 93 years, averaging 59 years. In one series, patients with low-grade tumors tended to be younger (average age, 46 years) than those with high-grade tumors (average age, 64 years) (63).

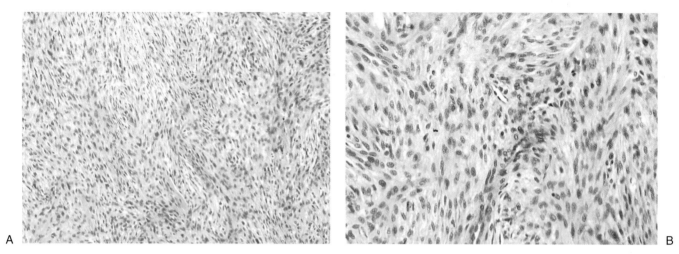

**FIG. 41.9.** *Malignant fibrous histiocytoma.* **A,B:** The characteristic storiform pattern is shown.

## Pathology

The tumors reportedly have measured from 1.0 to 20 cm, averaging 7.0 cm. In a patient with multiple tumors, the two largest tumors were each 7.0 cm. The excised lesion may have a circumscribed or an ill-defined border. The neoplasm is firm to hard with a gray, tan, or white cut surface. Necrosis, mucoid change, and calcification are infrequent.

The microscopic hallmark of malignant fibrous histiocytoma is the storiform growth pattern in which the spindle cells are arranged in a pinwheel pattern (Fig. 41.9). Capillaries or small blood vessels may be found at the center of the storiform complex. Giant cells, usually with multiple nuclei, myxoid change, and a chronic inflammatory cell infiltrate are variably present (Fig. 41.10). High-grade lesions are characterized by easily identified mitoses, generally numbering

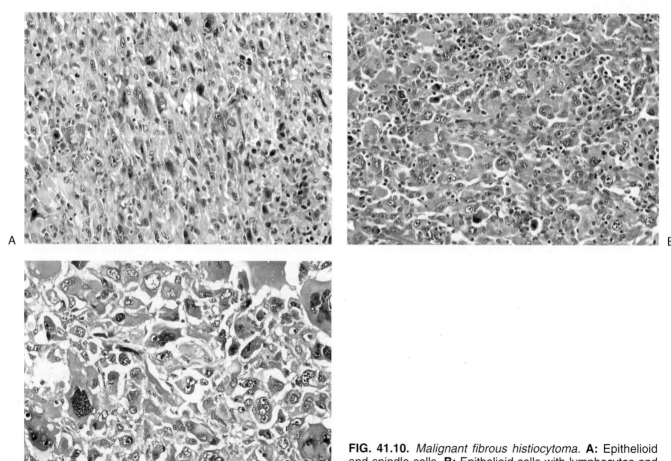

**FIG. 41.10.** *Malignant fibrous histiocytoma.* **A:** Epithelioid and spindle cells. **B:** Epithelioid cells with lymphocytes and plasma cells are present. **C:** Bizarre giant cells in a part of the tumor are depicted.

more than 3/10 hpf, cellular pleomorphism, and necrosis. Low-grade tumors have little mitotic activity as well as minimal pleomorphism or necrosis. Cellularity alone is not a reliable criterion for distinguishing between low- and high-grade malignant fibrous histiocytomas of the breast.

Immunohistochemical stains are not specific. The tumors are reactive for vimentin and occasionally for actin (63) or rarely cytokeratin (Fig. 41.11). All pathologic and clinical features must be given careful consideration when a tumor with storiform growth displays cytokeratin reactivity because these lesions are usually metaplastic carcinomas, but rarely aberrant cytokeratin expression is present in various sarcomas. Immunoreactivity for $\alpha_1$-antitrypsin has been reported in malignant fibrous histiocytomas of the breast (70) and other sites (82,83). The electron microscopic features of mammary malignant fibrous histiocytoma have been reported (66,67,77,78). Aspiration cytology yields spindle cells, giant cells, and conspicuous capillaries (84).

### Treatment and Prognosis

With few exceptions, treatment has been by mastectomy with or without axillary dissection. A small minority of patients have been managed successfully by local excision alone. Local recurrence has been reported after mastectomy and local excision. The choice between mastectomy and local excision depends on the individual clinical presentation. This determines the likelihood of obtaining complete excision, negative margins, and a cosmetically satisfactory result. Axillary lymph node dissection is not indicated for malignant fibrous histiocytoma unless necessitated to obtain an adequate margin or if nodal metastases are suggested by clinical findings.

Recurrence and death from disease have been reported in about 40% of patients. The most frequent sites of metastases are the lungs and bones. Tumors that developed metastases have been high-grade histologically. Local recurrence is not infrequent among low-grade tumors. Systemic recurrences

and deaths usually occurred within 3 years and rarely more than 5 years after diagnoses (63,65,66).

## FIBROSARCOMA

Tumors in which the dominant growth pattern is composed of elongated spindle cells arranged in broad interdigitating sheets, bands, or fascicles (so-called herringbone pattern) are classified as *fibrosarcoma* (Fig. 41.12). Some fibrosarcomas lacking the classic herringbone pattern consist of a more loosely structured fibroblastic proliferation (Fig. 41.13). Sarcomas with a storiform structure are termed *malignant fibrous histiocytomas,* but many of these lesions were probably classified as fibrosarcoma in the past. Consequently, the relative frequency in the breast of these types of sarcoma is difficult to determine from published reports. In two institutional series, Terrier et al. classified 11 sarcomas as malignant fibrous histiocytoma and 2 as fibrosarcomas (85), and Callery et al. reported 9 fibrosarcomas and 5 malignant fibrous histiocytomas (86). Jones et al. reported that 17 of 32 tumors in the malignant fibrous histiocytomas/fibrosarcoma group had a storiform growth pattern (87). In the latter series, tumors with the fibrosarcomatous herringbone pattern tended to be histologically low grade and to have a better prognosis than sarcomas with the malignant fibrous histiocytoma pattern, which were more often high-grade. Local recurrences were observed in 60% of low-grade sarcomas with no significant difference in relation to growth pattern, and no deaths from sarcomas occurred. Among patients with high-grade tumors, recurrence and death from sarcoma occurred with nearly the same frequency among patients with both growth patterns. The higher local recurrence rate in patients with low-grade lesions in this series probably is related to more frequent treatment by local excision alone.

Most instances of postradiation fibrosarcoma involving patients treated for breast carcinoma have arisen in the chest wall after mastectomy. Rare examples of parenchymal origin after breast conservation and radiotherapy have been reported (88).

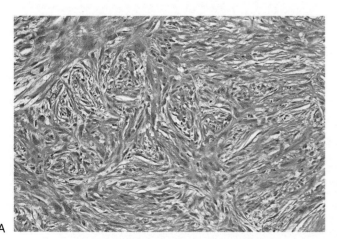
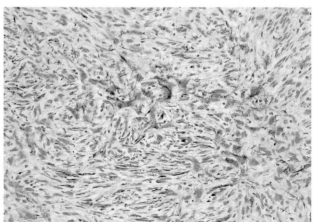

A        B

**FIG. 41.11.** *Malignant fibrous histiocytoma.* **A:** A low-grade tumor from a 22-year-old woman. Mitotic figures were infrequent. **B:** The tumor displayed immunoreactivity for cytokeratin (shown) and vimentin but not for actin (anti-CK7; avidin-biotin).

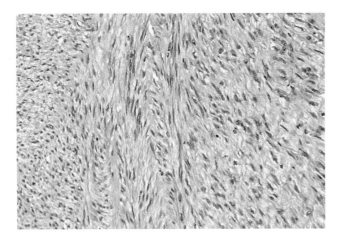

**FIG. 41.12.** *Fibrosarcoma.* The tumor consists of spindle cells with elongated nuclei arranged in interwoven bundles. The gross appearance of this tumor is shown in Fig. 41.1B.

If surgery is limited to excision, careful evaluation of the margins is mandatory. Reexcision, mastectomy, or adjuvant radiotherapy are indicated if fibrosarcoma is present at the resection margin. Total mastectomy is the recommended surgical treatment for high-grade fibrosarcoma.

## RHABDOMYOSARCOMA

Primary rhabdomyosarcoma of the breast is an uncommon and poorly characterized neoplasm (Fig. 41.14). Most tumors with rhabdomyosarcomatous features in the breast are variants of metaplastic carcinoma, malignant phyllodes tumor (89), or metastatic from nonmammary primary sites (90–93). Evidence for origin in the breast parenchyma or for myomatous differentiation is questionable in most published cases. For example, three rhabdomyosarcomas classified as *mammary sarcomas* in one report (94) "superficially infiltrated skeletal muscle but the tumors were centered in the breast." Striations were identified microscopically in only

one of the three neoplasms. The other two tumors had "racquet" and "strap" cells with peripherally placed nuclei. Two of the tumors recurred locally, with chest wall invasion in one case. Striations were also absent from another sarcoma, which had "strap" and "racquet" cells (89). None of these tumors were examined by electron microscopy, and the reports predate immunohistochemistry.

Evans described a 4 × 6 × 12-cm circumscribed tumor in the upper outer quadrant of a 41-year-old woman as a rhabdomyosarcoma (95). "Primitive" cross striations were detected by special stains. The report predated immunohistochemistry and electron microscopy to confirm myogenous origin. Recurrence in the muscles of the ipsilateral upper arm that occurred 32 months after mastectomy was treated by forequarter amputation. The patient was alive 4 years after diagnosis, with recurrent tumor in the supraclavicular region.

A mammary neoplasm with well-documented rhabdomyosarcomatous differentiation was reported by Woodard et al. (96). The tumor was a 5-cm mass located in the central part of the breast of a 16-year-old girl. The patient remained well 11 years after mastectomy. Microscopic examination revealed rhabdomyosarcoma and a 2.3-cm fibroadenoma "immediately adjacent without capsular separation." The fibroadenoma was described as having "cell-poor stroma." Cross striations were seen in routine sections, and rhabdomyosarcomatous differentiation was confirmed by electron microscopy. In this instance, origin from the associated fibroepithelial neoplasm cannot be excluded.

Herrera and Lugo-Vicente reported a 13-year-old girl with a 6-cm tumor that was classified as rhabdomyosarcoma with positive immunostains for desmin, myoglobin, and actin (97). The tumor was confined to the breast clinically and pathologically. After a simple mastectomy, the patient received chemotherapy and remained well 1 year later. This child had a strong history of malignant tumors in her family, including a brother with osteogenic sarcoma.

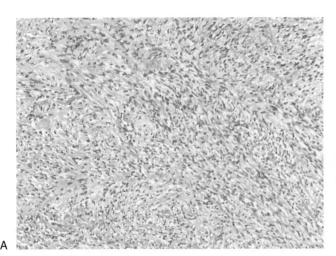

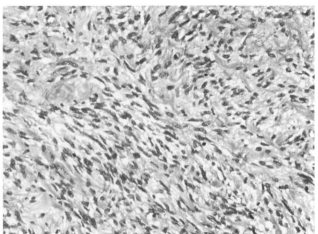

A

B

**FIG. 41.13.** *Fibrosarcoma.* **A,B:** Loosely organized groups of spindle cells are present in the collagenous stroma.

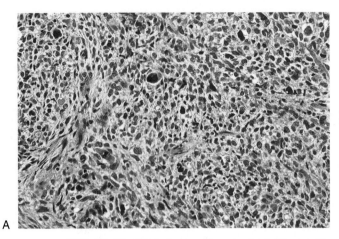
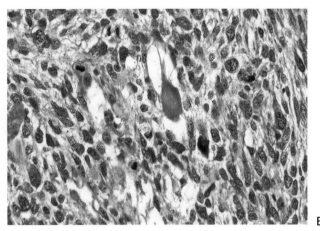

A                                                                                                                                          B

**FIG. 41.14.** *Rhabdomyosarcoma.* **A,B:** Strap cells with eosinophilic cytoplasm are distributed in the tumor.

A review of rhabdomyosarcomas involving the breast entered in the Intergroup Rhabdomyosarcoma Study identified seven female patients who had primary breast tumors (93). They ranged in age from 13.6 to 16.9 years with tumors 3 to 21 cm in diameter. Six tumors were histologically alveolar, and one was embryonal. Three of the patients died of metastatic sarcoma, and four were disease free after 150 to 365 weeks of follow-up.

Metastatic rhabdomyosarcoma in the breast is usually the alveolar type in children and young adults (90,91,98–100). Mammary involvement is most often a manifestation of widespread metastases (see Chapter 35). Five patients with mammary metastases had primary tumors of the perineum (90,92,98). A review of 19 patients whose initial site of metastasis was the breast revealed the following distribution of initial primary tumors: extremity, eight cases; nasopharynx/paranasal sinuses, seven cases; and trunk, four cases (93). The histologic subtype was alveolar in 18 determinate cases. The median age at diagnosis of the primary tumor was 15.0 years. Three patients were alive and disease free after follow-up of 7.6, 15.7, and 17 years. Rarely, the breast metastasis is the presenting manifestation of a previously undiagnosed nonmammary rhabdomyosarcoma (100).

Histologically, metastatic alveolar rhabdomyosarcoma is composed of small, round to oval cells that form poorly defined aggregates in the mammary parenchyma. Mitoses are easily identified. The differential diagnosis, which includes malignant lymphoma and invasive lobular carcinoma, can be readily resolved with immunohistochemical studies for myoid, epithelial, and lymphoid differentiation. In one report, two tumors with clinical and histologic features compatible with metastatic alveolar rhabdomyosarcoma in children were immunoreactive for vimentin and α-sarcomeric actin; negative for desmin, myoglobin, and α–smooth-muscle actin; and did not have "distinct crossbanding" when studied by electron microscopy (100).

The cytologic appearance of rhabdomyosarcoma in the breast of an adolescent has been reported (101). Myoid dif-

ferentiation was confirmed with a positive myoglobin stain. The patient had bilateral mammary and axillary involvement as well as left inguinal metastases. Clinical workup did not exclude a nonmammary primary.

## HEMANGIOPERICYTOMA

Hemangiopericytoma, an uncommon mesenchymal neoplasm, derived from the pericytes of blood vessels, was characterized in 1942 by Stout and Murray (102). These tumors arise in the soft tissues at numerous locations throughout the body. The breast is an uncommon site, with fewer than 20 cases documented in published reports (103–107).

### Clinical Presentation

With the exception of a 7-year-old girl and a 5-year-old boy (108), the patients were adults, including one man (104) and women 22 to 67 years of age. Patients presented with an enlarging painless mass that occurred with equal frequency in the left and right breast. Mammography in one case revealed a well-circumscribed dense mass that was hypoechogenic with posterior enhancement on sonography (109).

### Gross Pathology

The well-circumscribed, round to oval tumor consists of firm to hard homogeneous pale yellow, gray, or white tissue. The cut surface may have a whorled texture with dilated vascular spaces and a nodular contour. The diameter ranges from 1 to 19 cm.

### Microscopic Pathology

The histologic features are identical to those of hemangiopericytoma in other sites. The tumor is composed of round, plump, oval, and spindle cells oriented around vascular channels of varying caliber (Fig. 41.15). The vessels

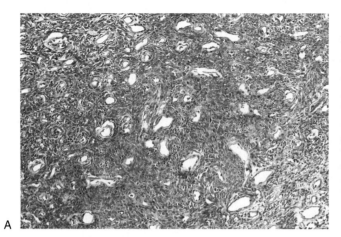

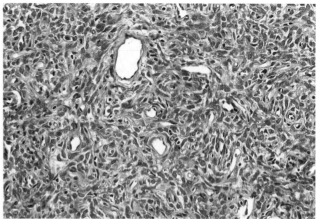

**FIG. 41.15.** *Hemangiopericytoma.* **A,B:** Many small capillaries are present in the storiform structure of the tumor.

often have a branching or "staghorn" configuration. More compact zones have a spongiform appearance. The endothelium is supported by a reticulin-rich stroma without appreciable collagen or actin-positive cells (Fig. 41.16). Focal fibrosis occurs in scattered patches and may be especially prominent at the tumor margin, where atrophic breast tissue compressed by the expanding tumor tends to form a pseudocapsule. Perivascular fibrosis is variably present (Fig. 41.17). Areas of necrosis rarely occur in mammary hemangiopericytomas.

The tumor cells are distributed in compact sheets, bands, and trabeculae around and between the vascular spaces. Mitoses are infrequent in most mammary hemangiopericytomas, and the cells lack other cytologic features of high-grade sarcomas, such as anaplasia and pleomorphic cells.

The cytologic specimen obtained by FNA contains clumps of tissue, spindle to oval cells with hyperchromatic nuclei, and abundant capillaries. The appearance is suggestive of a mesenchymal neoplasm but is not specific for hemangiopericytoma (104).

Electron microscopy of one breast tumor revealed neoplastic pericytic cells closely opposed to the endothelial cells (105). An incomplete basal lamina surrounded tumor cells characterized by complex interdigitating cytoplasmic processes with pinocytotic vesicles. Fine microfilaments were scattered in the cytoplasm. Dense bodies and plaques were absent. Evidence of smooth-muscle differentiation is variably present (105). The electron microscopic appearance is the same as that of hemangiopericytoma at other sites (110).

Endothelial cells of the capillaries are immunoreactive for *Ulex europaeus* I lectin, factor VIII, CD34, and CD31, but no reactivity has been found in the tumor cells. Reactivity for vimentin (103,105) has been observed in tumor cells, and variable staining for actin has been reported (103,105).

The diagnosis of hemangiopericytoma as a specific tumor in the breast is important because of the favorable prognosis of this neoplasm. Other malignant tumors may have vascular areas that resemble hemangiopericytoma. High-grade leiomyosarcoma and malignant fibrous histiocytoma have readily identifiable mitotic figures and structural features

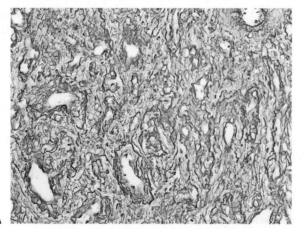

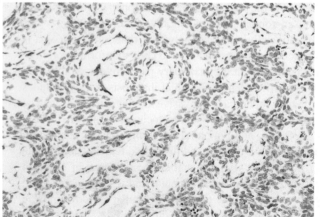

**FIG. 41.16.** *Hemangiopericytoma.* **A:** Cellular elements and vascular spaces are outlined by a reticulin network. **B:** Scant actin immunoreactivity is limited to cells lining small blood vessels (anti–smooth-muscle actin; avidin-biotin).

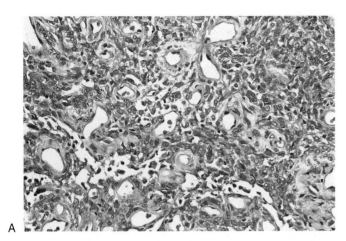
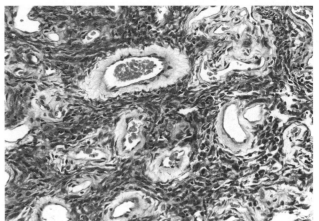

**FIG. 41.17.** *Hemangiopericytoma.* **A:** Thin bands of collagen outline some vascular structures. **B:** Conspicuous collagen bands surround the larger vascular channels.

that distinguish these tumors from hemangiopericytoma. Metastatic sarcomatous renal carcinoma in the breast may mimic mammary hemangiopericytoma, and rarely hemangiopericytoma originating at another site may metastasize to the breast (111).

### Prognosis and Treatment

Reported follow-up in 15 cases varies from less than a year to 276 months. Approximately equal numbers of patients have been treated by mastectomy and local excision. No patient had metastases detected in an axillary dissection. None of the patients described in published reports has developed local recurrence or systemic metastases, whether treated by local excision or mastectomy, with follow-up as long as 23 years and averaging 5 years. However in the author's experience, a mitotically active high-grade hemangiopericytoma of the breast resulted in pulmonary metastases (Fig. 41.18). Mammary hemangiopericytomas that lack

high-grade features, such as necrosis or numerous mitoses, should be considered low-grade neoplasms. Treatment can be conservative, with emphasis on wide local excision rather than mastectomy if an adequate margin can be achieved with an acceptable cosmetic result. Axillary dissection and systemic adjuvant therapy are not indicated for these low-grade lesions.

### DERMATOFIBROSARCOMA PROTUBERANS

Dermatofibrosarcoma protuberans, a tumor that arises in the skin and subcutaneous tissue is technically not a primary breast neoplasm. The distinction is not always readily apparent clinically, however, and treatment may involve mastectomy.

### Clinical Presentation

These tumors tend to enlarge slowly, and there may be ulceration of the overlying skin (112–114). The relatively

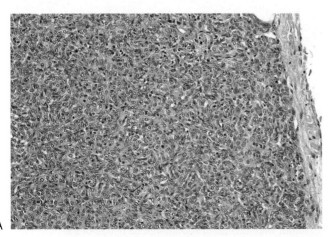
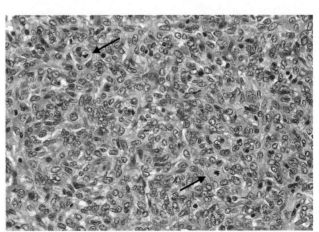

**FIG. 41.18.** *Hemangiopericytoma with metastases.* **A:** The primary tumor had a well-circumscribed border. **B:** The growth pattern was compact, and few distinct open vascular channels were present. Mitotic figures were identified *(arrows). (continued)*

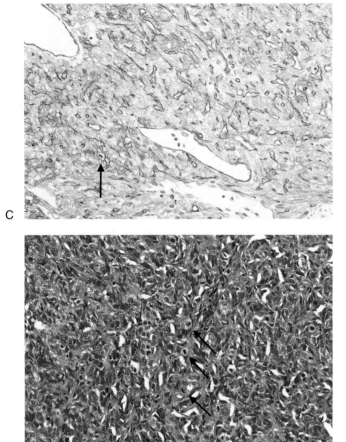

C

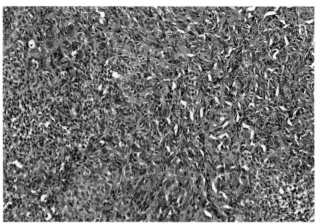

D

E

**FIG. 41.18.** *Continued.* **C:** A network of vascular channels is highlighted in the primary tumor by the immunostain for CD34 (avidin-biotin). *Arrow* indicates a mitotic figure. **D,E:** The appearance of a pulmonary metastasis approximately 2 years after excision of the breast tumor. Mitoses are present *(arrows).*

superficial involvement of the breast may suggest dermatofibrosarcoma protuberans.

## Pathology

The excised tumor consists of firm, white to tan tissue with a grossly well-defined border. Microscopically, the neoplasm is composed of uniform spindle cells arranged in a

very prominent storiform pattern (Fig. 41.19). Rare mitoses may be encountered. Giant cells are not a characteristic feature of this neoplasm.

## Treatment and Prognosis

Local excision may be attempted for smaller lesions, but mastectomy may be necessary for large tumors. These tu-

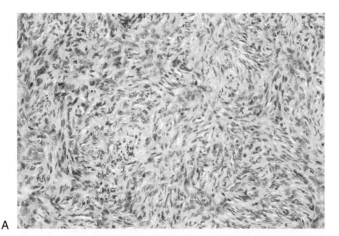

A

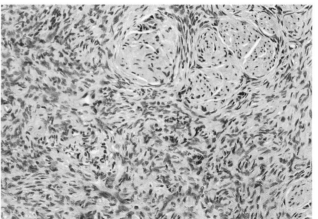

B

**FIG. 41.19.** *Dermatofibrosarcoma protuberans.* **A:** The tumor was located in subcutaneous tissue of the breast near the areola and invaded the nipple. The prominent storiform pattern is shown. **B:** The tumor surrounds smooth-muscle bundles in the nipple. An actin immunostain was reactive in the normal smooth muscle but not in the tumor.

mors do not metastasize, but local recurrence may occur. Long-term recurrence-free survival of up to 15 years has been reported (112,113).

## SARCOMAS OF PERIPHERAL NERVE SHEATH

This term applies to sarcomas arising from or exhibiting differentiation in the form of cells that constitute the supporting sheath of peripheral nerves. Most of these tumors arise from Schwann cells, but origin from perineurial fibroblasts also may be detected. In patients with von Recklinghausen's disease, multiple neurofibromas may be present in the breast and give rise to sarcoma. Concurrent tubular carcinoma and malignant schwannoma in the breast of a woman with von Recklinghausen's disease has been reported (115). A patient with separate malignant schwannomas of the breast and ulnar nerve did not have clinical stigmata of von Recklinghausen's disease (116). Spontaneous malignant peripheral nerve sheath tumors rarely occur in the breast (117). Isolated cases were mentioned in two series (118,119), the latter in a man.

## MISCELLANEOUS SARCOMAS

*Alveolar soft-part sarcoma* involving the right breast of a 16-year-old girl was described by Luna Vega et al. (120). The patient presented with a 4-cm painless subareolar mass that was reportedly "present without change for years." The tumor involved underlying pectoral muscle, necessitating total mastectomy and partial resection of the pectoralis major muscle.

A *malignant mesenchymoma* in a 61-year-old woman was treated by simple mastectomy, and the patient died of lung metastases 7 months after diagnosis (121). Histologically, the tumor consisted of myxoid stroma, spindle cell sarcoma with osteoid, bone, cartilage, and liposarcomatous elements.

Several tumors with a plexiform growth pattern and the histologic appearance of *angioblastic sarcoma* have been encountered in the breast (Fig. 41.20). A *malignant myofibroblastoma* was reported by Taccagni et al. (122). The diagnosis was confirmed by electron microscopy and immunohistochemistry, including demonstration of fibronexus junctions and fibronectin fibrils. The patient died of

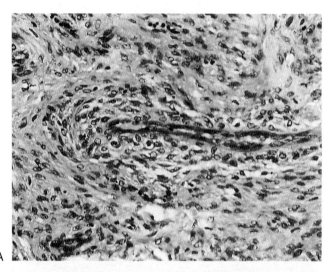

A

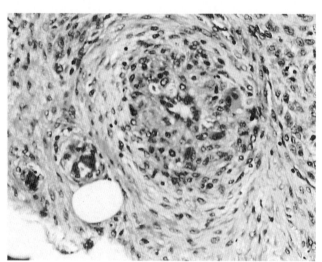

B

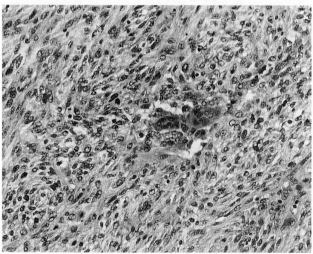

C

**FIG. 41.20.** *Angioblastic sarcoma.* **A:** A conspicuous feature of this sarcoma is the perivascular proliferation of atypical cells and the prominence of endothelial cells with hyperchromatic nuclei **B:** A transverse section of a vessel similar to the one in **A** showing the circumferential orientation of neoplastic cells and small multinucleated cells. **C:** A capillary obscured by multinucleated histiocytoid cells is shown in the *center.*

metastatic tumor 11 months after diagnosis. A male patient with myofibroblastic sarcoma described by González-Palacios et al. presented as a 2.5-cm tumor in a 60-year-old man (123). Histologic examination revealed a spindle cell neoplasm in which the tumor cells had "faintly eosinophilic cytoplasm" and a mitotic rate of 10/hpf. A mastectomy was performed. There were no nodal metastases. During the ensuing 10 years, the patient had five local recurrences that were treated by excisional surgery. Invasion of skeletal muscle was documented in a recurrence. Low-grade myofibroblastic sarcoma features pleomorphic hyperchromatic inva-

sive spindle cells associated with areas of pseudoangiomatous stromal growth and sparse mitoses (Fig. 41.21), whereas high grade myofibroblastic sarcomas have more abundant mitoses and a less well defined pseudoangiomatous structure.

*Kaposi's sarcoma* is exceedingly uncommon as a primary tumor of the breast. Ng et al. reported secondary involvement of the breast in a 33-year-old human immunodeficiency virus (HIV)-positive man who initially presented with skin lesions on the abdomen and hip (124). The mammary lesions consisted of a cutaneous rash and an underlying

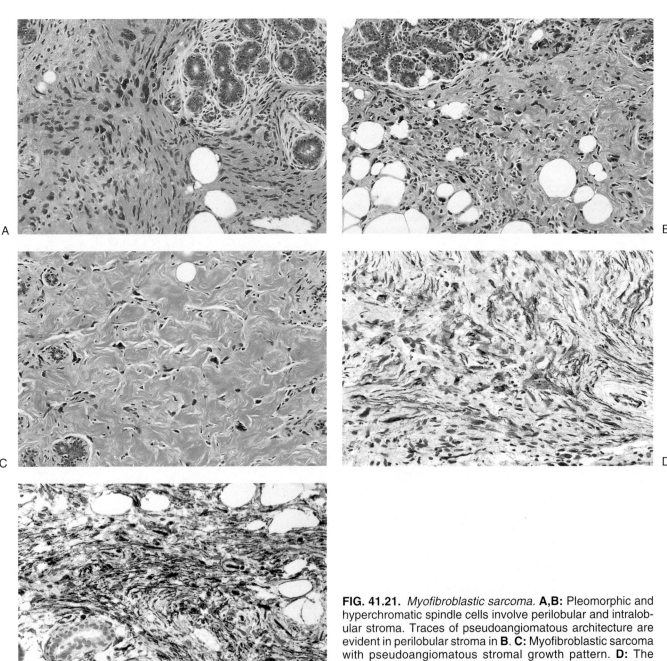

**FIG. 41.21.** *Myofibroblastic sarcoma.* **A,B:** Pleomorphic and hyperchromatic spindle cells involve perilobular and intralobular stroma. Traces of pseudoangiomatous architecture are evident in perilobular stroma in **B**. **C:** Myofibroblastic sarcoma with pseudoangiomatous stromal growth pattern. **D:** The tumor cells are immunoreactive for smooth-muscle actin (avidin-biotin). **E:** Immunoreactivity for CD34 is shown in tumor surrounding a small duct (avidin-biotin).

2-cm mass in the breast as well as in the axilla. The diagnosis of Kaposi's sarcoma in the breast was confirmed by biopsy.

## ANGIOSARCOMA

Angiosarcoma arises in the breast more often than in any other organ. Until recently, angiosarcoma of the breast was regarded as almost always fatal (125–127). Subsequent studies have shown it to be a morphologically heterogeneous group of neoplasms in which grade is prognostically significant (128,129).

### Clinical Presentation

With rare exceptions, the initial clinical finding is a painless mass. Blue or purple discoloration of the skin reflecting hemorrhage and vascularity of the lesion accompanies large or superficial tumors, but in many cases there are no external features to suggest angiosarcoma. Mammographic examination of palpable angiosarcomas revealed ill-defined, lobulated tumors, with areas of high and low echogenicity on sonography (130,131). In one study, 7 of 21 lesions were inapparent on mammography (131). Others also reported nonspecific findings with mammography and ultrasonography (132,133). Rarely, nonpalpable angiosarcomas measuring less than 3 cm have been detected by mammography, but most small nonpalpable vascular lesions have proven to be hemangiomas (134). Magnetic resonance imaging (MRI) revealed markedly enhancing masses in a patient with bilateral angiosarcomas measuring 10.0 and 1.5 cm, respectively (135). Because patients with angiosarcoma in one breast may develop asynchronous contralateral lesions, MRI of the opposite breast should be obtained at the time of diagnosis and periodically during follow-up.

Age at diagnosis ranges from the teens (126,128,129) to 91 years (135), with a mean of 34 (128) and a median of 38 years (129). A statistically significant correlation between age at diagnosis and tumor grade was reported in one study (129). The median ages of patients with low-, intermediate, and high-grade tumors were 43, 34, and 29 years, respectively.

Because of the relative youth of patients with mammary angiosarcoma, it is not unexpected that a number of the patients were also pregnant (129,136–138). Coexistent pregnancy was present in 4 of 63 cases (6%) in one series (129). Patients with angiosarcoma diagnosed during pregnancy seem to have an especially poor prognosis, apparently because most have high-grade tumors. This probably reflects their youth rather than a particular association between high-grade angiosarcoma and pregnancy. One woman who reportedly had a 15-cm low-grade angiosarcoma during pregnancy developed a local recurrence 2 years later and remained well for 5 years after excision of the recurrence (137). The earlier age at diagnosis of patients with high-grade lesions also may explain the relatively high frequency

of bilateral involvement because the contralateral breast lesions are often metastases (127,136). Some mammary angiosarcomas have low or negligible levels of hormone receptors (139–141), but there is no evidence that these tumors are hormone dependent.

The left and right breast are involved with equal frequency. Concurrent bilateral angiosarcomas are extremely uncommon (128,142). Only three well-documented cases of angiosarcoma of the male breast have been reported (129,141,143). A fourth case is questionable because the patient had systemic metastases as well as tumor in the breast, there was clinical evidence of bone metastases 2 years earlier, and photographic support for the diagnosis is not convincing (144).

*Postmastectomy angiosarcoma* of the chest wall has been described in patients who received postoperative radiotherapy in this anatomic region (145–148). These tumors are part of the spectrum of mesenchymal neoplasms that have been documented in the radiated chest wall. Virtually all sarcomas that have occurred in the mammary gland itself after breast-conserving surgery and irradiation for carcinoma have been angiosarcomas (149–155). The interval between radiation and diagnosis of angiosarcoma ranges from 3 to 12 years, with most occurring within 6 years after radiotherapy (156). With few exceptions, these women were more than 50 years of age when treated for mammary carcinoma (156–158). One patient had recurrent carcinoma as well as angiosarcoma in the same breast (154), and in another case angiosarcoma developed coincidentally in a breast reconstructed with a silicone implant after breast-conserving surgery and radiotherapy (157).

Cutaneous presentation of *postradiation angiosarcoma* of the breast occurs more frequently than postradiation parenchymal angiosarcoma in the conserved breast (153,159–165). The initial skin changes may be subtle. In one reported case, "a little bit of purplish discoloration" was interpreted as postradiotherapy telangiectasia, and a later ecchymotic area was attributed to trauma (166). Many patients who present with angiosarcoma in the skin also have parenchymal involvement. A review of the comprehensive national database of the Netherlands identified 21 patients with postradiation angiosarcoma of the conserved breast diagnosed between 1987 and 1995 (167). Origin was described as cutaneous in 17 cases (81%).

Published case reports have not shown a consistent relationship between cutaneous angiosarcoma of the breast and mammary edema following radiation of the breast or chronic edema after treatment of the breast and axilla (160,164,167). The amount of radiation or the use of a boost dose has not been associated with the development of postradiation angiosarcoma of the breast or the location of the tumor (164,167). The interval to diagnosis of angiosarcoma after radiotherapy appears to be inversely related to the age at treatment for breast carcinoma, decreasing with advancing age (167).

Low-grade (158,161,162,165,167), moderately differentiated (153,158,167), and high-grade (160,164,167) postradiation angiosarcomas have been described. The high-grade lesions usually exhibit the same heterogeneous mixture of low- and high-grade components seen in spontaneous parenchymal angiosarcomas. High-grade foci typically form multiple subcutaneous and dermal tumor nodules. Cytogenetic analysis of one postradiation mammary cutaneous angiosarcoma revealed clonal rearrangements involving 14 different chromosomes (168).

The estimated risk of cutaneous or parenchymal angiosarcoma of the breast after breast conservation and radiation for carcinoma is 0.3% (169) to 0.4% (153). In one report, subsequent angiosarcoma of the breast was detected in 2 of 3,295 (0.06%) women treated for breast carcinoma by conservative surgery and radiotherapy (154). Analysis of data from the Netherlands cancer database revealed the estimated incidence of angiosarcoma to be 1.35% in patients who were treated by breast conservation and radiotherapy for mammary carcinoma and 1.59% in women who survived 5 years (167). This incidence of mammary angiosarcoma after breast irradiation was equivalent to a relative risk of 3,200 compared with the incidence of spontaneous mammary angiosarcoma in the Dutch population (0.0005%).

The prognosis of postirradiation angiosarcoma of the breast parenchyma or skin of the breast is influenced by tumor grade and is most favorable in women with low-grade tumors (167). In a series of 21 women from the Netherlands, the 3- and 5-year overall survival rates were 72% and 55%, respectively, with a disease-free survival at 5 years of 35% (167). In this series, patients treated by complete tumor resection, usually mastectomy, had a more favorable outcome.

Rarely, angiosarcoma has been found in a breast affected by mammary carcinoma without a history of radiotherapy. In one unusual case, mastectomy revealed coexistent, concurrent adenocarcinoma and angiosarcoma in a breast that had chronic lymphedema 4 years after segmental mastectomy without radiotherapy for carcinoma (135). Coincidental angiosarcoma and infiltrating lobular carcinoma in the same breast were reported in a 59-year-old woman (170). Asynchronous contralateral mammary carcinoma has been described in two women. One of these patients had contralateral carcinoma treated by mastectomy prior the development of angiosarcoma (129). In the second case, right breast carcinoma had been treated by lumpectomy and radiotherapy 5 years before angiosarcoma was detected in the left breast (171). The author has reviewed slides from a 17-year-old girl with concurrent low-grade angiosarcoma and malignant phyllodes tumor in one breast.

Malignant neoplasms at sites other than the breast have been found only rarely in patients with mammary angiosarcoma. These neoplasms include malignant lymphoma (129,141), Hodgkin's disease (129), and pulmonary adenocarcinoma (129). One series described nonneoplastic thyroid disease in 30% of mammary angiosarcoma patients (141). Antecedent trauma has been noted by some investigators, but there is no convincing evidence to implicate injury as an etiologic factor. Trauma may draw attention to an already existing tumor, especially if hemorrhage in the lesion causes it to enlarge. Angiosarcomas at various somatic sites have been associated with foreign-body material retained for many years (172), but angiosarcoma of the breast has not been described as having arisen at the site of a prosthetic implant.

The Kasabach-Merritt syndrome has been attributed to angiosarcoma of the breast in one case report (173). This condition, characterized by consumptive thrombocytopenia, usually complicates angiomas in infants and children and only rarely has been observed as a complication of angiosarcoma.

## Gross Pathology

The tumors vary in size from 1 cm to 20 cm or larger, averaging about 5 cm. Few angiosarcomas are smaller than 2

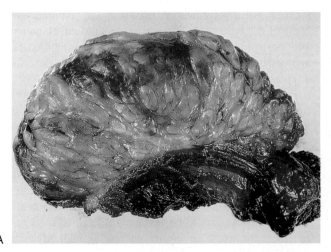
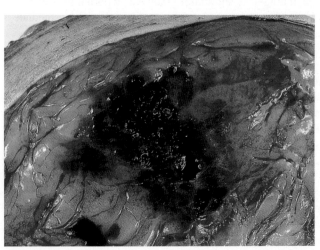

A      B

**FIG. 41.22.** *Angiosarcoma, gross appearance.* **A:** An ill-defined red tumor mass in the central part of the breast. **B:** A circumscribed tumor with cystic hemorrhagic foci.

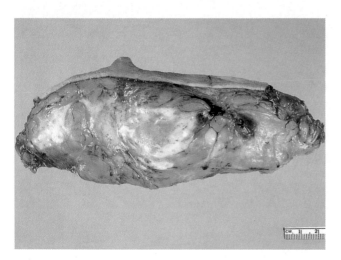

**FIG. 41.23.** *Angiosarcoma, gross appearance.* Punctate red foci of sarcoma are present throughout much of the pale fibrous and fatty breast tissue. The stellate hemorrhagic focus on the *right* is a biopsy site.

cm. There is no significant difference in the average size of high- and low-grade lesions.

In many cases, angiosarcoma forms a friable, firm or spongy hemorrhagic tumor (Fig. 41.22). Areas of cystic hemorrhagic necrosis are commonly evident in large, high-grade lesions. Focal hemorrhage or hemorrhagic discoloration in the surrounding breast is usually an indication of tumor extending beyond the grossly evident mass. Some angiosarcomas exhibit little or no hemorrhage grossly (Fig. 41.23). Angiosarcomas that do not appear to be vascular grossly are generally described as poorly defined areas of thickening or induration.

**Microscopic Pathology**

Microscopically, angiosarcoma consists of a heterogenous group of lesions, a phenomenon recognized as early as 1942 by Hill and Stout (174). They stated that "malignant hemangioendothelioma can be divided into three general classes." One group consisted of cases in which the primary tumor and its metastases resembled a "simple angioma." In the intermediate type, the primary tumor appeared "well differentiated and innocent," but recurrent or metastatic lesions were clearly malignant. Tumors in the third group were "recognizable as malignant from the beginning."

Three histologic patterns of growth in the primary tumor have been described (Table 41.1). These reflect the degree of differentiation and have proven to correlate with prognosis (128,129,175).

Low-grade or type I tumors are composed of open, anastomosing vascular channels that proliferate diffusely in mammary glandular tissue and fat (Fig. 41.24). Infiltration into lobules is characterized by spread of the vascular channels within the intralobular stroma, a process that leads to separation and atrophy of the lobular glandular units (Fig. 41.25). Some prominent hyperchromatic endothelial nuclei may be found, but the endothelial cells often have inconspicuous nuclei (Fig. 41.26). Endothelial cells are distributed in a flat single-cell layer around the vascular spaces. Papillary formations are absent or at most extremely infrequent. Mitotic figures are rarely seen in the neoplastic endothelial cells of a low-grade tumor (Fig. 41.27). If mitotic figures are encountered with regularity in a histologically low-grade appearing area in a biopsy specimen, high-grade areas are likely to be present elsewhere in the tumor. The vascular lumens are usually large, open, and anastomosing. Red blood cells are typically present in small numbers, but occasional lesions are congested.

Several unusual structural variants of low-grade angiosarcoma may be difficult to recognize. One of these is composed predominantly of capillary-like vascular spaces (Fig. 41.28). Another type of lesion consists of small, often narrow vascular channels without a conspicuous anastomosing structure (Fig. 41.29). The manner in which the neoplastic vessels are dispersed in the stroma may be mistaken for pseudoangiomatous stromal hyperplasia. Diffusely infiltrating low-grade angiosarcoma composed predominantly of spindle cells may be mistaken for an angiolipoma if only a limited sample is available to examine (Fig. 41.30).

The amount of stroma formed in low-grade angiosarcomas varies to a considerable degree. In most cases, little

**TABLE 41.1.** *Histologic characteristics of mammary angiosarcoma*

| Histologic features | Grade | | |
| --- | --- | --- | --- |
| | Low | Intermediate | High |
| Lesions involving breast parenchyma | Present | Present | Present |
| Anastomosing vascular channels | Present | Present | Present |
| Hyperchromatic endothelial cells | Present | Present | Present |
| Endothelial tufting | Minimal | Present | Prominent |
| Papillary formations | Absent | Focally present | Present |
| Solid and spindle cell foci | Absent | Absent or minimal | Present |
| Mitoses | Rare or absent | Present in papillary areas | Numerous; present even in structurally low-grade areas |
| "Blood lakes" | Absent | Absent | Present |
| Necrosis | Absent | Absent | Present |

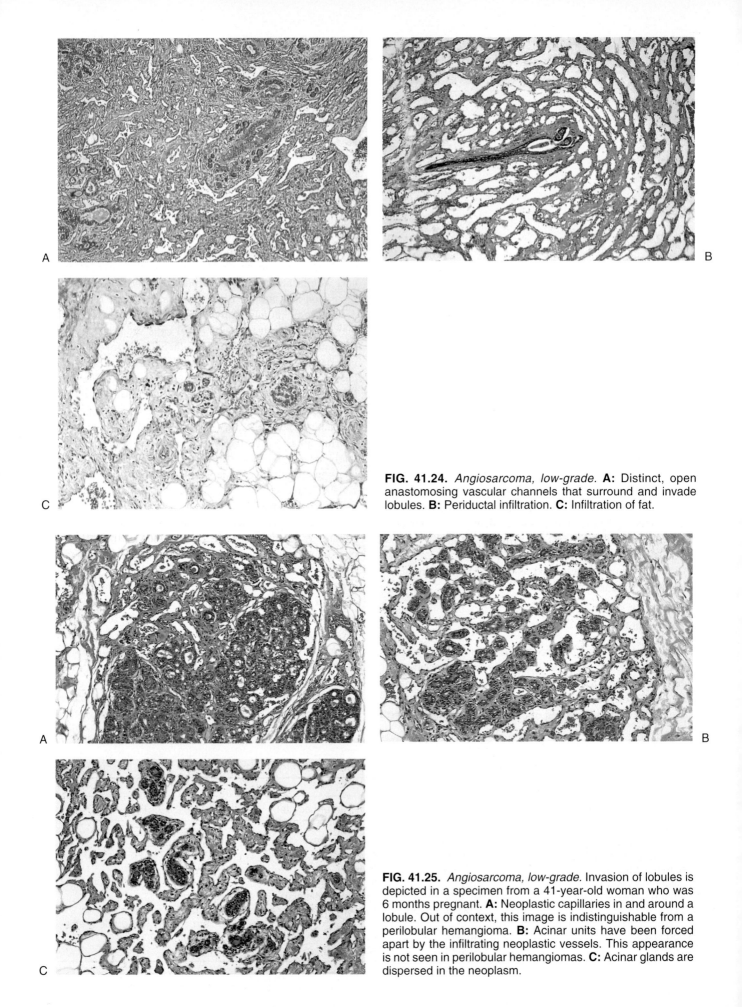

**FIG. 41.24.** *Angiosarcoma, low-grade.* **A:** Distinct, open anastomosing vascular channels that surround and invade lobules. **B:** Periductal infiltration. **C:** Infiltration of fat.

**FIG. 41.25.** *Angiosarcoma, low-grade.* Invasion of lobules is depicted in a specimen from a 41-year-old woman who was 6 months pregnant. **A:** Neoplastic capillaries in and around a lobule. Out of context, this image is indistinguishable from a perilobular hemangioma. **B:** Acinar units have been forced apart by the infiltrating neoplastic vessels. This appearance is not seen in perilobular hemangiomas. **C:** Acinar glands are dispersed in the neoplasm.

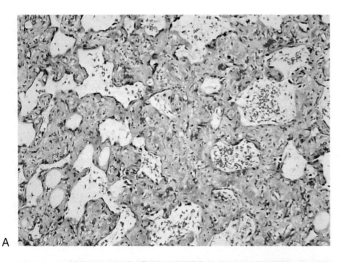

A

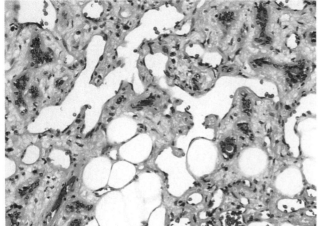

B

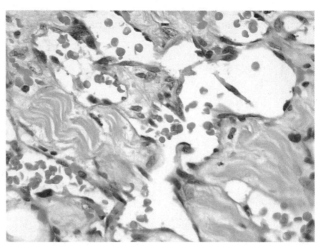

C

**FIG. 41.26.** *Angiosarcoma, low-grade.* **A:** The endothelial cells are flat, and have hyperchromatic nuclei. **B:** The endothelial cell nuclei are inconspicuous. Remnants of lobular glands are present. **C:** Most of the nuclei are pale and small.

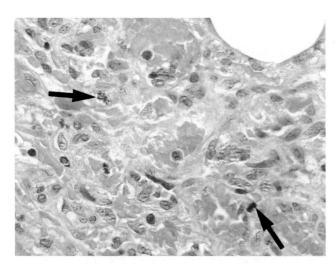

**FIG. 41.27.** *Angiosarcoma with mitoses.* Two mitotic figures are shown in one high-power field *(arrows).* The nuclei of the tumor cells are pleomorphic. This finding in a structurally low-grade appearing tumor is likely to be associated with high-grade foci elsewhere in the tumor.

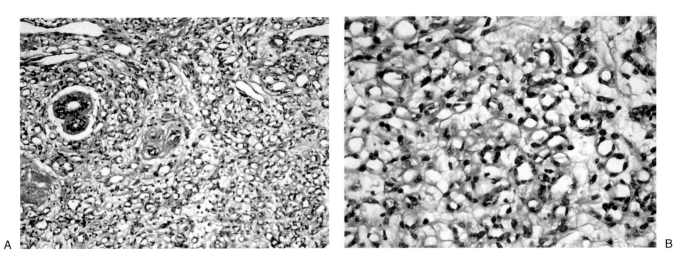

**FIG. 41.28.** *Angiosarcoma, low-grade, capillary type.* **A,B:** The neoplasm is composed of small, closely packed round capillaries that have hyperchromatic nuclei.

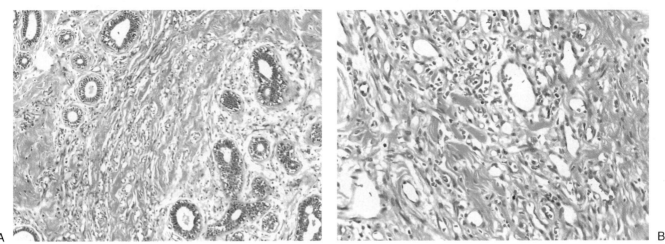

**FIG. 41.29.** *Angiosarcoma, low-grade, resembling pseudoangiomatous stromal hyperplasia.* **A:** Small round and elongated vascular structures infiltrating the collagenous stroma and lobules are shown. There is a tendency to spare lobules. **B:** The vascular spaces vary in size and shape. Anastomoses are not conspicuous.

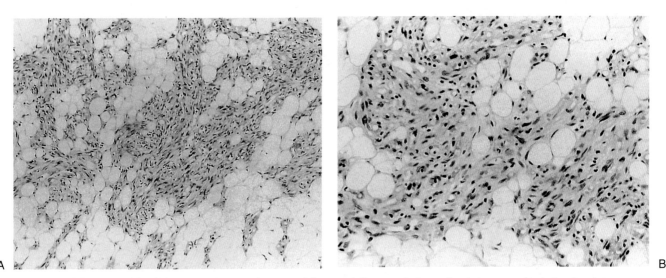

**FIG. 41.30.** *Angiosarcoma, low-grade, resembling angiolipoma.* **A:** Irregular, interconnected sheets of small spindle cells infiltrating fat form the basic structure. *(continued)*

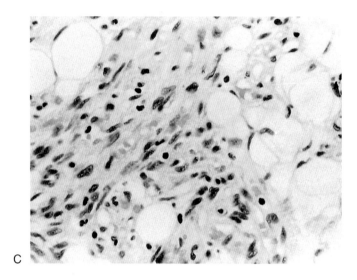

C

FIG. 41.30. *Continued.* **B,C:** Ill-defined small vascular lumens that contain red blood cells are present among the spindle cells.

stroma is formed and the lesion consists largely of vascular channels permeating mammary parenchyma. A minority of low-grade angiosarcomas have collagenous stroma focally or diffusely (Fig. 41.31). Despite their more dense appearance, these lesions qualify as low-grade tumors if no endothelial proliferation is found.

Low-grade components are found in intermediate and high-grade lesions, sometimes constituting the bulk of the tumor. This is particularly true for type II or intermediate-grade angiosarcomas, which are distinguished from low-grade tumors by having scattered focal areas of more cellular proliferation (Figs. 41.32 and 41.33). The latter tumors

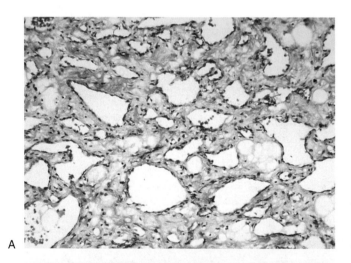

A

FIG. 41.31. *Angiosarcoma, low-grade, stromal fibrosis.* **A:** A few spindle cells are seen in the myxoid stroma. **B:** The moderately cellular stroma is composed of spindle cells. **C:** In some areas, the stroma tends to obscure the neoplastic vascular pattern.

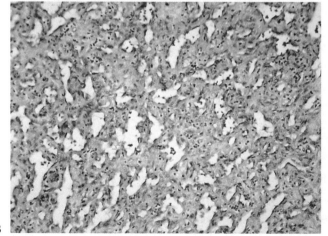

B

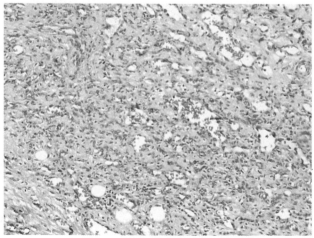

C

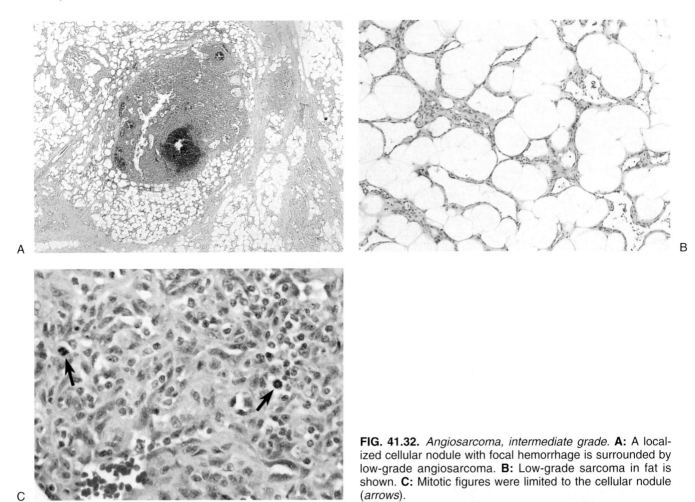

**FIG. 41.32.** *Angiosarcoma, intermediate grade.* **A:** A localized cellular nodule with focal hemorrhage is surrounded by low-grade angiosarcoma. **B:** Low-grade sarcoma in fat is shown. **C:** Mitotic figures were limited to the cellular nodule (*arrows*).

**FIG. 41.33.** *Angiosarcoma, intermediate grade.* **A,B:** The pictures show a localized focus of neoplastic papillary endothelial growth.

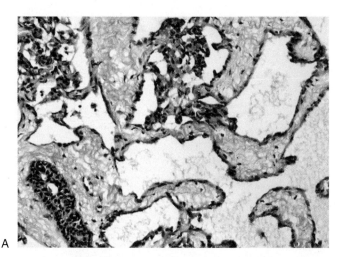
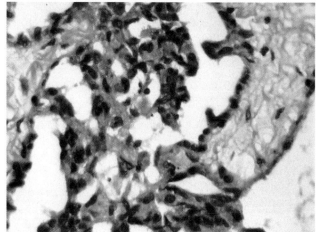

A                                                                                          B

**FIG. 41.34.** *Angiosarcoma, intermediate grade.* **A,B:** A focus of well-developed papillary endothelial proliferation is depicted.

usually consist of small buds or papillary fronds of endothelial cells that project into the vascular lumens (Figs. 41.34 and 41.35). Less often, the focally cellular areas feature polygonal and spindle cells, or there are foci that combine spindle cell and papillary elements. Infrequent mitoses may be found in papillary or spindle cell areas. Some spindle cell foci resemble lesions encountered in Kaposi's sarcoma (Fig. 41.36). At least 75% of type II or intermediate grade angiosarcomas consist of low-grade elements with cellular foci scattered throughout the tumor. Transitions to cellular foci occur abruptly. An unusual variant of intermediate-grade angiosarcoma features numerous nodules composed of spindle cells with a swirling pattern (Fig. 41.37). The distribution of these nodules suggests perithelial origin.

Type III or high-grade angiosarcoma exhibits the malignant histologic features usually attributed to angiosarcomas. Part of the lesion is composed of low- and intermediate-grade elements, but in many cases more than half of the tumor has high-grade malignant features. These consist of prominent endothelial tufting and solid papillary formations that contain cytologically malignant endothelial cells (Fig. 41.38). In some lesions, conspicuous solid and spindle cell areas with sparse vascular elements are seen (Fig. 41.39). Mitoses usually are identified without difficulty in the cellular components. Areas of hemorrhage, often accompanied by necrosis, have been referred to as *blood lakes* (Figs. 41.40 and 41.41). Necrosis and blood lakes are seen only in high-grade angiosarcomas. Epithelioid angiosarcoma is an uncommon high-grade variant, with histologic features similar to angiosarcoma in the Stewart-Treves syndrome (176). The epithelioid appearance of the cells may be mistaken for mammary adenocarcinoma. Immunohistochemistry and electron microscopy are helpful in the differential diagnosis (176).

With few exceptions, angiosarcomas have infiltrative borders that feature well-formed or low-grade vascular

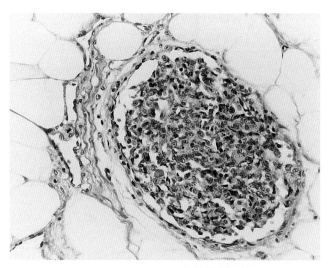

**FIG. 41.35.** *Angiosarcoma, intermediate grade.* An intravascular papillary focus is illustrated.

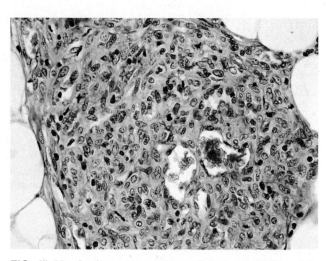

**FIG. 41.36.** *Angiosarcoma, intermediate grade.* This nodule is composed of spindle cells around small vascular spaces.

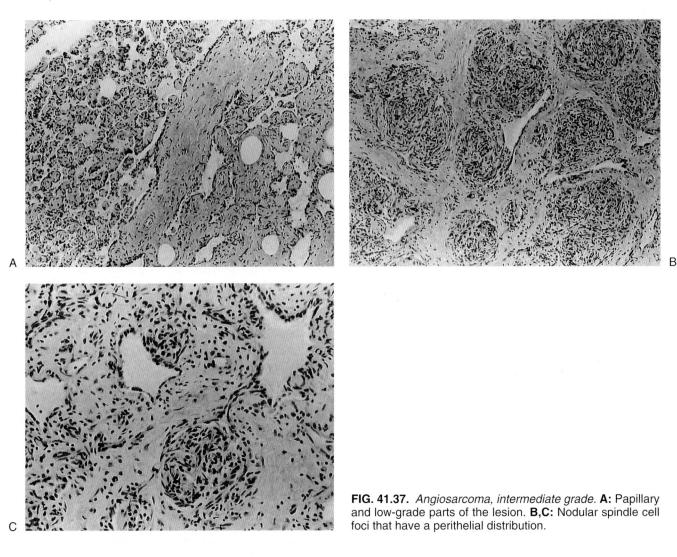

**FIG. 41.37.** *Angiosarcoma, intermediate grade.* **A:** Papillary and low-grade parts of the lesion. **B,C:** Nodular spindle cell foci that have a perithelial distribution.

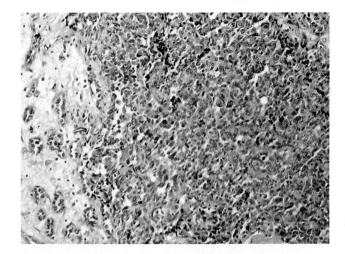

**FIG. 41.38.** *Angiosarcoma, high-grade.* The tumor had extensive densely cellular areas like the one shown here, composed of cells with hyperchromatic pleomorphic nuclei.

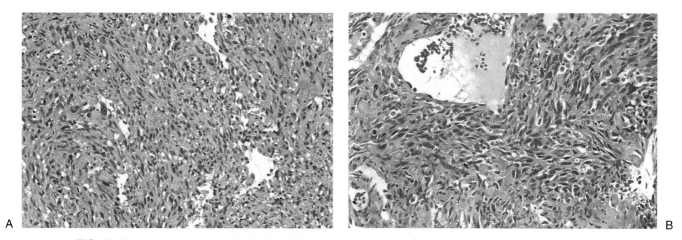

**FIG. 41.39.** *Angiosarcoma, high-grade.* **A,B:** A hemorrhagic spindle cell area with few vascular spaces.

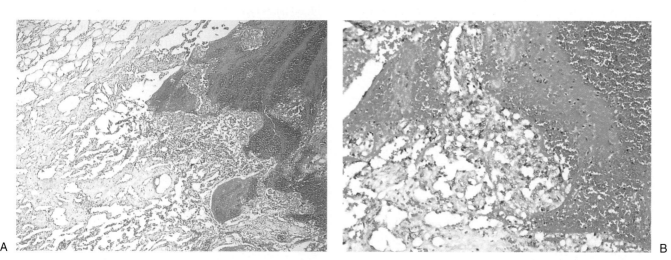

**FIG. 41.40.** *Angiosarcoma, high-grade.* **A,B:** Hemorrhagic foci referred to as "blood lakes" are shown.

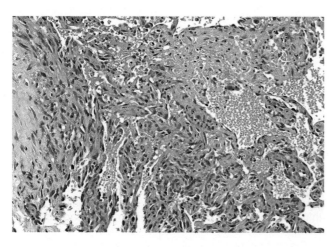

**FIG. 41.41.** *Angiosarcoma, high-grade.* Focal necrosis is shown in the *upper right corner* in a tumor with spindle cell growth.

channels. In some cases, the peripheral vascular component is so orderly that the neoplastic vascular channels are structurally indistinguishable from existing capillaries in the normal parenchyma or resemble angiolipoma (Fig. 41.42).

Because of the varied microscopic structure of intermediate and high-grade lesions, it is not possible to classify accurately a tumor as a low-grade angiosarcoma unless it has been excised and generously sampled. The tendency for peripheral portions to have a low-grade structure is likely to be misleading when a superficial biopsy has been obtained from an intermediate or high-grade tumor, which also may lead to a mistaken diagnosis of hemangioma (129) and in part explains references to lesions classified as *metastasizing hemangiomas* (177,178).

It is not difficult to distinguish between a high-grade angiosarcoma and a hemangioma, but problems may be encountered with low- and intermediate-grade tumors. Some general guidelines are helpful in these situations (128,134). Hemangiomas are rarely larger than 2 cm, and few angiosarcomas measure less than 2 cm. Hemangiomas tend to have well-circumscribed borders grossly and microscopically, whereas angiosarcomas have invasive margins. Some angiomas are divided into lobules or nodules by fibrous septae, a feature not seen in angiosarcomas, which lack an internal

structure. Many angiomas consist of isolated, largely unconnected vascular channels, such as those typically seen in cavernous hemangiomas. Anastomosing vascular spaces may be found in angiomas; but, except for angiomatosis (179), anastomoses are not nearly as numerous or serpiginous as in angiosarcomas. In the mammary parenchyma, the vascular proliferation in angiosarcomas invades into and expands lobules, whereas angiomas other than perilobular hemangiomas tend to surround lobules and ducts (180). A thick-walled nonneoplastic "feeding" blood vessel sometimes is found at the periphery of hemangiomas; this is not a feature of angiosarcomas.

The histologic characteristics of *postradiation angiosarcoma* of the skin, subcutaneous tissue, and breast differ in some details from primary parenchymal angiosarcoma not associated with radiotherapy (160). High-grade areas, found in most of these cases, are composed of solid epithelioid or solid spindle cell foci, with variable numbers of slit-like spaces containing intraluminal or extravasated red blood cells (Fig. 41.43). Hemorrhage resulting in the formation of blood lakes typically is distributed in these sarcomatous foci. Lesions with low- and intermediate-grade structural patterns exhibit variable vasoformative growth and papillary endothelial hyperplasia (Fig. 41.44). In contrast to spontaneous

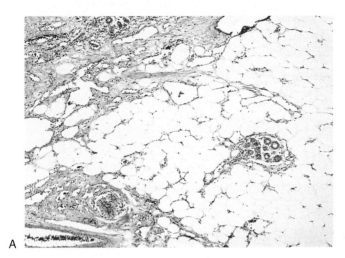

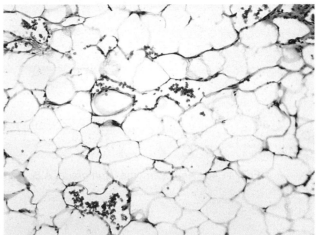

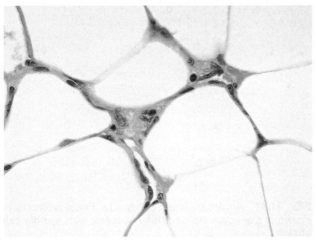

**FIG. 41.42.** *Angiosarcoma, high-grade with low-grade component invading fat.* All images are from a single tumor. **A:** Angiosarcoma involving glandular parenchyma and fat. **B:** Irregular dilated neoplastic vascular channels with an inconspicuous endothelium are shown. **C:** Capillaries in the fat that could be traced to the angiosarcomatous part of the lesion.

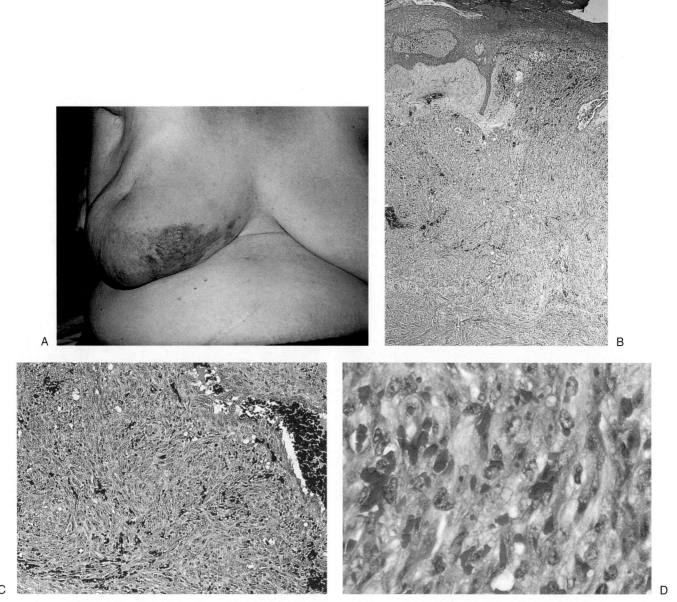

**FIG. 41.43.** *Angiosarcoma of mammary skin after breast-conserving surgery and radiation for carcinoma.* **A:** Angiosarcoma involves the skin and much of the lower half of the right breast. The retracted area in the upper outer quadrant is the site of a prior lumpectomy. **B:** Solid masses of high-grade angiosarcoma in the dermis. **C:** The sarcoma is composed of spindle cells and dilated vascular channels lined by plump malignant endothelial cells. **D:** The nuclei have vesicular chromatin and one or more prominent nucleoli.

parenchymal angiosarcomas, in which nuclear grade frequently parallels structural differentiation, regardless of the microscopic pattern, malignant cells in postradiation angiosarcoma typically have poorly differentiated nuclei that have vesicular chromatin, prominent nucleoli, and mitotic activity (Fig. 41.45). Unusual histologic variants of cutaneous angiosarcoma include a perithelial arrangement of neoplastic cells (Fig. 41.46), storiform spindle cell growth (Fig. 41.47), and tumors with cavernous elements (Fig. 41.48).

Angiosarcoma arising in the skin and breast after radio-

therapy must be distinguished from benign vascular lesions that can arise in these tissues in the same clinical setting (160) (Table 41.2). The latter have been referred to as *atypical vascular lesions* (AVL) because they were initially mistaken for angiosarcoma and their prognostic significance has not been fully evaluated. Presently, there is no evidence that these benign vascular lesions evolve into angiosarcoma in patients who have had follow-up for as long as 10 years (160). Recurrence of AVL has been observed. One patient developed a another AVL 17 months after excision of the first lesion (160). A second patient had a 1-cm lesion in her

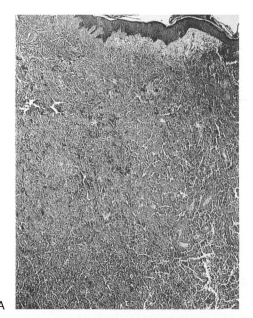

A

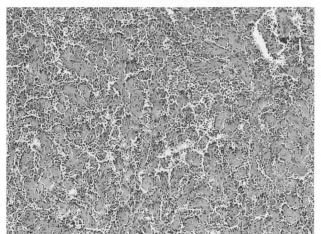

B

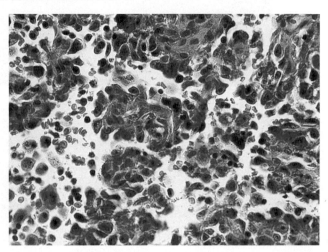

C

**FIG. 41.44.** *Angiosarcoma of the mammary skin and breast after lumpectomy and radiation for carcinoma.* **A:** This sarcoma has extensive anastomosing vascular channels that create a papillary configuration in areas. **B,C:** The papillary structures are composed of malignant endothelial cells supported by slender cores of fibrovascular stroma.

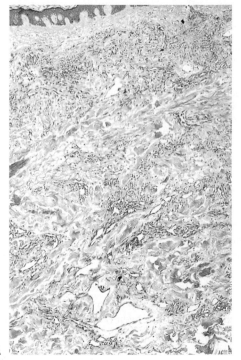

A

**FIG. 41.45.** *Angiosarcoma of the mammary skin after breast-conserving surgery and radiation for carcinoma.* **A:** This low-grade angiosarcoma was composed of small capillary-size vascular structures involving the full thickness of the dermis. The mammary parenchyma also was involved. *(continued)*

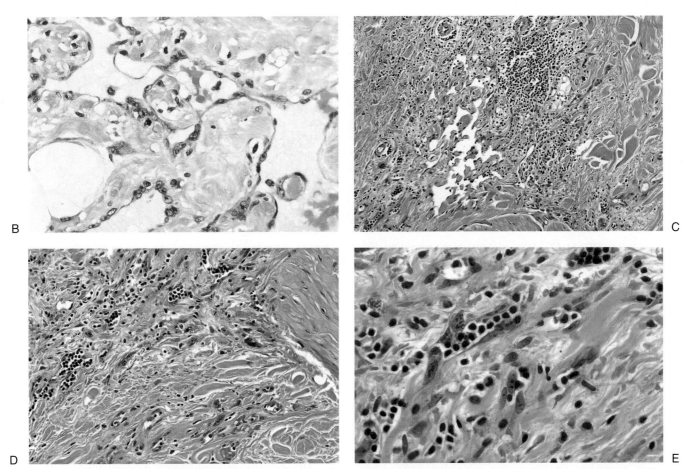

**FIG. 41.45.** *Continued.* **B:** Nuclei are vesicular with punctate nucleoli. A mitosis is shown. **C:** Images **C–E** are from another patient who developed cutaneous angiosarcoma 9 years after radiotherapy. This field shows ectatic vascular channels and atypical cells in the stroma. **D,E:** Tumor cells with pleomorphic nuclei and multiple nucleoli.

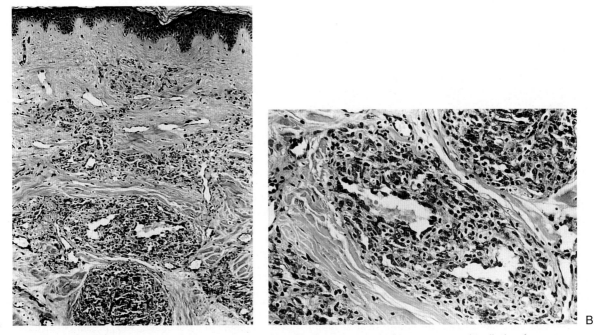

**FIG. 41.46.** *Angiosarcoma of the mammary skin after breast-conserving surgery and radiation for carcinoma.* **A,B:** This sarcoma has an unusual nodular perithelial structure.

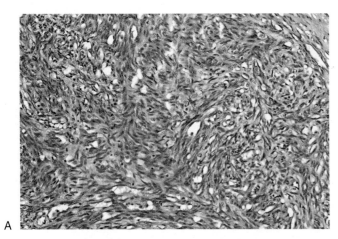 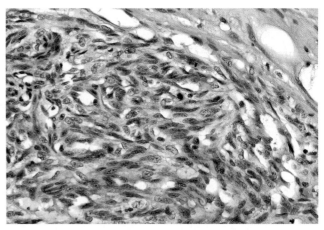

**FIG. 41.47.** *Angiosarcoma of the mammary skin after breast-conserving surgery and radiation for breast carcinoma.* **A:** The tumor is composed of swirling spindle cells with a storiform architecture. **B:** Vesicular nuclei are shown.

mastectomy scar 35 months after radiotherapy, accompanied by smaller satellite nodules (181). Fourteen months later, a second crop of lesions appeared nearby. Both areas were diagnosed as acquired progressive lymphangioma. In a third

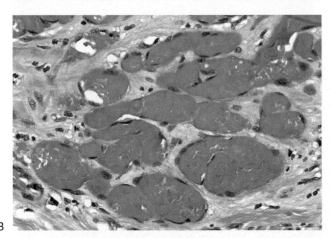

**FIG. 41.48.** *Angiosarcoma of the mammary skin after breast-conserving surgery and radiation for breast carcinoma.* **A:** Dilated, cavernous vascular spaces are shown next to tumor with a capillary structure. **B:** Note the vesicular nuclei with punctate nucleoli in this cavernous area.

case, multiple lesions arose in the parasternal area and axilla 10 years after mastectomy and axillary lymph node dissection followed by radiotherapy (182). Additional lesions appeared in the same area and on the arm outside the radiation field 4 years later. Biopsies on both occasions were interpreted as lymphangiosarcoma. The lesions continued "waxing and waning" thereafter, and on subsequent review the diagnosis was revised to a "lymphedema-related dilatation or proliferation of lymph vessels, resembling lymphangioma circumscripta" (H. Peterse, personal communication, 1996).

The diagnosis of postradiation angiosarcoma can be suggested in the specimen obtained by FNA cytology (183). Epithelioid forms of angiosarcoma may resemble recurrent carcinoma in a cytologic specimen and require immunohistochemical studies to distinguish these lesions (184).

*Atypical vascular lesions* typically develop 2 to 5 years after radiotherapy as single or multiple pink papules in the skin measuring 5 mm or less in diameter (Figs. 41.49 and 41.50). Rarely, AVLs develop in the breast parenchyma (Fig.

**TABLE 41.2.** *Histopathologic characteristics of atypical vascular lesions and cutaneous angiosarcoma*

| Characteristic | AVL | AS |
|---|---|---|
| Infiltration of subcutis | − | +++ |
| "Blood lakes" | − | +++ |
| Papillary endothelial hyperplasia | − | +++ |
| Prominent nucleoli | − | +++ |
| Mitotic figures | − | +++ |
| Marked cytologic atypia | − | +++ |
| Anastomotic vessels | ++ | +++ |
| Chronic inflammation | +++ | + |
| Hyperchromatic endothelial cells | +++ | ++ |
| Dissection of dermal collagen | +/− | +++ |
| Relative circumscription | +++ | − |
| Projection of stroma into lumen | +++ | − |

−, Absent; +/−, rare focal finding; +, occasionally present; ++, present in most cases; +++, present in all cases.

*AS*, cutaneous angiosarcoma; *AVL*, atypical vascular lesions.

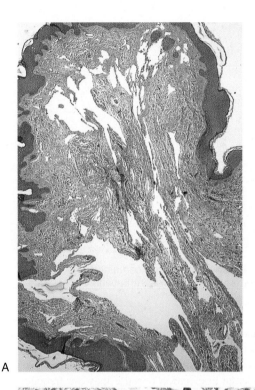

**FIG. 41.49.** *Atypical vascular lesion, skin.* This lesion appeared clinically to be a cutaneous papilloma. **A:** A whole-mount histologic section showing dilated vascular spaces in the dermis of the skin. **B:** Smooth-muscle proliferation is present in the stroma with a mild lymphocytic infiltrate between serpiginous vascular spaces. **C:** The endothelial cells have prominent hyperchromatic nuclei.

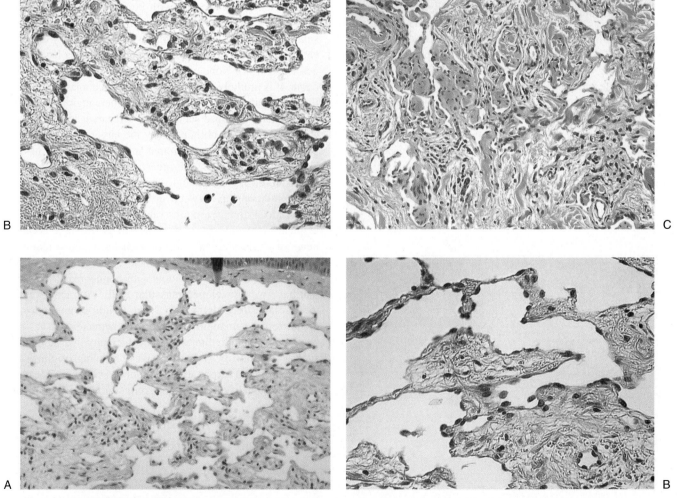

**FIG. 41.50.** *Atypical vascular lesion, skin.* **A,B:** Empty, dilated anastomosing vascular spaces are shown in the superficial dermis.

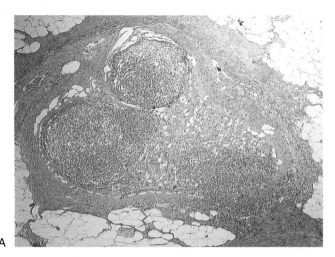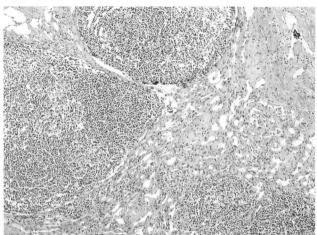

A                                                                    B

FIG. 41.51. *Atypical vascular lesion, breast.* **A:** This tumor was well circumscribed and contained lymphoid follicles with germinal centers. **B:** Open, serpiginous vascular spaces are present between the lymphoid follicles.

41.51). Histologic examination reveals a focal proliferation in the papillary and reticular dermis of dilated, anastomosing vascular channels lined for the most part by a single layer of endothelial cells that may have hyperchromatic nuclei (Table 41.2). The vascular spaces are usually empty, but occasionally there are lymphocytes in the stroma and in the vascular lumens (Fig. 41.52). An unusual postradiation AVL consists of compressed vascular spaces that appear to be capillaries (Fig. 41.53). This vascular proliferation may extend into middle and deep dermal areas. The endothelial cells lack the cytologic characteristic of postradiation angiosarcoma.

A few patients with mammary angiosarcoma also have had hemangiomas (129). One patient with low-grade angiosarcoma had a hemangioma of her scalp diagnosed at the same time her breast tumor was detected. Because she was disease free 5 years after mastectomy, the diagnosis of a coincidental cutaneous hemangioma was substantiated not only by differences in the histologic appearance of the le-

sions, but also by clinical follow-up. Incidental perilobular hemangiomas have been found in mastectomy specimens from patients with mammary angiosarcoma, which is probably a coincidental association because they are frequent in breast tissue from women with benign breast lesions and mammary carcinoma. A few perilobular hemangiomas and small nonpalpable hemangiomas with cytologically atypical endothelial cells and irregularly shaped margins have been described (134). None of these patients developed angiosarcoma. It is unlikely that origin of angiosarcoma from a perilobular hemangioma or microscopic hemangioma will be demonstrable because such a small precursor lesion almost certainly would be obliterated by the larger malignant neoplasm. Perilobular hemangiomas may be multifocal in one breast or may involve both breasts (180) and should not be mistaken for metastatic angiosarcoma in these situations.

The relationship between grossly evident hemangiomas and angiosarcomas remains obscure. Hemangiomas with atypical cytologic and structural features resemble components of angiosarcomas, but all such lesions also retain at least some hemangiomatous elements, such as circumscription, lobulation, or association with nonneoplastic vessels that have well-developed muscular walls. Atypical hemangiomas are rarely larger than 2 cm. Origin of an angiosarcoma from a hemangioma or atypical hemangioma has not been reported in the literature. The difficulty in establishing such a relationship is akin to that of proving origin of liposarcoma from a lipoma. The author has seen only one case that might qualify as an angiosarcoma arising in a hemangioma.

### Immunohistochemistry and Electron Microscopy

Immunoreactivity for factor VIII-related antigen has been detected in angiomas and angiosarcomas originating in the breast and in other organs (175,185–187)(Fig. 41.54). Two studies of mammary angiosarcomas reported more intense

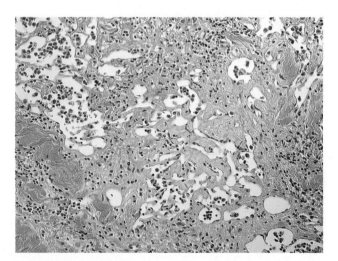

FIG. 41.52. *Atypical vascular lesion, skin.* Lymphocytes are present in the stroma and in the vascular spaces.

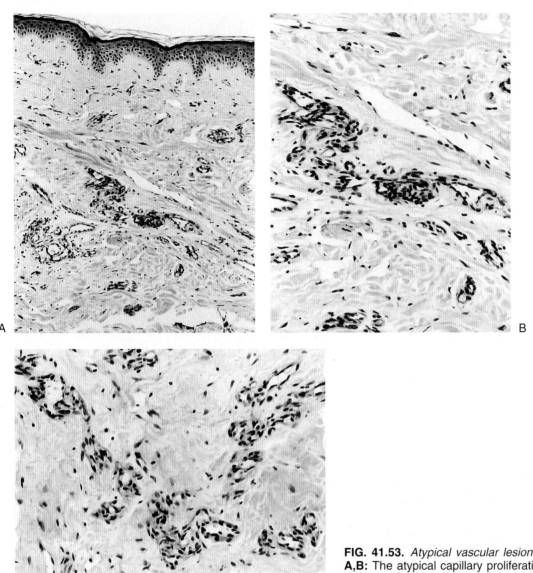

**FIG. 41.53.** *Atypical vascular lesion of skin, capillary type.* **A,B:** The atypical capillary proliferation stands out from the surrounding tissue. **C:** Loosely connected capillaries in which endothelial cells have hyperchromatic nuclei are shown.

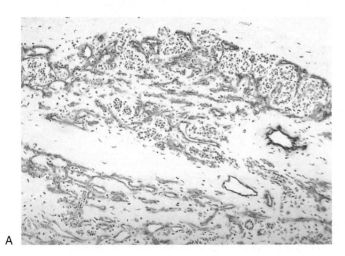

**FIG. 41.54.** *Angiosarcoma, immunoreactivity with vascular markers.* **A:** This low-grade angiosarcoma infiltrating lobules is immunoreactive for factor VIII (avidin-biotin). *(continued)*

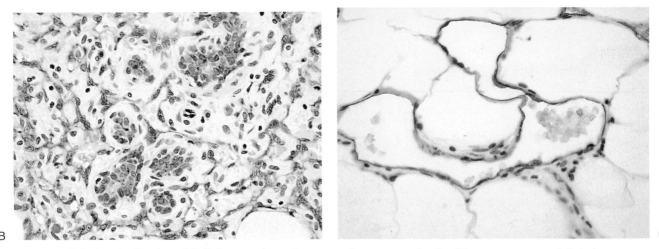

**FIG. 41.54.** *Continued.* **B,C:** Low-grade angiosarcoma immunoreactive for *Ulex europaeus* agglutinin-I is shown in a lobule and in fat (avidin-biotin).

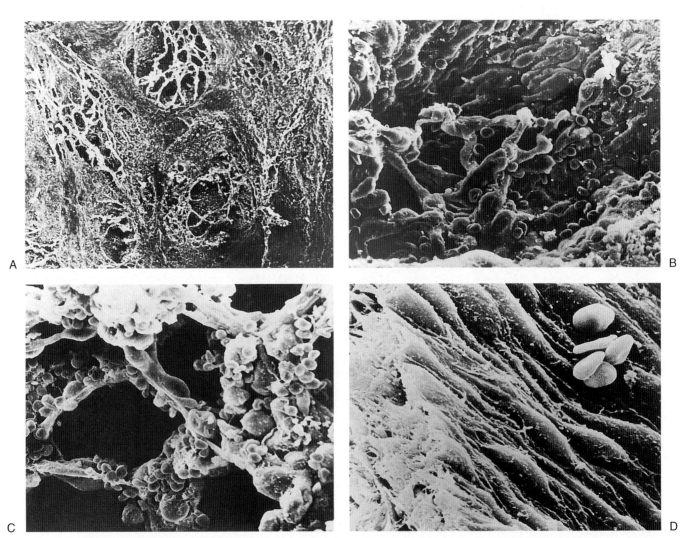

**FIG. 41.55.** *Angiosarcoma, scanning electron microscopy.* **A:** Endothelial cells lining a large neoplastic space ("blood sinus") form a network of cytoplasmic processes between anastomosing vascular channels. **B:** A magnified view of cords of neoplastic endothelial cells. **C:** Bulging nuclei are responsible for protrusions on the surfaces of the cells. **D:** The endothelial surface of a normal submucosal gastric vein showing elongated bulging nuclei. (**A–D:** From Toth B, Malick L. Scanning electron-microscopic study of the surface characteristics of neoplastic endothelial cells in blood vessels. *J Pathol* 1976;118:59–64, with permission.)

staining for factor VIII in well-differentiated than in poorly differentiated portions of the tumor (175,186). Sparse or absent reactivity for factor VIII has been reported more commonly in nonmammary angiosarcomas (185,187). Variable staining for *Ulex europaeus* agglutinin-I (UEA-I) also has been described in angiosarcomas (187). In one series, the neoplastic endothelium in 6 of 14 angiosarcomas was reactive for factor VIII and 11 stained for UEA-I (187). Immunoreactivity for tumor-associated glycoprotein-72 demonstrated with antibody B72.3 was reported to be highly specific for angiosarcoma (188). Angiosarcomas also exhibit reactivity for CD34 and CD31 (188,189). These reagents are especially useful for distinguishing epithelioid forms of angiosarcoma from carcinoma and other neoplasms.

Several investigators have reported on the ultrastructural features of mammary angiosarcoma (171,175,190,191). Weibel-Palade bodies were described in neoplastic endothelial cells in most of the lesions, although they may be inconspicuous or absent in areas of solid growth. Neoplastic endothelial cells contain pinocytotic vesicles at the luminal and basal surface. Small cytoplasmic projections or papillae have been noted projecting into the vascular lumen. The neoplastic endothelium and basal lamina are frequently discontinuous. Pericytic cells have been found associated with endothelial cells in some tumors.

Scanning electron microscopy of mammary angiosarcomas revealed a structure similar to chemically induced angiosarcoma of the murine liver (191,192) (Fig. 41.55). Compared with normal vessels, endothelial cells in the sarcoma were oriented in an overlapping disorderly fashion, sometimes projecting into the vascular lumen to form bridges or cord-like structures. Along the vascular wall these cells were arranged in a spiderweb pattern. Although a disorderly and lace-like arrangement of endothelial cells was found in vessels in reactive lesions and in benign vascular tumors, none of these entities had clusters and cords of atypical endothelial cells protruding into the vascular lumen.

### Prognosis and Treatment

In 1980, Chen (126) reviewed 87 published cases and reported that 14% of the patients were disease free at 3 years and only 7% (127,193,194) survived disease free after 5 years. An additional patient treated initially by excisional surgery underwent a mastectomy 2 years later for a local recurrence and remained well 11 years after the mastectomy (195). Additional case reports of patients who survived longer than 5 years were subsequently published (142,196,197).

Because of the poor survival results in reports through 1980, little information could be obtained about prognostic factors. Steingaszner et al. reviewed 10 cases from the Armed Forces Institute of Pathology and concluded that a high mitotic rate and relatively long pretreatment duration were associated with a poor prognosis (127). Subsequently, it was reported that patients who were aware of the tumor and delayed obtaining medical care had significantly (*p*

<0.01) larger tumors (median size, 6 cm) than those who sought treatment at first awareness (median size, 3 cm) (129). Size and duration of symptoms, however, were not significantly correlated with tumor grade, the likelihood of recurrence, or with survival.

Donnell et al. studied 40 patients with mammary angiosarcoma and found that the overall disease-free survival was 41% at 3 years and 33% at 5 years (128). Tumor grade was the most important prognostic factor. Most patients with orderly or low-grade lesions remained disease free, whereas virtually all women with high-grade tumors died of recurrent sarcoma within 5 years (Fig. 41.56).

An expanded series of 87 patients confirmed the statistically significant correlation between the grade of angiosarcoma and prognosis (129). Twenty-five of the patients (40%) had low-grade lesions, 12 had intermediate grade tumors (19%), and 26 (41%) had high-grade angiosarcomas. Analysis of survival curves for these patients revealed the following estimated probabilities of disease-free survival 5 and 10 years after treatment: low-grade: 76%; intermediate grade: 70%; and high-grade: 15%. The median duration of disease-free survival also was correlated with tumor grade (low, >15 years; intermediate, >12 years; high, 15 months). The longest survival in this series was 18 years, with no evidence of disease in a patient who was 23 years of age when she was treated for a high-grade mammary angiosarcoma.

The prognosis of angiosarcoma arising in the breast after radiotherapy is determined by the degree of differentiation of the tumor and, when stratified for grade, does not appear to differ substantially from that of spontaneous parenchymal angiosarcoma unassociated with radiotherapy.

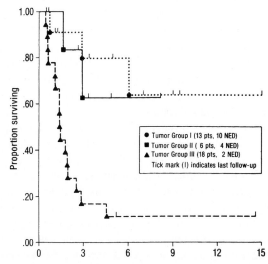

**FIG. 41.56.** *Angiosarcoma, survival analysis.* The patients were stratified by histologic group (grade). Patients with high-grade sarcomas (group 3) had a significantly lower survival rate compared with women with low-grade (group 1) and intermediate-grade (group 2) tumors. (From Donnell RM, Rosen PP, Lieberman PH, et al. Angiosarcoma and other vascular tumors of the breast: pathologic analysis as a guide to prognosis. *Am J Surg Pathol* 1981;5:629–642, with permission.)

Despite the fact that low-grade angiosarcoma has a relatively favorable prognosis, these patients can develop local and systemic recurrences (128,129). Patients who initially have low-grade angiosarcoma may have intermediate or high-grade areas in recurrent lesions. Recurrence and metastases that originate from high-grade sarcomas can be composed in part or entirely of low-grade components.

The prognosis of intermediate grade angiosarcoma is slightly less favorable than, but not significantly different from, that of low-grade tumors. It is interesting that the median age of these patients falls between the median ages of women with low- and high-grade lesions. These tumors are relatively infrequent, constituting 20% or fewer of mammary angiosarcomas. For the present, one should identify patients with intermediate-grade sarcomas to assemble a larger group that will make it possible to determine more accurately the prognosis for patients in this category.

The most frequent sites of metastases, other than local recurrences at the mastectomy site, are bone, the lungs, the liver, the contralateral breast, and the skin (129). Spread to the opposite breast may be a manifestation of the apparent cutaneous tropism of these tumors. The distinction between metastatic tumor in the contralateral breast and a new primary contralateral angiosarcoma is quite difficult. The histologic grade of the first tumor, a comparison of the histologic features of the tumors, and the interval between the lesions are factors to consider. Experience has shown that bilateral primary angiosarcoma is uncommon and that contralateral breast involvement is usually evidence of metastatic spread, often the first metastasis to be identified (126). Two unusual instances of clinically significant metastases in the gingiva have been reported (198,199). Metastatic angiosarcoma has been described in the ovary and placenta (200), and rarely metastases may present in remote subcutaneous sites (201,202).

Total mastectomy is the recommended primary surgical therapy. Axillary dissection is not indicated because metastases rarely involve these lymph nodes (126,129). Radical mastectomy is not appropriate unless the tumor is close to or involves the deep fascia. Rarely, a small lesion might be encompassed by quadrantectomy.

A diagnosis of angiosarcoma may be suggested in a specimen obtained by FNA if it contains malignant spindle cells and papillary clusters (203). An incisional biopsy can provide sufficient material for the diagnosis of mammary angiosarcoma, but unless it contains a high-grade lesion, the findings may be misleading with respect to grade. Peripheral portions of these tumors often have a low-grade pattern.

The role of radiation in the primary treatment of mammary angiosarcoma has not been determined. In one series, individual patients with low- and intermediate-grade lesions remained disease free after excision and radiotherapy (129). One patient with a high-grade tumor developed a mammary recurrence after breast-conserving surgery.

Following surgery, systemic adjuvant chemotherapy may be offered, but the effectiveness of this treatment remains

**TABLE 41.3.** *Mammary angiosarcoma: adjuvant chemotherapy and prognosis*

| Tumor grade (No. of patients) | Frequency of recurrence | |
| --- | --- | --- |
| | After adjuvant chemotherapy No. (%) | After no adjuvant chemotherapy No. (%) |
| Low (25) | 2/10 (20) | 4/15 (27) |
| Intermediate (12) | 2/7 (29) | 2/5 (40) |
| High (26) | 10/14 (71) | 12/12 (100) |
| Total | 14/31 (45) | 18/32 (56) |

Based on Nanus D, Kaufman R. Angiosarcoma of the breast: adjuvant chemotherapy with antinumyein. *Proc Am Soc Clin Oncol* 1986;5:73, with permission.

uncertain. Donnell et al. reported that 9 of 15 patients who remained disease free had been treated with adjuvant chemotherapy after surgery (14 patients) or excisional biopsy (1 patient) (128). Most of these patients were treated with actinomycin D (128,204). It also was noted that nearly 50% (8 of 14) of patients who died of recurrent sarcoma had not had adjuvant therapy. Adjuvant therapy with cyclophosphamide and vincristine (192), velban (194), adriamycin-containing regimens (205), and various other drugs (141) also was reported in a few cases without proving to be particularly effective.

Rosen et al. compared 32 patients who received adjuvant chemotherapy with 31 women who were not so treated (129) (Table 41.3). The drugs most often used were doxorubicin hydrochloride (adriamycin) or actinomycin D. Eleven patients also received chest-wall radiation. Among patients not treated with adjuvant chemotherapy, four had chest-wall irradiation. The median size of tumors among women given adjuvant chemotherapy (5 cm) was not significantly different from that of patients not so treated (4 cm). Recurrences developed in 14 of 31 (45%) patients who received adjuvant chemotherapy and in 18 of 32 (56%) who were not treated. When stratified by tumor grade, recurrences were consistently less frequent among women treated with adjuvant chemotherapy, although the differences were not statistically significant. Because high-grade lesions have such a poor prognosis and most of the few long-term survivors had adjuvant chemotherapy, this treatment should be considered for these patients.

## POSTMASTECTOMY ANGIOSARCOMA (STEWART-TREVES SYNDROME)

Angiosarcoma arising in the lymphedematous upper extremity is not a primary breast neoplasm, but most cases have developed as a complication of the treatment of mammary carcinoma. Since the report by Stewart and Treves in 1948, the relationship of postmastectomy angiosarcoma to lymphedema of the upper arm has been referred to as the

*Stewart-Treves syndrome* (206). It was subsequently noted that angiosarcomas can arise in extremities rendered lymphedematous by conditions not associated with mammary carcinoma, including congenital lymphedema and parasitic infestation (207–209). Origin of the tumors in lymphedematous limbs is the reason that the term *lymphangiosarcoma* has been used; however, the lesions are similar to high-grade angiosarcomas that arise at other sites, and microscopically they most closely resemble angiosarcomas that occur in the mammary skin and breast after lumpectomy and radiotherapy.

The pathogenesis of angiosarcoma in areas of chronic lymphedema is unknown. It is unlikely that irradiation contributes directly to this process because the lesion develops in the absence of radiotherapy, and, in irradiated patients, it originates outside of the treated field. Impaired immune responsiveness has been demonstrated in anatomic areas affected by lymphatic obstruction (210,211). Hence, the lymphedematous limb may be a relatively privileged site immunologically, subject to neoplastic transformation (212,213), a situation that also may contribute to the development of malignant lymphoma in this setting (214,215).

### Clinical Presentation

The estimated frequency of postmastectomy angiosarcoma in the lymphedematous extremity ranges from 0.07% (216) to 0.45% (217). A population-based study of sarcomas in Swedish women with breast carcinoma found that 30 angiosarcomas arose in an edematous arm, and two were present in a conserved breast (218). Most of the patients were treated in the era before widespread breast conservation. The development of angiosarcoma in the ipsilateral arm was not significantly associated with the amount of radiation. Compared with that of control women who did not have lymphedema, the odds ratio for developing Stewart-Treves angiosarcoma was 12.0 [95% confidence interval (CI), 3.5–41.0].

Age at diagnosis averaged about 65 years (range, 44–84 years). Nearly 65% of patients who developed Stewart-Treves syndrome had irradiation of the chest wall and axilla after a radical mastectomy.

A distinction should be made between angiosarcoma in the Stewart-Treves syndrome and postirradiation angiosarcoma of the skin and soft tissue of the chest wall (219–221). The latter arises after mastectomy on the chest wall in the irradiation field and is one of several types of radiation-induced sarcoma (222). Most patients with radiation-induced angiosarcoma of the chest wall have not had lymphedema of the ipsilateral arm (219,220), but this complication was present in one case (221). The interval to onset of postirradiation angiosarcoma of the chest wall has been less than 10 years, with most tumors having arisen in 3 to 6 years. Also excluded from the Stewart-Treves syndrome are patients who develop angiosarcoma of the mammary skin or mammary parenchyma following breast-conserving surgery and

irradiation. These forms of angiosarcoma, discussed earlier in this chapter, are not specifically related to postirradiation edema of the breast.

The average interval between treatment of mammary carcinoma and the clinical appearance of Stewart-Treves angiosarcoma in the arm is about 10 years (209,223), although periods as short as 1 year (224,225) and as long as 49 years (226) have been reported. The initial lesions appear on the upper inner or medial arm in at least 75% of cases (209), but they also have been found on the forearm and elbow. They often consist of purplish discoloration of the skin that may be mistaken for an ecchymosis. These subtle changes evolve into plaques that enlarge into blue or blue–red nodules (Fig. 41.57). Superficial vesicles or bullae that contain hemorrhagic fluid tend to develop before the surface ulcerates, leading to oozing of serosanguinous fluid or hemorrhage. Usually, there is rapid progression from the initial lesion with spread in the skin to involve the chest wall and forearm, but rarely the evolution of the disease can have a chronic course.

### Gross Pathology

Biopsies obtained at an early stage before the development of nodules and plaques reveal lesions limited to the dermis of the skin and the superficial subcutaneous tissues. These usually consist of punctate hemorrhagic foci with little or no induration. When surgery is performed in a more advanced case, there are usually hemorrhagic tumor nodules involving muscle as well as the subcutaneous fat and skin (Fig. 41.58). The gross distribution of satellite cutaneous and deep soft tissue lesions suggests that they develop from in-transit metastases or that there may be multiple sites of origin. Stewart and Treves (206) noted that deep tumors were associated with blood vessels and that in some instances tumor was present in large veins.

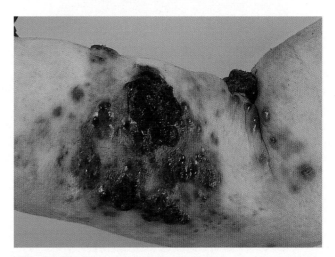

**FIG. 41.57.** *Postmastectomy angiosarcoma.* Hemorrhagic tumor masses involving the distal upper arm and proximal forearm are shown.

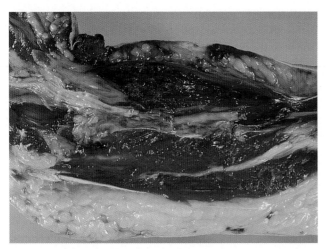

**FIG. 41.58.** *Postmastectomy angiosarcoma.* In this hemisected amputation specimen, angiosarcoma involves the subcutaneous tissue and underlying muscle.

## Microscopic Pathology

The histologic appearance of angiosarcoma arising in the lymphedematous limb is heterogeneous. Biopsies of flat discolored or faintly infiltrated skin lesions reveal inconspicuous lesions. Diffuse alterations related to the underlying chronic lymphedema consist of edema and collagenization of the dermis and focal lymphocytic infiltrates in the superficial dermis that tend to have a perivascular distribution (Fig. 41.59). A subtle proliferation of small vessels in the superficial dermis commonly occurs in chronic lymphedema (Fig. 41.60). The earliest evidence of angiosarcoma usually consists of the focal proliferation of irregularly shaped vascular channels lined by somewhat prominent endothelial cells that have hyperchromatic nuclei (Fig. 41.61). Erythrocytes can be seen in these vessels and also in the surrounding dermal stroma. These early lesions may be indistinguishable from Kaposi's sarcoma, a diagnostic problem emphasized by Stewart and Treves (206).

The formation of interconnecting vascular channels, papillary endothelial proliferation, and hemorrhage are indicative of more fully developed lesions (Figs. 41.62 and 41.63). In advanced cases, endothelial growth may be so exuberant that the accumulated cells form nodules (Fig. 41.64). When such foci have an epithelial appearance, the lesions can be difficult to distinguish from carcinoma by light microscopy (Fig. 41.65). A diagnosis of retrograde metastasis of mammary carcinoma may be suggested by such lesions, but it is usually possible to identify areas with a distinct vascular component, often with a prominent papillary configuration. Spindle cell sarcomatous elements may be found in association with lesions that have an epithelial growth pattern or as independent lesions. Larger veins appear to become involved most often as a result of intramural neoplastic proliferation rather than as a consequence of transmural invasion by extrinsic tumor foci. Embolic spread of angiosarcoma has been found at distant sites such as the lung and kidney.

## Immunohistochemistry and Electron Microscopy

The distinction between Stewart-Treves angiosarcoma and recurrent mammary carcinoma is usually not difficult clinically, but biopsies of undifferentiated tumor nodules can present a problem to the pathologist. Poorly differentiated recurrent carcinoma generally contains little or no mucin, but the tumor cells are reactive immunohistochemically for cytokeratin (227). Vimentin reactivity is absent from many carcinomas and present in angiosarcomas (228) (Fig. 41.66).

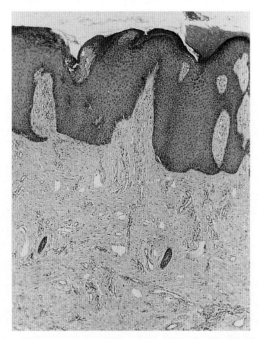

**FIG. 41.59.** *Chronic lymphedema.* Collagenization of the dermis, increased dermal vascularity, and lymphangiectasia are shown. Pseudoepitheliomatous hyperplasia of the epidermis is present.

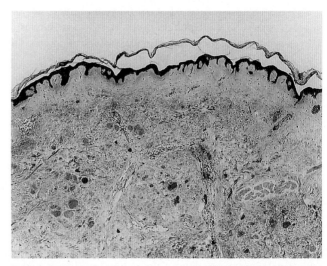

**FIG. 41.60.** *Chronic lymphedema.* Dilated, congested capillaries and a band-like dermal lymphocytic infiltrate are shown.

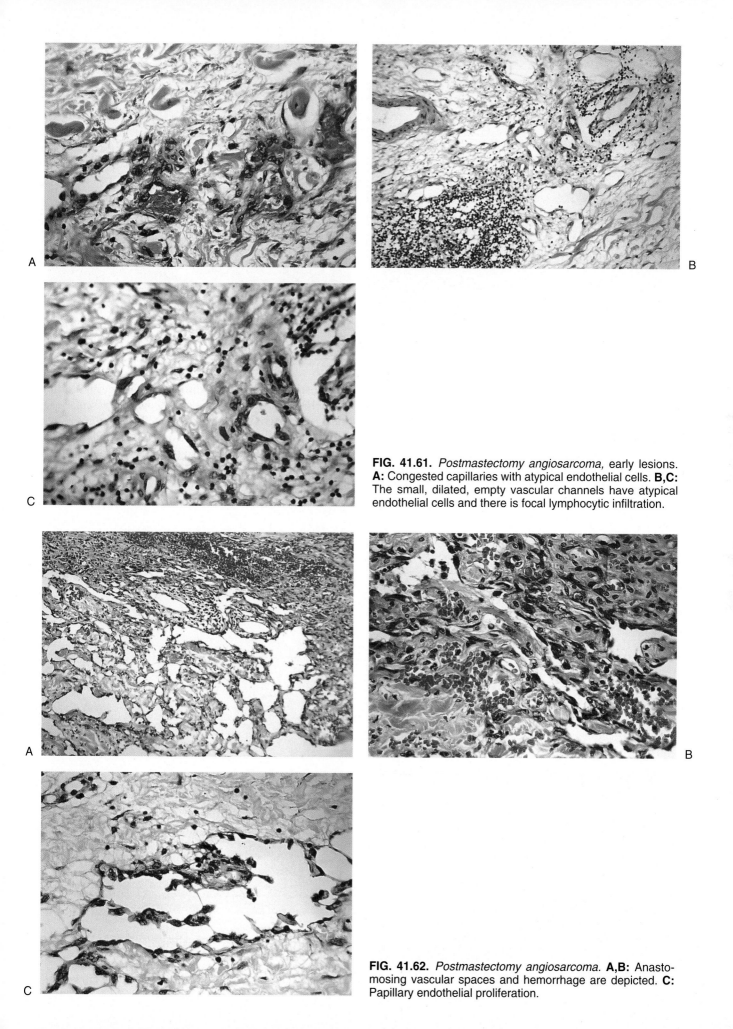

**FIG. 41.61.** *Postmastectomy angiosarcoma,* early lesions. **A:** Congested capillaries with atypical endothelial cells. **B,C:** The small, dilated, empty vascular channels have atypical endothelial cells and there is focal lymphocytic infiltration.

**FIG. 41.62.** *Postmastectomy angiosarcoma.* **A,B:** Anastomosing vascular spaces and hemorrhage are depicted. **C:** Papillary endothelial proliferation.

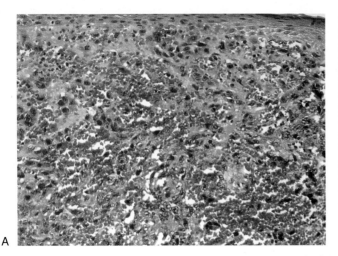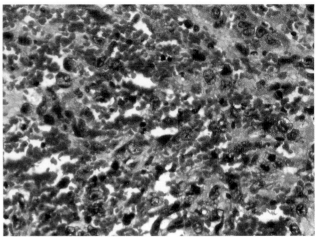

**FIG. 41.63.** *Postmastectomy angiosarcoma.* **A:** A hemorrhagic tumor nodule that developed in the soft tissue of the arm. **B:** The tumor cells have poorly differentiated nuclei with vesicular chromatin and prominent nucleoli.

Immunoreactivity for the blood group antigen UEA-I has been reported to be strong in vascular components and variable in solid undifferentiated areas of Stewart-Treves angiosarcoma (228,229). Immunoreactivity for UEA-I also has been found in mammary carcinomas (230).

Factor VIII has been detected in cells lining well-formed neoplastic vascular channels (228,229,231), but it has been absent (228,231) or minimally expressed (219) in poorly dif-

ferentiated foci. It is often difficult to distinguish histologically between well-differentiated neoplastic vascular channels and reactive vessels associated with chronic lymphedema. Both may be factor VIII immunoreactive. Anti-CD34 and CD31 are also reactive with most angiosarcomas, but they are less specific because they also stain other types of sarcoma (Fig. 41.67).

Immunohistochemical studies are also helpful in the

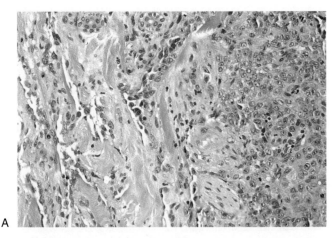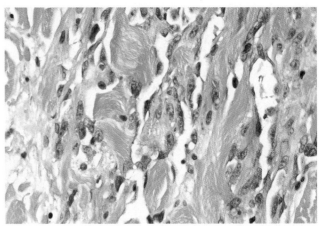

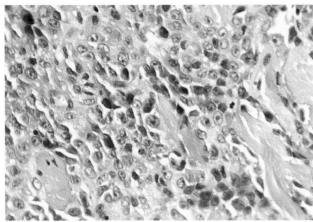

**FIG. 41.64.** *Postmastectomy angiosarcoma.* **A:** This tumor nodule has slit-shaped vascular spaces and a solid epithelioid component. **B:** The vascular area. **C:** The epithelioid area. Nucleoli are more prominent in this part of the lesion.

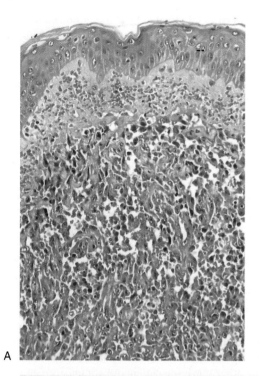

A

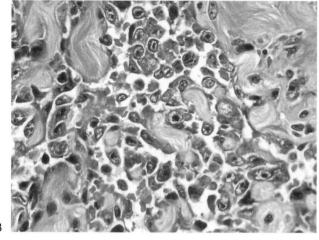

B

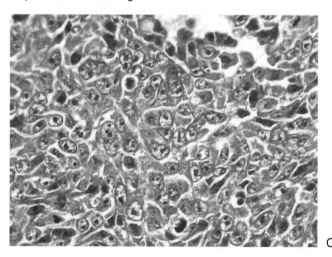

C

**FIG. 41.65.** *Postmastectomy angiosarcoma, epithelioid type.* **A,B:** The tumor composed of epithelioid cells had a vascular pattern in this region. **C:** Part of the sarcoma had epithelioid cells arranged in a sheet.

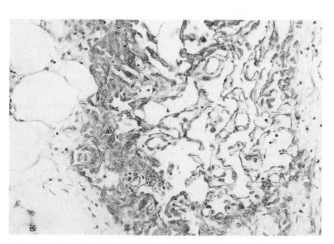

**FIG. 41.66.** *Postmastectomy angiosarcoma, vimentin.* The tumor cells are immunoreactive for vimentin (avidin-biotin).

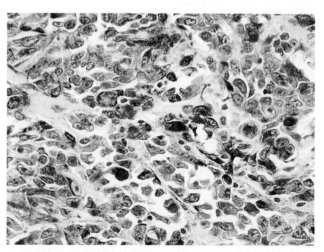

**FIG. 41.67.** *Postmastectomy angiosarcoma, CD31.* Intense immunostaining for CD31 is shown (avidin-biotin).

diagnosis of other malignant neoplasms that may arise in the lymphedematous limb. Two reported instances of malignant lymphoma were immunoreactive for markers of lymphoid origin, including L26, which is indicative of B-cell origin (214,215). An example of malignant melanoma that arose in the skin of an arm with postmastectomy lymphedema predated modern immunohistochemistry, but one would expect melanoma to be reactive for S-100 protein, HMB-45 antigen, and possibly vimentin (232). After careful evaluation of the clinical presentation and a thorough assessment of histologic sections, it is usually possible to distinguish between Stewart-Treves angiosarcoma and the exceedingly rare retrograde metastatic carcinoma or other malignant neoplasm.

Several studies established the heterogeneous ultrastructural features of Stewart-Treves angiosarcoma (228,229,231, 233,234). The electron microscopic findings were typical for a malignant vascular lesion characterized by a proliferation of endothelial cells. In angiomatous areas, endothelial cells resting on a basement membrane were joined by well-formed junctional complexes. The cytoplasm contained pinocytotic vesicles, clusters of intermediate filaments, and Weibel-Palade bodies. With loss of differentiation, Weibel-Palade bodies and pinocytotic vesicles became less numerous. Solid portions of the tumors were composed of round and spindle cells arranged in a loosely cohesive fashion, joined by primitive and well-formed desmosomes. Erythrocytes were seen in neoplastic vascular lumens and between neoplastic cells in poorly differentiated areas. Pericytic cells were reportedly not evident (229) or were present only in well-differentiated areas (233–235).

Immunohistochemical and ultrastructural observations led to the widely held conclusion that the neoplastic cells in Stewart-Treves angiosarcoma have properties more typically associated with blood vascular than with lymphatic endothelium. The features that characterize blood vascular endothelium include fenestrated cells, Weibel-Palade bodies, pinocytotic activity, and pericytic cells.

## Prognosis and Treatment

No reliable treatment for Stewart-Treves angiosarcoma has been found, and most patients died of metastatic sarcoma less than 2 years after diagnosis. Ten to 15% of reported patients have survived for 5 years. Amputation may offer the best chance for cure. Local recurrence occurs more frequently after treatment by excisional surgery, radiation, or chemotherapy alone than after amputation. Systemic metastases invariably involve the lungs and often occur in bone, the liver, or other sites. The brain is rarely involved by metastases. Other malignant neoplasms, particularly contralateral mammary carcinoma, may occur in patients with postmastectomy angiosarcoma (223).

Woodward et al. (209) assembled survival data on 129 patients from the literature before 1972, including their series of women treated at the Mayo Clinic. The median survival was 19 months. Eleven patients (9%) survived 5 years, in-

cluding seven of 61 (11%) treated by amputation and four of 48 (8%) treated with radiation and other methods without amputation.

A subsequent study from the M.D. Anderson Hospital (236) reported that 8 of 22 patients were treated by forequarter amputation and that four of the eight remained disease-free from 6 months to 7 years after surgery. Systemic chemotherapy consisting of various regimens administered to 11 patients yielded a 42% response rate. The median survival of responders, 26.5 months, was substantially longer than that of nonresponders, 4 months. Local infusional chemotherapy administered to six patients resulted in two complete responses and one partial response.

Sordillo et al. (223) reported that 6 of 44 patients (14%) with "lymphangiosarcoma" survived disease free for 5 to 19 years (median, 13 years). Five of the six were surviving patients treated for postmastectomy Stewart-Treves angiosarcoma (four by amputation, one by radiation). Two women survived 13 and 19 years. After amputation and actinomycin D chemotherapy, one of these women had a chest-wall recurrence. The recurrence was treated with radiotherapy and further actinomycin D, after which the patient remained disease free. The other surviving patient did not undergo amputation but had irradiation of the arm and actinomycin D chemotherapy (237).

## REFERENCES

### Sarcoma

1. Gutman H, Pollock RE, Ross MI, et al. Sarcoma of the breast: implications for extent of therapy. The MD Anderson experience. *Surgery* 1994;116:505–509.
2. McGregor GI, Knowling MA, Este FA. Sarcoma and cystosarcoma phyllodes tumors of the breast—a retrospective review of 58 cases. *Am J Surg* 1994;167:477–480.
3. Glenn J, Kinsella T, Glatstein E, et al. A randomized, prospective trial of adjuvant chemotherapy in adults with soft tissue sarcomas of the head and neck, breast, and trunk. *Cancer* 1985;55:1206–1214.
4. Mazanet R, Antman KH. Sarcomas of soft tissue and bone. *Cancer* 1991;68:463–473.

### Stromal Sarcoma

5. Berg JW, DeCrosse JJ, Fracchia AA, et al. Stromal sarcomas of the breast: a unified approach to connective tissue sarcomas other than cystosarcoma phyllodes. *Cancer* 1962;13:419–424.
6. Christensen L, Schiodt T, Blichert-Toft M, et al. Sarcomas of the breast: a clinico-pathologic study of 67 patients with long term follow-up. *Eur J Surg Oncol* 1988;14:214–247.
7. Terrier Ph, Terrier-Lacombe MJ, Mouriesse H, et al. Primary breast sarcoma: a review of 33 cases with immunohistochemistry and prognostic factors. *Breast Cancer Res Treat* 1989;13:39–48.
8. Callery CD, Rosen PP, Kinne DW. Sarcoma of the breast: a study of 32 patients with reappraisal of classification and therapy. *Ann Surg* 1985;201:527–532.

### Leiomyosarcoma

9. Allison JG, Dodds HM. Leiomyoma of the male nipple: a case report and literature review. *Am Surg* 1989;55:501–502.
10. Nasciemento AG, Rosen PP, Karas M. Leiomyoma of the nipple. *Am J Surg Pathol* 1979;3:151–154.

11. Tsujoka K, Kashihara M, Imamura S. Cutaneous leiomyoma of the male nipple. *Dermatology* 1985;170:98–100.
12. Hernandez FJ. Leiomyosarcoma of the male breast originating in the nipple. *Am J Surg Pathol* 1978;2:299–304.
13. Parham DM, Robertson AJ, Hussein KA, et al. Leiomyosarcoma of the breast: cytological and histological features, with a review of the literature. *Cytopathology* 1992;3:245–252.
14. Alessi E, Sala F. Leiomyosarcoma in ectopic areola. *Am J Dermatopathol* 1992;14:165–169.
15. Cameron HM, Stamperl H, Warambo W. Leiomyosarcoma of the breast originating from myothelium (myoepithelium). *J Pathol* 1974;114:89–92.
16. Pardo-Mindan J, Garcia-Julian G, Altuna ME. Leiomyosarcoma of the breast. *Am J Clin Pathol* 1974;62:477–480.
17. Visfeldt J, Sheike O. Male breast cancer. I. Histologic typing and grading of 187 Danish cases. *Cancer* 1973;32:985–990.
18. Crocker DJ, Murad TM. Ultrastructure of fibrosarcoma in a male breast. *Cancer* 1969;29:891–899.
19. Barnes L, Pietruszka M. Sarcomas of the breast: a clinicopathologic analysis of 10 cases. *Cancer* 1977;40:1577–1585.
20. Falconieri G, Della Libera D, Zanconati F, et al. Leiomyosarcoma of the female breast: report of two new cases and a review of the literature. *Am J Clin Pathol* 1997;108:19–25.
21. Arista-Nasr J, Gonzalez-Gomez I, Angeles-Angeles A, et al. Primary recurrent leiomyosarcoma of the breast: case report with ultrastructure and immunohistochemical study and review of the literature. *Am J Clin Pathol* 1989;92:500–505.
22. Terrier PH, Terrier-Lacombe MJ, Mouriesse H, et al. Primary breast sarcoma: a review of 33 cases with immunohistochemistry and prognostic factors. *Breast Cancer Res Treat* 1989;13:39–48.
23. Bouropoulou V, Markaki S, Prevedorou D, et al. Sarcomas of the breast. A clinicopathologic, histochemical and immunohistochemical study of ten cases. *Breast Dis* 1989;2:59–70.
24. Waterworth PD, Gompertz RHK, Hennessy C, et al. Primary leiomyosarcoma of the breast. *Br J Surg* 1992;79:169–170.
25. González-Palacios F. Leiomyosarcoma of the female breast. *Am J Clin Pathol* 1998;109:650–651.
26. Nielsen BB. Leiomyosarcoma of the breast with late dissemination. *Virchows Arch* 1984;403:241–245.
27. Falconieri G. Leiomyosarcoma of the female breast [Letter]. *Am J Clin Pathol* 1999;109:651.
28. Callery CD, Rosen PP, Kinne DW. Sarcoma of the breast: a study of 32 patients with reappraisal of classification and therapy. *Ann Surg* 1985;201:527–532.
29. Pollard SG, Marks PV, Temple LN, et al. Breast sarcoma: a clinicopathologic review of 25 cases. *Cancer* 1990;66:941–944.
30. Christensen L, Schiodt T, Blichert-Toft M, et al. Sarcomas of the breast: a clinico-pathologic study of 67 patients with long term follow-up. *Eur J Surg Oncol* 1988;14:214–247.
31. Chen KTK, Kuo T, Koffman KD. Leiomyosarcoma of the breast: a case report of long survival and late hepatic metastases. *Cancer* 1981;47:1883–1886.

## Liposarcoma

32. Austin RM, Dupree WB. Liposarcoma of the breast: a clinicopathologic study of 20 cases. *Hum Pathol* 1986;17:906–913.
33. Powell CM, Rosen PP. Adipose differentiation in cystosarcoma phyllodes. *Am J Surg Pathol* 1994;18:720–727.
34. Vivian JB, Tan EGC, Frayne JR, et al. Bilateral liposarcoma of the breast. *Aust N Z J Surg* 1993;63:658–659.
35. Hummer CD, Burkart TJ. Liposarcoma of the breast: a case of bilateral involvement. *Am J Surg* 1967;113:558–561.
36. Arbabi L, Warhol HJ. Pleomorphic liposarcoma following radiotherapy for breast carcinoma. *Cancer* 1982;49:878–880.
37. Barnes L, Pietruszka M. Sarcomas of the breast. A clinicopathologic analysis of 10 cases. *Cancer* 1977;40:1577–1585.
38. Bouropoulou V, Markaki S, Prevedorou D, et al. Sarcomas of the breast. A clinicopathologic, histochemical and immunohistochemical study of ten cases. *Breast Dis* 1989;2:59–70.
39. Callery CD, Rosen PP, Kinne DW. Sarcoma of the breast: a study of 32 patients with reappraisal of classification and therapy. *Ann Surg* 1985;201:527–532.
40. Kanemoto K, Nakamura T, Matsuyama S, et al. Liposarcoma of the

breast, review of the literature and a report of a case. *Jpn J Surg* 1981;11:381–384.
41. Odom JW, Mikhailova B, Pryce E, et al. Liposarcoma of the breast: report of a case and review of the literature. *Breast Dis* 1991;4:293–298.
42. Pollard SG, Marks PV, Temple LN, et al. Breast sarcoma: a clinicopathologic review of 25 cases. *Cancer* 1990;66:941–944.
43. Rasmussen J, Jensen H. Liposarcoma of the breast: case report and review of the literature. *Virchows Arch* 1979;385:117–124.
44. Christensen L, Schiodt T, Blichert-Toft M, et al. Sarcomas of the breast: a clinico-pathologic study of 67 patients with long term follow-up. *Eur J Surg Oncol* 1988;14:214–247.

## Osteogenic and Chondrosarcoma

45. Remadi S, Doussis-Anagnostopoulu I, Mac Gee W. Primary osteosarcoma of the breast. *Pathol Res Pract* 1995;191:471–474.
46. Brown AL, Holwill SD, Thomas VA, et al. Case report: primary osteosarcoma of the breast: imaging and histological features. *Clin Radiol* 1998;53:920–922.
47. Savage AP, Sagor GR, Dovey P. Osteosarcoma of the breast: a case report with an unusual diagnostic feature. *Clin Oncol* 1984;10:295–298.
48. Lee JK, Sun SS. Primary osteogenic sarcoma of the breast demonstrated by Tc-99m MDP scintigraphy. *Clin Nucl Med* 1998;23:619.
49. Barnes L, Pietruszka M. Sarcomas of the breast: a clinicopathologic analysis of 10 cases. *Cancer* 1977;40:1577–1585.
50. Beltaos E, Banerjee TK. Chondrosarcoma of the breast. *Am J Clin Pathol* 1979;71:345–349.
51. Benediktsdottir K, Lagerberg F, Lundell L, et al. Osteogenic sarcoma of the breast. *Acta Pathol Microbiol Scand [A]* 1980;88:161–165.
52. Bouropoulou V, Markaki S, Prevedorou D, et al. Sarcomas of the breast: a clinicopathologic, histochemical and immunohistochemical study of ten cases. *Breast Dis* 1989;2:59–70.
53. Callery CD, Rosen PP, Kinne DW. Sarcoma of the breast: a study of 32 patients with reappraisal of classification and therapy. *Ann Surg* 1985;201:527–532.
54. Going JJ, Lumsden AB, Anderson JJ. A classical osteogenic sarcoma of the breast: histology, immunohistochemistry and ultrastructure. *Histopathology* 1986;10:631–641.
55. Ladefaged C, Nielsen BB. Primary chondrosarcoma of the breast: a case report and review of the literature. *Breast* 1984;10:26–28.
56. Lumsden AB, Harrison D, Chetty U, et al. Osteogenic sarcoma—a rare primary tumour of the breast. *Eur J Surg Oncol* 1985;11:83–86.
57. Mufarrij AA, Feiner HD. Breast sarcoma with giant cells and osteoid: a case report and review of the literature. *Am J Surg Pathol* 1987;11:225–230.
58. Muller AGS, Van Zyl JA. Primary osteosarcoma of the breast. *J Surg Oncol* 1993;52:135–136.
59. Teich S, Brecher IN. Osteogenic sarcoma of the breast: a case report. *Breast* 1985;11:11–15.
60. Meunier B, Leveque J, Le Prise E, et al. Three cases of sarcoma occurring after radiation therapy of breast cancers. *Eur J Obstet Gynecol Reprod Biol* 1994;57:33–36.
61. Gonzalez-Licea A, Yardley JH, Hartmann WH. Malignant tumor of the breast with bone formation: studies by light and electron microscopy. *Cancer* 1967;20:1234–1247.
62. Aubrey DA, Andrews GS. Mammary osteogenic sarcoma. *Br J Surg* 1971;58:472–474.

## Malignant Fibrous Histiocytoma

63. Jones MW, Norris HJ, Wargotz ES, et al. Fibrosarcoma—malignant fibrous histiocytoma of the breast. A clinicopathologic study of 32 cases. *Am J Surg Pathol* 1992;16:667–674.
64. Bouropoulou V, Markaki S, Prevedorou D, et al. Sarcomas of the breast: a clinicopathologic, histochemical and immunohistochemical study of ten cases. *Breast Dis* 1989;2:59–70.
65. Callery CD, Rosen PP, Kinne DW. Sarcoma of the breast: a study of 32 patients with reappraisal of classification and therapy. *Ann Surg* 1985;201:527–532.
66. Langham MR, Mills AS, DeMay RM, et al. Malignant fibrous histiocytoma of the breast: a case report and review of the literature. *Cancer* 1984;54:558–563.

67. Niekerk JLM, Wobbes T, Holland R, et al. Malignant fibrous histio-cytoma of the breast with axillary lymph node involvement. *J Surg Oncol* 1987;34:32–35.

68. Ostyn C, Spector I, Bremner CG. Malignant fibrous histiocytoma of the breast: a case report. *S Afr Med J* 1987;71:665–666.

69. Remer S, Tartter PI, Schwartz IS. Malignant fibrous histiocytoma of the breast: a case report and review of the literature. *Breast Dis* 1987;1:37–45.

70. Rossen K, Stamp I, Sorensen IM. Primary malignant fibrous histio-toma of the breast. A report of four cases and review of the literature. *APMIS* 1991;99:696–702.

71. Christensen L, Schiodt T, Blichert-Toft M, et al. Sarcomas of the breast: a clinico-pathologic study of 67 patients with long term follow-up. *Eur J Surg Oncol* 1988;14:214–247.

72. Kraft R, Altermatt HJ, Nguyen-Tran Q, et al. Primäres malignes fi-brüses Histiocytom einer mamma virilis. *Pathologie* 1988;9:334–339.

73. Dirix LY, Fierens H, Langerock G, et al. Radiation related malignant fibrous histiocytoma. *Acta Clin Belg* 1988;43:204–208.

74. Meunier B, Leveque J, Le Prise E, et al. Three cases of sarcoma oc-curring after radiation therapy of breast cancers. *Eur J Obstet Gynecol Reprod Biol* 1994;57:33–36.

75. Brady MS, Garfein CF, Petrek JA, et al. Post-treatment sarcoma in breast cancer patients. *Ann Surg Oncol* 1994;1:66–72.

76. Laskin WB, Silverman TA, Enzinger FM. Postradiation soft tissue sarcomas: an analysis of 53 cases. *Cancer* 1988;62:2330–2340.

77. Tsuneyoshi M, Enjoji M. Postirradiation sarcoma (malignant fibrous histiocytoma) following breast carcinoma: an ultrastructural study of a case. *Cancer* 1979;45:1419–1423.

78. Vera-Sempere F, Llombart-Bosch A. Malignant fibrohistiocytoma (MFH) of the breast: primary and postirradiation variants—an ultra-structural study. *Pathol Res Pract* 1984;178:289–296.

79. Hardy TJ, An T, Brown PW, et al. Postirradiation sarcoma (malignant fibrous histiocytoma) of axilla. *Cancer* 1978;42:118–124.

80. Kuten A, Sapir D, Cohen Y, et al. Postirradiation soft tissue sarcoma occurring in breast cancer patients: reports of seven cases and results of combination chemotherapy. *J Surg Oncol* 1985;28:168–171.

81. Luzzatto R, Grossmann S, Scholl JG, et al. Postradiation pleomorphic malignant fibrous histiocytoma of the breast. *Acta Cytol* 1986;30:48–50.

82. Leader M, Patel J, Collins M, et al. Anti-alpha-1-antichymotrypsin staining in 194 sarcomas, 38 carcinomas and 17 malignant melanomas. *Am J Surg Pathol* 1987;11:133–139.

83. Lentini M, Grosso M, Carozza G. Fibrohistiocytic tumors of the soft tissue. An immunohistochemical study of 183 cases. *Path Res Pract* 1986;181:713–717.

84. Stanley MW, Tani EM, Horwitz CA, et al. Primary spindle-cell sar-comas of the breast: diagnosis by fine-needle aspiration. *Diagn Cy-topathol* 1988;4:244–249.

## Fibrosarcoma

85. Terrier P, Terrier-Lacombe MJ, Mouriesse H, et al. Primary breast sar-coma: a review of 33 cases with immunohistochemistry and prognos-tic factors. *Breast Cancer Res Treat* 1989;13:39–48.

86. Callery CD, Rosen PP, Kinne DW. Sarcoma of the breast: a study of 32 patients with reappraisal of classification and therapy. *Ann Surg* 1985;201:527–532.

87. Jones MW, Norris HJ, Wargotz ES, et al. Fibrosarcoma—malignant fibrous histiocytoma of the breast: a clinicopathologic study of 32 cases. *Am J Surg Pathol* 1992;16:667–674.

88. Borman H, Safak T, Ertoy D. Fibrosarcoma following radiotherapy for breast carcinoma: a case report and review of the literature. *Ann Plast Surg* 1998;41:201–204.

## Rhabdomyosarcoma

89. Barnes L, Pietruszka M. Sarcomas of the breast. A clinicopathologic analysis of 10 cases. *Cancer* 1977;40:1577–1585.

90. Hadju SI, Urban JA. Cancers metastatic to the breast. *Cancer* 1972;29:1691–1696.

91. Howarth GB, Caces JN, Pratt CB. Breast metastases in children with rhabdomyosarcoma. *Cancer* 1980;46:2520–2524.

92. Wakely Jr PE, Powers CN, Frable WJ. Metachronous soft-tissue

masses in children and young adults with cancer: correlation of his-tology and aspiration cytology. *Hum Pathol* 1990;21:669–677.

93. Hays DM, Donaldson SS, Shimada H, et al. Primary and metastatic rhabdomyosarcoma in the breast: neoplasms of adolescent females, a report from the Intergroup Rhabdomyosarcoma Study. *Med Pediatr Oncol* 1997;29:181–189.

94. Obermann HA. Sarcomas of the breast. *Cancer* 1965;18:1233–1243.

95. Evans RW. Rhabdomyosarcoma of breast. *J Clin Pathol* 1953;6:140–144.

96. Woodard BH, Farnham R, Mossler JA, et al. Rhabdomysarcoma of the breast. *Arch Pathol Lab Med* 1980;104:445–446.

97. Herrera LJ, Lugo-Vicente H. Primary embryonal rhabdomyosarcoma of the breast in an adolescent female: a case report. *J Pediatr Surg* 1998;33:1582–1584.

98. Copeland LJ, Sneige N, Stringer A, et al. Alveolar rhabdomyosarcoma of the female genitalia. *Cancer* 1985;56:849–855.

99. Deeley TJ. Secondary deposits in the breast. *Br J Cancer* 1965;19:738–743.

100. Pappo I, Zamir O, Ron N, et al. Alvelar rhabdomyosarcoma in young females presenting as breast tumor: two case reports and review of the literature. *Breast Dis* 1994;7:69–77.

101. Torres V, Ferrer R. Cytology of fine needle aspiration biopsy of pri-mary breast rhabdomyosarcoma in an adolescent girl. *Acta Cytol* 1985;29:430–444.

## Hemangiopericytoma

102. Stout AP, Murray MR. Hemangiopericytoma: a vascular tumor fea-turing Zimmerman's pericytes. *Ann Surg* 1942;116:26–33.

103. Arias-Stella J, Rosen PP. Hemangiopericytoma of the breast. *Mod Pathol* 1988;1:98–103.

104. Jiménez-Ayala M, Dìez-Nau MD, Larrad A, et al. Hemangiopericy-toma in a male breast: report of a case with cytologic, histologic and immunochemical studies. *Acta Cytol* 1991;35:234–238.

105. Mittal KR, Gerald W, True LD. Hemangiopericytoma of breast: report of a case with ultrastructural and immunohistochemical findings. *Hum Pathol* 1986;17:1181–1183.

106. Tavassoli FA, Weiss S. Hemangiopericytoma of the breast. *Am J Surg Pathol* 1981;5:745–752.

107. Volmer J, Pickartz H, Jautzke G. Vascular tumors in the region of the breast. *Virchows Arch* 1980;385:201–214.

108. Kaufman SL, Stout AP. Hemangiopericytoma in children. *Cancer* 1960;13:695–710.

109. van Kints MJ, Tjon A Tham RTO, et al. Hemangiopericytoma of the breast: mammographic and sonographic findings. *AJR Am J Roentgenol* 1994;163:61–63.

110. Battifora H. Hemangiopericytoma: ultrastructural study of five cases. *Cancer* 1973;31:1418–1432.

111. Panda A, Dayal Y, Singhal V, et al. Hemangiopericytoma. *Br J Opthalmol* 1984;64:124–127.

## Dermatofibrosarcoma Protuberans

112. Callery CD, Rosen PP, Kinne DW. Sarcoma of the breast: a study of 32 patients with reappraisal of classification and therapy. *Ann Surg* 1985;201:527–532.

113. Obermann HA. Sarcomas of the breast. *Cancer* 1965;18:1233–1243.

114. Karcnik TJ, Miller JA, Fromowitz F, et al. Dermatofibrosarcoma pro-tuberans of the breast: a rare malignant tumor simulating benign dis-ease. *Breast J* 1999;5:262–263.

## Sarcomas of Peripheral Nerve Sheath

115. Malas S, Krawitz HE, Sur RK, et al. Von Recklinghausen's disease as-sociated with a primary malignant schwannoma of the breast. *J Surg Oncol* 1995;59:273–275.

116. Hauser H, Beham A, Steindorfer P, et al. Malignant schwannoma of the breast. *Langenbecks Arch Chir* 1995;380:350–353.

117. Catania S, Pacifico E, Zurrida S, et al. Malignant schwannoma of the breast. *Eur J Surg Oncol* 1992;18:80–81.

118. Pollard SG, Marks PV, Temple LN, et al. Breast sarcoma: a clinico-pathologic review of 25 cases. *Cancer* 1990;66:941–944.

119. Visfeldt J, Sheike O. Male breast cancer. I. Histologic typing and grading of 187 Danish cases. *Cancer* 1973;32:985–990.

## Miscellaneous Sarcomas

120. Luna Vega AR, Vetto JT, Kinne DW. Primary sarcomas of the breast in women under 20 years of age. *N Y State J Med* 1992;92:497–498.
121. Obermann HA. Sarcomas of the breast. *Cancer* 1965;18:1233–1243.
122. Taccagni G, Rovere E, Masullo M, et al. Myofibroblastoma of the breast: review of the literature on myofibroblastic tumors and criteria for defining myofibroblastic differentiation. *Am J Surg Pathol* 1997;21:489–496.
123. González-Palacios F, Enriquez JL, San Miguel P, et al. Myofibroblastic tumors of the breast: a histologic spectrum with a case of recurrent male breast myofibrosarcoma. *Int J Surg Pathol* 1999;7:11–17.
124. Ng CS, Taylor CB, O'Donnell PJ, et al. Case report: mammographic and ultrasound appearances of Kaposi's sarcoma of the breast. *Clin Radiol* 1996;51:735–736.

## Angiosarcoma

125. Barber KW, Harrison EG, Clagett T, Pratt JH. Angiosarcoma of the breast. *Surg Gynecol Obstet* 1960;48:869–878.
126. Chen KTK, Kirkeguard DD, Bocian JJ. Angiosarcoma of the breast. *Cancer* 1980;46:368–371.
127. Steingaszner LG, Enzinger FM, Taylor HB. Hemangiosarcoma of the breast. *Cancer* 1965;18:352–361.
128. Donnell RM, Rosen PP, Lieberman PH, et al. Angiosarcoma and other vascular tumors of the breast: pathologic analysis as a guide to prognosis. *Am J Surg Pathol* 1981;5:629–642.
129. Rosen PP, Kimmel M, Ernsberger D. Mammary angiosarcoma: the prognostic significance of tumor differentiation. *Cancer* 1988;62:2145–2151.
130. Grant EG, Holt RW, Chung B, et al. Angiosarcoma of the breast sonographic, xeromammographic and pathologic appearance. *AJR Am J Roentgenol* 1983;141:691–692.
131. Liberman L, Dershaw DD, Kaufman RJ, et al. Angiosarcoma of the breast. *Radiology* 1992;183:649–654.
132. Schnarkowski P, Kessler M, Arnholdt H, et al. Angiosarcoma of the breast: mammographic, sonographic and pathological findings. *Eur J Radiol* 1997;24:54–56.
133. Marchant LK, Orel SG, Perez-Jaffe LA, et al. Bilateral angiosarcoma of the breast on MR imaging. *AJR Am J Roentgenol* 1997;169:1009–1010.
134. Jozefczyk MA, Rosen PP. Vascular tumors of the breast. II. Perilobular hemangiomas and hemangiomas. *Am J Surg Pathol* 1985;9:491–503.
135. Benda JA, Al-Jurf AS, Benson AJB III. Angiosarcoma of the breast following segmental mastectomy complicated by lymphedema. *Am J Clin Pathol* 1987;87:651–655.
136. Batchelor GB. Hemangioblastoma of the breast associated with pregnancy. *Br J Surg* 1959;46:647–649.
137. Horne WI, Percival WT. Hemangiosarcoma of the breast. *Can J Surg* 1975;18:81–84.
138. Khanna SD, Manchanda RL, Saigal RK, et al. Hemangioendothelioma (angiosarcoma) of the breast. *Arch Surg* 1964;88:807–809.
139. Brentani MM, Pacheco MM, Oshima CTF, et al. Steroid receptors in breast angiosarcoma. *Cancer* 1983;51:2105–2111.
140. Hunter TB, Martin PC, Dietzen CD, et al. Angiosarcoma of the breast: two case reports and a review of the literature. *Cancer* 1985;56:2099–2106.
141. Rainwater LM, Martin JK Jr, Gaffey TA, et al. Angiosarcoma of the breast. *Arch Surg* 1986;121:669–672.
142. Bundred NJ, O'Reilly K, Smart JG. Long term survival following bilateral breast angiosarcoma. *Eur J Surg Oncol* 1989;15:263–264.
143. Schackelford RT. Surgical disorders of the breast. In: Schakelford RT, ed. *Diagnosis of surgical disease,* vol 1. Philadelphia: WB Saunders, 1968:439–551.
144. Yadav RVS, Sahariah S, Mittal VK, et al. Angiosarcoma of the male breast. *Int J Surg* 1976;61:463–464.
145. Davies JD, Rees GJG, Mera SL. Angiosarcoma in irradiated postmastectomy chest wall. *Histopathology* 1983;7:947–956.
146. Hamels J, Blondiau P, Mirgaux M. Cutaneous angiosarcoma arising in

a mastectomy scar after therapeutic irradiation. *Bull Cancer* 1981;68:353–356.
147. Maddox JC, Evans HL. Angiosarcoma of skin and soft tissue: a study of forty-four cases. *Cancer* 1981;48:1907–1921.
148. Otis CN, Peschel R, McKhann C, et al. The rapid onset of cutaneous angiosarcoma after radiotherapy for breast carcinoma. *Cancer* 1986;57:2130–2134.
149. Del Mastro L, Garrone O, Guenzi M, et al. Angiosarcoma of the residual breast after conservative surgery and radiotherapy for primary carcinoma. *Ann Oncol* 1994;5:163–165.
150. Givens SS, Ellerbroek NA, Butler JJ, et al. Angiosarcoma arising in an irradiated breast: a case report and review of the literature. *Cancer* 1989;64:2214–2216.
151. Stokkel MPM, Peterse HL. Angiosarcoma of the breast after lumpectomy and radiation therapy for adenocarcinoma. *Cancer* 1992;69:2965–2968.
152. Turner WH, Greenall MJ. Sarcoma induced by radiotherapy after breast conservation surgery. *Br J Surg* 1991;78:1317–1318.
153. Wijnmaalen A, van Ooijen B, van Geel BN, et al. Angiosarcoma of the breast following lumpectomy, axillary lymph node dissection, and radiotherapy for primary breast cancer: three case reports and a review of the literature. *Int J Radiat Oncol Biol Phys* 1993;26:135–139.
154. Zucali R, Merson M, Placucci M, et al. Soft tissue sarcoma of the breast after conservative surgery and irradiation for early mammary cancer. *Radiother Oncol* 1994;30:271–273.
155. Pendlebury SC, Bilous M, Langlands AO. Sarcomas following radiation therapy for breast cancer: a report of three cases and a review of the literature. *Int J Radiat Oncol Biol Phys* 1994;31:405–410.
156. Cafiero F, Gipponi M, Peressini A, et al. Radiation-associated angiosarcoma: diagnostic and therapeutic implications—two case reports and a review of the literature. *Cancer* 1996;77:2496–2502.
157. Perin T, Massarut S, Roncadin M, et al. Radiation-associated angiosarcoma. Diagnostic and therapeutic implications—two case reports and a review of the literature. *Cancer* 1997;80:519–520.
158. Molitor JL, Spielmann M, Contesso G. Angiosarcoma of the breast after conservative surgery and radiation therapy for breast carcinoma: three new cases. *Eur J Cancer* 1996;32A:1820.
159. Badwe RA, Hanby AM, Fentiman IS, et al. Angiosarcoma of the skin overlying an irradiated breast. *Breast Cancer Res Treat* 1991;19:69–72.
160. Fineberg S, Rosen PP. Angiosarcoma and atypical cutaneous vascular lesions after radiation therapy for breast carcinoma. *Am J Clin Pathol* 1994;102:757–763.
161. Moshaluk CA, Merino MJ, Danforth DN, et al. Low grade angiosarcoma of the skin of the breast: a complication of lumpectomy and radiation therapy for breast carcinoma. *Hum Pathol* 1992;23:710–714.
162. Rubin E, Maddox WA, Mazur MT. Cutaneous angiosarcoma of the breast 7 years after lumpectomy and radiation therapy. *Radiology* 1990;174:258–260.
163. Taat CW, van Toor BSJ, Slors JFM, et al. Dermal angiosarcoma of the breast: a complication of primary radiotherapy? *Eur J Surg Oncol* 1992;18:391–395.
164. Timmer SJ, Osuch JR, Colony LH, et al. Angiosarcoma of the breast following lumpectomy and radiation therapy for breast carcinoma: case report and review of the literature. *Breast J* 1997;3:40–47.
165. Bolin DJ, Lukas GM. Low-grade dermal angiosarcoma of the breast following radiotherapy. *Am Surg* 1996;62:668–672.
166. Deutsch M, Rosenstein MM. Angiosarcoma of the breast mimicking radiation dermatitis arising after lumpectomy and breast irradiation. A case report. *Am J Clin Oncol* 1998;21:608–609.
167. Strobbe LJ, Peterse HL, van Tinteren H, et al. Angiosarcoma of the breast after conservation therapy for invasive cancer, the incidence and outcome: an unforseen sequela. *Breast Cancer Res Treat* 1998;47:101–109.
168. Gil-Benso R, López-Ginés C, Soriano P, et al. Cytogenetic study of angiosarcoma of the breast. *Genes Chromosomes Cancer* 1994;10:210–212.
169. Slotman BJ, van Hattum AH, Meyer S, et al. Angiosarcoma of the breast following conserving treatment for breast cancer. *Eur J Cancer* 1994;30A:416–417.
170. Britt LD, Lambert P, Sharma R, et al. Angiosarcoma of the breast. Initial misdiagnosis is still common. *Arch Surg* 1995;130:221–223.
171. Gentile-Fradet A, Pallud C, LeDoussal V, et al. Hèmangioendothéliosarcome mammaire: a propos de deux observations, dont une avec étude ultrastructurale. *Arch Anat Cytol Pathol* 1981;29:149–153.

172. Jennings TA, Peterson L, Axiotis CA, et al. Angiosarcoma associated with foreign body material. A report of three cases. *Cancer* 1988; 62:2436–2444.
173. Mazzocchi A, Foschini MP, Marconi F, et al. Syndrome associated to angiosarcoma of the breast: a case report and review of the literature. *Tumori* 1993;79:137–140.
174. Hill RP, Stout AP. Sarcoma of the breast. *Arch Surg* 1942;44: 723–729.
175. Merino MJ, Berman M, Carter D. Angiosarcoma of the breast. *Am J Surg Pathol* 1983;7:53–60.
176. Macías-Martínez V, Murrieta-Tiburcio L, Molina-Cérdenas H, et al. Epithelioid angiosarcoma of the breast: clinicopathological, immuno-histochemical and ultrastructural study of a case. *Am J Surg Pathol* 1997;21:599–604.
177. Borrmann R. Metastasenbildung bei histologisch gutartigen Geschwülsten (Fall von metastasierendem Angiom). *Beitr Z Pathol Anat U Z Allg Pathol* 1907;40:372–392.
178. Ewing J. *Neoplastic diseases: a textbook on tumors.* Philadelphia: WB Saunders, 1919:223–224.
179. Rosen PP. Vascular tumors of the breast. III. Angiomatosis. *Am J Surg Pathol* 1985;9:652–658.
180. Rosen PP, Ridolfi RL. The perilobular hemangioma. *Am J Clin Pathol* 1977;68:21–23.
181. Rosso R, Gianelli U, Carnevali L. Acquired progressive lymphan-gioma of the skin following radiotherapy for breast carcinoma. *J Cu-tan Pathol* 1995;22:164–167.
182. Janse AJ, van Coevorden F, Peterse H, et al. Lymphedema-induced lymphangiosarcoma. *Eur J Surg Oncol* 1995;21:155–158.
183. Layfield LJ, Dodd LG. Cytologic findings in a case of postirradiation angiosarcoma of the breast. *Acta Cytol* 1997;41:612–614.
184. Vesoulis Z, Cunliffe C. Fine-needle aspiration biopsy of postradiation epithelioid angiosarcoma of breast. *Diagn Cytopathol* 2000;22: 172–175.
185. Burgdorf WHC, Mukai K, Rosai J. Immunohistochemical identifica-tion of Factor VIII-related antigen in endothelial cells of cutaneous le-sions of alleged vascular nature. *Am J Clin Pathol* 1989;75:167–171.
186. Guarda LA, Ordonez NG, Smith JL Jr, et al. Immunoperoxidase lo-calization of Factor VIII in angiosarcomas. *Arch Pathol Lab Med* 1982;106:515–516.
187. Yonezawa S, Maruyama I, Sakae K, et al. Thrombomodulin as a marker for vascular tumors: comparative study with Factor VIII and *Ulex europaeus* I lectin. *Am J Clin Pathol* 1987;88:405–411.
188. Sirgi KE, Wick MR, Swanson PE. B72.3 and CD34 immunoreactiv-ity in malignant epithelioid soft tissue tumors: adjuncts in the recog-nition of endothelial neoplasms. *Am J Surg Pathol* 1993;17:179–185.
189. De Young BR, Wick MR, Fitzgibbon JF, et al. CD31: an immunospe-cific marker for endothelial differentiation in human neoplasms. *Appl Immunohistochem* 1993;1:97–100.
190. Alvarez-Fernandez E, Salinero-Paniagua E. Vascular tumors of the mammary gland: a histochemical and ultrastructural study. *Virchows Arch* 1981;394:31–47.
191. Hamazaki M, Tanaka T. Hemangiosarcoma of the breast: case report with scanning electron microscopic study. *Acta Pathol Jpn* 1978;28:605–613.
192. Toth B, Malick L. Scanning electron-microscopic study of the surface characteristics of neoplastic endothelial cells in blood vessels. *J Pathol* 1976;118:59–64.
193. Masser SR, Mongeau CJ, Rioux A. Angiosarcoma of the breast. *Can J Surg* 1977;20:341–343.
194. Myerowitz RL, Pietruszka M, Barnes EL. Primary angiosarcoma of the breast. *JAMA* 1978;239:403.
195. Ryan JF, Kealy WF. Concommitant angiosarcoma and carcinoma of the breast: a case report. *Histopathology* 1985;9:893–899.
196. Rosner D. Angiosarcoma of the breast: long-term survival following adjuvant chemotherapy. *J Surg Oncol* 1988;39:90–95.
197. Savage R. The treatment of angiosarcoma of the breast. *J Surg Oncol* 1981;18:129–134.
198. Epstein JB, Knowling MA, LeRiche JC. Multiple gingival metastases from angiosarcoma of the breast. *Oral Surg Oral Med Oral Pathol* 1987;64:554–557.
199. Win KKS, Yasuoka T, Kamiya H, et al. Breast angiosarcoma metastatic to the maxillary gingiva: case report. *Int J Oral Maxillofac Surg* 1992;21:282–283.
209. Sedgely MG, Oster AG, Fortune DW. Angiosarcoma of breast metastatic to the ovary and placenta. *Aust N Z J Obstet Gynecol* 1985;25:229–230.
201. Baum JK, Levine AJ, Ingold JA. Angiosarcoma of the breast with re-port of unusual site of first metastasis. *J Surg Oncol* 1990;43:125–130.
202. Kessler E, Kozenitzky IL. Hemangiosarcoma of the breast. *J Clin Pathol* 1971;24:530–532.
203. Gupta RK, Naran S, Dowle C. Needle aspiration cytology and im-munocytochemical study in a case of angiosarcoma of the breast. *Di-agn Cytopathol* 1991;7:363–365.
204. Nanus D, Kaufman R. Angiosarcoma of the breast: adjuvant chemotherapy with actinomycin D (abstract). *Proc Am Soc Clin On-col* 1986;5:73.
205. Antman KH, Corson J, Greenberger J, et al. Multimodality therapy in the management of angiosarcoma of the breast. *Cancer* 1982;20: 2000–2003.

## Postmastectomy Angiosarcoma (Stewart-Treves Syndrome)

206. Stewart FW, Treves N. Lymphangiosarcoma in postmastectomy lym-phedema. *Cancer* 1949;1:64–81.
207. Merrick TA, Erlandson RA, Hajdu SI. Lymphangiosarcoma of a con-genitally lymphedematous arm. *Arch Pathol Lab Med* 1971;91: 365–371.
208. Muller R, Hajdu SI, Brennan MF. Lymphangiosarcoma associated with chronic filarial lymphedema. *Cancer* 1987;59:179–183.
209. Woodward AH, Ivins JC, Soule EH. Lymphangiosarcoma arising in chronic lymphedematous extremities. *Cancer* 1972;30:562–572.
210. Lambert PB, Frank HA, Bellman S, et al. The role of the lymph trunks in the response to allogeneic skin transplants. *Transplantation* 1965;3:62–73.
211. Stark RB, Dwyer EM, DeForest M. Effect of surgical ablation of re-gional lymph nodes on survival of skin homografts. *Ann NY Acad Sci* 1960;87:140–145.
212. Futrell JW, Albright NI, Myers GH. Prevention of tumor growth in an "immunologically privileged site" by adoptive transfer of tumor spe-cific transplantation immunity. *J Surg Res* 1972;12:62–69.
213. Schreiber H, Barry FM, Russell WC, et al. Stewart-Treves syndrome: a lethal complication of post-mastectomy lymphedema and regional immune deficiency. *Arch Surg* 1979;114:82–85.
214. d'Amore ESG, Wick MR, Geisinger KR, et al. Primary malignant lymphoma arising in postmastectomy lymphedema: another facet of the Stewart-Treves syndrome. *Am J Surg Pathol* 1990;14:456–463.
215. Waxman M, Fatteh S, Elias JM, et al. Malignant lymphoma of the skin associated with post mastectomy lymphedema. *Arch Pathol Lab Med* 1984;108:206–208
216. Fitzpatrick PJ. Lymphangiosarcoma and breast cancer. *Can J Surg* 1969;12:172–177.
217. Schirger A. Post-operative lymphedema: etiologic and diagnostic fac-tors. *Med Clin North Am* 1962;46:1045–1050.
218. Karlsson P, Holmberg E, Samuelsson A, et al. Soft tissue sarcoma af-ter treatment for breast cancer—a Swedish population-based study. *Eur J Cancer* 1998;34:2068–2075.
219. Davies JD, Rees GJG, Mera SL. Angiosarcoma in irradiated post-mastectomy chest wall. *Histopathology* 1983;7:947–956.
220. Hamels J, Blondiau P, Mirgaux M. Cutaneous angiosarcoma arising in a mastectomy scar after therapeutic irradiation. *Bull Cancer* 1981;68:353–356.
221. Lo TCM, Silverman ML, Edelstein A. Post-irradiation hemangiosar-coma of the chest wall. *Acta Radiol Oncol* 1985;24:237–240.
222. Chen KTK, Hoffman KD, Hendricks EJ. Angiosarcoma following therapeutic irradiaion. *Cancer* 1979;44:2044–2048.
223. Sordillo PP, Chapman R, Hajdu SI, et al. Lymphangiosarcoma. *Can-cer* 1981;48:1674–1679.
224. Birge RF, Peisen CJ, Thornton FE, et al. Angiosarcoma in post-mas-tectomy lymphedema. *J Iowa Med Soc* 1957;47:491–495.
225. Sternby NH, Gynning I, Hogeman KE. Post-mastectomy angiosar-coma. *Acta Chir Scand* 1961;121:420–432.
226. Scott RB, Nydick I, Conway H. Lymphangiosarcoma arising in lym-phedema. *Am J Med* 1960;28:1008–1012.
227. Hashimoto K, Matsumoto M, Eto H, et al. Differentiation of metastatic breast carcinoma from Stewart-Treves angiosarcoma. *Arch Dermatol* 1985;121:742–746.
228. Miettinen M, Lehto V-P, Virtanen I. Postmastectomy angiosarcoma

(Stewart-Treves syndrome): light microscopic, immunohistological, and ultrastructural characteristics of two cases. *Am J Surg Pathol* 1983;7:329–339.

229. Capo V, Ozzello L, Fenoglio CM, et al. Angiosarcomas arising in edematous extremities: immunostaining for Factor VIII-related antigen and ultrastructural features. *Hum Pathol* 1985;16:144–150.

230. Lee AK, DeLellis RA, Rosen PP, et al. ABH blood group isoantigen expression in breast carcinomas—an immunohistochemical evaluation using monoclonal antibodies. *Am J Clin Pathol* 1985;83:308–319.

231. Tomita K, Yokogawa A, Oda Y, et al. Lymphangiosarcoma in postmastectomy lymphedema (Stewart-Treves syndrome): ultrastructural and immunohistologic characteristics. *J Surg Oncol* 1988;38:275–282.

232. Sarkany I. Malignant melanomas in lymphedematous arm following radical mastectomy for breast carcinoma (an extension of the syndrome of Stewart and Treves). *J Soc Med* 1972;65:253–254.

233. McWilliam LJ, Harris M. Histogenesis of post-mastectomy angiosarcoma—an ultrastructural study. *Histopathology* 1985;9:331–343.

234. Lagac R, Leroy J-P. Comparative electron microscopic study of cutaneous and soft tissue angiosarcomas, post-mastectomy angiosarcoma (Stewart-Treves syndrome) and Kaposi's sarcoma. *Ultrastruct Pathol* 1987;11:161–173.

235. Silverberg SG, Kay S, Koss LG. Post-mastectomy lymphangiosarcoma; ultrastructural observations. *Cancer* 1971;27:100–108.

236. Yap B-S, Yap H-Y, McBride CM, et al. Chemotherapy for post-mastectomy lymphangiosarcoma. *Cancer* 1981;47:853–856.

237. Kaufmann T, Chu F, Kaufman R. Post-mastectomy lymphangiosarcoma (Stewart-Treves syndrome): report of two long-term survivals. *Br J Radiol* 1991;64:867–860.

# CHAPTER 42

# Lymphoid and Hematopoietic Tumors

## NON-HODGKIN'S LYMPHOMA

The diagnosis of primary mammary lymphoma should be limited to patients without evidence of systemic lymphoma or leukemia at the time that the breast lesion is detected (1). Clinically, the disease should involve only the breast or the breast and ipsilateral lymph nodes. Less than 0.5% of all malignant lymphomas involve the breast primarily (2–4). Lymphomas constitute approximately 0.15% of malignant mammary neoplasms (5). The occurrence of synchronous and metachronous lymphoma and breast carcinoma has been described (6,7). Mammary involvement by lymphoma occurs in some but not all of these patients.

### Clinical Presentation

With rare exceptions, patients described in the literature have been women (7–12). The women range from 13 to 90 years of age at diagnosis (average, 55 years) (4,7,11,13–15). A bimodal age distribution with peaks in the mid 30s and mid 60s has been described (11,15–17). Mammary lymphoma has been diagnosed in pregnant and recently postpartum women (1,14,15) who may be prone to bilateral involvement (7). In contrast to breast carcinoma, which is more frequent on the left, unilateral primary lymphoma has affected the right breast more often, with a ratio of approximately 60:40 (1,4,6,7,14,17,18). Analysis of a series of published cases revealed that the right side predominance was statistically significant (17). Bilateral disease occurs in about 10% of patients at the time of diagnosis (1,6,7,11,14,15,19), and contralateral involvement may develop with progression (17,19,20), leading to a total frequency of bilaterality of 15% to 20% (21). Infiltration of the nipple may occur (11,22).

The presenting symptom in virtually all cases is a mass, sometimes painful, located most often in the upper outer quadrant. A history of recent onset and rapid growth is not unusual (1,17,19). The tumor often is solitary, but patients with multiple lesions (17,19,20) and diffuse infiltration have been described. Skin fixation, sometimes with cutaneous inflammatory changes, may occur, resulting in a clinical pattern resembling inflammatory carcinoma (10,19,20,23–25). Enlarged axillary lymph nodes have been described clinically in 30% to 50% of patients (5,17,20,23,26). Systemic symptoms are infrequent (5,17). Mammary cutaneous T-cell lymphoma (27) and follicular lymphoma (28) have been described in women with silicone breast implants. Mammary involvement by large cell lymphoma has been reported in a patient with a "lymphoproliferative disorder," and there have been rare patients with autoimmune disease preceding breast lymphoma (18). Association with bilateral gynecomastia was noted in a male patient who had B-cell lymphoma localized to one breast (12). In two studies, 3% and 17%, respectively, of the patients were treated for another malignant neoplasm diagnosed before, coincident with, or after the lymphoma (13,17).

Mammographically, the tumor may be well defined and circumscribed, or irregular and thus difficult to distinguish from other lesions (4,19,24,29,30). It has been suggested that diffuse infiltration and multiple ill-defined lesions are radiologic clues to the diagnosis of lymphoma. Multiple lesions are not uncommon (31), and rarely they have a miliary distribution (32). There is no association between specific subtypes of lymphoma and radiologic findings on mammography (24,29). Mammary lymphoma differs somewhat from carcinoma on ultrasonography (30,31,33). The tumors are hypoechoic when studied by ultrasonography (12,24). Magnetic resonance imaging in one case showed rapid, strong multicentric lesion enhancement (34). Diffuse tumor uptake of technetium 99m methylene diphosphonate (Tc-99m MDP) in a breast lymphoma was found in the course of a bone scan study (25).

### Gross Pathology

The tumors have measured 1 to 12 cm (average, 3.0 cm). The excised specimen usually contains a circumscribed, fleshy tumor that may have a nodular configuration (Fig. 42.1). The cut surface is gray-white to pink. Areas of softening and brown discoloration tend to be regions of necrosis in the tumor.

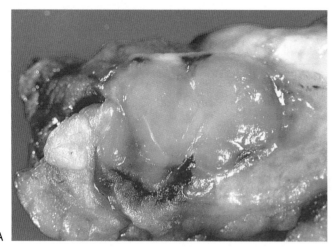
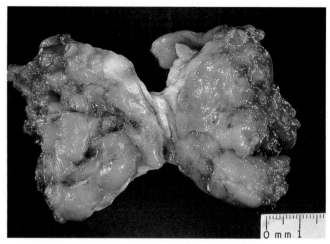

**FIG. 42.1.** *Malignant lymphoma, gross appearance.* **A:** A fleshy, bulging oval tumor with a well-circumscribed border. **B:** Bisected multinodular lymphoma.

## Microscopic Pathology

Histologic examination usually reveals that the lymphomatous infiltrate extends into the breast parenchyma beyond the grossly evident mass. Because of changes in diagnostic terms and classification schemes in the past three decades, it is difficult to compare the distribution of lymphoma types among the different studies published during this time period. The largest subgroup of primary mammary lymphomas was described as diffuse histiocytic when classified by the Rappaport system (1,4,14,17,18) or as diffuse large cell (Fig. 42.2) (7,18). Poorly differentiated lymphocytic lymphomas, the majority of which are diffuse (Fig. 42.3), and mixed lymphomas, equally nodular and diffuse (Fig. 42.4), are the second and third most common, respectively (4,17,20). Well-differentiated lymphocytic (Fig. 42.5), lymphoblastic, undifferentiated, and Burkitt's lymphomas account for 5% to 10% of mammary lymphomas in most series. However, 62% of lymphomas in one study (14)

were classified as undifferentiated, and Burkitt's lymphomas were prominent in a series of African women diagnosed during pregnancy and lactation (35). Burkitt's lymphoma with a similar pattern of clinical presentation has been described in a series of Japanese patients (13). Patients with mammary Burkitt's lymphoma often present with massive bilateral breast enlargement (15). A study of two Danish sisters with Burkitt's lymphoma diagnosed at age 18 and 21 years revealed no evidence of Epstein-Barr virus in their tumors when studied by *in situ* hybridization (36).

Studies presented in terms of the Kiel classification have characterized the majority of tumors as centroblastic-centrocytic diffuse or centroblastic diffuse (5,17,19). Immunoblastic lymphoma, lymphoplasmacytic immunocytoma, and lymphocytic lymphomas are uncommon. The scarcity of lymphoplasmacytic lymphomas of the breast distinguishes extranodal lymphoma in the breast from lymphomas arising in the stomach, gastrointestinal tract, and lung, which exhibit plasmacytic differentiation more often (Fig. 42.6) (5,37,38).

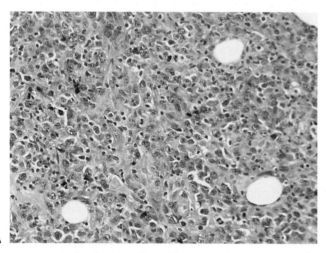
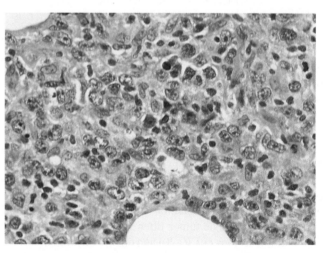

**FIG. 42.2.** *Malignant lymphoma, large cell type, diffuse.* **A,B:** Tumor cells diffusely infiltrate the fibrofatty breast tissue.

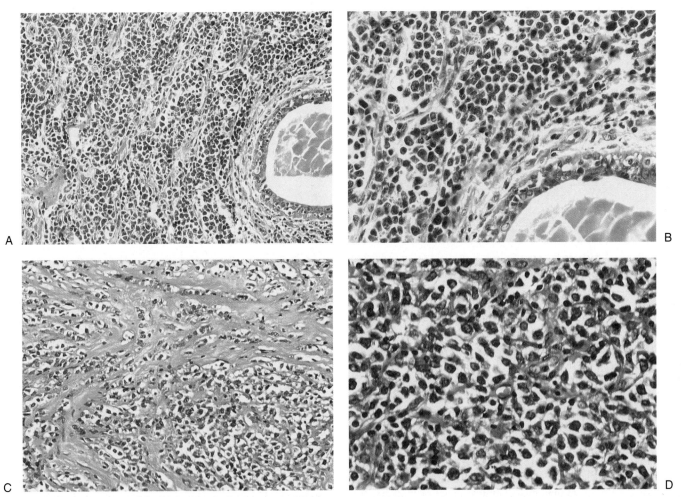

**FIG. 42.3.** *Malignant lymphoma, poorly differentiated lymphocytic, diffuse.* **A,B:** Periductal infiltrate is present. **C,D:** Stromal infiltrate displays shrinkage artifact.

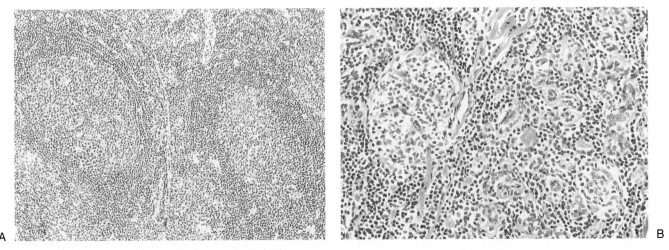

**FIG. 42.4.** *Malignant lymphoma, mixed.* **A,B:** Lesion has a nodular pattern.

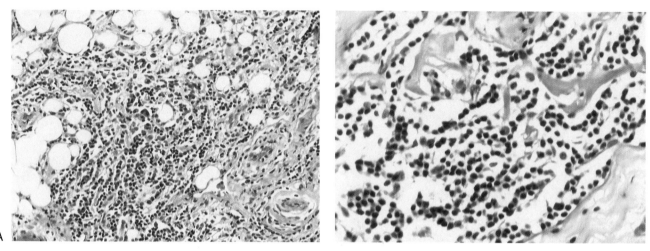

**FIG. 42.5.** *Malignant lymphoma, small cell lymphocytic.* **A,B:** Tumor cells are arranged in a linear pattern that resembles infiltrating lobular carcinoma.

In the Lukes-Collins scheme, the majority of mammary lymphomas are the large noncleaved diffuse and large cleaved diffuse types (5,13,17). Diffuse large cleaved, diffuse small cleaved, and diffuse or follicular mixed cell lymphomas were the three most common cell types according to the Working Formulation (17,39).

A few reports characterized mammary lymphomas beyond standard histologic classifications. Most lymphomas of the female breast are B-cell type (7,13,39–42), with only rare examples of T-cell (7,13,18,43–45,45a) and histiocytic lymphoma (46) described. A series of 11 primary breast tumors studied with an immunohistochemical panel of markers included five diffuse large B-cell lymphomas, two follicular center lymphomas, two marginal zone B-cell lymphomas (MALT-type), one lymphoplasmacytoid lymphoma, and one "unclassified peripheral B-cell neoplasm" (43). Very few instances of Ki1 (CD30)-positive B and T lymphomas have been identified in the breast (18,45a). Most T-cell lymphomas of the breast are monoclonal for T-cell receptor β and/or T-cell receptor γ (45a). One T-cell lymphoma had the clinical features of inflammatory carcinoma (42). When studied by electron microscopy, a T-cell lymphoma was composed of multilobulated cells (43). This tumor was positive for intracytoplasmic immunoglobulin M (IgM) but negative for immunoglobulin G (IgG) and immunoglobulin A (IgA) heavy chains. Jeon et al. (13) reported monotypical staining for kappa light chains in one of seven non-Hodgkin's lymphomas examined by frozen section.

A lymphoma of the male breast marked for IgG heavy chains and kappa light chains (9) and four male lymphomas have been characterized as B-cell type (10–12). Two tumors with plasmacytic features that marked for cytoplasmic IgM kappa were characterized by Telesinghe and Anthony (47) as follicle center lymphomas. Cohen and Brooks (48) reported that IgM was the most frequent heavy chain type found in B-cell lymphomas of the breast. Mammary lymphomas that

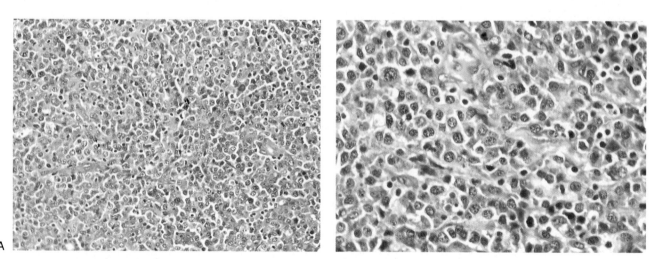

**FIG. 42.6.** *Malignant lymphoma, lymphoplasmacytic.* **A:** This diffuse infiltrate is composed of tumor cells with amphophilic cytoplasm. **B:** Nuclear and cytoplasmic features suggest plasmacytoid differentiation.

marked for IgA have been described less often. One tumor classified as a polymorphic immunocytoma was immunoreactive for IgA (49). The serum contained a monoclonal peak for IgA kappa that was reduced after treatment. A second tumor characterized as lymphoplasmacytic immunocytoma contained amyloid deposits, marked for IgA and kappa, and was associated with elevated serum IgA. Epstein-Barr virus RNA was detected in only one of 27 mammary lymphomas studied by *in situ* hybridization (7).

Lymphoma in the breast typically consists of a uniform population of tumor cells that diffusely infiltrate the mammary parenchyma. Ducts and lobules in the central portion of the lesion may be partly or totally obliterated. In some cases, the stroma develops a dense sclerotic reaction that may be mistaken for amyloid (Fig. 42.7). Ducts and lobules are better preserved away from the center of the lesion, but there is a tendency for the lymphomatous infiltrate to concentrate in and around these structures. Extension of lymphoma cells into ductal epithelium may mimic pagetoid spread of carcinoma. This growth pattern has been referred to as a lym-

phoepithelial lesion (23,40). Lymphomatous infiltration into the epithelium of ducts and lobules simulating *in situ* carcinoma has been described, particularly in poorly differentiated lymphocytic lymphomas. When this occurs, the malignant lymphoid cells expand ducts and lobular glands, displacing the epithelial cells that may be clustered in the lumen simulating *in situ* carcinoma (Fig. 42.8). The frequency of lymphoepithelial lesions among mammary lymphomas varies from 0% (13,46) to 75% (23) in different series. This broad range suggests that the criteria for the recognition of lymphoepithelial lesions in the breast are not well defined.

A reactive lymphoid infiltrate composed of small lymphocytes is very commonly present at the periphery of the tumor. The lymphoid infiltrate tends to localize around epithelial elements and blood vessels. Germinal centers may be formed in these reactive infiltrates, but they also occur in nodular lymphomas. Areas in some nodular lymphomas have an epithelioid appearance that mimics a granulomatous reaction (Fig. 42.9).

In some instances, the linear pattern assumed by

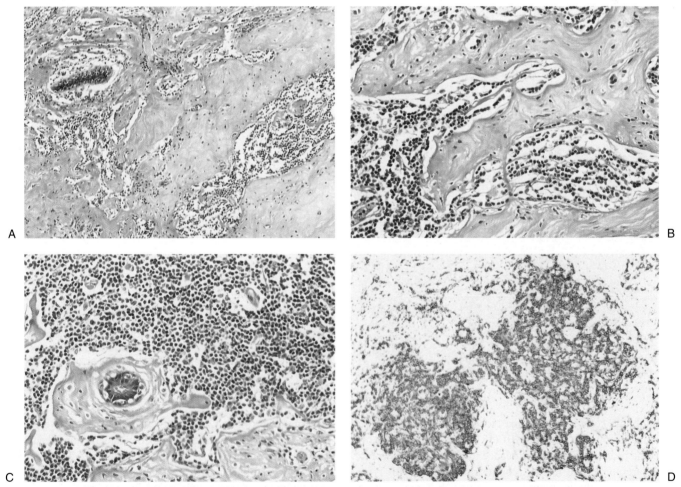

**FIG. 42.7.** *Malignant lymphoma, stromal sclerosis.* **A,B:** The lymphomatous infiltrate in this 48-year-old patient is growing in collagenized pseudoangiomatous stroma that does not have the staining properties of amyloid. **C:** Atrophic duct in the tumor. **D:** Tumor cells were immunoreactive for L26 (CD20) in this B-cell lymphoma (avidin-biotin).

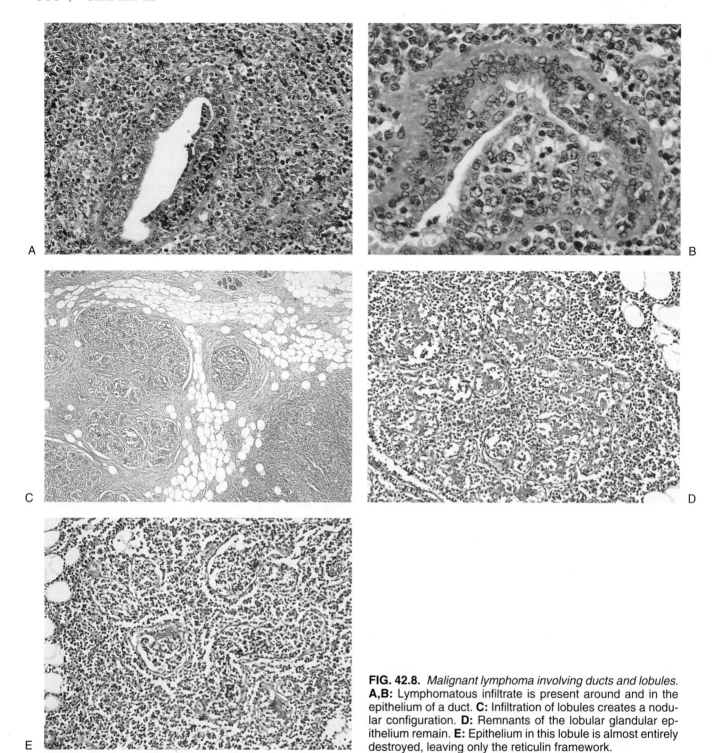

**FIG. 42.8.** *Malignant lymphoma involving ducts and lobules.*
**A,B:** Lymphomatous infiltrate is present around and in the epithelium of a duct. **C:** Infiltration of lobules creates a nodular configuration. **D:** Remnants of the lobular glandular epithelium remain. **E:** Epithelium in this lobule is almost entirely destroyed, leaving only the reticulin framework.

lymphoma cells in the stroma closely resembles invasive lobular carcinoma (Fig. 42.10) (18). Signet-ring cell lymphoma bears a striking resemblance to signet-ring cell lobular carcinoma, and it may require immunostains for lymphoid and epithelial markers to distinguish between these entities (Fig. 42.11).

The appearance of lymphoma involving mammary stroma that is altered by pseudoangiomatous stromal hyperplasia is

striking (Figs. 42.7, 42.12). The presence of a reactive lymphoid infiltrate offers little assistance in these lesions because it occurs in carcinomas as well as in lymphomas. The pattern of vascular dilation with central necrosis caused by angiotrophic lymphoma involving the breast is easily mistaken for intraductal carcinoma (Fig. 42.13). Calcification is not a characteristic feature of lymphoma, but it may be found coincidentally in epithelial lesions or in fat necrosis (Fig. 42.14).

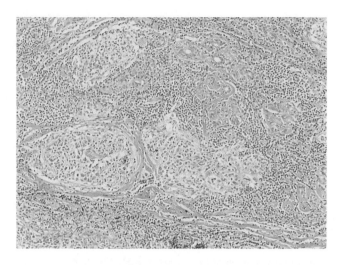

**FIG. 42.9.** *Malignant lymphoma, nodular.* The epithelioid appearance of the lesion in and around a lobule resembles a granuloma.

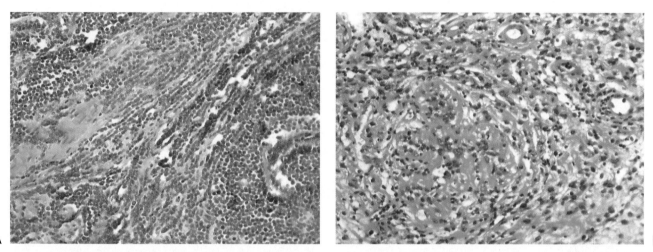

A

B

**FIG. 42.10.** *Malignant lymphoma, resembling infiltrating lobular carcinoma.* **A:** Linear growth. **B:** Circumferential growth around a sclerotic lobule.

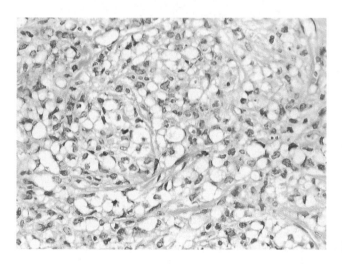

**FIG. 42.11.** *Malignant lymphoma, signet-ring cell.*

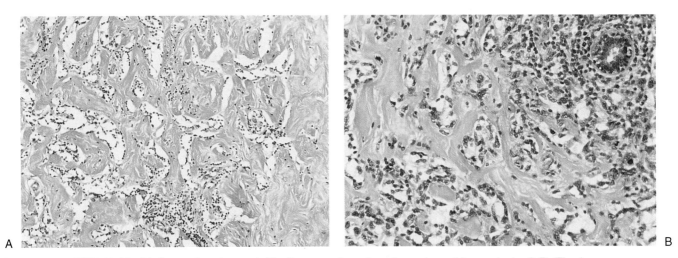

**FIG. 42.12.** *Malignant lymphoma, infiltrating pseudoangiomatous stromal hyperplasia.* **A,B:** The lymphomatous infiltrate occupies pseudoangiomatous spaces in the stroma.

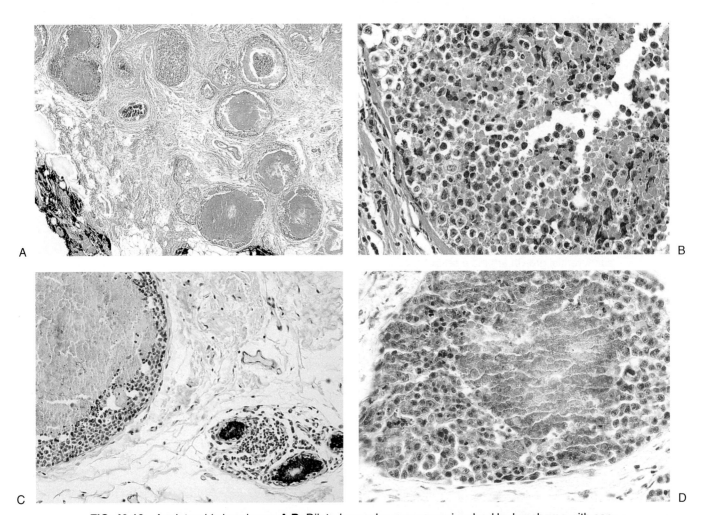

**FIG. 42.13.** *Angiotrophic lymphoma.* **A,B:** Dilated vascular spaces are involved by lymphoma with central necrosis. The pattern resembles comedocarcinoma. **C:** Immunostain for cytokeratin shows reactivity limited to the epithelium of a small lobule (anti-CAM5.2, avidin-biotin). **D:** Tumor cells are immunoreactive for lymphocyte common antigen (LCA) (avidin-biotin).

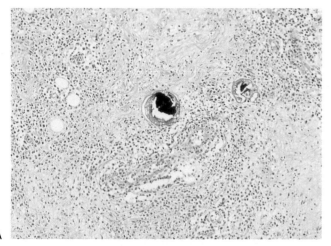

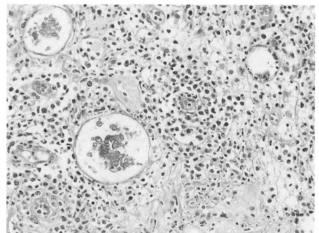

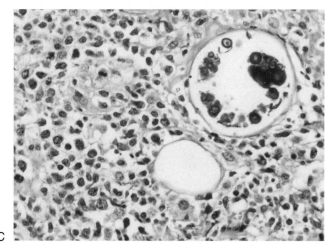

**FIG. 42.14.** *Lymphoma with calcifications in fat necrosis.* **A:** Large calcification is present in the *center.* **B:** Note stages of calcification in the fat cells. **C:** Multiple discrete calcified granules in this fat cell resemble the contents of a parasitic egg.

When faced with these diagnostic problems, it is useful to recall that the reactive lymphoid infiltrate that accompanies most lymphomas is rarely found in invasive lobular carcinoma (see Chapter 34). Many lobular carcinomas exhibit glandular features evidenced by intracytoplasmic mucin secretion, which can be demonstrated with Alcian blue, periodic acid-Schiff (PAS), and mucicarmine stains. Cells with signet-ring cell features have been described in lymphomas, and these may contain PAS-positive material (18). If these procedures are not definitive, immunohistochemical markers for epithelial and lymphoid differentiation generally resolve the issue. Biochemical analysis for estrogen and progesterone receptors reportedly has been positive in some lymphomas (16), whereas others reported finding only estrogen receptors (46) or no receptors (13). These results could reflect inclusion of varying proportions of glandular tissue in the specimens analyzed. Strong, diffuse nuclear immunoreactivity for hormone receptors is indicative of carcinoma. Electron microscopy also may be used, but for the most part it has been supplanted by immunohistochemistry for resolving this problem. Rarely, carcinoma and lymphoma may coexist in the same breast (Fig. 42.15).

Distinguishing large cell lymphoma from poorly differen-

tiated carcinoma sometimes is difficult, especially when the tumor lacks a classic intraductal component. Large cell lymphoma may assume solid, diffuse, and sometimes alveolar growth patterns that resemble carcinoma (Fig. 42.16). In one instance, diffuse large cell lymphoma was interpreted as medullary carcinoma (18). The limited samples of needle core biopsies provide a setting where there is a risk of mistaking lymphoma for carcinoma. The differential diagnosis of large cell lymphoma in the breast also includes malacoplakia (50).

The tendency of mammary lymphomas to localize in and around glandular structures has been regarded by some authors as evidence that some of these tumors arise from mucosa-associated lymphoid tissue, so-called MALT lymphomas (23,51). Lymphocytes are commonly found in normal resting mammary epithelium and in the pregnant state (52). Their numbers often are increased in tissues affected by inflammatory, hyperplastic, and neoplastic conditions (53–55). Antibodies secreted by these cells are detectable in colostrum (53). Many mucosa-associated lymphomas exhibit plasmacytoid differentiation and other MALT features that characterize these low-grade B-cell lymphomas (Fig. 42.17). They account for 25% to 50% of lymphomas of the intestinal tract, salivary glands, and lungs.

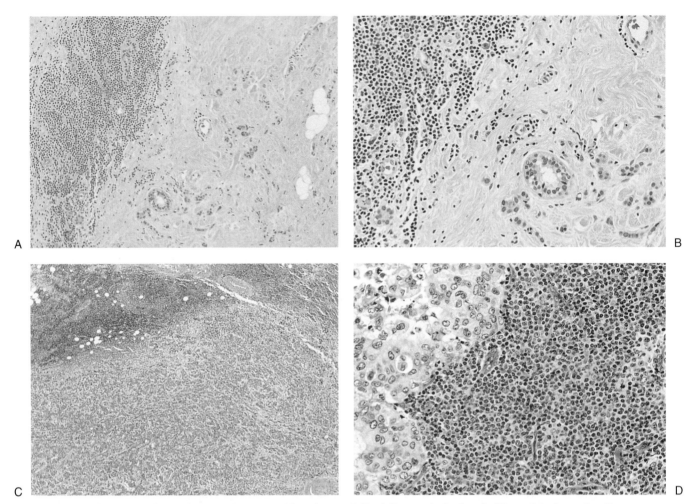

**FIG. 42.15.** *Coexisting carcinoma and lymphoma.* **A,B:** Adjacent foci of well-differentiated small cell lymphocytic lymphoma *(left)* and tubulolobular carcinoma *(right)*. **C,D:** Metastatic poorly differentiated duct carcinoma in an axillary lymph node involved by lymphocytic lymphoma. This is a different patient from the one whose specimen is depicted in **A** and **B**.

That this cytologic pattern is uncommon in the breast suggests that the majority of mammary lymphomas do not arise from mucosa-associated lymphoid tissue (7,17). It has not been possible to study a sufficient number of breast lym-

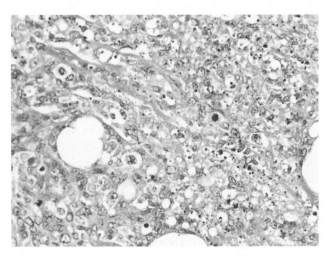

**FIG. 42.16.** *Lymphoma resembling poorly differentiated carcinoma.*

phomas exhibiting plasmacytoid differentiation to determine if they have a particular epithelial tropism.

Aozasa et al. (40) reported finding evidence of lymphocytic mastopathy in 42% of lymphomas, and this association has been described by others (40,56). Lymphocytic mastopathy has been associated with juvenile type I diabetes mellitus, thyroiditis, and immunologic disorders (57). Histologic features include lymphocytic infiltrates composed largely of B cells with admixed T cells involving lobules and with a perivascular distribution. Lymphoid follicles are formed, sometimes with germinal centers. Human leukocyte antigen (HLA)-DR antigen is expressed by ductal epithelium in the absence of the pathologic changes of periductal mastitis or duct ectasia. Because some of these histopathologic features are seen in many mammary lymphomas, further study will be necessary to determine if there is a specific relationship of HLA-DR expression, lymphocytic mastopathy, and mammary lymphoma, and if these features characterize a variant of MALT lymphoma (see Chapter 3).

The term *pseudolymphoma* has been applied to tumor-forming lymphoid lesions that are thought to be benign reac-

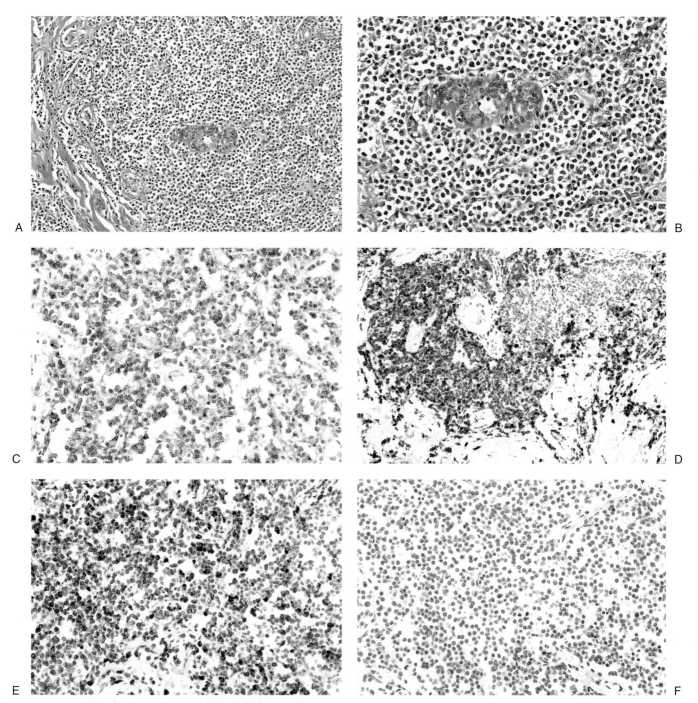

**FIG. 42.17.** *MALT lymphoma.* **A,B:** Lymphomatous infiltrate around a mammary duct consists of small cells with plasmacytic features. **C:** Tumor cells are reactive for CD43. **D:** Immunoreactivity for CD79. **E:** Immunoreactivity for kappa. **F:** There was no reactivity for lambda (all immunostains avidin-biotin).

tive conditions. This diagnosis has been made most often in organs that contain mucosa-associated lymphoid tissue, such as the lungs, stomach, and intestines. The concept of pseudolymphoma has been questioned by a number of investigators, because some patients initially thought to have this condition have proven on further follow-up to develop systemic malignant lymphoma (38,58,59). In a review of the literature, Marchevsky et al. (59) found that five of 33 patients with pseudolymphoma of the lung developed lymphoma or leukemia. They concluded that "pulmonary pseudolym-

phomas do not necessarily follow a benign course." Some features that are said to characterize "pseudolymphomas," such as germinal center formation and the absence of nodal involvement, may be found in mammary lymphomas. The specificity of this diagnosis when applied to lymphoid tumors of the breast remains questionable.

The number of unreported patients initially diagnosed as having mammary pseudolymphoma who later developed malignant lymphoma is not known. Few cases have been reported with this diagnosis (1,26,60–63). Some of the lesions

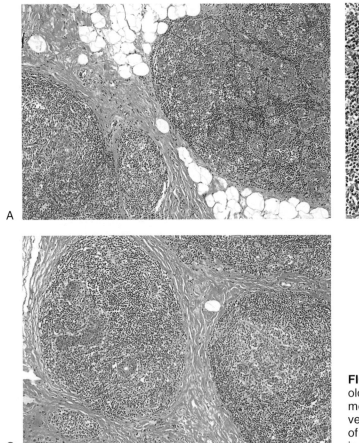

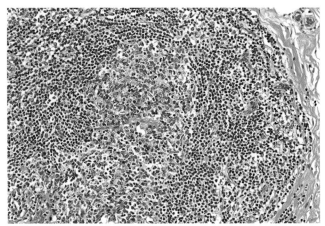

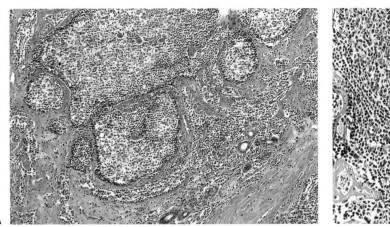

FIG. 42.18. *"Pseudolymphoma."* The patient was a 26-year-old woman, 4 months postpartum, with a unilateral breast tumor. Gene rearrangement studies and immunostains revealed a polyclonal B-cell infiltrate. **A,B:** Lesion is composed of small lymphocytes and has germinal centers. **C:** Infiltrate involves lobular glands.

appeared after trauma, and clinically they have consistently measured about 3 cm in diameter. Axillary nodal enlargement was absent in all cases. The patients were 26 to 77 years old, and they reportedly did not have systemic symptoms. Serum immunoglobulin studies in three cases revealed polyclonal elevation of IgG in two and a normal IgG level in the third (61). Mammography in one case revealed a circumscribed lobulated mass (60). Coexistent Graves' disease was reported in one case (62).

The distinction between pseudolymphoma and lymphoma is based on histologic and marker analysis. Tumors described as pseudolymphomas have been characterized by an infiltrate composed largely of mature lymphocytes (Figs. 42.18 and 42.19). Germinal centers often are present, espe-

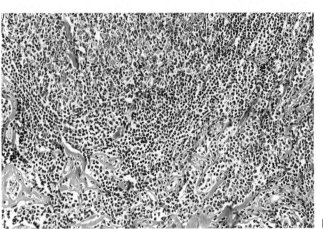

FIG. 42.19. *"Pseudolymphoma."* **A:** Lobules were largely spared in this lesion. **B:** Lymphoid cells proved to have a polyclonal immunophenotype. The specimen is from a patient who presented with bilateral lesions.

cially at the periphery, and sometimes they are numerous. The infiltrate tends to concentrate in the stroma, on occasion accompanied by fat necrosis and fibrosis. The epithelium of ducts and lobules is largely spared, although these structures can be surrounded by the infiltrative process. Small numbers of eosinophils, plasma cells, and histiocytes are scattered throughout the lesion. Follicular hyperplasia has been described in ipsilateral axillary lymph nodes (26,60). Immunofluorescent study in one case revealed approximately equal numbers of B and T cells, with the presence of kappa and lambda light chains on the surface of B cells indicating a polyclonal, reactive process (60). Flow cytometry in another case revealed a normal distribution of B and T cells and of kappa and lambda light chains (62).

Follow-up of most patients with a diagnosis of mammary pseudolymphoma exceeds 2 years and extends to 10 (1) and 15 (26) years in individual cases. None of the women had a recurrence in the breast or developed systemic lymphoma following treatment by various modalities including local excision alone (61), excision followed by radiotherapy (1,60), and mastectomy with axillary dissection (26).

The term *pseudolymphoma* now seems to be entrenched in the literature. Unusual lesions composed of a polymorphic lymphoid population proven to be polyclonal by appropriate laboratory studies, including molecular genetic analysis, are best referred to as atypical lymphoid infiltrates with an uncertain clinical course.

The differential diagnosis of lymphohistiocytic infiltrative disease in the breast also includes *extranodal sinus histiocytosis with massive lymphadenopathy (Rosai-Dorfman's disease)*. Involvement of virtually every organ including the breast has been described (Fig. 42.20) (64). Mammography reveals a dense mass that may be nodular or ill defined (65,66). Axillary adenopathy is present in some but not all patients. Lymph node infiltration is characterized histologically by diffuse expansion of sinuses due to a histiocytic infiltrate. Subcutaneous lesions have been described in the breast, and there are rare examples of nodular unilateral or bilateral mammary parenchymal involvement (65,67). The lesion may have plasma cells and germinal centers, and appear to be a reactive process when spindled histiocytic cells are associated with collagen deposition in a storiform pattern (Fig. 42.20). The infiltrating histiocytic cells have single or multiple nuclei that contain one or more nucleoli, and there may be occasional mitotic figures. The histiocytes exhibit lymphophagocytosis or erythrophagocytosis. Aspiration cytology of the breast lesion is likely to suggest an inflammatory process or lymphoma (67). The infiltrating histiocytic cells are reactive for S-100 and histiocytic markers such as CD68 in almost all cases, but there usually is an inverse relationship in the intensity of staining for these markers. The immunohistochemical phenotype will rule out most metastatic tumors, but lesions with strong S-100 staining and weak or absent histiocytic markers (CD68) may require more extensive study for HMB45, lysozyme, and other markers.

## Molecular Genetics

Limited information is available from genetic analyses of mammary non-Hodgkin's lymphomas. Bobrow et al. (46) failed to find evidence for t(14;18) translocation in six lymphomas when DNA extracted from paraffin-embedded tissue was studied by the polymerase chain reaction. This result is consistent with other studies that detected t(14;18) translocation more frequently in nodal than in extranodal lymphomas (68). These observations suggest that different genetic mechanisms may be involved in the pathogenesis of these types of lymphoma. Gene rearrangement studies of bone marrow samples are helpful in staging patients who appear to have primary mammary lymphoma, especially when lymphoid aggregates are present in the marrow (42).

## Treatment and Prognosis

A review published in 1984 of 132 reported cases found that 41% of the patients underwent a mastectomy with axillary dissection and that a simple mastectomy was performed in 16% (69). Adjuvant radiation and/or chemotherapy were given to 40% of women treated by mastectomy. Surgery was limited to excision in 43% of cases, usually supplemented by radiation and/or chemotherapy. In some instances, mastectomy was performed because the biopsy was erroneously interpreted as carcinoma.

Until fairly recently, there has been a tendency to treat patients with "primary" lymphoma clinically limited to the breast and axillary lymph nodes by mastectomy and to reserve excision for women with systemic disease. However, it has now been demonstrated that excellent local control in the breast and regional lymph nodes can be achieved with radiation after partial mastectomy and, as a consequence, mastectomy is only recommended for specific clinical problems such as bulky local disease or infected, ulcerated lesions (70–72).

Regardless of the type of local therapy, the majority of recurrences occur at distant sites or in the opposite breast. Terminal leukemic transformation is infrequent (13,40). Systemic therapy must be considered in all cases. The role of various staging procedures, including laparotomy, in the selection of adjuvant systemic treatment remains uncertain. No prospective randomized trial has been performed to determine if any type of chemotherapy deemed effective for lymphoma given in an adjuvant setting improves the prognosis of patients with mammary lymphoma, although some success has been reported generally with adjuvant chemotherapy in non-Hodgkin's lymphomas (70,73).

A review of 205 patients with all stages of mammary lymphoma reported prior to 1984 revealed a disease-free survival of 3.4% at 5 years and 2% at 10 years (69). However, subsequent analyses of patients with stage I and IIE disease limited to the breast or breast and axillary lymph nodes revealed more favorable results. DeBlasio et al. (71) reported a 50% disease-free survival at 4 years, with 66% of patients surviving. In another series, 72% of patients were alive after a median follow-up of 55 months, with 44% disease free

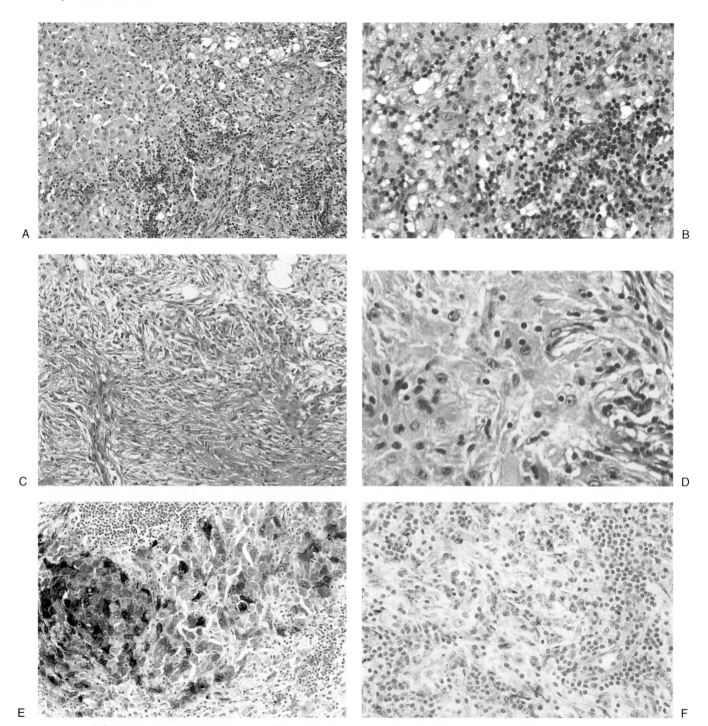

**FIG. 42.20.** *Idiopathic histiocytosis (Rosai-Dorfman disease).* **A,B:** Diffuse infiltrate of histiocytic cells is mixed with small lymphocytes. Cytoplasmic vacuoles are present in some histiocytes. **C:** Area with a spindle cell storiform pattern. **D:** Lymphophagocytosis. **E:** Strong S-100 immunoreactivity. **F:** Weak reactivity for CD68. *(continued)*

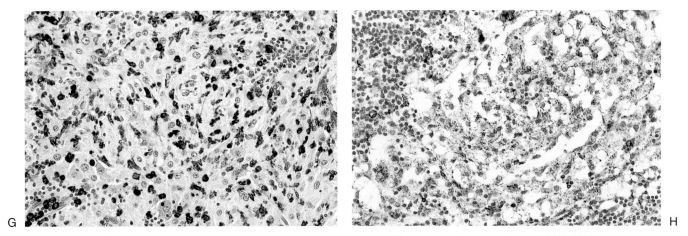

**FIG. 42.20.** *Continued.* **G:** Strong reactivity for lysozyme. **H:** Finely granular reactivity for PGM1 (all immunostains avidin-biotin).

(72). Brustein et al. (17) reported that 41% of stage I and IIE patients survived 10 years. In the combined data from three other series (4,14,20), these authors found that 47% of patients survived 10 years. Tumor size and bilaterality do not appear to have a significant effect on prognosis (5,13). Patients with stage I disease and those with histologically low-grade lesions have the most favorable prognosis (5,13).

Ha et al. (39) analyzed 23 patients with primary mammary non-Hodgkin's lymphoma (stage IE: 17 patients; IIE: 5 patients; and IV: 1 patient with bilateral disease limited to breasts). Overall and disease-free 5-year survival rates were 74% and 73%, respectively, for the entire group, and 65% and 70%, respectively, for 17 patients with diffuse large cell lymphoma. An aggressive clinical course was reported in a small series of patients with mammary T-cell lymphomas (45a).

## HODGKIN'S DISEASE

Hodgkin's disease is very rarely found in the breast. Mammary infiltration is usually the result of direct extension from axillary or mediastinal lymph nodes (74), part of regional disease with discontinuous axillary nodal involvement (75), or a manifestation of systemic disease (75,76). Wood and Coltman (77) reviewed 354 reported examples of extranodal Hodgkin's disease published prior to 1973 and found eight (2%) that involved the breast. Another patient with primary Hodgkin's disease of the breast was included in a series reported by Ariad et al. (45). Most of the patients were women, and almost all ultimately developed systemic disease. Recurrent Hodgkin's disease presenting as a breast mass has been reported (Fig. 42.21) (78). In one series, four women with recurrent tumor limited to the breast were found among 2,365 patients with Hodgkin's disease (79). Two other patients had breast lesions at the time of diagnosis. Nodular sclerosis and mixed cellularity Hodgkin's disease have been reported in the breast.

The diagnosis of Hodgkin's disease in the breast is best made by surgical biopsy, although the sample obtained by fine needle aspiration may prove satisfactory. The aspirate contains a mixed population of cells including leukocytes,

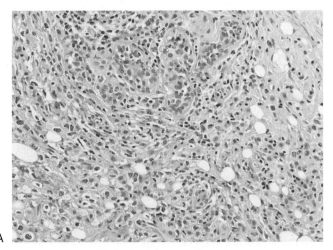
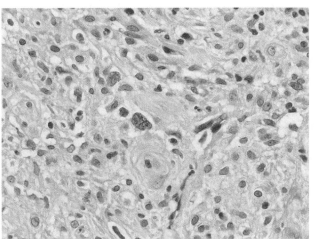

**FIG. 42.21.** *Hodgkin's disease.* **A,B:** Breast involvement in a patient with a diagnosis previously established in a cervical lymph node.

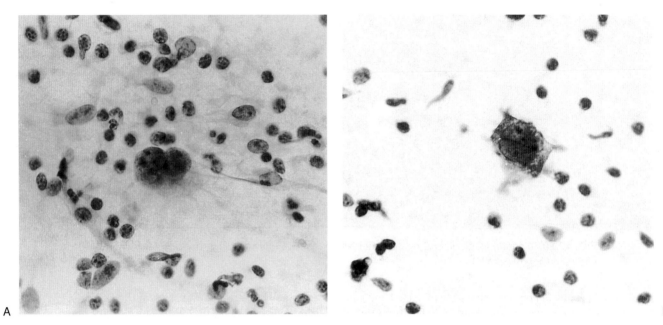

A                                                                                                          B

**FIG. 42.22.** *Hodgkin's disease.* **A,B:** Reed-Sternberg cells, stromal cells, and lymphocytes in a fine needle aspiration smear from recurrent Hodgkin's disease in the breast. (Courtesy of C. Corrigan, C. Sewell, and A. Martin.)

mature lymphocytes, and plasma cells. Giant cells with the nuclear characteristics of Reed-Sternberg cells are a diagnostic feature. The identification of Reed-Sternberg cells can be confirmed by immunohistochemical staining for Leu-M1. A number of patients have developed mammary carcinoma following the treatment of Hodgkin's disease with radiation and/or chemotherapy (6,80,81). On average, the interval between diagnosis of Hodgkin's disease and carcinoma has been about 14 years. The distinction between recurrent Hodgkin's disease and mammary carcinoma must be considered in the interpretation of an aspiration cytology specimen in this setting (Fig. 42.22).

## PLASMACYTIC TUMORS

### Clinical Presentation

Extramedullary neoplastic plasmacytic infiltrates can occur at many sites as part of disseminated multiple myeloma. The mammary gland is infrequently involved clinically when patients present with typical osseous manifestations. No breast infiltrates were found in two large autopsy studies of myeloma patients (82,83), and only one patient had a breast lesion in a third series (84). Asynchronous mammary plasmacytomas that developed 1.5 to 5 years after the diagnosis of multiple myeloma have been described in four patients with kappa light-chain myeloma. Three were women 40 (85), 50 (86), and 75 years old (87), and the fourth was a man 65 years old (87). A fifth patient was reported by Craft (88).

Plasmacytoma of the breast presenting as an isolated initial manifestation of systemic disease was described in 1934 by Cutler (89). One year after a 5-cm plasmacytoma was excised from her breast, the 49-year-old woman reported by Cutler developed plasmacytomas of the larynx, maxillary antrum, and supraclavicular area. Osseous involvement was not detected during the brief reported follow-up. A second case report documented a 42-year-old woman who presented with multiple unilateral mammary plasmacytomas measuring up to 2.5 cm (90). Coincidentally, the diagnosis of multiple myeloma was established by finding immature plasma cells in the bone marrow, Bence Jones proteinuria, and a serum myeloma protein spike. There are reports of three additional patients who each presented with a single unilateral breast tumor as the first manifestation of multiple myeloma (91,92). One was a 50-year-old woman with a 2-cm right breast lesion who proved on clinical evaluation to have osseous and other soft tissue myelomatous infiltrates, amyloidosis, and plasma cell leukemia with IgG lambda paraproteinemia. The second woman was 49 years old when she presented with a 2-cm plasmacytoma of the right breast. Workup revealed IgG kappa paraproteinemia and osseous lesions. The third patient was an 85-year-old woman with monoclonal kappa gammopathy, a 5-cm breast tumor, and no clinical evidence of lesions outside the breast (92). Two instances of synchronous bilateral mammary plasmacytoma, serum IgA paraproteinemia, and multiple myeloma have been described in a 13-year-old (93) and a 61-year-old (94) patient, respectively. The latter patient had multiple nodules in both breasts that were no longer evident when mammography was repeated 9 weeks after the initiation of treatment.

Approximately 4% of plasmacytomas are entirely extramedullary tumors, with the majority occurring in the respiratory tract (84,95). Extramedullary plasmacytoma limited to the breast has been described in five patients. Innes and Newall (84) referred to a 43-year-old woman with bilateral breast lesions and no evidence of systemic involvement. Serum electrophoresis was not performed. Proctor et al. (96)

described a 63-year-old woman with normal serum protein and immunoglobulin levels, who remained disease free 46 months after excision and local radiotherapy of a solitary right breast tumor.

Three women with mammary plasmacytomas had abnormal serum proteins. In one case, a 70-year-old woman with a solitary tumor had mildly increased serum IgG and IgM levels but no monoclonal spike or urinary Bence Jones protein (97). Nine years following a radical mastectomy, she remained well except for excision of a nasal plasmacytic polyp 6 years after treatment of the breast tumor. A second patient was a 73-year-old woman with a single tumor and elevated serum IgG with a monoclonal lambda peak (98). IgM and IgA levels were normal. Bone marrow aspiration revealed that "plasma cells were present but not conspicuously increased." Forty months after excision and local mammary radiation, the patient remained well. A third woman was 49 years old when she presented with two tumors in the left breast measuring 3 and 4 cm in largest diameter, respectively (99). Immunoglobulin D (IgD) and lambda were demonstrated in the tumor cells by immunohistochemistry, and the serum contained IgD lambda monoclonal protein. The bone marrow contained only normal plasma cells. Two weeks after a mastectomy, a plasmacytoma of the nasal cavity was

identified, and this regressed after combination chemotherapy. The patient reportedly had no evidence of myeloma 12 months later.

Mammography revealed a circumscribed mass that was hypoechoic and solid on ultrasound (85,99).

### Gross Pathology

Solitary plasmacytomas of the breast have generally measured between 2 and 4 cm in diameter. Tumors less than 1 cm have been described in patients who have multiple lesions. The masses typically are well circumscribed and tan or brown. Plasmacytomas that developed in patients with multiple myeloma usually were described as firm and rubbery, whereas solitary extramedullary tumors typically were soft.

### Microscopic Pathology

The histologic features of breast lesions in systemic and solitary plasmacytomas are similar. In patients with multiple myeloma, the tumors have been composed of "abnormal" or "immature" plasma cells, whereas solitary plasmacytomas contain "a mixture of mature and immature plasma cells" (Fig. 42.23). The diagnosis of mammary plasmacytoma can

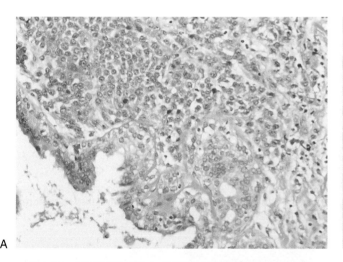

A

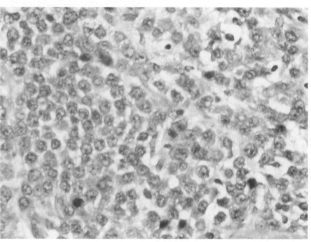

B

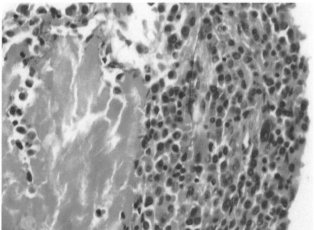

C

**FIG. 42.23.** *Plasmacytoma, multiple myeloma.* **A,B:** Immature plasma cells that formed a tumor in the breast of a 66-year-old woman. The tumor cells stained for lambda chains but not for kappa, and they were positive with the methyl green pyronine stain. **C:** Biopsy of the bone marrow revealed mature and immature plasma cells.

be established with a fine needle aspiration, which yields material suitable for clonality analysis by flow cytometry and immunohistochemistry (Fig. 42.24) (100). Mitoses, nuclear pleomorphism, and multinucleated plasma cells may be seen in solitary plasmacytomas. Mammary glandular structures are largely effaced in the region where the plasma cell infiltrate is most concentrated. However, the neoplastic cells spread microscopically in the mammary parenchyma and fat beyond the grossly evident mass.

Histologically, mammary plasmacytoma should be distinguished from plasma cell mastitis, amyloid tumor, and plasma cell granuloma (101). If appropriate samples are available, immunohistochemical studies for immunoglobulins may be performed on the tissue to determine if the infiltrate has the monoclonal character of a neoplastic process or if it is a reactive polyclonal lesion. Plasma cell mastitis is a periductal process that features duct dilatation, a mixed inflammatory infiltrate, and abscess formation (see Chapter 3). Amyloid that characterizes mammary amyloid tumor is absent from mammary plasmacytoma, and the plasma cells associated with amyloid tumor are mature (see

Chapter 3). Plasma cell granuloma is a well-circumscribed, lobulated tumor predominantly composed of mature plasma cells embedded in hyalinized myofibroblastic stroma (Fig. 42.25) (101). A lymphocytic infiltrate tends to form nodules with germinal centers at the periphery of the tumor. Russell bodies are present, and the cells exhibit polyclonal immunoreactivity for kappa and lambda light-chain immunoglobulins.

### Treatment and Prognosis

Following the histologic diagnosis of a plasmacytic tumor of the breast, the patient should be evaluated for evidence of systemic involvement. Prognosis and treatment will depend on the type and extent of the underlying disorder. Treatment may consist of excision and local radiation in patients who prove to have a lesion limited to the breast. The prognosis for patients with solitary mammary plasmacytoma appears to be excellent, but extended follow-up and study of more cases will be necessary to determine whether these patients are at risk to ultimately develop systemic disease.

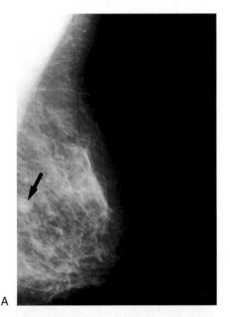

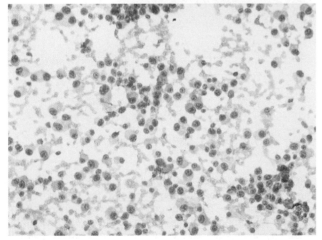

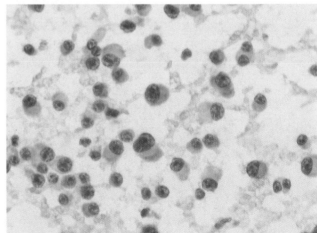

**FIG. 42.24.** *Multiple myeloma.* **A:** Mammogram of a 64-year-old woman with multiple myeloma revealed a discrete parenchymal nodule. **B,C:** Fine needle aspiration smear revealed mature and immature plasma cells.

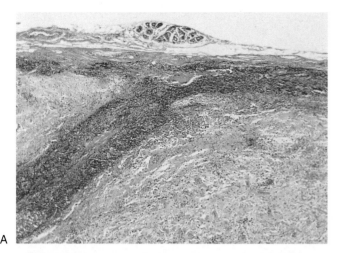

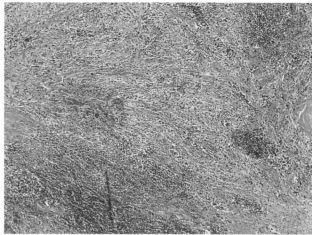

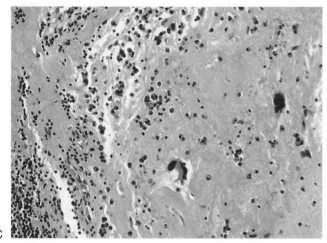

**FIG. 42.25.** *Plasmacytic granuloma.* **A:** At low magnification, a lobule is present at the circumscribed border of this tumor, which is demarcated by a lymphoplasmacytic infiltrate. **B:** Localized aggregate of lymphocytes and diffuse infiltrate of lymphocytes and plasma cells. **C:** Lymphocytes, plasma cells, and atypical myofibroblasts in collagenous stroma that did not have staining properties of amyloid. (Courtesy of Dr. G. Pettinato, J.C. Manivel, L. Insabato, A. DeChiara, and G. Petrella.)

## LEUKEMIC INFILTRATION

Leukemic infiltration of the breast occurs not uncommonly at an advanced stage, but only rarely as the initial manifestation of the disease or as the site of localized recurrence (102).

### Granulocytic Sarcoma

Granulocytic leukemia may present with tumoral breast involvement, also referred to as granulocytic sarcoma (103,104). The term *chloroma* has been used to describe extramedullary tumor-forming granulocytic leukemia infiltrates that develop a green color as a result of the enzymatic action of myeloperoxidase (verdoperoxidase) contained in the neoplastic cells (105). In the past, tumors that do not have a green color have been termed *myeloblastoma*. Green and colorless tumors may occur at different sites in one patient, and presently the diagnosis of granulocytic sarcoma should be used for either form of the disease. Hematogenous evidence of myelogenous leukemia usually appears less than 1 year after the initial parenchymal lesion. Mammary infiltrates have been described as a secondary manifestation in patients with established leukemia (106). The rarity of this

event is evidenced by the absence of breast involvement in a large series of patients with granulocytic leukemia collected by the Eastern Cooperative Oncology Group (107). Leukemic infiltration may be mistaken for a breast abscess clinically and pathologically (108).

The patients range in age from 21 to 56 years, with rare instances of patients pregnant at the time of diagnosis. One patient found to have acute myelocytic leukemia when 32 weeks pregnant went into remission after delivery of the baby by cesarean section. Bilateral breast infiltrates were the first sign of recurrence 3 months later (109). Unilateral and bilateral tumors have been reported, and the lesions may be multifocal (110,111). Physical examination reveals one or more unilateral or bilateral masses. Concurrent chloromatous infiltration of axillary lymph nodes was found in one patient (104). The mammographic appearance of mammary chloromas is nonspecific (110,111). Mixed echogenicity is observed on ultrasonography (112,113).

Microscopically, the growth pattern may simulate invasive lobular carcinoma or malignant lymphoma (18, 106,114). The neoplastic cells forming broad sheets or cords invade into and around normal mammary parenchymal structures. Intraepithelial extension of the leukemic infiltrate simulates *in situ* carcinoma. The diagnosis of granulocytic

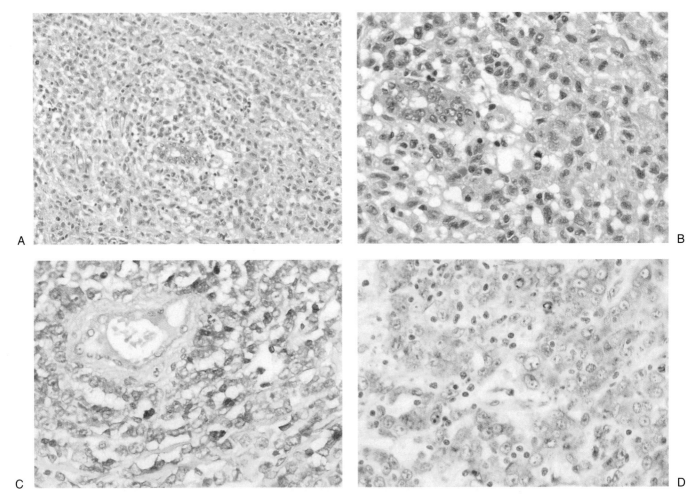

**FIG. 42.26.** *Granulocytic sarcoma.* **A,B:** This periductal infiltrate of undifferentiated granulocytic cells could be mistaken for carcinoma. **C:** A few tumor cells are reactive *(red)* with the naphthol-ASD-chloroacetate esterase stain. Undifferentiated cells are not stained. **D:** Differentiated cells are positive with the immunostain for muramidase (avidin-biotin).

sarcoma may be suggested by cytoplasmic granules in maturing myeloid cells or by the presence of relatively numerous mature myeloid cells scattered throughout the lesion (Fig. 42.26).

Special stains are especially helpful to establish the diagnosis. The tumor cells do not contain mucin, and they give a negative reaction for immunocytochemical epithelial markers such as cytokeratin and epithelial membrane antigen. Myeloid granules are reactive histochemically with the naphthol-ASD-chloroacetate esterase stain and immunohistochemically for lysozyme (muramidase). The diagnosis of granulocytic sarcoma can be established by fine needle aspiration biopsy if immature myelocytic cells are recognized in the cytologic specimen (104,111,115). Mammary chloroma is effectively treated with radiation therapy (110).

### Lymphocytic Leukemia

Mammary infiltration has been described in patients with chronic lymphocytic leukemia (116–118). The lesions tend to be bilateral. Coincidental bone marrow and hematogenous involvement usually are present, and recurrence may be manifested by mammary involvement (117). The mammographic and ultrasonographic findings in a 19-year-old patient with acute lymphoblastic leukemia have been reported (119).

### MYELOID METAPLASIA

Breast masses formed by myeloid metaplasia have been reported in elderly female patients 6 to 16 years after diagnosis of myelofibrosis (120–123). The tumors measured 1.8 to 8 cm. One patient reportedly had no other tumorous manifestations of myeloid metaplasia except hepatic enlargement (121). The other patients had splenomegaly. Mammography revealed bilateral confluent densities in one case (122). The lesions were smooth, homogeneous, and hypoechoic on sonography. Microscopic examination reveals a diffuse infiltrate of mature and maturing hematopoietic cells, including megakaryocytes (Fig.

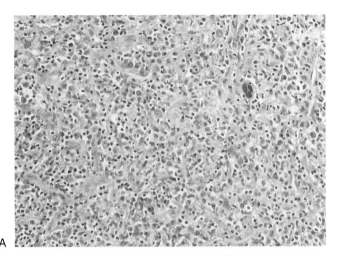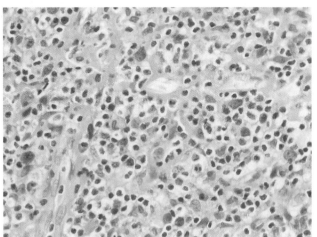

**FIG. 42.27.** *Myeloid metaplasia.* **A:** Diffuse infiltrate of hematopoietic cells includes a conspicuous megakaryocyte with a bilobed nucleus. **B:** Immature and mature hematopoietic cells in the mammary stroma.

42.27). Mammary extramedullary hematopoiesis has been described in postmortem examinations of patients with myelofibrosis (123).

## REFERENCES

### Non-Hodgkin's Lymphoma

1. Wiseman C, Liao KT. Primary lymphoma of the breast. *Cancer* 1972;29:1705–1712.
2. Cutler SJ, Young JL, eds. Third national cancer survey: incidence data. *NCI Monograph No. 41* 1975:413–414.
3. Kim H. Extranodal lymphomas. In: van den Tweel JG, ed. *Malignant lymphoproliferative diseases.* Boston: Martinus Nijhoff, 1980:459–467.
4. Schouten JT, Weese JL, Carbone P. Lymphoma of the breast. *Ann Surg* 1981;194:749–753.
5. Giardini R, Piccolo C, Rilke F. Primary non-Hodgkin's lymphomas of the female breast. *Cancer* 1992;69:725–735.
6. Sanford DB, Yeomans-Kinney A, McLaughlin PW, et al. Ninety-one cases of breast cancer and chronic lymphoproliferative neoplasm: a retrospective review of a population at high risk for multiple malignancies. *Breast J* 1996;2:312–319.
7. Arber DA, Simpson JF, Weiss LM, et al. Non-Hodgkin's lymphoma involving the breast. *Am J Surg Pathol* 1994;18:288–295.
8. Talvalkar GV. Primary lymphosarcoma of the breast: a report of ten cases. *Indian J Cancer* 1973;10:322–329.
9. Tanino M, Tatsuzawa T, Funada T, et al. Lymphosarcoma of the male breast: a case report. *Breast* 1984;10:13–15.
10. Murata T, Kuroda H, Nakahama T, et al. Primary non-Hodgkin malignant lymphoma of the male breast. *Jpn J Clin Oncol* 1996; 26:243–247.
11. Abbondanzo SL, Seidman JD, Lefkowitz M, et al. Primary diffuse large B-cell lymphoma of the breast. A clinicopathologic study of 31 cases. *Pathol Res Pract* 1996;192:37–43.
12. Sashiyama H, Abe Y, Miyazawa Y, et al. Primary non-Hodgkin's lymphoma of the male breast: a case report. *Breast Cancer* 1999;6:55–58.
13. Jeon HJ, Akagi T, Hoshida Y, et al. Primary non-Hodgkin malignant lymphoma of the breast. An immunohistochemical study of seven patients with breast lymphoma in Japan. *Cancer* 1992;70:2451–2459.
14. Mambo NC, Burke JS, Butler JJ. Primary malignant lymphomas of the breast. *Cancer* 1977;39:2033–2040.
15. Shepherd JJ, Wright DH. Burkitt's tumor presenting as bilateral swelling of the breast in women of child-bearing age. *Br J Surg* 1967;54:776–780.
16. Hugh JC, Jackson FI, Hanson J, et al. Primary breast lymphoma. An immunohistologic study of 20 new cases. *Cancer* 1990;66: 2602–2617.
17. Brustein S, Filippa DA, Kimmel M, et al. Malignant lymphoma of the breast: a study of 53 patients. *Ann Surg* 1987;205:144–150.
18. Lin Y, Govindan R, Hess JL. Malignant hematopoietic breast tumors. *Am J Clin Pathol* 1997;107:177–186.
19. Dixon JM, Lumsden AB, Krajewski A, et al. Primary lymphoma of the breast. *Br J Surg* 1987;74:214–217.
20. DeCosse JJ, Berg JW, Fracchia AA, et al. Primary lymphosarcoma of the breast. A review of 14 cases. *Cancer* 1962;15:1264–1268.
21. Freedman SJ, Kagan AR, Friedman NB. Bilaterality in primary lymphosarcoma of the breast. *Am J Clin Pathol* 1971;55:82–87.
22. Bundred NJ, Whitfield BCS, Parker AC, et al. Nipple oedema: an unusual presenting sign of non-Hodgkin's lymphoma. *Eur J Surg Oncol* 1985;11:61–63.
23. Lamovec J, Jancar J. Primary malignant lymphoma of the breast. Lymphoma of the mucosa-associated lymphoid tissue. *Cancer* 1987;60:3033–3041.
24. DiPiro PJ, Lester S, Meyer JE, et al. Non-Hodgkin lymphoma of the breast: clinical and radiologic presentations. *Breast J* 1996;2: 380–384.
25. Goyal M, Bang D. Tc-99m MDP uptake in primary breast lymphoma. *Clin Nucl Med* 1998;23:614–615.
26. Oberman HA. Primary lymphoreticular neoplasms of the breast. *Surg Gynecol Obstet* 1966;123:1047–1051.
27. Duvic M, Moore D, Menter A, et al. Cutaneous T-cell lymphoma in association with silicone breast implants. *J Am Acad Dermatol* 1995;32:939–942.
28. Cook PD, Osborne BM, Connor RL, et al. Follicular lymphoma adjacent to foreign body granulomatous inflammation and fibrosis surrounding silicone breast prosthesis. *Am J Surg Pathol* 1995; 19:712–717.
29. Meyer JE, Kopans DB, Long JC. Mammographic appearance of malignant lymphoma of the breast. *Radiology* 1980;135:623–626.
30. Pope Jr, TL, Brenbridge ANAG, Sloop FB Jr, et al. Primary histiocytic lymphoma of the breast: mammographic, sonographic and pathologic correlation. *J Clin Ultrasound* 1985;13:667–670.
31. Liberman L, Giess CS, Dershaw DD, et al. Non-Hodgkin lymphoma of the breast: imaging characteristics and correlation with histopathologic findings. *Radiology* 1994;192:157–160.
32. Pameijer FA, Beijerinck D, Hoogenboom HHVM, et al. Non-Hodgkin's lymphoma of the breast causing miliary densities on mammography. *AJR Am J Roentgenol* 1995;164:609–610.
33. Derchi LE, Rizzatto G, Giuseppetti GM, et al. Metastatic tumors in the breast: sonographic findings. *J Ultrasound Med* 1985;4:69–74.
34. Mussurakis S, Carleton PJ, Turnbull LW. MR imaging of primary non-Hodgkin's breast lymphoma. A case report. *Acta Radiol* 1997;38:104–107.
35. Aghadiuno PU, Ibeziako PA. Clinicopathologic study of breast

carcinoma occurring during pregnancy and lactation. *Int J Gynaecol Obstet* 1983;21:17–26.

36. Poulsen LO, Christensen JH, Sorensen B, et al. Immunologic observations in close relatives of two sisters with mammary Burkitt's lymphoma. *Cancer* 1991;68:1031–1034.

37. Filippa DA, Lieberman PH, Weingrad DN, et al. Primary lymphomas of the gastrointestinal tract. Analysis of prognostic factors with emphasis on histological type. *Am J Surg Pathol* 1983; 7: 363–372.

38. L'hoste R, Filippa DA, Lieberman PH, et al. Primary pulmonary lymphoma. A clinicopathologic analysis of 36 cases. *Cancer* 1984; 54:1397–1406.

39. Ha CS, Dubey P, Goyal LK, et al. Localized primary non-Hodgkin lymphoma of the breast. *Am J Clin Oncol* 1998;21:376–380.

40. Aozasa K, Ohsawa M, Saeki K, et al. Malignant lymphoma of the breast. Immunologic type and association with lymphocytic mastopathy. *Am J Clin Pathol* 1992;97:699–704.

41. Elavathil LJ, Kahn HJ, Hanna W. Primary multilobulated B-cell lymphoma of the breast. *Arch Pathol Lab Med* 1989;113:1081–1084.

42. Topalovski M, Crisan D, Mattson JC. Lymphoma of the breast. A clinicopathologic study of primary and secondary cases. *Arch Pathol Lab Med* 1999;123:1208–1218.

43. Kosaka M, Tsuchihashi N, Takishita M, et al. Primary adult T-cell lymphoma of the breast. *Acta Haematol* 1992;87:202–205.

44. Narasimhan P, Holzman RS, Weiser SM, et al. T-cell lymphoma of the breast presenting as inflammatory carcinoma. *Breast Dis* 1994;7:367–371.

45. Ariad S, Lewis D, Cohen R, et al. Breast lymphoma. A clinical and pathological review and 10-year treatment results. *S Afr Med J* 1995;85:85–89.

45a. Aguilera NSI, Tavassoli FA, Chu W, et al. T-cell lymphoma presenting in the breast: a histologic, immunophenotypic and molecular genetic study of four cases. *Mod Pathol* 2000;13:599–605.

46. Bobrow LG, Richards MA, Happerfield LC, et al. Breast lymphomas: a clinicopathologic review. *Hum Pathol* 1993;24:274–278.

47. Telesinghe PU, Anthony PP. Primary lymphoma of the breast. *Histopathology* 1985;9:297–307.

48. Cohen PL, Brooks JJ. Lymphomas of the breast. A clinicopathologic and immunohistochemical study of primary and secondary cases. *Cancer* 1991;67:1359–1369.

49. Alm P, Brandt L, Olsson H. Immunoglobulin-A producing probably primary lymphoma of the breast. *Virchows Arch [A]* 1983; 399:355–360.

50. Pérez-Guillermo M, Sola-Pérez J, Rodríguez-Bermejo M. Malacoplakia and Rosai-Dorfman disease: two entities of histiocytic origin infrequently localized in the female breast—the cytologic aspect in aspirates obtained via fine-needle aspiration cytology. *Diagn Cytopathol* 1993;9:698–704.

51. Isaacson P, Wright DH. Extranodal malignant lymphoma arising from mucosa-associated lymphoid tissue. *Cancer* 1984;53: 2515–2524.

52. Ferguson DJP. Intraepithelial lymphocytes and macrophages in the normal breast. *Virchows Arch [A]* 1985;407:369–378.

53. Goldblum RM, Ahlstedt S, Carlsson B, et al. Antibody-forming cells in human colostrum after oral immunization. *Nature* 1975;257: 797–798.

54. Jackson DE, Lally ET, Nakamura MC, et al. Migration of IgA-bearing lymphocytes into salivary glands. *Cell Immunol* 1981;63: 203–209.

55. Weisz-Carrington P, Roux ME, McWilliams M, et al. Organ and isotype distribution of plasma cells producing specific antibody after oral immunization: evidence for a generalized secretory immune system. *J Immunol* 1979;123:1705–1708.

56. Rooney N, Snead D, Goodman S, et al. Primary breast lymphoma with skin involvement arising in lymphocytic lobulitis. *Histopathology* 1994;24:81–84.

57. Schwartz IS, Strauchen JA. Lymphocytic mastopathy: an autoimmune disease of the breast? *Am J Clin Pathol* 1990;93:725–730.

58. Greenberg SD, Heisler JG, Gyorkey F, et al. Pulmonary lymphoma versus pseudolymphoma: a perplexing problem. *South Med J* 1972;65:775–784.

59. Marchevsky A, Padilla M, Kaneko M, et al. Localized lymphoid nodules of lung: a reappraisal of the lymphoma versus pseudolymphoma dilemma. *Cancer* 1983;51:2070–2077.

60. Fisher ER, Palekar AS, Paulson JD, et al. Pseudolymphoma of the breast. *Cancer* 1979;44:258–263.

61. Lin JJ, Farha GJ, Taylor RJ. Pseudolymphoma of the breast I. In a study of 8,654 consecutive tylectomies and mastectomies. *Cancer* 1980;45:973–978.

62. Jeffrey KM, Pantazis CG, Wei JP. Pseudolymphoma of the breast associated with Graves' thyrotoxicosis. *Breast Dis* 1994;7:169–173.

63. Nakano A, Hamada Y, Hirono M, et al. Differentiation between pseudo and malignant lymphoma of the breast—a case report. *Jpn J Surg* 1982;12:76–78.

64. Foucar E, Rosai J, Dorfman R. Sinus histiocytosis with massive lymphadenopathy (Rosai-Dorfman disease): review of the entity. *Semin Diagn Pathol* 1990;7:19–73.

65. Green I, Dorfman RF, Rosai J. Breast involvement by extranodal Rosai-Dorfman disease: report of seven cases. *Am J Surg Pathol* 1997;21:664–668.

66. Hammond LA, Keh C, Rowlands DC. Rosai-Dorfman disease in the breast. *Histopathology* 1996;29:582–584.

67. Soares FA, Llorach-Velludo MA, Andrade JM. Rosai-Dorfman's disease of the breast. *Am J Surg Pathol* 1999;23:359–360.

68. Raghoebier S, Kramer MHH, Van Krieken JHJM, et al. Essential differences in oncogenic involvement between primary nodal and extranodal large cell lymphoma. *Blood* 1991;78:2680–2685.

69. Fischer MG, Chideckel NJ. "Primary" lymphoma of the breast. *Breast* 1984;10:7–9.

70. Monfardini S, Banfi A, Bonadonna G, et al. Improved five year survival after combined radiotherapy-chemotherapy for stage I–II non-Hodgkin's lymphoma. *Int J Radiat Oncol Biol Phys* 1980;6:125–134.

71. DeBlasio D, McCormick B, Straus D, et al. Definitive irradiation for localized non-Hodgkin's lymphoma of breast. *Int J Radiat Oncol Biol Phys* 1989;17:843–846.

72. Smith MR, Brustein S, Straus DJ. Lozalized non-Hodgkin's lymphoma of the breast. *Cancer* 1987;59:351–354.

73. Nissen NI, Ersboll J, Hansen HS, et al. A randomized study of radiotherapy versus radiotherapy plus chemotherapy in stage I–II non-Hodgkin's lymphoma. *Cancer* 1983;52:1–7.

## Hodgkin's Disease

74. Yarhold JR, Jelliffee AM, Hudson V, et al. The response of treatment of nodular sclerosing Hodgkin's disease with extranodal involvement. *Clin Radiol* 1982;33:141–144.

75. Shehata WM, Pauke TW, Schleuter JA. Hodgkin's disease of the breast. A case report and review of the literature. *Breast* 1985;11:19–21.

76. Schouten JT, Weese JL, Carbone PP. Lymphoma of the breast. *Ann Surg* 1981;194:749–753.

77. Wood NL, Coltman CA Jr. Localized primary extranodal Hodgkin's disease. *Ann Intern Med* 1973;78:113–118.

78. Meis JM, Butler JJ, Osborne BM. Hodgkin's disease involving the breast and chest wall. *Cancer* 1986;57:1859–1865.

79. Corrigan C, Sewell C, Martin A. Recurrent Hodgkin's disease in the breast. Diagnosis of a case by fine needle aspiration and immunocytochemistry. *Acta Cytol* 1990;34:669–672.

80. Janjan NA, Wilson JF, Gillin M, et al. Mammary carcinoma developing after radiotherapy and chemotherapy for Hodgkin's disease. *Cancer* 1988;61:252–254.

81. Carey RW, Linggood RM, Wood WM, et al. Breast cancer developing in four women cured of Hodgkin's disease. *Cancer* 1984; 54:2234–2236.

## Plasmacytic Tumors

82. Hayes DW, Bennett WA, Heck FJ. Extramedullary lesions in multiple myeloma. *Arch Pathol* 1952;53:262–272.

83. Pasmantier M, Azar H. Extraskeletal spread in multiple plasma cell myeloma. *Cancer* 1969;23:167–174.

84. Innes J, Newall J. Myelomatosis. *Lancet* 1961;1:239–245.

85. Kim EE, Sawwaf ZW, Sneigej N. Multiple myeloma of the breast: magnetic resonance and ultrasound imaging findings. *Breast Dis* 1996;9:229–233.

86. Ross JS, King TM, Spector JI, et al. Plasmacytoma of the breast. An unusual case of recurrent myeloma. *Arch Intern Med* 1987;147: 1838–1840.

87. Greene FL, Branham G, McFarland J, et al. Breast lesions in a male and female with multiple myeloma. *Breast* 1981;11:30–31.

88. Craft IL. The late appearance of extra-medullary lesions in myelomatosis. *Br J Cancer* 1967;21:501–504.

89. Cutler CW Jr. Plasma cell tumor of the breast with metastases. *Ann Surg* 1934;100:392–395.

90. Rosenberg B, Attie JN, Mandelbaum HL. Breast tumor as the presenting sign of multiple myeloma. *N Engl J Med* 1963;269:359–361.

91. Ben-Yehuda A, Steiner-Saltz D, Libson E, et al. Plasmacytoma of the breast. Unusual initial manifestation of myeloma: report of two cases and review of the literature. *Blut* 1989;58:169–170.

92. Alhan E, Calik A, Kucuktulu U, et al. Solitary extramedullary plasmacytoma of the breast with kappa monoclonal gammopathy. *Pathol* 1995;87:71–73.

93. Maeda K, Abesamis CM, Kuhn LM. Multiple myeloma in childhood: report of a case with breast tumors as a presenting manifestation. *Am J Clin Pathol* 1973;60:552–558.

94. Bassett WB, Weiss RB. Plasmacytomas of the breast: an unusual manifestation of multiple myeloma. *South Med J* 1979;72:1492–1494.

95. Dolin S, Dewar SP. Extramedullary plasmacytoma. *Am J Pathol* 1956;32:83–103.

96. Proctor NS, Rippey JJ, Shulman G, et al. Extramedullary plasmacytoma of the breast. *J Pathol* 1975;116:97–100.

97. Merino MJ. Plasmacytoma of the breast. *Arch Pathol Lab Med* 1984;108:676–678.

98. Kirshenbaum G, Rhone DP. Solitary extramedullary plasmacytoma of the breast with serum monoclonal protein: a case report and review of the literature. *Am J Clin Pathol* 1985;83:230–232.

99. Momiyama N, Ishikawa T, Doi T, et al. Extramedullary plasmacytoma of the breast with serum IgD monoclonal protein: a case report and review of the literature. *Breast Cancer* 1999;6:217–221.

100. Cangiarella J, Waisman J, Cohen JM, et al. Plasmacytoma of the breast. A report of two cases diagnosed by aspiration biopsy. *Acta Cytol* 2000;44:91–94.

101. Pettinato G, Manivel JC, Insabato L, et al. Plasma cell granuloma (inflammatory pseudo-tumor) of the breast. *Am J Clin Pathol* 1988;90:627–632.

## Leukemic Infiltration

102. Weinblatt ME, Kochen J. Breast nodules as the initial site of relapse in childhood leukemia. *Med Pediatr Oncol* 1990;18:510–512.

103. Pettinato G, DeChiara A, Insabato L, et al. Fine needle aspiration biopsy of granulocytic sarcoma (chloroma) of the breast. *Acta Cytol* 1988;32:67–71.

104. Sears HF, Reid J. Granulocytic sarcoma. Local presentation of a systemic disease. *Cancer* 1976;37:1808–1813.

105. Wiernick PH, Serpick AA. Granulocytic sarcoma (chloroma). *Blood* 1970;35:361–369.

106. Pascoe RH. Tumors composed of immature granulocytes occurring in breast in chronic granulocytic leukemia. *Cancer* 1970;25:697–704.

107. Neiman RS, Barcos M, Berard C, et al. Granulocytic sarcoma. A clinicopathologic study of 61 biopsied cases. *Cancer* 1981;48:1426–1437.

108. Gelin G, Gomez P, Gross G. Leucose tumorale simulant un abces de sein. *Bull Soc Med Hop Paris* 1952;68:376–379.

109. Antunez de Mayolo J, Ahn YS, Temple JD, et al. Spontaneous remission of acute leukemia after the termination of pregnancy. *Cancer* 1989;63:1621–1623.

110. Barloon TJ, Young DC, Bass SH. Multicentric granulocytic sarcoma (chloroma) of the breast: mammographic findings. Case report. *AJR Am J Roentgenol* 1993;161:963–964.

111. Gartenhaus WS, Mir R, Pliskin A, et al. Granulocytic sarcoma of breast: a leukemic bilateral metachronous presentation and literature review. *Med Pediatr Oncol* 1985;13:22–29.

112. Hiorns MP, Murfitt J. Granulocytic sarcoma (chloroma) of the breast: sonographic findings. *AJR Am J Roentgenol* 1997;169:1639–1640.

113. Son HJ, Oh KK. Multicentric granulocytic sarcoma of the breast: mammographic and sonographic findings. *AJR Am J Roentgenol* 1998;171:274–275.

114. Blackwell B. Acute leukemia presenting as a lump in the breast. *Br J Surg* 1963;50:769–771.

115. Barker TH. Granulocytic sarcoma of the breast diagnosed by fine needle aspiration (FNA) cytology. *Cytopathology* 1998;9:135–137.

116. Desablens B, Quang TN, Claisse JF, et al. Localisation mammaire au cours de la leucemie lymphoide chronique. *Presse Med* 1985;14:2301.

117. Gogoi PK, Stewart ID, Keane PF, et al. Chronic lymphocytic leukemia presenting with bilateral involvement. *Clin Lab Haemat* 1989;11:57–60.

118. Seale DL, Riddervoid HO, Tears CD, et al. Roentgenographic appearance of chronic lymphatic leukemia involving the female breast. *AJR Am J Roentgenol* 1972;115:808–810.

119. Memis A, Killi R, Orguc S, et al. Bilateral breast involvement in acute lymphoblastic leukemia: color doppler sonography findings. *AJR Am J Roentgenol* 1995;165:1011.

120. Brooks JJ, Krugman DT, Damjanov I. Myeloid metaplasia presenting as a breast mass. *Am J Surg Pathol* 1980;4:281–285.

121. Martinelli G, Santini D, Bazzocchi F, et al. Myeloid metaplasia of the breast. A lesion which clinically mimics carcinoma. *Virchows Arch [A]* 1983;401:203–207.

122. Zonderland HM, Michiels JJ, Tenkate FJW. Mammographic and sonographic demonstration of extramedullary hematopoiesis of the breast. *Clin Radiol* 1991;44:64–65.

123. Glew RH, Haese WH, McIntyre PA. Myeloid metaplasia with myelofibrosis. The clinical spectrum of extramedullary hematopoiesis and tumor formation. *Johns Hopkins Med J* 1973;132:253–270.

# CHAPTER 43

# Pathologic Effects of Therapy

## RADIATION

The breasts may be exposed secondarily to radiation during diagnostic procedures such as mammography and fluoroscopy (1,2) or in the course of radiotherapy administered to another organ, such as during mediastinal radiotherapy for Hodgkin's disease (3–6). The radiation exposure in these situations has been associated with an increased risk for the subsequent development of breast carcinoma (1–3,7). It remains to be determined whether this risk is lower when exposure to low-dose irradiation is fractionated (7,8).

Data from four studies reviewed by Cutuli included 175 patients who developed a total of 200 breast carcinomas and two sarcomas after radiotherapy for Hodgkin's disease (9,10). The median age at diagnosis of Hodgkin's disease ranged form 24 to 27 years. The median age of diagnosis of breast carcinoma was 40 to 43 years, with a median interval of 15 to 17 years. The frequency of bilaterality was about 15%, representing a threefold to fourfold increase over expected. Among the four studies, 17% to 62% of carcinomas had axillary lymph node metastases. In one study, the relative risk (RR) for developing breast carcinoma was 136 [95% confidence interval (CI), 34–371] in patients younger than 15 years of age who underwent radiation for Hodgkin's disease compared with the RR for the general population; for those treated at ages 15 to 19, 20 to 24, and 25 to 29 years, the RRs were 19, 19, and 7.3, respectively (11). Others reported the cumulative probability of developing breast carcinoma was estimated to be 35% by age 40 (95% CI, 17.4–52.6) (6). A third study of women with Hodgkin's disease treated before age 21 found a RR of 26.2 (95% CI, 15.0–42.6) with a 20-year actuarial risk of 9.2% (12).

Estimates of radiation dosage to the breasts during the treatment of Hodgkin's disease indicate that the effects are at a potentially carcinogenic level (13,14). Kowalski and Smith studied the distribution of radiation with an anthropomorphic phantom (15). Some regions of the breast in the treatment fields had greater than 70% of the prescribed therapeutic dose, whereas blocked regions received 2% to 29% of the prescribed dose.

Mastectomy has been recommended for the primary surgical treatment of breast carcinoma that develops after Hodgkin's disease treated with radiotherapy (16); however, Karasek and Deutsch have reported on six patients successfully treated with lumpectomy and radiation with "good to excellent cosmetic results" and "no significant acute adverse reactions and no late sequelae" after a median follow-up of 60 months (17).

No structural changes attributable to this level of incidental radiation are evident when the mammary glandular tissue is examined histopathologically. Except for a trend to less desmoplastic reaction in carcinomas that arose in irradiated women, Dvoretsky et al. found no histologic difference between tumors in women previously radiated for postpartum mastitis and a control group (18). Patients treated for Hodgkin's disease have carcinomas that tend to be poorly differentiated but that in other respects are not significantly different pathologically from tumors that arise in women without prior irradiation (5). Virtually all detected carcinomas have been ductal, with rare examples of infiltrating lobular and special types such as mucinous carcinoma (10). About 15% of the carcinomas are intraductal.

Radiation of the breast for mammary carcinoma in the course of breast-conserving treatment involves levels of exposure that produce alterations in nonneoplastic as well as neoplastic tissues. A study of noncancerous breast tissue samples obtained before and after adjuvant radiotherapy for breast carcinoma revealed increased immunohistochemical expression of p53 and increased proliferative activity assessed by Ki67 expression in the posttreatment tissues (19). This effect was observed as long as 10 years after radiotherapy. The risk of second malignant neoplasms that develop after therapeutic radiotherapy as part of breast-conservation therapy was studied by Obedian et al. (20). The analysis was based on a comparison of 1,029 patients treated by lumpectomy with radiation (LRT) and 1,387 patients treated by mastectomy (MAST). The median follow-up was 14.6 years and 16 years, respectively, for the LRT and MAST patients. The risk of contralateral carcinoma was 10% in both cohorts. For women 45 years or younger at the time of treatment, the

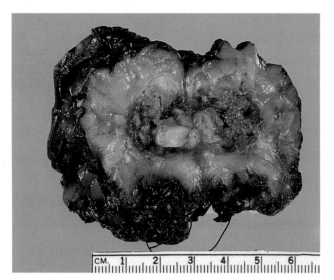

**FIG. 43.1.** *Radiation-induced fat necrosis.* Cystic fat necrosis at the site of prior interstitial and external beam radiation therapy after lumpectomy for invasive duct carcinoma.

risks for contralateral carcinoma were not significantly different (LRT, 10%; MAST, 7%) after 15 years of follow-up. The frequency of contralateral carcinoma was lower in women who received adjuvant hormonal therapy (HT), but the difference was not statistically significant. Nonmammary malignant neoplasms were diagnosed at 15 years in 11% of LRT patients and in 10% after mastectomy. The risk of lung carcinoma was higher among smokers than among nonsmokers who received radiotherapy ($p = 0.06$).

Long-term clinical effects of therapeutic mammary radiation on the normal breast evolve over months to years (21). The extent to which these occur varies among individual patients. Some women ultimately exhibit diffuse increased firmness or sclerosis of the breast, but in most women, this effect is mild and the tissue remains elastic. Ptosis, a natural change of aging, is less pronounced in the irradiated breast (21). Cutaneous atrophy and telangiectasia are likely to be more conspicuous in areas that received a radiation boost. The radiated breast is usually unable to lactate, but the untreated breast is unaffected (22,23). Radiation can be delivered effectively to the breast that contains an implant for cosmesis or reconstruction, although there may be a tendency for more frequent fibrous encapsulation of the prosthesis (24). The adverse clinical effects of radiation may be exaggerated in patients who have a collagen vascular disease, such as scleroderma, and radiation is contraindicated in most women with these conditions (25).

Clinical abnormalities that suggest recurrent carcinoma following radiation and breast-conserving therapy may be detected by mammography or by physical examination. Holli et al. reported that the interpretation of mammograms following breast conservation with radiotherapy was more difficult than in women who underwent surgical excision without radiation (26). Fat necrosis, parenchymal distortion, and fibrosis in the irradiated group led to more frequent false-positive interpretations and a greater frequency of additional diagnostic tests.

The most common mammographic indications for biopsy after breast conservation include a new mass lesion, a change in an existing postoperative scar, and the appearance of calcifications (27–29). Coarse, scattered benign-appearing calcifications may be found in 25% of irradiated breasts and are generally of little concern (30). On the other hand, clustered calcifications present a significant problem (31). Calcified sutures in the biopsy site may mimic the pattern of calcifications associated with carcinoma, although rarely suture calcifications have a distinctive knotted configuration (32). Fat necrosis, which often has a stellate configuration and may contain calcifications, can be easily mistaken for recurrent carcinoma radiologically (33,34). Overall, about 50% of these biopsies reveal carcinoma (27,29,31–35). Localized,

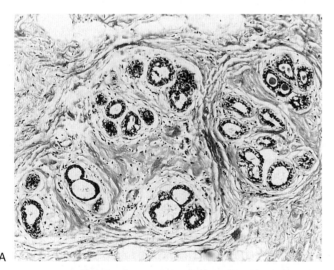

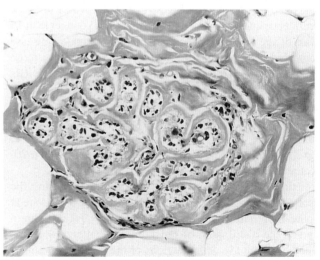

**FIG. 43.2.** *Radiation effect in normal breast.* **A:** A normal lobule in 52-year-old woman prior to external radiotherapy. **B:** A lobule from the same patient 6 months after treatment exhibiting epithelial atrophy, thickening of basement membranes, and intralobular sclerosis.

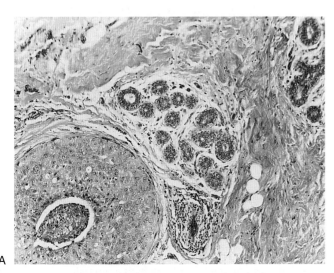 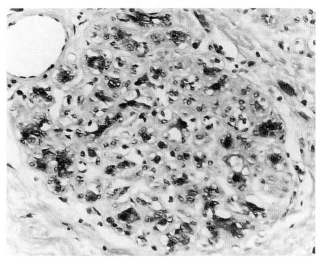

A                                                     B

**FIG. 43.3.** *Radiation effect in normal breast.* **A:** Intraductal carcinoma and adjacent normal lobules in a 37-year-old woman. **B:** A lobule from the same patient after external beam radiotherapy exhibiting epithelial atrophy and intralobular sclerosis. Persisting epithelial nuclei are hyperchromatic and pleomorphic.

encapsulated fat necrosis with a cystic appearance has been described at the site of iridium implantation (30) (Fig. 43.1).

Radiation-induced histologic changes must be distinguished from recurrent carcinoma in the interpretation of a posttreatment biopsy. Compared with a preradiation specimen, the major changes in a normal breast are apparent in terminal duct–lobular units (36) (Figs. 43.2 and 43.3). These include the following: (a) collagenization of intralobular stroma; (b) thickening of periacinar and periductular basement membranes; (c) severe atrophy of acinar and ductular epithelium; (d) cytologic atypia of residual epithelial cells; and (e) relatively prominent acinar myoepithelial cells that seem to be preserved to a greater extent than the epithelial cells. In a minority of specimens, one also may find atypical

fibroblasts in the interlobular stroma (Fig. 43.4). When studied *in vitro,* atypical fibroblasts isolated from irradiated human mammary stroma expressed oncofetal fibronectin and an α-actin isoform specific for smooth-muscle cells indicative of myofibroblastic differentiation (37).

Generally, the effects on the larger ducts are less pronounced following primary radiotherapy than are those in lobules (Fig. 43.5). Substantial variation can be observed from one patient to another in the severity of changes in the lobules, and on occasion they may be so slight as to be virtually indistinguishable from physiologic atrophy. In any one patient, most of the glandular tissue responds in a uniform fashion if the entire breast has been radiated. Extreme variations in different parts of the breast are not common. In one study, dif-

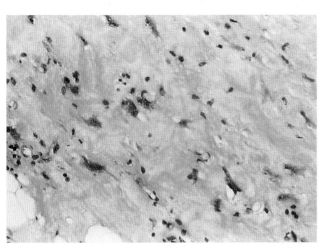

**FIG. 43.4.** *Radiation atypia in stromal fibroblasts.*

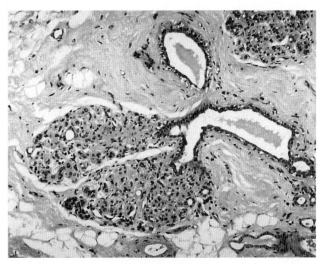

**FIG. 43.5.** *Duct and lobule in radiated breast.* In contrast to lobular sclerosis, the ducts in this postradiation breast appear to be unaffected.

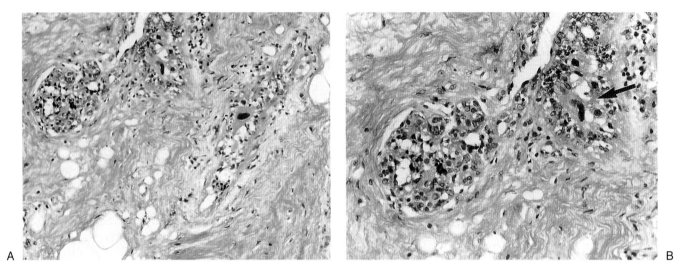

**FIG. 43.6.** *Radiation atypia in ducts.* **A:** Individual ductal cells are enlarged and have hyperchromatic nuclei in this biopsy from a patient who had external beam radiotherapy with a boost. **B:** A magnified view of the atypical epithelial cells in the duct lumen *(arrow).*

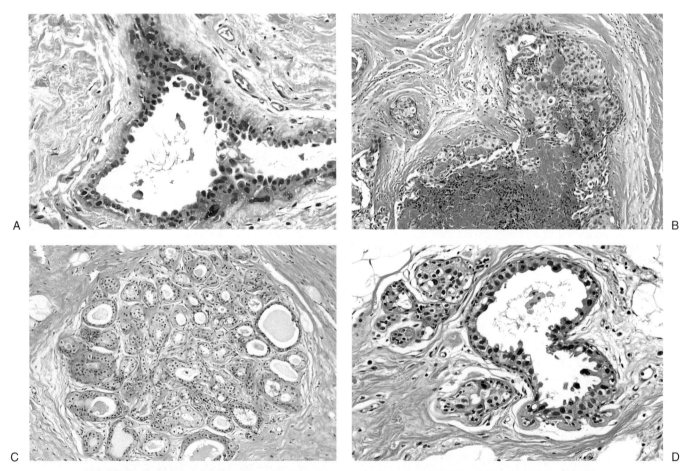

**FIG. 43.7.** *Radiation atypia in duct with apocrine metaplasia.* **A:** Epithelial nuclei are enlarged and hyperchromatic. Images **B–D** are from the same patient. **B:** In 1994, the patient underwent breast-conserving surgery and radiotherapy for intraductal carcinoma shown here. **C:** Coincidental with intraductal carcinoma in 1994, the breast also had foci of apocrine metaplasia shown here in a lobule. **D:** Biopsy performed in 1998 showed apocrine metaplasia with cytological atypia. There was no recurrent carcinoma.

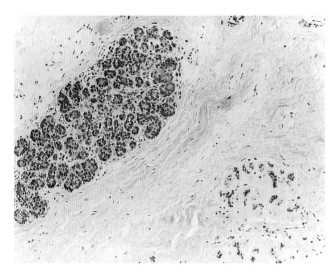

**FIG. 43.8.** *Lobular carcinoma* in situ *after radiation therapy.* The *in situ* carcinoma appears to be unaffected by the treatment. A lobule not involved by carcinoma showing radiation atrophy is present in the *lower right corner.*

ferences in radiation effect between individual patients were not correlated with radiation dosage, patient age, posttreatment interval, or the use of adjuvant chemotherapy (36).

When a radioactive implant or external boost has been used to give more intense treatment to the biopsy site, histologic changes in this area may be more severe than in the surrounding breast. Fat necrosis and atypia of stromal fibroblasts are more common in proximity to such "boosted" or implanted areas (30). Radiation-induced vascular changes are not ordinarily seen after external beam radiotherapy, but they may occur where a boost dose has been delivered. Cytologic and architectural indications of radiation effect in larger blood vessels include fragmentation of elastica, endothelial atypia, and myointimal proliferation that leads to vascular sclerosis. Prominent, cytologically atypical en-

dothelial cells are also apparent in capillaries. In boosted areas, epithelial atypia may occur in the larger ducts of the breast and even may be superimposed on existing hyperplastic changes (Fig. 43.6) or apocrine metaplasia (Fig. 43.7).

Cytologic atypia can create diagnostic problems even if one is aware of the typical appearance of radiation-induced atrophy of the breast (38–40). False-positive fine needle aspiration (FNA) cytology diagnoses have been attributed to radiation atypia (41). In one series, the diagnostic yield with incisional or needle core biopsy was considerably higher than with aspiration cytology (29). The aspirate from a breast with radiation changes alone tends to be sparsely cellular because of treatment-induced atrophy. Filomena et al. reported that all carcinomas recurrent in radiated breasts that they diagnosed by FNA had at least five epithelial cell clusters and more than 15 single epithelial cells on the available slides (42). Usually, there were two diagnostic slides per case. Cytologic features of radiated epithelial cells were frequently extremely atypical, including nuclear enlargement, increased nuclear:cytoplasmic ratio, and prominent nucleoli. Loss of cohesion, irregular nuclear borders, and necrosis are features associated with carcinoma in this setting (43).

*In situ* lobular and intraductal carcinomas persisting after radiation therapy are largely intact so that the affected lobules and ducts are filled and often expanded with a neoplastic cell population. Comparison with the histologic appearance of the tumor and noncancerous tissue before treatment may be helpful in difficult cases. Apocrine metaplasia is sensitive to radiation effect and tends to exhibit cytologic atypia, which can be striking after radiation treatment. Knowledge that apocrine metaplasia was present in the pretreatment specimen can be helpful in correctly interpreting the posttreatment biopsy with radiation atypia in apocrine metaplasia. Frequently, little or no microscopic change attributable to treatment is evident when preradiation and postradiation samples of *in situ* carcinoma are compared (Figs. 43.8 and 43.9). From time to time,

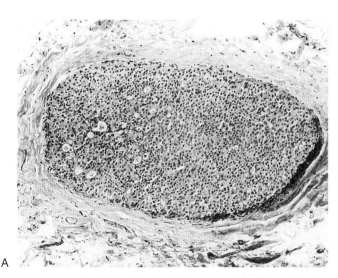

A

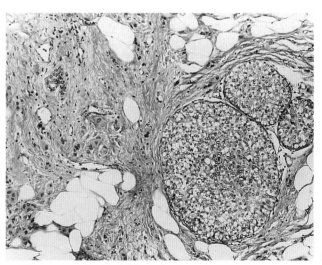

B

**FIG. 43.9.** *Intraductal carcinoma before and after radiation.* **A:** Intraductal carcinoma prior to radiotherapy. **B:** Recurrent carcinoma in the same patient 2 years after treatment. The intraductal carcinoma closely resembles the pretreatment lesion. Invasive carcinoma is present on the *left.*

radiated invasive tumor contains cells with multiple hyperchromatic nuclei or there is focal necrosis not seen in the pretreatment biopsy, and it may be suspected that these are radiation effects in residual tumor.

## CHEMOTHERAPY

Treatment-related histologic changes may be detected in mammary carcinoma and in nonneoplastic breast tissue examined after patients have received chemotherapy. Early reports described the effects of alkylating compounds on normal tissues (44). Striking cytologic atypia with the formation of giant cells is most pronounced in the epithelium of the urinary bladder and lung. Less severe cellular changes also can be found in the breast. Breast carcinomas arising during treatment with alkylating agents do not exhibit these cytologic abnormalities.

Chemotherapy effect is now most often encountered in the breast when patients with locally advanced or inflammatory carcinoma have been given high-dose systemic therapy preoperatively, so-called neoadjuvant therapy (45). The morphologic changes in the tumor are often the result of the combined effect of multiple chemotherapeutic agents, sometimes complicated by radiation therapy.

In general, the histopathologic effects of systemic chemotherapy can be correlated with the extent of clinical response. The greatest histopathologic alterations usually are found in patients who appear clinically to have complete resolution of their neoplasm (46,47). It is possible to observe dissociation between the clinical picture after therapy and the histologic findings when the patient seems to have a complete response, but histologic examination of the breast reveals a substantial amount of residual tumor. In one study of 43 patients who received preoperative chemotherapy, only about 50% of the tumors had histopathologic changes of treatment effect (48). Mammography may suggest a response in patients treated with neoadjuvant chemotherapy, but this procedure is not reliable for predicting the pathological status of the breast. Vinnicombe et al. reported that five of eight patients judged by mammography to have had a complete response had residual carcinoma pathologically (49). Magnetic resonance imaging (MRI) may be a more effective method than mammography for detecting residual carcinoma in the breast after neoadjuvant chemotherapy (50). Positron emission tomography (PET) appears to be a sensitive method for identifying patients who respond early in the course of chemotherapy treatment, but it remains to be determined whether this procedure can discriminate between patients with complete and partial response after treatment has been concluded (51,52). Placement of a clip at the tumor site is useful as a guide for following tumor regression radiographically and for locating the position of a tumor after complete regression (53).

The clinical assessment of the axillary lymph nodes after neoadjuvant chemotherapy can be difficult. Patients who have a response in the breast usually exhibit decreased clinical evidence of axillary disease, which may manifest as smaller metastases in fewer lymph nodes in the axillary dissection specimen than were present before treatment (54,55). The resultant clinical down-staging actually may suggest an absence of nodal metastases, leading to a decision not to perform an axillary dissection (56). Kuerer et al. found that ultrasonography was significantly more sensitive (62%) than physical examination (45%) for detecting persistent axillary metastases after neoadjuvant therapy (57). Physical examination, which is correct in 84% of cases, had a higher specificity than ultrasonography (70%), but the difference was not statistically significant. In this study, 55 patients with locally advanced carcinoma were considered to have negative lymph nodes when evaluated clinically and by ultrasonography. Histologic examination revealed nodal metastases in 29 of the 55 patients after axillary dissection. Metastases were found in either one to three lymph nodes or were limited to foci 2 to 5 mm in diameter in 28 of these cases.

Usually, similar chemotherapy effects are found in the primary tumor and in axillary nodal metastases from inflammatory or locally advanced carcinoma. When no residual tumor is detectable grossly in the breast, about 60% of patients are found to have persistent carcinoma histologically. Prognosis is related to the completeness of response and appears to be especially favorable at 5 years in patients with the least evidence of tumor in the breast after therapy. Feldman et al. reported a 93% 5-year survival in patients with no gross tumor in the breast or axillary lymph nodes compared with a 30% 5-year survival in those with grossly evident residual tumor (47). Others found a 5-year disease-free survival of 87% after complete clinical regression and 65% when regression was incomplete (58).

A study of 372 patients with locally advanced breast carcinoma found that 60 patients (16%) had a complete pathologic tumor response after neoadjuvant therapy and that 43 (12%) had no histologic evidence of carcinoma in the breast or axillary nodes (56). There was a significant correlation between complete pathologic response in the tumor and in the axillary lymph nodes. Factors predictive of complete pathologic response were poorly differentiated nuclear grade, negative estrogen receptors and anaplastic or poorly differentiated histologic grade. Patients with a complete pathologic response had significantly better 5-year overall and disease-free survival rates (89% and 87%, respectively) than those with a partial pathologic response (64% and 58%, respectively).

Residual carcinoma may be detected by cytokeratin immunohistochemistry in lymph nodes that appear to show complete histologic response in routine histologic sections. Kuerer et al. studied 191 patients with locally advanced carcinoma treated with neoadjuvant chemotherapy after axillary metastases were documented by FNA (55). Routine histologic sections of lymph nodes obtained in axillary dissections after treatment revealed no metastases in 43

(23%). Factors associated with conversion to negative nodal status were estrogen receptor-negative tumors and complete pathologic response in the primary tumor. The 5-year disease-free survival was 87% for patients with histologically negative nodes and 51% for those with residual nodal disease. Cytokeratin immunostaining of histologically negative lymph nodes in 39 cases revealed occult micrometastases in four cases (10%). Patients without occult micrometastases had a better 5-year disease-free survival (87%) than those with occult metastases (75%).

The histologic effects of chemotherapy can be appreciated most easily by comparing samples taken before and after treatment. The fundamental manifestation of treatment effect is a decrease in tumor cellularity (Fig. 43.10). In the most extreme situation, no residual carcinoma may be detectable, an occurrence reported in 6.7% (47) and 10% (59) of cases. If the breast of a patient who has a complete histologic and clinical response is examined histologically soon after treatment, residual degenerated and infarcted necrotic

invasive carcinoma may be recognized by the loss of normal staining properties and decreased architectural detail. With the passage of time, the degenerated invasive carcinoma is absorbed. Healed sites of previous infiltrating carcinoma may be appreciated because of residual architectural distortion characterized by fibrosis, stromal edema, increased vascularity composed largely of thin-walled vessels, and a chronic inflammatory cell infiltrate (Fig. 43.10) (60). Fibrosis and atrophy of lymphoid tissue are characteristic features of chemotherapy effect at sites of metastatic carcinoma in lymph nodes (61) (Figs. 43.11 and 43.12).

There is some evidence that foci of intraductal carcinoma and lymphatic tumor emboli may be relatively more resistant to treatment than invasive carcinoma. In a minority of instances, the only residual carcinoma found after complete clinical response is in one or both of these sites. Sharkey et al. reported finding "unusually prominent intraductal and/or intralymphatic tumor" in 40% of specimens obtained after preoperative doxorubicin/cyclophosphamide consistent with

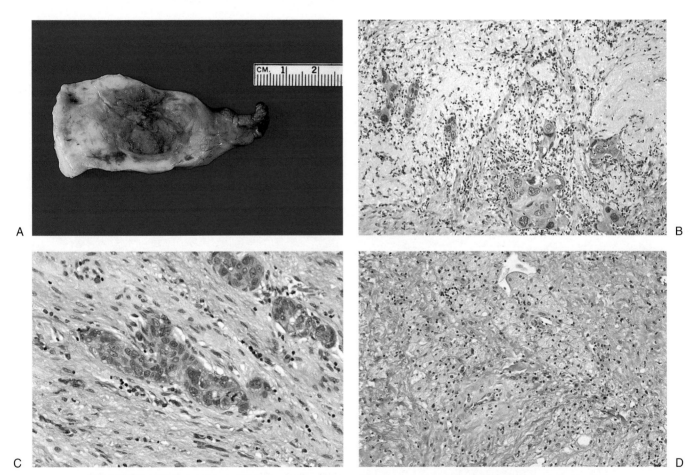

**FIG. 43.10.** *Chemotherapy effect.* **A:** This excisional biopsy performed after neoadjuvant therapy reveals a persistent 2-cm mass. Before treatment, the carcinoma measured nearly 5 cm. **B:** Residual invasive carcinoma and stromal elastosis that has replaced tumor destroyed by the treatment. Carcinoma cells that remain have large vesicular and pleomorphic nuclei. **C:** Residual carcinoma after chemotherapy showing mitotic activity and modest cytologic atypia. **D:** Complete histologic response characterized by histiocytes, elastosis, inflammation, and fibrosis.

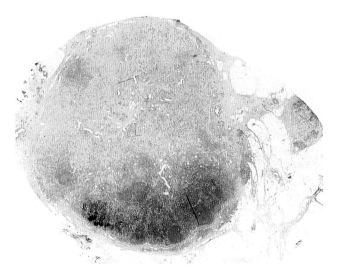

**FIG. 43.11.** *Postchemotherapy fibrosis in a lymph node.* Much of the lymph node architecture is effaced by fibrosis in the area occupied by metastatic carcinoma.

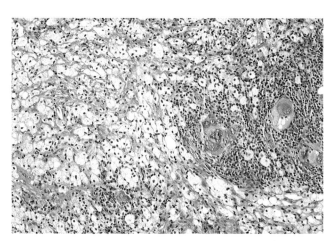

**FIG. 43.12.** *Postchemotherapy effect, lymph node.* Small groups of carcinoma cells with pleomorphic nuclei persist in this lymph node where most of the tumor, destroyed by treatment, has been replaced by histiocytes. This is from the case shown in Fig. 43.10 **A** and **B**.

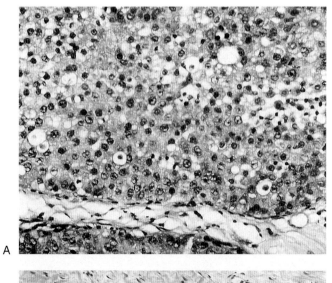

A

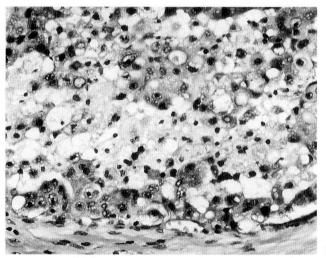

B

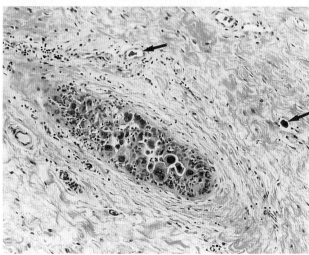

C

**FIG. 43.13.** *Chemotherapy effect in intraductal carcinoma.* **A:** Pretreatment intraductal carcinoma. **B:** Persistent intraductal carcinoma after chemotherapy showing necrosis and cytologic atypia. **C:** Marked epithelial atypia is shown in this intraductal carcinoma after chemotherapy. Clusters of carcinoma cells are present in lymphatic spaces *(arrows).*

relative resistance of carcinoma in these tissue compartments (48).

Residual intraductal and invasive carcinoma cells can appear morphologically unaltered after neoadjuvant therapy, but in most cases they exhibit cytologic changes that reflect treatment effect (46,58). The effects may be more pronounced after combined chemoradiotherapy than following either form of treatment alone (62). The cells are enlarged because of increased cytoplasmic volume (Figs. 43.10, 43.13, and 43.14). The cytoplasm often contains vacuoles or eosinophilic granules (61). Cellular borders are typically well defined, and the cells tend to shrink away from the stroma. Some carcinoma cells feature enlargement, pleomorphism, and hyperchromasia of nuclei (45). Multinucleated cells and abnormal mitotic figures are not conspicuous chemotherapy effects. The altered carcinoma cells may resemble histiocytes, especially when present individually, but they retain immunohistochemical reactivity for cytokeratin and epithelial membrane antigen.

Aneuploid carcinomas are more likely than diploid tumors to exhibit histologic and cytologic changes resulting from chemotherapy (46). The effect of chemotherapy on tumor cell proliferation as measured with the Ki67 antibody and mitotic counts is variable (45). Proliferative rates may be increased, decreased, or remain unchanged. A tendency to increased immunoreactivity for p53 and HER2/neu oncogenes after chemotherapy has been reported (45). Carcinomas that were not immunoreactive before therapy may become positive after treatment, or expression of the marker may be enhanced in the posttherapy specimen. An analysis comparing the components of histologic grading in a small series of prechemotherapy and postchemotherapy specimens did not reveal significant differences in nuclear pleomorphism, tubule formation, or mitotic count (59). Others reported that nuclear grade was increased in 32% of cases (48). Because the cytologic effects of chemotherapy on the appearance of carcinoma cell nuclei are not clearly correlated with differentiation in a clinically meaningful way, grading of treated carcinomas may not be predictive of prognosis after chemotherapy. Molecular changes in p53 reflected in loss of heterozygosity have been reported in tumors after neoadjuvant chemotherapy with increased immunoreactivity for p53 and HER2/neu in tumor and normal tissue (63).

Nonneoplastic breast parenchyma also is altered following cytotoxic chemotherapy, but the changes are more subtle than those induced in the tumor. The glandular elements undergo diffuse atrophy, causing a reduction in the number of lobules and in the size of existing lobules (48,61,64). Cytologic atypia may be seen in duct and lobular epithelial cells, but in many cases these changes are not attributable specifically to treatment effect. Comparison with a pretreatment specimen is particularly helpful in this situation and in the interpretation of aspiration cytology specimens. Regressive changes may also be found in the lymphoid tissue of axillary lymph nodes (48).

## HORMONE TREATMENT EFFECT

Estrogens and androgens have been used to treat mammary carcinoma for approximately 50 years. In 1949, Adair et al. (65) described the pathologic effects of sex steroid hormones, noting that changes in the tumor tissue attributed to treatment consisted of "degenerative changes in the nucleus and cytoplasm of the cancer cells and fibroblastic proliferation and sclerosis of the connective tissue." It also was observed that the vaginal mucosa exhibited cytologic changes of maturation in response to estrogen, whereas androgens caused atrophy. Similar effects of hormones on breast carcinoma were illustrated by Taylor et al. (66). Watson and Fetterman were unable to detect changes attributable to testosterone in two cases that underwent biopsy before and after treatment (67). Coincidentally, Lowenhaupt and Steinbach reported that low-grade carcinomas were more likely to respond to treatment with estrogens (68). Godwin and Escher concluded that fibrosis and cytoplasmic vacuolization appeared to be more prominent in some hormone-treated cases, but the changes were not regarded as specific (69).

The results of a detailed examination of the effects of therapeutic doses of estrogen on noncancerous mammary glandular tissue were reported by Huseby and Thomas in 1954 (70). In postmenopausal women, normal breast epithelium was stimulated to proliferate with the elongation of small terminal ducts and the formation of lobules. Epithelial changes were accompanied by the accumulation of interlobular connective tissue. These investigators also commented "that the reaction to estrogen administration of certain abnormal, but nonmalignant, epithelial structures was one of proliferation and thus more like that of the normal breast epithelium than like that of the cancerous epithelium." The clinical and pathologic responses of the carcinomas to treatment did not correlate with the extent or degree of change that occurred in normal breast tissue because it was observed that two pa-

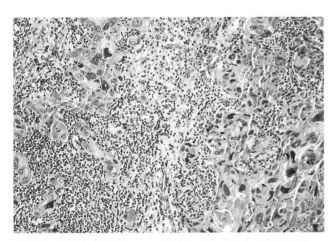

**FIG. 43.14.** *Chemotherapy effect in invasive carcinoma.* The tumor cells have extremely pleomorphic nuclei. Some nuclei are hyperchromatic or have nucleoli. Note focal necrosis in the tumor *(lower right)*.

tients with "excellent regressions of breast cancer" showed "no evidence of stimulation of the normal breast epithelium."

Further studies of the morphologic changes associated with tumor regression in hormone-treated patients were reported by Emerson et al. (71). They confirmed the observation that low-grade tumors were more likely to respond to treatment and also noted that the duration of regression was longer. Apparently viable tumor cells were found in mammary lymphatics of patients whose primary tumors were undergoing regression. Persistent intraductal carcinoma also was noted in some of these cases. These findings suggest that tumor cells at these sites might be less responsive or that they may be exposed to less effective levels of hormone.

Epidemiologic studies have shown that an antiestrogen such as tamoxifen can be effective in reducing the frequency of breast carcinoma in high-risk women. This conclusion is based in part on the reduced occurrence of contralateral carcinoma among breast carcinoma patients who received adjuvant tamoxifen therapy. Further evidence has come from a prospective randomized clinical trial involving women at high risk of developing carcinoma with a strong positive family history or a biopsy that demonstrated atypical hyperplasia or lobular carcinoma in situ (72).

The effects of tamoxifen on normal breast tissue have received little attention. Walker et al. examined tissues from breast carcinoma patients treated with tamoxifen for 4 days to 3 weeks before surgery and observed increased immunoreactivity for estrogen receptor in ductal and lobular epithelium compared with untreated normals (73). This effect did not appear to be influenced by the duration of treatment. No differences in immunoreactivity for progesterone receptor, epidermal growth factor receptor, and Ki67 were found. These investigators did not describe histologic findings associated with tamoxifen beyond the immunohistochemical results.

## REFERENCES

### Radiation

1. Boice JD, Manson RR, Rosenstein M. Breast cancer in women after repeated fluoroscopic examinations of the chest. *J Natl Cancer Inst* 1977;159:823–832.
2. Hildreth NG, Shore RE, Dvoretsky PM. The risk of breast cancer after irradiation of the thymus in infancy. *N Engl J Med* 1989;321:1281–1284.
3. Anderson N, Lokich J. Bilateral breast cancer after cured Hodgkin's disease. *Cancer* 1990;65:221–223.
4. O'Brien PC, Barton MB, Fisher R, for Australian Radiation Oncology Lymphoma Group (AROLG). Breast cancer following treatment for Hodgkin's disease: the need for screening in a young population. *Australas Radiol* 1995;39:271–276.
5. Yahalom J, Petrek JA, Biddinger PW, et al. Breast cancer in patients irradiated for Hodgkin's disease: a clinical and pathological study of 45 events in 37 patients. *J Clin Oncol* 1992;10:1674–1681.
6. Bhatia S, Robison LL, Oberlin O, et al. Breast cancer and other second neoplasms after childhood Hodgkin's disease. *N Engl J Med* 1996;334:745–751.
7. Little MP, Boice JDJ. Comparison of breast cancer incidence in the Massachusetts tuberculosis fluoroscopy cohort and in the Japanese

8. Ullrich RL. Risks for radiation-induced breast cancer: the debate continues. *Radiat Res* 1999;151:123–124.
9. Cutuli B. Radiation-induced breast cancer after treatment for Hodgkin's disease. *J Clin Oncol* 1998;16:2285–2287.
10. Cutuli B, Dhermain F, Borel C, et al. Breast cancer in patients treated for Hodgkin's disease: clinical and pathological analysis of 76 cases in 63 patients. *Eur J Cancer* 1997;33:2315–2320.
11. Hancock SL, Tucker MA, Hoppe RT. Breast cancer after treatment of Hodgkin's disease. *J Natl Cancer Inst* 1993;85:25–31.
12. Wolden SL, Lamborn KR, Cleary SF, et al. Second cancers following pediatric Hodgkin's disease. *J Clin Oncol* 1998;16:536–544.
13. Janjan NA, Zellmer DL. Calculated risk of breast cancer following mantle irradiation determined by measured dose. *Cancer Detect Prev* 1992;16:273–282.
14. Janjan NA, Wilson JF, Gillin M, et al. Mammary carcinoma developing after radiotherapy and chemotherapy for Hodgkin's disease. *Cancer* 1988;61:252–254.
15. Kowalski A, Smith S. Measurement of radiation dose delivered to breast tissue during mantle field irradiation for Hodgkin's disease. *Med Dosim* 1998;23:31–36.
16. Wolden SL, Hancock SL, Carlson RW, et al. Management of breast cancer after Hodgkin's disease. *J Clin Oncol* 2000;18:765–772.
17. Karasek K, Deutsch M. Lumpectomy and breast irradiation for breast cancer after radiotherapy for lymphoma. *Am J Clin Oncol* 1996;19:451–454.
18. Dvoretsky PM, Woodard E, Bonfiglio TA, et al. The pathology of breast cancer in women irradiated for acute postpartum mastitis. *Cancer* 1980;46:2257–2262.
19. Poeze M, von Meyenfeldt MF, Peterse JL, et al. Increased proliferative activity and p53 expression in normal glandular breast tissue after radiation therapy. *J Pathol* 1998;185:32–37.
20. Obedian E, Fischer DB, Haffty BG. Second malignancies after treatment of early-stage breast cancer: lumpectomy and radiation therapy versus mastectomy. *J Clin Oncol* 2000;18:2400–2412.
21. Pierquin B, Grimard L, Marinello G. Normal-tissue tolerance in the irradiation of female breast. In: Vaerth JM, Meyer JL, eds. *Tolerance of normal tissues.* Basel: Karger, 1989:341–348.
22. Higgins S, Haffty BG. Pregnancy and lactation after breast-conserving therapy for early stage breast cancer. *Cancer* 1994;73:2175–2180.
23. Varsos G, Yahalom J. Lactation following conservation surgery and radiotherapy for breast cancer. *J Surg Oncol* 1991;46:141–144.
24. Ryu J, Yahalom J, Shank B, et al. Radiation therapy after breast augmentation or reconstruction in early or recurrent breast cancer. *Cancer* 1990;66:844–847.
25. Robertson JM, Clark DH, Pevzner MM, et al. Breast conservation therapy: severe breast fibrosis after radiation therapy in patients with collagen vascular disease. *Cancer* 1991;68:502–508.
26. Holli K, Saaristo R, Isola J, et al. Effect of radiotherapy on the interpretation of routine follow-up mammography after conservative breast surgery: a randomized study. *Br J Cancer* 1998;78:542–545.
27. Dershaw DD, Shank B, Reisinger S. Mammographic findings after breast cancer treatment with local excision and definitive irradiation. *Radiology* 1987;164:445–461.
28. Solin LJ, Fowble BL, Troupin RH, et al. Biopsy results of new calcifications in the postirradiated breast. *Cancer* 1989;63:1956–1961.
29. Solin LJ, Fowble BL, Schultz DJ, et al. The detection of local recurrence after definitive irradiation for early stage carcinoma of the breast: an analysis of the results of breast biopsies performed in previously irradiated breasts. *Cancer* 1990;65:2497–2502.
30. Girling AC, Hanby AM, Millis RR. Radiation and other pathological changes in breast tissue after conservation treatment for carcinoma. *J Clin Pathol* 1990;43:152–156.
31. Rebner M, Pennes DR, Adler DD, et al. Breast microcalcifications after lumpectomy and radiation therapy. *Radiology* 1989;170:691–693.
32. Davis SP, Stomper PC, Weidner N, et al. Suture calcification mimicking recurrence in the irradiated breast: a potential pitfall in mammographic evaluation. *Radiology* 1989;172:247–248.
33. Clarke D, Curtis JL, Martinez A, et al. Fat necrosis of the breast simulating recurrent carcinoma after primary radiotherapy in the management of early breast cancer. *Cancer* 1983;52:442–445.
34. Rostom AY, El-Sayed ME. Fat necrosis of the breast: an unusual complication of lumpectomy and radiotherapy in breast cancer. *Clin Radiol* 1987;38:31.
35. Stomper PC, Recht A, Berenberg AL, et al. Mammographic detection

of recurrent cancer in the irradiated breast. *AJR Am J Roentgenol* 1987;148:39–43.

36. Schnitt SJ, Connolly JL, Harris JR, et al. Radiation-induced changes in the breast. *Hum Pathol* 1984;15:545–550.

37. Brouty-Boyè D, Raux H, Azzarone B, et al. Fetal myofibroblast-like cells isolated from post-radiation fibrosis in human breast cancer. *Int J Cancer* 1991;47:697–702.

38. Pedio G, Landolt V, Zobeli L. Irradiated benign cells of the breast: a potential diagnostic pitfall in fine needle aspiration cytology. *Acta Cytol* 1989;32:127–128.

39. Bondeson L. Aspiration cytology of radiation-induced changes of normal breast epithelium. *Acta Cytol* 1987;31:309–310.

40. Peterse JL, Thunnissen FBJM, van Heerde P. Fine needle aspiration cytology or radiation-induced changes in non-neoplastic breast lesions: possible pitfalls in cytodiagnosis. *Acta Cytol* 1989;33:176–180.

41. Dornfield JM, Thompson SK, Shurbaji MS. Radiation-induced changes in the breast: a potential diagnostic pitfall on fine-needle aspiration. *Diagn Cytopathol* 1992;8:79–81.

42. Filomena CA, Jordan AG, Ehya H. Needle aspiration cytology of the irradiated breast. *Diagn Cytopathol* 1992;8:327–332.

43. Peterse JL, Koolman-Schellekens MA, van de Peppel-van de Ham T, et al. Atypia in fine-needle aspiration cytology of the breast: a histologic follow-up study of 301 cases. *Semin Diagn Pathol* 1989;6:126–134.

## Chemotherapy

44. Nelson BM, Andrews GA. Breast cancer and cytologic dysplasia in many organs after busulfan. *Am J Clin Pathol* 1964;43:37–44.

45. Rasbridge SA, Gillett CE, Seymour A-M, et al. The effects of chemotherapy on morphology, cellular proliferation, apoptosis and oncoprotein expression in primary breast carcinoma. *Br J Cancer* 1994;70:335–341.

46. Brifford M, Spyratos F, Tubiana-Huhn M, et al. Sequential cytopunctures during pre-operative chemotherapy for primary breast cancer. *Cancer* 1989;63:631–637.

47. Feldman LD, Hortobagyi GN, Buzdar AU, et al. Pathological assessment of response to induction chemotherapy in breast cancer. *Cancer Res* 1986;46:2578–2581.

48. Sharkey FE, Addington SL, Fowler LJ, et al. Effects of preoperative chemotherapy on the morphology of resectable breast carcinoma. *Mod Pathol* 1996;9:893–900.

49. Vinnicombe SJ, MacVicar AD, Guy RL, et al. Primary breast cancer: mammographic changes after neoadjuvant chemotherapy, with pathologic correlation. *Radiology* 1996;198:333–340.

50. Abraham DC, Jones RC, Jones SE, et al. Evaluation of neoadjuvant chemotherapeutic response of locally advanced breast cancer by magnetic resonance imaging. *Cancer* 1996;78:91–100.

51. Schelling M, Avril N, Nährig J, et al. Positron emission tomography using [$^{18}$F]-fluorodeoxy-D-glucose for monitoring primary chemotherapy in breast cancer. *J Clin Oncol* 2000;18:1689–1695.

52. Smith IC, Welch AE, Hutcheon AW, et al. Positron emission tomography using [$^{18}$F]-fluorodeoxy-D-glucose to predict the pathologic response of breast cancer to primary chemotherapy. *J Clin Oncol* 2000;18:1676–1688.

53. Baron LF, Baron PL, Ackerman SJ, et al. Sonographically guided clip placement facilitates localization of breast cancer after neoadjuvant chemotherapy. *AJR Am J Roentgenol* 2000;174:539–540.

54. Lenert JT, Vlastos G, Mirza NQ, et al. Primary tumor response to induction chemotherapy as a predictor of histological status of axillary nodes in operable breast cancer patients. *Ann Surg Oncol* 1999;6:762–767.

55. Kuerer HM, Sahin AA, Hunt KK, et al. Incidence and impact of documented eradication of breast cancer axillary lymph node metastases before surgery in patients treated with neoadjuvant chemotherapy. *Ann Surg* 1999;230:72–78.

56. Kuerer HM, Newman LA, Smith TL, et al. Clinical course of breast cancer patients with complete pathologic primary tumor and axillary lymph node response to doxorubicin-based neoadjuvant chemotherapy. *J Clin Oncol* 1999;17:460–469.

57. Kuerer HM, Newman LA, Fornage BD, et al. Role of axillary lymph node dissection after tumor downstaging with induction chemotherapy for locally advanced breast cancer. *Ann Surg Oncol* 1998;5:673–680.

58. McCready DR, Hortobagyi GN, Kau SW, et al. The prognostic significance of lymph node metastases after preoperative chemotherapy for locally advanced breast cancer. *Arch Surg* 1989;124:21–25.

59. Frierson Jr HF, Fechner RE. Histologic grade of locally advanced infiltrating ductal carcinoma after treatment with induction chemotherapy. *Am J Clin Pathol* 1994;102:154–157.

60. Addington S, Sharkey L, Fowler C, et al. Effects of preoperative chemotherapy on the morphology of resectable breast carcinoma. *Lab Invest* 1994;70:12A.

61. Aktepe F, Kapucuoglu N, Pak I. The effects of chemotherapy on breast cancer tissue in locally advanced breast cancer. *Histopathology* 1996;29:63–67.

62. Rilke F, Veronesi U, Luini A, et al. Preoperative chemotherapy alone and combined with preoperative radiotherapy in small-size breast cancer. *Breast J* 1996;2:176–180.

63. Merino MJ, San't Ambrogio S, Bryant B, et al. Genetic alterations of tumoral and non-tumoral breast tissues after chemotherapy treatment. *Mod Pathol* 2000;13:27A.

64. Kennedy S, Merino MJ, Swain SM, et al. The effects of hormonal and chemotherapy on tumoral and non-neoplastic breast tissue. *Hum Pathol* 1990;21:192–198.

## Hormone Treatment Effect

65. Adair FE, Mellors RC, Farrow JH, et al. The use of estrogens and androgens in advanced mammary cancer: clinical and laboratory study of one hundred and five female patients. *JAMA* 1949;140:1193–1200.

66. Taylor SG III, Slaughter DP, Smejkal W, et al. The effect of sex hormones on advanced carcinoma of the breast. *Cancer* 1948;1:604–617.

67. Watson JR, Fetterman, GH. Testosterone propionate in the treatment of advanced carcinoma of the breast. *Surg Gynecol Obstet* 1949;88:702–710.

68. Lowenhaupt E, Steinbach HL. Clinical response of metastatic lesions of carcinoma of the female breast to hormonal therapy as related to histologic grade of malignancy. *Surg Gynecol Obstet* 1949;88:291–294.

69. Godwin JT, Escher GC. Hormone-treated primary operable breast carcinoma. A pathological study of thirty-three cases. *Cancer* 1951;4:136–140.

70. Huseby RA, Thomas LB. Histological and histochemical alterations in the normal breast tissues of patients with advanced breast cancer being treated with estrogenic hormones. *Cancer* 1954;7:54–74.

71. Emerson WJ, Kennedy BJ, Taft EB. Correlation of histological alterations in breast cancer with response to hormone therapy. *Cancer* 1960;13:1047–1052.

72. Fisher B, Costantino JP, Wickerham DL, et al. Tamoxifen for prevention of breast cancer: report of the National Surgical Adjuvant Breast and Bowel Project P-1 Study. *J Natl Cancer Inst* 1998;90:1371–1388.

73. Walker KJ, Price-Thomas JM, Candlish W, et al. Influence of the antiestrogen tamoxifen on normal breast tissue. *Br J Cancer* 1991;64:764–768.

## CHAPTER 44

# Cutaneous Neoplasms

## MALIGNANT MELANOMA AND MELANOCYTIC LESIONS OF THE MAMMARY SKIN AND BREAST

Malignant melanoma of the skin of the breast occurs more often in men than in women (1–4). Patients have been 16 to 72 years of age, with the average age of women in their midthirties and men in their forties. Any region may be affected but origin in the nipple–areola complex is relatively uncommon (5).

Approximately two-thirds of lesions arise medial to the midclavicular line or in the central region. Metastases occur in axillary lymph nodes in about 50% of patients, and this is more likely to occur with a lateral than with a medial lesion. Supraclavicular lymph node metastases derive from tumors of the infraclavicular region or the upper half of the breast. Internal mammary lymph node metastases were not found in 20 patients subjected to dissection of these nodes (2,3). Only 6 of 16 patients with widely disseminated malignant melanoma at autopsy had metastases in internal mammary lymph nodes (3). The frequency of regional lymph node involvement and 5-year disease-free survival are inversely related to the thickness of the primary lesion as determined by Clark's level of invasion (3).

There is no predilection for any histologic type of malignant melanoma to arise in the skin of the breast. Nodular, superficial spreading, and ulcerated lesions have been described. An antecedent nevus is suggested clinically in many cases when the patient reports a recent change in a longstanding pigmented lesion, and this often is confirmed histologically. Some patients with malignant melanoma of the nipple or areola report change in an existing "mole," but in most cases, a new pigmented lesion is described (5). Origin of a malignant melanoma of the mammary skin at the site of a tattoo has been described (6).

The histologic diagnosis of malignant melanoma of the skin of the breast is based on the same criteria used to assess nonmammary cutaneous lesions. Malignant melanoma of the nipple–areola complex presents a special problem. The presence of melanin pigment is not sufficient to distinguish malignant melanoma from Paget's disease because Paget's cells

may acquire such pigment (7,8). This phenomenon is not a unique property of the skin, having been described in other epithelial tissues such as the oral mucosa and minor salivary glands (9), and in an anorectal adenocarcinoma (10). Melanin pigmentation of carcinoma cells also can occur when the primary tumor extends to the epidermis and at sites of cutaneous metastases of mammary carcinoma (11,12) or in locally recurrent carcinoma at the site of a mastectomy (13). The presence of intraductal or invasive carcinoma or both in the breast (14) and reactivity for one or more epithelial markers such as cytokeratin, epithelial membrane antigen, or mucin are convincing evidence for Paget's disease rather than melanoma. Malignant melanoma is S-100 positive in virtually all instances, and it is usually reactive for HMB-45, but not for HER2/*neu*, which stains more than 90% of Paget's disease. A strongly positive S-100 stain is suggestive of malignant melanoma, but confirmatory evidence is necessary to confidently establish the diagnosis (Fig. 44.1).

The prognosis of malignant melanoma of the mammary skin or nipple–areola complex depends on the stage at diagnosis. In the largest series, about 60% of all patients remained disease free 5 years after treatment. When axillary lymph nodes were uninvolved, the 5-year disease-free survival was nearly 90%, and it dropped to about 25% when there were axillary nodal metastases (3). When stratified by stage, no significant differences in the outcome were found between men and women or between patients with medial and lateral lesions.

Most patients in retrospective series were treated by mastectomy and axillary dissection regardless of the location of the primary lesion. Although mastectomy might be necessary in some cases, many patients can be treated by wide excision that may include some underlying breast parenchyma (3,4). Origin in the nipple–areola complex is not considered a contraindication to wide excision if a cosmetically acceptable result can be obtained (5). Axillary dissection, when performed, should include the tail of Spence to ensure excision of all lymph nodes. Sentinel lymph node mapping is presently a reliable method for assessing the axilla in patients with malignant melanoma of the mammary skin.

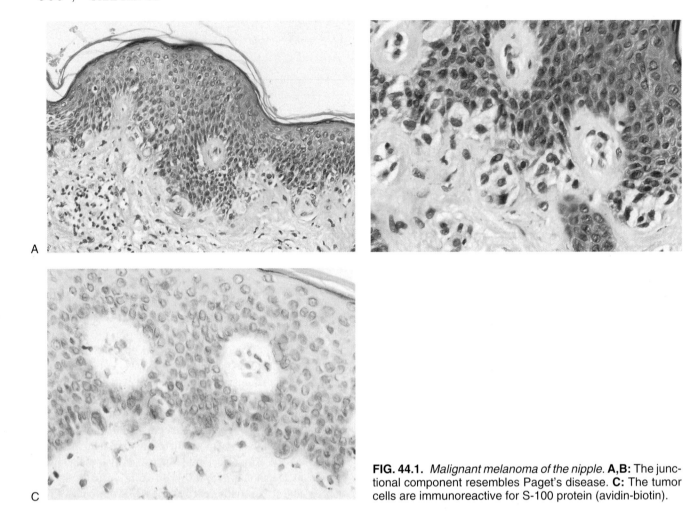

FIG. 44.1. *Malignant melanoma of the nipple.* **A,B:** The junctional component resembles Paget's disease. **C:** The tumor cells are immunoreactive for S-100 protein (avidin-biotin).

Pigmented melanocytic lesions of the mammary parenchyma are very uncommon. Blue nevi have been found in the breast (Fig. 44.2) and they may be associated with axillary lymph nodes (see Chapter 45). An exceedingly unusual example of a cellular blue nevus of the breast has been studied by the author (Fig. 44.3). The lesion was identical to cellular blue nevi described by Rodriquez and Ackerman in a series that included two tumors of the "chest and breast" (15) and to a case reported by Busam et al. (16). Malignant melanoma has arisen from cellular blue nevi in other organs and this lesion could conceivably be the substrate for primary malignant melanoma of the breast (17,18). Geschickter

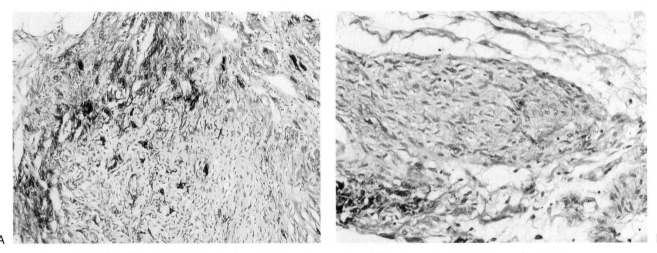

FIG. 44.2. *Blue nevus of the breast.* **A:** A heavily pigmented blue nevus found in the breast. **B:** The lesion was associated with a nerve.

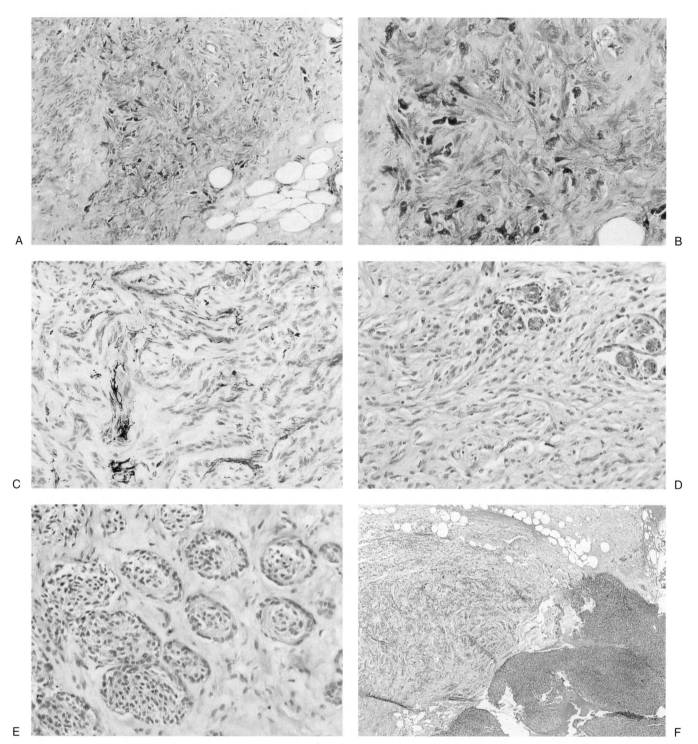

**FIG. 44.3.** *Cellular blue nevus of the breast.* **A,B:** A portion of the lesion was composed of heavily pigmented spindle cells. **C:** The pigment was black with the Fontana-Masson stain. **D:** The spindle cell portion of the tumor invaded mammary glandular parenchyma. **E:** Alveolar nests were formed by the spindle cells. **F:** The cellular portion of the tumor on the *right* contrasts sharply with the blue nevus component. *(continued)*

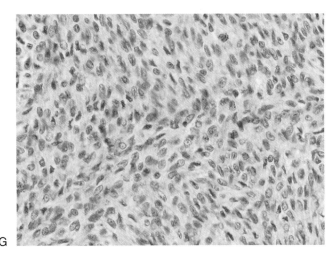
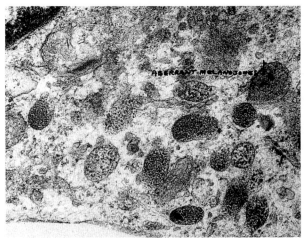

G

H

**FIG. 44.3.** *Continued.* **G:** In the cellular region, the cells have oval nuclei, inconspicuous nucleoli, and few mitoses. **H:** Electron microscopy revealed aberrant melanosomes. (**H:** Courtesy of Dr. R. A. Erlandson.)

referred to a malignant mammary tumor with melanin pigment as a melanosarcoma (19).

Primary malignant melanoma of the breast parenchyma has been reported, but the precise nature of these lesions has not been well documented, and they could be further instances of melanocytic differentiation in carcinomas (20–22). Two of these patients died within a year of detection of the breast lesion, with widespread metastatic melanoma leaving considerable doubt as to the primary site (20,22). A third patient had a solitary metastasis in the ileum resected 3 years after mastectomy for the melanocytic breast lesion, and she remained well 14 years after mastectomy (21). An intriguing aspect of the later case is the notation that the patient was aware of the breast tumor for 2 years and that "it has grown steadily" before she presented for treatment. The microscopic description does not mention any nevus-like features in the primary lesion. Before a diagnosis of primary malignant melanoma of the breast can be established with confidence, an extramammary malignant melanoma that could be the source of a metastasis in the breast should be excluded, and a predisposing associated lesion in the breast should be identified (see Chapter 36).

The possibility that melanin pigment could be formed directly by neoplastic mammary glandular epithelium is suggested by a reported example of a "pigmented papillary carcinoma of the male breast" that arose in the subareolar region and "did not affect the overlaying skin" (23). Further evidence for aberrant or metaplastic melanocytic differentiation of an epithelial neoplasm is represented by melanin-containing mammary carcinomas, studied by the author (Fig. 44.4). Melanosomes were demonstrated in one of these tumors by electron microscopy.

Several case reports documented other examples of melanocytic metaplasia in breast carcinoma. One patient was 72 years of age when she underwent mastectomy for a T2N1 tumor with lymph node metastases documented by axillary dissection (24). The neoplasm was composed of nonpig-

mented invasive ductal carcinoma with intraductal carcinoma and an invasive heavily pigmented melanocytic component. Epithelial markers (CAM5.2 and CA19-9) were expressed only in the adenocarcinoma, whereas HMB45 and vimentin were limited to the melanocytic regions. S-100 was detected in both portions of the tumor. The pigment was stained black with the Fontana-Masson method and bleached with $KMnO_4$. Melanosomes and premelanosomes were demonstrated by electron microscopy. The patient died of metastatic tumor about 18 months after diagnosis, and at autopsy some metastases were "brown–black" grossly. No evidence of an extramammary melanoma primary was detected. Microdissected samples of intraductal and invasive ductal carcinoma from areas with melanocytic differentiation and from metastases were obtained for polymerase chain reaction-based microsatellite analysis with 37 markers. Loss of heterozygosity was detected on multiple chromosome arms, with similar patterns in all components. This result suggests that the adenocarcinomatous and melanocytic aspects of the tumor derived from a single neoplastic clone and that the genetic alterations leading to melanocytic metaplasia occurred in the *in situ* phase of the neoplasm.

Padmore et al. studied melanocytic tumors from two women, 41 and 44 years of age at diagnosis (25). The older of these patients had a 3-cm tumor and no axillary metastases. She remained disease free 1 year after mastectomy. The second patient had a 3-cm cystic tumor and two lymph nodes with metastases that exhibited carcinomatous and melanomatous features. Cells with an epithelial phenotype were immunoreactive for cytokeratin (CAM5.2) and S-100 protein, whereas reactivity for HMB45 was limited to melanin-containing spindle cells in both tumors. Ruffolo et al. described a 4-cm tumor from a 34-year-old woman treated by breast-conservation surgery (26). Metastatic carcinoma without melanomatous features involved two axillary lymph nodes. The patient died of metastases after

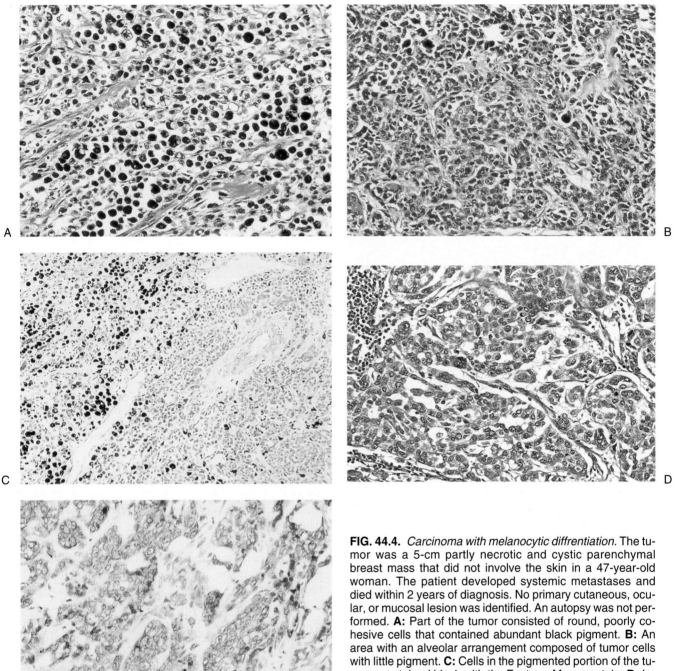

**FIG. 44.4.** *Carcinoma with melanocytic diffrentiation.* The tumor was a 5-cm partly necrotic and cystic parenchymal breast mass that did not involve the skin in a 47-year-old woman. The patient developed systemic metastases and died within 2 years of diagnosis. No primary cutaneous, ocular, or mucosal lesion was identified. An autopsy was not performed. **A:** Part of the tumor consisted of round, poorly cohesive cells that contained abundant black pigment. **B:** An area with an alveolar arrangement composed of tumor cells with little pigment. **C:** Cells in the pigmented portion of the tumor are stained black with the Fontana-Masson stain. **D:** Invasive poorly differentiated carcinoma in the tumor. **E:** The tumor cells shown in **D** were immunoreactive for cytokeratin. (AE1/AE3; avidin-biotin). (Courtesy of B. Shmookler.)

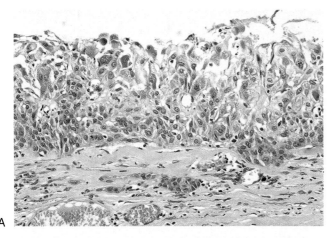

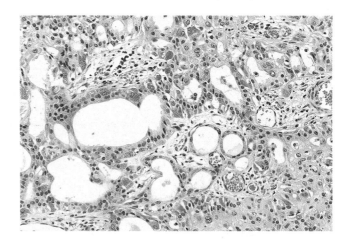

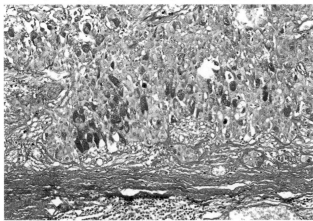

**FIG. 44.5.** *Carcinoma with lipofuscin pigment.* **A:** The cavity of the cystic tumor was lined by a thick layer of *in situ* carcinoma with apocrine and clear cell differentiation. Brown granular pigment was present in some tumor cells. **B:** Part of the tumor showing cribriform growth and pigmented cells. **C:** The brown granular pigment is stained magenta with the periodic acid-Schiff reaction. The tumor cells were reactive for cytokeratin and S-100 but not for HMB-45 or other melanocytic markers.

chemotherapy. Nonpigmented cells with an epithelial phenotype in this tumor were reactive for cytokeratin but not for S-100 or HMB45, whereas the pigmented cells stained with S-100 and HMB45.

Pigmentation suggestive of melanocytic differentiation in breast carcinoma can be encountered in other circumstances. Saitoh et al. described a pigmented tumor excised from the right nipple of a 63-year-old man (27). The tumor was located in the breast and dermis without Paget's disease of the epidermis. Histologically, the tumor was described as a ductal carcinoma infiltrated by pigment-containing dendritic cells. Immunoreactivity for S-100 and HMB45 was limited to the dendritic cells, which were not stained by markers of epithelial differentiation.

A potential source of melanin-like pigmentation is the accumulation of abundant lipofuscin in carcinoma cells (Fig. 44.5). Grossly, the tumor may appear tan or light brown, but it will not have the dark brown or black color of a melanocytic lesion (28). Cutaneous xanthogranulomatous lesions at sites other than the breast can also mimic malignant melanoma (28a).

## NONMELANOMATOUS CUTANEOUS MAMMARY TUMORS

Benign and malignant neoplasms that arise at various cutaneous sites may be found in the skin and subcutaneous tis-

sue of the breast (29). The upper medial skin of the female breasts in the "cleavage" area receives more sun exposure than other parts of the breast and may be predisposed to develop neoplasms such as basal cell carcinoma (30). Metastatic neoplasms in the mammary skin, especially carcinomas, can mimic primary cutaneous carcinomas of the breast (31).

Because the morphologic spectrum of *adnexal (sweat gland) carcinomas* is similar to that of breast carcinoma, these tumors can present a difficult problem in differential diagnosis (Figs. 44.6–44.9). Adnexal carcinomas of the mammary skin are occasionally large enough to impinge on the breast tissue, thereby obscuring origin from the skin. If it is present, the distribution of an *in situ* component can be helpful in determining the primary tissue of origin (Figs. 44.10 and 44.11). When ectopic mammary glandular tissue mingles with skin appendage glands in the dermis of the axillary skin, it is especially difficult to pinpoint the origin of a carcinoma found in these structures, even if an *in situ* element is identified.

For the most part, immunohistochemical markers give similar results in mammary and sweat gland carcinomas (Figs. 44.12 and 44.13) (32). A particularly vexing problem arises if a patient had a prior carcinoma or has a concurrent carcinoma of the mammary glandular parenchyma and adenocarcinoma in the skin of the axilla or at a distant site. Wallace et al. studied a series of skin lesions that included

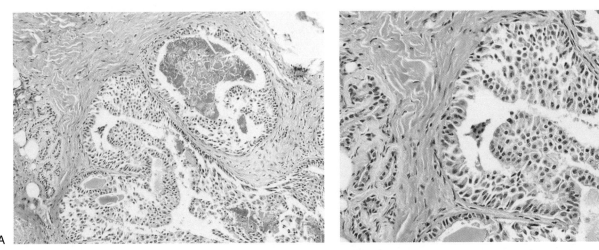

**FIG. 44.6.** *Adnexal gland carcinoma, papillary type.* **A,B:** Orderly papillary carcinoma. An uninvolved sweat gland is shown on the *left.*

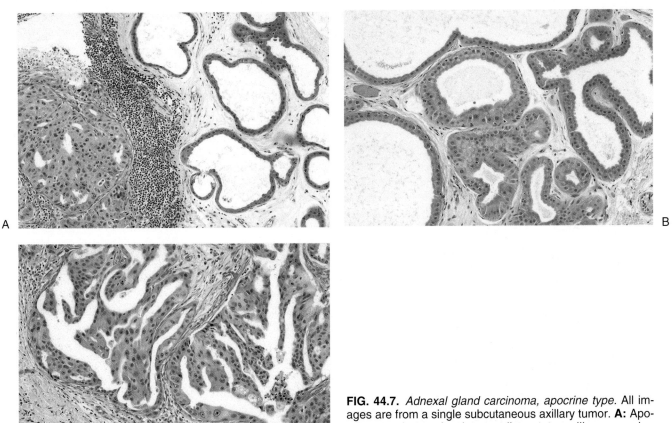

**FIG. 44.7.** *Adnexal gland carcinoma, apocrine type.* All images are from a single subcutaneous axillary tumor. **A:** Apocrine carcinoma is shown adjacent to axillary apocrine glands. **B:** Mild epithelial hyperplasia in apocrine glands. **C:** Papillary apocrine carcinoma.

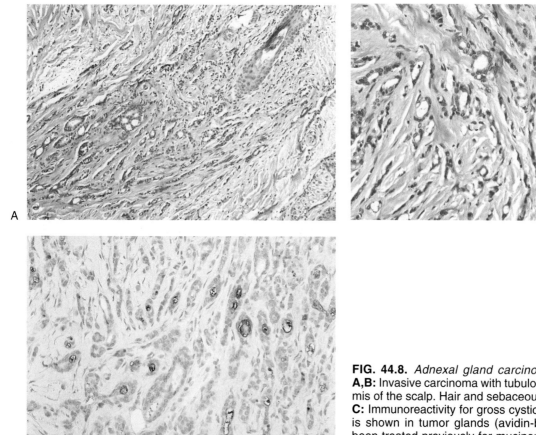

A
B
C

**FIG. 44.8.** *Adnexal gland carcinoma, tubulolobular type.*
**A,B:** Invasive carcinoma with tubulolobular growth in the dermis of the scalp. Hair and sebaceous structures are present.
**C:** Immunoreactivity for gross cystic disease fluid protein-15 is shown in tumor glands (avidin-biotin). This patient had been treated previously for mucinous mammary carcinoma. The scalp lesion was interpreted as a primary adnexal tumor.

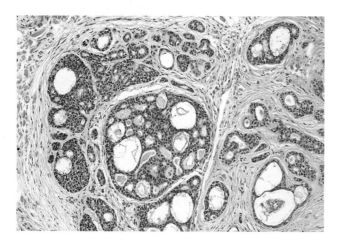

**FIG. 44.9.** *Adnexal gland carcinoma, cribriform.* This image is from a 1-cm discrete tumor in the dermis of the axillary skin.

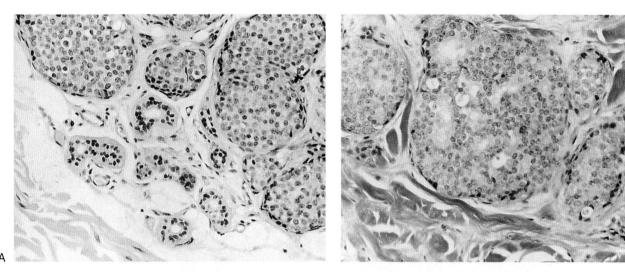

**FIG. 44.10.** *Adnexal gland carcinoma.* **A:** The *in situ* portion of this neoplasm resembles mammary lobular carcinoma *in situ*. Uninvolved sweat gland structures are shown in the *center*. **B:** The invasive component among dermal collagen fibers has a cribriform structure.

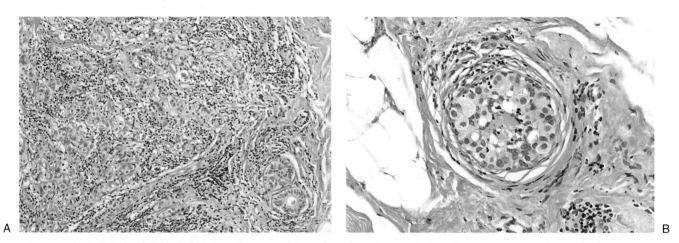

**FIG. 44.11.** *Adnexal gland carcinoma with intraductal carcinoma.* **A:** Invasive carcinoma is shown next to two skin adnexal gland structures. One of these glands has hyperplastic epithelium. **B:** Intraductal carcinoma in an adnexal gland duct.

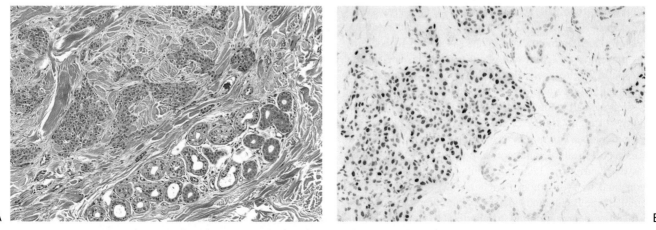

**FIG. 44.12.** *Adnexal gland carcinoma in the axillary skin.* **A:** The histologic appearance of this carcinoma shown next to a sweat gland is indistinguishable histologically from mammary carcinoma. **B:** Nuclear reactivity for estrogen receptors is present only in the carcinoma (avidin-biotin).

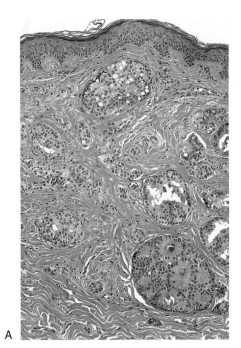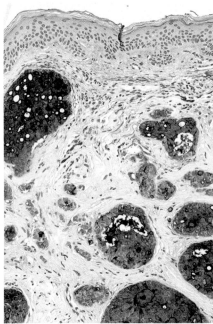

**FIG. 44.13.** *Adnexal gland carcinoma of chest wall skin.* The lesion was an 8-mm cutaneous nodule in the upper midchest. No breast tissue was present. **A:** Carcinoma, partly cribriform. Calcifications are present in the gland at the *bottom.* A trace of sebaceous differentiation is evident in the gland beneath the epidermis. **B:** The tumor was strongly reactive for gross cystic disease protein 15 (shown) as well as estrogen and progesterone receptors (not shown) (avidin-biotin).

metastatic mammary carcinoma and carcinomas of skin adnexal gland origin (33). The patterns of immunoreactivity for estrogen and progesterone receptors and gross cystic disease fluid protein-15 (GCDFP-15) were not sufficiently different to distinguish reliably between the two groups of lesions. Wick et al. detected GCDFP-15 significantly more often in breast than in eccrine sweat gland carcinoma but also reported finding GCDFP-15 reactivity in sweat gland carcinomas of apocrine type (32). In the same study, carcinoembryonic antigen was expressed more often by sweat gland than by breast carcinomas.

Busam et al. analyzed immunoreactivity of estrogen (ER) and progesterone (PR) receptors and epidermal growth factor receptor (EGF-R) in 42 primary sweat gland carcinomas and in breast carcinoma specimens (34). EGF-R reactivity was present in 81% of sweat gland carcinomas and in only 17% and 22%, respectively, of the primary and metastatic breast carcinoma samples. The expression of ER and PR in sweat gland carcinoma and breast carcinoma was not significantly different. Hanby et al. studied 12 examples of primary mucinous carcinoma of the skin and found all the tumors to be strongly immunoreactive for ER (35). PR also was detected in the 12 tumors, but staining was heterogeneous and weak in some instances. Two of the tumors resembled type B mucinous mammary carcinoma, which tends to manifest neuroendocrine differentiation. Both type B cutaneous mucinous carcinomas were argyrophilic with the Grimelius stain. The 12 tumors were also immunoreactive

for the mucous-associated peptide TFF1 but not for TFF2, and they expressed TFF1 and TFF3 mRNA. TFF1 and TFF3 of the trefoil factor family are peptides up-regulated by ER, thereby indicating the functionality of ER in these tumors.

When the differential diagnosis includes carcinoma of skin adnexal gland or mammary origin, the biopsy sample should be thoroughly examined for evidence of mammary glandular tissue and for the presence of an *in situ* component in skin appendages or breast parenchyma. In some of these situations, the distinction between primary or metastatic mammary carcinoma and sweat gland carcinoma cannot be made with absolute certainty, and a judgment must be made that takes into consideration clinical factors as well as the location and histopathology of the lesion.

The skin of the nipple gives rise on rare occasions to neoplasms that commonly develop in sun-exposed skin. About 17 examples of *basal cell carcinoma* of the nipple have been reported (36–40). Most patients were men ranging in age from 43 to 80 years (median, 60); the women ranged from 49 to 75 years of age. This sex distribution probably reflects the much greater exposure to the sun of the male breast. One woman with bilateral cutaneous lesions has been reported (40).

The lesion presents as a scaling red, eczematous condition that may have been noted by the patient for as long as 10 years before seeking medical attention. Ulceration, plaque-like thickening of the skin, and nodular lesions have been described. Occasionally, involvement extends to the areola.

Clinically, the differential diagnosis of basal cell carcinoma of the nipple includes inflammatory conditions, florid papillomatosis of the nipple, Bowen's disease, and Paget's disease. Biopsy is necessary to establish the diagnosis. Calcifications may be evident in the lesion on mammography (40a).

Microscopically, there does not appear to be a predilection for a particular type of basal cell carcinoma to arise in the nipple since various patterns have been described. Basaloid proliferation originating in the epidermis is a diagnostic feature that is accompanied by lateral growth within the dermis and the nipple stroma. Intraepithelial extension into or invasion of lactiferous ducts is sometimes observed (Fig. 44.14). Keratinization occurs in solid as well as cystic foci. Rarely, the entire tumor may exhibit basal–squamous differentiation (Fig. 44.15).

Most patients with basal cell carcinoma of the nipple have been treated successfully by wide excision occasionally supplemented by irradiation. Mastectomy may be performed when patients develop axillary nodal metastases, an event that has been reported on two occasions. In one instance, a 46-year-old man had a single lymph node metastasis detected after a mastectomy was performed for a 1.5-cm tumor (36). In the second case, axillary nodal enlargement became apparent 4 years after a basal cell carcinoma of the nipple was treated by excision and radiation. Axillary dissection revealed metastatic tumor in three lymph nodes (39).

*Nevoid hyperkeratosis* is a unilateral or bilateral condition characterized by pigmented hyperkeratotic thickening of the skin of the nipple and areola (41,42). The clinical appearance resembles acanthosis nigricans (Fig. 44.16). In some women, nevoid hyperkeratosis has been associated with pregnancy occurring in the second or third decade of life (41,43). A number of male patients developed nevoid hyperkeratosis during treatment with diethylstilbestrol for prostatic carcinoma (42,44). A patient with bilateral nevoid hyperkeratosis and generalized cutaneous T-cell lymphoma was described by Ahn et al. (45). Histologically, nevoid hyperkeratosis is characterized by papillary hyperplasia with hyperkeratosis. Basal hyperpigmentation is variably present. Treatment with topical lactic acid or retinoic acid and cryotherapy have been recommended.

Benign adnexal neoplasms found in the mammary region include *eccrine spiradenoma* and *hidradenoma* of the axillary skin (Fig. 44.17) and sebaceous adenoma of the nipple (Fig. 44.18). Tumors with the histologic appearance of *nodular hidradenoma* also have been described superficially beneath the skin or areola of the breast (Fig. 44.19) (46).

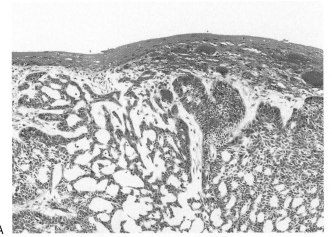
A

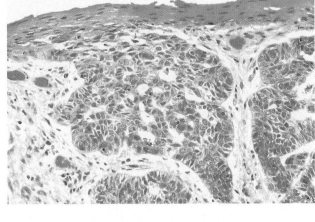
B

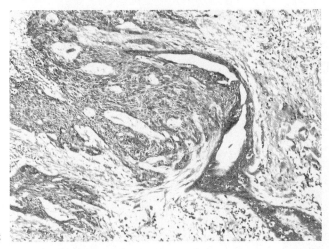
C

**FIG. 44.14.** *Basal cell carcinoma of the nipple.* **A:** Basal cell carcinoma with an adenoid pattern growing beneath the attenuated epidermis. **B:** Carcinoma attached to the epidermis. **C:** Basal cell carcinoma invading a major lactiferous duct. All images are from a single case.

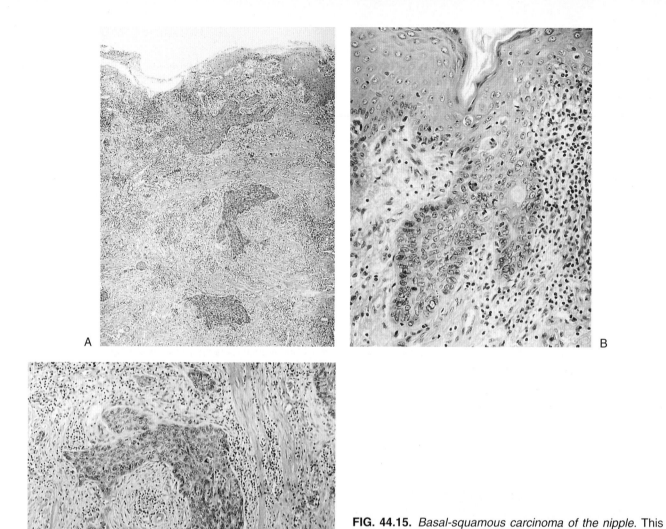

**FIG. 44.15.** *Basal-squamous carcinoma of the nipple.* This ulcerated lesion in the nipple of a woman was thought to be Paget's disease clinically. **A:** In the center of the lesion, carcinoma involves the full thickness of the epidermis and invades the stroma of the nipple. **B:** *In situ* carcinoma arising from the basal layer of the epidermis. **C:** Invasive carcinoma with squamous differentiation.

**FIG. 44.16.** *Nevoid hyperkeratosis of the areola.* **A:** The skin of the areola is thickened and focally pigmented. **B:** This biopsy from a nonpigmented area shows papillary hyperplasia of the epidermis with hyperkeratosis and a mild dermal lymphocytic reaction. The patient was 29 years of age. The skin changes were present for "several years."

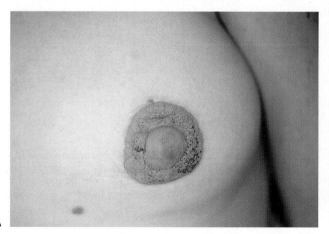

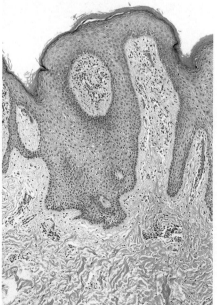

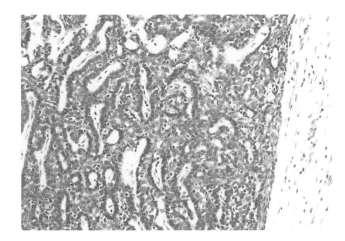

**FIG. 44.17.** *Eccrine spiradenoma of axillary skin.*

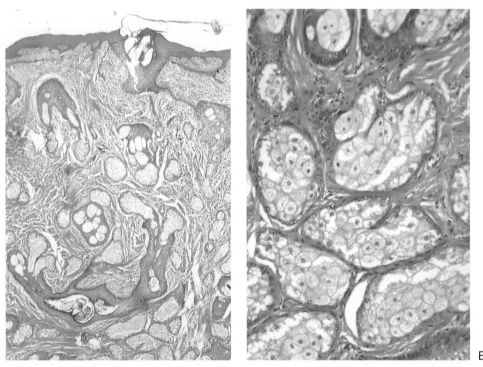

**FIG. 44.18.** *Sebaceous adenoma of the nipple.* **A,B:** A nodular tumor formed by adenomatous proliferation of sebaceous glands.

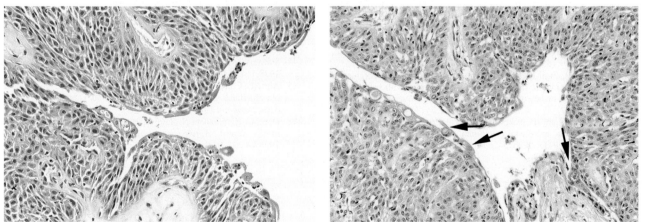

**FIG. 44.19.** *Hidradenoma, subareolar.* **A,B:** The tumor was solid and cystic. Note vacuolated superficial cells that contain mucin demonstrated with the mucicarmine stain in **B** (*arrows*).

# REFERENCES

## Malignant Melanoma and Melanocytic Lesions of the Mammary Skin and Breast

1. Jochimsen PR, Pearlman NW, Lawton RL, et al. Melanoma of skin of the breast: therapeutic considerations based on six cases. *Surgery* 1977;81:583–587.
2. Lee YTN, Sparks FC, Morton DL. Primary melanoma of skin of the breast region. *Ann Surg* 1977;185:17–22.
3. Papachristou DN, Kinne DW, Rosen PP, et al. Cutaneous melanoma of the breast. *Surgery* 1979;85:322–328.
4. Roses DF, Harris MN, Stern JS, et al. Cutaneous melanoma of the breast. *Ann Surg* 1979;189:112–115.
5. Papachristou DN, Kinne DW, Ashikari R, et al. Melanoma of the nipple and areola. *Br J Surg* 1979;66:287–288.
6. Lee Y-TN, Craig JR. Melanoma in a tattoo of the breast. *J Surg Oncol* 1984;25:100–101.
7. Sau P, Solis J, Lupton GP, et al. Pigmented breast carcinoma. A clinical and histologic simulator of malignant melanoma. *Arch Dermatol* 1989;125:536–539.
8. Culbertson JD, Horn RC. Paget's disease of the nipple: review of 25 cases with special reference to melanin pigmentation of 'Paget cells'. *Arch Surg* 1956;72:224–231.
9. Dunlap CL, Tomich CE. Melanocyte colonization of oral squamous cell carcinoma. *Oral Surg* 1981;52:524–530.
10. Chumas JC, Lorelle CA. Melanotic adenocarcinoma of the anorectum. *Am J Surg Pathol* 1981;5:711–717.
11. Azzopardi JG, Eusebi V. Melanocyte colonization and pigmentation of breast carcinoma. *Histopathology* 1977;1:21–30.
12. Poiares-Baptista A, Abreu de Vasconcelos A. Cutaneous pigmented metastasis from breast carcinoma simulating malignant melanoma. *Int J Dermatol* 1988;27:124–125.
13. Gadkari R, Pangarkar MA, Lele VR, et al. Florid melanocytic colonization in a metastasis of breast carcinoma: a case report. *Acta Cytol* 1997;41:1353–1355.
14. Fernàndez-Figueras MT, Puig L, Casanova JM, et al. Pigmented epidermotropic ductal carcinoma of the breast in a male. *J Cutan Pathol* 1995;22:176–180.
15. Rodriguez HA, Ackerman LV. Cellular blue nevus: clinicopathologic study of forty-five cases. *Cancer* 1968;21:393–405.
16. Busam KJ, Woodruff JM, Erlandson RA, et al. Large plaque-type blue nevus with subcutaneous cellular nodules. *Am J Surg Pathol* 2000;24:92–99.
17. Connelly J, Smith Jr LJ. Malignant blue nevus. *Cancer* 1991;67:2653–2657.
18. Löffler KU, Witschel H. Primary malignant melanoma of the orbit arising in a cellular blue naevus. *Br J Ophthalmol* 1989;73:388–393.
19. Geschickter CF. Mammary sarcoma. In: *Diseases of the breast: diagnosis, pathology, treatment.* 2nd ed. Philadelphia: JB Lippincott, 1943:390.
20. Bernardo MM, Mascarenbas MJ, Lopes DP. Primary malignant melanoma of the breast. *Acta Med Port* 1980;2:39–43.
21. Gatch WD. A melanoma, apparently primary in a breast. Its single known metastasis in the small bowel. *AMA Arch Surg* 1956;73:266–268.
22. Stephenson SE Jr, Byrd BF Jr. Malignant melanoma of the breast. *Am J Surg* 1959;97:232–235.
23. Romanelli R, Toncini C. Pigmented papillary carcinoma of the male breast. *Tumori* 1986;72:105–108.
24. Nobukawa B, Fujii H, Hirai S, et al. Breast carcinoma diverging to aberrant melanocytic differentiation: a case report with histopathologic and loss of heterozygosity analyses. *Am J Surg Pathol* 1999;23:1280–1287.
25. Padmore RF, Lara JF, Ackerman DJ, et al. Primary combined malignant melanoma and ductal carcinoma of the breast: a report of two cases. *Cancer* 1996;78:2515–2525.
26. Ruffolo EF, Koerner FC, Maluf HM. Metaplastic carcinoma of the breast with melanocytic differentiation. *Mod Pathol* 1997; 10: 592–596.
27. Saitoh K, Saga K, Okazaki M, et al. Pigmented primary carcinoma of the breast: a clinical mimic of malignant melanoma. *Br J Dermatol* 1998;139:287–290.
28. Shin SJ, Kanomata N, Rosen PP. Mammary carcinoma with prominent cytoplasmic lipofuscin granules mimicking melanocytic differentiation. *Histopathology* 2000;37:456–459.
28a. Busam KJ, Rosai J, Iversen KBS, et al. Xanthogranulomas with inconspicuous foam cells and giant cells mimicking malignant melanoma. *Am J Surg Pathol* 2000;24:864–869.

## Nonmelanomatous Cutaneous Mammary Tumors

29. Ilie B. Neoplasms in skin and subcutis over the breast simulating breast neoplasms: case reports and literature review. *J Surg Oncol* 1986;31:191–198.
30. Nunez M, Marques A, de las Heras E, et al. Bilateral basal cell carcinoma of the breasts in a woman. *J Dermatol* 1995;22:226–228.
31. Hajdu SI, Urban JA. Cancers metastatic to the breast. *Cancer* 1972;29:1691–1696.
32. Wick MR, Ockner DM, Mills SE, et al. Homologous carcinomas of the breast, skin, and salivary glands: a histologic and immunohistochemical comparison of ductal mammary carcinoma, ductal sweat gland carcinoma, and salivary duct carcinoma. *Am J Clin Pathol* 1998; 109:75–84.
33. Wallace ML, Longacre TA, Smoller BR. Estrogen and progesterone receptors and anti-gross cystic disease fluid protein 15 (BRST-2) fail to distinguish metastatic breast carcinoma from eccrine neoplasms. *Mod Pathol* 1995;8:897–901.
34. Busam KJ, Tan L, Granter SR, et al. Epidermal growth factor, estrogen, and progesterone receptor expression in primary sweat gland carcinomas and primary and metastatic mammary carcinomas. *Mod Pathol* 1999;12:786–793.
35. Hanby AM, McKee P, Jeffery M, et al. Primary mucinous carcinomas of the skin express TFF1, TFF3, estrogen receptor, and progesterone receptors. *Am J Surg Pathol* 1998;22:1125–1131.
36. Baker M, Kim H-K, Todd M. Basal cell carcinoma masquerading as breast cancer in a male. *Breast* 1985;11:25–27.
37. Benharroch D, Geffen DB, Peiser J, et al. Basal cell carcinoma of the male nipple: case report and review of the literature. *J Dermatol Surg Oncol* 1993;19:137–139.
38. Robinson H. Rodent ulcer of the male breast. *Trans Pathol Soc London* 1893;44:147–148.
39. Shertz WT, Balogh K. Metastasizing basal cell carcinoma of the nipple. *Arch Pathol Lab Med* 1986;110:761–762.
40. Wong SW, Smith JG Jr, Thomas WO. Bilateral basal cell carcinoma of the breasts. *J Am Acad Dermatol* 1993;28:777.
40a. Cooper RA, Ellers DB. Mammographic findings in basal cell carcinoma of the male nipple. *AJR Am J Roentgenol* 2000;175:1065–1066.
41. Revert A, Banuls J, Montesinos E, et al. Nevoid hyperkeratosis of the areola. *Int J Dermatol* 1993;32:745–746.
42. Mold DE, Jegasothy BV. Estrogen-induced hyperkeratosis of the nipple. *Cutis* 1980;26:95–96.
43. Vestey JP, Bunney MH. Unilateral hyperkeratosis of the nipple: the response to cryotherapy. *Arch Dermatol* 1986;122:1360–1361.
44. Schwartz RA. Hyperkeratosis of nipple and areola. *Arch Dermatol* 1978;114:1844–1845.
45. Ahn SK, Chung J, Lee WS, et al. Hyperkeratosis of the nipple and areola simultaneously developing with cutaneous T-cell lymphoma. *J Am Acad Dermatol* 1995;32:124–125.
46. Domoto H, Terahata S, Sato K, et al. Nodular hidradenoma of the breast: report of two cases with literature review. *Pathol Int* 1998;48:907–911.

# CHAPTER 45

# The Pathology of Axillary and Intramammary Lymph Nodes

This chapter is devoted to diverse pathologic changes, other than metastatic breast cancer, that affect the axillary lymph nodes. The final section is a discussion of the pathology of intramammary lymph nodes. Additional information about axillary lymph nodes can be found in Chapter 12 (staging), Chapter 14 (prognosis), and Chapter 46 (pathologic examination) as well as various chapters that discuss the pathology of lymph nodes in relation to specific pathologic conditions.

## HETEROTOPIC GLANDS

Heterotopic benign glandular tissue has been found in or associated with lymph nodes at various sites. At sites other than the axilla, heterotopic glands typically occur in the affected lymph node. A frequent example of this phenomenon is inclusion of salivary gland tissue in cervical lymph nodes (1). These glands usually appear to be histologically normal except for their aberrant location, but they may undergo squamous metaplasia and become cystic. Glandular inclusions in pelvic and periaortic lymph nodes are derived from the mesothelial lining of the peritoneum, which undergoes glandular metaplasia (2–4). Heterotopic glandular inclusions in the axillary lymph nodes are derived from the breast or skin appendage glands (5–12).

In contrast to the sites described already, heterotopic glands in the axilla occur in the capsule of a lymph node or in perinodal tissue as well as in the lymphoid tissue. With the exception of extremely uncommon heterotopic intranodal inclusions, the finding of orderly glands distributed singly or in small groups within a subcapsular sinus or in the substance of an axillary lymph node should be regarded as evidence of metastatic carcinoma. Well-differentiated metastatic carcinoma in axillary lymph nodes that has been mistakenly diagnosed as glandular heterotopia usually occurs in patients with well-differentiated ductal carcinoma or in patients with intraductal carcinoma who have undergone a needling procedure resulting in epithelial displacement

(13). Rarely, well-differentiated nodal metastases represent a minor, inconspicuous component of a primary tumor, most of which is histologically different and less differentiated (Figs. 45.1 and 45.2).

The histogenesis of glandular heterotopia associated with axillary lymph nodes is unknown, but the phenomenon is most likely due to an embryologic maldevelopment. There is no association between glandular heterotopia and the presence of accessory breast tissue in the axilla.

### Clinical Presentation

At least 10 reported examples of heterotopic glandular tissue associated with axillary lymph nodes have occurred in women. Among those with age recorded, five were 23 to 53 years of age, and one was 90. Most of the patients presented with an axillary mass, but in two cases (5,10), the affected lymph nodes were clinically inapparent. One of the patients had been treated by mastectomy for carcinoma of the left breast 10 years before an enlarged right axillary lymph node that contained heterotopic glandular tissue was excised (8). None of the other women was known to have mammary carcinoma, but two underwent mastectomies for benign proliferative disease.

### Gross Pathology

Enlarged lymph nodes with grossly apparent cysts were described in three cases. In one case, the cysts contained "colorless or brownish fluid" (6), whereas in another the cysts contained "cottage-cheese-like material" (12).

### Microscopic Pathology

Cystic epithelial inclusions in lymph nodes have been lined by squamous and apocrine epithelium (5–7,12) (Fig. 45.3). Discharge of keratin from squamous cysts can elicit a granulomatous reaction (12). Some inclusions appear to be

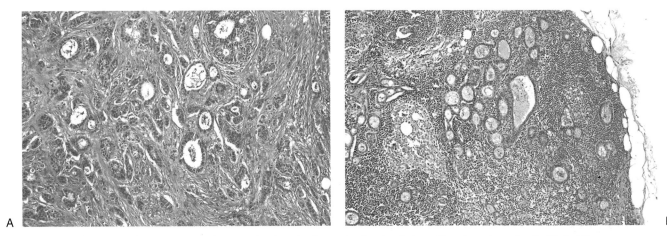

**FIG. 45.1.** *Metastatic carcinoma mistaken for heterotopic glands in axillary lymph node.* **A:** Well-differentiated glandular elements with open lumens are distributed in the midst of moderately differentiated infiltrating duct carcinoma in the primary tumor. **B:** The nodal metastasis consisting only of the well-differentiated glands was diagnosed mistakenly as glandular heterotopia.

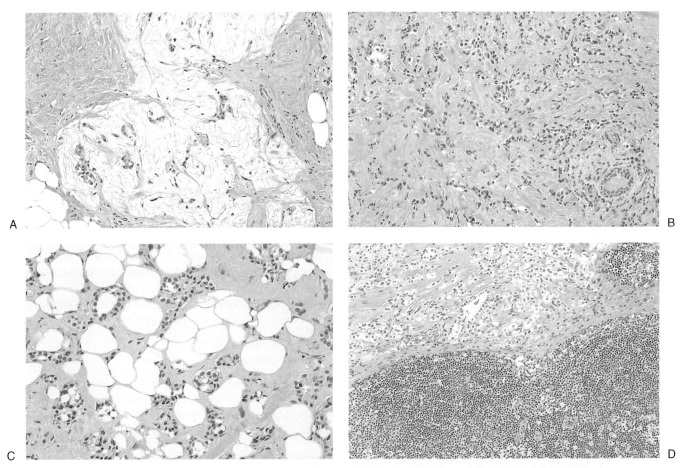

**FIG. 45.2.** *Metastatic carcinoma in the capsule of a sentinel lymph node mistaken for a heterotopic gland inclusion.* **A,B:** The primary tumor had a mixed growth pattern consisting almost entirely of mucinous **(A)** and classic **(B)** infiltrating lobular carcinoma. **C:** Less than 5% of the tumor had this well-differentiated structure. **D:** Metastatic carcinoma, found only in the capsule and adjacent tissue of this sentinel lymph node, had well-differentiated glands, which were misdiagnosed as heterotopic inclusions.

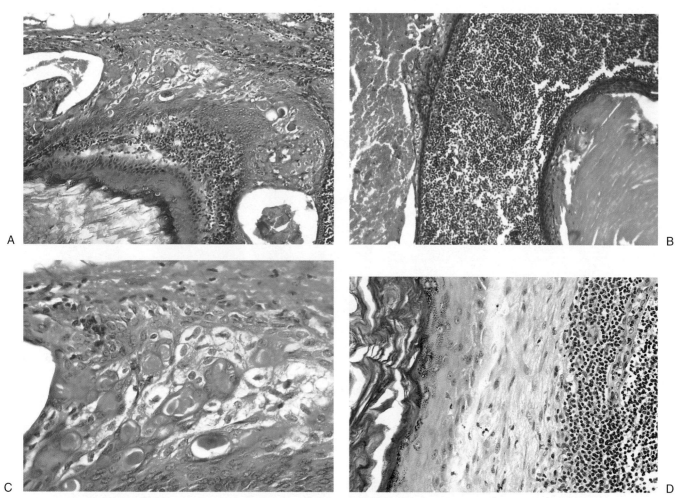

**FIG. 45.3.** *Heterotopic glands in axillary lymph node.* This glandular complex may be of sweat gland origin. **A:** Cystic glands with squamous metaplasia in a lymph node. The lymph node capsule is at the *upper border* of the picture. **B:** Cysts within the lymph node. **C:** Sebaceous metaplasia in the nodal inclusion. **D:** Squamous epithelium in a cyst with hyperkeratosis and pigmentation.

derived from skin appendage glands. Sebaceous differentiation may be present. Proliferative changes in the glandular inclusions have included apocrine metaplasia and duct hyperplasia (10). The differential diagnosis of cystic lesions in axillary lymph nodes includes bursal cyst (14).

One case report described papillary carcinoma that seemed to arise from a benign intranodal mammary glandular inclusion because some glands that appeared nonneoplastic were found to be associated with the intranodal carcinoma (11). The patient also had in one breast "a small intraductal papillary carcinoma . . . differing cytologically and architecturally from the nodal carcinoma." Because of the noninvasive character of the mammary lesion, and differences in the histologic appearance of the two processes, they were regarded as independent lesions, but metastatic involvement of the axillary lymph node is also possible.

The distinction between heterotopic mammary glands and metastatic carcinoma is usually not difficult (Fig. 45.4). The glandular structures typically occur outside of or within the lymph node capsule or in the lymphoid tissue rather than in nodal sinusoids. Myoepithelial cells and specialized intralobular stroma are evident in some heterotopic mammary lobules associated with lymph nodes. In the absence of myoepithelial cells, glands in axillary lymph nodes should be regarded as metastatic carcinoma, even if the growth pattern is well differentiated. Typically, these metastatic foci are distributed as isolated glands or as small groups of glands in the lymphoid tissue of the lymph node, in the capule, or in capsular and subcapsular lymphatic spaces (Figs. 45.1 and 45.2). A collagenous band that resembles a basement membrane may be found around part or all of such metastatic glands. Metastatic tubular carcinoma mistakenly diagnosed as "benign epithelial lined tubules within" a lymph node has been illustrated in a published report (15). Benign ductal structures can occur in the lymph node capsule, and these constitute an extremely rare form of heterotopia (Fig. 45.5).

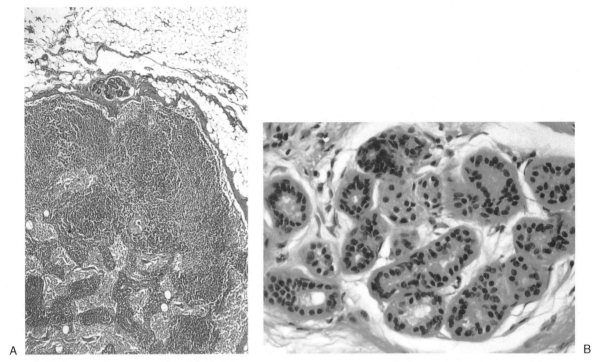

**FIG. 45.4.** *Heterotopic gland associated with an axillary lymph node.* This gland complex resembles a mammary lobule. **A:** The glandular structure is located in the lymph node capsule. **B:** A basement membrane is evident around each gland.

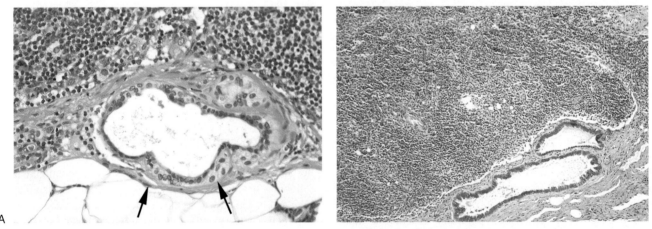

**FIG. 45.5.** *Heterotopic ducts associated with lymph nodes.* **A:** Myoepithelial cells (*arrows*) outline this benign duct in the capsule of an axillary lymph node. The 39-year-old patient had fibromatosis. **B:** Columnar cell hyperplasia is shown in these duct structures in the capsule of an intramammary lymph node.

## NEVUS CELL AGGREGATES

Collections of cells that resemble cutaneous nevi can be found in the capsules of lymph nodes in various areas of the body, including the axilla. Because of their association with the lymph node capsule rather than the lymphoid parenchyma in almost all cases, these groups of cells should be termed capsular "nevus cell aggregates" (NCAs) rather than the more often used nevus cell inclusion (16). The histogenesis of this anatomic variation is unknown, but origin in the lymph node capsule has been suggested. One investigator presented evidence of origin from cells in the walls of vessels in the lymph node capsule (17). This observation is consistent with the view that NCAs are angioglomic structures derived from perithelial cells with glomus properties around vessels in the lymph node capsule (18). It has also been hypothesized that NCAs arise by a process of "benign metastasis," in which cells are transported from benign cutaneous nevi to the lymph node. Rarely, these patients have a notable contiguous cutaneous nevus (19). The fact that a few patients have had prominent nevi or melanoma in the nearby skin suggests that some factor or factors may predispose particular patients to develop NCAs and melanocytic skin lesions. It is not known whether such patients have NCAs in nodal areas anatomically unrelated to the known cutaneous lesion. If NCAs were "benign metastases" from clinically inapparent or inconspicuous cutaneous nevi, it is difficult to envision the mechanism by which such "metastases" would be localized to the nodal capsule because one expects that cellular elements transported via the lymphatics should be deposited in nodal sinuses. The most likely explanation for the histogenesis of NCAs is that they are the result of embryologic maldevelopment.

Although NCAs have some glomoid structural features, the presence of melanin pigment verified by electron microscopy and the existence of heavily pigmented NCAs with a blue nevus configuration are indicative of nevocellular differentiation. As will be discussed subsequently, electron microscopy has documented many similarities between the cells of NCAs and cutaneous nevi, but it has failed to detect features of smooth-muscle differentiation commonly seen in glomus cells (20). Consequently, it seems more likely that NCAs develop from melanocytic cells arrested in migration from the neural crest to the skin or from undifferentiated neurocristic cells, which may be normally present in the capsules of superficial lymph nodes (21).

Stewart and Copeland first described NCAs in the hilar region of an axillary lymph node obtained from a patient with von Recklinghausen's disease, a bathing trunk nevus, and malignant melanoma (22). Stewart commented on three additional axillary NCAs in 1960 (23). A series of six cases was reported by Johnson and Helwig, who noted that NCAs often contain pigment with the staining properties of melanin (24). Two patients were women who had axillary lymph nodes removed in the treatment of breast carcinoma, and a third woman had fibrocystic mastopathy. NCAs also were found in axillary lymph nodes obtained from men with basal cell carcinoma and malignant melanoma and a cervical lymph node from a man with an epidermal inclusion cyst. Pigmented NCAs subsequently were described in an inguinal lymph node from an 8-year-old child with juvenile melanoma (25) and in a cervical lymph node from a man with squamous carcinoma of the larynx (26).

In 1974, McCarthy et al. described 24 patients who had NCAs, including 15 treated for malignant melanoma (27). Most NCAs were associated with axillary lymph nodes, but inguinal nodes were affected in seven and cervical nodes in two cases. The ages of the patients ranged from 17 to 70 years. The series included four women with axillary NCAs who had been treated for breast carcinoma. Pigmented nevi were present in the skin drained by the lymph nodes in 21 cases. McCarthy et al. reported that NCAs were present in 6.2% of 129 axillary and in 4.0% of 50 inguinal lymph node dissections. No NCAs were found in 130 dissections of thoracic, abdominal, or iliac lymph nodes.

Ridolfi et al. reviewed 909 consecutive mastectomy specimens from patients with mammary carcinoma and found a single NCA in each of three cases (0.33%) affecting 0.017% (3/17,504) of the lymph nodes examined (16). One hundred lymph node dissections from patients with malignant melanoma obtained from various sites also were reviewed. Three of 2,607 lymph nodes contained NCAs (0.12%). Another study in which lymph nodes were examined by immunohistochemistry as well as by routine histology reported that NCAs were present in 49 of 226 (22%) lymph node dissections (28). Seventy-eight percent of NCAs were detected by routine histology and 22% by staining for S-100 protein. Axillary lymph nodes were the most frequent site of NCA (22%), followed by cervical (18%) and inguinal (11%) nodes. Bautista et al. also used the stain for S-100 protein to study 300 axillary dissections (29). They reported finding NCAs in 7.3% of the specimens and in 0.54% of 5,186 lymph nodes examined.

Several conclusions can be drawn from the foregoing data:

1. NCAs occur in association with superficial lymph node groups that drain the skin as well as other organs. If they ever occur in visceral lymph nodes, it is extraordinarily unusual.

2. Lymph nodes that contain NCAs are most frequent in the axilla and less often in the groin and cervical regions.

3. NCAs have been found in lymph nodes from men, women, and children. Most patients have had malignant neoplasms, but NCAs have been found in lymph nodes from patients with benign neoplasms and nonneoplastic conditions. They may be more frequent in lymph nodes from patients with malignant melanoma than in the axillary lymph nodes of women with mammary carcinoma.

4. Although some patients with NCAs have a contiguous skin lesion such as malignant melanoma or a conspicuous nevus, most of these patients have no notable skin lesions.

## Clinical Presentation

Nevus cell aggregates are small, often microscopic structures that do not cause palpable enlargement of lymph nodes or any other clinical symptoms. Consequently, their presence is unsuspected until resected lymph nodes have been examined microscopically after excision.

## Gross Pathology

Rarely are NCAs visible grossly. Heavily pigmented NCAs have been described grossly on three occasions (19,28,29). In one instance, the gross findings suggested anthracotic pigment (30). The second example occurred in an inguinal lymph node removed incidentally during treatment of varicose veins consisting of "3 darkly pigmented nodules, the largest being 0.3 cm in diameter" (31). A third 0.8-cm lymph node from the axilla of a woman with breast carcinoma contained "a golden-brown crescentic lesion . . . that occupied approximately one-third of the perimeter" (21) (Fig. 45.6). In each of these instances, the microscopic configuration of the NCAs was that of a blue nevus.

## Microscopic Pathology

Two distinct microscopic patterns of NCAs have been described: NCAs that resemble intradermal nevi and NCAs with the appearance of blue nevi. The former are much more common, with fewer than 10% of NCAs having the blue nevus structure. Patients with the two types of NCAs do not differ appreciably with respect to age distribution, associated diseases, or the frequency of multinodal involvement; however, the absence of a difference may reflect the indications for nodal dissection rather than the true distribution of NCAs.

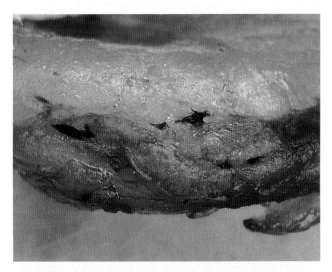

**FIG. 45.6.** *Nevus cell aggregate, gross appearance.* This blue nevus-type lesion had abundant black melanin pigment. (From Epstein JI, Erlandson RA, Rosen PP. Nodal blue nevi: a study of three cases. *Am J Surg Pathol* 1984;8:907–915, with permission.)

Nevus cell aggregates of the intradermal nevus type have a flat or nodular configuration in the lymph node capsule (Fig. 45.7). In most cases, a single lymph node is affected, but in rare instances, NCAs are found in two or more lymph nodes from a nodal group (18,24,32–34). In a single plane of section, NCAs occupy a fraction of the perimeter of a lymph node. They often appear to have a discontinuous distribution and may extend into the node itself along fibrous trabeculae. Any portion of the capsule may be affected; there does not seem to be a predilection to involve the hilar region. Rarely, the capsular stroma accompanying the NCA into the nodal substance is so sparse that the NCA appears to lie entirely in the cortical parenchyma of the lymph node. NCAs have not been encountered as isolated structures in the peripheral sinus of a lymph node.

The architecture of NCA is demonstrated in sections prepared with the reticulin stain. The cells that form an NCA are cytologically quite similar to cells of an ordinary intradermal nevus. They tend to be tightly clustered into poorly defined masses separated by, or sometimes seemingly centered about, thin-walled capillaries. When they have a particularly angular configuration, these capillaries may be mistaken for artifactual spaces. The outer peripheral portion of NCAs is usually sharply defined, whereas at the inner margin, NCA cells often merge with capsular tissue.

Cytologically, NCA cells are usually oval and have indistinct borders (Fig. 45.8). Polygonal cells are found in some cases. The central nuclei have fine, diffuse chromatin and are surrounded by pale or clear cytoplasm. Nucleoli are small and indistinct or absent. Mitoses are not seen. Multinucleated cells of the type sometimes found in intradermal nevi are not a feature of NCAs.

Fine brown pigment granules may be detected in the cytoplasm of a few scattered cells in a minority of NCAs. This pigment gives a negative Perls reaction for iron, and it is blackened with the Fontana-Masson and Grimelius stains (Fig. 45.9). NCAs contain no mucin when studied with mucicarmine, periodic acid-Schiff, or Alcian blue stains. Immunohistochemical studies revealed strong reactivity for S-100 protein, variable staining for HMB-45, and an absence of staining for cytokeratin or epithelial membrane antigen (Fig. 45.10).

The NCAs of the blue nevus variety have poorly defined borders. These heavily pigmented lesions, which occupy the lymph node capsule and radiate into surrounding fat, also may extend into the nodal lymphoid tissue (21,30,31,35) (Fig. 45.11). The finely granular pigment is golden or dark brown. It fills and often obscures the cytoplasm of many cells in the lesion, especially the closely packed elongated cells with dendritic processes. At the outer, peripheral edges of the NCA, these slender cells extend into the perinodal fat. It is unusual for a blue nevus NCA to extend along trabeculae into the substance of a lymph node. Scattered singly and in small groups among the spindle cells are polygonal cells with pale cytoplasm that contains coarsely clumped pigment. These epithelioid NCA cells resemble pigmented

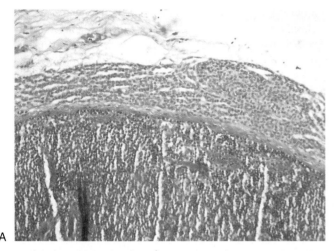

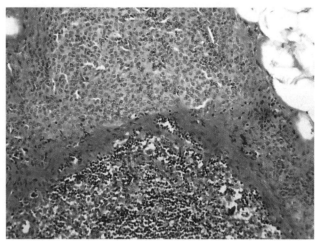

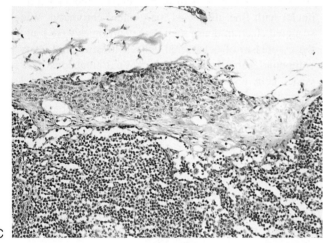

**FIG. 45.7.** *Nevus cell aggregate (NCA), flat and nodular types.* **A:** This flat lesion forms a band along the outer border of the lymph node capsule. **B:** A nodular NCA that protrudes away from the capsule of the lymph node. A flat extension of the NCA is shown on the *right.* **C:** A relatively inconspicuous oval NCA with a few pigment-containing cells.

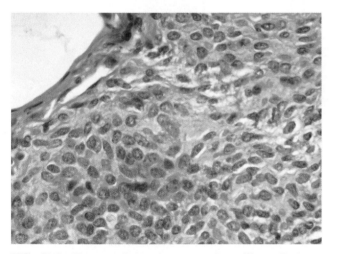

**FIG. 45.8.** *Nevus cell aggregate, cytology.* The cells have oval nuclei with finely granular chromatin. They are identical to cells typically found in a cutaneous dermal nevus.

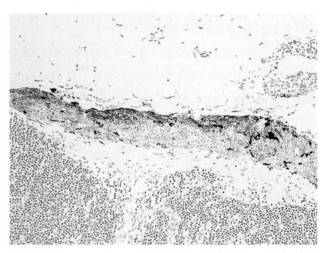

**FIG. 45.9.** *Nevus cell aggregate, Fontana-Masson stain.* The pigment stains black.

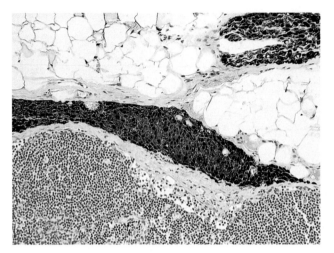

**FIG. 45.10.** *Nevus cell aggregate (NCA), S-100 stain.* The cells in the NCA and an adjacent nerve are immunoreactive for S-100 protein (avidin-biotin).

histiocytes. Mitotic figures and multinucleated giant cells are absent from the blue nevus type of NCA.

Because the indication for a lymph node dissection is almost always a contiguous malignant neoplasm, it is important that NCA not be mistakenly interpreted as metastatic tu-

mor (36). In patients with mammary carcinoma, NCAs most closely resemble metastatic lobular carcinoma. Features that help to distinguish NCAs from mammary carcinoma include the capsular location, the presence of brown pigment with the staining properties of melanin, an absence of mucin, and immunohistochemical reactivity consistent with neuroepithelial rather than glandular histogenesis. Rarely, the same lymph node may contain an NCA and metastatic tumor.

## Electron Microscopy

Ultrastructural studies of two NCAs have been published. The first report described a dermal nevus type of NCA obtained from the axillary lymph node of an 82-year-old woman treated by mastectomy for mammary carcinoma (20). The NCA consisted of nests of round cells that contained round nuclei with fine, dispersed marginated chromatin. Widely scattered electron-dense mature melanosomes were found in the cytoplasm of occasional cells. Ultrastructural study of compound, intradermal, and junctional cutaneous nevi revealed cells resembling those in NCA. Ultrastructural features of smooth-muscle differentiation were not identified. A blue nevus type of NCA contained round and elongated cells with abundant cytoplasmic spherical electron-dense mature

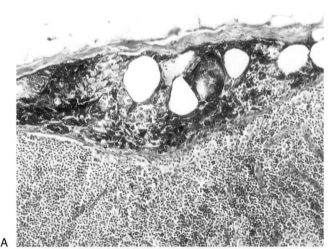

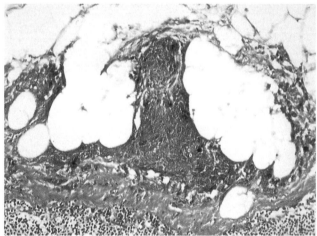

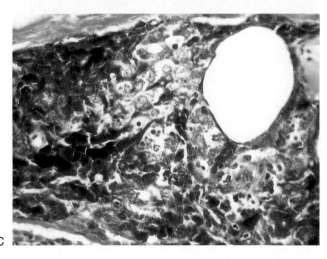

**FIG. 45.11.** *Nevus cell aggregate (NCA), blue nevus type.* **A,B:** Two heavily pigmented NCAs that radiate into the perinodal fat. The border along the lymph node capsule is smooth. **C:** Most of the cells are obscured by dense brown pigment.

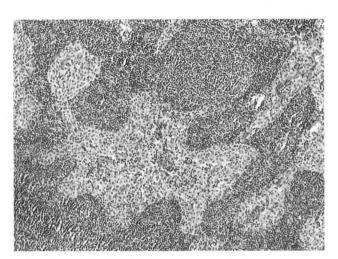

**FIG. 45.12.** *Sinus histiocytosis.* The lymph sinuses are distended by broad syncytial sheets of histiocytes.

stage IV melanosomes, as well as smaller, membrane-limited melanosomes in clusters (21).

### Prognosis

Theoretically, NCA could be the source of some malignant melanomas detected in lymph nodes in the absence of a demonstrable cutaneous primary. There is no evidence that the presence of NCAs in the lymph nodes of patients with an associated malignant neoplasm affects the prognosis of the neoplasm or that such patients are predisposed to developing any particular type of neoplasm subsequently.

### SINUS HISTIOCYTOSIS

*Sinus histiocytosis* has been defined as the "distention of the sinusoids of the lymph nodes by elongated histiocytes that have finely granular, eosinophilic-staining cytoplasm in a syncytial arrangement" (37) (Fig. 45.12). Various schemes have been devised to grade or subclassify the intensity of si-

nus histiocytosis, including 3-point (37), 5-point (38), and 2-point scales (39). In a 3-point grading, system sinus histiocytosis is described as minimal or absent, intermediate when sinusoids are widened by three to four histiocytes, and marked when the breadth of sinusoids is greater than four cells (37). Grading has been determined from the most severe change seen among the lymph nodes on a single slide (37), by assessing each lymph node separately and then calculating the mean intensity of reaction (38), or on the basis of the lymph node that showed the most extreme sinus histiocytosis (39). Lymph nodes exhibiting inflammatory sinus histiocytosis consisting of sinusoidal edema or erythrophagocytosis and polymorphonuclear leukocytes should be excluded from evaluation (Fig. 45.13). Lipid transported from the lactating breast to axillary lymph nodes accumulates in histiocytes, causing a variant of inflammatory sinus histiocytosis referred to as lactational histiocytosis (Fig. 45.14).

It has been suggested that sinus histiocytosis is a manifestation of cell-mediated immune reaction. Marked sinus histiocytosis in the ipsilateral axillary lymph nodes of patients with breast carcinoma has been associated with an enhanced cellular response to autologous breast cancer tissue (40) and to clinically evident enlargement of contralateral axillary lymph nodes (38). Several studies, largely carried out by Black and colleagues, reported a correlation between the grade of sinus histiocytosis and survival (37,38,41). Patients with the most intense, high-grade reaction had the most favorable prognosis. Marked sinus histiocytosis was associated with a better prognosis in node-negative and node-positive patients (42,43), with the effect more pronounced when nodal metastases were present (44). Silverberg et al. found that marked sinus histiocytosis indicated a favorable prognosis in women with moderately or poorly differentiated tumors and in those with fewer than nine positive lymph nodes (39). No correlation was found between outcome in women who had well-differentiated tumors, negative lymph nodes, or more than eight positive nodes.

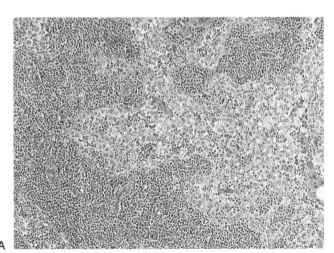

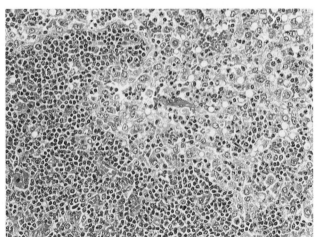

A                             B

**FIG. 45.13.** *Sinus histiocytosis, inflammatory.* **A:** Red blood cells are dispersed in the sinusoids. **B:** Red blood cells, leukocytes, and lymphocytes mingle with the histiocytes. Erythrophagocytosis is apparent.

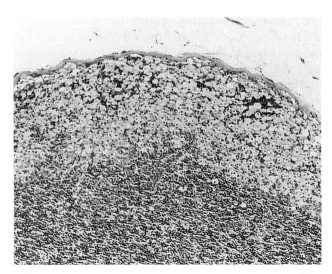

**FIG. 45.14.** *Sinus histiocytosis, lactational.* Histiocytes filled with lipid have accumulated in the sinusoids.

Friedell et al. found that the axillary lymph nodes of Japanese women with breast carcinoma had marked sinus histiocytosis more often than the lymph nodes from British women, regardless of the presence or absence of nodal metastases, and suggested that this phenomenon contributed to racial differences in survival (45). Survival analysis was not reported for the patients studied, however.

Others have not been able to confirm the association between sinus histiocytosis and prognosis. Berg concluded that nodal status and factors associated with lymph node metastases were more significant for prognosis (46). Moore et al. were unable to find a difference in the pattern of sinus histiocytosis between patients who survived and those who died of metastatic breast carcinoma (47). DiRe and Lane (48), Schiodt (49), and Kister et al. (50) also concluded that sinus histiocytosis was not a significant indicator of prognosis.

Failure of investigators to find a consistent relationship between sinus histiocytosis and prognosis in breast cancer may reflect significant technical problems in the histologic evaluation of this phenomenon. A major difficulty is the growing trend to biopsy the breast tumor days or weeks prior to the axillary dissection. As a consequence, the lymph nodes exhibit inflammatory alterations resulting from recent surgery. It is also necessary to have good quality sections of well-fixed tissue, and such preparations are not always available. Investigators have not used consistent grading schemes, and there is no consensus on the measurement, grading, or reporting of sinus histiocytosis. Finally, the evaluation of sinus histiocytosis has proven to be a highly subjective endeavor with considerable interobserver and intraobserver variability. In one study, an "experienced observer" achieved 70% self-reproducibility in two separate reviews of the same lymph nodes (37). Two less experienced pathologists agreed with the average grade of the two reviews of the "experienced observer" in 55% and 61% of cases, respectively.

## SILICONE LYMPHADENITIS

### Clinical Presentation

Reaction to silicone transported to lymph nodes has been described in association with orthopedic prostheses (51,52), cosmetic injection of silicone in the breast and other sites, and leakage from intact or ruptured silicone gel-containing breast implants (53,54). In the mammary region, clinically symptomatic adenopathy is manifested by nontender or painful axillary nodal enlargement. Asymptomatic silicone lymphadenitis may be encountered when a patient with a silicone-containing prosthesis undergoes an axillary dissection or lymph node biopsy for another condition, such as mammary carcinoma (53). Involvement of an intramammary lymph node can produce mammographic changes that mimic carcinoma (55). In one case, enlargement of an internal mammary lymph node because of silicone lymphadenitis mimicked recurrent carcinoma in a woman who had a total mastectomy for T1N0 breast carcinoma and reconstruction with a silicone outside/saline inside implant (56).

### Gross Pathology

Affected lymph nodes generally do not manifest specific or distinctive gross features. In some cases, the lymph nodes are enlarged and firmer than normal. In extreme examples of silicone lymphadenitis, the cut surface reveals a distorted nodal architecture and fibrosis (51). The gross appearance of lymph nodes with silicone lymphadenitis also is affected by concurrent diseases, such as metastatic carcinoma or malignant lymphoma.

### Microscopic Pathology

Considerable variation has been found in the extent of lymph node involvement in a given case. Some may be diffusely affected and others spared entirely. In most instances, silicone lymphadenitis has a patchy distribution in involved lymph nodes.

Histologic examination reveals diffuse follicular hyperplasia. Histiocytes with clear, vacuolated cytoplasm are scattered throughout the lymphoid tissue but tend to be concentrated in sinusoidal regions. Coalescent groups of clear cells are associated with the formation of empty vacuoles and the accumulation of foreign-body giant cells (53,54) (Fig. 45.15). Refractile and nonbirefringent particles may be present in the giant cells. Silicone lymphadenitis caused by material from orthopedic devices typically is characterized by a prominent granulomatous reaction with clumps of granular yellowish refractile material; silicone gel from mammary prostheses ordinarily produces finer vacuolated deposits that resemble soap suds. Asteroid bodies have been observed in lymphadenitis associated with silicone-containing orthopedic prostheses (51).

The differential diagnosis includes various causes of granulomatous lymphadenitis, adenitis associated with lymphangiography, and congenital storage diseases. The presence of

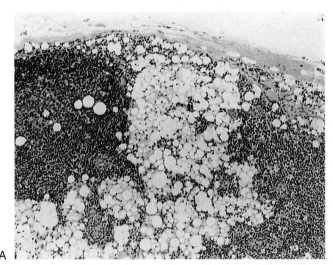
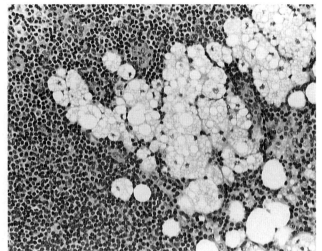

**FIG. 45.15.** *Silicone lymphadenitis.* **A,B:** The lymph node architecture is distorted by histiocytes with clear, vacuolated cytoplasm.

silicone compounds in lymph nodes and other tissues can be confirmed by electron microprobe analysis using transmission or scanning electron microscopy (51,54,57) and other techniques for microanalysis (58). A method for detecting silica in lymph nodes and other tissue samples by incineration has been described (59).

Routine histochemical and immunohistochemical procedures do not stain silicone in tissue sections. Most specific granulomatous reactions and sarcoidosis lack the vacuolated histiocytic reaction seen in silicone lymphadenitis. The distinction between lymphangiogram effect and storage diseases usually can be made on the basis of clinical information. One lymph node from a patient with silicone

lymphadenitis reportedly exhibited histologic features of Kikuchi's necrotizing lymphadenitis (60).

## PIGMENT DEPOSITS IN AXILLARY LYMPH NODES AND THE BREAST

Several types of pigmented material have been detected in axillary lymph nodes. Histiocytes may contain black anthracotic pigment, which apparently accumulates as a result of retrograde flow from thoracic to axillary lymphatics (Fig. 45.16). The pigment is usually not abundant and tends to be more prominent in apical rather than in low axillary lymph nodes. Cserni described a patient in whom anthracotic

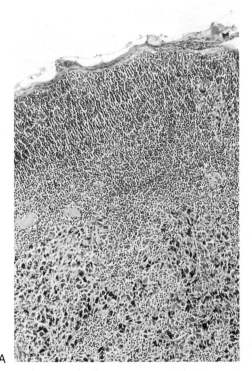

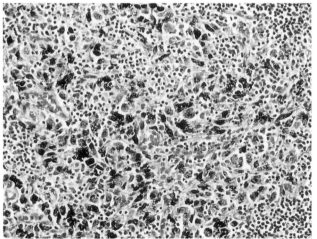

**FIG. 45.16.** *Anthracotic pigment.* **A,B:** Coarse black pigment in sinusoidal histiocytes that has elicited a granulomatous reaction. The histologic appearance of this axillary lymph node resembles a typical pulmonary lymph node.

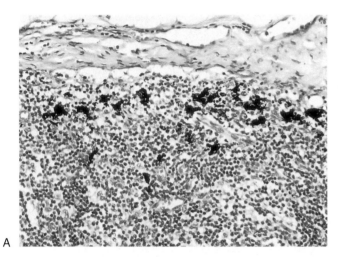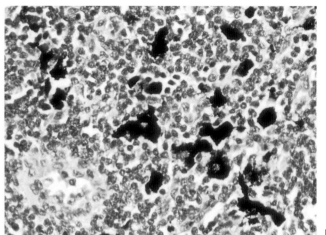

A
B

**FIG. 45.17.** *Tattoo pigment.* **A,B:** Pigment-laden histiocytes are scattered in the parenchyma of the lymph node. Two turquoise-colored particles are visible in **B**.

pigment in a lymph node was mistaken during surgery for staining with dye injected for sentinel lymph node mapping (61). Anthracotic and melanin pigment may not be grossly distinguishable in an axillary lymph node.

Prior surgical trauma or an underlying systemic condition, such as hemosiderosis, can cause accumulation of brown iron pigment. Dermatopathic lymphadenitis features melanin pigment transported from inflammatory skin lesions. Pigment from cutaneous tattoos also can be transported to axillary lymph nodes (Fig. 45.17). Patients who received systemic gold therapy for rheumatoid arthritis have reportedly developed gold deposits in lymph nodes that were visualized by mammography (62,63). In one case, the particles appeared to be within the breast radiologically and were thought to be microcalcifications that suggested carcinoma (63). At operation, however, the gold deposits were found within an intraparenchymal lymph node.

Ochronotic pigment is deposited in connective tissues of various types of in patients with ochronosis. The condition is caused by an autosomal recessive genetic defect, which results in the accumulation of homogentisic acid detectable in the urine as alcaptonuria. Ochronotic pigment in synovium is associated with the development of arthritis. Tumorous lesions resulting from ochronotic pigment deposition in the mammary stroma are brown to black, grossly resembling malignant melanoma (64). Histologic examination reveals dense fibrous tissue containing yellow–brown pigment, which stains black with the Fontana and methenamine silver stains (64). The lesions are hypocellular and lack the cytologic features of malignant melanoma.

## VASCULAR LESIONS

Hemangiomas are the most frequent benign vascular neoplasms encountered in axillary lymph nodes. Most are found in lymph nodes removed in the course of axillary dissections for various conditions and are chance findings, although they

may measure up to 0.5 cm (65). They may occupy the nodal hilum or parenchyma and sometimes extend to perinodal tissues. Nodal hemangiomas are typically of the capillary variety, but cavernous features may also be present (Fig. 45.18). Although usually solitary, multiple microscopic nodal hemangiomas occasionally are encountered. Breast tissue removed at the same time or previously may contain one or more perilobular hemangiomas, and in this setting care should be exercised to avoid misinterpreting the findings as evidence of angiosarcoma. Clinically evident nodal enlargement caused by an hemangioma has been reported (66).

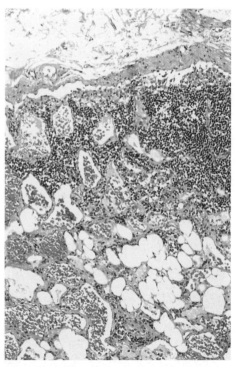

**FIG. 45.18.** *Nodal hemangioma.* A capillary hemangioma fills the center of this lymph node.

Kaposi's sarcoma may arise primarily in lymph nodes, including those in the axilla (67,68). This phenomenon was described before the recognition of the association between Kaposi's sarcoma and acquired immunodeficiency syndrome (AIDS) and probably constitutes a separate disease process. These patients usually exhibit evidence of systemic Kaposi's sarcoma with involvement of several nodal sites, although rarely the condition is clinically limited to one lymph node.

A Kaposi-like proliferative lesion, termed *vascular transformation* or *nodal angiomatosis*, is sometimes found incidentally in one or more lymph nodes removed from the axilla and other sites (69,70). This condition features the formation of complex capillary and cavernous vascular channels in the lymph sinuses. In most instances, vascular transformation is an incidental microscopic finding in lymph nodes removed during an operation for another disease; however, the condition can cause nodal enlargement that is clinically apparent (71). Common sites include the cervical, axillary, and supraclavicular lymph nodes. Involvement of mediastinal, inguinal, and various abdominal lymph node groups also has been reported. Vascular transformation has been found in axillary lymph nodes from patients with breast carcinoma (71,72). Rarely, there have been hemangiomas in the skin and other tissues drained by the lymph nodes affected by vascular transformation. The author has seen an unusual instance in which there was a vasoproliferative condition in the dermis of the skin overlying an infiltrating breast carcinoma in a patient with vascular transformation of the ipsilateral axillary lymph nodes. The cutaneous lesion was identical to the nodal vascular abnormality.

The histologic features of nodal vascular transformation are variable. The condition occurs mainly in lymphoid sinuses, largely sparing the lymph node capsule. Blood vessels in perinodal tissues may have a thickened muscular layer. Several vasoformative patterns found in differing proportions in individual cases include the formation of narrow vascular slits, open round spaces, solid foci composed of spindle and polygonal cells, and a plexiform pattern of interconnecting vascular spaces (Fig. 45.19). Red blood cells are found in many but not all vascular channels. Extravasation of red blood cells, fibrin deposits, and thrombosis are variably present. Endothelial cells display little or no cytologic atypia, papillary endothelial hyperplasia is absent, and there is minimal mitotic activity.

The cause of nodal vascular transformation is not known, but the appearance of the lesions suggests a proliferative response to an angiogenic stimulus that may be derived from an associated neoplasm in some cases.

## INTRAMAMMARY LYMPH NODES

Intramammary lymph nodes most often are located deep in the outer quadrants of the breast (73). Mammographic examination usually reveals a well-circumscribed mass that may have a lucent center and a peripheral "hilar" notch (74) (Figs. 45.20 and 45.21). Lymphoid hyperplasia in intramammary lymph nodes has been associated with rapid contrast uptake in contrast-enhanced magnetic resonance imaging (MRI) studies, a result that may suggest carcinoma (75). Fine needle aspiration of a benign intramammary lymph node yields a heterogeneous cellular specimen similar to material from a lymph node at any other site (76). Lymphocytes are the dominant cellular elements. Needle core biopsy samples usually include portions of the lymph node capsule and subcapsular sinuses as diagnostic features.

Enlargement of intramammary lymph nodes may be caused by inflammatory conditions, such as sinus histiocytosis (77), reaction to dermatitis (78), tuberculosis (79), foreign material such as gold (80), or neoplasms, including lymphoma (81,82) (Fig. 45.22), metastatic melanoma (77), and metastatic carcinoma (77,83,84). The distinction between medullary carcinoma and metastatic carcinoma in an intramammary lymph node is sometimes difficult. The

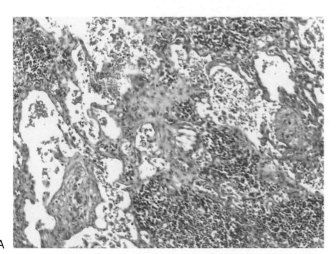
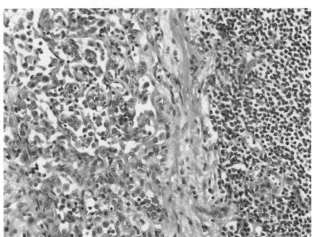

**FIG. 45.19.** *Vascular transformation of axillary lymph nodes.* **A:** The lymph sinuses have been transformed into dilated vascular channels separated by fibrous stroma. Red blood cells are present in the vascular spaces. **B:** An area in which angioendothelial proliferation fills a lymph sinus.

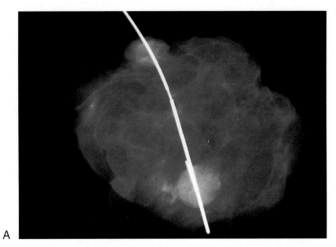
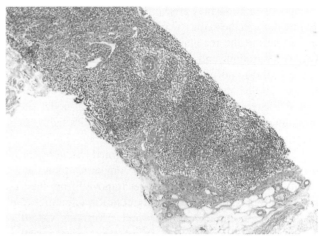

A

B

**FIG. 45.20.** *Intramammary lymph node detected by mammography.* **A:** A radiograph of a breast biopsy specimen that contains a lymph node with a localization wire in place. Note the "notch" in the contour of the lymph node in the 5 o'clock radius. **B:** The tissue sample obtained by needle core biopsy of a radiologically detected intramammary lymph node.

underlying architecture of a lymph node usually is revealed by a reticulin stain, whereas the presence of intraductal carcinoma, a prominent plasmacytic reaction, syncytial growth, and necrosis characterize medullary carcinoma.

Dawson et al. reviewed 18 patients with clinically palpable intramammary lymph nodes seen at one institution over a 6-year period (85). The patients ranged in age from 22 to 58 years (mean, 32 years). Three lumps were painful. The number of lymph nodes in the palpable lesions varied from

one to six, with a mean diameter of 0.8 cm. Pathologic findings in the lymph nodes included fibrosis, lymphoid hyperplasia, sinus histiocytosis, melanin pigmentation (seven cases), fatty infiltration, and a capsular nevus cell aggregate (one case).

McSweeney and Egan found intramammary lymph nodes in 52 of 173 (30%) breasts examined by whole-organ serial sectioning, specimen radiography, and pathologic examination (84). A lymph node was classified as intramammary

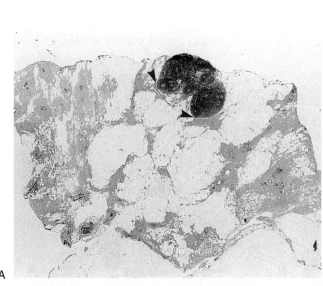
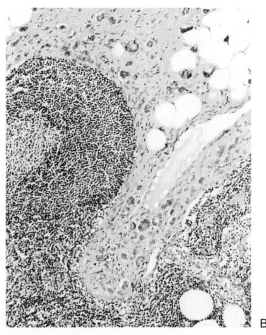

A

B

**FIG. 45.21.** *Intramammary lymph node.* **A:** Whole-mount histologic section of breast tissue from a mastectomy specimen. A bean-shaped lymph node with a hilar "notch" is located next to invasive carcinoma *(arrows).* **B:** Carcinoma invading the lymph node capsule. (**A:** From Rosen PP, Oberman HA. Tumors of the mammary gland. In: *Atlas of tumor pathology.* Washington, DC: Armed Forces Institute of Pathology, 1993.)

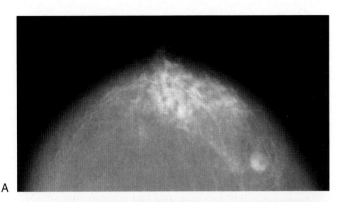

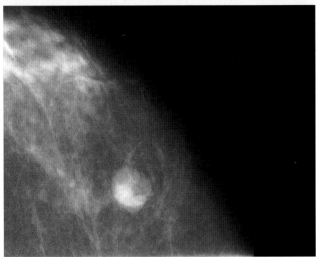

**FIG. 45.22.** *Enlarged intramammary lymph node mammogram.* **A,B:** The lymph node detected as a discrete mass contained malignant lymphoma. (Courtesy of Bela Ben-Dor, M.D.)

only if "completely surrounded by breast tissue." Lymph nodes were identified in 45 of 158 (29%) breasts removed for primary operable breast carcinoma. The size of lymph nodes ranged from 3 to 15 mm. A total of 72 lymph nodes was found, with nine being the largest number in a single case. This patient had at least one lymph node in each of three quadrants. The distribution of lymph nodes in the breast was as follows: upper outer, 26 (36%); lower outer, 21 (29%); upper inner, 11 (15%); central, 8 (11%); lower inner, 6 (8%). Seven breasts with carcinoma had one or more lymph nodes in the same quadrant as the primary tumor, and eight had nodes in other quadrants. A subareolar intramammary lymph node detected by mammography has been described (86).

Metastatic carcinoma was found in an intramammary lymph node in 10% of breasts with carcinoma and in 33% of breasts that had an intramammary lymph node and carcinoma (84). Lymph nodes that contained metastatic carcinoma were not especially enlarged, measuring 3 to 10 mm. Positive intramammary lymph nodes were found in six patients who were otherwise clinically stage I and in nine who were stage II. Twelve stage I patients with invasive carcinoma and negative intramammary lymph nodes had a 66% survival at 10 years, which was similar to the 74% survival

of 49 stage I patients with invasive carcinoma and no detectable intramammary lymph nodes. On the other hand, only 33% of six stage I patients with a positive intramammary lymph node survived 10 years. All carcinomas associated with intramammary lymph node metastases were invasive ductal type, including two with mucinous differentiation and two with associated Paget's disease.

Changes in intramammary lymph nodes documented in serial mammograms may be an indication of otherwise clinically inapparent carcinoma (87). These alterations include enlargement, increased density, and loss of the hilar notch resulting from metastatic carcinoma in the lymph node.

## REFERENCES

### Heterotopic Glands

1. Brown RB, Gaillard RA, Turner JA. The significance of aberrant or heterotopic parotid gland tissue in lymph nodes. *Ann Surg* 1953; 138:850–856.
2. Karp LA, Czernobilsky B. Glandular inclusions in pelvic and abdominal para-aortic lymph nodes. *Am J Clin Pathol* 1969;52:212–218.
3. Kempson RL. Consultant case: benign glandular inclusions in iliac lymph nodes. *Am J Surg Pathol* 1978;2:321–325.
4. Schnurr RC, Delgado G, Chun B. Benign glandular inclusions in para-aortic lymph nodes in women undergoing lymphadenectomies. *Am J Obstet Gynecol* 1978;130:813–816.
5. Edlow DW, Carter D. Heterotopic epithelium in axillary lymph nodes: report of a case and review of the literature. *Am J Clin Pathol* 1973;59:666–673.
6. Garret R, Ada AEW. Epithelial inclusion cysts in an axillary lymph node: report of a case simulating metastatic adenocarcinoma. *Cancer* 1957;10:173–178.
7. Haagensen CD. Heterotopic apocrine cysts in axillary lymph nodes. In: Haagensen CD. *Diseases of the breast,* 2nd ed. Philadelphia: WB Saunders, 1971;491.
8. Holdsworth PJ, Hopkinson JM, Leveson SH. Benign axillary epithelial lymph node inclusions—a histological pitfall. *Histopathology* 1988;13:226–228.
9. McDivitt RW, Stewart FW, Berg JW. Tumors of the breast. In: *Atlas of tumor pathology,* 2nd Series, Fascicle 2. Washington, DC: Armed Forces Institute of Pathology, 1969:116.
10. Turner DR, Millis RR. Breast tissue inclusions in axillary lymph nodes. *Histopathology* 1980;4:631–636.
11. Walker AN, Fechner RE. Papillary carcinoma arising from ectopic breast tissue in an axillary lymph node. *Diagn Gynecol Obstet* 1982;4:141–145.
12. Layfield LJ, Mooney E. Heterotopic epithelium in an intramammary lymph node. *Breast J* 2000;6:63–67.
13. Silton RM. More glandular inclusions. *Am J Surg Pathol* 1979; 3:285–286.
14. Graham D, Resnick JM. Bursal cyst: an unusual axillary mass. *Tenn Med* 1999;92:269–270.
15. Fisher CJ, Hill S, Millis RR. Benign lymph node inclusions mimicking metastatic carcinoma. *J Clin Pathol* 1994;47:245–247.

### Nevus Cell Aggregates

16. Ridolfi RL, Rosen PP, Thaler H. Nevus cell aggregates associated with lymph nodes: estimated frequency and clinical significance. *Cancer* 1977;39:164–171.
17. Nodl F. Uber anastomosen und epitheloide Gefaswandzellen hautnaher Lymphknoten. *Arch Dermatol Res* 1977;257:319–326.
18. Micheau C, Contesso G. Formations d'aspect angioglomique dans les ganglions lymphatiques axillaires. *Arch Anat Pathol* 1971;19:167–175.
19. Lambert WC, Brodkin RH. Nodal and subcutaneous cellular blue nevi. *Arch Dermatol* 1984;120:367–370.
20. Erlandson RA, Rosen PP. Electron microscopy of a nevus cell aggregate associated with an axillary lymph node. *Cancer* 1982;49:269–272.

21. Epstein JI, Erlandson RA, Rosen PP. Nodal blue nevi: a study of three cases. *Am J Surg Pathol* 1984;8:907–915.

22. Stewart FW, Copeland MM. Neurogenic sarcoma. *Am J Cancer* 1931;15:1235–1320.

23. Stewart FW. Early Cancer (Thayer lecture. The Johns Hopkins University, 1960), as cited by Wood Jr, S, Holyoke ED, Yardley JH. New York: Academic Press. *Canad Cancer Conf* 1960;4:167–223.

24. Johnson WT, Helwig EB. Benign nevus cells in the capsule of lymph nodes. *Cancer* 1969;23:747–753.

25. Lerman RI, Murray D, O'Hara JM, et al. Malignant melanoma of childhood. *Cancer* 1970;25:436–449.

26. Hart WR. Primary nevus of a lymph node. *Am J Clin Pathol* 1971; 55:88–92.

27. McCarthy SW, Palmer AA, Bale PM, et al. Nevus cells in lymph nodes. *Pathology* 1974;6:351–358.

28. Carson K, Wen D-R, Cochran AJ. Nodal nevi are frequent and selectively located in melanoma-draining nodes: implications for their etiology. *Lab Invest* 1994;70:44A.

29. Bautista NC, Cohen S, Anders KH. Benign melanocytic nevus cells in axillary lymph nodes: a prospective incidence and immunohistochemical study with literature review. *Am J Clin Pathol* 1994;102:102–108.

30. Azzopardi JG, Ross CM, Frizzera G. Blue naevi of lymph node capsule. *Histopathology* 1977;1:451–461.

31. Gray GF Jr, Dineen P. Benign nevus in lymph node. *N Y State J Med* 1976:754–755.

32. Bertrand G, Rabreau M, George P. Presence de cellules naeviques dans les ganglions lymphatiques. *Arch Anat Cytol Pathol* 1980;28:58–62.

33. Goldman RL. Blue nevus of lymph node capsule: report of a unique case. *Histopathology* 1981;5:445–450.

34. Nodl F. Spindelzelliger blauer Naevus mit Lymphknoten-"Metastasen." *Arch Dermatol* 1979;264:179–184.

35. Lamovec J. Blue nevus of the lymph node capsule: report of a new case with review of the literature. *Am J Clin Pathol* 1984;81:367–372.

36. Douglas-Jones AG. Benign lymph node inclusions mimicking metastatic carcinoma. *J Clin Pathol* 1994;47:868–869.

## Sinus Histiocytosis

37. Cutler SJ, Black MM, Friedell GH, et al. Prognostic factors in cancer of the female breast. II. Reproducibility of histopathologic classification. *Cancer* 1966;19:75–82.

38. Black MM, Asire AJ. Palpable axillary lymph nodes in cancer of the breast. Structural and biologic considerations. *Cancer* 1969;23: 251–259.

39. Silverberg SG, Chitale AR, Hind AD, et al. Sinus histiocytosis and mammary carcinoma: study of 366 radical mastectomies and an historical review. *Cancer* 1970;26:1177–1185.

40. Black MM, Leis HP Jr. Cellular responses to autologous breast cancer tissue. Correlation with stage and lymphoreticular reaction. *Cancer* 1971;28:263–273.

41. Black MM, Opler SR, Speer FD. Survival in breast cancer cases in relation to structure of primary tumor and regional lymph nodes. *Surg Gynecol Obstet* 1955;100:543–551.

42. Black MM, Speer FD. Sinus histiocytosis of lymph nodes in cancer. *Surg Gynecol Obstet* 1958;106:163–175.

43. Cutler SJ, Black MM, Goldenberg IS. Prognostic factors in cancer of the female breast. I. An investigation of some interrelations. *Cancer* 1963;16:1589–1597.

44. Cutler SJ, Black MM, Mork T, et al. Further observations on prognostic factors in cancer of the female breast. *Cancer* 1969;24:653–667.

45. Friedell GH, Soto EA, Kumaoka S, et al. Sinus histiocytosis in British and Japanese patients with breast cancer. *Lancet* 1974;II:1228–1229.

46. Berg JW. Sinus histiocytosis: a fallacious measure of host resistance to cancer. *Cancer* 1956;9:935–939.

47. Moore RD, Chapnick R, Schoenberg MD. Lymph nodes associated with carcinoma of the breast. *Cancer* 1960;13:545–549.

48. DiRe JJ, Lane M. The relation of sinus histiocytosis in axillary lymph nodes to surgical curability of carcinoma of the breast. *Am J Clin Path* 1963;40:508–515.

49. Schiodt T. *Breast carcinoma: a histologic and prognostic study of 650 followed-up cases.* Copenhagen: Munksgaard; 1966.

50. Kister SJ, Sommers SC, Haagensen CD, et al. Nuclear grade and sinus histiocytosis in cancer of the breast. *Cancer* 1969;23:570–575.

## Silicone Lymphadenitis

51. Benjamin E, Ahmed A, Rashid ATMF, et al. Silicone lymph adenopathy: a report of two cases one with concomitant malignant lymphoma. *Diagn Histopathol* 1982;5:133–141.

52. Harvey T, Leahy M. Silicone lymphadenopathy: a complication of silicone elastomer finger joint prostheses. *J Rheumatol* 1984;11:104–105.

53. Hausner RJ, Schoen FJ, Mendez-Fernandez MA, et al. Migration of silicone gel to axillary lymph nodes after prosthetic mammoplasty. *Arch Pathol Lab Med* 1981;105:371–372.

54. Wintsch W, Smahel J, Clodius L. Local and regional lymph node responses to ruptured gel-filled mammary prostheses. *Br J Plast Surg* 1978;31:349–352.

55. Rivero MA, Schwartz DS, Mies C. Silicon lymphadenopathy involving intramammary lymph nodes: a new complication of silicone mammaplasty. *AJR Am J Roentgenol* 1994;162:1089–1090.

56. Kao CC, Rand RP, Holt CA, et al. Internal mammary silicone lymphadenopathy mimicking recurrent breast cancer. *Plast Reconstr Surg* 1997;99:225–229.

57. Truong LD, Cartwright J Jr, Goodman MD, et al. Silicone lymphadenopathy associated with augmentation mammaplasty. Morphologic features in nine cases. *Am J Surg Pathol* 1988;12:484–491.

58. Greene WB, Raso DS, Walsh LG, et al. Electron probe microanalysis of silicon and the role of the macrophage in proximal (capsule) and distant sites in augmentation mammaplasty patients. *Plast Reconstr Surg* 1995;95:513–519.

59. Vaamonde R, Cabrera JM, Vaamonde-Martin RJ, et al. Silicone granulomatous lymphadenopathy and siliconomas of the breast. *Histol Histopathol* 1997;12:1003–1011.

60. Sever CE, Leith CP, Appenzeller J, et al. Kikuchi's histiocytic necrotizing lymphadenitis associated with ruptured silicone breast implant. *Arch Pathol Lab Med* 1996;120:380–385.

## Pigment Deposits in Axillary Lymph Nodes and the Breast

61. Cserni G. Misidentification of an axillary sentinel lymph node due to anthracosis. *Eur J Surg Oncol* 1998;24:168.

62. Bruwer A, Nelson GW, Spark RP. Punctate intranodal gold deposits simulating microcalcifications on mammograms. *Radiology* 1987; 163:87–88.

63. Carter TR. Intramammary lymph node gold deposits simulating microcalcifications on mammogram. *Hum Pathol* 1988;19:992–994.

64. Lefer LG, Rosier PP. Ochronosis in the breast. *Am J Clin Pathol* 1979;71:349–352.

## Vascular Lesions

65. Chan JKC, Grizzera G, Fletcher CD, et al. Primary vascular tumors of lymph nodes other than Kaposi's sarcoma: analysis of 39 cases and delineation of two new entities. *Am J Surg Pathol* 1992;16:335–350.

66. Kasznica J, Sideli RV, Collins MH. Lymph node hemangioma. *Arch Pathol Lab Med* 1989;113:804–807.

67. Lubin J, Rywlin AM. Lymphoma-like lymph node changes in Kaposi's sarcoma. *Arch Pathol Lab Med* 1971;92:338–341.

68. Ramos CV, Taylor HB, Hernandez BA, et al. Primary Kaposi's sarcoma of lymph nodes. *Am J Clin Pathol* 1976;66:998–1003.

69. Haferkamp O, Rosenau W, Lennert K. Vascular transformation of lymph node sinuses due to venous obstruction. *Arch Pathol* 1971;92:81–83.

70. Ostrowski ML, Siddiqui T, Barners RE, et al. Vascular transformation of lymph node sinuses, a process displaying a spectrum of histological features. *Arch Pathol Lab Med* 1990;114:656–660.

71. Chan JKC, Warnke RA, Dorfman R. Vascular transformation of sinuses in lymph nodes: a study of its morphological spectrum and distinction for Kaposi's sarcoma. *Am J Surg Pathol* 1991;15:732–743.

72. Fayemi AO. Nodal angiomatosis. *Arch Pathol* 1975;99:170–172.

## Intramammary Lymph Nodes

73. Kalisher L. Xeroradiography of axillary lymph node disease. *Radiology* 1975;114:67–71.

74. Meyer JE, Kopans DB, Lawrence WD. Normal intramammary lymph nodes presenting as occult breast masses. *Breast* 1982;40:30–32.

75. Gallardo X, Sentis M, Castaner E, et al. Enhancement of intramammary lymph nodes with lymphoid hyperplasia: a potential pitfall in breast MRI. *Eur Radiol* 1998;8:1662–1665.

76. Layfield LJ, Glasgow BJ, Hirschcowitz S, et al. Intramammary lymph nodes: cytologic findings and implications for fine-needle aspiration cytology diagnosis of breast nodules. *Diagn Cytopathol* 1997; 17:223–229.

77. Hyman LJ, Abellera M. Carcinomatous lymph nodes within breast parenchyma. *Arch Surg* 1974;109:759–761.

78. Kopans DB, Meyer JE, Murphy GF. Benign lymph nodes associated with dermatitis presenting as breast masses. *Radiology* 1980; 137:15–19.

79. Arnaout AH, Shousha S, Metaxas N, et al. Intramammary tuberculous lymphadenitis. *Histopathology* 1990;17:91–93.

80. Carter JR. Intramammary lymph node gold deposits simulating microcalcifications on mammogram. *Hum Pathol* 1988;19:992–994.

81. Meyer JE, Kopans DB, Long JC. Mammographic appearance of malignant lymphoma of the breast. *Radiology* 1980;135:623–626.

82. Laforga JB, Chorda D, Sevilla F. Intramammary lymph node involvement by mycosis fungoides diagnosed by fine-needle aspiration biopsy. *Diagn Cytopathol* 1998;19:124–126.

83. Lindfors KK, Kopans DB, McCarthy KA, et al. Breast cancer metastasis to intramammary lymph nodes. *AJR Am J Roentgenol* 1986; 146:133–136.

84. McSweeney MB, Egan RL. Prognosis of breast cancer related to intramammary lymph nodes. *Recent Results Cancer Res* 1984; 90:166–172.

85. Dawson PM, Shousha S, Burn JI. Lymph nodes presenting as breast lumps. *Br J Surg* 1987;74:1167–1168.

86. Shamlou KK. Intramammary lymph node in the lower outer quadrant detected by mammography. *AJR Am J Roentgenol* 1992;159:899.

87. Cawson J, Rose AK. Intramammary lymph node metastases—a rare presenting sign of breast cancer. *The Breast* 1995;4:122–126.

# CHAPTER 46

# Pathologic Examination of Breast and Lymph Node Specimens

The purpose of this chapter is to highlight clinically important aspects of the gross pathologic examination of breast specimens. This is not intended to be a comprehensive presentation of differing points of view, nor should this material be regarded as sufficiently detailed to serve as a laboratory "workbook."

The complexity of pathology reports has increased substantially in the past two decades to accommodate the need for more detailed individualized information about breast and related specimens. This has been necessitated by the availability of an array of primary and adjuvant therapy options and the desire to choose a course of treatment most likely to be beneficial for a given patient. Consequently, a greater number of observations is now recorded for each specimen, especially in regard to the microscopic characteristics of benign and carcinomatous breast specimens. With the advent of sentinel lymph node mapping, greater attention is also given to the diagnosis of specific lymph nodes. Immunohistochemical (IH) procedures have extended the pathologist's role in assessing biologic as well as morphologic prognostic markers; the results of these procedures also appear in the pathology report.

Various structured forms of pathology reports have been devised to present the array of data that a pathologist documents by gross and microscopic examination. These reports have the advantage of ensuring that important observations are noted and reported. They assist the clinical staff by providing comprehensive documentation and can be the source of a database for studies. One disadvantage of most structured reports is that they are inflexible with respect to the order in which information is presented so that, regardless of its importance, a particular finding always appears in the same part of the report. This requires that the entire report be read carefully to ensure that an important finding that might appear near the end of the report is not overlooked. Some pathology departments have addressed this issue by offering a free text summary diagnosis that highlights the most significant findings as well as a formatted comprehensive listing of findings. Additional information about pathology reporting may be found in several reviews and position papers (1–6).

## BREAST BIOPSY

### Small or Incisional Biopsy Specimens

Small needle or incisional biopsy specimens generally will be processed for histologic examination in their entirety. The physician performing the biopsy should exercise care not to crush the specimen. An electrocautery-type scalpel must not be used in obtaining such a biopsy. These samples can be examined by frozen section, but it must be understood that limited information about the characteristics of a lesion is obtained from small specimens. The histologic details can be altered by the frozen section process, and this may impede interpretation of subsequent permanent sections. Consequently, frozen section examination is not recommended unless there are exceptional clinical circumstances. The samples are suitable for IH hormone receptor analysis if they are not damaged by cautery and are promptly fixed in formaldehyde. Unless frozen section or some other study that requires fresh tissue is intended, small biopsy specimens should be placed immediately in fixative for transport to the laboratory.

### Excisional Biopsy Specimens

Many factors may influence the manner in which excisional biopsies are handled in a given situation. Paramount among these are logistic considerations relating to when and where the biopsy is performed and the particular clinical circumstances. Hence, the material presented in this section should be regarded as guidelines that may need to be modified in some situations.

## Gross Examination of Excisional Biopsy

The pathologist is responsible for describing the dimensions and character of the tissue removed from the patient. This can be accomplished most accurately if the excised specimen is delivered intact, promptly, and unfixed to the pathology laboratory.

The size of an excisional biopsy specimen should be recorded in centimeters in three dimensions, and the general shape (e.g., ovoid, spherical) should be recorded. Because the overall dimensions of an excisional biopsy cannot be determined after the tissue has been sliced open and dissected by the operator, the specimen should be intact when delivered to the laboratory. Specimen weight should be documented in grams.

The intact excisional biopsy specimen should be delivered to the pathology laboratory promptly. It is preferable that the tissue be unfixed so as not to preclude the possibility of performing a frozen section or to obtain material for electron microscopy and other studies. If a delay is anticipated, the tissue may be chilled, but freezing the entire specimen will compromise histologic examination. Even if a frozen section is not requested, the tissue should be dissected expeditiously to determine whether a grossly identifiable lesion is present. If a tumor is found, the size should be recorded in centimeters. Because of the critical prognostic significance of tumor size, this measurement should be made before tissue is removed for any purpose. It may be difficult to measure the tumor accurately if the specimen is received sliced previously by the surgeon. The gross character of the tumor (shape, consistency, appearance of cut surface) should be described. Whether or not a distinct lesion is found, the appearance of the breast parenchyma should be noted (consistency, relative proportions of fat and fibrous tissue, cysts or other lesions).

## Frozen Section

In the absence of a grossly apparent mass, routine frozen section examination of a seemingly benign breast biopsy specimen is not recommended. Although a small proportion of such specimens harbor grossly inapparent *in situ* or invasive carcinoma, these foci usually will not be detected in random frozen section (7,8).

The appropriateness of frozen section examination for the diagnosis of mammographically detected lesions has been the subject of controversy. Some reports encompassing large groups of cases have described little difficulty in using frozen sections in this setting (9–11). Others recommended that frozen sections not be routinely performed on such specimens because they are likely to present problems in diagnosis, the tissue may be distorted by freezing artifacts, interpretation may be more difficult in paraffin sections, and portions of the tissue may be lost in the process of making frozen sections (1).

Those who recommend using frozen sections to evaluate

nonpalpable lesions caution that a frozen section diagnosis of *in situ* carcinoma or of a benign lesion should be regarded as "preliminary" because of the potential for sampling error and that consequently ". . . definitive therapeutic decisions should be postponed until the final diagnosis on permanent sections has been made" (9). This issue was studied by Niemann et al., who compared the results in 440 consecutive biopsies, of which 98% were examined by frozen section to 604 biopsies, among which only 310 with gross lesions larger than 1.0 cm were submitted for frozen section (12). In the first group, the false-negative rate was 3.3%, with a sensitivity of 84%, whereas in the second, more selected series, the false-negative rate was 1% and the sensitivity 96%. These investigators concluded "that frozen section examination should be limited to cases with distinct gross lesions >1.0 cm." Presently, frozen section is recommended only if the resultant diagnosis will have an immediate effect on treatment, and it is not recommended for the diagnosis of nonpalpable mammographically detected lesions or biopsy specimens in which the pathologist cannot identify a distinct lesion. It is preferable to limit frozen section examination to tumors approximately 1 cm or larger, and a portion of the lesion should be set aside and not frozen.

## Sampling the Biopsy

The number of samples that should be taken from an excisional biopsy for histologic examination varies greatly with the clinical circumstances, the gross appearance of the tissue, and the results of frozen section, if it is performed. No fixed rule (e.g., "x" number of specimens should be examined per 5 g of tissue) can be reasonably applied. The tissue used for frozen section must be saved, processed into a paraffin section, and identified by a term such as the *frozen-section control*. Distinct tumors that appear grossly to be carcinomas 2 or 3 cm or smaller in diameter should be entirely submitted for histology, with samples taken to demonstrate peripheral features of the tumor. Adjacent breast tissue also must be examined microscopically for evidence of lymphatic tumor emboli, *in situ* carcinoma outside the lesion, and the status of the resection margins.

When no distinct tumor is present, some laboratories advocate processing the entire specimen, which may be appropriate in selected situations because of clinical or pathologic findings; however, the cost of applying this approach indiscriminately can become prohibitive, and judgment must be exercised here as well as in the choice of other clinical or laboratory diagnostic procedures. To establish criteria for sampling grossly negative breast biopsies, Schnitt and Wang carried out a retrospective study of 384 specimens entirely submitted for histologic examination from biopsies performed for clinically palpable lesions in which no distinct tumor was evident on gross pathologic examination (13). The paraffin-embedded samples were labeled sequentially. One to 80 blocks were required to submit entire specimens, resulting in 3,342 blocks (average, 8.7/case; median, 6/case).

Carcinoma was found in 23 (6%) specimens, and atypical hyperplasia was found in three others (0.8%). Eighty percent of the blocks consisting of fibrous parenchyma contained all carcinomas and two of the three atypical hyperplasias (AHs). One focus of atypical lobular hyperplasia was present among the 20% of specimens that consisted entirely of fat. If sampling had been limited to five blocks per case, 41% fewer blocks would have been prepared, but six of the 26 (23%) significant lesions would have been missed. By submitting up to 10 blocks of fibrous parenchyma per case, it would have been possible to detect 25 of the 26 significant lesions with an 18% reduction in blocks. Only a single microscopic focus of lobular carcinoma *in situ* was overlooked by this selection. Mathematic analysis of the relationship between specimen size and the number of samples needed to find carcinoma or AH indicated that ". . . it is not necessary to increase proportionately the actual number of blocks submitted to achieve the same probability of detecting carcinoma or AH in larger specimens as for smaller specimens (13). These researchers recommended submitting up to 10 samples of fibrous parenchyma or, if the specimen is entirely fat, a similar number of samples. If carcinoma or AH is found in the first set of slides, the remaining tissue may be processed.

Owings and colleagues also investigated the problem of tissue sampling from needle localization breast biopsies (14). They examined 157 consecutive specimens, among which 32% contained carcinoma. All specimens were submitted in their entirety for histologic examination. Forty-nine of 50 carcinomas (98%) and 14 of 19 AHs (74%) were directly related to mammographically detected foci of calcification and would have been found if histologic sampling had been limited to these foci. All carcinomas and 17 of 19 AHs (89%) were detected in samples selected from regions of calcification and all fibrous parenchyma. Although these data provide useful guidelines for initial tissue examination, it may be necessary to obtain further samples to determine the extent of the lesion if initial sections show carcinoma or atypia. The margins of excision should be examined at the time of initial tissue evaluation. These samples may, of necessity, consist of fatty, nonfibrous breast tissue.

Reexcision specimens obtained because a prior biopsy had microscopically positive or close margins usually do not have grossly apparent tumor. Abraham et al. reviewed 97 grossly negative reexcision specimens, from which all tissue was submitted for histologic examination to develop guidelines for processing such specimens (15). Overall, 1,867 tissue blocks were processed (range, 3–74; mean, 19.2). Ten or more blocks were prepared in 67% of the cases. Residual *in situ* or invasive carcinoma was present in 47 reexcisions (48%). The number of blocks with residual carcinoma ranged from 1 to 41, representing 2.4% to 100% of blocks of reexcision tissue. These investigators calculated that submitting two sections per centimeter of maximal tissue dimension from grossly benign reexcision specimens detected 97% of lesions having a major clinical impact on treatment with 315 (17%) fewer paraffin blocks.

## Gross Description as an Index of Samples Taken

The gross description of a biopsy is part of the pathology report. Included in this section must be a listing or index of the tissue samples taken for microscopic examination from each specimen, indicating the number of tissue blocks and providing a key to explain abbreviations used to designate individual samples. Each sample taken from a specimen should be identified with a unique letter or number, which appears on the corresponding paraffin block and histologic slide. All samples taken from a specimen should be identified with a common number or letter, and each should be further labeled with a subnumber, subletter, or other specific designation. For example, in this system, a left breast biopsy would be recorded as specimen "#1" and the samples in paraffin blocks and corresponding histologic slides designated as "#1A," "#1B," and so on. A second biopsy of the right breast would be listed as "#2," with samples designated "#2A," "#2B," and so on. Specific designations, such as "#1MM" instead of consecutive letters that might indicate "medial margin" should be recorded in the index of samples. This information is essential to understanding the significance of individual slides and the relationship of the findings in these slides to the overall diagnosis.

A substantial number of pathology reports prepared presently in the United States do not provide an adequate index of samples (slides) from a specimen or do so in a confusing manner. Because of the increasing mobility of patients and their slides, it is no longer permissible to adhere to idiosyncratic, obscure labelling practices unique to a given facility. One especially *unsatisfactory* method is to label samples taken for histology with consecutive letters without using numbers to designate individual specimens. In this scheme, the gross description will typically state, for example, that "samples A–H are from the left breast," "samples I–K, N–P are from the right breast," and "samples L, M are from the left inferior margin." If presented with the corresponding slides labeled "A–P," a pathologist has no indication that they represent three separate specimens. Even with a copy of the pathology report in hand, it requires close attention to segregate the slides corresponding to each specimen. This task would be greatly facilitated by numbering specimens separately as described above. For the example given here, "A–H" would be indicated as "left breast—#1A–#1H," samples "L, M" as "left breast inferior margin—#2A #2B," and samples "I–K, N–P" as "right breast—#3A–#3F."

## Assessing Margins of Excision

Technical factors complicate the microscopic evaluation of margins. The surface is often extremely irregular and has a large area relative to the sampling that can be accomplished in histologic sections. The uneven surface sometimes contains defects or crevasses that are not part of the true margin. Definitions of positive and "close" margins have not been standardized.

Because the contours and orientation of tissue slices may be altered in the course of preparing histologic sections, it is necessary to mark the surfaces so that they can be identified microscopically. This is most easily accomplished with finely particulate reagents, such as india ink or other dyes that remain adherent to the tissue throughout processing and are visible on the edge of the tissue under the microscope. Various colors can be used to designate specified surfaces or margins. If applied carefully with a cotton applicator, the ink or dye is unlikely to seep appreciably into crevasses in the tissue surface. The tissue should not be dipped into ink or dye because to do so would saturate the surface and lead to seepage into crevices in the surface that can be mistaken for margins microscopically. There is also a risk of contamination on the surface by tissue from a prior specimen. The pigments adhere better to fresh tissue that has been blotted free of blood and moisture than to formalin-fixed tissue. If properly applied to the intact specimen, the surface pigment should not contaminate the interior of the specimen (Fig. 46.1). An excisional biopsy that has been sliced by the operator cannot be reliably reassembled to "ink" the margins. This is another important reason why it is necessary that excisional biopsy specimens be submitted intact to the pathologist.

Once "inked," the specimen should be split in a plane, which will bisect the longest palpable diameter if a tumor can be appreciated (Fig. 46.1). The gross impression of the relationship of an evident tumor to the margins may be reported, although this can underestimate the frequency of involved margins because microscopic invasive and *in situ* carcinoma at the margins may not be apparent to gross inspection (16,17). Specimen radiography has not proven to be a reliable method for assessing the margins of excision at the time of operation (18). Frozen sections of margins are not indicated unless the tumor appears grossly close to a margin, and confirming this intraoperatively will have an immediate impact on treatment. Random frozen sections of margins that appear grossly unremarkable are not recommended. In one study, the sensitivity of this procedure was only 77% (19).

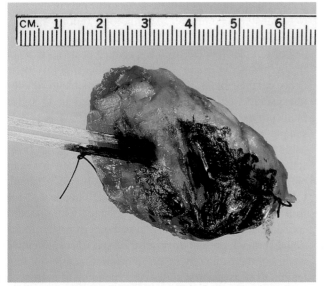

A

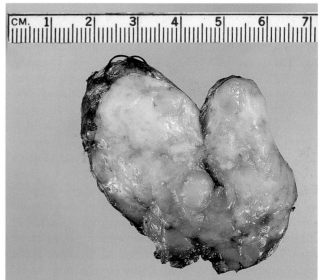

B

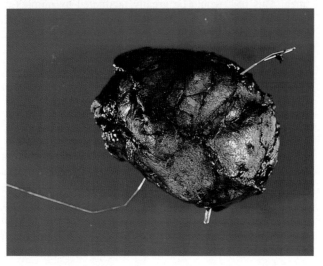

C

**FIG. 46.1.** *Inking an excisional biopsy specimen.* **A:** India ink is being applied to the external fatty surface with cotton-tipped applicators. Ink has not yet been applied to the pale portion of the surface. The long suture behind the applicators designates the lateral margin, and the short suture on the *right* indicates the superior surface. **B:** The specimen has been bisected showing ink limited to the outer surface of the tissue. No gross lesion is evident. **C:** The external surface of an intact needle localization excisional biopsy after the application of india ink. The localizing wire remains in place. A clip at the lower border of the specimen is an orientation marker.

Weber et al. described the results of a study in which frozen sections were performed on samples obtained from the surface of the cavity left after an excisional biopsy (20). Five samples were taken from each biopsy cavity in 140 cases with a mean subsequent follow-up of 57 months. Carcinoma was found in one or more biopsy cavity samples from 21 (15%) of the patients. In 14 of the 21 cases, negative margins were achieved by reexcision. Three patients found to have persistent involvement of margins underwent immediate mastectomy. This procedure has been questioned for several reasons presented by Esserman and Weidner (21). The cost-effectiveness is marginal at best, and in most institutions exceeds the cost of reoperation in the minority of cases with positive margins if the cavity biopsies are submitted only for paraffin section. The difficulty of distinguishing atypical hyperplasia from intraductal carcinoma in cavity biopsies is also a concern. Finally, conversion of planned excisional surgery to an immediate mastectomy without consultation with the patient is presently acceptable to relatively few women.

It is important to distinguish between *shaved* and *inked* margins when reporting the margin status of a biopsy. A shaved margin is a thin slice of tissue taken parallel to the surface of the specimen or biopsy cavity as a separate sample. Shave samples are sectioned *en face,* and the margin is considered positive if any carcinoma cells are detected. Because shave samples are likely to be at least 2 mm thick, it is possible for carcinoma detected in an *en face* histologic section to be 2 mm or farther from the true margin, a significant limitation of this method. Samples designated as inked margins are taken perpendicular to the surface and considered positive when carcinoma cells are seen microscopically at the inked edge.

Guidi et al. found that 39% of patients with a positive shave margin had negative inked margins and that the likelihood of having a positive inked margin increased with more frequent positive shave margins in a given case (22). Rubin et al. reported finding carcinoma in 9% of tumor-bed biopsies from 135 consecutive patients with histologically negative margins in lumpectomy specimens (23).

It is not possible to orient accurately the margins of an excisional biopsy specimen without guidance from the surgeon. This can be easily accomplished if the operator places a short suture at the superior margin and a long stitch laterally (Fig. 46.1). One widely accepted approach to evaluating margins histologically uses samples taken perpendicular to each of the six inked surfaces (superior, inferior, medial, lateral, superficial, and deep) with additional samples of margins determined by the gross findings. At least two perpendicular sections are taken from each surface. Carter recommended "peeling" the entire external surface from the specimen, a procedure that is technically difficult and likely to obscure orientation of the margin (24).

Cytologic methods for examining the margins of resection also have been investigated. Cox et al. used touch preparations from the surfaces of lumpectomy specimens to assess the margins (19) and had three false-positive interpretations. Frozen section examination yielded five false-negative and no false-positive results in the same series of specimens. Veronesi et al. explored the use of the monoclonal antibody B72.3 as a means of detecting carcinoma cells at the margins of excisional biopsies (25). Cytospin preparations were made from specimens obtained by scraping the biopsy surface. One significant limitation of this procedure was the fact that only 57% of the primary carcinomas were B72.3 positive. Immunoreactive cells were detected in 33% of the cytospin specimens containing a B72.3-positive tumor examined by using this investigative approach, whereas only 12% had positive margins histologically. The clinical significance of finding B72.3-positive cells cytologically on the surface of a specimen with histologically negative margins has not been determined. England et al. also described a method for evaluating the margins of a lumpectomy specimen by cytologic examination of cells obtained by scraping the surface of the tissue (26).

There is no standardized system for reporting the microscopic appearance of margins. Interpretation is directed at the distribution of intraductal or invasive carcinoma in relation to the margin. The proximity of lobular carcinoma *in situ* or proliferative lesions to the margin of resection has not proven to be a risk factor for local breast recurrence after conservation therapy.

Tumor transected at an inked surface represents a positive margin (Fig. 46.2). This criterion applies equally to *in situ* ductal and to any invasive carcinoma. Borderline situations occur in which tumor closely approaches the margin but is not transected (Fig. 46.3). One useful convention in these situations is to regard foci within one high-power microscopic field (2 mm) as being "close to the margin." Others defined tumor as close to the margin when it is within 3 mm of the inked surface (27). The actual microscopic distance in millimeters between carcinoma and a margin can be reported. The nature of the carcinoma at or close to the margin (*in situ* or invasive) should be stated and some estimate of the extent given. It is possible to describe the quantity of carcinoma at or near the margins by specifying the histologic findings in the relevant slides. For example, the report can be worded as follows: "Invasive duct carcinoma involves the inked medial margin in one 40× microscopic field (slide #1MM3) and intraductal carcinoma cribriform type is present in isolated ducts at the superior (#1SM2) and lateral (#1LM2) margins. Invasive carcinoma is close (within a 40× microscopic field) to the lateral margin (#1LM3)."

## Clinical Significance of Margin Assessment

The clinical importance of making a distinction between tumor transected at the margin or close to the margin is uncertain. Schnitt et al., who defined a close margin as carcinoma within 1 mm of the inked margin, reported local recurrence rates at 5 years after lumpectomy and radiation for patients with negative and close margins to be 0% and 4%,

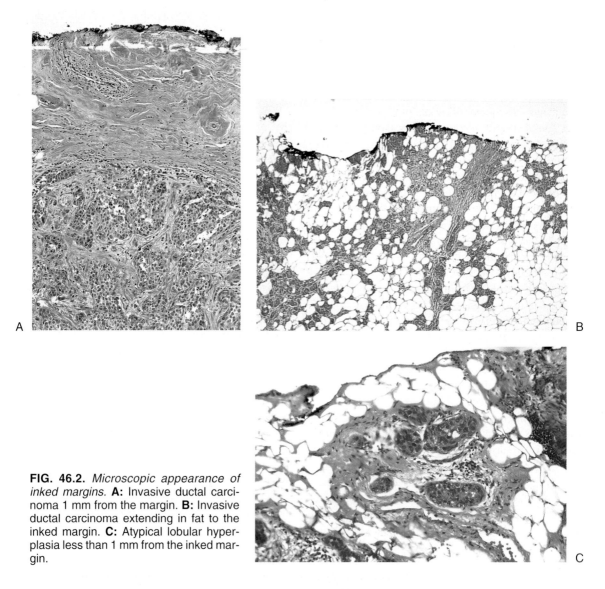

**FIG. 46.2.** *Microscopic appearance of inked margins.* **A:** Invasive ductal carcinoma 1 mm from the margin. **B:** Invasive ductal carcinoma extending in fat to the inked margin. **C:** Atypical lobular hyperplasia less than 1 mm from the inked margin.

**FIG. 46.3.** *Carcinoma close to the inked margins.* **A:** Intraductal carcinoma at various distances from the inked margin. **B:** Intraductal carcinoma less than 1 mm from the inked margin. *(continued)*

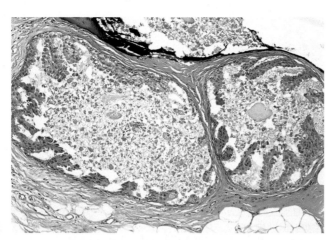
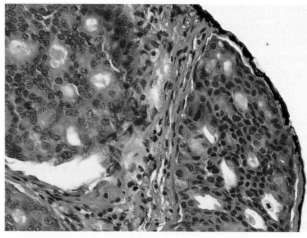

C

D

**FIG. 46.3.** *Continued.* **C:** About 0.1 mm of collagen and the basement membrane separate this intraductal carcinoma from the inked margin. **D:** Only basement membrane lies between the inked margin and intraductal carcinoma.

respectively (28). In this series, the margin was considered to be "focally" positive when carcinoma was "present at the margin in three or fewer low-power microscopic fields using a 4× objective" and "more than focally" positive if greater than three low-power fields were involved. The local recurrence rates for "focal" and "more than focal" involvement were 6% and 21%, respectively. The presence of an extensive component of intraductal carcinoma did not significantly increase the risk of local recurrence in patients with negative, close, or focally involved margins; however, the combination of extensive intraductal carcinoma and more than focal margin involvement was associated with a 50% local failure rate. These observations were confirmed in a subsequent analysis of a larger series by these investigators (29).

The number of margins with carcinoma is significantly related to the likelihood of finding residual tumor at the time of reexcision. Di Biase et al. reported that the number of positive margins diagnosed in biopsy cavity samples was a significant factor for local tumor control and overall survival (30). Local control was inferior for women with two or more positive margins compared with those with negative or only one positive margin. An assessment of the inked margins of excisional biopsy specimens yielded similar data in a study by Papa et al. (31). Residual carcinoma was found in 70% of reexcisions after excision with positive margins (tumor at inked surface) and in 25% after excisions with close margins (tumor <2 mm from inked surface). Residual tumor was found in 12.5%, 37.5%, and 47.9% of reexcision specimens after initial biopsies with one, two, or three positive margins, respectively. In other reports, residual carcinoma was found in 32% to 62% of reexcision specimens (32–36). The likelihood of finding residual carcinoma and the amount of carcinoma in the reexcision specimen were usually a function of the size of the initial tumor and the status of the original resection margins.

A related study of margin status and outcome was re-

ported by Pittinger et al. (27). In this analysis, a *close margin* was defined as tumor detected microscopically within 3 mm of the inked margin of the initial excisional biopsy. When reexcision was performed, residual carcinoma was found in 0%, 24%, 44%, and 48% of patients whose margin status for the initial biopsy was negative, close, positive, or unknown, respectively. Among patients with a follow-up of 3 years or longer, the frequency of breast recurrence after excision and radiotherapy was the same in those with negative and close margins. These investigators concluded that "reexcision of close margins is not necessary in patients" treated by breast-conservation therapy.

The status of lumpectomy margins is an important prognostic indicator for breast recurrence after breast-conservation therapy. Multivariate analysis of 869 stage I and II breast carcinoma patients treated by breast conservation with radiotherapy revealed that margin status was the only significant predictor for local control (37). Among women with positive margins, local control was improved when the dose of radiation to the tumor bed was increased ("boosted"). Mansfield et al. also found positive margin status to be a significant predictor of local failure in a multivariate analysis of stage I and II patients after a median follow-up of 40 months (38).

The local recurrence rate is lower if margins are negative than if they are positive or unknown (27,39,40), but it is well documented that margins reported to be negative do not provide complete assurance that local recurrence will not occur in patients given equivalent treatment (41). The breast recurrence rates for patients treated for "small" invasive carcinomas in a trial comparing lumpectomy to quadrantectomy, in which all patients received radiotherapy, were 4.5% and 8.6% and respectively (25). In a subsequent report, the 10-year estimated breast recurrence rate after lumpectomy was 18.6%, and 7.4% after quadrantectomy (42). Margin status, reported to be positive in 16.3% of lumpectomy cases and in 4.5% who underwent quadrantectomy, was not significantly related to recurrence in the breast, despite the fact that reexcision was not performed when margins were involved.

A study by the National Surgical Adjuvant Breast Project revealed a breast recurrence rate of nearly 40% in women with negative margins treated by lumpectomy without radiotherapy (43). Comparable negative margin patients who received radiotherapy had a 10% local recurrence rate at 8 years. Others reported local recurrence rates after radiation therapy of 28% (44), 13% (45) or 9% (46), 3.7% (40), 3% (27), 2% (19), and 0% (28) when margins were negative. Final margin status that takes account of reexcision is a much more reliable predictor of local control than original excision margins alone (39).

The relationship of local recurrence in the breast to the occurrence of distant metastases and death from breast carcinoma is controversial. Several studies showed no significant difference in distant disease-free survival between women who did or did not have a breast recurrence after conservation therapy. Others reported a less favorable outcome after local recurrence, which has been attributed to an initially more aggressive primary tumor causing local as well as distant metastases rather than the local recurrence giving rise to systemic disease (47–52).

Fortin et al. evaluated survival in patients treated by breast conservation with radiotherapy and concluded that local failure could be a source of distant metastases (53). The study included 2,030 patients with a median follow-up of 6 years. The local control rate at 10 years was 87%. Patients with local failure had a significantly less favorable 10-year survival rate (55%) than those who did not experience a breast recurrence. Local failure was a significant predictor of poor survival in multivariate analysis. Compared with those who did not experience local failure, the relative risk for death from breast carcinoma was 3.6 for those with local recurrence; their relative risk for systemic metastases was 5.6. Evidence for local recurrence as a possible source of distant metastases came from analysis of the timing of systemic recurrences. Among women with local breast recurrence, the rate of systemic recurrences was higher than in those without local failure, but the rates were parallel for 2 years after treatment. The rate of systemic recurrence rose thereafter among those with local recurrence reaching a peak around 6 years, whereas the group with local control had a declining rate of systemic spread more than 2 years after treatment (Fig. 46.4). Consequently, the mean time until systemic recurrence was significantly shorter among women with local control (1,050 days) than in the group with local failure (1,650 days). In this series, patients with close or positive margins had a higher local failure rate (15.7%) than those with negative margins. The presence of tumor at or close to the margin was associated with more frequent systemic recurrence (28%) than negative margins (17%).

Studies of margin status as a predictor of local control vary greatly in terms of the uniformity of surgical procedures performed, the completeness of pathologic evaluation, the methods of irradiation, and the length of follow-up. Differ-

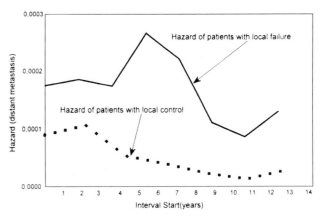

**FIG. 46.4.** *Local breast recurrence after conservation therapy and the hazard rate of distant metastases.* Patients with local control after primary therapy had a lower risk of systemic metastases than those with local failure. (From Fortin A, Larochelle M, Laverdiere J, et al. Local failure is responsible for the decrease in survival for patients with breast cancer treated with conservative surgery and postoperative radiotherapy. *J Clin Oncol* 1999;17:101–109, with permission.)

ences can be found in these variables between studies and also in the selection of treatment for patients within a given study. For example, Solin et al. used mastectomy to treat patients with grossly positive or diffusely positive microscopic margins (54). Among patients selected for breast conservation, there were significant differences in the total radiation dosages administered respectively to women with negative, positive, close, or unknown margins, with the lowest doses given to those with negative margins.

Mammography is an important element in the clinical follow-up of patients after breast-conservation therapy (55). In one study, 47 of 189 (25%) breast recurrences in patients without systemic metastases were detected by mammography alone. Mammographically detected lesions were smaller than those detected by palpation or other signs. Patient outcome was correlated significantly with the size of recurrent tumors. The 5-year frequencies of death and of systemic metastases were 38% and 30.7%, respectively, for patients with tumors 10 mm or smaller in diameter, whereas for patients with recurrent tumors larger than 10 mm, the frequencies were 46% and 54.4%, respectively. These results suggest that early detection of breast recurrence might be beneficial to overall prognosis in women treated by breast-conservation therapy.

## Reexcision of the Biopsy Site

Reexcision of the biopsy site is indicated when the margins of the initial excision are involved grossly by carcinoma, if breast conservation is desired, and if an acceptable cosmetic result can be achieved. Other relative indications for reexcision are the finding of residual microcalcifications at the biopsy site in the postbiopsy mammogram, extensive involvement of the margins by carcinoma microscopically, the presence of "extensive" intraductal carcinoma (defined later) in the initial excision specimen, and inability to assess the margin status of the first excision. Reexcision is less often recommended if involvement is limited to microscopic carcinoma at one focus or in one of multiple margins or if carcinoma is extensive and close to (variously defined as 1, 2, or 3 mm) but does not involve the margin. The likely cosmetic effect of reexcision and whether radiation will be used can influence the decision to recommend reexcision.

The reexcision specimen should be handled by the surgeon and pathologist in the same fashion as the primary lumpectomy is handled. The specimen should be submitted intact with orientation markers such as sutures. Frozen section examination of the margins of reexcision specimens is rarely indicated except to confirm a gross impression of carcinoma extending to a margin. The gross assessment of the amount of carcinoma, if any, remaining at the biopsy site is unreliable because fat necrosis, fibrosis, and hemorrhage in this region can produce a palpable alteration that may be mistaken for carcinoma. Most reexcision specimens, especially those 3 cm or smaller in diameter, can be submitted in their entirety. The extent of sampling of larger specimens depends on the gross findings and the indications for reexcision but generally should follow the guidelines for a primary lumpectomy discussed previously in this chapter.

## Extensive Intraductal Carcinoma

*Extensive intraductal carcinoma* (EIC) has been defined as the presence of intraductal carcinoma, making up more than 25% of the area of the entire invasive carcinoma and the presence of intraductal carcinoma in the surrounding breast tissue (2). Residual carcinoma, especially intraductal, is more likely to be found in the reexcision if the primary invasive carcinoma was accompanied by EIC (34). Among patients with a microscopically positive margin in the primary excision, there is a substantially greater likelihood of finding residual carcinoma in the reexcision if the initial specimen has EIC (2). The presence of EIC has been shown to be a predictor of increased risk for local recurrence in the breast by some investigators (2,28,44,56–58). Sinn et al. defined extensive intraductal carcinoma as being present if the extent of the intraductal component was at least twice the size of the invasive carcinoma or if the tumor was predominantly intraductal (56). The presence of EIC in this study was associated with low tumor grade, positive resection margins, and multifocal invasive carcinoma. In multivariate analysis, the factors associated with local recurrence were EIC [relative risk (RR) = 1.9], high-grade tumor (RR = 1.76), lobular carcinoma (RR = 1.65), age at diagnosis 40 years or younger (RR = 1.39), and "angioinvasion" (RR = 1.34). The risk of local breast recurrence at 5 years was 79.1 ± 3.6% when two or more of these risk factors were present, 95.4 ± 1.2% when one factor was present, and 99 ± 0.6% when none of the factors was present. Other investigators, however, have not reported a higher local recurrence rate in women with EIC or found that it was a significant predictor in univariate but not in multivariate analysis (28,29,39,45).

Ohtake et al. developed a unique method for mapping the distribution of intraductal carcinoma in patients with invasive carcinoma (59). The procedure used computer graphics to create a three-dimensional reconstruction of the ductal system using information obtained from subgross serial sections of the specimen. In most cases, intraductal extension tended to be distributed centrally from the invasive lesion toward the nipple. Less often, intraductal carcinoma extended only peripherally or both centrally and to the periphery. Anastomosing ductal branches connecting otherwise independent ductal systems were found in breast tissue not involved by intraductal carcinoma, and in one case such a connecting branch provided the bridge for extension of intraductal carcinoma beyond a single duct system. Further development of such computer graphic systems could provide a method for more accurately describing the distribution of intraductal carcinoma in clinical practice.

Many breast tumors are now diagnosed initially by needle core biopsy, especially when the lesion is not palpable. The samples obtained by this procedure typically include portions of the main lesion as well as peripheral tissue. Jimenez et al. reported that the relative proportions of intraductal and invasive carcinoma in needle biopsy samples correlated significantly with the distribution of these components in corresponding surgical excisions (60). A needle core biopsy was deemed to have EIC if the ratio of ducts with intraductal carcinoma to the number of cores was greater than 0.5. A specimen with a ratio of 0.5 or less was considered EIC negative. EIC was present in 70% of excisions after core biopsies with a ratio greater than 0.5 and in 36% when the ratio was 0.5. or less. EIC was present in only 2 of 29 (7%) excisional biopsies obtained after the core biopsy specimen had no intraductal carcinoma.

## TNM Staging

TNM staging according to criteria of the American Joint Committee on Cancer (AJCC) (see Chapter 12) may be inaccurate when based only on the initial excision if the patient has positive margins and residual tumor is detected in a reexcision specimen. Evidence to support this supposition was presented by Brenin and Morrow, who found a significantly greater frequency of nodal metastases in patients who had residual invasive tumor in a reexcision than when no tumor remained (61). The analysis was controlled for major predictors of lymph node metastases and compared patients on the basis of tumor size measured only in the initial excision. These researchers concluded that understaging may occur, especially among patients with T1a–b tumors, if invasive carcinoma remains in a reexcision, and they suggested that this possibility be considered in planning treatment. No method was offered for arriving at a tumor size based on measurements from both specimens. This issue is difficult to resolve because breast carcinomas are rarely spherical, and it is uncertain whether the diameter of residual tumor should be added to the largest diameter of the primary lesion. A small size increment could have a major impact on treatment, for example, by changing staging from T1a to T1b, making axillary staging probable, or from T1b to T1c, rendering the patient a candidate for adjuvant therapy.

Radiographic techniques offer promise for preoperative staging, and they may improve the accuracy of surgical excision. Magnetic resonance imaging (MRI) has proven more useful than conventional mammography for evaluating possible invasion of the pectoral muscle in patients with a deep or posterior tumor. A study of 19 patients with this clinical presentation revealed that 12 patients had mammographic findings suggestive of muscle involvement (62). MRI images showed extension to the prepectoral fat plane and muscle enhancement in five of these cases, which proved to be the only ones with muscle invasion demonstrated surgically.

Magnetic resonance imaging (MRI) has the potential for detecting the presence and distribution of EIC or multifocal and multicentric carcinoma. Esserman et al. analyzed 44 cases in which MRI and mammography had been performed (63). The MRI interpretation was in concordance with the pathologic findings in each of 19 patients with a unicentric tumor, all 10 patients with multifocal or multicentric carcinoma, and in seven of eight patients (88%) with EIC. The false-positive rate, representing an MRI determination of more extensive tumor than was detected pathologically, and the false-negative rate were each about 3%. Ultrasonography has also proven effective for detecting multifocal or multicentric carcinoma that was not apparent in conventional mammograms (64).

The presence of lymphatic tumor emboli associated with a primary carcinoma or in a reexcision specimen was associated with a significantly increased risk for local recurrence in patients treated by lumpectomy and radiotherapy (24,25) in some reports (31,43,44), but others reported no association (29,55).

## Biopsy Specimen Radiography

The radiologic examination of excised breast tissue has been used for nearly 75 years (65). As early as 1913, Albert Salomon, a surgeon at the University of Berlin, reported on the use of radiography to study mastectomy specimens (66). Salomon used serial sections of specimens to correlate histologic and radiologic features of breast carcinoma. He described radiologically detected calcifications in breast carcinomas, but the clinical significance of this finding was not appreciated until several decades later when clinical mammography had been substantially improved (67). In 1951, Leborgne commented on a case in which "roentgenographic study of the operative specimen also permitted the localization of the tiny calcifications for histopathologic study, and thus aided in finding a small cancer" (68).

The increasing use of clinical mammography is a major factor in the progressively earlier stage of breast carcinomas detected in the past two decades (69). Carcinomas are detected because of an abnormal soft-tissue structure, the presence of calcifications, or as a result of both findings. Soft-tissue alterations in the breast may be distorted in the excised specimen, rendering them less suited to specimen radiographic study. Changes in the relationships of structures in the compressed breast at the time of mammography and the altered orientation in an excised specimen make it difficult to compare these features accurately in clinical and specimen radiographs. Clinical mammographic findings, which do not lend themselves to specimen radiography, are alterations in parenchymal pattern, skin changes, vascular abnormalities, and ill-defined mass lesions (70,71). Specimen compression devices are useful for localizing noncalcified lesions in specimen radiographs (72), and image quality may be improved further if the specimen is immersed in water (72–74) (Fig. 46.5). Sonography also has been used to assess biopsy spec-

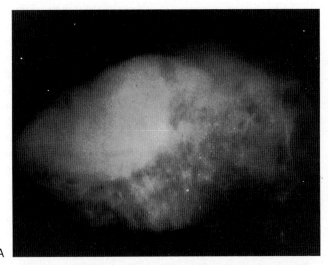
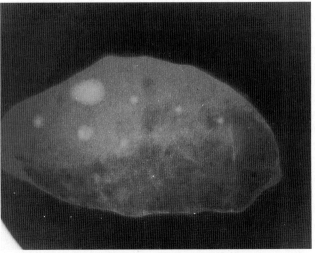

A

B

**FIG. 46.5.** *Specimen radiography with compression.* **A:** A specimen radiograph taken without compression. No discrete lesions are apparent. **B:** A radiograph of the specimen shown in **A** taken with compression. Seven discrete, circumscribed nodules can be seen. The largest nodule was a fibroadenoma; the others were cysts.

imens obtained after preoperative sonographic localization of nonpalpable lesions (75).

Specimen radiography has been particularly helpful for lesions with calcifications. The presence of calcifications in the lesion or close to it provides an intrinsic marker that can be seen in the clinical and specimen radiograph (Fig. 46.6). Specimen radiography provides a method for proving that a nonpalpable lesion has been removed, and it is an efficient technique for pinpointing the area for histologic examination (76) (Fig. 46.7). Carcinoma is found in about 25% of nonpalpable lesions biopsied because the mammogram reveals a pattern of calcification that suggests carcinoma (70,71,77).

To evaluate a breast specimen radiograph effectively, it is necessary to have the clinical mammogram simultaneously available. A variety of procedures have been described in the literature for specimen radiography, and this presentation will not address their advantages or disadvantages, which often depend on the availability of personnel and other resources in a given institution. Thus, the processing or interpretation of specimen radiographs may be the responsibility of a pathologist, surgeon, or radiologist; however, certain principles apply in most situations.

A radiograph should be made of the intact excisional biopsy, and the film should be compared with the mammogram before the specimen is moved or dissected. If the tissue is dissected before obtaining a specimen radiograph, a fortuitous cut may disrupt the pattern of calcifications and interfere with comparison of the clinical and specimen films. Changes in the position of the specimen make it difficult to pinpoint the location of calcifications.

It is recommended that nonpalpable mammographically detected lesions be processed solely for paraffin sections and that frozen sections be performed only in exceptional situations (1). In one study of 359 mammographically detected lesions, frozen section yielded a correct diagnosis in 68% of cases, 17.3% did not have a frozen section, 1.9% of frozen sections yielded false-negative results, and 0.6% were false-positive diagnoses (78).

The immediate goal of specimen radiography is to confirm that a nonpalpable lesion has been excised, which should be determined intraoperatively. If the lesion is not present in the specimen, the surgeon may elect to obtain more tissue. Postoperative mammography is reportedly useful for evaluating patients with a negative or inconclusive

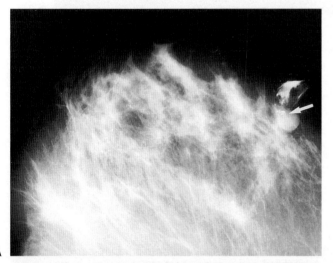

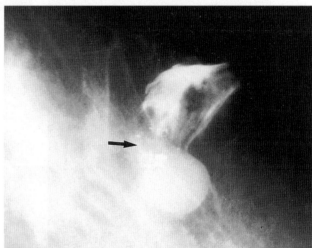

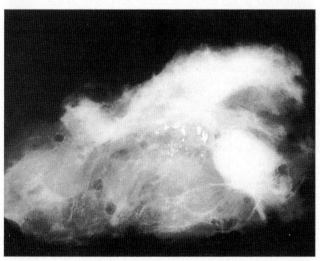

A

B

C

**FIG. 46.6.** *Mammography-specimen radiography correlation.* **A,B:** This craniocaudad mammogram of the left breast from a 71-year-old woman reveals a circumscribed oval mass. In this view, calcifications are seen overlying the density *(arrows)*. An irregular area of density *(white)* above the mass is dye injected for localization. **C:** The calcifications are shown to be separate from the oval mass in this specimen radiograph. The radiopaque localizing dye has been absorbed and is not visible. The mass was a fibroadenoma and the calcifications were at the site of intraductal carcinoma.

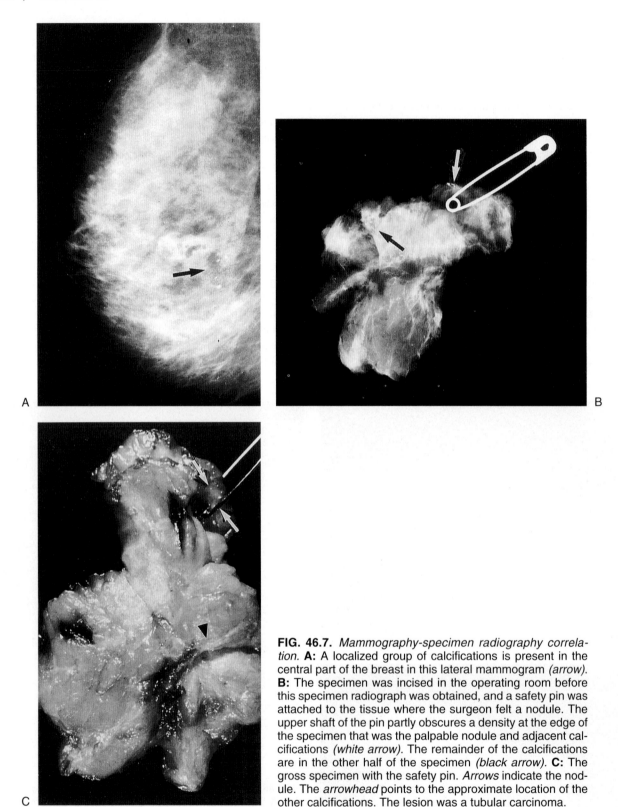

**FIG. 46.7.** *Mammography-specimen radiography correlation.* **A:** A localized group of calcifications is present in the central part of the breast in this lateral mammogram *(arrow).* **B:** The specimen was incised in the operating room before this specimen radiograph was obtained, and a safety pin was attached to the tissue where the surgeon felt a nodule. The upper shaft of the pin partly obscures a density at the edge of the specimen that was the palpable nodule and adjacent calcifications *(white arrow).* The remainder of the calcifications are in the other half of the specimen *(black arrow).* **C:** The gross specimen with the safety pin. *Arrows* indicate the nodule. The *arrowhead* points to the approximate location of the other calcifications. The lesion was a tubular carcinoma.

specimen radiograph following biopsy of a lesion without calcifications (79). Others recommend delaying operative mammography for 6 to 12 weeks after biopsy to minimize discomfort associated with the procedure and to allow subsidence of postsurgical inflammation that may obscure the

mammogram (80). Missed lesions have been reported in up to 13.6% of needle localization biopsies (81), but in most series, this occurred in 5% or less of cases (82–84).

False-negative specimen radiographs may occur because the lesion has been distorted by the operation, by dissection after excision, or as a result of positioning the specimen so that it obscured the lesion when the image was obtained. The specimen radiograph also may be negative because of inaccurate preoperative localization or loss of localization resulting from displacement of a needle or wire used in this procedure. Finally, the position of calcifications may be misjudged in conventional mammographic views if localization has not been performed. Cutaneous calcifications can be misinterpreted as an intraparenchymal lesion (85). Tangential views and stereotactic imaging are useful for confirming the cutaneous position of such calcifications (86). One unusual cutaneous abnormality that may mimic calcifications in the breast is a skin tattoo (87). Tattoo powder applied to specimens inadvertently or purposefully to mark margins can be an iatrogenic source of microcalcifications that may interfere with the interpretation of a specimen radiograph (88).

A variety of procedures are available to mark areas in the breast preoperatively to assist the surgeon in excising the lesion and to minimize the size of the specimen required. These procedures include placement of one or more needles or hooked wires in proximity to the lesion (89,90) and the injection of dyes, usually a combination of visible and radiopaque components (91,92) (Fig. 46.8). Presently, almost all localization procedures use a wire or needle placement technique with ultrasound or stereotactic guidance.

Localization assists the pathologist in finding the lesion for pathologic study. Before the position of the specimen is changed, the site of the radiographically detected calcifications or a density should be identified grossly. This portion of the tissue should be excised from the specimen and labeled. The remainder of the tissue also must be dissected because occasionally the calcifications have proven to be in a benign process near an unanticipated carcinoma fortuitously included in the excisional biopsy.

It is essential that the localization wire be left within the excisional biopsy specimen (Figs. 46.1 and 46.9). The pathologist must describe the wire in the gross specimen report. It is advisable that the segment of wire be measured. Localization wires occasionally have been transected intraoperatively, or they may retract into the breast preoperatively and migrate from the lesion in question (93,94). In one remarkable case, a retracted wire migrated to the subcutaneous tissue of the ipsilateral buttock (94).

Most of the lesions that are the target of a wire localization biopsy are microscopic in size. Unless there is a compelling clinical need, frozen section examination is not recommended in these cases (1). If a decision is made to attempt a frozen section and the diagnosis is not readily apparent in the initial slides from the tissue block, further sectioning should not be carried out and the remaining tissue must be fixed for paraffin sections. The surgeon must defer to the pathologist's judgment as to the feasibility of obtaining a diagnosis by frozen section.

## Pathology of Mammary Calcifications

Microcalcifications found in breast tissue were thoroughly described and classified by Frappart et al. (95,96). Most of the calcifications detected in mammograms are basophilic concretions of varying size composed of calcium phosphates largely in the form of hydroxyapatite (97) (Fig. 46.10). These type II calcifications of Frappart are not birefringent. They react with the von Kossa stain and with alizarin red at pH 4.2 and 7.0 (98). A black precipitate is formed with silver nitrate/rubeanic acid but not after pretreatment with 5% acetic acid (98,99).

Foschini et al. described three patterns of calcium phosphate calcification in intraductal carcinoma (100). *Granular calcifications* were formed by deposition of calcium on nuclear debris or on secreted mucosubstances. *Lamellar*

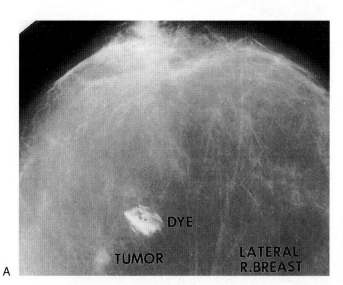
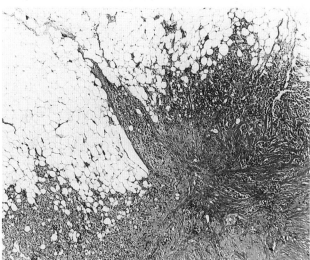

**FIG. 46.8.** *Mammography, nonpalpable tumor without calcification.* **A:** A craniocaudad mammogram of the right breast showing a nonpalpable tumor and dye injected for localization. **B:** The lesion was an invasive duct carcinoma.

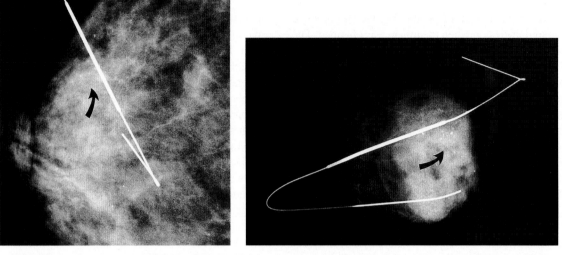

**FIG. 46.9.** *Specimen radiography with localizing wire.* The specimen is from a 55-year-old woman status post left mastectomy with new right breast calcifications. **A:** Craniocaudal mammogram of the right breast shows the localizing wire placed at the site of a new 5-mm cluster of calcifications *(arrow)* in the medial retroareolar region. **B:** The specimen radiograph confirms retrieval of the calcifications *(arrow)* and the localizing wire. Histologic analysis showed intraductal and invasive ductal carcinoma with calcifications in the *in situ* component. (Courtesy of Laura Liberman, M.D.)

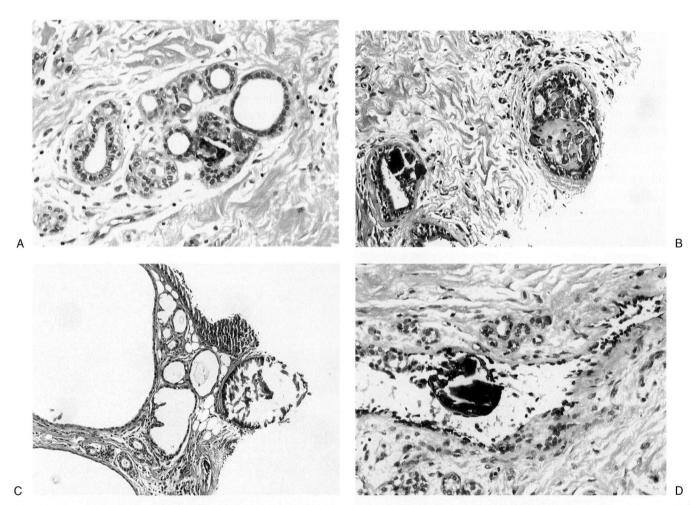

**FIG. 46.10.** *Calcification in benign breast.* Various configurations are depicted. **A:** Lobular microcalcification. **B:** Calcifications in atrophic terminal ducts. An "ossifying" calcification is shown on the *right* in this needle core biopsy specimen. **C:** A ring calcification in one of several cysts in a needle core biopsy sample. **D:** Intraductal calcification. *(continued)*

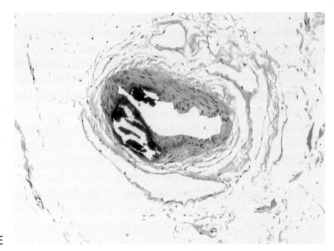
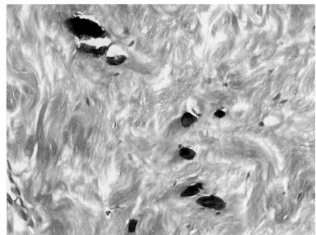

E

F

**FIG. 46.10.** *Continued.* **E:** Arterial calcification. **F:** Stromal calcifications.

*calcifications* resulted from deposits of calcium on proteinaceous or mucoid material arranged in concentric layers. Calcification on *nuclear debris* was found only in intraductal carcinoma with necrosis of intermediate or poorly differentiated grade, whereas the other types of calcification were present mainly in well to moderately differentiated lesions.

Type I microcalcifications composed of calcium oxalate dihydrate crystals (weddelite) are birefringent, nonbasophilic, von Kossa's-negative crystals (97,99,101) (Fig. 46.11). The term *weddelite* derives from the fact that calcium oxalate used commercially was originally extracted from the Weddell Sea, located in the vicinity of the Falkland Islands, named after the British explorer James Weddell (1787–1834) (102). Type I calcifications are not stained by alizarin red at pH 4.2, and at pH 7.0 alizarin red staining is weak or absent. Black staining is observed with silver nitrate/rubeanic acid with or without pretreatment with 5% acetic acid (99). Because they are colorless, calcium oxalate crystals are difficult to identify in hematoxylin and eosin

(H&E)–stained sections with regular light microscopy. They tend to fragment and sometimes are accompanied by multinucleated giant cells. Intact crystals assume various configurations, including overlapping plates, rosettes, sheaves, rods, and geometric shapes, such as pyramids or diamonds (Fig. 46.12).

In one series, 9 of 66 of mammographically detected calcifications (13.6%) identified histologically consisted of calcium oxalate crystals (type I), 72.7% were calcium phosphate (type II), and 13.6% were a mixture of types I and II (97). Similar frequencies of calcium phosphate and oxalate calcifications have been found by other investigators (103). Tornos et al. reported finding type I calcifications alone in 2% and in combination with type II calcifications in 10.4% of 153 specimens (99). Calcium oxalate crystals have been responsible for 7.3% (101) and 12% (104) of mammographically localized calcifications that led to biopsy.

Calcium phosphate calcifications (type II) and calcium oxalate crystals (type I) appear as conventional calcifications

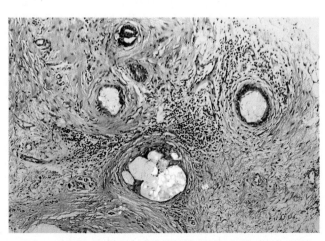
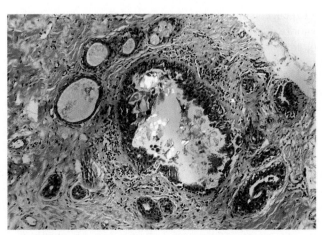

A

B

**FIG. 46.11.** *Calcium oxalate calcifications.* **A:** The calcifications appear as bright birefringent crystals in this section of mastitis examined with polarized illumination. **B:** Calcium oxalate crystals are birefringent in this duct with apocrine epithelium. The specimen is from a needle core biopsy. (Polarized illumination.)

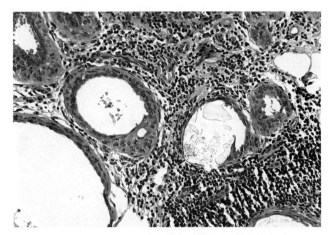

**FIG. 46.12.** *Calcium oxalate calcification.* The visibility of these crystals was enhanced when the tissue was examined with the microscope condenser lowered to heighten refractivity.

in specimen radiographs and in clinical mammograms. Type II calcifications are typically of high to medium density, and they may have irregular or distinct shapes suggestive of carcinoma in a mammogram, whereas type I crystals are likely to appear as polyhedral deposits of low to medium density (105). An analysis of 2,000 screening mammograms revealed that 3% of women examined had two or more polyhedral microcalcifications (106).

Calcium oxalate crystals are seen most frequently in benign microcysts, especially those with apocrine epithelium, and in dilated ducts (Figs. 46.11 and 46.12) (97,99,101, 103,107,108). This association suggests that apocrine epithelium can synthesize or concentrate and secrete oxalic acid or calcium oxalate. In some cases, type II calcium phosphate calcifications have been present coincidentally with calcium oxalate deposits in proliferative lesions. It is unusual for calcium oxalate crystals to develop in carcinoma (96,107). Calcium oxalate crystals have been described in papillary intraductal carcinoma (109).

Type I, calcium oxalate crystals, probably account for the majority of instances in which "calcifications" are reportedly not present in histologic sections of breast biopsies obtained for calcifications found in a mammogram (110,111). In this situation, sections should be examined with polarized light. Fragments of birefringent material may be the only residual evidence of larger crystalline deposits, which sometimes are shattered or partially dissolved during processing of the tissue.

Radiographic examination of paraffin blocks is an essential procedure if a biopsy has been performed for calcifications, and they are not evident in the histologic sections (112). Calcifications are easily identified in the resultant radiographic images, thus allowing the pathologist to select tissue blocks for deeper sections. Radiographs should be obtained to document the presence of calcifications in needle core biopsy samples (113,114).

Image analysis has been applied to the classification of calcifications as they appear in mammograms to refine the characterization of calcification associated with benign and malignant lesions (115–118). Features studied include the number of particles in a cluster, the number of clusters, distances between calcifications in a cluster, and the area of clusters. Data from these analyses ultimately may lead to the development of automated image-screening systems for calcifications, but such procedures cannot replace other aspects of the visual examination of mammograms involving the interpretation of noncalcific parenchymal alterations.

The description of calcifications in clinical mammography is currently presented according to the American College of Radiology Breast Imaging Reporting and Data System (BI-RADS) classification (119). Calcifications classified as *ductal* are typically linear if associated with carcinoma and often branching, whereas benign ductal calcifications are described as "rod-like." *Nonductal* calcifications are typically punctate, pleomorphic, or coarse, irregular deposits. The distribution is usually reported as clustered, linear, segmental or regional.

The precise microanatomic distribution of calcifications is an important consideration when correlating imaging findings with the pathologic diagnosis. Although the presence of calcifications may contribute to the radiologic impression that leads to a biopsy and the finding of carcinoma, some of the calcifications may not be located in the carcinoma, which becomes a concern, especially when a needle core biopsy is performed to sample a lesion with intermediate (BI-RADS 3) or suspicious (BI-RADS 4) calcifications. In some instances, the needle biopsy shown to contain calcifications by specimen radiograph and histologic examination can be an unrepresentative sample of peritumoral tissue. To assess this issue, Selim and Tahan studied the distinction of calcifications in benign tissue surrounding and in carcinomas (120). Calcification was limited to the carcinoma in 31% of cases and was present only in benign components within 1 cm of the carcinoma in 34%. Calcifications were present in the carcinoma and adjacent benign tissue in 35%. These observations underscore the need for correlation between mammography and the diagnosis obtained by needle core biopsy to determine whether the sample is representative of the radiographic image. If the benign biopsy diagnosis is discordant with the mammographic impression, surgical biopsy should be considered, even if calcifications were obtained and documented in the needle core biopsy.

Calcifications are often an important clue to the presence of recurrent carcinoma in the breast after conservation therapy. Dershaw et al. found that at least 10 calcifications were present in 17 of 22 (77%) of breast recurrences (121). The patterns of calcification were classified as highly suspicious for carcinoma (BI-RADS 5) in 77% of the cases and as suggestive of carcinoma requiring biopsy (BI-RADS 4) in the remaining cases. Less worrisome punctate and coarse calcifications were also present in 36% and 14% of cases, respectively, but these were always coincidental with malignant patterns of calcification. Other investigators have not observed the same degree of specificity in calcifications that developed in a breast after conservation therapy (122,123). When a needle core biopsy from the site of a possible breast recurrence shows calcifications and benign histologic changes, the results must be integrated with the mammographic findings to determine whether surgical excision should be performed.

Spontaneous "disappearance" of calcifications has been documented *in vivo* by serial mammograms (124,125). The composition of calcifications prone to this process is not known, but follow-up studies suggested that the associated lesions are usually benign (124). A study of needle core biopsy specimens revealed that radiographically detectable calcifications no longer could be seen in radiographs of the specimens after several days of storage in aqueous solutions, including 10% formaldehyde, whereas the calcifications were preserved in samples stored in ethanol (126). An increase in the number and extent of calcifications raises concern for the presence of carcinoma.

Rapid expansion of the area of calcifications has been associated with *comedo* intraductal carcinoma, whereas slower growth of calcifications characterizes *noncomedo* intraductal carcinoma (127). The mean doubling time for all intraductal carcinomas based on the extent of calcifications was $118.0 \pm 111.2$ days (range, 18–539 days). The mean diameters of noncomedo and comedo intraductal carcinomas based on the distribution of calcifications were $255.8 \pm 71.1$ μm and $302.7 \pm 232.0$ μm, respectively, using a computerized image analysis system.

Mammographically detected calcifications are rarely a manifestation of systemic conditions. In one case, a diagnosis of Klippel-Trenaunay syndrome was made after calcifications found in a routine mammogram were shown to be localized to subcutaneous vascular structures (128). Chronic renal failure is associated with "metastatic" calcifications in soft tissues and blood vessels at various sites, including the breast (129,130).

Arterial calcifications were found in 9% of mammograms from women 50 to 68 years of age at entry into a screening program and in 15.4% of the women studied who had diabetes mellitus (131). An overall excess cardiovascular mortality of 40% was found after 16 to 19 years of follow-up among women with arterial calcifications [hazard ratio, 1.4; 95% confidence interval (CI), 1.1–1.8]; in the group with diabetes, excess mortality from cardiovascular disease was 90% (hazard ratio, 1.9; 95% CI, 1.1–3.2).

Noncalcified crystalloids found in the salivary gland ducts also occur rarely in mammary ducts or lobules, and they are usually associated with intraductal carcinoma (132). These deposits are not visualized in mammograms, and they are not birefringent. Histologic examination reveals eosinophilic, variously shaped crystal-like deposits (needles, rhomboid, hexagonal, plate, and tetrahedral) measuring up to 500 μm, with an average size of 20 μm (Fig. 46.13). Secretion on the surfaces of crystalloids is stained with Alcian blue, mucicarmine, periodic acid-Schiff (PAS), and the antibody for

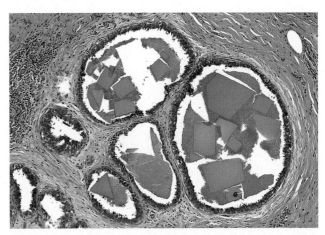

**FIG. 46.13.** *Noncalcified crystalloids.* Characteristic rectangular and triangular shapes are shown associated with proteinaceous secretion in small cysts. Intraductal carcinoma in contiguous ducts (not shown) also contained crystalloids.

epithelial membrane antigen. Crystalloids are electron-dense when examined by electron microscopy, and they do not contain calcium phosphate hydroxyapatite or calcium oxalate. The source of crystalloids in the mammary gland is not known, but it has been speculated that they are formed by crystallization of protein–carbohydrate complexes in abnormal secretions produced by the neoplastic epithelium.

### Needle Core Biopsy as a Diagnostic Procedure

The increasing use of stereotaxic guided core biopsies has made it possible to sample a growing number of nonpalpable radiographically detected lesions. In one series of 100 such lesions at least 5 mm in diameter, needle core biopsies correctly identified 35 of 36 carcinomas confirmed on open surgical biopsy (133). Five to six core biopsy specimens obtained with a 14-gauge needle provide adequate samples for the diagnosis of most lesions. Liberman et al. found that six cores proved to be diagnostic in 92% of mammographic lesions with calcifications, whereas five cores were sufficient for 99% of mass lesions (134).

There is generally a high level of concordance between the diagnosis obtained with stereotactic needle core biopsy and the subsequent surgical excision. Gisvold et al. reported a slightly higher concordance rate for benign (90%) than for malignant lesions (85%) when at least five cores were obtained (135). When there were fewer than five cores, the concordance rates decreased to 66% and 34% for benign and carcinomatous lesions, respectively. The positive predictive value of stereotactic needle core biopsy for the presence of invasion in patients with carcinoma was 98% in 48 cases (136). In the one discordant instance, a fragment of carcinoma displaced into fat in a core biopsy sample was mistakenly interpreted as invasive carcinoma (Fig. 46.14). Excisional biopsies revealed intrinsic invasive carcinoma in 3 of 15 specimens from other patients who had only intraductal carcinoma in needle biopsy samples.

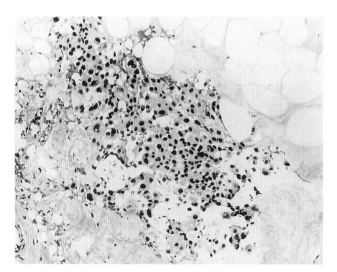

**FIG. 46.14.** *Displaced carcinoma in a stereotactic needle core biopsy.* This specimen was mistakenly interpreted as invasive carcinoma. The subsequent excisional biopsy showed only intraductal carcinoma with additional displaced epithelium.

## Pathologic Changes Attributable to Needling Procedures

The placement of localizing wires has become more precise with the widespread use of stereotactic procedures. Direct penetration of the lesion is sought when biopsy is combined with localization. Follow-up mammography performed 6 months after stereotactic 14-gauge biopsy revealed no architectural distortion attributable to the procedure in 24 patients studied by Kaye et al. (137). In two cases, there were fewer calcifications in postbiopsy mammograms and a 6-mm fibroadenoma contained a 2 × 3-mm defect.

Traumatic changes occur in the breast tissue as a result of needle localization and biopsy procedures (Figs. 46.15 and 46.16). Displacement of benign epithelium into the breast stroma can be found in subsequent excisional biopsies (Figs. 46.17–46.19). Displaced intraductal carcinoma has been observed in breast stroma and within vascular channels in

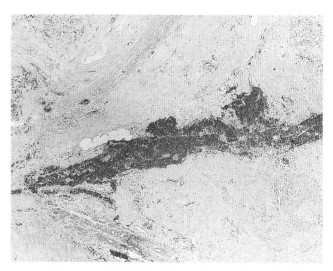

**FIG. 46.16.** *Traumatic effects of needle core biopsy.* Hemorrhage along a needle track is shown.

breast specimens obtained subsequent to needling procedures (Figs. 46.20–46.22). In patients with intraductal carcinoma, these displaced carcinoma fragments can mimic stromal invasion, and in some circumstances, they represent a potential source of misdiagnosis of intrinsic invasive carcinoma (Fig. 46.23). Histologic findings suggesting displacement of intraductal carcinoma include the presence of scattered, isolated fragments of carcinomatous epithelium in artificial spaces within breast stroma, accompanied by hemorrhage, fat necrosis, inflammation, hemosiderin-laden macrophages, or granulation tissue. Calcifications and "foamy" histiocytes of the type commonly seen in intraductal lesions may be associated with displaced carcinomatous epithelium. The extent to which breast needling procedures might contribute to the hematogenous or lymphatic dispersal of tumor cells has not been specifically determined. Methods for detecting carcinoma cells in the peripheral blood discussed later in this chapter, such as reverse transcriptase-polymerase chain reaction (RT-PCR) and immunomagnetic separation, may be useful for investigating this question.

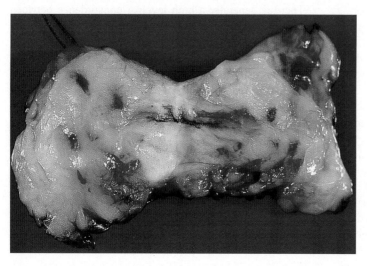

**FIG. 46.15.** *Traumatic effects of needle core biopsy.* This excisional biopsy specimen was obtained after stereotactic biopsies were performed. The specimen has been incised to expose the interior. The punctate red foci are needle tracks.

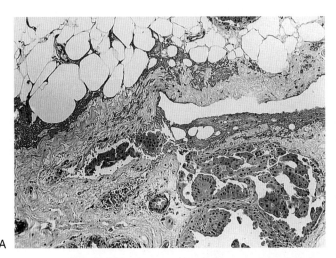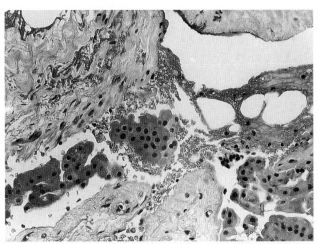

A                  B

**FIG. 46.17.** *Displaced benign epithelium.* **A:** A focus of cystic papillary apocrine metaplasia on the *lower right* has been disrupted, and fragments of apocrine epithelium have been displaced into the needle track, which is a defect running horizontally across the midportion of the photograph. **B:** Fragments of benign apocrine epithelium displaced in the needle track.

Studies addressing the incidence of the phenomenon of epithelial displacement following needling have been few. Boppana et al. reviewed 100 consecutive breast carcinomas that had been subjected to prior fine needle aspiration (FNA) and noted displaced epithelial fragments in 36% of cases (138). Youngson et al. reviewed slides from 43 consecutive cases in which surgical biopsy, mastectomy, or both had been performed following an initial stereotaxic 14-gauge core biopsy diagnosis of breast carcinoma and identified displaced epithelial fragments outside the primary lesion in 12 of 43 (28%) cases (139). Multiple needling procedures (e.g., local anesthetic injection in all 43 cases, needle localization in 22/43 cases, suture placement in 18/43 cases, and FNA in 1/43 cases), however, had been performed in each of the re-

viewed cases. Review of excisional biopsy specimens containing carcinoma from 43 patients after a prior stereotaxic core biopsy revealed displaced neoplastic epithelium outside the main tumor mass in 12 (28%) (140). In seven of these patients, the primary lesion was intraductal carcinoma; five had invasive tumors. The frequency of epithelial displacement has been reduced substantially since the introduction of vacuum-assisted stereotactic biopsy.

The clinical significance of epithelial displacement is unknown. These alterations present the pathologist with a challenging diagnostic problem. Eliciting a history of previous needling procedure may help to prevent histopathologic confusion and an erroneous tissue diagnosis. A malignant diagnosis should not be based solely on the appearance of

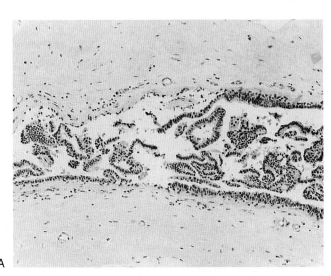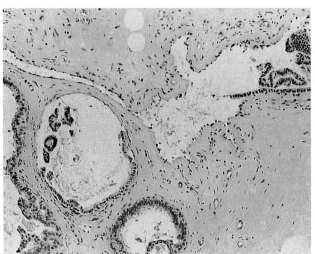

A                  B

**FIG. 46.18.** *Displaced epithelium within ducts.* These photographs illustrate benign duct epithelium displaced by a fine needle aspiration. **A:** Fragments of duct epithelium that were stripped from the basement membrane have been displaced into the duct lumen. The detached epithelium resembles a papillary proliferation. **B:** Part of the duct shown in **A** is present in the *upper right corner.* There is detached epithelium in the cyst on the *left.*

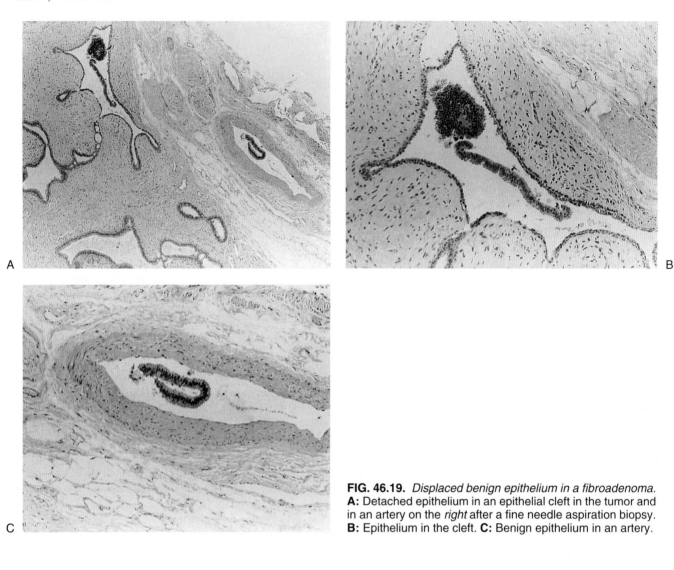

**FIG. 46.19.** *Displaced benign epithelium in a fibroadenoma.* **A:** Detached epithelium in an epithelial cleft in the tumor and in an artery on the *right* after a fine needle aspiration biopsy. **B:** Epithelium in the cleft. **C:** Benign epithelium in an artery.

**FIG. 46.20.** *Displaced intraductal carcinoma.* This biopsy was obtained after a stereotactic core biopsy. **A:** Detached fragments of micropapillary carcinoma in a duct lumen. The neoplastic epithelium has been stripped away from the myoepithelial cell layer *(arrows).* **B:** Detached fragments of micropapillary intraductal carcinoma are shown in the needle track.

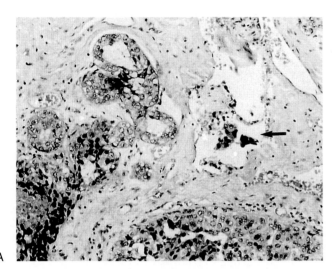
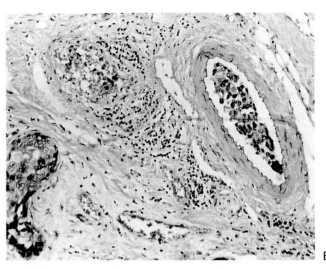

**FIG. 46.21.** *Displaced intraductal carcinoma.* **A:** High-grade intraductal carcinoma with comedonecrosis *(lower left corner)* in an excisional biopsy after a fine needle aspiration biopsy and stereotactic needle localization. Small clusters of carcinoma cells are present in a dilated lymphatic channel *(arrow).* **B:** Displaced intraductal carcinoma is shown in an artery.

epithelium within stroma because epithelial displacement has been observed following needling procedures in benign breast lesions, notably papillary duct hyperplasia and intraductal papilloma.

The significance of carcinomatous lymphovascular emboli remains uncertain in the setting described here. Until further information becomes available, we have interpreted the finding of lymphatic tumor emboli as evidence of invasion in patients with *in situ* carcinoma, even when conventional stromal invasion cannot be identified. We have also interpreted the finding of clusters of carcinoma cells in a lymph node capsule or subcapsular sinus as metastatic carcinoma, even when no intrinsic invasion has been found (Figs. 46.24 and 46.25). Such foci may be mistakenly diagnosed as benign ectopic mammary glands. These patients usually also have lymphatic tumor emboli in the breast parenchyma in the vicinity of the needling procedure. One unusual patient presented with a clinically enlarged axillary lymph node diffusely involved by metastatic carcinoma 7 years after a mastectomy for intraductal carcinoma that was diagnosed by needle biopsy (Fig. 46.26). Lymph nodes removed from the axilla at the time of mastectomy had no carcinoma identified in routine sections. On review, the site of the needle core biopsy in the breast exhibited epithelial displacement with

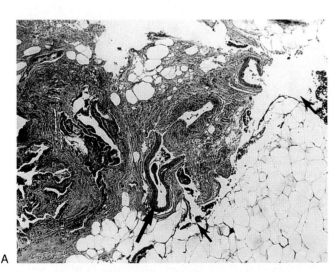
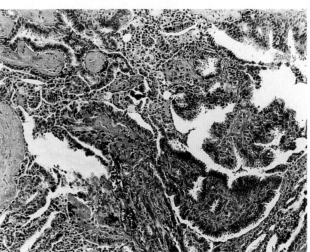

**FIG. 46.22.** *Displaced papillary carcinoma in an artery.* **A:** Part of the needle track resulting from a needle core biopsy is shown on the right and lower center *(small arrows).* Displaced carcinoma is present in an artery *(large arrow)* and in the stroma in the center. The papillary tumor is shown on the *left.* **B:** A portion of the papillary carcinoma that was disrupted by the needling procedure.

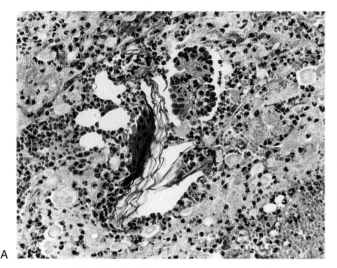
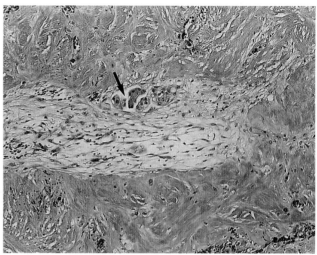

**FIG. 46.23.** *Displaced intraductal carcinoma in a needle track.* **A:** Detached fragments of papillary carcinoma and squamous epithelium (presumably from the skin) are shown surrounded by inflammatory cells in a needle track. **B:** Detached fragments of intraductal carcinoma *(arrow)* are shown in granulation tissue at the site of a healing needle track.

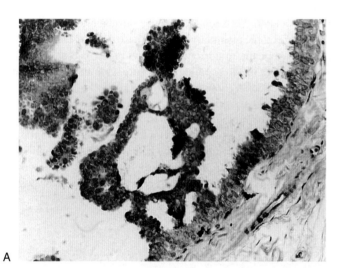
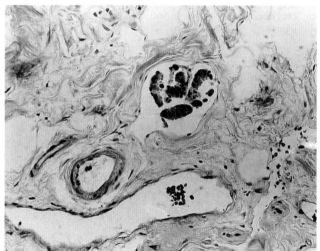
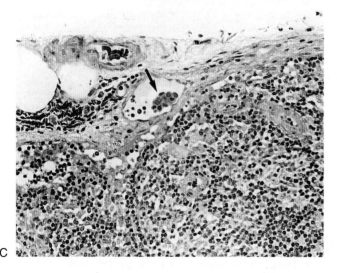

**FIG. 46.24.** *Displaced intraductal carcinoma in lymphatic spaces of the breast and carcinoma in axillary lymph nodes.* The patient had a fine needle aspiration biopsy and stereotactic localization before this excisional biopsy was performed. **A:** Micropapillary intraductal carcinoma. **B:** Clusters of intraductal carcinoma cells in a lymphatic channel. **C:** An axillary dissection, performed after intralymphatic carcinoma was found in the breast biopsy, revealed small clusters of carcinoma cells in the capsular lymphatics of lymph nodes such as the one shown here *(arrow)* and in peripheral sinusoids.

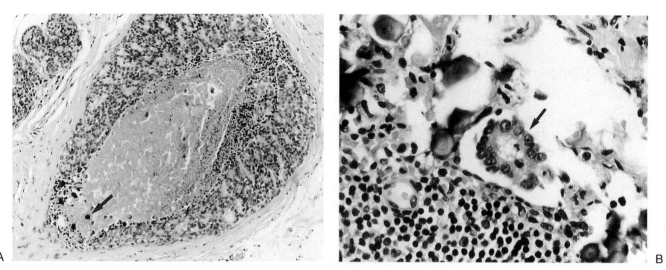

**FIG. 46.25.** *Displaced intraductal carcinoma in the breast and carcinoma in axillary lymph nodes.* **A:** Comedo intraductal carcinoma in an excisional biopsy performed after a stereotactic needle core biopsy and needle localization for nonpalpable mammographically detected calcifications. Small granular calcifications are present in the intraductal carcinoma *(arrow).* **B:** A cluster of carcinoma cells *(arrow)* and several calcifications in the peripheral sinus of an axillary lymph node.

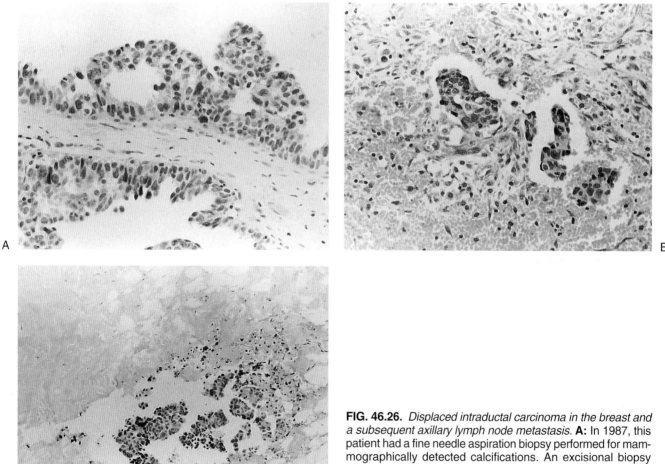

**FIG. 46.26.** *Displaced intraductal carcinoma in the breast and a subsequent axillary lymph node metastasis.* **A:** In 1987, this patient had a fine needle aspiration biopsy performed for mammographically detected calcifications. An excisional biopsy performed shortly thereafter revealed intraductal carcinoma, papillary and cribriform type, shown here. **B,C:** Fragments of displaced intraductal carcinoma were present in the stroma of the biopsy specimen. *(continued)*

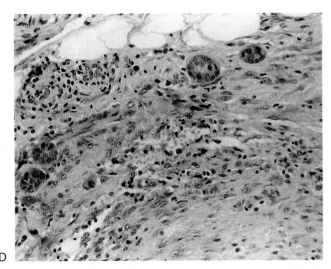
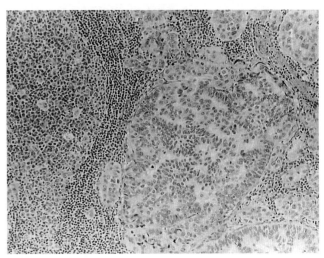

D                                                            E

**FIG. 46.26.** *Continued.* **D:** These clusters of displaced carcinoma cells were present in granulation tissue at the excisional biopsy site in the subsequent mastectomy specimen. No intrinsic invasive carcinoma was found in the breast, and no metastatic carcinoma was identified in eight axillary lymph nodes included with the mastectomy. **E:** In 1994, the patient presented with an ipsilateral axillary tumor that proved to be metastatic mammary carcinoma in a lymph node. The growth pattern duplicated that of the previous intraductal carcinoma. A likely explanation for this set of circumstances is that intraductal carcinoma cells displaced to the lymph node in 1987 persisted and were able to grow in the intervening 7 years, progressing to invasive carcinoma.

carcinoma cells in lymphatic channels. The viability of *in situ* carcinoma cells displaced into vascular channels and possibly deposited in sites outside the breast is unknown.

## INTRAOPERATIVE THERMAL (ELECTROCAUTERY) DAMAGE IN BIOPSY SPECIMENS

Electrocautery instruments used for the excision of tissue from the urinary bladder, prostate gland, breast, and other sites decrease blood loss from dissected tissues because the surfaces are coagulated as they are separated by the cutting edge. When used to perform an excisional breast biopsy, these instruments reduce the risk of hematoma formation in the biopsy cavity, and the operation can be completed in a shorter time (141).

The thermal effect may produce significant changes in the excised tissues. Reduced estrogen receptor activity has been described (142–144), with the decrease in receptor activity sufficient to result in a false-negative report (145). IH study of prostate and breast specimens after electrocautery treatment also reveals a decrease in steroid binding (142,143) (Fig. 46.27).

The histologic changes in the breast caused by thermal injury are similar to those seen at other sites. Thermal damage is most severe at the surface of the specimen generally penetrating not more than a millimeter. The manner in which the instrument is used, the character of the tissue, and the size of the specimen removed influence the intensity and depth of the effect. The most significant effect is severe alteration in cytologic detail. Microscopic architecture may be so distorted that the distinction between normal, hyperplastic, and

neoplastic tissues can no longer be determined (Figs. 46.28 and 46.29). Because the damage is maximal at the edges or surfaces of the tissues, electrocautery artifacts severely limit assessment of the margins of excision (Figs. 46.28 and 46.30). If an excision is carried out with little or no breast parenchyma surrounding a carcinoma, thermal damage may occur in the tumor itself. In addition to the risk for altering receptor activity, the histologic artifacts interfere with the diagnosis or classification of the tumor and with the assessment of microscopic prognostic features of the tumor such as nuclear and histologic grade (Figs. 46.29, 46.31, and 46.32).

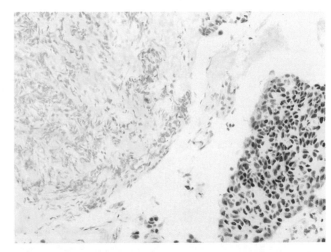

**FIG. 46.27.** *Cautery effect and estrogen receptors.* This biopsy sample shows nuclear reactivity in intact carcinoma on the *right*. No staining is present in cauterized carcinoma on the *left*.

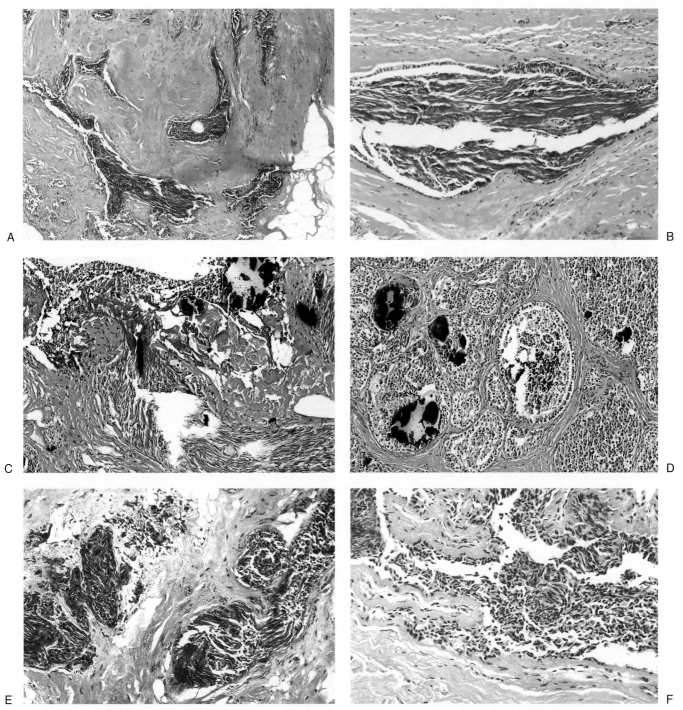

**FIG. 46.28.** *Cautery effect.* **A,B:** The smudged appearance of ductal epithelium and the stroma are typical changes resulting from severe thermal damage. No diagnosis can be given for this tissue. **C:** Calcifications and a duct with severe cautery effect are present at the inked margin. This part of the margin was not interpretable. **D:** Tissue deeper in the specimen shown in **C** shows cautery induced disruption of an intraductal proliferation, probably carcinoma, with calcifications. A definite diagnosis of intraductal carcinoma was not possible. **E:** The most severe cautery-associated changes in this biopsy specimen are on the *left*, near the surface of the tissue. **F:** A duct deeper in the specimen shown in **E** with less severe cautery effect. No diagnosis can be made on the tissues shown in **E** and **F**.

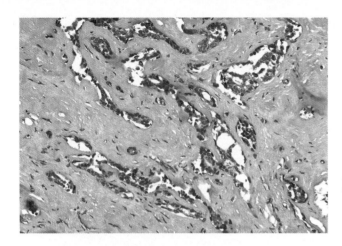

**FIG. 46.29.** *Cautery effect.* Loss of cellular cohesion, shrinkage of cells, and detachment of the epithelium characterize cautery effect in this glandular proliferation. Carcinoma could not be ruled out, but no specific diagnosis was made. Immunostaining was unreliable because of severe background reactivity and loss of specific cellular localization.

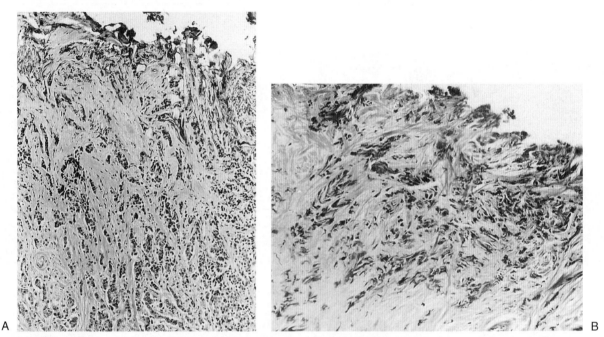

**FIG. 46.30.** *Cautery effect.* **A:** The tissue is distorted by cautery effect at the margin. This area can reasonably be interpreted as showing carcinoma at the margin because it is continuous with underlying carcinoma. **B:** This isolated distorted area at the margin of another specimen could be a benign lesion, such as sclerosing adenosis, or invasive carcinoma.

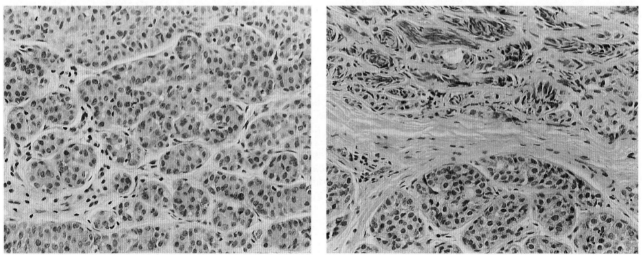

**FIG. 46.31.** *Cautery effect, lobular carcinoma* in situ. **A:** The patient had lobular carcinoma *in situ,* shown here in sclerosing adenosis. **B:** The area in the upper part of the photograph near the margin is uninterpretable due to cautery effect. *In situ* carcinoma in sclerosing adenosis is present *below. (continued)*

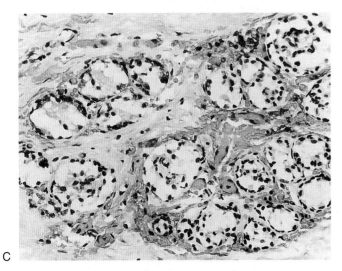

**FIG. 46.31.** *Continued.* **C:** A nondiagnostic lobule in which the epithelial cells were destroyed by thermal damage. All images are from a single specimen.

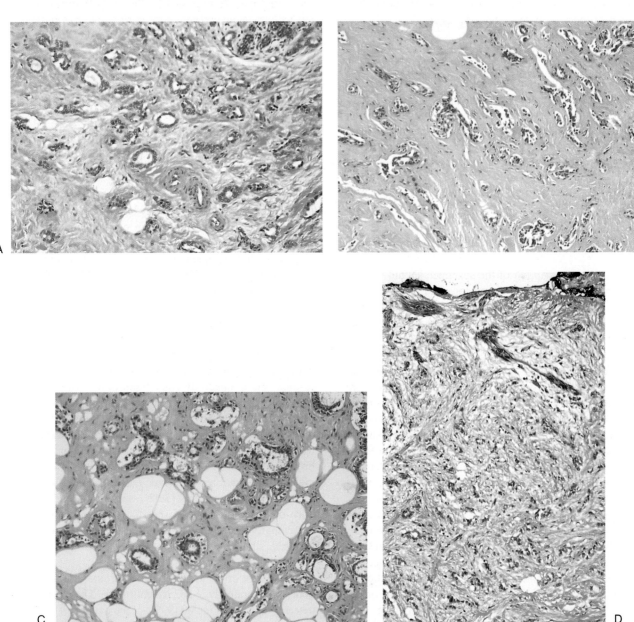

**FIG. 46.32.** *Cautery effect, tubular carcinoma.* **A:** Tubular carcinoma in the center of a biopsy specimen. **B,C:** Adjacent portions of the biopsy shown in **A** exhibiting cautery effect. The glandular configuration is evident in **C** and is probably part of the carcinoma. The interpretation of **B** is uncertain. **D:** Severe cautery effect at the surface of the specimen. No diagnosis can be made in the region of the inked margin at the top.

Thermal artefacts may make it impossible to determine whether intraductal carcinoma is present in tissue outside the tumor mass. I have encountered egregious instances in which cautery-induced changes were so severe that no diagnosis could be made and the presence of carcinoma could not be affirmed or denied (Figs. 46.28 and 46.29). In this situation, the patient may undergo a reexcision to determine whether carcinoma remains at the biopsy site. Because the features of the primary tumor are critical for assessing prognosis and determining therapy, such a patient is left not knowing whether she had carcinoma, what her prognosis might be, and how she should be treated. Fortunately, this scenario is infrequent, but it is a reminder that the primary purpose of a surgical biopsy is to obtain a specimen for histologic diagnosis and that the procedure should be performed in a manner most likely to achieve this goal.

## MASTECTOMY

The purpose of the gross description of a mastectomy is to document the extent of the operation and the appearance of tissue removed. A standard radical mastectomy usually can be oriented easily on the basis of landmarks in the specimen, especially the position of the muscle segments. This may not be accomplished so easily with various types of modified radical mastectomy, which have, for the most part, replaced the radical mastectomy. It is important that the surgeon indicate whether there is anything unusual about the specimen and that important landmarks such as levels of axillary lymph nodes and segments of muscle, if present, be identified.

The external description of the specimen should include the following: overall size, dimensions and appearance of the skin with measurement of scars or incisions, appearance of nipple and areola, presence of muscle and axillary tissue, and location of any distinct palpable lesion.

Dissection of the specimen is accomplished most easily by placing it skin side down anatomically oriented to identify the quadrants. One visualizes the findings as if one were looking through the patient from back to front. The external noncutaneous surfaces should be inspected and palpated for evidence of tumor involvement and inked. For a standard radical mastectomy, the cut edge of the sternal attachment of the pectoralis major muscle marks the medial side. In such a specimen, the fascia between the major and minor pectoralis muscles should be dissected to identify Rotter's nodes.

The breast is dissected by a series of parallel incisions approximately 5 mm apart through the posterior surface up to the skin. A tumor, if present, should be described in the same fashion as for a biopsy specimen. The size and character of a biopsy site should be noted, including areas of induration. It is preferable that these areas not be identified as tumor because the reaction in a healing biopsy cavity may be grossly indistinguishable from carcinoma. The appearance of the remaining breast parenchyma is also recorded, including relative proportions of fat and fibrous parenchyma; the size, location, and character of any discrete lesions; and the

presence or absence of cysts. Samples for histologic examination are taken from the tumor or biopsy site, nipple, skin quadrants, and margins, including the deep surface under the tumor, and in some instances the external surface not covered by skin that is close to the tumor.

A vertical section of the nipple usually suffices to detect Paget's disease or other involvement by carcinoma, even when it is not clinically suspected. With more elaborate sectioning of the nipple, unsuspected foci of Paget's disease or intraductal carcinoma may be detected which are of minor clinical significance for a patient treated by mastectomy. Hence, preparing multiple sections of the nipple is not cost-effective for routine use. Generally, two sections are taken randomly from the breast per quadrant, but more extensive sectioning may be indicated by the gross findings or if the mastectomy were performed for *in situ* lobular or intraductal carcinoma or as a "prophylactic" procedure.

## AXILLARY LYMPH NODES

Some aspects of the pathology of axillary lymph nodes are discussed in Chapter 45.

### Nonsurgical Imaging Methods for Staging of Axillary Lymph Nodes

Clinical methods for detecting metastatic carcinoma in axillary lymph nodes preoperatively have not been sufficiently effective to be used routinely in clinical practice (146). These procedures have involved injection of radioactive tracers, such as technetium-99m ($^{99m}$Tc) (147–151), computed tomography (CT) scanning (152), MRI (153–155), and positron emission tomography (PET) scanning with radiolabeled glucose analogues (156,157).

In a series of breast carcinoma patients studied by $^{99m}$Tc sestamibi scintigraphy, the imaging studies were interpreted as showing metastatic carcinoma in 7 of 11 (64%) patients with histologically proven nodal metastases (147). Similar results were obtained by Danielsson et al., who reported a sensitivity of 67% and specificity of 80% in a study of 58 patients (150). These investigators concluded that the procedure could not be "recommended as a routine method for the detection of axillary lymph node metastases in patients with breast carcinoma." A third study involving 100 patients yielded somewhat better results, correctly identifying 38 of 48 node-negative patients (79.2% sensitivity) and 44 of 52 node-positive cases (84.6% specificity) (149). Tolmos et al. detected 15 of 17 (88%) histologically confirmed axillary metastases but reported a false-negative rate of 5 of 14 cases (35.7%) (148).

Yoshimura et al. used MRI to evaluate axillary lymph nodes preoperatively in 202 patients (154). They were able to detect lymph nodes in 200 (99%) of the patients. The two patients with no MRI-detectable lymph nodes had histologically negative axillae. Histologically, 4,043 lymph nodes were identified at levels I and II, an average of 20 per case. Overall, 3,528 lymph nodes were negative, and 515 (12.7%) contained metastatic carcinoma. These investigators correlated histologic and MRI measured long- and short-axis dimensions for the largest lymph node in each case (mean long axis: histologic, 11.2 ± 5.3 mm; MRI, 11.9 ± 6.0 mm; mean short axis: histologically, 7.3 ± 4.0; MRI, 7.8 ± 4.6) and reported that the measurements were significantly related. A lymph node 10 mm or larger with a long:short ratio less than 1.6 on MRI was present in 59 of 80 (74%) histologically positive axillae.

Using these criteria, these researchers had a false-negative rate of 17 of 131 (13%) and a false-positive rate of 8 of 71 (12.2%). Ten of the 17 false-negative cases had micrometastases, and in 16 of the 17 cases, the largest lymph nodes were within the normal size range (<10 mm). Compared with clinical assessment, MRI was more accurate (88% vs. 79%) in predicting axillary nodal status. Computer programs have been developed to select lymph node regions of interest (ROI) for automated screening of MRI images, and in one study, the maximum enhancement ratio of automated ROI was a strong predictor of axillary nodal status (155).

Computed tomography scanning has been compared with sentinel lymph node mapping as a method for staging the axilla. Miyauchi et al. studied 51 women who had a full axillary dissection after CT scanning and sentinel lymph node (SLN) biopsy (151). False-negative SLN mapping occurred in 3 of 51 (6%) cases when non-SLNs contained metastatic carcinoma after the SLN was negative. False-negative CT interpretations were recorded in 10 cases (19.7%). CT scans were able to identify the SLN in 42 of 51 (82.4%) cases. Hata et al. investigated thin section CT as a method for improving the detection of axillary lymph node metastases and reported 93.8% sensitivity for detecting positive lymph nodes (152); however, specificity (detection of node-negative cases) remained relatively low (82.1%) because the procedure was unable to detect micrometastases.

In a series of 51 women studied after injection of 2-(fluorine-18)-fluoro-2-deoxy-D-glucose (F-18FDG), PET scanning detected 19 of 24 (79%) patients with histologically documented lymph node metastases (156). In this series, PET imaging was 96% correct in identifying women without axillary nodal metastases. Among women with tumors larger than 2 cm, PET accurately identified 94% of women with nodal metastases (sensitivity) and 100% with negative lymph nodes (specificity). In the pT1 group with tumors smaller than 2 cm, PET had a sensitivity of only 33%. The researchers concluded that PET imaging was not a "substitute for histopathologic analysis in detecting axillary lymph node metastases." Yutani et al. reported that dual-head coincidence gamma camera FDG imaging was not as reliable as FDG PET imaging for detecting axillary nodal metastases, especially metastases smaller than 1 cm (157).

## Axillary Staging Based on Clinicopathologic Factors

Clinical and pathologic factors have been studied extensively in an effort to define parameters that could identify patients with the lowest risk for axillary metastases. The goal of this effort has been to establish criteria that could serve as a basis for not performing axillary dissection if the probability of there being nodal metastases was sufficiently low. Silverstein emphasized the importance of distinguishing between palpable and nonpalpable tumors in these analyses (158). The frequency of nodal metastases was lower in every T-category when patients with nonpalpable tumors were compared with those with palpable tumors, with significant differences in T1b, T1c, and T2 cases. A comparison of the frequencies of nodal metastases in this review is shown in Table 46.1. Overall, nodal metastases were found in 45 of 364 (12.3%) patients with nonpalpable and in 450 of 1,217 (37%) with palpable T1 and T2 tumors, respectively.

By combining palpability with other tumor characteristics, Barth et al. identified a subset that represented 13% of more than 900 patients with T1 tumors, among whom 3% had axillary nodal metastases (159). The 117 women in the low-risk group had nonpalpable, non-high-grade tumors that measured 1 cm or smaller and lacked parenchymal lymphovascular invasion. These researchers concluded that axillary dissection should be omitted for patients with this clinicopathologic presentation, "especially if the decision for adjuvant treatment was not altered by the results of ALND" (axillary lymph node dissection). Other studies reported that lymphatic invasion was an important factor associated with nodal metastases in patients with small T1 tumors. In three separate studies, when lymphatic tumor emboli were absent, the reported frequency of positive axillary lymph nodes was 9% for tumors smaller than 10 mm (160), 7% for tumors 5 mm or smaller with low nuclear grade (161), and 4.8% for tumors smaller than 5 mm (162). Port et al. reported that 30 of 247 (12.1%) T1a and T1b patients had axillary lymph node metastases (T1a, 7.4%; T1b, 14.5%) (163). The presence of lymphovascular invasion was a significant predictor of nodal involvement (27.8% vs. 10.9%) for the entire group. These investigators did not believe these data defined "a subgroup at acceptably low risk of nodal positivity" who would not require axillary lymph node staging. Shoup et al. found axillary lymph node metastases in 4.3%, 16.4%, and 31.7% of patients with T1a, T1b, and T1c tumors, respectively (164). Other factors that contributed significantly to increased risk of nodal involvement were poorly differentiated nuclear grade and lymphovascular invasion.

**TABLE 46.1.** *Frequency of lymph node metastases in patients with nonpalpable and palpable carcinomas*

| T Group | Nonpalpable | | Palpable | | |
| | No. of patients | No. + (%) | No. of patients | No. + (%) | p value |
|---|---|---|---|---|---|
| T1a | 59 | 2 (3) | 45 | 3 (7) | NS |
| T1b | 116 | 7 (6) | 158 | 36 (23) | 0.0005 |
| T1c | 130 | 23 (18) | 506 | 160 (32) | 0.003 |
| T2 | 59 | 13 (22) | 508 | 251 (49) | 0.0001 |
| Total | 364 | 45 (12.3) | 1217 | 450 (37) | |

Based on Silverstein MJ. Predicting axillary nodal positivity in 1,787 patients with invasive breast carcinoma. *Breast J* 1998;4:324–329, with permission.

Morrow's review of the problem of identifying patients at low risk for axillary metastases led to the conclusion "that tumor size, whether alone or in combination with other prognostic factors, cannot reliably identify a group of breast cancers with a less than 5% risk of axillary nodal metastases" (165). She also noted that patients with a single focus of microinvasion and those without true tubular carcinomas 1 cm or smaller were at "extremely low risk of axillary metastases."

The issue of tumor size as a sole determinant of the risk of axillary lymph node metastases remains controversial. One group of investigators found axillary metastases in 3 of 66 women (4.5%) who had T1a tumors, and a literature review of combined data for single-institution trials reported axillary involvement in 3.9% of 256 patients (166). These researchers concluded that "our data support abandoning routine axillary dissection in T1a breast cancer." Similar results were reported by Pandelidis et al., who detected axillary lymph node metastases in 2 of 54 (3.7%) T1a cases (167). On the other hand, McGee et al. reviewed data from three large urban hospitals with a total series of 3,077 breast cancer cases and reported finding axillary lymph node metastases in 8 of 74 (12.2%) patients with T1a tumors (168). The authors believed that "these results justify axillary node dissections even for very small invasive cancers."

### Surgical Staging of the Axilla by Endoscopic Axillary Dissection

Endoscopic axillary lymph node dissection is an interesting and potentially valuable technique for clinical staging of the axilla. The procedure is currently regarded as investigational, but in the future it might be used in conjunction with sentinel lymph node mapping or other imaging procedures to provide a minimally invasive method for staging the axilla. In an investigational setting, endoscopic axillary dissections were performed in 12 cadavers, yielding an average of $9.9 \pm 7.2$ lymph nodes (range, 2–22) (169). These researchers identified the axillary vein in each case and important nerves in more than 80% of the procedures.

### Gross Pathologic Examination of Axillary Lymph Nodes

With the exception of standard radical mastectomy specimens, it is virtually impossible to determine, by anatomic orientation alone, the position or level of lymph nodes in axillary contents received with a mastectomy specimen. If this information is desired clinically, the lymph node groups should be tagged or submitted as separately identified specimens. In properly oriented, complete axillary dissection specimens, the distribution of lymph node metastases follows a consistent pattern in almost all cases. When lymph nodes are affected, metastases are found in a stepwise fashion in the low, middle, and upper or proximal axillary zones. Several researchers reported that discontinuous or "skip"

metastases, which do not follow this distribution, were found in 2% or fewer of all patients or in fewer than 5% of patients with axillary nodal metastases (170–172). Metastases limited to level II (mid-axilla) account for 30% to 50% of cases of discontinuous involvement (170,171). In a study of more than 1,000 patients with a mean follow-up of 97 months who underwent complete axillary dissection (levels I, II, and III tumor size), the number of involved lymph nodes and the level of involvement were independent predicative factors for survival (173). Rarely, isolated metastases are confined to the interpectoral lymph node of Rotter in the absence of any axillary nodal metastases (173a). This pattern of spread is equivalent to a "skip" metastasis at level II and it could be associated with false negative SLN mapping.

Careful manual dissection of the unfixed axillary fat is the most cost-effective method for isolating the lymph nodes for microscopic study. In this process, firm bits of fat and other tissue may be mistaken for lymph nodes. Although the gross description should include a count of tissue samples thought to be lymph nodes that were submitted for histology, the final number of nodes is determined from those counted in tissue sections. The overall gross character and dimensions of lymph nodes should be described. It is generally advisable to avoid stating that metastases are grossly present or absent because uncertainty arises when the results of microscopic study differ from the gross impression. Lymph nodes distorted by inflammation or hyperplasia, and in some cases enlarged by fatty infiltration, are a common cause of a false-positive interpretation on gross pathologic and clinical examination (Fig. 46.33).

Numerous procedures are available to facilitate the isolation of lymph nodes in the axillary fat. These methods include obtaining radiographs of the fat (174,175); fixing the fat in Bouin's solution, which stains fat intensely yellow but leaves the lymph nodes white; using Carnoy's fixative; and clearing the fat by a process that renders it relatively trans-

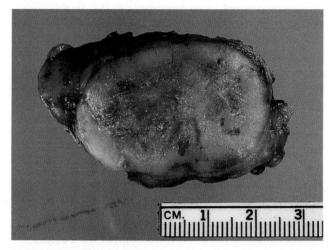

**FIG. 46.33.** *Fatty infiltration of a lymph node.* The lymph node is grossly enlarged by a lipomatous mass of fat that fills the hilum. Lymphoid tissue forms a thin brown band at the periphery.

parent so that solid structures, such as lymph nodes, stand out when the tissue is placed over a light source (176).

These techniques will increase the yield of lymph nodes obtained by locating small lymph nodes that may be missed on palpation. In a study of 42 axillary dissections, the mean number of lymph nodes found was increased by clearing from 20 to 26 in stage I cases, and from 22 to 30 in patients with stage II disease (177). Additional positive lymph nodes were found in the stage II group but not in cases originally assigned to stage I on the basis of manually dissected lymph nodes. Hartveit et al. cleared axillary tissue from 63 node-negative cases and found one lymph node that contained a micrometastasis that had not been found by routine processing (178). Although it is possible that an occasional patient may be incorrectly staged because a positive lymph node was missed in manual dissection, the likelihood of this is so small as not to justify the considerable time and expense required for clearing.

Many lymph nodes isolated from the axillary tissue that appear grossly to be uninvolved by metastatic carcinoma are 0.5 cm or smaller. These lymph nodes are usually submitted in entirety for histologic examination. Each of these lymph nodes appears as a single sample in the corresponding slide. Lymph nodes 0.5 to 1.0 cm are ordinarily bisected in the long axis, if this can be determined. Lymph nodes larger than 1 cm may be divided into more than two portions. There is no consensus on whether it is necessary to examine all lymph node tissue histologically. The gross description should state how this issue has been handled. All tissue from a lymph node divided into two or more parts should be processed together in one or more separately designated paraffin blocks. Consequently, each partitioned lymph node will require at least one cassette so that multiple portions of metastatic carcinoma from a single subdivided lymph node will not be mistakenly interpreted as two or more involved lymph nodes. If a lymph node contains grossly apparent metastatic carcinoma, it is not necessary to process the entire lymph node for histologic study, but the samples should be taken in a manner which would be most likely to demonstrate extranodal spread, if it is present.

There is no consensus as to the optimum procedure to use when submitting tissue from grossly benign lymph nodes too large to process entirely for histologic examination. This will generally apply to lymph nodes 5 mm or larger. Recommendations include submitting one half of a bisected lymph node, submitting a representative sample, or processing up to one full cassette of tissue per large lymph node (179–181).

An important concern in considering the need to process all tissue from large, grossly negative lymph nodes is the cost of this effort relative to the amount of useful additional information compared with more restricted sampling of these lymph nodes. This issue was addressed by Niemann et al. in a study of consecutive lymph node dissections from various anatomic regions, which yielded 2,915 lymph nodes from 149 patients (182). Lymph nodes too large to be processed intact were divided into two or more samples. Additional lymph node tissue representing material that would

not be been included if only one sample per lymph node had been examined histologically uncovered metastatic carcinoma in nine lymph nodes judged negative in the initial sample from seven patients. Each of these patients already had metastases detected in routine sections of other lymph nodes, and the additional information raised the stage in only two cases, both with cervical metastases from oropharyngeal carcinoma. No changes in staging occurred among the 50 women with mammary carcinoma included in the study. The estimated cost for preparing and examining the 808 additional tissue blocks needed for all lymph node tissue was estimated to be $5,935.62, or $847.94 per case with an additional positive lymph node. These investigators concluded that "whether these results justify the expense incurred remains an open question. We do not intend to make recommendations on the appropriate means of submitting lymph nodes; this is a decision that should be made by individual laboratories."

Portions of grossly negative lymph nodes may be reserved for ancillary studies and therefore not submitted for histologic examination. Presently, these are investigational procedures that attempt to detect evidence of submicroscopic metastases by RT-PCR. Increased interest in this approach has arisen as a result of the development of SLN mapping. Results of these studies are described later in this chapter. Smith et al. investigated the potential impact on axillary staging that might result from examining one half of each sentinel lymph node histologically if the other half were reserved for molecular analysis (183). The study was based on 227 patients included in an SLN mapping protocol in which all patients underwent a complete axillary dissection. As part of the study design, all lymph nodes larger than 8 mm were bisected and the two halves were submitted for histologic examination separately. Sixty patients had axillary nodal metastases, totalling 230 lymph nodes. On review, 107 (46.5%) of the positive lymph nodes were found to have been bisected. Carcinoma was present in both halves of 64 (59.8%) lymph nodes and only in one half of 43 (40.2%) lymph nodes. Both halves were more likely to be involved if a patient had metastases in multiple lymph nodes. In 12 patients (20% of those with nodal metastases), the only evidence of metastatic carcinoma was contained in one half of one lymph node. These data suggest that failing to process both halves of a bisected lymph node for histologic study could affect the accuracy of lymph node staging if the reserved portion contains the only evidence of metastatic carcinoma. Heterogeneous distribution of metastatic carcinoma documented in this study also may explain some of the discrepant results between RT-PCR and histologic examination of different portions of a single lymph node.

## Sentinel Lymph Node Mapping

Intraoperative mapping of the lymphatic drainage from the breast has proven an effective method for locating one or more lymph nodes most likely to harbor metastatic carcinoma, the so-called sentinel lymph node(s). An important advantage of SLN mapping compared with conventional axillary dissection is reduced postoperative morbidity (184). Patients experienced significantly more frequent and a greater degree of lymphedema as well as other symptoms after axillary dissection, leading the researchers to conclude that SLN biopsy was "associated with negligible morbidity compared with complete axillary lymph node dissection" (184).

The procedures now widely used involve injection of a vital blue dye, a radioactive tracer such as $^{99m}$Tc-sulfur colloid, or a combination of these reagents. Blue dye transported to the SLN can be identified visually. Allergic reactions to the blue dye are infrequent and generally mild. Retrograde migration of the dye may cause it to persist in dermal lymphatics, resulting in a bluish hue in the skin that can persist for months. Isosulfan blue absorbed systemically can cause transient false low oxygen saturation measurements when determined by pulse oximetry. Radiocolloid localization can be identified preoperatively by lymphoscintigraphy and intraoperatively using a probe to detect gamma irradiation (gamma probe). Lymphoscintigraphy is an important part of the procedure because it can alert the surgeon to the location of the SLN and to extraaxillary drainage.

*Extraaxillary 'hotspots'* usually represent SLNs outside the axillary lymphatic drainage, such as the internal mammary and supraclavicular lymph nodes, or in aberrant subcutaneous and intramammary lymph nodes. Involvement of internal mammary lymph nodes most often occurs in patients with medial tumors or who have axillary metastasis. In a review of 7,070 patients described in numerous studies, Morrow and Foster found that 347 (4.9%) had metastatic carcinoma limited to the internal mammary lymph nodes (185). Harlow et al. found extraaxillary hotspots in 44 of 680 patients (6.5%) who had SLN mapping, including nine (1.3%) whose only hotspot was extraaxillary (186). Three patients had more than one extraaxillary hotspot. The most common site of extraaxillary localization was in the internal mammary lymph nodes. Other locations of extraaxillary hotspots were supraclavicular, interpectoral, infraclavicular, intramuscular (pectoralis major), the thyroid gland, and the chest wall. Surgical biopsy revealed lymph nodes in 35 (79.5%) of the hotspot sites; no lymph nodes were found in nine sites. Three of the 35 (8.6%) extraaxillary lymph nodes contained metastatic carcinoma, including two patients with negative axillary SLNs. Krag reported that 8% of patients had extraaxillary hotspots and that 3% of positive SLNs were extraaxillary in location (187). Hill et al. reported extraaxillary hotspots in 35 of 195 patients (17%) examined by lymphoscintigraphy (188). All the extraaxillary sites had an internal mammary distribution. Five (2%) of these patients also had supraclavicular localizaton, and in eight (4%), the only activity was in the internal mammary lymph node region.

There is no consensus on the clinical management of ex-

traaxillary nodal hotspots, especially those with an internal mammary distribution. Harlow et al. recommended "removal of these nodes . . . to improve staging" (186). Cody suggested that internal mammary SLN biopsy be considered for "medially placed tumors smaller than 1 cm, if either lymphoscintigraphy or the interoperative gamma probe suggests internal mammary drainage of isotope" (189). Bobin et al. performed SLN mapping on 33 women with medial or inner quadrant tumors and reported locating SLNs in 26 (79%) (190). Veronesi reported that 6 of 380 patients (1.6%) had internal mammary hotspots and that these patients all had negative axillary lymph nodes (191). He noted that "their prognostic significance is as great as that of the axillary nodes." Internal mammary sentinel lymph nodes were detected in 10 of 80 (12%) patients evaluated by Johnson et al. (191a). Four tumors were in a medial quadrant, and six were in outer quadrants. Three of the ten patients had internal mammary nodal metastases.

Numerous articles have described the technical aspects of SLN mapping in breast carcinoma (189,192–196), and most describe successful identification, with experience, of one or more SLNs in 85% or more patients. Radioisotope localization appears to find SLNs more frequently than the blue-dye technique alone, and the combination of both procedures has proven superior to either alone. Cox et al. reported successful localization of one or more SLNs in 665 of 700 patients (95%) using a combined radiocolloid (Tc-labelled sulfur colloid) and isosulfan blue-dye method (195). A full axillary dissection was performed in the 35 cases with no identifiable SLNs yielding metastatic carcinoma in 8 (22.5%). They retrieved 1,348 SLNs from 665 patients, an average of two per case. In 26%, three or more SLNs were identified. These investigators reported that 374 of 1,348 (27.8%) of the lymph nodes were blue and hot, whereas 568 (42.1%) were only hot and 406 (30.1%) only blue. Overall, 69.9% of SLN were hot and 57.9% were blue. Guenther et al. also observed a substantial risk of nodal metastasis in women with no detectable SLN (197). Positive lymph nodes were found in 33.3% of these patients, including some women with five or more affected nodes.

In a review of 1,564 patients who underwent SLN mapping described in 16 reports, Cody found that SLNs were detected in 76% of cases by the blue-dye method, in 90% by an isotope procedure, and in 93% with a combined technique (189). The false-negative rate for SLN mapping among women who also had an axillary dissection was 5% (28/545), yielding a sensitivity of 95% (517/545). The false-negative rate was higher for SLN mapping with the blue-dye method alone (8%) than for the radioisotope alone or combined methods (each 4%). Among patients who had lymph nodes other than the SLNs examined, the SLN was the only positive lymph node in 45% of cases, with a slightly greater frequency using the combined technique (33/67, 49%) than with isotope alone (142/327, 43%) or the blue-dye technique alone (611/136, 45%).

Injections of blue dye and radiocolloid are performed separately into the breast parenchyma around the tumor sites in most studies. Prior excisional biopsy is not a contraindication to SLN mapping so long as the injection is placed in breast parenchyma around the biopsy cavity (189,196). A large biopsy cavity, however, especially in the upper outer quadrant, may compromise lymphatic drainage in the region and has been associated with unsuccessful or false-negative SLN mapping (189). Successful SLN mapping also has been reported after subdermal injection of radiocolloid (198,199) or intradermal injection of blue dye (200) over the tumor site.

Sentinel lymph note mapping is used most widely for patients with T1 and T2 invasive breast carcinoma. The frequency of detecting a positive SLN increases with tumor size. In one study, the frequency of positive SLN was 4.3%, 19.5%, and 23.8% for T1a, T1b, and T1c tumors, respectively, and 48.9% and 66.7% for T2 and T3 tumors (201). Bass et al. reported the following frequencies of positive SLN mapping in relation to tumor size: T1, 13 of 69 (18.8%); T2, 108 of 202 (53.5%); and T3, 22 of 25 (88%) (202).

Patients with nonpalpable invasive breast carcinoma diagnosed by percutaneous needle core biopsy are excellent candidates for SLN mapping. Compared with women who had carcinoma diagnosed by surgical excision or FNA, patients diagnosed by core needle biopsy have a similar success rate with sentinel lymph node mapping (203). Needle localization may be combined with intraparenchymal injection of the tracer and is necessary even if intradermal injection of the tracer is preferred (204). Liberman et al. reported that SLNs were identified in 30 of 33 women (91%) with nonpalpable infiltrating carcinomas (0.5–2.2 cm; median, 1 cm) who underwent SLN mapping with combined blue-dye and radiocolloid injection (204). Twenty-nine of the SLNs were at level I in the axilla, and one was intramammary. Three women without a detectable SLN had tumors that measured 0.8 to 1.5 cm. Complete axillary dissection yielded negative lymph nodes in two and three positive lymph nodes in the third patient with no detectable SLN. Twenty-three of the other 30 women (77%) had a negative SLN. Axillary dissection in the seven women (23%) with a positive SLN revealed no metastatic tumor in six and one positive non-SLN in the seventh patient. These data are consistent with the expected frequency of positive SLN in patients with T1 breast carcinoma.

Several reports presented data on the frequency of positive SLNs in *patients with intraductal carcinoma.* In 1998, Cox et al. reported finding positive sentinel lymph nodes in 11 of 150 patients (7.3%) with intraductal carcinoma (195). The intraductal carcinomas with positive lymph nodes were mainly of the comedo type. A subsequent analysis provided details on 86 patients with intraductal carcinoma who underwent SLN mapping (196). Cytokeratin (CK) staining revealed micrometastases in SLNs from five patients (6%), only one of which was evident on the H&E stain. Four of the five patients had comedo intraductal car-

cinoma, and the fifth had a 9.5-cm cribriform and micropapillary lesion. Axillary dissection in four of these cases did not detect other axillary lymph node metastases. A third report by Cox et al. described finding positive SLNs in 18 of 200 patients (9%) with intraductal carcinoma (202). Pendas et al. reported that 5 of 87 patients (6%) with intraductal carcinoma in their series had immunohistochemically positive SLNs, and they recommended SLN mapping for patients with relatively large high-grade intraductal carcinomas (205).

Results of SLN mapping also have been reported for a limited number of *patients with microinvasive carcinoma.* Dauway et al. described nine women with T1mic tumors (invasion ≤1 mm) who underwent SLN mapping with detection of micrometastases by IH in three (33%) (196). Complete axillary dissection in these three patients did not uncover additional positive lymph nodes. Zavotsky et al. performed SLN mapping in 14 women with "microinvasive" carcinoma (206). Invasive foci measured 1 mm in 11 cases and 2 mm in three others. Positive SLNs were identified in two cases (14%), both associated with 4.5-cm high-grade intraductal carcinomas that had invasion measuring ≥1 mm and 2 mm, respectively. Neither had additional positive axillary lymph nodes, but one later developed a malignant pleural effusion.

Sentinel lymph node mapping has been successful in *patients previously treated with neoadjuvant chemotherapy.* Cohen et al. (206a) found that the SLN accurately predicted axillary status in 28 of 31 patients (90%) studied, and that the reliability of the procedure was enhanced by submitting the SLN for serial sections and immunohistochemistry.

*Multifocal invasive carcinoma* may be a risk factor for SLN metastases. In one study, 15 of 25 patients (60%) with multifocal invasion (5 lobular, 10 ductal) had a positive SLN (207); however, the risk of having positive SLNs appears to depend on the size of the largest invasive focus and, when stratified on this basis, may not differ appreciably from patients with a unifocal tumor of equivalent size. The likelihood of there being positive non-SLNs was greater when the SLN was positive (53%) than if the SLN was negative (10%). Veronesi et al. reported finding positive axillary lymph nodes in 31 of 46 patients (67%) who had multicentric or extensively multifocal carcinomas (208). Three of these patients had a negative SLN, leading Veronesi et al. to conclude that "patients with multifocality should not be candidate for sentinel lymph node biopsy" as a substitute for axillary dissection.

*Radiation exposure* in the patient and in medical personnel is an issue of some concern when a radioactive tracer is used. The subject was thoroughly reviewed by Waddington et al., who concluded that "the radiation doses to staff groups involved in all aspects of the technique are low, and under normal circumstances and levels of workload, routine radiation monitoring will not be required. Standard biohazard precautions prevent direct intake of radioactive contamination" (208a). It has been estimated that the radiation dose to the tissue at the injection site is about 45 rads per mCi (209). Excision of the SLN, frequently concurrent with the tumor site, greatly reduces local radiation in the patient. Dosimetry studies obtained intraoperatively have measured exposure to the surgeon's hands to be 9.4 ± 3.6 mrem per operation (210). Stratmann et al. reported that average exposure to surgeons' hands was 34.25 mrem/h, 18.62 mrem/h, and 0.06 mrem/h at the injection site, at the lumpectomy site, and at the sentinel lymph node, respectively (210a). Exposure to pathologists' hands was 18.62 mrem/h and 0.06 mrem/h during handling of the lumpectomy and sentinel lymph node specimens, respectively. Lower exposure levels can be expected for pathology personnel even if tissue is submitted for diagnosis without a delay because contact with the specimens is brief at any stage in pathology processing. Veronesi et al. found that absorbed radiation dose for the surgeon, calculated in terms of exposure during 100 operations per year, was within the dose limits for the general population compared with the recommendation of the International Commission on Radiological Protection (208). The effective absorbed dose to the surgeon, expressed in microSieverts, during 100 operations per year was estimated to be 90 ± 25, which is about the recommended safe dose of 100 microSieverts for the general population. Recommendations for the handling of radioactive breast biopsy and sentinel lymph node specimens in the pathology laboratory have been published (210b).

### Intraoperative Diagnosis of Sentinel Lymph Nodes

Intraoperative histologic diagnosis of SLNs is appropriate outside of a research protocol only if management of the patients will be influenced during the operation by the result of this procedure. For example, permission to perform an axillary dissection may be dependent on detecting carcinoma in the SLN, or the operation may be terminated if the frozen section of the SLN is reported to be negative.

Intraoperative diagnosis of SLN can be accomplished by frozen section, imprint cytology, or a combination of the two techniques. Advocates of the imprint method feel that preparing a frozen section is wasteful because the frozen samples are trimmed in the microtome to obtain a surface suitable for sectioning. Some lymph nodes are difficult to cut for frozen section, especially when there is fatty infiltration. Imprint cytology not only spares tissue, but it also makes it possible to obtain specimens from multiple cut surfaces of a lymph node, thereby allowing wider sampling of the tissue than would be achieved by a single frozen section, and it is also less time consuming. A significant drawback is that many pathologists are not skilled in cytology diagnosis, and it may be difficult to recognize sparse carcinoma cells in the highly cellular background of lymph node imprints. Reactive histiocytes are a potential source of a false-negative diagnosis (see Chapter 45). Imprint preparations can be stained rapidly with H&E, Giemsa, or other procedures. The choice of staining procedure depends on the pathologist's preference for interpreting a particular preparation.

The feasibility of cytologic examination of axillary lymph nodes intraoperatively was investigated in a study of 127 stage I and II patients who did not undergo SLN mapping (211). Enlarged or hard lymph nodes excised before complete axillary dissection were used to prepare touch imprints, which were stained with Giemsa and H&E techniques. The mean number of lymph nodes sampled per patient was five, resulting in a total of 635 lymph nodes examined cytologically. The accuracy of imprint cytology compared with histologic diagnosis was 94% and 91% for Giemsa and H&E staining, respectively.

Several studies documented the use of cytologic preparations for the diagnosis of SLN with varying success (212–216). Two separate reports from different institutions each described results obtained in 55 patients who had SLN specimens diagnosed intraoperatively with H&E (213,214). The results for both studies were identical, with one false-negative interpretation (0.8%) in each report. The negative predictive value was 99.2%, sensitivity was 95.7%, specificity was 100%, and positive predictive value was 100%. Moes et al. reported on 66 patients who had 175 SLNs examined intraoperatively with H&E-stained cytologic preparations made by scraping the cut surfaces of bisected lymph nodes (216). The cytologic diagnosis corresponded to the histologic diagnosis in 167 of 175 SLNs (95.4%). There were six false-negative and one false-positive cytologic interpretation, but the latter patient had another lymph node that was cytologically and histologically positive. Litz et al. reported false-negative results in five of seven (71%) SLNs evaluated by imprint cytology with the H&E stain (215). Failure to detect metastatic carcinoma cytologically was attributed to micrometastases in four cases and inability to recognize metastatic lobular carcinoma in one case. These researchers considered this level of inaccuracy to be unacceptably high. In another study, "intraoperative touch imprint cytology was able to identify metastatic disease in 50% of the positive SLNs" (196). These investigators considered this result, albeit 50% false negative, to be beneficial because those with a positive SLN had the "advantage of converting the operation to a CLND (complete lymph node dissection), avoiding a second trip to the operating room." Ku et al. reported intraoperative false-negative diagnoses in 10 of 103 (10%) SLNs and one false-positive diagnosis, for an accuracy of 91% (212).

Frozen-section examination of the SLN has been evaluated in several studies, and the results have proven reliable in most cases. Hill et al. reported on a study of 405 patients who had an SLN examined by frozen section (188). Metastatic carcinoma was detected in 68 of the patients (17%), but final paraffin sections were positive in 78, yielding 10 false-negative frozen section reports (13%). False negative rates for frozen section examination of SLNs reported in other studies were 18 of 75 (17%) (198), 19 of 225 (8%) (217), and 3 of 50 (6%) (218). Turner et al. were able to detect only 28% of micrometastatic SLNs (≤2.0 mm) but were successful by frozen section in 98% of SLNs with macrometastases (>2.0 mm).

Rapid CK-IH staining has been applied to frozen sections to detect micrometastases and reduce the false-negative rate (219). Veronesi et al. described a procedure in which paired halves of SLNs had sections cut at 50-μm intervals, resulting in approximately 30 sections for each lymph node half (208). One section from each pair was immediately stained with H&E, and if these preparations did not demonstrate metastatic carcinoma, rapid CK-IH was done on the remaining sections. Using the combined H&E and IH process to examine SLN from 119 patients, these researchers had a false-negative rate of 5.5%, whereas in a prior series of 192 patients with SLN studied by frozen section alone, the false-negative rate obtained by the same investigators had been 32.1%. A subsequent report from the same institution described 155 patients who had SLN examined by frozen section and IH, apparently including the 119 patients reported by Veronesi et al. (208,220). The maximum time required to examined the SLN, including frozen section and IH was 65 minutes, during which interval surgery on the breast was completed. In 45 of 70 patients (64%) who had a positive SLN, the diagnosis was made on the first pair of sections, whereas in the other 25 cases, metastases were detected in subsequent levels. All metastatic foci were seen in the H&E and frozen section. IH on the frozen section was helpful for confirming the presence of metastatic carcinoma but did not detect carcinoma which was not evident in the H&E slides.

A direct comparison of the results of frozen section and imprint cytology was reported by van Diest et al. (221). False negative diagnosis were obtained in 4 of 31 (13%) SLNs examined by frozen section and in 10 of 26 (38%) examined by imprint cytology. In 11 cases, the imprint preparations were considered unsatisfactory for diagnosis. There was 88% concordance between imprints and frozen section, but 7 of 23 (30%) SLN diagnosed as positive on frozen section had a negative imprint. The sensitivity and overall accuracy of frozen section (87%; 95%) were substantially greater than for imprint cytology (62%; 83%). Turner et al. evaluated the results of combined frozen section and imprint cytology (222). The overall accuracy was 93.2%. The combined diagnostic approach detected 87% of SLNs with macrometastases (>2 mm) but only 28% of micrometastases found by H&E on paraffin sections.

Data from the various studies described in this section demonstrate that metastatic carcinoma can be detected in SLNs from many patients intraoperatively by either frozen section or imprint cytologic examination. These procedures are approximately equivalent for detecting micrometastases (<2 mm) in more than 90% of cases, and neither is especially reliable for identifying micrometastases, which are the major source of false-negative intraoperative diagnoses. In cases where the diagnosis may be difficult, having imprint cytology as well as frozen section available can be useful, and rapid CK-IH also has been helpful in this circumstance.

Despite these limitations, intraoperative diagnosis of an SLN makes an important contribution because patients with a positive SLN can have a complete axillary dissection without a second trip to the operating room.

## Histologic Examination of Sentinel Lymph Nodes

As noted in the preceding discussion, metastatic carcinoma is readily detected in a single routine H&E section of a SLN if it is involved by a macrometastasis (>2 mm). Additional procedures, such as obtaining multiple sections or CK-IH, contribute largely to the finding of micrometastases in SLNs that appear to be histologically negative in a routine H&E section and less frequently to the finding of a macrometastasis buried in a large lymph node or a macrometastasis that is eccentrically positioned. These procedures have assumed greater importance with the widespread use of SLN mapping, which identifies the lymph node or nodes most likely to harbor metastatic carcinoma. As experience has accumulated, there is growing evidence to support limiting axillary staging to SLN mapping in patients with T1 tumors and a clinically negative axilla and possibly other patient groups if the SLN mapping is negative. It is therefore essential to maximize the information obtained from pathologic examination of the SLN and reduce the likelihood of a false-negative SLN diagnosis.

Presently, intraoperative diagnosis of the SLN is obtained by cytology, frozen section, or both methods, as discussed already. A positive intraoperative diagnosis is confirmed from the paraffin-embedded frozen section tissue, with H&E sections supplemented by CK-IH if necessary. If the intraoperative examination does not detect metastatic carcinoma, more intensive studies of the SLN are indicated. In a substantial number of cases, metastatic carcinoma, if present, will be uncovered by one or more routine H&E sections without the necessity for IH. Nonetheless, the tissue is used most effectively if all sections are cut at one time according to a set plan for H&E and IH.

Various protocols combining multiple sections and CK-IH have been used to examine SLNs, but there is no consensus as to which is most cost-effective. The procedures used include two H&E levels separated by 40 μm and one CK-IH section (222); serial sectioning with every sixth level taken for H&E and the succeeding two levels for CK and epithelial membrane antigen (EMA) IH (223); H&E and CK-IH on paired sections separated by 40 μm (224); and CK-IH on serial sections taken at 0.25-mm intervals through the block (225); one H&E section and CK-IH at four additional levels not otherwise specified (226); three H&E levels "100–500 μm apart" (198); multiple H&E sections (4–20) without IH (199); at least four H&E levels and CK-IH (201); and serial sections of the entire lymph node at 0.5-mm intervals stained with H&E and CK-IH (223).

A study by Turner et al. provides some guidance for assessing these various protocols (224). These researchers studied 42 patients whose SLNs were negative on frozen section and two H&E paraffin section levels. CK-IH performed on sections consecutive with the 2 H&E levels revealed micrometastases in eight cases. CK-IH also done on eight additional levels cut at 40-μm intervals revealed a micrometastasis in one more lymph node. Overall, eight of nine (89%) SLNs with micrometastases were detected in the first two H&E and IH levels separated by 40 μm. Another study suggests that three H&E sections taken at levels 25%, 50%, and 75% into the tissue block would detect virtually all metastatic foci in a lymph node (227). On the basis of these reports, one practical protocol is to obtain three H&E levels separated by 40 μm with a CK-IH stain accompanying each level or corresponding to at least one of the levels.

In my experience, none of the commonly used CK reagents has a particular advantage or disadvantage; however, carcinoma cells sometimes display subtle differences in CK reactivity, and it may be helpful to use more than one antibody such as CAM5.2, CK-7, or AE1/AE3 separately on different sections.

### Relationship Between Sentinel and Nonsentinel Lymph Nodes

The histologic findings in the SLN are a strong predictor of the presence or absence of metastases in nonsentinel lymph nodes (NSLNs), a fact that validates the SLN concept. This was demonstrated convincingly by Turner et al., who studied 103 patients who underwent SLN mapping followed by dissection of level I–II lymph nodes (222). Routine H&E study of the SLN revealed metastatic carcinoma in 33 patients (32%). CK-IH detected micrometastases in an SLN from 10 of the remaining 70 patients (14.3%) whose SLN appeared negative with H&E staining, leaving 60 women with negative SLN after H&E and IH stains. None of the 1,087 NSLNs from these 60 patients was found to have metastatic carcinoma on H&E, and only 0.09% had micrometastases demonstrated by IH. Consequently, only 1 of 60 (1.7%) patients with an SLN negative on H&E and IH had a positive NSLN. On the other hand, 18 of 43 patients (41.9%) with a positive SLN had NSLN metastases.

The distinction between a true-positive SLN on frozen section and a false-negative SLN is also a significant predictor of the presence of metastases in NSLN because the true-positive group usually has macrometastases (>2 mm) and the false-negative group mainly has micrometastases (≤ 2 mm). Turner et al. reported that the frequency of positive NSLNs was 64% when the SLN was positive intraoperatively and 18% when the SLN diagnosis during surgery was falsely negative (228). Similar results were reported by Viale et al., who found NSLN metastases in 18.8% of patients with micrometastatic SLN and in 54.8% of women with SLN macrometastases (>2 mm) (229).

Veronesi et al. reported that NSLNs were positive in H&E sections from 5.9% of patients who had a negative SLN after H&E and IH stains. (208). The overall concordance between the SLN and final axillary lymph node status was 96.8%. Twelve patients with a negative SLN who had a positive NSLN represented 3.2% of all cases. In this study, NSLNs were not examined by IH. Comparable findings were reported by Weaver et al. in an analysis of 385 patients who underwent axillary dissection in conjunction with SLN mapping (230). When studied by H&E sections, 43 of 57 (75.4%) patients with positive NSLN also had positive SLN; the remaining 14 with positive NSLN were 5% of patients with negative SLN, indicating a negative predictive value of 95%. These researchers were able to perform CK-IH on SLNs and NSLNs from 214 cases that appeared to be negative in H&E sections. Micrometastases were detected in 19 SLNs (7.9%), and four of these cases also had positive NSLNs (1.9%). Another three patients (1.4%) had micrometastases in NSLN but not in SLN. These data confirm the reliability of routine H&E and IH studies of the SLN as a method for identifying patients with the greatest risk for positive NSLN.

The risk of NSLN metastases appears to be influenced not only by the size of the SLN metastasis but also by the number of positive SLNs. Chu et al. detected micrometastases by IH in H&E-negative NSLNs in 11.8% of cases where there was one positive SLN and in 29.4% when more than one SLN contained metastatic carcinoma (231). Other pathologic factors associated with NSLN metastases in univariate analysis were tumor size and angiolymphatic invasion, but only tumor size and the number of positive SLNs were significant risk factors in multivariate analysis. Turner et al. reported that the following factors were associated with NSLN metastases in patients with metastatic carcinoma in SLN: macrometastatic carcinoma in the SLN; extranodal extension of the SLN metastasis; the number of involved SLNs; primary tumor size; primary tumor grade; and the presence of lymphatic tumor emboli in the breast (231a).

### Histopathology of Sentinel Lymph Nodes

A deposit of metastatic carcinoma in a lymph node is described as a *micrometastasis* if it measures 2 mm or less in largest diameter and as a *macrometastasis* if larger than 2 mm. Multiple metastases in a single lymph node are usually characterized on the basis of the largest focus, and a lymph node may therefore be classified as having a micrometastases, although the aggregate diameters of the tumor deposits may appear to exceed 2 mm. These terms apply equally to SLN and NSLN.

Lymphatic flow into lymph nodes occurs through channels that drain predominantly into subcapsular sinusoids and thence to parenchymal sinusoids. This pattern of physiologic and anatomic function is responsible for the frequent observation that small metastatic deposits identified in H&E sections are usually located in the subcapsular sinusoids (Fig. 46.34). Consequently, pathologists devote particular attention to this region during histologic examination of SLNs. Isolated tumor cells, particularly those lacking pleomorphic cytologic features, can be difficult to separate from histio-

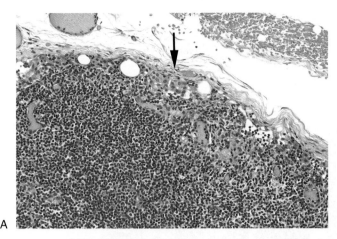

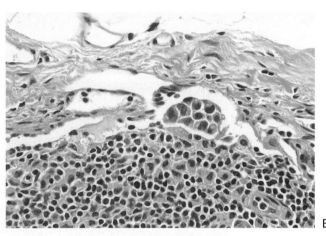

**FIG. 46.34.** *Sentinel lymph nodes, peripheral sinusoids.* **A,B:** Small deposits of metastatic carcinoma are present in peripheral sinusoids of two lymph nodes. The less distinct metastasis in **A** is indicated by an *arrow.* Cytokeratin immunostaining is usually not needed to detect such metastases.

cytes, which normally crowd the sinusoids (Fig. 46.35). Some metastatic carcinoma cells appear to undergo changes that suggest degenerative alterations represented by nuclear pyknosis and increased eosinophilia of the cytoplasm. These cells are quite likely to be indistinguishable from histiocytes, and it is usually necessary to rely on CK-IH to determine whether an epithelial cell is present (Fig. 46.36).

Clusters of carcinoma cells are recognized more readily in sinusoids than are isolated cells, in part because of a tendency for the cohesive carcinoma cells to separate from the surrounding histiocytes, causing them to appear to be located in a lacunar space (Figs. 46.34, 46.36, and 46.37). By itself, this is not a completely reliable diagnostic criterion because carcinoma cells vary in their cohesiveness. Metastatic

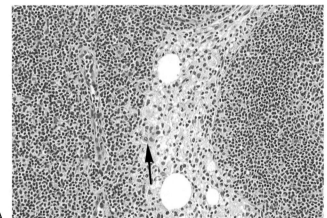

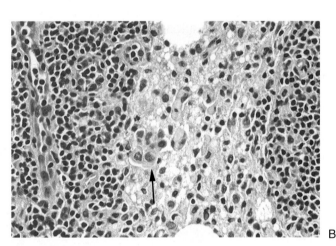

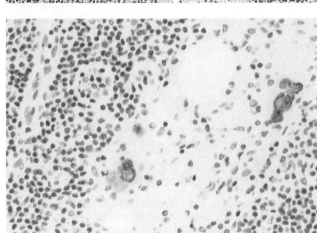

**FIG. 46.35.** *Sentinel lymph nodes, central sinusoids.* **A,B:** Two large lipid vacuoles are present among histiocytes that fill a central sinusoid. A cluster of "suspicious" cells located between the lipid vacuoles is indicated by the *arrow.* **C:** The immunostain for cytokeratin 7 (CK-7) on a replicate section discloses two clusters of immunoreactive cells near the upper lipid vacuole. The lower CK-7–positive cell group is in the location of the suspicious cells in **B** (avidin-biotin).

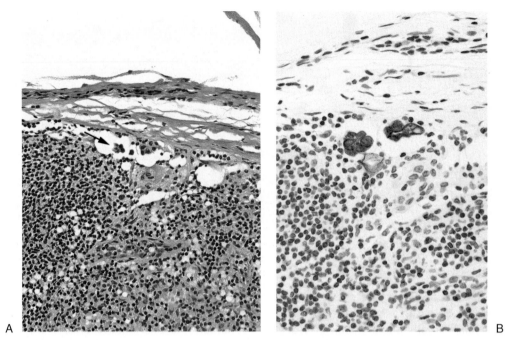

**FIG. 46.36.** *Sentinel lymph node.* **A:** The small cluster of cells in the peripheral sinusoid of this lymph is not clearly diagnostic of metastatic carcinoma *(arrow)*. Note the dark, pyknotic nuclei. **B:** Reactivity for CK-7 is shown, establishing the epithelial character of the cells shown in **A** (avidin-biotin). Unstained nuclei are evident in the cluster on the *right.*

lobular carcinoma is notorious in this regard because it is characterized by loss of cell surface adhesion proteins such as E-cadherin, and it tends to involve lymph nodes in a dispersed fashion without particular regard to sinusoidal distribution (Fig. 46.38).

One of the interesting observations to result from intense histologic examination of SLN with multiple sections and IH is that isolated micrometastases can be found in the core and lymphoid stroma without detectable subcapsular deposits (Figs. 46.35 and 46.39). These parenchymal micrometastases are particularly difficult to appreciate in H&E sections, and they usually are detected only after CK-IH sections have

been prepared. This distribution of metastatic carcinoma has been associated with, but is not specific for, lobular carcinoma.

Metastatic carcinoma in SLN and NSLN usually duplicates the cytologic and histologic features of the primary tumor. Knowledge of the appearance of the primary tumor is therefore useful in screening lymph nodes in general, and especially SLNs, for metastatic carcinoma. Comparison of cytologic features can be done with small micrometastases and even single cells, whereas architectural comparison frequently requires metastatic foci of 1 to 2 mm or larger. Because of the possibility of heterogeneity in the primary tu-

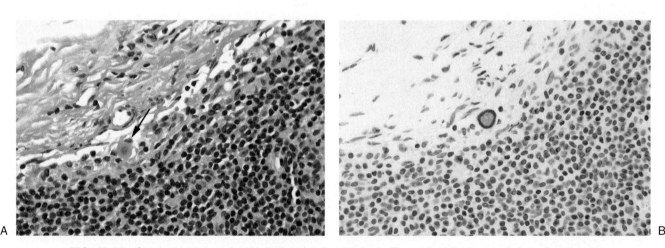

**FIG. 46.37.** *Sentinel lymph node with isolated cell metastasis.* The patient had comedo intraductal carcinoma with microinvasion. **A:** The nature of the solitary cell *(arrow)* identified in the peripheral sinus was uncertain. **B:** The cell was immunoreactive with the cytokeratin immunostain AE1/AE3 (avidin-biotin).

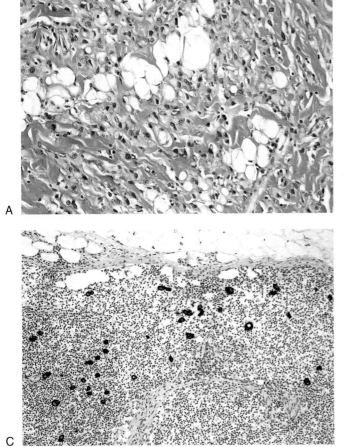

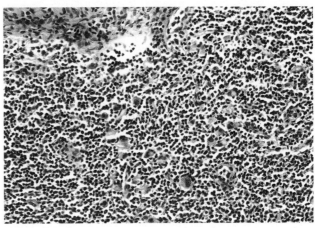

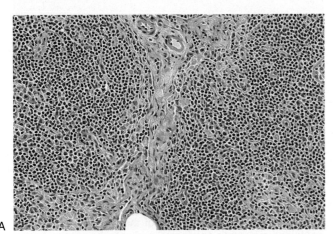

**FIG. 46.38.** *Sentinel lymph node in invasive lobular carcinoma.* **A:** A 7-mm invasive lobular carcinoma in the breast. **B:** Cells with hyperchromatic nuclei in the lymphoid tissue of the sentinel lymph node. **C:** Numerous cells in the lymphoid tissue are reactive for cytokerain 7 (CK-7) and the peripheral sinusoids are virtually devoid of CK-positive cells (avidin-biotin).

mor, it is preferable to have a substantial sample of tissue from an excisional biopsy than to rely on the limited material in a needle core biopsy (Fig. 46.40). Marked histologic disparity between the breast tumor and a lymph node metastasis can be indicative of a second, inapparent focus of carcinoma in the breast (Fig. 46.41). Despite the expectation that high-grade tumors are more likely than low-grade tumors to

be the source of axillary nodal metastases, the reverse situation can occur.

*Microinvasive carcinoma (T1mic),* defined as an invasive focus smaller than 1 mm, can be the source of metastatic carcinoma in axillary lymph nodes, especially the SLN. Data on the expected frequency of SLN metastases in patients with microinvasive carcinoma are limited. These patients are

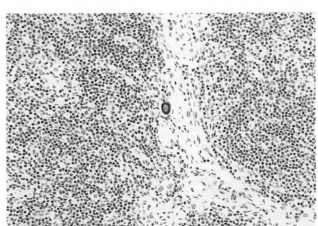

**FIG. 46.39.** *Sentinel lymph node.* **A,B:** Replicate sections of fibrous stroma within a lymph node. The immunostain for AE1/AE3 revealed a single cytokeratin-positive cell **(B)**, which was not evident in the hematoxylin and eosin section **(A)** (avidin-biotin).

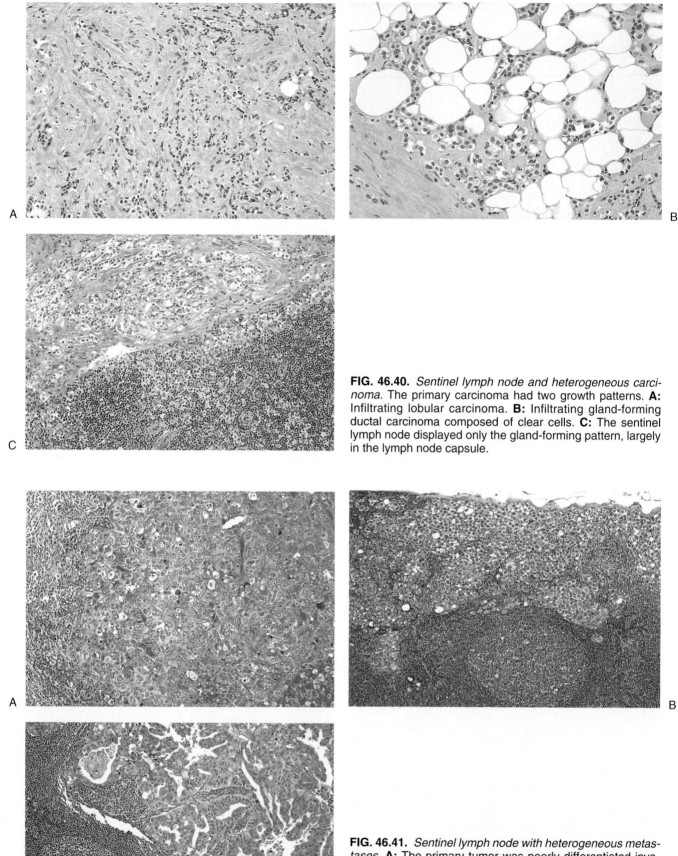

**FIG. 46.40.** *Sentinel lymph node and heterogeneous carcinoma.* The primary carcinoma had two growth patterns. **A:** Infiltrating lobular carcinoma. **B:** Infiltrating gland-forming ductal carcinoma composed of clear cells. **C:** The sentinel lymph node displayed only the gland-forming pattern, largely in the lymph node capsule.

**FIG. 46.41.** *Sentinel lymph node with heterogeneous metastases.* **A:** The primary tumor was poorly differentiated invasive ductal carcinoma. **B:** Part of the sentinel lymph node contained metastatic carcinoma similar to the primary tumor. **C:** The lymph node also contained metastatic papillary apocrine carcinoma. This pattern was not found in the primary breast tumor and presumably derived from a second undetected breast carcinoma.

excellent candidates for SLN mapping because of the specificity of the procedure and the exceptionally low probability of metastases in the NSLN. Involvement of the SLN is typically micrometastatic and often inapparent without CK-IH. Consequently, it is preferable to omit frozen section when the primary lesion has been found to have only microinvasive carcinoma after thorough histologic examination (Fig. 46.37).

The vast majority of metastatic foci in lymph nodes are readily identified as carcinoma and are distinguishable from rarely occurring noncarcinomatous glandular inclusion. Difficulty arises when glands in the lymph node or in perinodal tissue have a close resemblance to nonneoplastic mammary lobules or ducts. In most cases, these nodal foci are well-differentiated metastatic carcinoma, usually originating in a tubular or tubulolobular carcinoma (Fig. 46.42). These metastatic foci may be in the lymphoid stroma or in the lymph node sinuses. For a discussion of heterotopic glands in axillary lymph nodes and their distinction from metastatic carcinoma, see Chapter 45.

Another benign lesion encountered in SLN as well as in lymph nodes generally is the *nevus cell aggregate*. These neuroepithelial structures localized to the lymph node capsule, rarely extending into perinodal tissue or along fibrovascular tissue into the lymph node, are not immunoreactive for CK. Because of their cytologic features, the pathologist inexperienced in the appearance of nevus cell aggregates may interpret this finding as metastatic lobular carcinoma. A complete discussion of nevus cell aggregates can be found in Chapter 45.

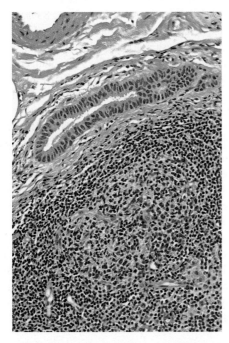

**FIG. 46.42.** *Sentinel lymph node, well-differentiated carcinoma.* Metastatic well-differentiated duct carcinoma in the capsule of a sentinel lymph node. Foci such as this sometimes are misinterpreted as benign ductal inclusions. Myoepithelial cells are not present in this metastatic gland.

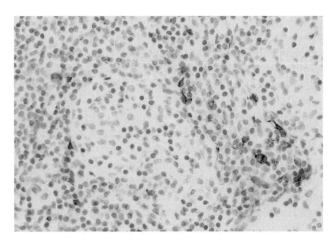

**FIG. 46.43.** *Sentinel lymph node, dendritic cells.* Dendritic cells in the lymphoid tissue are immunoreactive for CAM5.2 cytokeratin (avidin-biotin). By comparison with metastatic carcinoma, they have sparse cytoplasm and ill-defined cell borders.

The *pseudosentinel lymph node* is a source of concern. It is a lymph node with the clinical characteristics of an SLN (distinct labelling with blue-dye radiocolloid or both agents) that does not contain metastatic carcinoma or harbors micrometastases in a patient who proves to have macrometastases in NSLN. The lymph node found to act as a SLN has most likely assumed this function secondarily because lymphatic drainage in the original true SLN has been obstructed by metastatic carcinoma. Unfortunately, a "pseudosentinel" lymph node cannot be distinguished from a true SLN unless the status of the other lymph nodes is known.

*Dendritic cells,* CK-positive, interstitial reticulum cells, are elements in the reticulo-histiocytic system involved in presenting antigens to CD34(+) T cells (231b). Dendritic cells are present throughout the lymphoid tissue, especially in subcapsular paracortical and medullary regions. These cells are immunoreactive for CK8 and 18 but not CK19. Increased numbers of dendritic cells can be found in reactive lymph nodes. In contrast to most carcinoma cells, they are not located in the sinusoids, and they have irregular shapes with branching dendritic processes (Fig. 46.43). Dendritic reticulum cells are reported to be reactive with pan-CK and CAM5.2 but not with the AE1/AE3 antibody cocktail (231b).

## Molecular Studies of Sentinel Lymph Nodes to Detect Micrometastases

RT-PCR is an ultrasensitive method for detecting mRNA associated with specific markers at extremely low levels of expression. The technique is capable of detecting one CEA-positive cell among $1 \times 10^6$ mononuclear cells (232) or one carcinoma cell among $1 \times 10^6$ lymphocytes (233,234).

For several years, RT-PCR has been studied as a method for detecting micrometastases in axillary lymph nodes. Some of this work antedated the introduction of SLN mapping; therefore, the early results are not specific for the SLN. Noguchi et al. reported two studies of CK19 expression determined by RT-PCR in axillary lymph nodes from women with breast carcinoma. In one study, CK19 expression was seen in all lymph nodes with histologically documented metastatic carcinoma but in only 5 of 53 (9%) lymph nodes lacking metastatic carcinoma (235). These researchers also reported that mucin-1 (MUC-1) RNA was detectable in all lymph nodes that had metastatic carcinoma and in 6% of histologically negative lymph nodes. A second report documented similar results with CK19 detected in 90% of histologically positive lymph nodes and in 14% of histologically negative lymph nodes (236). Lymphatic invasion was present in primary tumors associated with histologically positive (70%) and CK19 RT-PCR positive/histologically negative (53%) lymph nodes significantly more often than when the lymph nodes were histologically and CK19 RT-PCR negative (18%).

Schoenfeld et el. studied 530 histologically negative lymph nodes from 75 consecutive patients for CK19 mRNA by RT-PCR (237). CK19 was detected in 20% of the 530 histologically negative lymph nodes. The presence of CK19 mRNA in histologically negative lymph nodes was significantly correlated with tumor size and histologic grade. CK19 mRNA was detected in all histologically positive lymph nodes. These investigators also studied 33 histologically negative/RT-PCR–positive lymph nodes by CK19 IH and detected immunoreactive cells in three (9%). Forty-one lymph nodes that were histologically and RT-PCR negative had no CK19 immunoreactive cells.

The value of a multimarker panel for the RT-PCR study of lymph nodes was explored by Lockett et al. (238). These investigators studied axillary lymph nodes for three markers: CK19, c-myc, and prolactin-inducible protein (PIP). Lymph nodes larger than 1 cm were bisected, with the halves used for histopathologic and molecular analysis, respectively. Metastatic carcinoma was detected in lymph nodes from 24 patients by routine histologic examination. RT-PCR detected at least one of the three tumors markers in 22 (92%) of the histologically positive lymph nodes; two histologically positive lymph nodes were RT-PCR negative. RT-PCR demonstrated one or more epithelial marker in 15 (40%) histologically negative cases. The distribution of RT-PCR positivity varied among the three molecular markers. In the 22 histologically positive, RT-PCR–positive cases, the frequencies of expression for c-myc, CK19, and PIP were 41%, 73%, and 32%, whereas in 15 histologically negative, RT-PCR–positive cases, the frequencies of expression were 93%, 13%, and 20%, respectively. Correlation with tumor size (T-stage) was weak because c-myc, CK19, and PIP were expressed in 100%, 50%, and 25% of the lymph nodes associated with T1 tumors and in 55%, 55%, and 35% associated with tumors T2 or larger. Multiple markers tended to be found more often in histologically positive than in histologically negative lymph nodes. The fact that no marker was positive in every histologically positive lymph node underscores the value of using a multigene panel for RT-PCR detection of micrometastases.

The specificity of CK19 mRNA as a marker for metastatic carcinoma was questioned by investigators who reported CK19 mRNA in lymph nodes from patients not known to have carcinoma (239). These researchers also reported that the frequency of CK19 mRNA in histologically negative axillary lymph nodes from patients with breast carcinoma (95/143, 66.4%) was nearly as high as in histologically positive lymph nodes (128/166, 77.1%). The discrepancies may relate to technical issues in RT-PCR methodology in that detectability of CK19 mRNA has been shown to be partly dependent on the number of cycles of amplification performed (240). Schoenfeld and Coombes reported that CK19 mRNA was not detectable in negative lymph nodes when amplification was maintained below 40 cycles but that it appeared in paired samples from these lymph nodes amplified beyond 40 cycles. These observations underscore the need for establishing standardized methods before these ultrasensitive techniques can be applied in clinical practice.

RT-PCR has been used in the study of SLN. Bostick et al. evaluated the expression of a panel of markers (CEA; CK19; CK20; gastrointestinal tumor-associated antigen 733.2, or GA732.2; and MUC-1) using RT-PCR to analyze frozen section samples of SLN (241). They reported that CK20 was the only marker not detected in control lymph nodes from patients who did not have carcinoma. In 12 SLNs classified as negative in H&E sections and by immunostaining for CK, marker expression by RT-PCR was detected for GA733.2, MUC-1, CK19, CEA, and CK20 in 92%, 83%, 67%, 42%, and 8%, respectively, of the samples analyzed. The frequencies of detecting these markers in histologically or IH-positive SLNs were 70%, 70%, 80%, 70%, and 20%, respectively, for GA733.2, MUC-1, CK19, CEA, and CK20. No single marker was expressed in all 10 histologically positive lymph nodes, but mRNA for at least one marker was detected in 9 of the 10 positive lymph nodes. Because of the high frequency of expression of most of these markers in lymph nodes from patients without cancer and in the negative SLNs in this study, the investigators concluded that MUC-1, CK19, CEA, and GA733.2 were not diagnostically useful for detecting SLN micrometastases. Another study by Bostick et al. explored the detection of three other mRNA tumor markers: c-met, P97, and 4GalNac-T (4-N-acetyl galactosaminyl transferase) (242). One of 17 SLNs with histologically documented metastases did not express any of these three mRNA markers. The markers were expressed individually in 53% to 83% of histologically negative SLNs, and all three markers were expressed in 43% of negative SLNs.

Failure to detect mRNA markers in histologically positive lymph nodes is probably due to sampling error. The significance of markers detected in SLN with no histologically identified carcinoma is unknown. Presently, an ideal mRNA marker expressed only by tumor cells and not in any normal lymph nodes has not been identified. Therefore, detection of mRNA markers in histologically negative lymph nodes cannot be interpreted as indicative of metastatic carcinoma, and these experimental results should not play a role in clinical staging at present. None of these procedures has been standardized to diminish or eliminate false-positive results, which might be due to extremely low levels of marker expression by normal cells or the result of some other mechanism.

## Clinical Significance of Axillary Lymph Node Micrometastases and Sentinel Lymph Node Mapping

In addition to detecting metastatic carcinoma in axillary lymph nodes and establishing the level of involvement, histologic examination can provide other information about the metastatic foci. The number of lymph nodes that contain metastases should be documented. Prognosis is significantly decreased as the number of affected lymph nodes increases. Patients are generally stratified in the following three categories: one to three, four to nine, and 10 or more affected lymph nodes (243).

Several investigators have assessed the prognostic significance of the size of metastatic foci in axillary lymph nodes. In these studies, micrometastases were 2 mm or smaller in diameter; larger metastases were macrometastases (244–247). Micrometastases may be detected in routine sections of lymph nodes, in serial sections of initially negative lymph nodes, or by CK-IH. Metastases found by the latter two methods have been referred to as *occult micrometastases.* The frequency with which occult micrometastases have been detected varies from 9% (248,249) to 33% (250), with a median of 17% in eight reports recently reviewed (249). Studies that did not take the number of involved lymph nodes or the size of the primary tumor into consideration led to the conclusion that patients with macrometastases had a less favorable prognosis than those with micrometastases (244–246). It has been further suggested that the prognosis for women with micrometastases did not differ significantly from that of women with negative lymph nodes (244, 251–253).

Analyses that evaluate the size of metastases and number of affected lymph nodes are difficult to perform and practical only when limited to patients with single nodal metastases classified as either a macrometastasis or micrometastasis. If two lymph nodes are involved, three categories are possible (2 micrometastases, 2 macrometastases, or 1 each); with more extensive metastases, the stratification becomes impractical. One study analyzed the prognostic significance of a solitary nodal metastasis in T1N1 and T2N1 patients with an average follow-up of 10 years (247). When the T1N1 and T2N1 patients with a single nodal metastasis were analyzed together, there was a significantly poorer prognosis among patients with a single macrometastasis compared with those who had a micrometastasis. A major prognostic

difference was apparent after stratification by tumor size. During the first 6 years of follow-up, T1 patients with negative nodes and those with a single micrometastasis had similar survival curves, significantly better than those with macrometastases. With additional follow-up, the disease-free survival of patients with a micrometastasis became nearly identical to that of patients with a macrometastasis and significantly worse than that of patients with negative lymph nodes. Conversely, T2 patients with negative lymph nodes or a single micrometastasis had survival rates that did not differ significantly throughout the 10-year follow-up. Both groups had an outcome significantly better than T2 patients with a macrometastasis. These observations demonstrate that tumor size, length of follow-up, and the number of involved lymph nodes influence the prognostic significance of axillary micrometastases.

de Mascarel et al. used a serial sectioning technique to restudy lymph nodes initially reported as negative (254). Disease-free and overall survival were similar for patients with a single micrometastasis and a single macrometastasis detected in this fashion and significantly less favorable than among the patients with negative lymph nodes.

The significance of occult micrometastases in axillary lymph nodes was also investigated in a Ludwig Breast Cancer Study Group prospective cooperative adjuvant chemotherapy trial that included 921 patients judged to have negative axillary lymph nodes in routine sections (249). Additional sections of the lymph nodes were prepared at six levels. Occult micrometastases in a single lymph node were found in 83 (9%) of the cases. Factors significantly associated with the detection of micrometastases were tumor size larger than 2 cm, peritumoral vascular invasion, and diagnosis before age 50. Occult micrometastases were detected with nearly equal frequency in patients with invasive ductal and lobular carcinoma. Five-year disease-free and overall survival were significantly lower in patients with a single micrometastasis, whether the metastasis was found in routine or in serial sections. Multivariate analysis revealed that the unfavorable prognostic effect of solitary occult micrometastases was significantly correlated with the following: invasive duct carcinoma, high-grade tumors, tumors larger than 2 cm, and peritumoral vascular invasion.

A second study of the Ludwig Breast Cancer Study Group patient database used CK immunostaining (AE1 and CAM5.2) as well as serial sectioning of histologically negative lymph nodes (255). Lymph node samples were available for 736 patients. Occult nodal metastases were found in 52 (7%) patients by serial sectioning and in 149 (20%) by IH. Both methods were positive in 45 (6%) cases, and both were negative in 581 (79%). Among the 110 (15%) discrepant cases, 103 were positive only by IH and seven only in serial sections. Immunostaining was more sensitive for detecting an occult metastasis than serial sections among all histologic types, especially for infiltrating lobular carcinoma, in which 39% (20/51) of patients with histologically negative lymph nodes were found to have occult metastases. The yield of IH detected occult metastases in patients with infiltrating ductal, special types, and mixed duct-lobular carcinomas was 13%, 16% and 38%, respectively. Occult metastases detected by serial sectioning or by IH were associated with a significantly less favorable disease-free and overall survival in postmenopausal but not in premenopausal women. Occult micrometastases detected by IH were a significant risk factor for recurrence in multivariate analysis.

The identification in routine sections of isolated metastatic cells or small groups of cells originating from infiltrating lobular carcinoma presents a particularly vexing problem. These small cells may be difficult to distinguish from histiocytes and reactive cells in a lymph node stained with H&E. To investigate this issue, Bussolati et al. prepared new sections of lymph nodes reported to be negative from 50 patients with infiltrating lobular carcinoma (256). By using antibodies to three epithelial-associated IH markers (EMA, HMFG-2, human milk fat globule membrane; and CK), these researchers were able to detect metastatic carcinoma in 26 lymph nodes from 12 of 50 patients (24%). Because carcinoma cells were evident in H&E-stained duplicate sections of seven lymph nodes from five patients, the net contribution of the IH studies was to detect tumor cells in 2.4% of the lymph nodes from 14% of the patients. For the most part, the positive cells were present individually in sinuses or in the lymphoid tissue. Although the tumor cells were stained most intensely and consistently with anti-EMA, there were rare instances in which cells proven to be histiocytes by chymotrypsin and $\alpha_1$-antitrypsin staining exhibited cytoplasmic staining with anti-EMA. Recurrences occurred in 2 of 12 (17%) immunocytochemically positive cases, and in 7 of 38 (18%) negative cases. It should be noted that plasma cells are also immunoreactive for EMA and this fact complicates the interpretation of studies using this reagent.

Trojani et al. applied a mixture of five monoclonal antibodies to existing histologic sections of lymph nodes reported to be negative from 150 consecutive patients with an average follow-up of 10 years (257). Overall, 21 patients (14%) were found to have occult micrometastases. The yield of positive lymph nodes was greater in patients with invasive lobular (38%) than in those with invasive ductal (11%) carcinoma. The finding of occult micrometastases was not related to tumor grade or lymphatic tumor emboli. Instances of plasma cells with positive staining with anti-EMA were noted, a phenomenon previously reported by Delsol et al. (258). Among patients with invasive duct carcinoma, death due to disease was significantly more frequent in the group with micrometastases (23%) than in those with IH-negative lymph nodes (6.3%).

de Mascarel et al. used the monoclonal antibody panel described by Trojani et al. (257) to study 218 lymph node-negative cases (254). Immunoreactive cells were detected in 37 of 89 (41%) lymph node dissections from patients with infiltrating lobular carcinoma and in 13 of 129 (10%) with invasive duct carcinoma. Micrometastases did not significantly influence prognosis in the patients with infiltrating lobular

carcinoma after a median follow-up of 9.3 years. There was a significant correlation with recurrence but not with survival among women with ductal carcinoma followed for a median of 15.6 years.

Elson et al. found occult nodal micrometastases in 20 of 97 histologically node-negative patients restudied by IH using a "cocktail" of CK (AE1/AE3) and tumor-associated glycoprotein (DF3) antibodies (259). In retrospect, nine patients had metastases that were overlooked initially in the original sections. New micrometastases were uncovered by serial sectioning and IH in 11 cases. The presence of micrometastases did not have a significant effect on disease-free or overall survival after a mean follow-up of 5.7 years. In another study by these investigators of 98 patients, occult metastases were detected in histologically negative lymph nodes from 9% of the women, but after follow-up of up to 14 years, the presence or absence of micrometastases did not significantly affect prognosis (260). On the other hand, Friedman et al. reported that the presence of a single occult nodal micrometastasis detected by serial resectioning of negative lymph nodes had the same prognostically unfavorable significance as a similar metastasis detected in routine sections when compared to node-negative patients (248).

Another retrospective study of axillary lymph nodes previously reported to be negative in 208 patients yielded occult metastases in 51 (24.5%) cases studied with a combination of resectioning and IH (261). Occult metastases were detected more often in lymph nodes from patients with lobular (38%) than with duct (25%) carcinoma and in women younger than 50 years (41%) than in women 50 years and older (19%). Although the presence and increasing size of occult metastases were significantly associated with decreased disease-free survival in multivariate analysis, these factors were not significant predictors of overall survival.

The weight of evidence from the foregoing retrospective studies indicates that the presence of micrometastases detected in routine H&E sections of axillary lymph nodes predicts an adverse prognosis compared with patients who have histologically negative lymph nodes (262–264). The same observation applies to occult micrometastases uncovered by serial sections or IH in histologically negative lymph nodes. The frequency of detecting occult micrometastases is higher for infiltrating lobular and duct-lobular carcinoma than for infiltrating duct carcinoma. Occult micrometastases, however, have been detected even in histologically negative lymph nodes from patients with prognostically favorable special types of carcinoma. The presence of peritumoral lymphovascular tumor emboli in the breast is a factor associated with occult micrometastases. The size of the primary tumor is directly correlated with detection of occult micrometastases.

Follow-up data on SLN patients will be needed to determine the significance of micrometastases and occult micrometastases detected only in SLNs. Prospective studies have been initiated to assess the prognostic significance of micrometastases in SLNs (189). Because of the overall favorable prognosis of many patients who undergo SLN mapping with the finding of histologically negative SLN, it will require large numbers of patients with long-term follow-up to determine the extent to which occult micrometastases in the SLN alter prognosis. If the aforementioned retrospective studies are a reliable guide, it is likely that SLN micrometastases will be prognostically meaningful. It is unfortunate that SLN cannot be identified retrospectively because they were inevitably included in the total axillary lymph node specimens submitted by prior investigators for serial sections and IH. The advantage of SLN mapping is that it identifies the lymph node(s) with the highest probability of harboring any metastases, including micrometastases detected by H&E sectioning and occult micrometastases uncovered by serial sections and IH. In view of the low probability of metastases in non-SLN when the SLN has only micrometastases, SLN mapping has proven to be a less morbid and more selective method than conventional axillary dissection for finding patients with micrometastases who are possibly at risk for recurrence and who might benefit from systemic adjuvant therapy. Follow-up studies yet to be completed are necessary to determine whether all SLN micrometastases are prognostically important.

Another issue is how to manage the axilla after SLN mapping uncovers micrometastatic disease. Options include completion of axillary dissection, radiotherapy, reliance on systemic adjuvant therapy, or no treatment (265,265a). A prospective study of 67 patients in whom negative SLN mapping was the only axillary staging procedure was reported by Giuliano et al. after a median follow-up of 39 months (265b). No axillary recurrences were observed.

The survival of metastatic carcinoma cells in lymph nodes depends on many factors, such as the angiogenic capacity of the cells and the cytotoxic microenvironment of the lymph node (266). The survivability of micrometastatic carcinoma cells has been questioned, a concern supported in some instances by the degenerated appearance of the cells in histologic sections. A method developed for isolating micrometastatic carcinoma cells for *in vitro* culture may prove useful for investigating this question (267). At present, the issue remains unsettled, and this dilemma is unlikely to be easily or speedily resolved. Clinical judgment is needed to decide currently how the finding of occult micrometastases in SLN should influence the management of an individual patient. Speculative opinions unsupported by follow-up information, such as the statement that "we believe that this phenomenon in itself, does not carry risk of future metastatic behavior," referring to epithelial cells in some lymph nodes as resulting from "benign transport," are premature (268).

Modification of the *tumor, node, metastasis (TNM) staging system* to distinguish the presence of "isolated tumor cells" from micrometastases has been suggested (269). The term *isolated tumor cells* was offered for situations in which evidence of epithelial cells comparable with metastatic carcinoma is detected in tissues such as bone marrow or lymph nodes or in the blood by nonmorphologic methods, such as flow cytometry or PCR. The term *isolated tumor cells* also was applied to "single tumor cells or small clusters" identified by morphologic methods such as CK-IH. Isolated tumor cells were said to differ from micrometastases in having no contact with a vascular or lymph sinus wall, showing no invasion of a vascular lymph sinus wall, an absence of stromal reaction, and no evidence of tumor cell proliferation. The term *isolated tumor cells* would apply to the rare circumstances in which tumor cells are found in lymphovascular channels at sites of intraductal carcinoma that exhibit epithelial disruption attributable to a needling procedure. An "optional proposal" for the classification of isolated tumor cells, which would incorporate morphologic and molecular data into the TNM staging system, is shown in Table 46.2. This terminology applies only to patients with axillary lymph nodes with no histologic evidence of metastases after routine H&E sections have been examined microscopically.

### Extranodal Extension

The prognostic significance of the spread of metastatic carcinoma from a lymph node to the surrounding axillary tissues, so-called extranodal extension, is uncertain (Fig. 46.44) It has been difficult to analyze this feature independently of other factors, such as the number of involved lymph nodes or the size of the primary tumor. The presence of extranodal extension is generally associated with tumors larger than 2 cm and the presence of carcinoma in four or more lymph nodes. Several studies reviewed here suggested that extranodal extension indicates a higher risk of systemic or local recurrence in patients already predisposed to these events because of unfavorable prognostic factors. The reports do not provide compelling evidence that extranodal extension is a high-risk factor for axillary recurrence in women who have a complete axillary dissection. Extranodal extension appears to have a negative effect on relapse-free and overall survival. In some studies, this effect is influenced by the number of lymph nodes involved by metastases (<4 or >4). There does not appear to be a consensus favoring axillary radiation in these patients.

**TABLE 46.2.** *An "optional proposal" for incorporating "isolated tumor cell" data into TNM staging for patients with histologically negative lymph nodes*

| N Stage Group | Definition |
|---|---|
| pNO | No regional lymph node metastases histologically; no examination for isolated tumor cells (ITC), morphologic (i) or nonmorphologic molecular (mol) studies |
| pNO (i–) | Negative morphologic findings for ITC |
| pNO (i+) | Positive morphologic findings for ITC |
| pNO (mol–) | Negative nonmorphologic findings for ITC |
| pNO (mol+) | Positive nonmorphologic findings for ITC |

ITC, isolated tumor cells; TNM, tumor, node, metastasis.
Based on Hermanek P, Huttler RV, Sobin LH, et al. International Union Against Cancer. Classification of isolated tumor cells and micrometastasis. *Cancer* 1999;86:2668–2673, with permission.

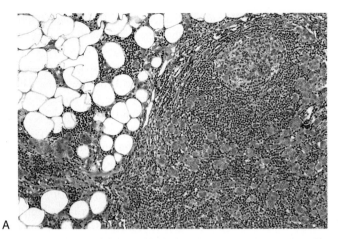
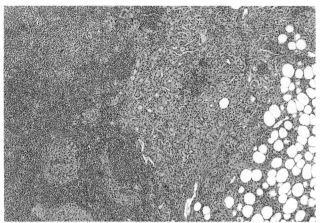

**FIG. 46.44.** *Extranodal extension.* **A:** Invasive lobular carcinoma surrounds a germinal center and invades perinodal fat. **B:** Invasive duct carcinoma has destroyed the lymph node capsule and extended into perinodal fat *(right).*

Several retrospective studies have found extranodal extension to be prognostically unfavorable in women treated by mastectomy and axillary dissection. Hultborn and Tornberg described a series of patients treated by mastectomy and postoperative radiotherapy (270). Among women with extranodal involvement, the 10-year survival (19%) was substantially lower than that of patients with metastases limited to their axillary nodes (52%). Pierce et al. reported that microscopic extranodal extension was significantly more frequent in women with four or more nodal metastases and that it was a significant predictor of systemic rather than local axillary recurrence (271). Fisher et al. also found that extranodal extension was significantly more frequent in patients who had four or more lymph nodes with metastases, infiltrating duct carcinoma, and carcinomas that had a stellate configuration (272). In this prospective study, patients with extranodal extension had a significantly higher frequency of short-term relapse, but the analysis did not demonstrate that the tendency to treatment failure was independent of the extent of nodal involvement.

A series of 308 patients with positive nodes treated by mastectomy without adjuvant radiation or chemotherapy with 10 years of follow-up was evaluated at the Milan National Cancer Institute (273). The frequency of extranodal extension was significantly related to the number of involved lymph nodes (one to three nodes positive, 27% extracapsular; four or more nodes positive, 51% extracapsular). Further analysis revealed that extracapsular extension of nodal metastases did not have an impact on prognosis when only one lymph node was involved, but if two or more lymph nodes were affected, extracapsular extension was associated with a significantly higher recurrence rate.

Leonard et al. reported that extranodal tumor extension was significantly more frequent in patients with tumors larger than 2 cm, high-grade carcinomas, when there were more than three lymph node metastases, and when there was lymphatic or vascular invasion at the primary tumor site (274). This study did not detect an increased risk of axillary recurrence associated with extranodal extension, regardless of treatment with axillary radiation or systemic chemother-

apy. Multivariate analysis revealed that the presence of extranodal extension and more than three nodal metastases were significant independent prognostic factors, with the number of involved lymph nodes having a stronger effect. In the study of Leonard et al., extracapsular spread was associated with a less favorable overall prognosis in patients with one to three nodal metastases but not when more than three lymph nodes were involved.

Stage II or III patients who had extracapsular nodal metastases had a high recurrence rate after treatment with surgery and chemotherapy without local–regional radiotherapy in a retrospective review of 82 cases (275). Overall, 78% of the women developed recurrent carcinoma, including 60% with a local–regional component. Compared with node-positive women who did not have extracapsular extension, the 82 patients with extracapsular extension had a higher local–regional failure rate and lower disease-free survival. In multivariate analysis with other prognostic factors, however, extracapsular extension did not remain an independent prognostic factor.

The issue of extracapsular extension as a risk factor for axillary recurrence was addressed in several reports. Mignano et al. found no axillary recurrences among 43 patients with extracapsular extension treated by mastectomy, axillary dissection, and chemotherapy without radiation (276). Fisher et al. reported axillary recurrences in 7% of stage II or III patients treated by surgery and chemotherapy without radiation and did not consider this to be a sufficient risk to warrant routine axillary radiation (275). Hetelekidis et al. analyzed the significance of extracapsular extension for axillary recurrence among women treated by breast-conserving surgery and radiotherapy (277). Compared with women without extracapsular extension, those with extracapsular tumor were significantly older (median age, 51 vs. 47) and had four or more involved lymph nodes more frequently (43% vs. 15%). Two of four patients with initial regional recurrences had axillary recurrences. This was an insufficient number for statistical analysis; however, one of the patients with axillary recurrence had received adjuvant postoperative regional radiotherapy that included the axilla.

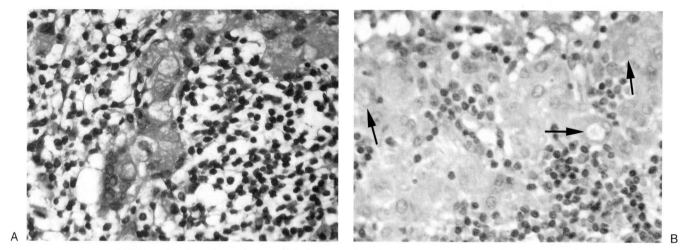

**FIG. 46.45.** *Vacuolated histiocytes.* **A:** The intracytoplasmic lumens suggest signet-ring cells. **B:** The vacuoles are weakly stained with the mucicarmine stain (*arrows*).

Although it is infrequent, extracapsular extension can be found associated with carcinomas 2 cm or smaller (T1). Goldstein et al. studied a highly selected group of 86 patients with T1N1 carcinoma and a single axillary lymph node metastasis that measured 0.5 cm or smaller in diameter (278). These women were identified among 650 T1N1 patients after excluding patients for multiple factors, which included a history of local recurrence, a positive surgical margin, axillary radiation, fewer than seven lymph nodes resected, more than one positive lymph node, and nodal metastasis larger than 0.5 cm. Extracapsular extension was identified in eight (13%) cases, and three of these women developed distant metastases. Invasion of hilar extranodal tissue also proved a significant risk factor for distant metastases. Because of case selection, the study could not assess the risk for local recurrence in the axilla.

### Pathologic Changes in Axillary Lymph Nodes that Mimic Metastatic Carcinoma

Vacuolated histiocytes that resemble signet-ring adenocarcinoma cells present a troublesome diagnostic problem

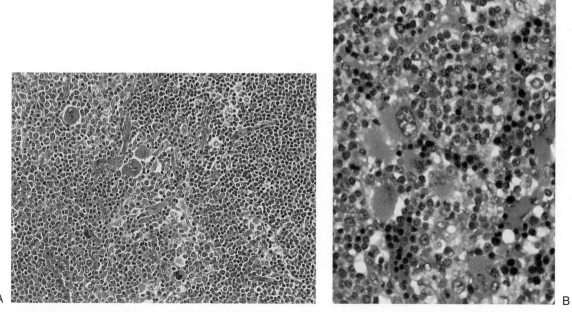

**FIG. 46.46.** *Extramedullary hematopoiesis in axillary lymph node.* The patient had invasive duct carcinoma and no hematologic disorder was detected. **A:** Immature hematopoietic cells and megakaryocytes are present among the lymphocytes. **B:** Megakaryocytes and erythroid precursors in the lymph node.

(279–281). The histiocytes stain positively with antichymotrypsin and anti-$\alpha_1$-trypsin and for lysozyme (281). They are weakly positive or negative with stains for mucin (mucicarmine, PAS) and IH epithelial markers such as CKs (AE1/AE3) and gross cystic disease fluid protein 15 (280,281) (Fig. 46.45). Electron microscopy in one case revealed a single cytoplasmic vacuole in each cell, which in some cells contained an amorphous electron-dense material interpreted to be lipid (280). The nature of the vacuolar material is unknown. This unusual form of histiocytic alteration does not appear to be specifically related to breast carcinoma. One patient was found to have signet-ring sinus histiocytosis after coronary bypass surgery with no documented evidence of mammary carcinoma (279).

The differential diagnosis of signet-ring histiocytes in axillary lymph nodes also includes a lymphangiogram effect (282), silicone lymphadenitis (283), Whipple's disease (284), signet-ring cell melanoma (285), and lymphoma (286).

Hematologic disorders involving axillary lymph nodes may be confused with or obscure metastatic carcinoma. These conditions include extramedullary hematopoiesis (Fig. 46.46) and coexisting lymphoma or leukemia (Fig. 46.47). Nevus cell aggregates usually occur in the lymph node capsule but may extend along stromal trabeculae into the lymph node (see Chapter 45).

## DETECTION OF MICROMETASTASES IN BONE MARROW

Another clinically important application of the IH detection of micrometastases is in the study of bone marrow (286a). In the absence of fibrosis or the finding of atypical cells in a paratrabecular distribution, this procedure is more

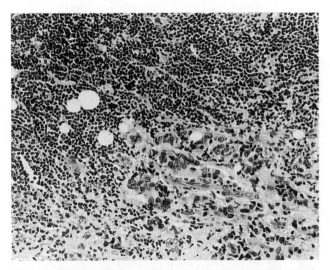

**FIG. 46.47.** *Metastatic carcinoma and chronic lymphocytic leukemia in an axillary lymph node.* The leukemic infiltrate is shown *above* merging with metastatic lobular carcinoma *below.*

likely to detect occult metastases in patients with lobular than with ductal carcinoma (287). IH with EMA has been used to identify micrometastases in tissue sections of bone marrow (288). The authors found alkaline-phosphatase conjugates preferable to horseradish peroxidase and were able to effectively block endogenous alkaline phosphatase with 20% acetic acid. EMA-positive cells were detected in 15 aspirates, but malignant cells were recognized in only eight Giemsa-stained samples from the same aspirates. Tumor cells were detected in routine smears from 2 of 11 aspirates, with fewer than 100 EMA-positive cells per smear. EMA-positive cells were found in marrow aspirates from 9 of 24 (38%) patients with known bone marrow metastases, 4 of 20 (20%) with nonosseous systemic metastases, and 2 of 30 (7%) not known to have metastatic disease.

Ginsbourg et al. studied bone marrow aspirates from 200 patients to detect occult micrometastases and to determine the proliferative activity of the metastatic cells (289). There was no significant difference in the frequency of positive bone marrow aspirates from the three groups examined (20 primary operable patients, 60% positive; 160 previously treated patients apparently disease free, 56% positive; 20 with known metastatic disease, 65% positive). S-phase was estimated by applying an antibromodeoxyuridine (BrdU) antibody to the bone marrow suspension after it was incubated with BrdU. By using fluorescein-conjugated antibodies, it was possible to visualize epithelial cells with cytoplasmic labeling using an anti-EMA antibody and nuclei that had incorporated BrdU. The proportion of epithelial cells with nuclear labeling (S-phase cells) was nearly identical, regardless of whether the patient had known metastatic disease or was clinically disease free. These results suggested that the proliferative rate of micrometastatic breast carcinoma cells in the bone marrow was not dependent on the clinical status of the patient.

Repeat follow-up bone marrow aspirations have been described in two series of patients. Positive aspirations were obtained initially in 21 (26%) of the cases studied by Mansi et al. (290). After a median follow-up of 18 months, only 2 of the 82 patients who remained clinically disease free (2.4%) had tumor cells detected in a second marrow aspirate, both having had carcinoma cells in their initial bone marrow sample. One of these women had received adjuvant chemotherapy, and the other had not been so treated. During the course of follow-up, 6 of the 82 patients developed a recurrence, four having had bone micrometastases initially, including one of the two women with a subsequent positive marrow. Among 16 additional patients with local recurrence, three (19%) had a positive bone marrow aspirate at the time of recurrence, whereas the aspirate was positive in 30% at the time of nonosseous systemic recurrence and in all patients with radiologically evident bone metastases.

A second study of patients with initial and follow-up bone marrow aspirations examined by immunocytochemistry involved 59 women with inflammatory or locally advanced carcinoma (291). CK immunostains detected CK-positive cells in bone marrow samples from 29 (49.2%) of the patients before systemic chemotherapy. Overall, 26 patients (41%) had a CK-positive bone marrow after chemotherapy, with no significant difference in the number of CK-positive cells before (17 per $2 \times 10^6$ leukocytes) and after (12 per $2 \times 10^6$ leukocytes) treatment. Approximately equal numbers of patients who were CK positive initially became CK negative as patients who were initially CK negative became CK positive. Bone marrow status was not significantly related to age at diagnosis or the number of lymph nodes with metastases. The presence of CK-positive cells in the bone marrow was significantly correlated with higher frequency of systemic metastases and shorter survival.

A larger study by Braun et al. presented data on bone marrow samples obtained from patients with stage I, II, and III breast carcinoma (292). CK-positive cells were detected in specimens from 199 of the 552 (36%) patients and also in 2 of 191 (1%) control samples from patients not known to have carcinoma. The presence or absence of axillary nodal metastases was not predictive of bone marrow status. After a follow-up of 4 years, systemic recurrence and death from breast carcinoma were significantly more frequent in women with a CK-positive marrow, regardless of axillary nodal status. After adjustment for systemic adjuvant chemotherapy, the relative risk of death due to breast carcinoma was 4.17 (95% CI, 2.51–6.94) for women with a CK-positive marrow compared with those who had a CK-negative specimen.

Another marker that has been investigated as a potential indicator of bone marrow micrometastases is the antigen TAG12, a polymorphic tumor-associated epithelial mucin, recognized by the monoclonal antibody 2E11. Diel et al. (293) reported that this reagent identified immunoreactive cells in bone marrow from 55% (203/367) lymph node-positive and 31% (112/360) lymph node-negative patients. Detection of 2E11-positive cells was significantly related to tumor size, nodal status, and tumor grade. In a multivariate analysis that controlled for adjuvant therapy and stage, bone marrow reactivity was an independent prognostic indicator for disease-free and overall survival after a short (median, 36 months) follow-up. Cross-reactivity of the antibody with basophilic myelocytes and monocytes was observed in a small number of cases.

Although the antibody to EMA reacts with epithelial tissues and neoplasms, heterogeneous staining is observed in tissue sections, and some epithelial cells are apparently not reactive. This observation led to concern that this reagent might not detect all tumor cells in marrow aspirates, thereby resulting in false-negative diagnoses. Dearnaley et al. did not detect EMA-positive cells in 25% of bone marrow aspirates that had carcinoma cells in Giemsa-stained smears (288). Thor et al., using the horseradish peroxidase technique, found that the antibody to high–molecular-weight CK (CAM 5.2) reacted with 83% of bone marrow samples known to contain tumor cells and that it did not cross-react with hematopoietic cells (294). With this procedure, the false-negative rate was 17%. Antibodies to EMA and two other epithelial-associated antigens were at least equally as effective for detecting epithelial cells, but they also sometimes stained marrow elements, especially plasma cells and immature hematopoietic cells. Others also reported cross reactivity of EMA with bone marrow mononuclear cells at a concentration of 24 per 1,000 normal bone marrow cells examined, whereas no cross reactivity was detected with CAM5.2, an antibody to keratins 8, 18, and 19 and with KL-1, an antibody that recognized keratins 1 to 4, 10, and 11 (295).

The possibility of using two or more antibodies to create a reagent "cocktail" has been investigated as a method for reducing false-negative marrow analyses. Cote et al. combined monoclonal antibodies C26 and T16, which react with surface glycoproteins and AE-1, which reacts with cytoplasmic acidic CK antigens (296). Using an immunofluorescent labeling system, the assay was sensitive enough to detect one tumor cell in $5 \times 10^5$ to $1 \times 10^6$ marrow cells with no false-positives in control specimens (297). Extrinsic cells were found in bone marrow aspirations from 18 of 51 (35%) patients examined by the monoclonal antibody method, but no extrinsic cells were seen when portions of the same specimens were studied by routine cytology (296). Positive bone marrow detected by immunofluorescence tended to be more frequent in patients who had axillary lymph node metastases and a more advanced stage at diagnosis. The presence of bone marrow micrometastases was significantly associated with earlier and more frequent relapse. The unfavorable prognostic effect of micrometastases in the bone marrow was independent of the stage of the primary tumor at diagnosis (298).

The multiple monoclonal antibody cocktail has been adapted to the immunoalkaline phosphatase method, which makes it possible to screen specimens by light microscopy (299). The procedure is sufficiently sensitive to detect one tumor cell among $1 \times 10^5$ bone marrow cells (300). Using this method, one group of investigators reported finding tumor cells in the bone marrow of 18% of breast carcinoma patients (301). Finding tumor cells in the bone marrow was not significantly related to tumor size or axillary lymph node status.

Molino et al. studied bone marrow specimens from 109 patients using a pool of five epithelial-associated monoclonal antibodies with the alkaline phosphatase antialkaline phosphatase method (302). The combined reagents showed no cross reactivity with normal bone marrow elements (303). The presence of immunoreactive cells in the bone marrow was not significantly related to tumor size, nodal status, estrogen receptor expression, or proliferative rate (Ki-67). The investigators found a greater frequency of bone marrow positivity when specimens were taken at the time of breast surgery (28/74 or 37.9% positive) than if the aspirate was taken sometime after surgery (6/29, 17.1%). Bone marrow status was not significantly related to recurrence or survival, regardless of nodal status after a median follow-up of 36 months. Because of the relationship between the timing of bone marrow sampling and bone marrow positivity, these investigators speculated that the bone marrow might contain circulating tumor cells rather than established metastatic deposits in some patients.

The techniques of molecular biology also have been applied to the detection of micrometastases in the bone marrow of patients with breast carcinoma. Datta et al. used RT-PCR to study peripheral blood and bone marrow samples for the CK19 mRNA (304). *In vitro* experiments revealed that the procedure was able to detect 10 mammary carcinoma cells added to $10^6$ peripheral blood cells. Evidence of a CK19 transcript was found in five of six histologically negative bone marrow samples from stage IV patients.

Using RT-PCR for CK19, Slade et al. reported positive results in peripheral blood samples from 20 of 37 (54%) patients with metastatic carcinoma and in bone marrow samples from 14 of 23 (61%) with primary operative carcinoma (305). Immunoreactive cells were detected by IH in bone marrow samples from 10 of 23 (43.7%) primary operative patients. These investigators concluded that RT-PCR is a promising method for monitoring the presence of tumor cells in peripheral blood and bone marrow to assess prognosis and response to therapy.

## DETECTION OF CARCINOMA IN PERIPHERAL BLOOD

Various techniques, ranging from basic cytologic examination to RT-PCR, have consistently demonstrated the presence of tumor cells circulating in the peripheral blood in the absence of known metastatic disease in patients with carcinoma of the breast and other organs. The clinical significance of this observation has not been determined. With the availability of ultrasensitive detection systems such as RT-PCR, it is not possible to distinguish between the presence of a small number of tumor cells in transit within vascular spaces of a tissue sample and a true micrometastatic deposit. As noted previously, this issue has been raised with respect to bone marrow, but it might also be relevant to molecular analysis of lymph nodes such as SLN.

Various markers used to assay peripheral blood for epithelial cells by RT-PCR include epidermal growth factor receptor (306), CEA (233,241), mammaglobin (307,307a); CKs (241), and MUC-1 (241). Bostick et al. reported that CEA, CK19, and MUC-1 had limited usefulness as markers for carcinoma cells in peripheral blood because they were detected by RT-PCR in samples from patients who did not have carcinoma, whereas CK20 was not found in cancer-free patients (241).

Zach et al. screened peripheral blood samples for human mammaglobin mRNA (hMAM) by RT-PCR and reported that the procedure was capable of detecting one tumor cell in $10^6$ to $10^7$ leukocytes (307). All samples of peripheral blood from healthy volunteers were negative, whereas hMAM was detected in blood from 3 of 53 (6%) patients with no evidence of metastases and in 21 of 43 (49%) with metastatic carcinoma. hMAM appears to have specificity for mammary carcinoma because it was not detected in peripheral blood samples from 39 of 41 patients with other types of carcinoma. The two exceptional patients had malignant lymphomas, neoplasms characterized by translocations involving the chromosomal region that includes the mammaglobin gene. Grünewald et al. reported mammaglobin gene expression in peripheral blood was a more reliable marker for detecting breast carcinoma cells than epidermal growth factor receptor or cytokeratin 19 (307a).

Smith et al. used a quantitative RT-PCR method to analyze CK19 in the peripheral blood of women with locally advanced or metastatic breast carcinoma (308). Three of five patients who responded to treatment showed a corresponding decrease in peripheral blood CK19 expression. Samples examined by IH showed decreased numbers of cells in four of the five responders.

Epidermal growth factor receptor (EGFR) is present in numerous varieties of malignant neoplasms, including breast carcinoma. EGFR mRNA was detected in peripheral blood from 4 of 18 (22%) patients with known metastatic carcinoma but not in samples from patients with locally recurrent carcinoma or receiving adjuvant therapy and negative results were obtained in normal controls (306). Although not specific for breast carcinoma, this study suggests that RT-PCR detection of EGFR mRNA could be a useful marker for metastatic carcinoma.

Immunomagnetic cell sorting is a technique that makes it possible to separate epithelial cells selectively from peripheral blood for RT-PCR analysis and for cytologic examination. The procedure makes use of magnetic antibodies directed at surface antigens of tumor cells. The antibody and abherent cells can be isolated from the blood by immunoglobulin G (IgG)-coated magnetic beads and exposure to a magnetic field (309–312).

Using immunomagnetic separation, Brandt et al. were able to isolate HER2/*neu*-positive cells from the peripheral blood and demonstrate immunoreactivity to cytokeratin as well as HER2/*neu* in the captured cells (309). Krag et al. used this technique to examine the temporal relationship of tumor cells in the peripheral blood before and after surgical excision of the primary tumor (313). Cells removed by immunomagnetic selection were fixed on histologic slides for CK staining and microscopic counting. Tumor cells were present in the peripheral blood of 18 of 19 (95%) patients before excision of the primary tumor. The incidence of tumor cells in the peripheral blood declined rapidly within 48 hours postoperatively, but about 30% of patients continued to have positive samples up to 14 days postoperatively. These researchers hypothesized that persistence of tumor cells in the peripheral blood might indicate the presence of clonogenic tumor cells at a site remote from the primary carcinoma and that this finding could identify patients with subclinical metastases.

## EXAMINATION OF PROSTHETIC BREAST IMPLANTS

A written policy for the handling of breast prosthetic devices should be established and implemented. The prosthetic device should be accessioned as a specimen by the pathology laboratory. The patient should be informed by the surgeon that this will occur and that the prosthesis will be retained for a standard period as stated in the institutional or pathology department procedure manual before being discarded. The patient may request return of the device during this period of storage; however, the device may not be given to the patient before it has been accessioned and described in the pathology department. Documentation that the patient has been advised about this procedure for handling the device may be incorporated into the operative consent form or in some other record.

Prostheses with adherent tissue visible on gross inspection require storage in a standard laboratory fixative, such as 10% buffered formalin. It is preferable that the patient be notified after surgery of the policy regarding disposal of prosthetic devices. Implants returned to the patient should be sealed in a labeled biohazard container. A release form signed by the patient should be used to document receipt of the specimen by the patient and that the patient has been instructed about the biohazard risks associated with the specimen.

The pathology report for an explanted prosthetic device should follow the format used for tissue specimens. The written report should include all clinical history and information supplied in the accompanying laboratory requisition. It is preferable that photographic documentation be obtained for an explanted device, although this may not be done in every instance. When any photograph is taken, it is advantageous to include in the photograph the identity of the patient as well as the serial number, brand name, or other visible identifying markings pertaining to the specimen in question. These markings also should be stated in the written report.

The gross description should include salient features of the device. The weight of the prosthesis should be recorded

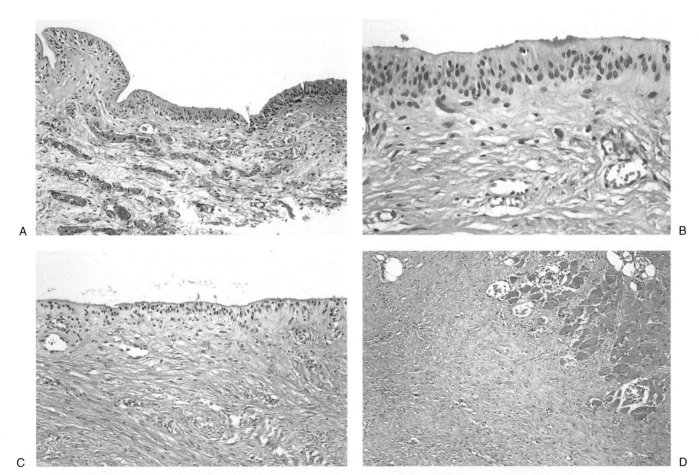

**FIG. 46.48.** *Implant capsule with fibromatosis in a 19-year-old girl.* **A,B:** Part of the implant capsule with typical reactive changes and synovial metaplasia on the surface. **C,D:** Fibromatosis involving the wall of the implant capsule below synovial metaplasia and invasion of adjacent pectoral muscle.

in grams, and the shape should be reported. The appearance of the external surface (smooth, textured, and so on) should be recorded, and a statement should be made about the apparent integrity of the surface. The prosthesis may appear to be intact, or if it is disrupted, the extent of rupture should be reported. The character of the contents should be described if visible.

Any tissue received with the prosthesis must be described grossly and examined histologically, whether it is a separate specimen or it is adherent to the prosthesis. In most instances, the tissue constitutes the capsule around the device. To the extent possible, which may vary in different circumstances, the weight in grams and dimensions in centimeters of the tissue should be recorded. The character of the inner surface of capsular tissue, if identifiable, should be described. Significant gross features, such as hemorrhage, calcification, or foreign nontissue material attached to the specimen, should be reported.

Samples of the capsule and any breast parenchyma removed with the prosthetic device must be examined microscopically. The report should describe the general histologic features of the specimen, such as fibrosis, type of inflammatory reaction, and calcification. Changes on the capsule surface, including the presence or absence of synovial metaplasia, should be reported (see Chapter 3). Foreign material also should be described, but the specific identification of the material is best reserved for spectroscopic analysis and other procedures (314,315). Fibromatosis can arise in the tissues around a prosthetic breast implant (Fig. 46.48) and very rarely clinically occult carcinoma is found in periprosthetic tissue.

## OTHER FOREIGN BODIES

A number of foreign bodies may be found in the breast. Some of these are the consequence of medical procedures. Included in this category are localizing wires or needles, which can be broken during a procedure or transected intra-operatively (316,317). Portions of catheters used for drainage of abscesses or after surgery may be inadvertently detached, unknowingly retained, and detected mammographically as asymptomatic abnormalities (318–320) (Fig. 46.49). In one case, a retained folded Penrose drain caused localized inflammation without a palpable mass 7 years following a biopsy for "benign disease" (321). Linear calcifications were seen mammographically. Calcifications in retained gauze sponges or in sutures may mimic the mammographic appearance of calcifications in carcinoma (Fig. 46.50). Suture calcifications may suggest recurrent carcinoma at the site of prior lumpectomy in a patient treated by breast conservation (322). The nature of such calcifications can be appreciated more readily if they have a knotted configuration or a smooth linear distribution. Scarring and old suture material detected histologically in the absence of mammographic calcifications should alert the pathologist to the fact that the tissue being examined is the site of a prior surgical procedure. The surgeon may fail to inform the pathologist that a biopsy was previously performed in a given case, and sometimes the surgeon is unaware of the procedure. Tattoo pigments in the skin of the breast (323) and soap crystals on the skin containing calcium (324) also can mimic intramammary calcifications. An unusual case report described the finding of metallic fragments and a suspicious 2-cm mass with calcifications in the baseline mammogram of a 38-year-old woman (325). A needle core biopsy revealed metallic particles and fibrous material composed of cotton fibers with a giant cell foreign-body reaction. By history, the patient had sustained a gunshot wound in the breast causing a portion of her clothing to be embedded in the wound.

Various nonmedical foreign bodies of known or factitious origin have been described in the breast. These include glass (326), needles (317), hairpins (327), and stones (328). Chinese herbal treatment of breast abscess has been associated with punctate lead-containing deposits on mammography (329).

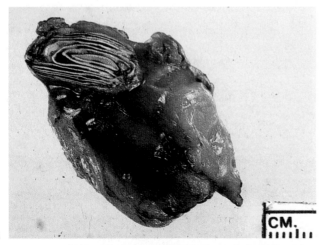
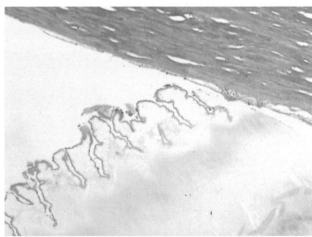

A                                                                                                    B

**FIG. 46.49.** *Unusual foreign body.* **A:** This mammographically detected foreign body is a retained, sequestered drain inserted 35 years earlier to evacuate an abscess. **B:** The histologic appearance of the degenerated drain and surrounding fibrous capsule.

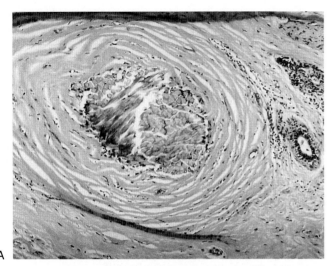
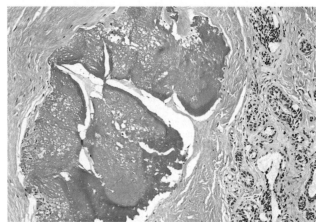

A                                                         B

**FIG. 46.50.** *Suture granuloma.* **A:** A nonabsorbable suture surrounded by a fibrous reaction. This site was detected by mammography because of calcification associated with the suture material. The sutures remained from an operation performed 10 years earlier. **B:** Calcified suture material in a healed biopsy site.

## REFERENCES

1. Association of Directors of Anatomic and Surgical Pathology. Immediate management of mammographically detected breast lesions. *Am J Surg Pathol* 1993;12:850–851.
2. Connolly JL, Schnitt SJ. Evaluation of breast biopsy specimens in patients considered for treatment by conservative surgery and radiation therapy for early breast cancer. *Pathol Annu* 1988;23:1–23.
3. National Cancer Institute. Standardized management of breast specimens: recommended by Pathology Working Group. Breast Cancer Task Force. *Am J Clin Pathol* 1973;60:789–798.
4. Schmidt WA. The breast. In: *Principles and techniques of surgical pathology.* MA: Butterworth, 1983:362–388.
5. Schnitt SJ, Connolly JL. Processing and evaluation of breast excision specimens: a clinically oriented approach. *Am J Clin Pathol* 1992;98:125–137.
6. Association of Directors of Anatomic and Surgical Pathology. Recommendations for the reporting of breast carcinoma. *Am J Clin Pathol* 1995;104:614–619.
7. Rosen PP, Senie R, Schottenfeld D, et al. Noninvasive breast carcinoma: frequency of unsuspected invasion and implication for treatment. *Ann Surg* 1979;89:98–103.
8. Speights VO Jr. Evaluation of frozen sections in grossly benign breast biopsies. *Mod Pathol* 1994;7:762–765.
9. Bianchi S, Palli D, Ciatto S, et al. Accuracy and reliability of frozen section diagnosis in a series of 672 nonpalpable breast lesions. *Am J Clin Pathol* 1995;103:199–205.
10. Ferreiro JA, Gisvold JJ, Bostwick DG. Accuracy of frozen-section diagnosis of mammographically directed breast biopsies. Results of 1,490 consecutive cases. *Am J Surg Pathol* 1995;19:1267–1271.
11. Tinnemans JG, Wobbes T, Holland R, et al. Mammographic and histopathologic correlation of nonpalpable lesions of the breast and the reliability of frozen section diagnosis. *Surg Gynecol Obstet* 1987;165:523–529.
12. Niemann TH, Lucas JG, Marsh WL Jr. To freeze or not to freeze. A comparison of methods for the handling of breast biopsies with no palpable abnormality. *Am J Clin Pathol* 1996;106:225–228.
13. Schnitt S, Wang HH. Histologic sampling of grossly benign breast biopsies: how much is enough? *Am J Surg Pathol* 1989;13:505–512.
14. Owings DV, Hann L, Schnitt SJ. How thoroughly should needle localization breast biopsies be sampled for microscopic examination? A prospective mammographic/pathologic correlative study. *Am J Surg Pathol* 1990;14:578–583.
15. Abraham SC, Fox K, Fraker D, et al. Sampling of grossly benign breast reexcisions: a multidisciplinary approach to assessing adequacy. *Am J Surg Pathol* 1999;23:316–322.
16. Pezner RD, Terz J, Ben-Ezra J, et al. Now there are two effective conservation approaches for patients with stage I and II breast cancer: how pathological assessment of inked resection margins can provide valuable information for the radiation oncologist. *Am J Clin Oncol* 1990;13:175–179.
17. Sauter ER, Hoffman JP, Ottery FD, et al. Is frozen section analysis of reexcision lumpectomy margins worthwhile? Margin analysis in breast reexcisions. *Cancer* 1994;73:2607–2612.
18. Aitken RJ, Going JJ, Chetty U. Assessment of surgical excision during breast conservation surgery by intraoperative two-dimensional specimen radiology. *Br J Surg* 1990;77:322–323.
19. Cox CE, Ku NN, Reintgen D, et al. Touch preparation cytology of breast lumpectomy margins with histologic correlation. *Arch Surg* 1991;126:490–493.
20. Weber S, Storm FK, Stitt J, et al. The role of frozen section analysis of margins during breast conservation surgery. *Cancer J Sci Am* 1997;3:273–277.
21. Esserman L, Weidner N. Is routine frozen section assessment feasible in the practice environment of the 1990s? *Cancer J Sci Am* 1997;3:266–267.
22. Guidi AJ, Connolly JL, Harris JR, et al. The relationship between shaved margin and inked margin status in breast excision specimens. *Cancer* 1997;79:1568–1573.
23. Rubin P, O'Hanlon D, Browell D, et al. Tumour bed biopsy detects the presence of multifocal disease in patients undergoing breast conservation therapy for primary breast carcinoma. *Eur J Surg Oncol* 1996;22:23–26.
24. Carter D. Margins of "lumpectomy" for breast cancer. *Hum Pathol* 1986;17:330–332.
25. Veronesi U, Farante G, Galimberti V, et al. Evaluation of resection margins after breast conservative surgery with monoclonal antibodies. *Eur J Surg Oncol* 1991;17:338–341.
26. England DW, Chan SY, Stonelake PS, et al. Assessment of excision margins following wide local excision for breast carcinoma using specimen scrape cytology and tumour bed biopsy. *Eur J Surg Oncol* 1994;20:425–429.
27. Pittinger TP, Maronian NC, Poulter CA, et al. Importance of margin status in outcome of breast-conserving surgery for carcinoma. *Surgery* 1994;116:605–609.
28. Schnitt SJ, Abner A, Gelman R, et al. The relationship between microscopic margins of resection and the risk of local recurrence in patients with breast cancer treated with breast-conserving surgery and radiation therapy. *Cancer* 1994;74:1746–1751.
29. Gage I, Schnitt SJ, Nixon AJ, et al. Pathologic margin involvement and the risk of recurrence in patients treated with breast-conserving therapy. *Cancer* 1996;78:1921–1928.

30. DiBiase SJ, Komarnicky LT, Schwartz GF, et al. The number of positive margins influences the outcome of women treated with breast preservation for early stage breast carcinoma. *Cancer* 1998; 82:2212–2220.

31. Papa MZ, Zippel D, Koller M, et al. Positive margins of breast biopsy: is reexcision always necessary? *J Surg Oncol* 1999;70:167–171.

32. Gwin JL, Eisenberg BL, Hoffman JP, et al. Incidence of gross and microscopic carcinoma in specimens from patients with breast cancer after re-excision lumpectomy. *Ann Surg* 1993;218:729–734.

33. McCormick B, Kinne D, Petrek J, et al. Limited resection for breast cancer: a study of inked specimen margins before radiotherapy. *Int J Radiat Oncol Biol Phys* 1987;13:1667–1671.

34. Schnitt SJ, Connolly JL, Khettry U, et al. Pathologic findings on re-excision of the primary site in breast cancer patients considered for treatment by primary radiation therapy. *Cancer* 1987;59:675–681.

35. Solin LJ, Fowble B, Martz K, et al. Results of re-excisional biopsy of the primary tumor in preparation for definitive irradiation of patients with early stage breast cancer. *Int J Radiat Oncol Biol Phys* 1986;12:721–725.

36. Stotter AT, McNeese MD, Ames FC, et al. Predicting the rate and extent of locoregional failure after breast conservative therapy for early breast cancer. *Cancer* 1989;64:2217–2225.

37. Heimann R, Powers C, Halpern HJ, et al. Breast preservation in stage I and II carcinoma of the breast: the University of Chicago experience. *Cancer* 1996;78:1722–1730.

38. Mansfield CM, Komarnicky LT, Schwartz GF, et al. Ten-year results in 1070 patients with stages I and II breast cancer treated by conservative surgery and radiation therapy. *Cancer* 1995;75:2328–2336.

39. Smitt MC, Nowels KW, Zdeblick MJ, et al. The importance of the lumpectomy surgical margin status in long term results of breast conservation. *Cancer* 1995;76:259–267.

40. Spivack B, Khanna MM, Tafra L, et al. Margin status and local recurrence after breast-conserving surgery. *Arch Surg* 1994;129:952–957.

41. Veronesi U. How important is the assessment of resection margins in conservative surgery for breast cancer? *Cancer* 1994;74:1660–1661.

42. Mariani L, Salvadori B, Marubini E, et al. Ten year results of a randomised trial comparing two conservative treatment strategies for small size breast cancer. *Eur J Cancer* 1998;34:1156–1162.

43. Fisher ER, Sass R, Fisher B, et al., and collaborating NSABP investigators. Pathologic findings from the National Surgical Adjuvant Breast Project (Protocol 6). II. Relation of local breast recurrence to multicentricity. *Cancer* 1986;57:1717–1724.

44. Fourquet A, Campana F, Zafrani B, et al. Prognostic factors of breast recurrence in the conservative management of early breast cancer: a 25-year follow-up. *Int J Radiat Oncol Biol Phys* 1989;17:719–725.

45. Ryoo MC, Kagan AR, Wollin M, et al. Prognostic factors for recurrence and comesis in 393 patients after radiation therapy for early mammary carcinoma. *Radiology* 1989;172:555–559.

46. Anscher MS, Jones P, Prosnitz LR, et al. Local failure and margin status in early-stage breast carcinoma treated with conservation surgery and radiation therapy. *Ann Surg* 1993;218:22–28.

47. Veronesi U, Marubini E, Del Vecchio M, et al. Local recurrences and distant metastases after conservative breast cancer treatments: partly independent events. *J Natl Cancer Inst* 1995;87:19–27.

48. Haffty BG, Reiss M, Beinfield M, et al. Ipsilateral breast tumor recurrence as a predictor of distant disease: implications for systemic therapy at the time of local relapse. *J Clin Oncol* 1996;14:52–57.

49. Noguchi S, Koyama H, Kasugai T, et al. A case-control study on risk factors for local recurrences or distant metastases in breast cancer patients treated with breast-conserving surgery. *Oncology* 1997; 54:468–474.

50. Fisher B, Anderson S, Fisher ER, et al. Significance of ipsilateral breast tumour recurrence after lumpectomy. *Lancet* 1991;338: 327–331.

51. Silvestrini R, Daidone MG, Luisi A, et al. Biologic and clinicopathologic factors as indicators of specific relapse types in node-negative breast cancer. *J Clin Oncol* 1995;13:697–704.

52. Francis M, Cakir B, Ung O, et al. Prognosis after breast recurrence following conservative surgery and radiotherapy in patients with node-negative breast cancer. *Br J Surg* 1999;86:1556–1562.

53. Fortin A, Larochelle M, Laverdiere J, et al. Local failure is responsible for the decrease in survival for patients with breast cancer treated with conservative surgery and postoperative radiotherapy. *J Clin Oncol* 1999;17:101–109.

54. Solin LJ, Fowble BL, Schultz DJ, et al. The significance of the pathol-

55. Voogd AC, van Tienhoven G, Peterse HL, et al. Local recurrence after breast conservation therapy for early stage breast carcinoma: detection, treatment, and outcome in 266 patients. Dutch Study Group on Local Recurrence after Breast Conservation (BORST). *Cancer* 1999;85:437–446.

56. Sinn HP, Anton HW, Magener A, et al. Extensive and predominant *in situ* component in breast carcinoma: their influence on treatment results after breast-conserving therapy. *Eur J Cancer* 1998;34:646–653.

57. Peterse JL, van Dongen JA, Bartelink H. Recurrence of breast carcinoma after breast conserving treatment. *Eur J Surg Oncol* 1988;14:123–126.

58. Zafrani B, Vielh P, Fourquet A, et al. Conservative treatment of early breast cancer: prognostic value of the ductal *in situ* component and other pathological variables on local control and survival. Long-term results. *Eur J Cancer Clin Oncol* 1989;25:1645–1650.

59. Ohtake T, Abe R, Kimijima I, et al. Intraductal extension of primary invasive breast carcinoma treated by breast-conservation surgery: computer graphic three-dimensional reconstruction of the mammary duct-lobular systems. *Cancer* 1995;76:32–45.

60. Jimenez RE, Bongers S, Bouwman D, et al. Clinicopathologic significance of ductal carcinoma *in situ* in breast core needle biopsies with invasive cancer. *Am J Surg Pathol* 2000;24:123–128.

61. Brenin DR, Morrow M. Accuracy of AJCC staging for breast cancer patients undergoing re-excision for positive margins. American Joint Committee on Cancer. *Ann Surg Oncol* 1998;5:719–723.

62. Morris EA, Schwartz LH, Drotman MB, et al. Evaluation of pectoralis major muscle in patients with posterior breast tumors on breast MR images: early experience. *Radiology* 2000;214:67–72.

63. Esserman L, Hylton N, Yassa L, et al. Utility of magnetic resonance imaging in the management of breast cancer: evidence for improved preoperative staging. *J Clin Oncol* 1999;17:110–119.

64. Berg WA, Gilbreath PL. Multicentric and multifocal cancer: whole-breast US in preoperative evaluation. *Radiology* 2000;214:59–66.

65. Rosen PP. Specimen radiography and the diagnosis of clinically occult mammary carcinoma. *Pathol Annu* 1980;15:225–237.

66. Salomon A. Beitrag zur Pathologie und Klinik der mammacarcinome. *Arch Kiln Chir* 1918;101:573–668.

67. Gershon-Cohen J, Colcher AE. An evaluation of the roentgen diagnosis of early carcinoma of the breast. *JAMA* 1937;108:867–871.

68. Leborgne R. Diagnosis of tumors of the breast by simple roentgenography: calcifications in carcinoma. *AJR Am J Roentgenol* 1951; 65:1–11.

69. Cody III HS. The impact of mammography in 1096 consecutive patients with breast cancer, 1979–1993. *Cancer* 1995;76:1579–1584.

70. Rosen PP, Snyder RE, Urban JA, et al. Correlation of suspicious mammograms and x-rays of breast biopsies during surgery. Results in 60 cases. *Cancer* 1973;31:656–659.

71. Snyder RE, Rosen PP. Radiography of breast specimens. *Cancer* 1971;28:1608–1611.

72. Chilcote WA, Davis GA, Suchy P, et al. Breast specimen radiography: evaluation of a compression device. *Radiology* 1988;168:425–427.

73. Eastgate RJ, Gilchrist KW, Matallana RH. Enhancement of tissue structure visualization in breast specimen radiography. *Radiology* 1979;132:744–746.

74. Philip J, Harris WG, Rustage JH. Radiography of breast biopsy specimens. *Br J Surg* 1982;69:126–127.

75. Birdwell RL, Ikeda DM, Jeffrey SS. Value of sonographic identification of breast masses in excised specimens in the breast imaging department: report of 7 cases. *Breast Dis* 1996;9:93–99.

76. Bauermeister DE, Hall MH. Specimen radiography—a mandatory adjunct to mammography. *Am J Clin Pathol* 1973;59:782–788.

77. Meyer JE, Eberlein TJ, Stomper PC, et al. Biopsy of occult breast lesions. Analysis of 1261 abnormalities. *JAMA* 1990;263:2341–2343.

78. Tinnemans JG, Wobbes T, Holland R, et al. Mammographic and histopathologic correlation of nonpalpable lesions of the breast and the reliability of frozen section diagnosis. *Surg Gynecol Obstet* 1987;165:523–529.

79. Pastakia B, Chang V, McDonald H, et al. Immediate post-excision mammography for occult noncalcified breast lesions. *South Med J* 1990;83:30–33.

80. Reid SE Jr, Scanlon EF, Bernstein JR, et al. An alternative approach to nonpalpable breast biopsies. *J Surg Oncol* 1990;44:93–96.

81. Norton LW, Zeligman BF, Pearlman NW. Accuracy and cost of needle localization breast biopsy. *Arch Surg* 1988;123:945–950.

82. Leis HP, Cammarata A, LaRaja RD, et al. Breast biopsy and guidance for occult lesions. *Int Surg* 1985;70:115–118.

83. Meyer JE, Sonnenfeld MR, Greene RA, et al. Preoperative localization of clinically occult breast lesions: experience at a referral hospital. *Radiology* 1988;169:627–628.

84. Symmonds RF Jr, Roberts JW. Management of nonpalpable breast abnormalities. *Ann Surg* 1987;205:520–528.

85. Kopans DB, Meyer JE, Homer MJ, et al. Dermal deposits mistaken for breast calcifications. *Radiology* 1983;149:592–594.

86. Linden SS, Sullivan DC. Breast skin calcifications: localization with a stereotactic device. *Radiology* 1989;171:570–571.

87. Brown RC, Zuehlke RL, Ehrhardt JC, et al. Tattoos simulating calcifications on xeroradiography of the breast. *Radiology* 1981;138:583–584.

88. Lager DJ, O'Connor JC, Robinson RA, et al. Factitious microcalcifications in breast biopsy material: laboratory-induced error by use of tattoo powder for specimen mammography. *J Surg Oncol* 1989;40:281–282.

89. Frank HA, Hall FM, Steer ME. Preoperative localization of nonpalpable breast lesions demonstrated by mammography. *N Engl J Med* 1976;295:259–260.

90. Silverstein MJ, Gamagami P, Rosser RJ, et al. Hooked-wire-directed breast biopsy and overpenetrated mammography. *Cancer* 1987;59:715–722.

91. Czarmecki DJ, Feider HK, Splittgerber GF. Toluidine blue dye as a breast localization marker. *Am J Radiol* 1989;153:261–263.

92. Hirsch JI, Banks WL Jr, Sullivan JS, et al. Noninterference of isosulfan blue on estrogen-receptor activity. *Radiology* 1989;171:109–110.

93. Davis PS, Wechler RJ, Feig SA, et al. Migration of breast biopsy localization wire. *AJR Am J Roentgenol* 1988;150:787–788.

94. Owen AWMC, Kumer EN. Migration of localizing wires used in guided biopsy of the breast. *Clin Radiol* 1991;43:251.

95. Frappart L, Boudeulle M, Boumendil J, et al. Structure and composition of microcalcifications in benign and malignant lesions of the breast. *Hum Pathol* 1984;15:880–889.

96. Frappart L, Remy I, Hu CL, et al. Different types of microcalcifications observed in breast pathology: correlations with histopathologic diagnosis and radiologic examination of operative specimens. *Virchows Arch* 1986;410:179–187.

97. Radi MJ. Calcium oxalate crystals in breast biopsies: an overlooked form of microcalcification associated with benign breast disease. *Arch Pathol Lab Med* 1989;113:1367–1369.

98. Symonds DA. Use of the von Kossa stain in identifying occult calcifications in breast biopsies. *Am J Clin Pathol* 1990;94:44–48.

99. Tornos C, Silva E, El-Naggar A, et al. Calcium oxalate crystals in breast biopsies. The missing microcalicifications. *Am J Surg Pathol* 1990;14:961–968.

100. Foschini MP, Fornelli A, Peterse JL, et al. Microcalcifcations in ductal carcinoma *in situ* of the breast: histochemical and immunohistochemical study. *Hum Pathol* 1996;27:178–183.

101. Going JJ, Anderson TJ, Crocker PR, et al. Weddellite calcification in the breast: eighteen cases with implications for breast cancer screening. *Histopathology* 1990;16:119–124.

102. Ortiz-Hidalgo C. Dihydrate birefringent calcium oxalate or Weddellite calcification [Letter]. *J Clin Pathol.* 2000;53:84–85.

103. Winston JS, Yeh I-T, Evers K, et al. Calcium oxalate is associated with benign breast tissue. *Am J Clin Pathol* 1993;100:488–492.

104. Truong LD, Cartwright J Jr, Alpert L. Calcium oxalate in breast lesions biopsied for calcification detected in screening mammography: incidence and clinical significance. *Mod Pathol* 1992;5:146–152.

105. Frouge C, Meunier M, Guinebretière J-M, et al. Polyhedral-shaped microcalcification on mammography: histologic correlation with calcium oxalate. *Radiology* 1993;186:681–684.

106. Frouge C, Guinebretière J-M, Juras J, et al. Polyhedral microcalcifcations on mammograms: prevalence and morphometric analysis. *AJR Am J Roentgenol* 1996;167:621–624.

107. Gonzalez JEG, Caldwell RG, Valaitis JO. Calcium oxalate crystals in the breast. Pathology and significance. *Am J Surg Pathol* 1991;15:586–591.

108. Feirt N, Vazquez MF. Indeterminate microcalcifications (BIRAD 3): what do they represent pathologically? *Mod Pathol* 2000;13:21A.

109. Singh N, Theaker JM. Calcium oxalate crystals (Weddellite) within the secretions of ductal carcinoma *in situ*—a rare phenomenon. *J Clin Pathol* 1999;52:145–146.

110. Stein MA, Karlan MS. Calcification in breast biopsy specimens: discrepancies in radiologic—pathologic identification. *Radiology* 1991;179:111–114.

111. Surratt JR, Monsees BS, Mazoujian G. Calcium oxalate microcalcifications in the breast. *Radiology* 1991;181:141–142.

112. Rebner M, Helvie MA, Pennes DR, et al. Paraffin tissue block radiography: adjunct to breast specimen radiography. *Radiology* 1989;173:695–696.

113. Brem RF, Askin FB, Gatewood OM. Selection of core biopsy specimens for pathologic evaluation of targeted microcalcifications. *AJR Am J Roentgenol* 1999;173:901–902.

114. Liberman L, Evans III WP, Dershaw DD, et al. Specimen radiography of microcalcifications in stereotactic mammary core biopsies. *Radiology* 1994;190:223–225.

115. Wu YC, Freedman MT, Hasegawa A, et al. Classification of microcalcifications in radiographs of pathologic specimens for the diagnosis of breast cancer. *Acad Radiol* 1995;2:199–204.

116. Wu Y, Doi K, Giger ML, et al. Computerized detection of clustered microcalcifications in digital mammograms: applications of artificial neural networks. *Med Phys* 1992;19:555–560.

117. Ng KH, Looi LM, Bradley DA. Microcalcification clustering parameters in breast disease: a morphometric analysis of radiographs of excision specimens. *Br J Radiol* 1996;69:326–334.

118. Zhang W, Doi K, Giger ML, et al. Computerized detection of clustered microcalcifications in digital mammograms using a shift-invariant artificial neural network. *Med Phys* 1994;21:517–524.

119. American College of Radiology (ACR). *Breast imaging reporting and data system (BI-RADS)*, 2nd ed. Reston, VA: American College of Radiology, 1995.

120. Selim A, Tahan SR. Microscopic localization of calcifications in and around breast carcinoma: a cautionary note for needle core biopsies. *Ann Surg* 1998;228:95–98.

121. Dershaw DD, Giess CS, McCormick B, et al. Patterns of mammographically detected calcifications after breast-conserving therapy associated with tumor recurrence. *Cancer* 1997;79:1355–1361.

122. Rebner M, Helvie MA, Pennes DR, et al. Paraffin tissue block radiography: adjunct to breast specimen radiography. *Radiology* 1989;173:695–696.

123. Mitnick JS, Vazquez MF, Roses DF, et al. Recurrent breast cancer: stereotaxic localization for fine-needle aspiration biopsy: work in progress. *Radiology* 1992;182:103–106.

124. Homer MJ, Slowinski J. Spontaneously disappearing calcifications in the breast: incidence appearance and implications. *Breast Dis* 1992;5:251–258.

125. Parker MD, Clark RL, McLelland R, et al. Disappearing breast calcifications. *Radiology* 1989;172:677–680.

126. Moritz JD, Luftner-Nagel S, Westerhof JP, et al. Microcalcifications in breast core biopsy specimens: disappearance at radiography after storage in formaldehyde. *Radiology* 1996;200:361–363.

127. Matsunaga T, Nakamura Y, Mimuro M, et al. Chronological changes of microcalcifications of breast carcinoma. *Breast Cancer* 1998;5:269–277.

128. Apestegía L, Pina L, Inchusta M, et al. Klippel-Trenaunay syndrome: a very infrequent cause of microcalcifications in mammography. *Eur Radiol* 1997;7:123–125.

129. Evans SE, Whitehouse GH. Extensive calcification in the breast in chronic renal failure. *Br J Radiol* 1991;64:757–759.

130. Resnikoff LB, Mendelson EB, Tobin CE, et al. Breast imaging case of the day. Metastatic calcification in the breast from secondary hyperparathyroidism induced by chronic renal failure. *Radiographics* 1996;16:1512–1513.

131. Kemmeren JM, Beijerinck D, van Noord PA, et al. Breast arterial calcifications: association with diabetes mellitus and cardiovascular mortality. Work in progress. *Radiology* 1996;201:75–78.

132. Ro JY, Ngadiman S, Sahin A, et al. Intraluminal crystalloids in breast carcinoma. Immunohistochemical, ultrastructural, and energy-dispersive x-ray element analysis in four cases. *Arch Pathol Lab Med* 1997;121:593–598.

133. Elvecrog EL, Lechner MC, Nelson MT. Nonpalpable breast lesions: correlation of stereotaxic large-core needle biopsy and surgical biopsy results. *Radiology* 1993;188:453–455.

134. Liberman L, Dershaw DD, Rosen PP, et al. Stereotaxic 14-gauge breast biopsy: how many core biopsy specimens are needed? *Radiology* 1994;192:793–795.

135. Gisvold JJ, Goellner JR, Grant CS, et al. Breast biopsy: a comparative

study of stereotaxically guided core and excisional techniques. *AJR Am J Roentgenol* 1994;162:815–820.

136. Liberman L, Dershaw DD, Rosen PP, et al. Stereotaxic core biopsy of breast carcinoma: accuracy at predicting invasion. *Radiology* 1995;194:379–381.

137. Kaye MD, Vicinanza-Adami CA, Sullivan ML. Mammographic findings after stereotaxic biopsy of the breast performed with large-core needles. *Radiology* 1994;192:149–151.

138. Boppana S, May M, Hoda S. Does prior fine-needle-aspiration cause diagnostic difficulties in histologic evaluation of breast carcinomas? *Lab Invest* 1994;70:13A.

139. Youngson BJ, Cranor M, Rosen PP. Epithelial displacement in surgical breast specimens following needling procedures. *Am J Surg Path* 1994;18:896–903.

140. Youngson BJ, Liberman L, Rosen PP. Displacement of carcinomatous epithelium in surgical breast specimens following stereotaxic core biopsy. *A m J Clin Pathol* 1995;103:598–602.

141. Pilnik S, Steichen F. The use of the hemostatic scalpel in operations upon the breast. *Surg Gynecol Obstet* 1986;162:589–591.

142. Bloom ND, Johnson F, Pertshuck L, et al. Electrocautery: effects on steroid receptors in human breast cancer. *J Surg Oncol* 1984; 25:21–24.

143. Pertshuck LP, Tobin EH, Tanapat P, et al. Histochemical analyses of steroid hormone receptors in breast and prostate carcinoma. *J Histochem Cytochem* 1980;28:799–810.

144. Rosenthal LJ. Discrepant estrogen receptor protein levels according to surgical technique. *Am J Surg* 1979;138:680–681.

145. Rosen PP. Electrocautery induced artifacts in breast biopsy specimens: an iatrogenic source of diagnostic difficulty. Letter to the editor *Ann Surg* 1986;204:612–613.

146. Bombardieri E, Crippa F, Maffioli L, et al. Nuclear medicine approaches for detection of axillary lymph node metastases. *Q J Nucl Med* 1998;42:54–65.

147. Lam WWM, Yang WT, Chan YL, et al. Detection of axillary lymph node metastases in breast carcinoma by technetium-99m sestamibi breast scintigraphy, ultrasound and conventional mammography. *Eur J Nucl Med* 1996;23:498–503.

148. Tolmos J, Khalkhali I, Vargas H, et al. Detection of axillary lymph node metastasis of breast carcinoma with technetium-99m sestamibi scintimammography. *Am Surg* 1997;63:850–853.

149. Taillefer R, Robidoux A, Turpin S, et al. Metastatic axillary lymph node technetium-99m-MIBI imaging in primary breast cancer. *J Nucl Med* 1998;39:459–464.

150. Danielsson R, Bone B, Perbeck L, et al. Evaluation of planar scintimammography with 99mTc-MIBI in the detection of axillary lymph node metastases of breast carcinoma. *Acta Radiol* 1999;40:491–495.

151. Miyauchi M, Yamamoto N, Imanaka N, et al. Computed tomography for preoperative evaluation of axillary nodal status in breast cancer. *Breast Cancer* 1999;6:243–248.

152. Hata Y, Ogawa Y, Nishioka A, et al. Thin section computed tomography in the prone position for detection of axillary lymph node metastases in breast cancer. *Oncol Rep* 1998;5:1403–1406.

153. Harika L, Wessleder R, Poss K, et al. Macromolecular intravenous contrast agent for MR lymphography: characterization and efficacy studies. *Radiology* 1996;198:365–370.

154. Yoshimura G, Sakurai T, Oura S, et al. Evaluation of axillary lymph node status in breast cancer with MRI. *Breast Cancer* 1999; 6:249–258.

155. Mussurakis S, Buckley DL, Horsman A. Prediction of axillary lymph node status in invasive breast cancer with dynamic contrast-enhanced MR imaging. *Radiology* 1997;203:317–321.

156. Avril N, Dose J, Jünicke F, et al. Assessment of axillary lymph node involvement in breast cancer patients with positron emission tomography using radiolabeled 2-(fluorine-18)-fluoro-2-deoxy-D-glucose. *J Natl Cancer Inst* 1996;88:1204–1209.

157. Yutani K, Tatsumi M, Shiba E, et al. Comparison of dual-head coincidence gamma camera FDG imaging with FDG PET in detection of breast cancer and axillary lymph node metastasis. *J Nucl Med* 1999;40:1003–1008.

158. Silverstein MJ. Predicting axillary nodal positivity in 1787 patients with invasive breast carcinoma. *Breast J* 1998;4:324–329.

159. Barth A, Craig PH, Silverstein MJ. Predictors of axillary lymph node metastases in patients with T1 breast carcinoma. *Cancer* 1997; 79:1918–1922.

160. Chadha M, Chabon AB, Friedmann P, et al. Predictors of axillary lymph node metastases in patients with T1 breast cancer: a multivariate analysis. *Cancer* 1994;73:350–353.

161. Mustafa IA, Cole B, Wanebo HJ, et al. The impact of histopathology on nodal metastases in minimal breast cancer. *Arch Surg* 1997; 132:384–390.

162. Olivotto IA, Jackson JS, Mates D, et al. Prediction of axillary lymph node involvement of women with invasive breast carcinoma: a multivariate analysis. *Cancer* 1998;83:948–955.

163. Port ER, Tan LK, Borgen PI, et al. Incidence of axillary lymph node metastases in T1a and T1b breast carcinoma. *Ann Surg Oncol* 1998;5:23–27.

164. Shoup M, Malinzak L, Weisenberger J, et al. Predictors of axillary lymph node metastasis in T1 breast carcinoma. *Am Surg* 1999; 65:748–752.

165. Morrow M. Management of the axillary nodes. *Breast Cancer* 1999;6:1–12.

166. Chontos AJ, Maher DP, Ratzer ER, et al. Axillary lymph node dissection: is it required in T1a breast cancer? *J Am Coll Surg* 1997; 184:493–498.

167. Pandelidis SM, Peters KL, Walusimbi MS, et al. The role of axillary dissection in mammographically detected carcinoma. *J Am Coll Surg* 1997;184:341–345.

168. McGee JM, Youmans R, Clingan F, et al. The value of axillary dissection in T1a breast cancer. *Am J Surg* 1996;172:501–504.

169. Brunt LM, Jones DB, Wu JS, et al. Endoscopic axillary lymph node dissection: an experimental study in human cadavers. *J Am Coll Surg* 1998;187:158–163.

170. Lloyd LR, Waits RK, Schroder D, et al. Axillary dissection for breast carcinoma: the myth of skip metastases. *Ann Surg* 1989;55:381–384.

171. Rosen PP, Lesser ML, Kinne DW, et al. Discontinuous or "skip" metastases in breast carcinoma: Analysis of 1228 axillary dissections. *Ann Surg* 1983;197:276–283.

172. Veronesi U, Rilke F, Luini A, et al. Distribution of axillary node metastases by level of invasion: an analysis of 539 cases. *Cancer* 1987;59:682–687.

173. Zurrida S, Morabito A, Galimberti V, et al. Importance of the level of axillary involvement in relation to traditional variables in the prognosis of breast cancer. *Int J Oncol* 1999;15:475–480.

173a. Bale A, Gardner B, Shende M, et al. Can interpectoral nodes be sentinel nodes? *Am J Surg* 1999;178:360–361.

174. Anderson J, Jensen J. Lymph node identification: specimen radiography of tissue predominated by fat. *Am J Clin Pathol* 1977; 68:511–572.

175. Groote AD, Oosterhuis JW, Molenaar WM, et al. Radiographic imaging of lymph nodes in lymph node dissection specimens. *Lab Invest* 1985;52:326–329.

176. Durkin K, Haagensen CD. An improved technique for the study of lymph nodes in surgical specimens. *Ann Surg* 1980;191:419–429.

177. Morrow M, Evans J, Rosen PP, et al. Does clearing of axillary lymph nodes contribute to accurate staging of breast carcinoma? *Cancer* 1984;53:1329–1332.

178. Hartveit F, Samonsen G, Tanqen M, et al. Routine histological investigation of the axillary lymph nodes in breast cancer. *Clin Oncol* 1982;8:121–126.

179. Schmidt WA. In: *Principles and techniques of surgical pathology.* Menlo Park, CA: Addison-Wesley, 1983:362–388.

180. Silverberg SG, Masood S. The breast. In: *Principles and practice of surgical pathology and cytopathology.* New York: Churchill Livingston, 1997:579.

181. Rosai J. In: *Ackerman's surgical pathology.* St. Louis: Mosby, 1996:2682.

182. Niemann TH, Yilmaz AG, Marsh WLJ, et al. A half a node or a whole node: a comparison of methods for submitting lymph nodes. *Am J Clin Pathol* 1998;109:571–576.

183. Smith PA, Harlow SP, Krag DN, et al. Submission of lymph node tissue for ancillary studies decreases the accuracy of conventional breast cancer axillary node staging. *Mod Pathol* 1999;12:781–785.

184. Schrenk P, Rieger R, Shamiyeh A, et al. Morbidity following sentinel lymph node biopsy versus axillary lymph node dissection for patients with breast carcinoma. *Cancer* 2000;88:608–614.

185. Morrow M, Foster RS Jr. Staging of breast cancer: a new rationale for internal mammary node biopsy. *Arch Surg* 1981;116:748–751.

186. Harlow S, Krag D, Weaver D, et al. Extra-axillary sentinel lymph nodes in breast cancer. *Breast Cancer* 1999;6:159–165.

187. Krag DN. The sentinel node for staging breast cancer: current review. *Breast Cancer* 1999;63:233–236.

188. Hill AD, Tran KN, Akhurst T, et al. Lessons learned from 500 cases of lymphatic mapping for breast cancer. *Ann Surg* 1999;229:528–535.

189. Cody HL. Sentinel lymph node mapping in breast cancer. *Breast Cancer* 1999;6:13–22.

190. Bobin JY, Zinzindohoue C, Isaac S, et al. Tagging sentinel lymph nodes: a study of 100 patients with breast cancer. *Eur J Cancer* 1999;35:569–573.

191. Veronesi U. The sentinel node and breast cancer. *Br J Surg* 1999;86:1–2.

191a. Johnson N, Soot L, Nelson J, et al. Sentinel node biopsy and internal mammary lymphatic mapping in breast cancer. *Am J Surg* 2000:179:386–388.

192. Miltenburg DM, Miller C, Karamlou TB, et al. Meta-analysis of sentinel lymph node biopsy in breast cancer. *J Surg Res* 1999; 84:138–142.

193. Haigh PL, Hsueh EC, Giuliano AE. Sentinel lymphadenectomy in breast cancer. *Breast Cancer* 1999;6:139–144.

194. McMasters KM, Giuliano AE, Ross MI, et al. Sentinel-lymph-node biopsy for breast cancer—not yet the standard of care. *N Engl J Med* 1998;339:990–995.

195. Cox CE, Haddad F, Bass S, et al. Lymphatic mapping in the treatment of breast cancer. *Oncology* 1998;12:1283–1292.

196. Dauway EL, Giuliano R, Pendas S, et al. Lymphatic mapping: a technique providing accurate staging for breast cancer. *Breast Cancer* 1999;6:145–154.

197. Guenther JM, Krishnamoorthy M, Tan LR. Sentinel lymphadenectomy for breast cancer in a community managed care setting. *Cancer J Sci Am* 1997;3:336–340.

198. Veronesi U, Paganelli G, Galimberti V, et al. Sentinel-node biopsy to avoid axillary dissection in breast cancer with clinically negative lymph-nodes. *Lancet* 1997;349:1864–1867.

199. Sandrucci S, Mussa A. Sentinel lymph node biopsy and axillary staging of T1-T2 N0 breast cancer: a multicenter study. *Semin Surg Oncol* 1998;15:278–283.

200. Borgstein PJ, Meijer S, Pijpers R. Intradermal blue dye to identify sentinel lymph-node in breast cancer. *Lancet* 1997;349:1668–1669.

201. Reynolds C, Mick R, Donohue JH, et al. Sentinel lymph node biopsy with metastasis: can axillary dissection be avoided in some patients with breast cancer? *J Clin Oncol* 1999;17:1720–1726.

202. Bass SS, Lyman GH, McCann CR, et al. Lymphatic mapping and sentinel lymph node biopsy. *Breast J* 1999;5:288–295.

203. Haigh PI, Hansen NM, Qi K, et al. Biopsy method and excision volume do not affect success rate of subsequent sentinel lymph node dissection in breast cancer. *Ann Surg Oncol* 2000;7:21–27.

204. Liberman L, Cody HS, Hill AD, et al. Sentinel lymph node biopsy after percutaneous diagnosis of nonpalpable breast cancer. *Radiology* 1999;211:835–844.

205. Pendas S, Dauway E, Giuliano R, et al. Sentinel node biopsy in ductal carcinoma in situ patients. *Ann Surg Oncol* 2000;7:15–20.

206. Zavotsky J, Hansen N, Brennan MB, et al. Lymph node metastasis from ductal carcinoma in situ with microinvasion. *Cancer* 1999; 85:2439–2443.

206a. Cohen LF, Breslin TM, Kuerer HM, et al. Identification and evaluation of axillary sentinel lymph nodes in patients with breast carcinoma with neoadjuvant chemotherapy. *Am J Surg Pathol* 2000; 24:1266–1272.

207. Kaptain S, Montgomery LL, Son T, et al. Sentinel lymph node (SLN) metastases in multifocal invasive breast carcinoma (MIBC). *Mod Pathol* 2000;13:24A.

208. Veronesi U, Paganelli G, Viale G, et al. Sentinel lymph node biopsy and axillary dissection in breast cancer: results in a large series. *J Natl Cancer Inst* 1999;91:368–373.

208a. Waddington WA, Keshtgar MRS, Taylor I, et al. Radiation safety of the sentinel lymph node technique in breast cancer. *Eur J Nucl Med* 2000;27:377–391.

209. Glass EC, Essner R, Giuliano AE. Sentinel node localization in breast cancer. *Semin Nucl Med* 1999;29:57–68.

210. Miner T, Shriver C, Flicek P, et al. Additional guidelines for the safe management of radiation associated with sentinel lymph node biopsy. In: *Proceedings of 51st Annual Cancer Symposium of Society of Surgical Oncology and World Congress of Surgical Oncology,* 1998:13.

210a. Stratmann SL, McCarty TM, Kuhn JA. Radiation safety with breast sentinel node biopsy. *Am J Surg* 1999;178:454–457.

210b. Fitzgibbons PL, LiVolsi VA. Recommendations for handling radioactive specimens obtained by sentinel lymphadenectomy. Surgical

Pathology Committee of the College of American Pathologists, and the Association of Directors of Anatomic and Surgical Pathology. *Am J Surg Pathol* 2000;24:1549–1551.

211. Anastasiadis PG, Koutlaki NG, Liberis VA, et al. Cytologic diagnosis of axillary lymph node metastasis in breast cancer. *Acta Cytol* 2000;44:18–22.

212. Ku NK, Ahmad N, Smith PV, et al. Intraoperative imprint cytology of sentinel lymph nodes in breast cancer. *Acta Cytol* 1997;41: 1606–1607.

213. Rubio IT, Korourian S, Cowan C, et al. Use of touch preps for intraoperative diagnosis of sentinel lymph node metastases in breast cancer. *Ann Surg Oncol* 1998;5:689–694.

214. Ratanawichitrasin A, Biscotti CV, Levy L, et al. Touch imprint cytological analysis of sentinel lymph nodes for detecting axillary metastases in patients with breast cancer. *Br J Surg* 1999;86:1346–1348.

215. Litz C, Miller R, Ewing G, et al. Intraoperative sentinel lymph node touch imprints are not sensitive in detecting metastatic carcinoma. *Mod Pathol* 2000;13:26A.

216. Moes GS, Guibord RS, Weaver DL, et al. Intraoperative cytologic evaluation of sentinel lymph node in breast cancer patients. *Mod Pathol* 2000;13:28A.

217. Turner RR, Giuliano AE. Intraoperative pathologic examination of the sentinel lymph node. *Ann Surg Oncol* 1998;5:670–672.

218. Flett MM, Going JJ, Stanton PD, et al. Sentinel node localization in patients with breast cancer. *Br J Surg* 1998;85:991–993.

219. Chilosi M, Lestani M, Pedron S, et al. A rapid immunostaining method for frozen sections. *Biotech Histochem* 1994;69:235–239.

220. Viale G, Bosari S, Mazzarol G, et al. Intraoperative examination of axillary sentinel lymph nodes in breast carcinoma patients. *Cancer* 1999;85:2433–2438.

221. van Diest PJ, Torrenga H, Borgstein PJ, et al. Reliability of intraoperative frozen section and imprint cytological investigation of sentinel lymph nodes in breast cancer. *Histopathology* 1999;35:14–18.

222. Turner RR, Ollila DW, Krasne DL, et al. Histopathologic validation of the sentinel lymph node hypothesis for breast carcinoma. *Ann Surg* 1997;226:271–276.

223. Cserni G. Metastases in axillary sentinel lymph nodes in breast cancer as detected by intensive histopathological work up. *J Clin Pathol* 1999;52:922–924.

224. Turner RR, Ollila DW, Stern S, et al. Optimal histopathologic examination of the sentinel lymph node for breast carcinoma staging. *Am J Surg Pathol* 1999;23:263–267.

225. Dowlatshahi K, Fan M, Bloom KJ, et al. Occult metastases in the sentinel lymph nodes of patients with early stage breast carcinoma: a preliminary study. *Cancer* 1999;86:990–996.

226. Czerniecki BJ, Scheff AM, Callans LS, et al. Immunohistochemistry with pancytokeratins improves the sensitivity of sentinel lymph node biopsy in patients with breast carcinoma. *Cancer* 1999;85:1098–1103.

227. Zhang PJ, Reisner RM, Nangia R, et al. Effectiveness of multiple-level sectioning in detecting axillary nodal micrometastasis in breast cancer: a retrospective study with immunohistochemical analysis. *Arch Pathol Lab Med* 1998;122:687–690.

228. Turner RR, Hansen NM, Stern SL, et al. Intraoperative examination of the sentinel lymph node for breast carcinoma staging. *Am J Clin Pathol* 1999;112:627–634.

229. Viale G, Renne G, Pruneri G, et al. The axillary lymph node status in breast carcinoma patients with micrometastatic sentinel nodes. *Mod Pathol* 2000;13:49A.

230. Weaver DL, Krag DN, Ashikaga T, et al. Pathologic analysis of sentinel and nonsentinel lymph nodes in breast carcinoma: a multicenter study. *Cancer* 2000;88:1099–1107.

231. Chu KU, Turner RR, Hansen NM, et al. Sentinel node metastasis in patients with breast carcinoma accurately predicts immunohistochemically detectable nonsentinel node metastasis. *Ann Surg Oncol* 1999;6:756–761.

231a. Turner RR, Chu KU, Qi K. et al. Pathologic features associated with nonsentinel lymph node metastases in patients with metastatic breast carcinoma in a sentinel lymph node. *Cancer* 2000;89:574–581.

231b. Xu X, Roberts SA, Pasha TL, et al. Undesirable cytokeratin immunoreactivity of native nonepithelial cells in sentinel lymph nodes from patients with breast carcinoma. *Arch Pathol Lab Med* 2000;124:1310–1313,

232. Burchill SA, Bradbury MF, Pittman K, et al. Detection of epithelial cancer cells in peripheral blood by reverse transcriptase-polymerase chain reaction. *Br J Cancer* 1995;71:278–281.

233. Mori M, Mimori K, Inoue H, et al. Detection of cancer micrometastases in lymph nodes by reverse transcriptase-polymerase chain reaction. *Cancer Res* 1995;55:3417–3420.

234. Noguchi S, Aihara T, Nakamori S, et al. The detection of breast carcinoma micrometastases in axillary lymph nodes by means of reverse transcriptase-polymerase chain reaction. *Cancer* 1994;74:1595–1600.

235. Noguchi S, Aihara T, Motomura K, et al. Detection of breast cancer micrometastases in axillary lymph nodes by means of reverse transcriptase-polymerase chain reaction: comparison between MUC1 mRNA and keratin 19 mRNA amplification. *Am J Pathol* 1996;148:649–656.

236. Noguchi S, Aihara T, Motomura K, et al. Histologic characteristics of breast cancers with occult lymph node metastases detected by keratin 19 mRNA reverse transcriptase-polymerase chain reaction. *Cancer* 1996;78:1235–1240.

237. Schoenfeld A, Luqmani Y, Sinnett HD, et al. Keratin 19 mRNA measurement to detect micrometastases in lymph nodes in breast cancer patients. *Br J Cancer* 1996;74:1639–1642.

238. Lockett MA, Baron PL, O'Brien PH, et al. Detection of occult breast cancer micrometastases in axillary lymph nodes using a multimarker reverse transcriptase-polymerase chain reaction panel. *J Am Coll Surg* 1998;187:9–16.

239. Yun K, Gunn J, Merrie AE, et al. Keratin 19 mRNA is detectable by RT-PCR in lymph nodes of patients without breast cancer. *Br J Cancer* 1997;76:1112.

240. Schoenfeld A, Coombes RC. Keratin 19 mRNA is detectable by RT-PCR in lymph nodes of patients without breast cancer [Reply]. *Br J Cancer* 1997;76:1112–1113.

241. Bostick PJ, Chatterjee S, Chi DD, et al. Limitations of specific reverse-transcriptase polymerase chain reaction markers in the detection of metastases in the lymph nodes and blood of breast cancer patients. *J Clin Oncol* 1998;16:2632–2640.

242. Bostick PJ, Huynh KT, Sarantou T, et al. Detection of metastases in sentinel lymph nodes of breast cancer patients by multiple-marker RT-PCR. *Int J Cancer* 1998;79:645–651.

243. Jatoi I, Hilsenbeck SG, Clark GM, et al. Significance of axillary lymph node metastasis in primary breast cancer. *J Clin Oncol* 1999;17:2334–2340.

244. Attiyeh FF, Jensen M, Huvos AG, et al. Axillary micrometastases and macrometastases in carcinoma of the breast. *Surg Gynecol Obstet* 1977;144:839–842.

245. Fisher ER, Palekar A, Rockette H, et al. Pathologic findings from the National Surgical Adjuvant Breast Project (Protocol No.4). V. Significance of axillary nodal micro- and macrometastases. *Cancer* 1978;42:2032–2038.

246. Huvos AG, Hutter RVP, Berg JW. Significance of axillary macrometastases and micrometastases in mammary cancer. *Ann Surg* 1971;173:44–46.

247. Rosen PP, Saigo PE, Braun DW, et al. Axillary micro- and macrometastases in breast cancer. Prognostic significance of tumor size. *Ann Surg* 1981;194:585–591.

248. Friedman S, Bertin F, Mouriesse H, et al. Importance of tumor cells in axillary node sinus margins ("clandestine" metastases) discovered by serial sectioning in operable breast carcinoma. *Acta Oncol* 1988;27:483–487.

249. International (Ludwig) Breast Cancer Study Group. Prognostic importance of occult axillary lymph node micrometastases from breast cancers. *Lancet* 1990;1:1565–1568.

250. Saphir O, Amromin GD. Obscure axillary lymph-node metastasis in carcinoma of the breast. *Cancer* 1948;1:238–241.

251. Fisher ER, Swamidos S, Lee CH, et al. Detection and significance of occult axillary node metastases in patients with invasive breast cancer. *Cancer* 1978;45:2025–2031.

252. Pickren JW. Significance of occult metastases: a study of breast cancer. *Cancer* 1961;14:1266–1271.

253. Wilkinson EJ, Hause LL, Hoffman RG, et al. Occult axillary lymph node metastases in invasive breast carcinoma: characteristics of the primary tumor and significance of the metastases. *Pathol Annu* 1982;17:67–91.

254. de Mascarel I, Bonichon F, Coindre JM, et al. Prognostic significance of breast cancer axillary lymph node micrometastases assessed by two special techniques: reevaluation with longer follow-up. *Br J Cancer* 1992;66:523–527.

255. Cote RJ, Peterson HF, Chaiwun B, et al. Role of immunohistochemical detection of lymph-node metastases in management of breast cancer. International Breast Cancer Study Group. *Lancet* 1999;354:896–900.

256. Bussolati G, Gugliotta P, Morra I, et al. The immunohistochemical detection of lymph node metastases from infiltrating lobular carcinoma of the breast. *Br J Cancer* 1986;54:631–636.

257. Trojani M, de Mascarel I, Bonichon F, et al. Micrometastases to axillary lymph nodes from carcinoma of breast: detection by immunohistochemistry and prognostic significance. *Br J Cancer* 1987;55:303–306.

258. Delsol G, Gatter KC, Stein H, et al. Human lymphoid cells express epithelial membrane antigen: implications for diagnosis of human neoplasms. *Lancet* 1984;II:1124–1128.

259. Elson CE, Kufe D, Johnston WW. Immunohistochemical detection and significance of axillary lymph node micrometastases in breast carcinoma. *Anal Quant Cytol Histol* 1993;15:171–178.

260. Galea MH, Athanassiou E, Bell J, et al. Occult regional lymph node metastases from breast carcinoma: immunohistological detection with antibodies CAM 5.2 and NCRC-11. *J Pathol* 1991;165:221–227.

261. McGuckin MA, Cummings MC, Walsh MD, et al. Occult axillary node metastases in breast cancer: their detection and prognostic significance. *Br J Cancer* 1996;73:88–95.

262. Dowlatshahi K, Fan M, Snider HC, et al. Lymph node micrometastases from breast carcinoma: reviewing the dilemma. *Cancer* 1997;80:1188–1197.

263. Siziopikou KP, Schnitt SJ, Connolly JL, et al. Detection and significance of occult axillary metastatic disease in breast cancer patients. *Breast J* 1999;5:221–229.

264. Steinhoff MM. Axillary node micrometastases detection and biologic significance. *Breast J* 1999;5:325–329.

265. Recht A. Should irradiation replace dissection for patients with breast cancer with clinically negative axillary lymph nodes? *J Surg Oncol* 1999;72:184–192.

265a. Galper S, Recht A, Silver B, et al. Is radiation alone adequate treatment to the axilla for patients with limited axillary surgery? Implications for treatment after a positive sentinel node biopsy. *Int J Radiat Oncol Biol Phys* 2000;48:125–132.

265b. Giuliano AE, Haigh PI, Brennan MB, et al. Prospective observational study of sentinel lymphadectomy without further axillary dissection in patients with sentinel node-negative breast cancer. *J Clin Oncol* 2000;18:2553–2559.

266. Santin AD. Lymph node metastases: the importance of the microenvironment. *Cancer* 2000;88:175–179.

267. Scheunemann P, Izbicki JR, Pantel K. Tumorigenic potential of apparently tumor-free lymph nodes. *N Engl J Med* 1999;340:1687.

268. Carter BA, Jensen RA, Simpson JF, et al. Benign transport of breast epithelium into axillary lymph nodes post biopsy. *Am J Clin Pathol* 2000;113:259–265.

269. Hermanek P, Hutter RV, Sobin LH, et al. International Union Against Cancer. Classification of isolated tumor cells and micrometastasis. *Cancer* 1999;86:2668–2673.

270. Hultborn KA, Tornberg B. Mammary cancer: the biologic character of mammary carcinoma studied in 517 cases by a new form of malignancy grading. *Acta Radiol* 1960;Suppl.196:1–146.

271. Pierce LJ, Oberman HA, Strawderman MH, et al. Microscopic extracapsular extension in the axilla: is this an indication for axillary radiotherapy? *Int J Radiation Oncol Biol Phys* 1995;33:253–259.

272. Fisher ER, Gregorio RM, Redmond C, et al. Pathologic findings from the National Surgical Adjuvant Breast Project (Protocol No.4). III. The significance of extranodal extension of axillary metastases. *Am J Clin Pathol* 1976;65:439–449.

273. Cascinelli N, Greco M, Bufalino R, et al. Prognosis of breast cancer with axillary node metastases after surgical treatment only. *Eur J Cancer Clin Oncol* 1987;23:795–799.

274. Leonard C, Corkill M, Tompkin J, et al. Are axillary recurrence and overall survival affected by axillary extranodal tumor extension in breast cancer? Implications for radiation therapy. *J Clin Oncol* 1995;13:47–53.

275. Fisher BJ, Perera FE, Cooke AL, et al. Extracapsular axillary node extension in patients receiving adjuvant systemic therapy: an indication for radiotherapy? *Int J Radiat Oncol Biol Phys* 1997;38:551–559.

276. Mignano JE, Zahurak ML, Chakravarthy A, et al. Significance of axillary lymph node extranodal soft tissue extension and indications for postmastectomy irradiation. *Cancer* 1999;86:1258–1262.

277. Hetelekidis S, Schnitt SJ, Silver B, et al. The significance of extracap-

sular extension of axillary lymph node metastases in early-stage breast cancer. *Int J Rad Oncol Biol Phys* 2000;46:31–34.

278. Goldstein NS, Mani A, Vicini F, et al. Prognostic features in patients with stage T1 breast carcinoma and a 0.5-cm or less lymph node metastasis: significance of lymph node hilar tissue invasion. *Am J Clin Pathol* 1999;111:21–28.

279. Cappellari J, Islandar S, Woodruff R. Signet ring cell sinus histiocytosis. *Am J Clin Pathol* 1990;94:800–801.

280. Frost AR, Shek YH, Lack EE. "Signet ring" sinus histiocytosis mimicking metastatic adenocarcinoma: a report of two cases with immunohistochemical and ultrastructural study. *Mod Pathol* 1992; 5:497–500.

281. Gould E, Perez J, Albores-Saavedra J, et al. Signet ring cell sinus histiocytosis: a previously unrecognized histologic condition mimicking metastatic adenocarcinoma in lymph nodes. *Am J Clin Pathol* 1989;92:509–512.

282. Ravel R. Histopathology of lymph nodes after lymphangiography. *Am J Clin Pathol* 1966;46:335–340.

283. Truong L, Cartwright J, Goodman D, et al. Silicone lymphadenopathy associated with augmentation mammoplasty: morphologic features in nine cases. *Am J Surg Pathol* 1988;12:484–491.

284. Chears W, Smith A, Ruffin J. Diagnosis of Whipple's disease by peripheral lymph node biopsy: report of a case. *Am J Med* 1959; 27:351–353.

285. Livolsi VA, Brooks JJ, Soslow R, et al. Signet cell melanocytic lesions. *Mod Pathol* 1992;5:515–520.

286. Kim K, Dorfman RF, Rappaport H. Signet ring cell lymphoma: a rare morphologic and functional expression of nodular (follicular) lymphoma. *Am J Surg Pathol* 1978;2:119–132.

286a. Müller P, Schlimo K. Bone marrow "micrometastases" of epithelial tumors: detection and clinical relevance. *J Cancer Res Clin Oncol* 2000;126:607–618.

287. Dunphy CH. The role of wide-spectrum cytokeratin staining of bone marrow cores in patients with ductal carcinoma of the breast. *Mod Pathol* 1996;10:955–958.

288. Dearnaley DP, Sloane JP, Ormerod MG, et al. Increased detection of mammary carcinoma cells in marrow smears using antisera to epithelial membrane antigen. *Br J Cancer* 1981;44:85–90.

289. Ginsbourg M, Musset M, Misset JL, et al. Simultaneous detection in the bone marrow of mammary cancer metastatic cells and of their labelling index as respective markers of the residual minimum submacroscopic disease and its proliferative condition (preliminary results). *Biomed Pharmacother* 1986;40:386–388.

290. Mansi JL, Berger U, McDonnell T, et al. The fate of bone marrow micrometastases in patients with primary breast cancer. *J Clin Oncol* 1989;7:445–449.

291. Braun S, Kentenich C, Janni W, et al. Lack of effect of adjuvant chemotherapy on the elimination of single dormant tumor cells in bone marrow of high-risk breast cancer patients. *J Clin Oncol* 2000;18:80–86.

292. Braun S, Pantel K, Muller P, et al. Cytokeratin-positive cells in the bone marrow and survival of patients with stage I, II, or III breast cancer. *N Engl J Med* 2000;342:525–533.

293. Diel IJ, Kaufmann M, Costa SD, et al. Micrometastatic breast cancer cells in bone marrow at primary surgery: prognostic value in comparison with nodal status. *J Natl Cancer Inst* 1996;88:1652–1658.

294. Thor A, Viglione MJ, Ohuchi N, et al. Comparison of monoclonal antibodies for the detection of occult breast carcinoma metastases in bone marrow. *Breast Cancer Res Treat* 1988;11:133–145.

295. Okumura A, Tokuda Y, Tanaka M, et al. Immunohistochemical detection of tumor cells in the bone marrow of breast cancer patients. *Jpn J Clin Oncol* 1998;28:480–485.

296. Cote RJ, Rosen PP, Hakes TB, et al. Monoclonal antibodies detect occult breast carcinoma metastases in the bone marrow of patients with early stage disease. *Am J Surg Pathol* 1988;12:333–340.

297. Osborne MP, Asina S, Wong GY, et al. Immunofluorescent monoclonal antibody detection of breast cancer in bone marrow: sensitivity in a model system. *Cancer Res* 1989;49:2510–2513.

298. Cote RJ, Rosen PP, Lesser ML, et al. Prediction of early relapse in patients with operable breast cancer by detection of occult bone marrow micrometastases. *J Clin Oncol* 1991;9:1749–1756.

299. Cordell JL, Falini B, Erber WN, et al. Immunoenzymatic labeling of monoclonal antibodies using immune complexes of alkaline phosphatase and monoclonal anti-alkaline phosphatase (APAAP complexes). *J Histochem Cytochem* 1984;32:219–229.

300. Taha M, Ordonez NG, Kulkarni S, et al. A monoclonal antibody cocktail for detection of micrometastatic tumor cells in the bone marrow of breast cancer patients. *Bone Marrow Transplant* 1989;4:297–303.

301. Schlimok G, Funke I, Holzmann B, et al. Micrometastatic cancer cells in bone marrow: in vivo detection with anti-cytokeratin and in vivo labelling with anti-17-1A monoclonal antibodies. *Proc Natl Acad Sci USA* 1987;84:8672–8676.

302. Molino A, Pelosi G, Turazza M, et al. Bone marrow micrometastases in 109 breast cancer patients: correlations with clinical and pathological features and prognosis. *Breast Cancer Res Treat* 1997;42:23–30.

303. Tagliabue E, Porro G, Barbanti P, et al. Improvement of tumor cell detection using a pool of monoclonal antibodies. *Hybridoma* 1986; 5:107–115.

304. Datta YH, Adams PT, Drobyski WR, et al. Sensitive detection of occult breast cancer by the reverse transcriptase polymerase chain reaction. *J Clin Oncol* 1994;12:475–482.

305. Slade MJ, Smith BM, Sinnett HD, et al. Quantitative polymerase chain reaction for the detection of micrometastases in patients with breast cancer. *J Clin Oncol* 1999;17:870–879.

306. Leitzel K, Lieu B, Curley E, et al. Detection of cancer cells in peripheral blood of breast cancer patients using reverse transcription-polymerase chain reaction for epidermal growth factor receptor. *Clin Cancer Res* 1998;4:3037–3043.

307. Zach O, Kasparu H, Krieger O, et al. Detection of circulating mammary carcinoma cells in the peripheral blood of breast cancer patients via a nested reverse transcriptase polymerase chain reaction assay for mammaglobin mRNA. *J Clin Oncol* 1999;17:2015–2019.

307a. Grünewald K, Haun M, Urbanek M, et al. Mammaglobin gene expression: a superior marker of breast cancer cells in peripheral blood in comparison to epidermal-growth-factor-receptor and cytokeratin-19. *Lab Invest* 2000;80:1071–1077.

308. Smith BM, Slade MJ, English J, et al. Response of circulating tumor cells to systemic therapy in patients with metastatic breast cancer: comparison of quantitative polymerase chain reaction and immunocytochemical techniques. *J Clin Oncol* 2000;18:1432–1439.

309. Brandt B, Roetger A, Heidl S, et al. Isolation of blood-borne epithelium-derived c-*erb*B-2 oncoprotein-positive clustered cells from the peripheral blood of breast cancer patients. *Int J Cancer* 1998; 76:824–828.

310. Eaton MC, Hardingham JE, Kotasek D, et al. Immunobead RT-PCR: a sensitive method for detection of circulating tumor cells. *Biotechniques* 1997;22:100–105.

311. Hildebrandt M, Mapara MY, Korner IJ, et al. Reverse transcriptase-polymerase chain reaction (RT-PCR)-controlled immunomagnetic purging of breast cancer cells using the magnetic cell separation (MACS) system: a sensitive method for monitoring purging efficiency. *Exp Hematol* 1997;25:57–65.

312. Naume B, Borgen E, Beiske K, et al. Immunomagnetic techniques for the enrichment and detection of isolated breast carcinoma cells in bone marrow and peripheral blood. *J Hematother* 1997;6:103–114.

313. Krag DN, Ashikaga T, Moss TJ, et al. Breast cancer cells in the blood: a pilot study. *Breast J* 1999;5:354–358.

314. Raso DS, Greene WB, Metcalf JS. Synovial metaplasia of a periprosthetic breast capsule. *Arch Pathol Lab Med* 1994;118:249–251.

315. Raso DS, Crymes LW, Metcalf JS. Histological assessment of fifty breast capsules from smooth and textured augmentation and reconstruction mammoplasty prostheses with emphasis on the role of synovial metaplasia. *Mod Pathol* 1994;7:310–316.

316. O'Doherty AJ. Spontaneous fracture of the wire tip during breast localization. *Br J Radiol* 1991;64:1154–1156.

317. Homer MJ. Transection of localization hooked wire during breast biopsy. *AJR Am J Roentgenol* 1983;141:929–930.

318. Barzilai M, Roisman I. Foreign bodies in the breast. *Breast Dis* 1995;8:179–183.

319. Hoda SA, Borgen P, Rosen PP. Unanticipated clinical presentation of unusual foreign body in the breast. *Breast Dis* 1994;7:227–230.

320. Holt RW, Potter JF. Retained Groshong catheter cuff presenting as a breast mass. *Breast Dis* 1993;6:153–155.

321. de Souza GA. Penrose drain as a foreign body in the breast. *Breast J* 1999;5:208–210.

322. Davis SP, Stomper PC, Weidner N, et al. Suture calcification mimicking recurrence in the irradiated breast: a potential pitfall in mammographic evaluation. *Radiology* 1989;172:247–248.

323. Brown RC, Zuehlke RL, Ehrhardt JC, et al. Tattoos simulating calcifications on xeroradiographs of the breast. *Radiology* 1981;138: 583–584.

324. Thomas DR, Fisher MS, Caroline DF. Case report: soap—another artefact that can mimic intramammary calcifications. *Clin Radiol* 1995;50:64–66.

325. Wakabayashi M, Reid JD, Bhattacharjee M. Foreign body granuloma caused by prior gunshot wound mimicking malignant breast mass. *AJR Am J Roentgenol* 1999;173:321–322.

326. Kupic EA. Glass foreign body in the breast simulating a hyperdense nodule on mammography. *AJR Am J Roentgenol* 1992;159:1125.

327. Schwartz DL, So HB, Schneider KM, et al. Chronic insertion of foreign bodies into the mature breast. *J Pediatr Surg* 1977;12:743–744.

328. Sampson D. Unusual self-inflicted injury of the breast. *Postgrad Med* 1975;51:116–118.

329. Moon WK, Park JM, Im J-G, et al. Metallic punctate densities in the breast after Chinese herbal treatment: mammographic findings. *Radiology* 2000;21:890–894.

# Subject Index

Page numbers followed by "f" indicate figures; page numbers followed by "t" indicate tabular material.

## A

Aberrant breast tissue, 26
  ectopic carcinoma in, 676, 676f
Abscesses
  breast, 73, 73f
  in granulomatous lobular mastitis, 40, 40f
  subareolar, 73–74
Acantholytic carcinoma, 432, 434, 435f, 436f
Actinomycosis, 65
Adenocarcinoma, with spindle cell carcinoma, 431, 434f
Adenoid cystic carcinoma, 535–548
  aspiration cytology of, 536, 541, 541f
  clinical features of, 535–536, 535f
  electron microscopy of, 547
  histochemistry and cytology of, 547
  metastatic, 548, 548f
  pathology of, gross, 536, 536f
  pathology of, microscopic, 536–547, 537f–546f
    basaloid, 541, 544f
    collagenous spherulosis, 545, 546f
    cylindromatous, 536, 539f
    cystic, 536, 537f
    duct involvement, 536, 538f
    ductular differentiation, 541, 543f
    high-grade, 541, 543f, 544f, 545
    intraductal, 536, 539f
    invasive growth pattern, 536, 537f
    lobular, 536, 538f
    metaplasia, 541, 542f
    Paget's disease and, 546f, 547
    reticular, 541, 541f
    *vs.* scirrhous carcinoma, 536, 540f
    shrinkage artifact, 536, 538f
    solid, 541, 541f
    stromal differentiation, unusual, 545, 545f
    structural heterogeneity, 536, 540f
    syringomatous differentiation, 541, 542f
    tubular, 541, 542f
    tubular carcinoma and, 546f, 547
  prognosis and treatment of, 547–548, 548f
Adenoid cystic hyperplasia. *See* Collagenous spherulosis
Adenoleiomyoma, 781
Adenolipoma, 779–781, 780f
Adenoma(s). *See also* specific types, e.g., Fibroadenoma, Syringomatous adenoma of the nipple
  apocrine, 167
  ductal, 77, 167
  lactating, *vs.* fibroadenoma, 171, 172f, 173f
  of nipple, syringomatous, 111–114 (*See also* Syringomatous adenoma of the nipple)
  pleomorphic, 130, 132f, 167

in adenomyoepithelioma, 130, 132f
  pure, 167, 167f (*See also* Fibroadenoma)
  tubular, 167, 167f (*See also* Fibroadenoma)
Adenomyoepithelioma, 77, 121–134
  in adenosquamous carcinoma, low-grade, 445, 446f–447f
  clinical presentation of, 121–123, 122f
  cytology of, 133–134
  electron microscopy of, 133
  histochemistry of, 132–133, 133f
  malignant, 127, 130, 131f
  pathology of, gross, 122f, 123
  pathology of, microscopic, 123–132, 123f–133f
    from adenosis, 123, 124f
    with apocrine metaplasia, 124, 126f, 127
    with cartilaginous metaplasia, 127, 127f
    clear cytoplasm, 124, 124f
    cystic papillary, 127, 129f
    glandular component, 127, 129f
    growth pattern, 124, 124f
    infarction and calcification, 127, 128f
    from lobular proliferation, 123, 123f
    malignant, 127, 130, 131f
    mixed tumors, 130, 132f
    mucoepidermoid differentiation, 127, 128f
    myoepithelial carcinoma in, 130, 131f
    myoepithelial cell nuclei, 127, 130f
    myoepithelial cells, 124, 126f, 130f
      prominent, 124, 125f
      with trabecular pattern, 124, 126f
    nodules, aggregated, 123, 123f
    pleomorphic adenomas, 130, 132f
    with sebaceous metaplasia, 127, 127f
    spindle cell myoid growth, 127, 129f
    with squamous metaplasia, 127, 127f
  prognosis and treatment of, 134
Adenosis, 139–151
  apocrine, 145, 146f, 147f
  blunt duct, 149, 149f
  clinical presentation of, 139, 140f
  differential diagnosis of, 149–151, 150f, 151f
  in fibroadenomas, 149, 149f
  florid, 139, 141, 141f–143f
    in pregnancy, 141, 143f
  neural invasion by, 145, 149f
  pathology of
    gross, 139, 140f, 141f
    microscopic, 139, 141–149, 142f–149f (*See also* Adenosis, sclerosing)
  treatment and prognosis of, 151
  tubular, 145, 149, 149f
Adenosis, microglandular, 152–160
  atypical, 154–155, 156f, 157f
  carcinoma in
    with basaloid differentiation, 158, 159f

intraductal, 155, 156f
    invasive, high-grade, 155, 157f, 158
    with secretory differentiation, 158, 158f
  clinical presentation of, 152
  immunoreactivity of, 153–154, 153f, 154f
  metastases of, 159, 160f
  oncocytic differentiation in, 154
  pathology of, gross, 152
  pathology of, microscopic, 152–155, 152f–159f, 158
    atypical, 154–155, 156f
    carcinoma in, 155, 157f
      with basaloid differentiation, 158, 159f
      with matrix-forming chondroid metaplasia, 155, 157f
      with secretory differentiation, 158, 158f
    eosinophilic cytoplasmic granules, 154, 155f
    epithelial cells, flat-to-cuboidal, 153, 153f
    immunoreactivity, 153–154, 153f–154f
    intraductal carcinoma in, 155, 156f
    myoepithelial cells, 154, 154f
    PAS and mucicarmine staining of, 153, 153f
    *vs.* sclerosing adenosis, 154, 155f
    small glands in fibrous/fatty stroma, 152, 152f
  prognosis and treatment of, 158–160, 160f
  with sclerosing adenosis, 154, 155f
  variations in, 154, 155f
Adenosis, sclerosing, 141, 143f–145f, 145
  apocrine metaplasia in, 141, 146f, 147f
  with atrophy, marked, 141, 145f
  clear cell apocrine metaplasia in, 141, 147f
  collagenous spherulosis in, 141, 148f
  in fat, 141, 144f
  fibroadenoma with, 149, 149f, 170, 171f
  intraductal carcinoma in, 150, 150f, 151f, 282f–284, 283–284
  lobular carcinoma *in situ* in, 149, 150f
  with microglandular adenosis, 154, 155f
  variants of, 145, 147f, 148f
Adenosquamous carcinoma, 431, 431t–432t
  low-grade, 443–448, 443f–447f
    immunoreactivity in, 446, 448f
    recurrent, 446, 448f
Adnexal gland, Paget's disease in, 570, 572f–573f
Adnexal gland carcinoma
  apocrine, 904, 905f
  in axillary skin, 904, 907f, 908
  cribriform, 904, 906f
  with intraductal carcinoma, 904, 907f
  papillary, 904, 905f
  *in situ,* 904, 907f
  tubulolobular, 904, 905f
Adolescent breast development
  female, 2, 3f
  male, 2, 3f

Adolescent giant fibroadenomas, 165
Adolescent macromastia, 23–24, 24f
Age. *See also* Children; Juvenile
  carcinoma and, 654–656
Alveolar soft-part sarcoma, 827
Amastia, 23, 24f
Amyloid tumor, 56–58, 57f, 58f
Amyloidosis, 56–58, 57f
Anatomy, breast
  adolescent, 2, 3f
  adult gross, 2–3
    functional, 4–5
  adult microscopic, 5–8, 5f–8f
  clear cell change in, 18–19, 18f, 19f
  embryology in, 1
  fatty *vs.* fibroglandular tissue in, 5
  infantile, 1, 2f
  lymphatic drainage in, 4
  in menopause, 14–15, 14f
  menstrual cycle on, 8–11, 9f, 10f
  in pregnancy, 11–14, 12f, 13f
  pregnancy-like change in, 15–18, 16f–18f
Androgen receptors, in apocrine carcinoma,
  493–494
Androgen treatment, effects of, 895
Aneurysm, 806
Angioblastic sarcoma, 827, 827f
Angiogenesis, 345–348, 346f, 347f
  in intraductal carcinoma, 290–291, 291f
Angiogenesis factor, atypical hyperplasia with, 243
Angiolipoma
  *vs.* angiosarcoma, 831, 834f–835f
  nonparenchymal, 803, 803f, 804f
Angioma, 787
Angiomatosis, 797–800
  clinical presentation of, 798
  pathology of
    gross, 798, 798f
    microscopic, 798–800, 798f, 799f
  prognosis and treatment of, 800, 800f
  recurrent, 800, 800f
Angiosarcoma, 829–850
  clinical presentation of, 829–830
  electron microscopy of, 848f, 849
  histologic characteristics of, 831, 831t
  immunohistochemistry of, 846–849, 847f–848f
  pathology of, gross, 830–831, 830f, 831f
  pathology of, microscopic, 831–846, 832f–847f
    *vs.* atypical vascular lesions, 841, 844–846,
      844t, 845f–847f
    breast, 844, 846f
    skin, 844, 845f, 846, 846f
    skin, capillary type, 846, 847f
    blood lakes, 837, 839f
    *vs.* hemangioma, 840
    high grade, 837, 838f–840f, 840
      with low-grade, in fat, 840, 840f
    intermediate grade, 835–837, 836f–838f
    low grade, 831, 832f–835f
      angiolipoma-like, 831, 834f–835f
      capillary type, 831, 834f
      with mitoses, 831, 833f
      pseudoangiomatous stromal
        hyperplasia–like, 831, 834f
      with stromal fibrosis, 831, 835, 835f
    postradiation, 840–841, 841f–844f
  in phyllodes tumor, 183, 187f
  postmastectomy, 829, 850–856, 851f–855f
    clinical presentation of, 851, 851f
    electron microscopy of, 856
    immunohistochemistry of, 852, 854–856, 855f
    pathology of, gross, 851, 852f
    pathology of, microscopic, 852, 852f–855f
      chronic lymphedema, 852, 852f
      early lesions, 852, 853f
      epithelioid, 852, 855f
      hemorrhage, 852, 853f, 854f
    prognosis and treatment of, 856
  postradiation, 829
  prognosis and treatment of, 849–850, 849f, 850t

Anti-estrogen, treatment effects of, 896
Anticoagulant therapy, hemorrhagic necrosis from,
  30
Apocrine adenoma, 167
Apocrine adenosis, 145, 146f, 147f, 167
Apocrine carcinoma, 483–495
  clinical presentation of, 484–485, 485f
  definition of, 483
  electron microscopy of, 493
  immunohistochemistry of, 493–494, 494f
  molecular pathology of, 494
  origin of, 483–484
  pathology of, gross, 485, 485f
  pathology of, microscopic, 486–493, 486f–493f
    architecture, 487, 488f–489f
    calcification, 487, 489f
    cribriform, 487, 488f
    cystic papillary, 487, 489f
    with granulomatous reaction, 487, 491, 491f
    histiocytoid, 492, 492f
    infiltrating, 491–492, 492f
    invasive, 492–493, 493f
    with lobular extension, 487, 490f
    lymphatic tumor emboli, 492–493
    with lymphocytic reaction, 487, 491f
    micropapillary, 487, 488f
    necrosis, 487, 489f
    nuclear grade, 487, 490f
    in sclerosing adenosis, 486, 486f–487f
  treatment and prognosis of, 494–495, 494f
Apocrine intraductal carcinoma, 487. *See also*
  Apocrine carcinoma
  lobular carcinoma *in situ* in, 600, 600f
Apocrine metaplasia, 483, 483f–484f. *See also*
  Apocrine carcinoma
  with calcium oxalate, 483, 484f
  cystic and papillary, 96–101
    clinical presentation of, 96–97
    electron microscopy of, 100
    immunohistochemistry of, 100
    pathology of, gross, 97
    pathology of, microscopic, 97–100, 98f–100f
    prognosis and treatment of, 100–101
  in phyllodes tumor, 192, 192f
Apoptosis, 339
Apoptotic index, 295
AREDYLD (acrorenal ectodermal dysplasia with
  lipotropic diabetes), 23
Areola, 5
  nevoid hyperkeratosis of, 909, 910f
Arterial circulation, 3–4
Aspergillosis, 66
Atypical duct hyperplasia, juvenile, 739–741,
  739f–742f
Atypical hyperplasia. *See under* Precancerous
  breast disease, proliferative (fibrocystic)
  breast changes
  *vs.* hyperplasia and carcinoma *in situ,* 238–239
Atypical lobular hyperplasia, 610–617
  clinical presentation of, 610
  E-cadherin in, 614
  management of, clinical, 621–623
  pathology of, 610f–614f, 611, 613–614
    borderline, 613, 613f
    *vs.* duct hyperplasia with lobular extension,
      614, 615f
    in ducts, 614, 615f–616f
    cloverleaf, 613–614, 614f
  prognosis with, 614, 617
Atypical medullary carcinoma, 410, 421. *See also*
  Medullary carcinoma
Atypical vascular lesions, *vs.* angiosarcoma, 841,
  844–846, 844t, 845f–847f
  breast, 844, 846f
  skin, 844, 845f, 846, 846f
  capillary type, 846, 847f
Axillary lymph nodes, 254

pathology of, 913–925
  pigment deposits in, 923–924, 923f, 924f
  staging of, 958–960
Axillary lymph node metastases, in occult
  carcinoma, 661–673. *See also* Lymph node
  metastases, axillary

**B**

Basal cell carcinoma, of nipple, 909, 909f
Basal-squamous carcinoma, of nipple, 909, 910f
*bcl-2* gene, 340, 340f
  with atypical hyperplasia, 241
  in intraductal carcinoma, 279f, 295
    expression of, 279, 279f
*bcl-2* protein, in fetal breast, 1
Becker's nevus, mammary hypoplasia with, 23
Benign mesenchymal neoplasms, 749–806
  aneurysms, 806
  angiomas, 787
  angiomatosis, 797–800
    clinical presentation of, 798
    pathology of, gross, 798, 798f
    pathology of, microscopic, 798–800, 798f,
      799f
    prognosis and treatment of, 800, 800f
    recurrent, 800, 800f
  fibromatosis, 749–757 (*See also* Fibromatosis)
  fibrous tumor, 757, 757f
  giant cell fibroblastoma, 775
  granular cell tumor, 775–778
    clinical presentation of, 775–776
    malignant, 777, 778f
    pathology of, gross, 776, 777f
    pathology of, microscopic, 776–777, 777f,
      778f
    prognosis and treatment of, 777–778, 778f
  hamartoma, 779–781, 780f
  hemangiomas, 789–797, 790f–797f (*See also*
    Hemangiomas)
    nonparenchymal, of mammary region,
      803–806, 803f–806f
      clinical presentation of, 803
      pathology of, 803–806, 803–806f
      prognosis and treatment of, 806
    perilobular, 787–789, 787t, 788f
    venous, 800–803, 801f, 802f (*See also*
      Hemangiomas, venous)
  leiomyoma, 781–782, 781f, 782f
  lipoma, 786, 786f–787f
  mucinosis, 784–786, 785f
  myeloid metaplasia, 784
  myofibroblastoma, 766–774, 767f–773f (*See
    also* Myofibroblastoma)
  "myoid hamartoma," 782–783, 783f
  myxoma, 784, 784f
  nerve and nerve sheath tumors, 778–779, 779f
  perivascular myoid differentiation, 774–775,
    774f–775f
  pseudoangiomatous stromal hyperplasia,
    757–766, 758f–765f (*See also*
    Pseudoangiomatous stromal hyperplasia)
  vascular lesions, 787, 787t
Bilaterality
  in invasive duct carcinoma, 327
  and prognosis, 327
Biopsy. *See also* specific cancers, e.g., Intraductal
  carcinoma, needle core biopsy of
  after breast conservation, 891–892
  for proliferative (fibrocystic) breast changes, 232
    breast carcinoma after, 233–234, 234t
Biopsy specimens
  excisional, 932
  frozen section, 932
  incisional, 931
  margin assessment in, 933–938, 933f, 936f
  pathologic examination of, 931–982
  thermal (electrocautery) damage in, 954–958,
    954f–957f

Blastomycosis, 66
Blood vessel invasion, 344–345, 344f
Bloom-Richardson histologic grading, 337, 338t
Blue nevus, of breast, 899, 900f–902f
Blunt duct adenosis, 149, 149f
Bone marrow, micrometastases in, 978–980
Border, tumor. See Tumor border
Borderline lesions, 237–238
   uncertainty about, 238
BRCA1 gene, 229–230
   with atypical hyperplasia, 241
   in invasive duct carcinoma, 327
BRCA2 gene, 229–230
   in invasive duct carcinoma, 327
Breast augmentation pathology, 49–53. See also
      Silicone mastitis
Breast carcinoma. See Carcinoma
Breast conservation, biopsy after, 891–892
Breast-conserving surgery, for intraductal
      carcinoma, 311–316
   risk factors for recurrences after, 313–316, 314t
Breast examination, self- vs. clinical, 655
Breast implants. See Implants, breast
Breast infarct, 30–32, 31f, 32f
Breast self-examination, 655
Breast tissue, ectopic, 25–26, 26f
   carcinoma in, 673–676, 673f–676f (See also
      Ectopic breast tissue)
Bromodeoxyuridine (BrdU), 354–355

C
Calcification(s)
   in adenomyoepithelioma, 127, 128f
   in apocrine carcinoma, 487, 489f
   in ductal hyperplasia, columnar cell, 217,
      218f–221f, 222–223, 223f
   in fibromatosis, myxoid, 753, 754f
   in intraductal carcinoma, 259–260, 260f
      dystrophic, 276f, 278
      micro-, 259–260, 260f
   in mucinous carcinoma, papillary, 467–468, 469f
   in mucocele-like tumor, 474, 476f
   in non-Hodgkin's lymphoma, 868, 871, 871f
   in pregnancy-like change, 15, 17f
   in tubular carcinoma, 373, 373f
   pathology of, 943–947, 944f–947f
Calcium oxalate, in apocrine metaplasia, 483, 484f
CAM5.2, 448–449
Carcinoembryonic antigen (CEA), in apocrine
      carcinoma, 493
Carcinoma(s)
   acantholytic, 432, 434, 435f, 436f
   adeno-, with spindle cell carcinoma, 431, 434f
   adenoid cystic, 535–548 (See also Adenoid
      cystic carcinoma)
   adenosquamous, 431, 431t–432t
      low-grade, 443–448, 443f–447f
         immunoreactivity in, 446, 448f
         recurrent, 446, 448f
   adnexal gland (See Adnexal gland carcinoma)
   age extremes of, 654–656
   apocrine, 483–495 (See also Apocrine
      carcinoma)
   apocrine intraductal, 487 (See also Apocrine
      carcinoma)
      lobular carcinoma in situ in, 600, 600f
   atypical medullary, 410, 421 (See also Medullary
      carcinoma)
   basal cell, of nipple, 909, 909f
   basal-squamous, of nipple, 909, 910f
   in children (See Children; Juvenile)
   chondroosseous, 437, 437f–439f
   chorio-, 425, 426f
   colonic, breast metastases from, 690, 691f
   comedo, 257–258
      grade of, 288
   comedo intraductal, 276–278, 276f–278f
      grade of, 288

cribriform, 257
   classic, 551–553, 552f
   intraductal, 257, 264, 265f–268f, 271f,
      273–276, 273f–276f, 503f–504f (See also
      Intraductal carcinoma)
cystic hypersecretory, 527–534 (See also Cystic
      hypersecretory carcinoma)
cystic hypersecretory intraductal, 273
cystic papillary mucinous, 467, 467f
in ectopic breast tissue, 673–676, 673f–676f
   in aberrant breast, 676, 676f
   in axilla, 674, 674f
      with invasive lobular carcinoma, 673, 673f
   in mediastinal teratoma, 674, 675f, 676
   in residual breast after mastectomy, 674, 674f,
      675f
in elderly, 654–656
endocrine features in, 497–501, 498f–500f (See
      also Mammary carcinoma with endocrine
      features)
endocrine intraductal, 281
endometrial, breast metastases from, 697, 698f
in fibroadenoma, 656–661 (See also
      Fibroadenoma)
   clinical presentation of, 656–657
   pathology of, gross, 657
   pathology of, microscopic, 657–660,
      657f–659f
   prognosis and treatment of, 661
flat micropapillary, 269f, 273
gastric, breast metastases from, 690, 691f
glycogen-rich, 557–559, 557f, 558f
with granulomatous reaction, 523, 523f
infiltrating duct, 463
   in children and adolescents, 745, 746f
   with endocrine features, 500
   with medullary features, 410 (See also
      Medullary carcinoma)
   with mucinous component, 463, 465, 466f
infiltrating lobular, vs. non-Hodgkin's
      lymphoma, 867–868, 869f
inflammatory, 676–683 (See also Inflammatory
      carcinoma)
   recurrent, 681, 681f, 682f (See also
      Inflammatory carcinoma)
intraductal, 257–317 (See also Intraductal
      carcinoma)
   medullary, 416f, 417
invasive duct, 325–356 (See also Invasive duct
      carcinoma)
invasive lobular, 627–648 (See also Invasive
      lobular carcinoma)
invasive micropapillary, 561–564 (See also
      Invasive micropapillary carcinoma)
invasive tubulolobular, small cell carcinoma
      with, 503, 505f
juvenile (See Secretory carcinoma)
in lactation, 653–654
laciform, 257
lipid-rich, 555–556, 555f
with lipofuscin, 904, 904f (See also Malignant
      melanoma)
lobular, 426, 427f
   historical perspective on, 627
   invasive (See Invasive lobular carcinoma)
   with juvenile papillomatosis, 733, 734f
   Paget's disease with, 569, 569f
   signet-ring cells in, 372f
   in situ (See Lobular carcinoma in situ)
lymph node metastases in, axillary, 661–673
      (See also Lymph node metastases, axillary)
of male breast (See Male breast, carcinoma of)
mammary
   with endocrine features (See Mammary
      carcinoma with endocrine features)
   with osteoclast-like giant cells, 517–525 (See
      also Mammary carcinoma with
      osteoclast-like giant cells)
   resembling carcinoma with osteoclast-like
      giant cells, 517–518, 518f–519f

matrix-producing, 440, 441f, 442, 442f
medullary, 405–422 (See also Medullary
      carcinoma)
   atypical, 410, 421
   intraductal, 416f, 417
melanin in, 904, 904f
metaplastic, 425–452 (See also Metaplastic
      carcinoma)
microinvasive, 303
micropapillary
   flat, 269f, 273
   intraductal (See Intraductal carcinoma)
   invasive, 561–564 (See also Micropapillary
      carcinoma, invasive)
minimally invasive, 303
mucinous, 463–480 (See also Mucinous
      carcinoma)
multicentric, 301
multifocal, 301
myoepithelial, 137, 137f
and non-Hodgkin's lymphoma, 871, 872f
nonmedullary, 413, 414f
oat cell, 503–508
   microscopic pathology of, 503–508,
      503f–507f (See also Small cell
      carcinoma)
   treatment and prognosis of, 507–508
occult
   inflammatory, 681 (See also Inflammatory
      carcinoma)
   with lymph node metastases, axillary,
      661–673 (See also Lymph node
      metastases, axillary)
oncocytic, 483
osseous, 437, 438f
   metaplastic, 437, 438f
ovarian, breast metastases from, 696, 697, 697f
papillary, 381–403 (See also Papillary
      carcinoma)
   intraductal, 281
   in situ, vs. invasive papillary carcinoma, 401,
      402f
   solid, mucinous carcinoma in, 467, 468f
in phyllodes tumor, 656–661 (See also Phyllodes
      tumor)
in pregnancy, 653–654
preinvasive, 249
primary, 668–669, 669t
prostatic, breast metastases from, 693, 696, 696f
pseudoangiomatous, 432, 434, 436f
renal
   clear cell, breast metastases from, 697, 699f
   sarcomatoid, breast metastases from, 697,
      698f–699f
sarcoid-like granulomas in, 41, 42f
scirrhous, vs. adenoid cystic carcinoma, 536,
      540f
secretory, 509–515 (See also Secretory
      carcinoma)
in situ (intraepithelial), 249–250
   with ductal-lobular features, 284, 286, 287f
   vs. hyperplasia and atypical hyperplasia,
      238–239
in situ lobular
   with intraductal carcinoma, 284, 286f
   tubular carcinoma with, 374–375, 375f
small cell, 503–508 (See also Small cell
      carcinoma)
   intraductal, 281–283, 282f
spindle and squamous, 426, 428f, 431–432, 432f,
      433f
spindle cell, 431–432, 432f, 433f
   with adenocarcinoma, 431, 434f
   with chondroid differentiation, 437, 439f
   intraductal, 281, 281f
spindle cell–keloidal, 432, 435f
squamous (See Squamous carcinoma)
staging of, 253–256
   clinical, 253–254
   histopathologic, 255

Carcinoma(s) (*contd.*)
history of, 254
lymph nodes in, 254
pathologic, 254
rules for, 253–254
stage grouping in, 255–256
TNM and pTNM, 253–255
sweat gland (*See* Apocrine carcinoma)
tubular, 365–379 (*See also* Tubular carcinoma)
tubulolobular, 370, 372f
invasive, small cell carcinoma with, 503, 505f
in young, 654–656
Carcinosarcomas, 428. *See also* Metaplastic
carcinoma
Carney's syndrome, 170
Cat scratch disease, 72–73
Cathepsin D, in papillary carcinoma, 382, 382f
CD44, 449
Cell polarity, atypical hyperplasia with, 242
Cervical intraepithelial neoplasia (CIN), 239
Chemotherapy, pathological effects of, 892–895
in aneuploid carcinomas, 895
histological, 893, 893f, 894
in intraductal carcinoma, 893, 894f, 895
in invasive carcinoma, 895, 895f
in lymph node, 893, 894f
lymph node fibrosis in, 893, 894f
from neoadjuvant therapy, 892
residual carcinoma in, 892–893
from systemic therapy, 892
Children, breast tumors in, 729–747. *See also*
Juvenile
atypical duct hyperplasia, 739–741, 739f–742f
carcinoma, 745–747, 745f–747f
fibroadenoma, 742, 742f, 743f
juvenile papillomatosis, 729–735 (*See also*
Juvenile papillomatosis)
papilloma and papillary duct hyperplasia,
735–739, 736f–738f
clinical presentation of, 735
pathology of, gross, 735, 736f
pathology of, microscopic, 735, 736f–738f,
737
treatment and prognosis with, 737, 739
phyllodes tumor, 743–745, 743f–745f
Chloroma, 881
Chondroid differentiation, in spindle cell
carcinoma, 437, 439f
Chondrolipoma, 779–781, 780f
Chondroosseous carcinoma, 437, 437f–439f
Chondrosarcoma, 818–819, 819f
Choriocarcinoma, 425, 426f
Chromomycosis, 66, 66f
Chrondrosarcoma, in phyllodes tumor, 183, 187f
Circulation, arterial and venous, 3–4
Clear cell apocrine metaplasia, in sclerosing
adenosis, 141, 147f
Clear cells
in breast, 18–19, 18f, 19f
in breast metastases, from nonmammary
malignant neoplasms, 693, 693f
in intraductal carcinoma, 264, 266f–267f, 272f,
273
micropapillary, 272f, 273
in lobular carcinoma *in situ*, 594, 594f, 609, 609f
in lobules, 18–19, 18f, 19f
in lymph node metastases, axillary, 663, 665f
in myoepithelial cells, 18, 19f
in Paget's disease of the nipple, 571, 573f, 574f
in papillary carcinoma, solid, 391, 392f
in renal carcinoma, breast metastases from, 697,
699f
in squamous carcinoma, 459, 459f
Coccidioidomycosis, 66
Coenurosis, 69
Collagenous spherulosis, 114–117
clinical presentation of, 114–115
intraductal carcinoma in, 273, 273f
lobular carcinoma *in situ* in, 598, 598f–599f, 600
pathology of, 114–117, 114f–116f
in sclerosing adenosis, 145, 148f

Colonic carcinoid tumor, breast metastases from,
690, 692f
Colonic carcinoma, breast metastases from, 690,
691f
Columnar cell change, in tubular carcinoma,
373–374, 374f
Columnar cell ductal hyperplasia, 215–217,
217f–223f, 222–223
atypical, 217, 219f–222f
calcification in, 217, 218f–221f, 222–223, 223f
lobular carcinoma *in situ* with, 217, 222f
Comedo intraductal carcinoma, 276–278,
276f–278f
grade of, 288
Comedocarcinoma, 257–258
grade of, 288
Configuration, tumor, 332f–335f, 334. *See also*
specific tumors
Cooper's ligaments, 2–3
Coumadin, hemorrhagic necrosis from, 30
Cribriform, 239
Cribriform carcinoma, 257, 551–553, 552f
classic, 551–553, 552f
intraductal (*See also* Intraductal carcinoma)
historical background on, 257
pathology of, microscopic, 264, 265f–268f,
271f, 273–276, 273f–276f, 503f–504f
Cryptococcosis, 66
Cutaneous neoplasms, 899–911
malignant melanoma, 899–904, 900f, 902f
melanocytic lesions, 899, 900f–902f
nonmelanomatous mammary tumors, 904,
905f–911f, 908–909
adnexal gland carcinoma, 904, 905f–908f, 908
apocrine, 904, 905f
in axillary skin, 904, 907f, 908
of chest wall skin, 904, 908, 908f
cribriform, 904, 906f
with intraductal carcinoma, 904, 907f
papillary, 904, 905f
*in situ*, 904, 907f
tubulolobular, 904, 906f
basal cell carcinoma, 909, 909f
basal-squamous carcinoma, 909, 910f
eccrine spiradenoma, 909, 910f
hidradenoma
of nipple axillary skin, 909, 910f
subareolar, 909, 910f
immunohistochemical markers of, 904, 907f,
908, 908f
immunoreactivity of, 908
nevoid hyperkeratosis, 909, 910f
of nipple, 908–909, 909f–910f
sebaceous adenoma of nipple, 909, 910f
Cyclin D1, 355–356
with atypical hyperplasia, 241
Cylindroma, 535. *See also* Adenoid cystic
carcinoma
Cystadenomas, papillary, 77
Cystic apocrine metaplasia, 96–101
clinical presentation of, 96–97
immunohistochemistry and electron microscopy
of, 100
pathology of
gross, 97
microscopic, 97–100, 98f–100f
prognosis and treatment of, 100–101
Cystic fibrosis, 56
Cystic hypersecretory carcinoma, 527–534
age distribution of, 527
fine needle aspiration of, 534, 534f
pathology of, gross, 527–528, 527f–528f
pathology of, microscopic, 528–534, 528f–534f
cysts with flat epithelium, 528, 528f–529f
histiocytes, 528, 529f
intraductal, 529, 530f–532f, 532
invasive, 532–533, 533f
invasive lobular carcinoma and, 533–534,
533f

in lobules, 529, 532f
prognosis and treatment of, 534
Cystic hypersecretory hyperplasia, 15, 18f,
527–534
pathology of, microscopic, 528–529, 529f–530f
with atypia, 528–529, 530f
with pregnancy-like hyperplasia, 529, 532,
532f
Cystic hypersecretory intraductal carcinoma, 273
Cystic papillary mucinous carcinoma, 467, 467f
Cystic papilloma
metaplastic carcinoma in, 426, 427f–428f
mucocele-like tumor in, 470, 473f
Cysticercosis, 69–70, 69f
Cytogenetics
of fibroadenoma, 164
of intraductal carcinoma, 295–296
Cytokeratin(s)
atypical hyperplasia with, 243–244
in metastatic carcinoma, 448–450, 448f–450f
*vs.* vimentin expression, 449–450
Cytokeratin AE1/AE3 reactivity, 448–449, 448f,
449f
Cytokeratin CK, 449, 450f
Cytosarcoma phyllodes, 176–197. *See also*
Phyllodes tumor

**D**

Dermatofibrosarcoma protuberans, 825–827, 826f
Dermatomyositis, 46–47
Developmental abnormalities, mammary, 23–26
aberrant breast tissue, 26
ectopic breast tissue, 25–26, 26f
hypoplasia and amastia, 23, 24f
macromastia, 23–25, 24f
transsexual breast, 26
Diabetic mastopathy, 53–56
clinical presentation of, 54, 54t
etiology of, 53
pathology of
gross, 54, 55f
microscopic, 54–56, 55f, 56f
prognosis and treatment of, 56
*Dracunculus medinensis,* 70
Duct carcinoma, invasive. *See* Invasive duct
carcinoma
Duct ectasia, of male breast, 703
Duct stasis, 35–36, 36f, 37f
Ductal adenoma, 77, 167
Ductal hyperplasia, 201–226
atypical, 213–215, 214f–216f
borderline lesions, 223–225, 224f, 225f
clinical presentation of, 203
columnar cell, 215–217, 217f–223f, 222–223
atypical, 217, 219f–222f
calcification in, 217, 218f–221f, 222–223,
223f
lobular carcinoma *in situ* with, 217, 222f
genetic abnormalities in, 201–202
investigational studies of, 201–203
with lobular extension, 614, 615f
needle core biopsy of, 225–226
ordinary (usual), 203–212
cytology of, 204–205, 205f
fenestrated, 212, 212f
florid, 205f, 207–208, 210–212, 210f–212f
histiocytes in, 210, 212f
micropapillary, 207, 207f, 208f
mild, 206f, 207–208
moderate, 206f, 207–208
"streaming," 207, 208f
in terminal duct lobular unit, 204, 205f
pathology of, gross, 203
pretubular, 216
prognosis and treatment of, 226
subareolar sclerosing, 94–96, 94f, 95f
Ductal intraepithelial neoplasia, 201. *See also*
Ductal hyperplasia

**E**

E-cadherin
  in atypical lobular hyperplasia, 614
  in distinction between ductal and lobular
    carcinoma, 609, 610
  in gastric carcinoma, 645
  in intraductal carcinoma, 294, iif
  in invasive lobular carcinoma, 638
  in lobular carcinoma *in situ*, 581, 589, 590, 594,
    600, 608, 609, iif
Eccrine spiradenoma, of axillary skin, 909, 910f
*Echinococcus granulosus,* 70
Ectopic breast tissue, 25–26, 26f
  carcinoma in, 673–676, 673f–676f
    in aberrant breast, 676, 676f
    in axilla, 674, 674f
      with invasive lobular carcinoma, 673, 673f
    in mediastinal teratoma, 674, 675f, 676
    in residual breast after mastectomy, 674, 674f,
      675f
Elastic tissue fibers, 6–7
Elastosis
  in invasive duct carcinoma, 351, 351f
  in tubular carcinoma, 373, 373f
Elderly, carcinoma in, 654–656
EMA, 448
Embryology, 1
Embryonal rhabdomyosarcoma, breast metastases
  from, 692f, 693
Endocrine features, of mammary carcinoma,
  497–501, 498f–500f. *See also* Mammary
  carcinoma with endocrine features
Endocrine intraductal carcinoma, 281
Endometrial carcinoma, breast metastases from,
  697, 698f
Epidermal growth factor receptor (EGF-R)
  with atypical hyperplasia, 241–242
  in intraductal carcinoma, 294, 294f
Epithelial cells. *See also* specific types, e.g.,
  Fibroepithelial, Myoepithelial
  mesenchymal conversion of, 426, 428
Epithelial hyperplasia, in phyllodes tumor
  atypical, 188, 190f
  florid, 188, 190f
Epithelial–stromal junction, 6–7, 8f
Epitheliosis, 204. *See also* Ductal hyperplasia
Estrogen receptor(s)
  in breast, 11
  in intraductal carcinoma, 291–292, 292f
  nuclear immunoreactivity of, 82, 84f
    in atypical hyperplasia, 242
  in papillary carcinoma, 382, 382f, 396, 398f
Estrogen replacement, effect on breast lobule,
  14–15, 14f
Estrogen treatment, effects of, 895–896
Examination
  breast, tumors detected by, 655
  of breast and lymph node specimens, 931–982
Extranodal sinus histiocytosis, with massive
  lymphadenopathy, 875, 876f–877f


**F**

Fat necrosis, 29–30, 30f
  with calcification, in non-Hodgkin's lymphoma,
    868, 871, 871f
  from radiation, 888f, 889
Fibroadenoma, 163–176
  adenosis in, 149, 149f
  adolescent giant, 165
  angiomatosis in, 798, 799f
  carcinomas in, 656–661
    clinical presentation of, 656–657
    pathology of, gross, 657
    pathology of, microscopic, 657–660,
      657f–659f
    prognosis and treatment of, 661
  in children and adolescents, 742, 742f, 743f

clinical presentation of, 164–167, 165f
complex, 170, 171f
cystic, 166f, 167
cytogenetic abnormalities in, 164
cytology of, 175–176
giant, 742
incidence of, 163
intracanalicular, 168
origin of, 167–168
pathology of, gross, 166f, 167
pathology of, microscopic, 167–175, 167f–176f
  complex, 170, 171f
  epithelial–stromal balance in, 168, 168f, 169f
  histologic hallmark in, 168
  with invasive duct carcinoma, 171, 172f
  juvenile, 171, 173–175, 173f–176f
  with lactating adenoma, 171, 172f, 173f
  with lobular carcinoma *in situ,* 171, 172f
  myoid stroma, 169, 169f
  myxoid stroma, 169–170, 170f
  with sclerosing adenosis, 170, 171f
  stromal giant cells, 169, 170f
pericanalicular, 168
risk factors for, 163–164
treatment and prognosis of, 176
Fibroadenomatoid gynecomastia, male, 703, 704f
Fibroadenomatoid mastopathy, 163, 164f
Fibrocystic breast changes, 139, 170, 171f,
  231–244. *See also under* Precancerous
  breast disease
Fibrocystic disease, 231–232
Fibroepithelial neoplasms, 163–197
  fibroadenoma, 163–176 (*See also* Fibroadenoma)
  fibroadenomatoid mastopathy, 163, 164f
  of male breast, 703, 704f
  phyllodes tumor, 176–197 (*See also* Phyllodes
    tumor)
  sclerosing lobular hyperplasia, 163, 164f
Fibrolipoma, 786, 786f
Fibroma-type inclusions, in phyllodes tumor, 192,
  193f
Fibromatosis, 749–757, 813. *See also* Sarcoma(s)
  chest wall invasion, 756, 756f
  clinical presentation of, 749–750, 750f
  historical perspective on, 749
  pathology of, gross, 750, 750f, 751f
  pathology of, microscopic, 751–756, 751f–755f
    invasive border, 753, 754f, 755f
    keloidal, 751, 751f–752f
    lymphocytic aggregates, 753, 754f
    lymphocytic infiltrates, focal, 753, 755f
    myxoid, 753, 753f
      with calcifications, 753, 754f
    nuclear atypia, 751, 753f
    spindle cells
      with nuclear pleomorphism, 751, 752f
      without nuclear atypia, 751, 752f
    storiform and interlacing, 753, 753f
  treatment and prognosis with, 756–757
Fibrosarcoma, 821–823, 822f
Fibrous tumor, 757, 757f
Filariasis, 66–69, 67f, 68f
Fine needle aspiration (FNA)
  of medullary carcinoma, 420–421, 420f
  for proliferative (fibrocystic) breast changes,
    232–233
Flat micropapillary carcinoma, 269f, 273
Florid adenosis, 139, 141, 141f–143f
  in pregnancy, 141, 143f
Florid papillomatosis of the nipple, 94, 101–111
  clinical features of, 101–102
  historical perspective on, 101
  in male breast, 703
  mammary carcinoma and, 104–105, 107–109,
    107f–111f
    infiltrating, 109, 110f
    intraductal, 105, 107, 107f
    invasive, 107, 108f

occult, with lymph node metastases, 107–109,
  108f–109f
Paget's disease in, 109, 110f
pathology of, 102–104, 102f–106f
  adenosis, 104, 105f
  mixed proliferative, 104, 106f
  papilloma, 102, 104, 104f
  sclerosing papilloma, 102, 103f
as precancerous, 109
treatment and follow-up of, 109–110
Flow cytometry
  of DNA aneuploidy, with atypical hyperplasia,
    240
  of invasive lobular carcinoma, 639
  of mucinous carcinoma, 478
  of ploidy, 353–354
  of S-fraction, 353–354
Fodrin, atypical hyperplasia with, 242–243
Follicular phase, lobule in, 9, 9f
Foreign bodies, 982–983
Fungal infections, 65–66, 66f


**G**

Galactoceles, 33, 33f
Gastric carcinoma
  breast metastases from, 690, 691f
  E-cadherin in, 645
GCDFP-15, in apocrine carcinoma, 493
Genetic predisposition, to precancerous breast
  disease, 229–231
Genetics. *See also* Cytogenetics
  of atypical hyperplasia, 239–244
  of intraductal carcinoma, 295–296
  of invasive duct carcinoma, 326–327
  of invasive lobular carcinoma, 639
  of lobular carcinoma *in situ*, 609
  of medullary carcinoma, 421
  of non-Hodgkin's lymphoma, 875
  on prognosis, 326–327
Giant cell arteritis, 43–44, 44f
Giant cell fibroblastoma, 775
Giant cells, in medullary carcinoma, 418f, 419
Giant fibroadenoma, 742
Glands of Montgomery, 5
  duct of, 7, 8f
  histology of, 7, 8f
Glycogen-rich carcinoma, 557–559, 557f, 558f
Grading, 334–339. *See also* specific cancers, e.g.,
  Intraductal carcinoma, grading of
  Bloom-Richardson histologic, 337, 338t
  field areas in, 337
  field size in, 337
  histologic, 336, 336f
  of intraductal carcinoma, 288–290, 288f, 289f,
    289t, 290t
  mitotic figures in, 337, 337t
  mitotic rate in, 336–337
  nuclear, 334–336, 335f (*See also* Nuclear grade)
  prognosis and, 337–338
  reproducibility of, 338–339
Granular cell tumor, 775–778
  clinical presentation of, 775–776
  malignant, 777, 778f
  pathology of
    gross, 776, 777f
    microscopic, 776–777, 777f, 778f
  prognosis and treatment of, 777–778, 778f
Granulocytic sarcoma, 881–882, 882f
Granuloma
  plasmacytic, 880, 881f
  sarcoid-like, in carcinoma, 41, 42f
  silicone, 49–51, 50f
Granulomatous angiopanniculitis, 47, 47f
Granulomatous lobular mastitis, 38–40, 39f, 40f
Gravid macromastia, 24–25, 24f
Growth factors. *See also* specific factors, e.g.,
  Insulin-like growth factor
  with atypical hyperplasia, 241–242

Growth rate, tumor, in invasive duct carcinoma, 353–356
  clinical assessment of, 353
  immunohistochemical assessment of, 354–356
  nuclear morphometry of, 356
  S-fraction and ploidy in, 353–354
Guinea worm, 70
Gynecomastia, of male breast, 704–711, 705f–711f
  apocrine metaplasia, 707, 708f
  duct hyperplasia, atypical, 709, 709f–710f
  electron microscopy of, 711
  fine needle aspiration cytology of, 711
  florid, 705, 705f, 706f
  inactive, 706f, 707
  lobular differentiation, 707, 707f, 708f
  pseudoangiomatous stromal hyperplasia, 707, 707f
  pseudolactational hyperplasia, 707, 708f
  regression of, 711
  squamous metaplasia, 707–708, 709f
Gynecomastia-like hyperplasia
  in female breast, 706f, 707

**H**
Hamartoma, 779–781, 780f
  myoid (muscular), 135, 135f, 782–783, 783f
Hellenzellen, 18
Hemangiomas, 789–797, 790f–797f, 924–925
  vs. angiosarcoma, 840
  clinical presentation of, 789, 790f
  metastasizing, 840
  needle core biopsy of, 797, 797f
  nonparenchymal, of mammary region, 803–806, 803f–806f
    clinical presentation of, 803
    pathology of, 803–806, 803f–806f
    prognosis and treatment of, 806
  pathology of, gross, 789
  pathology of, microscopic, 789–797, 791f–797f
    capillary, 792, 793f–794f
      nonparenchymal, 803, 805f
    cavernous, 789, 791, 791f–792
      nonparenchymal, 803, 804f
    complex, 792, 795f
    necrosis, 792, 796f
    noncavernous, 791–792
    septal fibrosis, 796f, 797
  perilobular, 787–789, 787t, 788f
  treatment and prognosis with, 797
  venous, 800–803, 801f, 802f
    clinical presentation of, 800
    pathology of, gross, 800
    pathology of, microscopic, 800–802, 801f, 802f
    prognosis and treatment of, 802–803
Hemangiopericytoma, 823–825, 824f, 825f
  clinical presentation of, 823
  metastases of, 825, 825f
  pathology of
    gross, 823
    microscopic, 823–825, 824f–826f
  prognosis and treatment of, 825, 825f
Hemorrhagic necrosis, from anticoagulants, 30
HER-2/neu oncogene (HER2), 240
  in intraductal carcinoma, 292–293, 293f
Herpes simplex, 72
Heterologous metaplasia, 437, 437f–440f, 442–443, 443f
Heterotropic glands
  clinical presentation, 913
  pathology of, 913–916, 915f, 916f
Hibernoma, 786, 786f
Hidradenoma
  of axillary skin, 909, 910f
  of nipple, 909, 910f
  subareolar, 909, 910f
Histiocytoma, malignant fibrous, 819–821, 820f, 821f

clinical presentation of, 819
pathology of, 820–821, 820f, 821f
treatment and prognosis with, 821
Histiocytosis, idiopathic, 875, 876f–877f
Histogenesis, histologic phenotype and, 425
Histologic grading, 336, 336f
  Bloom-Richardson, 337, 338t
Histologic phenotype
  histogenesis and, 425
  tissue of origin and, 425
Histopathologic grade, 255
Histopathologic types, 255
Histoplasmosis, 65–66
HIV infection, of breast, 73
Hodgkin's disease, 877–878, 877f, 878f
  radiation therapy effects from, 887
Hormone-replacement therapy (HRT), breast design and, 242
Hormone treatment effect, 895–896
Hotspots, 346, 347f
Hyperplasia
  adenoid cystic (See Collagenous spherulosis)
  atypical (See under Precancerous breast disease, proliferative (fibrocystic) breast changes)
  atypical duct, juvenile, 739–741, 739f–742f
  vs. atypical hyperplasia and carcinoma in situ, 238–239
  atypical lobular, 610–617 (See also Atypical lobular hyperplasia)
  cystic hypersecretory, 15, 18f
  ductal, 201–226 (See also Ductal hyperplasia)
    subareolar sclerosing, 94–96, 94f, 95f
  epithelial, in phyllodes tumor
    atypical, 188, 190f
    florid, 188, 190f
  lobular
    atypical, 610–617 (See also Atypical lobular hyperplasia)
    in pregnancy, 11–13, 12f
    of nipple ducts, sclerosing papillary, 94–96, 94f, 95f
  papillary endothelial, in nonparenchymal hemangioma, 803, 804f
  pregnancy-like, 15, 16f, 17f
    atypical, 15, 17f, 18f
    laminated secretion in, 15, 17f
  pseudoangiomatous stromal, 757–766, 758f–765f (See also Pseudoangiomatous stromal hyperplasia)
    invasive duct carcinoma in, 348, 350f
  sclerosing lobular, 163, 164f
Hypoplasia, mammary, 23, 24f

**I**
Idiopathic histiocytosis, 875, 876f–877f
Immunoglobulin localization, cyclical variation in, 10–11
Immunohistochemistry. See also specific disorders, e.g., Phyllodes tumor, immunohistochemistry of
  proliferation assessment of, 354–356
Immunophenotype, tissue of origin and, 425
Implants, breast, 49–53. See also Silicone mastitis
  infections from, 74
  pathologic examination of, 981–982
In situ (intraepithelial) carcinoma, 249–250
  with ductal lobular features, 284, 286, 287f
  vs. hyperplasia and atypical hyperplasia, 238–239
In situ lobular carcinoma. See Lobular carcinoma in situ
Incidence. See also specific disorders, e.g., Fibroadenoma, incidence of
  changes in, 331
Infantile breast
  development of, 1–2, 2f
  with lobule, 1, 2f
Infarct
  in adenomyoepithelioma, 127, 128f

breast, 30–32, 31f, 32f
  mammary, 32–33
  in papillary carcinoma, 31–32, 32f
  in papilloma, 82, 85f
  in sclerosing adenosis, postpartum, 31, 31f, 32–33, 33f
Infections, 65–74
  abscesses
    breast, 73, 73f
    subareolar, 73–74
  cat scratch disease, 72–73
  fungal, 65–66, 66f
  HIV, 73
  mycobacterial, 70–72, 71f, 72f
  parasitic, 66–70
    coenurosis, 69
    cysticercosis, 69–70, 69f
    Dracunculus medinensis, 70
    Echinococcus granulosus, 70
    filariasis, 66–69, 67f, 68f
    Liesegang's rings, 70
    Schistosoma japonicum, 69
    sparganosis, 70
    Trichinella, 70
  typhoid mastitis, 72
  viral, 72
Infiltrating duct carcinoma, 463
  in children and adolescents, 745, 746f
  with endocrine features, 500
  with medullary features, 410 (See also Medullary carcinoma)
  with mucinous component, 463, 465, 466f
Infiltrating lobular carcinoma, vs. non-Hodgkin's lymphoma, 867–868, 869f
Inflammatory and reactive tumors, 29–58
  amyloid tumor, 56–58, 57f, 58f
  breast infarct, 30–32, 31f, 32f
  cystic fibrosis, 56
  diabetic mastopathy, 53–56
    clinical presentation of, 54, 54t
    etiology of, 53
    pathology of, gross, 54, 55f
    pathology of, microscopic, 54–56, 55f, 56f
    prognosis and treatment of, 56
  fat necrosis, 29–30, 30f
  galactoceles, 33, 33f
  granulomatous lobular mastitis, 38–40, 39f, 40f
  hemorrhagic necrosis, from anticoagulant therapy, 30
  inflammatory pseudotumor, 42–43, 43f
  mammary duct ectasia, 34–38, 35f–38f
    clinical presentation of, 35
    etiology of, 34–35
    pathology of, gross, 35
    pathology of, microscopic, 35–38, 36f–38f
    treatment and prognosis of, 38
  mammary infarcts, 32–33
  paraffinoma, 48–49
  plasma cell mastitis, 33–34, 34f
  puerperal mastitis, 32
  Raynaud's phenomenon, in nipple, 33
  sarcoid-like granulomas in carcinoma, 41, 42f
  sarcoidosis, 40–42, 41f, 42f
  silicone mastitis and breast augmentation pathology, 49–53
    clinical presentation of, 49
    etiology of, 49
    pathology of, gross, 49, 50f
    pathology of, microscopic, 49–53, 50f–52f
    treatment and prognosis of, 53
  vasculitis, 43–48 (See also Vasculitis)
Inflammatory carcinoma, 676–683
  chemotherapy effect in, 682f, 683
  clinical features of, 677–678, 677f, 678f
  historical perspective on, 676–677
  pathology of, gross, 679, 679f
  pathology of, microscopic, 679–681, 679f–682f
    occult, 681
    primary, 679–681, 679f, 680f

recurrent, 681, 681f, 682f
primary, 677–678, 677f, 678f
prognosis and treatment of, 681–683, 682f
secondary (recurrent), 677, 678, 678f
Inflammatory lesions
in lactation, 32–33
in pregnancy, 32–33, 33f
Inflammatory pseudotumor, 42–43, 43f
Inflammatory recurrent carcinoma, 681, 681f, 682f.
*See also* Inflammatory carcinoma
Initiation, 231
Insulin-like growth factor (IGF), with atypical
hyperplasia, 242
Insulin-like growth factor receptor (IGF-R), with
atypical hyperplasia, 242
Integrins, atypical hyperplasia with, 243
Internal mammary lymph nodes, 254
Interpectoral lymph nodes, 254
Intracanalicular fibroadenoma, 168. *See also*
Fibroadenoma
Intracystic papilloma, 77
Intraductal carcinoma, 257–317
adnexal gland carcinoma with, 904, 907f
age range for, 262
angiogenesis in, 290–291, 291f
bilaterality of, 262–263
calcifications with, 259–260, 260f
clinical presentation of, 258–263, 260f, 261f
in collagenous spherulosis, 273, 273f
cribriform, 503f
cytogenetics and molecular genetics in, 295–296
cytologic diagnosis of, 298, 299f
ductogram of, 261–262, 261f
E-cadherin in, 294, iif
epidermal growth factor receptor in, 294, 294f
estrogen receptors in, 291–292, 292f
frozen sections of, 262
grading of, 288–290, 288f, 289f, 289t, 290t
high grade, 288–290, 288f, 289f, 289t
historical background on, 257–258
hormone receptors in, 291–292, 292f
incidence of, 258–259
laciform, 257
lobular carcinoma *in situ* with, 600, 600f
low grade, 288–290, 289f, 289t
mammary carcinoma with osteoclast-like giant
cells in, 522, 522f
mammography of, 259–260, 260f
margins of excision of, 310
in microglandular adenosis, 155, 156f
microinvasion in, 301–310, 302f–308f
basement membrane in, 301, 302f
defined, 303–305, 303f, 304f, 309–310
determination of, difficulty in, 308–309
immunostains of, 305–306, 305f
*vs.* invasive duct carcinoma, 306–307, 307f,
308f
with lymphocytic accumulation, 305, 305f
*vs.* minimally invasive carcinoma, 303
with poorly defined duct walls, 303, 303f
MRI of, 261
mucocele-like tumor with, 474, 475f, 476f
multicentricity and multifocality of, 300–301
needle core biopsy of, 296–298, 297f, 298f
nm23 gene product in, 294
oncogenes in, 292–294
HER2-*neu,* 292–293, 293f
p53, 293–294, 294f
palpable tumors in, 261
pathology of, gross, 263, 263f
pathology of, microscopic, 264–287
apocrine, 264, 266f, 271f, 272f, 298f
cribriform, 274, 276f
apoptosis, 279
basal lamina, 264, 265f
*bcl-2* expression in, 279, 279f, 295
classification difficulties in, 276, 276f
clear cell, 264, 266f–267f, 272f, 273
comedo, 276–278, 276f–278f, 288

cribriform, 257, 264, 265f–268f, 271f,
273–276, 273f–276f, 299f, 503f–504f
apocrine, 274, 276f
microlumens in, 274, 274f, 275f, 299f
with necrosis and mitotic activity, 274, 276,
276f
crystalloids in, 272f, 278, 278f
cytologic features of, 268, 268f
dimorphic, 264, 267, 267f
duct diameter and necrosis in, 279
dystrophic calcification in, 276f, 278
endocrine, 281
"healing," 279, 280f
with LCIS in single duct–lobular unit, 286,
288f
lobular extension of, 284, 286, 286f
micropapillary, 264, 266f, 268, 268f–272f,
270, 373f
apocrine, 271f
clear cell, 272f, 273
cystic hypersecretory, 273
flat, 269f, 273
fronds in, 270, 270f, 271f
with intermediate-/high-grade cytology,
268f, 271f, 272f, 273
nuclei in, 270, 270f–271f, 273
with squamous metaplasia, 272f, 273
mixed histologic patterns, 267–268
monomorphic, 264
myoepithelial cells, 264, 265f
papillary, 281
periductal fibrosis, 279, 280f
in radial sclerosing lesions, 284, 285f, 286f
in sclerosing adenosis, 282f–284f, 283–284,
298f
signet-ring cells, 264, 265f
site of origin, 264
*vs. in situ* carcinoma with ductal lobular
features, 284, 286, 287f
with *in situ* lobular carcinoma, 284, 286f
small cell, 281–283, 282f
solid, 279–281, 280f, 281f
spindle cell, 281, 281f
ploidy in, 294–295
proliferative rate in, 295, 295f
radiation effect in, 891, 891f
revertant, 306–307, 307f
risk factors for, 259
size and quantity of, 299–300
treatment and prognosis of, 310–317
breast-conserving surgery and radiotherapy,
311–316
recurrences after, 313–316, 314t
mastectomy, 310–311
recommendations for, 316–317
in tubular carcinoma, 373, 373f–375f
Intraductal medullary carcinoma, 416f, 417
Intraepithelial *(in situ)* carcinoma, 249–250
with ductal lobular features, 284, 286, 287f
*vs.* hyperplasia and atypical hyperplasia,
238–239
Intraepithelial neoplasia, 250
Intramammary lymph nodes, pathology of,
925–927, 926f, 927f
Invasive duct carcinoma, 325–356
with basal lamina components, 307, 308f
definition of, 325
elastosis in, 351, 351f
with fibroadenoma, 171, 172f
incidence of, 325
with intraductal carcinoma pattern, 306–307,
307f
myofibroblastic reaction in, 350, 351f
prognosis assessment in, 326–331 (*See also*
Prognosis assessment, in invasive duct
carcinoma)
prognostic markers in, morphologic, 331–353
microscopic histopathologic, 334–353 (*See
also under* Prognostic markers, in
invasive duct carcinoma)

pathology, gross, 331–334, 332f, 333f
size and nodal status in, 333
tumor configuration/shape in, 332f–335f,
334
tumor size in, 331, 333
tumor size in, measurement of, 333–334
in pseudoangiomatous stromal hyperplasia, 348,
350f
tumor growth rate in, 353–356
clinical assessment of, 353
immunohistochemical assessment of, 354–356
nuclear morphometry of, 356
S-fraction and ploidy in, flow cytometry of,
353–354
Invasive lobular carcinoma, 627–648
clinical features of, 627–629
cystic hypersecretory carcinoma and, 533–534,
533f
cytology of, 639, 639f
E-cadherin in, 638
ectopic breast carcinoma in axilla with, 673, 673f
electron microscopy of, 639
flow cytometry of, 639
histochemistry of, 638
historical perspective on, 627
immunohistochemistry of, 638–639
metastasis patterns of, 640–645, 640f–644f
with appendiceal carcinoid tumor, 644f, 645
endometrial, 643, 643f
lymph node, 640, 640f, 641f
orbital, 642, 642f
ovarian, 643, 643f
signet-ring cell histiocytes, 640, 641f
sinus catarrh, 640
stomach, 643–645, 644f
molecular genetics of, 639
pathology of, gross, 629
pathology of, microscopic, 629–638, 630f–638f
classic, 629, 630f
invasive, 630, 631f, 633f
alveolar, 634–635, 634f
dispersed, 630, 633f
granulomatous, 630, 632f
lymphocytic, 630, 631f, 632f
with mucin, 635, 635f
needle core biopsy, 630, 634f
occult, 630, 633f
periductal, 630, 631f
perineural invasion, 636, 638f
pleomorphic, 636, 636f, 637f
signet-ring cells, 635, 636f
solid, 634, 634f
trabecular, 629, 630f, 634–635
prognosis and treatment of, 645–648, 645f–647f
Invasive micropapillary carcinoma, 561–564
clinical presentation of, 561
pathology of, gross, 561
pathology of, microscopic, 561–564, 562f, 563f
apocrine, 561, 562f
intraductal, 563, 563f
lymph node metastasis, 563, 563f
mucinous carcinoma and, 563, 563f
prognosis and treatment of, 564
Invasive tubulolobular carcinoma, small cell
carcinoma with, 503, 505f
Ipsilateral lymph nodes, 254

**J**

Juvenile. *See also* Children
Juvenile atypical duct hyperplasia, 739–741,
739f–742f
Juvenile carcinoma. *See* Secretory carcinoma
Juvenile papillomatosis, 729–735
age distribution of, 729, 729f
carcinoma and, 733–734, 733f–735f
clinical presentation of, 729–730, 729f
mammography of, 729, 729f
pathology of, gross, 730, 730f

Juvenile papillomatosis (*contd.*)
 pathology of, microscopic, 731–733, 731f–733f
  apocrine metaplasia, 731, 732f
  cysts, 731, 731f
  duct hyperplasia, 731, 731f, 732f
  epithelial necrosis, 731, 733f
  histiocytes, 731, 732f
 treatment and prognosis with, 734–735
 tumor size at diagnosis in, 730, 730f

**K**

K903, 448–449
Kaposi's sarcoma, 828–829
Ki67, 355
 in apocrine carcinoma, 494
 in medullary carcinoma, 420, 420f

**L**

Laciform carcinoma, 257
Lactating adenoma, *vs.* fibroadenoma, 171, 172f, 173f
Lactation
 carcinoma in, 653–654
 histology of, 12f, 13, 13f
 inflammatory lesions in, 32–33
Lactational mastitis, 73, 73f
Lactiferous duct, major, 5–6, 5f, 6f
Lamprocytosis, 18
LCIS, with intraductal carcinoma, in single duct–lobular unit, 286, 288f
Leiomyosarcoma, 815–816, 815f–817f
 breast metastases from, 697, 698f
Leukemia, lymphocytic, 882
Leukemic infiltration, 881–882, 882f
Lewis-X antigens, 231
Liesegang's rings, 70
Lipid-rich carcinoma, 555–556, 555f
Lipofuscin, carcinoma with, 904, 904f. *See also* Malignant melanoma
Lipoma, 786, 786f–787f
Lipomatous hamartoma, with phyllodes tumor, 183, 185f
Lipomatous metaplasia, with phyllodes tumor, 183, 184f
Liposarcoma, 817–818, 817f–818f
 in phyllodes tumor, 183, 187f
Lobular cancerization, 273, 296
Lobular carcinoma, 426, 427f
 historical perspective on, 627
 invasive (*See* Invasive lobular carcinoma)
 with juvenile papillomatosis, 733, 734f
 Paget's disease with, 569, 569f
 signet-ring cells in, 372f
Lobular carcinoma *in situ*, 581–609, 582f, 585t–610t
 bilaterality of, 583–584, 583t
  histological types in, 584, 584t
 clinical presentation of, 582–585
 differential diagnosis of, 609, 609f–610f
 electron microscopy of, 608
 with fibroadenoma, 171, 172f
 frequency of, 581–582
 historical perspective on, 581, 582f, 627
 immunohistochemistry of, 608
 with intraductal carcinoma, 284, 286f
 invasive carcinoma with
  concurrent, risk of, 621
  subsequent, risk of, 618–621, 620f
 with juvenile papillomatosis, 733, 733f
 management of
  clinical, 621–623
  mastectomy, 623
  radiation and chemotherapy, 623–624
 molecular genetics of, 609
 multicentricity of, 584–585
 pathology of, gross, 585
 pathology of, microscopic, 585–610, 585f–610f

*vs.* apocrine differentiation, 609, 610f
 in apocrine intraductal carcinoma, 600, 600f
 apocrine metaplasia, 609, 610f
 classic, 590, 591f
  small cell, 590, 591f
 clear cell change, 609, 609f
 clear cells, 594, 594f
 cloverleaf ductal, 596, 597f
 in collagenous spherulosis, 598, 598f–599f, 600
 degenerative changes, 590, 590f
 duct extension, 594, 596f
 E-cadherin in, 581, 589, 590, 594, 600, 608, 609, iif
 in fat, 606, 607f
 florid, with focal necrosis, 588f–589f, 589
 glandular distension
  absent, 585–586, 586f–587f
  marked, 585–586, 585f, 586f
 with intraductal carcinoma, 600, 600f
 lobular distension, 586, 589
 lobular involvement, partial, 586, 587f, 589–590, 590f
 microinvasive, 606, 606f, 608, 608f
 mosaic, 594, 595f
 mucin
  glandular lumen, 592, 593f
  intracytoplasmic, 592, 592f, 594
 myoid, 594, 595f
  pleomorphic, 594, 595f
 pagetoid
  duct involvement, 596, 597f, 598f
  lobular involvement, 596, 598f
  spread, 596
 in papilloma, 600, 601f
 pleomorphic, 590, 591f
  large cell, 590, 591f
 post-menopausal, 594, 596, 596f
 in radial sclerosing lesions, 600, 601f
 in sclerosing adenosis, 600, 602f–606f, 603, 606
 signet-ring cells, 592, 593f
 in tubular adenosis, 603, 603f–604f
 typical, 585, 585f
 prognosis with, 614, 617, 617t
 radiation effect in, 891, 891f
 small cell carcinoma with, 503, 505f
 tubular carcinoma with, 374–375, 375f
 tumor type in ipsilateral/contralateral breasts, 584, 584t
 untreated, subsequent risk with, 585, 585t
Lobular extension, in medullary carcinoma, 411, 411f
 secondary nodule from, 417–418, 417f
Lobular hyperplasia
 atypical, prognosis with, 614, 617
 in pregnancy, 11–13, 12f
Lobular hyperplasia, atypical, 610–617
 clinical presentation of, 610
 management of, clinical, 621–623
 pathology of, 610f–614f, 611, 613–614
  borderline, 613, 613f
  *vs.* duct hyperplasia with lobular extension, 614, 615f
  in ducts, 614, 615f–616f
  cloverleaf, 613–614, 614f
Lobular involution, postlactational, 13–14, 13f
Lobular lymphocytic reaction extension, in medullary carcinoma, 411, 411f
Lobular neoplasia, 250, 617. *See also* Lobular carcinoma *in situ*
 *vs.* lobular carcinoma *in situ*, 617–618
Lobule(s)
 clear cell change in, 18–19, 18f, 19f
 effect of estrogen replacement on, 14–15, 14f
 in follicular phase, 9, 9f
 in luteal phase, 10, 10f
 menopausal atrophy of, 14, 14f
 in menstrual phase, 10, 10f

myoid metaplasia in, 6, 7f
 in nipple, 6, 6f
 in proliferative phase, 9, 9f
 in rat breast, 6, 7f
 in secretory phase, 10, 10f
Loss of heterozygosity (LOH), 231
 in apocrine carcinoma, 494
 on cancer progression, 326–327
 in intraductal carcinoma, 296
Lung metastasis, 442, 443f
Lupus mastopathy, 47–48, 48f
Luteal phase, lobule in, 10, 10f
Lymph node(s)
 in carcinoma staging, 254, 255
 regional, 254
Lymph node metastases, axillary, in occult carcinoma, 661–673
 biopsy of, excisional, 668
 clinical presentation of, 661–662
 immunohistochemistry of, 668
 lymphocytic reaction in, 668, 669f
 mucicarmine stain of, 666
 pathology of, gross, 662–663, 663f
 pathology of, microscopic, 663–669, 664f–669f
  apocrine, 663, 664f–665f
  clear cell, 663, 665f
  cribriform, 666, 667f
  diffuse, 663, 665f–666f
  metastatic, 666, 668f
  tubular type, 663, 666, 667f
  patterns of, 663, 663t
 prognosis with, 670–673, 670t, 671f, 671t
  lymph node status and, 670, 672f
  overall survival, 670–671, 671f
  tumor size and, 670, 672f
 treatment of, 669–670
Lymphangioma, recurrent, as angiomatosis, 800, 800f
Lymphatic drainage, 4
Lymphatic tumor emboli, 342–343, 342f, 343f
Lymphoblastic infiltrate, 341–342, 341f
Lymphocytic leukemia, 882
Lymphomas. *See* specific types, e.g., Non-Hodgkin's lymphoma, Hodgkin's disease
Lymphoplasmacytic reaction, in medullary carcinoma, 410–411, 410f, 412f

**M**

Macromastia, 23–25, 24f
 adolescent, 23–24, 24f
 gravid, 24–25, 24f
 penicillamine-induced, 25
Male breast, benign proliferative lesions of, 703–711, 706f, 707
 benign proliferative changes, 703–704
 duct ectasia, 703
 fibroepithelial tumors, 703, 704f
 florid papillomatosis of the nipple, 703
 gynecomastia, 704–711, 705f–711f
  apocrine metaplasia, 707, 708f
  duct hyperplasia, atypical, 709, 709f–710f
  electron microscopy of, 711
  fine needle aspiration cytology of, 711
  florid, 705, 705f, 706f
  inactive, 706f, 707
  lobular differentiation, 707, 707f, 708f
  pseudoangiomatous stromal hyperplasia, 707, 707f
  pseudolactational hyperplasia, 707, 708f
  regression of, 711
  squamous metaplasia, 707–708, 709f
 gynecomastia-like hyperplasia, 705–706, 706f
 papilloma, 703, 704f
Male breast, carcinoma of
 clinical presentation of, 716–717, 716f
 epidemiology of, 713–715
 pathology of, gross, 717, 717f
 pathology of, microscopic, 717–724, 718f–723f

growth patterns, 718, 719f
infiltrating duct, 717–718, 718f
intraductal, 720, 721f–722f
with granulation tissue, 723, 723f
myoepithelial cells, 720, 722f
papillary intraductal, 720, 720f
tubular, 718, 718f
treatment and prognosis in, 724–725
Malignant fibrous histiocytoma, 819–821, 820f, 821f
clinical presentation of, 819
pathology of, 820–821, 820f, 821f
treatment and prognosis with, 821
Malignant melanoma
breast metastases from, 693, 694f
epithelioid, breast metastases from, 693, 694f–695f
of mammary skin and breast, 899–904, 900f, 902f
of nipple, vs. Paget's disease of nipple, 574, 574f–575f
MALT lymphoma, 871–872, 873f
Mammary carcinoma, resembling carcinoma with osteoclast-like giant cells, 517–518, 518f–519f
Mammary carcinoma with endocrine features, 497–501, 498–500f
clinical presentation of, 497
immunoreactivity of, 497
pathology of
gross, 497–498, 498f
microscopic, 498–500, 498f–500f
prognosis and treatment of, 500–501
Mammary carcinoma with osteoclast-like giant cells, 517–525
clinical presentation of, 517
fine needle aspiration cytology of, 523–524, 523f, 524f
immunohistochemistry of, 524–525
metastatic, 525, 525f
pathology of, gross, 517–518, 517f–519f
pathology of, microscopic, 519–523, 519f–524f
anaplastic, 519, 522, 522f
apocrine, 519, 522f
vs. carcinoma with granulomatous reaction, 523, 523f
colonic-type, 519, 522f
cribriform, 519, 519f
infiltrating lobular, 519, 520f
in intraductal carcinoma, 522, 522f
mucinous, 519, 522f
vs. multinucleated stromal giant cells, 523, 524f
solid, 519, 520f
stromal fibrosis, 522, 523f
well differentiated, 519, 520f
prognosis and treatment of, 525, 525f
ultrastructure of, 524, 524f
Mammary duct ectasia, 34–38, 35f–38f
clinical presentation of, 35
etiology of, 34–35
pathology of
gross, 35
microscopic, 35–38, 36f–38f
treatment and prognosis of, 38
Mammary gland formation, fetal, 1
Mammary infarcts, 32–33
Mammary intraepithelial neoplasia (MIN), 201, 239. See also Ductal hyperplasia
Mammographically detected tumors, risk of dying from, 655
Mammography, for proliferative (fibrocystic) breast changes, 233
Maspin, 368, 370
Mastectomy
for intraductal carcinoma, 310–311
pathologic examination of, 958
residual breast tissue after, ectopic breast carcinoma in, 674, 674f, 675f

Mastitis
granulomatous lobular, 38–40, 39f, 40f
lactational, 73, 73f
plasma cell, 33–34, 34f
puerperal, 32
silicone, 49–53 (See also Silicone mastitis)
clinical presentation of, 49
etiology of, 49
pathology of, gross, 49, 50f
pathology of, microscopic, 49–53, 50f–52f
treatment and prognosis of, 53
tuberculous, 70–72, 71f, 72f
typhoid, 72
Mastitis obliterans, 37–38, 38f
Mastopathy, diabetic, 53–56. See also Diabetic mastopathy
Matrix-producing carcinoma, 440, 441f, 442, 442f
Mediastinal teratoma, ectopic breast tissue carcinoma in, 674, 675f, 676
Medullary carcinoma, 405–422
atypical, 421
clinical presentation of, 405–406, 406f
cytology of, 420–421, 420f
defined, 405
genetics of, 421
immunohistochemistry of, 419–420, 420f
pathology of, gross, 406–409, 407f–409f
pathology of, microscopic, 410–419, 410f–419f
apical, 410
germinal center formation, 411, 412f–413f
giant cells, 418f, 419
glandular differentiation, 414, 415f
intraductal, 416f, 417
lobular extension, 411, 411f
secondary nodule from, 417–418, 417f
lobular lymphocytic reaction extension, 411, 411f
lymphoplasmacytic reaction, 410–411, 410f, 412f
metaplastic changes, 418–419, 418f
microscopic circumscription, 411, 413, 413f, 414f
necrosis, 419, 419f
nuclear grade poorly differentiated, 415, 415f, 416f
spindle cell change, 418f, 419
squamous metaplasia, 418–419, 418f
syncytial growth, 413–414, 414f, 415f
tumor border, 413, 413f, 414f
vs. in nonmedullary carcinoma, 413, 414f
prognosis and treatment of, 421–422, 421f
ultrastructural studies of, 419
Melanin, in carcinoma with lipofuscin, 904, 904f
Melanocytic lesions, 899, 900f–902f
Melanosarcoma, 902
Menopause, lobular atrophy in, 14, 14f
Menstrual cycle, on breast anatomy, 8–11, 9f, 10f
Menstrual phase, lobule in, 10, 10f
Mesenchymal neoplasms, benign. See Benign mesenchymal neoplasms
Mesenchymoma, malignant, 827
Metaplasia, 425. See also Metaplastic carcinoma; specific types, e.g, Cystic apocrine metaplasia
Metaplastic carcinoma, 425–452. See also specific types, e.g., Squamous carcinoma
cell types in, 428–429
choriocarcinoma, 425, 426f
clinical presentation of, 429–430, 429f–430f
in cystic papilloma, 426, 427f–428f
electron microscopy of, 450
frequency of, 425–426
histologic phenotype and histogenesis in, 425
immunohistochemical studies of, 428–429, 448–449, 448f–450f
lobular, 426, 427f
mammary gland tissue susceptibility to, 425
origin of, 425

osseous sarcomatoid, 429, 429f–430f
pathology of, gross, 430–431, 430f
pathology of, microscopic, 431–448
acantholytic, 432, 434, 435f, 436f
adenosquamous, 431, 431t–432t
adenosquamous, low-grade, 443–448, 443f–447f
in adenomyoepithelioma, 445, 446f–447f
immunoreactivity in, 446, 448f
recurrent, 446, 448f
in sclerosing papilloma, 445, 446f
chondroosseous, 437, 437f–439f
heterologous, 437, 437f–440f, 442–443, 443f
lung metastases of , 442, 443f
matrix-producing, 440, 441f, 442, 442f
myxoid change, 437
osseous, 437, 438f
with osteoclast-like giant cells, 437, 440, 440f
pseudoangiomatous, 432, 434, 436f
spindle cell, 431–432, 432f
with adenocarcinoma, 431, 434f
with chondroid differentiation, 437, 439f
and squamous, 426, 428f, 431–432, 432f, 433f, 434, 437
spindle cell–keloidal, 432, 435f
squamous, 425–426, 426f, 431, 431f, 432f
prognosis and treatment of, 450–452, 451f, 451t
variants of, 425
Metastases. See also under specific cancers, e.g., Endometrial carcinoma, breast metastases from
distant, 255
lymph node (See Lymph node metastases)
Metastases, in breast, from nonmammary malignant neoplasms, 689–700
clinical presentation of, 689–697, 690f–697f
clear cell, 693, 693f
colonic carcinoid tumor, 690, 692f
colonic carcinoma, 690, 691f
embryonal rhabdomyosarcoma, 692f, 693
gastric carcinoma, 690, 691f
malignant melanoma, 693, 694f
epithelioid, 693, 694f–695f
ovarian carcinoma, 696, 697f
prostatic carcinoma, 693, 696, 696f
salivary gland
acinic cell carcinoma, 690, 691f
mucoepidermoid carcinoma, 690, 690f
distinguishing, 696–697
pathology of, microscopic, 697–699, 697f–700f
endometrial carcinoma, 697, 698f
leiomyosarcoma, 697, 698f
ovarian carcinoma, 697, 697f
renal carcinoma
clear cell, 697, 699f
sarcomatoid, 697, 698f–699f
thyroid gland, 697, 700f
prognosis and treatment of, 700, 700f
Metastasizing hemangiomas, 840
MIB1, 355
Microcalcifications, in intraductal carcinoma, 259–260, 260f
Microglandular adenosis, 152–160
atypical, 154–155, 156f, 157f
carcinoma in
with basaloid differentiation, 158, 159f
intraductal, 155, 156f
invasive, high-grade, 155, 157f, 158
with secretory differentiation, 158, 158f
clinical presentation of, 152
immunoreactivity of, 153–154, 153f, 154f
metastases of, 159, 160f
oncocytic differentiation in, 154, 155f
pathology of, gross, 152
pathology of, microscopic, 152–155, 152f–159f, 158
atypical, 154–155, 156f
carcinoma in, 155, 157f
with basaloid differentiation, 158, 159f

Microglandular adenosis (*contd.*)
    with matrix-forming chondroid metaplasia, 155, 157f
      with secretory differentiation, 158, 158f
    eosinophilic cytoplasmic granules, 154, 155f
    epithelial cells, flat-to-cuboidal, 153, 153f
    immunoreactivity, 153–154, 153f–154f
    intraductal carcinoma in, 155, 156f
    myoepithelial cells, 154, 154f
    PAS and mucicarmine staining of, 153, 153f
    *vs.* sclerosing adenosis, 154, 155f
    small glands in fibrous/fatty stroma, 152, 152f
    prognosis and treatment of, 158–160, 160f
    with sclerosing adenosis, 154, 155f
    variations in, 154, 155f
Microinvasion, 303, 606, 606f, 608, 608f
    of intraductal carcinoma, 301–310, 302f–308f
      at basement membrane, 301, 302f
      defined, 303–305, 303f, 304f, 309–310
    *vs.* minimally invasive carcinoma, 303
    in TNM staging, 254
Microinvasive carcinoma, 303
Micropapillary, 239
Micropapillary carcinoma, invasive, 561–564
    clinical presentation of, 561
    pathology of, gross, 561
    pathology of, microscopic, 561–564, 562f, 563f
      apocrine, 561, 562f
      intraductal, 563, 563f
      lymph node metastasis, 563, 563f
      mucinous carcinoma and, 563, 563f
    treatment and prognosis of, 564
Micropapillary intraductal carcinoma, 264, 266f, 268, 268f–272f, 270, 373f. *See also* intraductal carcinoma
    apocrine, 271f
    clear cell, 272f, 273
    cystic hypersecretory, 273
    flat, 269f, 273
    fronds in, 270, 270f, 271f
    with intermediate-/high-grade cytology, 268f, 271f, 272f, 273
    nuclei in, 270, 270f–271f, 273
    with squamous metaplasia, 272f, 273
Microscopic circumscription, in medullary carcinoma, 411, 413, 413f, 414f
Minimally invasive carcinoma, 303
Mitosin, 356
Mitotic figures, 337, 337t
Mitotic rate, 336–337
Mixed tumors, 130, 132f, 428
Molecular genetics. See Genetics
Mondor's disease, 48
Mortality, changes in, 331
Mucin secretion, in papillary carcinoma, 395–396, 395f, 396f
Mucinosis, 784–786, 785f
Mucinous carcinoma, 463–480
    clinical presentation of, 463–464, 464f
    cytology of, 477–478, 477f–479f
    definition of, 463
    electron microscopy of, 477
    flow cytometry of, 478
    invasive micropapillary carcinoma and, 563, 563f
    morphometry of, 478
    pathology of, gross, 464f, 465
    pathology of, microscopic, 465–476, 465f–476f
      argyrophilic granules, 467, 468f
      cystic papillary, 467, 467f
      histochemistry, 476–477, 476f
      *vs.* infiltrating duct carcinoma with mucinous features, 465, 466f
      knobby contours, 468, 470f
      lymphatic tumor emboli, 468, 470, 470f
      margin of mucin, 468, 469f
      *vs.* mucocele-like tumor, 470–476, 470f–476f
        with calcifications, 474, 476f
        in cystic papilloma, 470, 473f

        with ductal hyperplasia, 470, 472f–473f
        with intraductal carcinoma, 474, 475f, 476f
        in lobules, 473–474, 474f
      papillary, with calcifications, 467–468, 469f
      patterns, 467–468, 469f
      solid and cribriform, 467–468, 469f
      in solid papillary carcinoma, 467, 468f
      trabecular, 467–468, 469f
    prognosis and treatment of, 479–480, 479t, 480f
Mucocele-like tumor
    with calcifications, 474, 476f
    in cystic papilloma, 470, 473f
    with ductal hyperplasia, 470, 472f–473f
    with intraductal carcinoma, 474, 475f, 476f
    in lobules, 473–474, 474f
    *vs.* mucinous carcinoma, 470–476, 470f–476f
      (See also under Mucinous carcinoma, pathology of)
    with mucinous carcinoma, 474, 475f
Multicentric carcinoma, 301
Multicentricity, 300–301
Multifocal carcinoma, 301
Multifocality, 300
Multiple myeloma, 879–880, 880f
    plasmacytoma in, 879–880, 879f
Multivariate analysis, on prognosis, 330–331
Muscular hamartoma, 782–783, 783f
MVD, 346–347
Mycobacterial infections, 70–72, 71f, 72f
Myeloblastoma, 881
Myeloid metaplasia, 784, 882–883, 883f
Myoepithelial carcinoma, 137, 137f
Myoepithelial cells, 121
    clear cell change in, 18, 19f
    myoid metaplasia of, 781, 781f
Myoepithelial neoplasms, 121–137
    adenomyoepithelioma, 121–134 (See also Adenomyoepithelioma)
    myoepithelioma, 134–137, 134f–137f
    terminology for, 121
Myoepitheliomas, 121, 134–137, 134f–137f
    alveolar structure of, 136, 136f
    clinical presentation of, 134–135, 134f, 135f
    infiltrative growth pattern in, 135, 136f
    myoepithelial carcinoma, 137, 137f
    polygonal cell, 136–137, 136f, 137f
    spindle cell, 135–136, 135f
Myofibroblastic reaction, in invasive duct carcinoma, 350, 351f
Myofibroblastic sarcoma, 827–828, 828f
Myofibroblastoma, 766–774, 767f–773f
    clinical presentation of, 766–767
    malignant, 827–828, 828f
    pathology of, gross, 767, 767f
    pathology of, microscopic, 767–774, 768f–773f
      cellular, 769, 770f
        plus fibrous, 769, 772f
      classic, 767, 768f
      collagenized or fibrous, 768f, 769
      epithelioid, 769, 769f–770f
      fine needle aspiration cytology, 772–773, 773f
      infiltrative, 769, 771f–772f, 772
      myoid and cartilaginous, 772, 772f
      myxoid, 772, 773f
    treatment and prognosis with, 774
Myofibromatosis-type perivascular myoma, 774–775
Myoid differentiation. See also specific cancers
    perivascular, in tumors, 774–775, 774f–775f
Myoid hamartoma, 135, 135f, 782–783, 783f
Myoid metaplasia
    in lobule, 6, 7f
    of myoepithelial cells, 781, 781f
    in terminal duct lobular unit, 6, 7f
Myomas, 121
Myopericytoma, 774–775
Myosarcoma, in phyllodes tumor, 183, 187f, 745, 745f
Myothelial sarcoma, 121
Myxoid change, 437. See also specific cancers
Myxoma, 784, 784f

**N**

Necrosis, 339, 339f. *See also* specific carcinomas
    defined, 289–290
    fat, 29–30, 30f
      with calcification, in non-Hodgkin's lymphoma, 868, 871, 871f
      from radiation, 888f, 889
    hemorrhagic, from anticoagulants, 30
    in medullary carcinoma, 419, 419f
Neoplasia
    defined, 250
    intraepithelial, 250
    lobular, 250
Neoplasm. See specific types, e.g., Myoepithelial neoplasms
Nerve sheath tumors, 778–779, 779f
    sarcoma, 827
Nerve tumors, 778–779, 779f
Neurilemmomas, 778–779
Nevoid hyperkeratosis, of nipple and areola, 909, 910f
Nevus cell aggregates, 917–921, 918f–920f
Nipple(s)
    anatomy of, 5 (See also Adnexal gland)
    basal cell carcinoma of, 909, 909f
    basal-squamous carcinoma of, 909, 910f
    cutaneous neoplasms of, 908–909, 909f
    florid papillomatosis of, 94, 101–111 (See also Florid papillomatosis of the nipple)
      in male breast, 703
    hidradenoma of
      axillary skin, 909, 910f
      subareolar, 909, 910f
    malignant melanoma of, 899, 900f
      *vs.* Paget's disease of the nipple, 574, 574f–575f
    nevoid hyperkeratosis of, 909, 910f
    Paget's disease of (See Paget's disease of the nipple)
    sebaceous adenoma of, 909, 910f
    supernumerary, 25–26
    syringomatous adenoma of, 111–114 (See also Syringomatous adenoma of the nipple)
    tubular carcinoma in, 365–367, 366f
Nipple hidradenoma, 909, 910f
nm23 gene product, in intraductal carcinoma, 294
Nocardia, 65
Non-Hodgkin's lymphoma
    clinical presentation of, 863
    molecular genetics of, 875
    pathology of, gross, 863, 864f
    pathology of, microscopic, 863–875, 864f–874f, 876f–877f
      angiotrophic, 868, 870f
      with calcifications, in fat necrosis, 868, 871, 871f
      with carcinoma, 871, 872f
      carcinoma-like, 871, 872f
      in ducts and lobules, 867, 868f
      *vs.* idiopathic histiocytosis, 875, 876f–877f
      infiltrating lobular carcinoma–like, 867–868, 869f
      large cell, diffuse, 863, 864f
      lymphocytic diffuse, poorly differentiated, 863, 865f
      lymphoplasmacytic, 863, 866, 866f
      MALT, 871–872, 873f
      mixed, 863, 865f
      nodular, 867, 869f
      in pseudoangiomatous stromal hyperplasia, 868, 870f
      pseudolymphoma, 872–875, 874f
      signet-ring cell, 868, 869f
      small cell lymphocytic, 863, 866f
      stromal sclerosis, 866, 867f
    treatment and prognosis in, 875, 877
Nonmedullary carcinoma, tumor border in, 413, 414f

Nonparenchymal hemangiomas of mammary
    region, 803–806, 803f–806f
  clinical presentation of, 803
  pathology of, 803–806, 803f–806f
  prognosis and treatment of, 806
Nuclear grade
  of apocrine carcinoma, 487, 490f
  of medullary carcinoma, 415, 415f, 416f
  of small cell carcinoma, 503, 504f
Nuclear grading, 334–336, 335f
Nuclear morphometry, 356

**O**

Oat cell carcinoma, 503–508
  microscopic pathology of, 503–508, 503f–507f
    (*See also* Small cell carcinoma)
  treatment and prognosis of, 507–508
Occult carcinoma
  axillary lymph node metastases in, 661–673 (*See
    also under* Lymph node metastases,
    axillary)
  inflammatory, 681 (*See also* Inflammatory
    carcinoma)
  invasive lobular, 630, 633f
Ochrocytes, 7, 8f
Oncocytic carcinoma, 483
Oncogenes. *See also* specific oncogenes, e.g.,
  HER-2/*neu* oncogene
  with atypical hyperplasia, 240
  in intraductal carcinoma, 292–294
    HER2/*neu*, 292–293, 293f
    p53, 293–294, 294f
Osseous metaplastic carcinoma, 437, 438f
Osteoclast-like giant cells
  carcinoma with (*See* Mammary carcinoma with
    osteoclast-like giant cells)
  in metaplastic carcinoma, 437, 440, 440f
Osteogenic sarcoma, 818–819, 819f
Ovarian carcinoma, breast metastases from, 696,
  697, 697f

**P**

p53
  in apocrine carcinoma, 494
  in intraductal carcinoma, 293–294, 294f
  in medullary carcinoma, 420, 420f
  nuclear expression of, 240–241
Paget's disease, adenoid cystic carcinoma and,
  546f, 547
Paget's disease of the nipple, 254, 564–577
  cell origin in, 565–566
  clinical presentation of, 566–567, 566f
  historical perspective on, 565, 565f
  immunohistochemistry of, 574–577, 575t, 576f
  pathology of, gross, 567
  pathology of, microscopic, 567–574, 568f–574f
    in adnexal glands, 570, 572f–573f
    characteristic, 567, 568f
    clear cell change, 571, 573f, 574f
    hyperplasia epidermis, 567, 569, 569f
    intraductal carcinoma of terminal lactiferous
      duct and, 570, 572f
    invasive carcinoma of nipple and, 570, 571f
    with lobular carcinoma, 569, 569f
    *vs.* malignant melanoma of nipple, 574,
      574f–575f
    prognosis and treatment of, 577
    secondary, 569, 570f
    in squamous metaplasia, 569, 570f
Papillary apocrine change, 235–236
Papillary apocrine metaplasia, 96–101
  clinical presentation of, 96–97
  immunohistochemistry and electron microscopy
    of, 100
  pathology of
    gross, 97
    microscopic, 97–100, 98f–100f
  prognosis and treatment of, 100–101

Papillary carcinoma, 381–403
  benign *vs.* malignant, 381–382
  in children and adolescents, 747, 747f
  clinical presentation of, 382–383, 382f
  cytology of, 402–403
  defined, 381
  electron microscopy of, 398
  histochemistry of, 395–398
    endocrine differentiation, 396, 397f
    estrogen receptors, 396, 398f
    mucin, 395–396, 395f, 396f
  incidence of, 381
  infarcted, 31–32, 32f
  invasive, 398–402, 398f–402f
    mucinous, 398, 399f, 401
    needle biopsy, 398, 400f
    *vs. in situ* carcinoma, 401, 402f
    solid, 398, 401, 401f
  microinvasive, 398, 398f, 400f
  *vs.* papilloma, 385, 385t, 389f
  pathology of, gross, 383, 383f, 384f
  pathology of, microscopic, 383–395, 384f–394f
    apocrine, 388, 388f
    cribriform, 384f, 386f, 388f, 389f
    dimorphic, 388–390, 389f, 390f
    epithelial cells, 386–388, 387f–388f
    fibrotic, 386, 387f
    frond forming, 383–385, 384f
    growth patterns, 385, 386f
    micropapillary, 386f, 388f
    myoepithelial cells, 388, 389f
    papillary, 386f
    in papilloma, 391, 393f–394f, 394
    reticular, 386f
    solid, 385, 385f, 389f, 390–391, 391f
      glycogen-rich clear cell, 391, 392f
      mucoepidermoid, 391, 393f
      spindle cell, 391, 392f
    solid papillary with cribriform glands, 386f,
      389f
  prognosis and treatment of, 403
  signet-ring cells in, 395, 395f
Papillary cystadenomas, 77
Papillary duct hyperplasia, in children and young
  women
  clinical presentation of, 735
  pathology of
    gross, 735, 736f
    microscopic, 735, 736f, 737, 738f
  treatment and prognosis with, 737, 739
Papillary endothelial hyperplasia, in
  nonparenchymal hemangioma, 803, 804f
Papillary *in situ* carcinoma, *vs.* invasive papillary
  carcinoma, 401, 402f
Papillary intraductal carcinoma, 281
Papillary synovial metaplasia, 51, 52f
Papilloma, 77–87, 381–382, 389f. *See also*
    Papillary carcinoma
  adenomyoepithelioma, 77
  in children and young women
    clinical presentation of, 735
    pathology of, gross, 735, 736f
    pathology of, microscopic, 735, 737, 737f,
      738f
    treatment and prognosis with, 737, 739
  clinical presentation of, 77–78
  ductal adenoma, 77
  intracystic, 77
  lobular carcinoma *in situ* in, 600, 601f
  in male breast, 703, 704f
  multiple, 77
  *vs.* papillary carcinoma, 385, 385t
  papillary carcinoma in, 391, 393f–394f, 394
  papillary cystadenomas, 77
  pathology of, gross, 78–79, 78f, 79f
  pathology of, microscopic, 80–85, 80f–86f
    apocrine metaplasia, 80, 82f
    benign, 80, 81f
    estrogen receptors, 82, 84f

    infarcted, 82, 85f
    myoepithelial cell hyperplasia, 82, 84f
    squamous metaplasia, 85, 86f
    stromal histiocytes, 80, 82f
    stromal sclerosis, 82, 83f, 84f
  solitary, 77
  treatment and prognosis of, 85–87, 87t
Papillomatosis, 204. *See also* Ductal hyperplasia
  in children and young women (*See also* Juvenile
    papillomatosis)
    pathology of, microscopic, 737f, 738f
  florid
    of male nipple, 703
    of nipple, 94, 101–111 (*See also* Florid
      papillomatosis of the nipple)
  juvenile, 729–735 (*See also* Juvenile
    papillomatosis)
Paraffinoma, 48–49
Parasitic infections, 66–70
  coenurosis, 69
  cysticercosis, 69–70, 69f
  *Dracunculus medinensis*, 70
  *Echinococcus granulosus*, 70
  filariasis, 66–69, 67f, 68f
  Liesegang's rings, 70
  *Schistosoma japonicum*, 69
  sparganosis, 70
  *Trichinella*, 70
Pathologic classification, 255
Penicillamine-induced macromastia, 25
Pericanalicular fibroadenoma, 168. *See also*
  Fibroadenoma
Periductal stromal tumor, 176–197. *See also*
  Phyllodes tumor
Perilobular hemangiomas, 787–789, 787t, 788f
Perineural invasion, 348, 349f
Peripheral nerve sheath sarcoma, 827
Perivascular myoid differentiation, tumors with,
  774–775, 774f–775f
Phenotype, histologic
  histogenesis and, 425
  tissue of origin and, 425
Phlebitis, 48
Phyllodes tumor, 176–197
  benign, 180, 180f–185f, 183
    apocrine metaplasia in, 192, 192f
    digital fibroma-type inclusions in, 192, 193f
    with lipomatous hamartoma, 183, 185f
    with lipomatous metaplasia, 183, 184f
    with pseudoangiomatous stroma, 180, 181f
    squamous metaplasia in, 188, 192, 192f
  carcinomas in, 656–661
    clinical presentation of, 656–657
    pathology of, gross, 657
    pathology of, microscopic, 660–661, 660f,
      661f
    prognosis and treatment of, 661
  in children and adolescents, 743–745, 743f–745f
  clinical presentation of, 176–179, 178f
  cystic, 179, 179f–180f
  cytology of, 194f, 195
  electron microscopy of, 192, 194
  epithelial hyperplasia in
    atypical, 188, 190f
    florid, 188, 190f
  immunohistochemistry of, 192, 194
  incidence of, 176
  locally recurrent, 196, 196f
  malignant
    high-grade, 183, 186f–188f
      angiosarcoma in, 183, 187f
      chondrosarcoma and myosarcoma in, 183,
        187f
      liposarcoma in, 183, 187f
      rhabdomyosarcoma in, 183, 188f
    low-grade, 183, 187f, 188, 189f, 194f
    with metastases, 192, 193f, 195f
  myosarcoma in, 745, 745f
  pathology of, gross, 178f, 179, 179f

Phyllodes tumor (*contd.*)
  treatment and prognosis of, 195–197, 195f, 196f
  variant, 188, 191f
Pigment deposits in axillary lymph nodes,
    923–924, 923f, 924f
Plasma cell mastitis, 33–34, 34f
Plasmacytic granuloma, 880, 881f
Plasmacytic tumors
  clinical presentation of, 878–879
  pathology of
    gross, 879
    microscopic, 879–880, 879f–881f
  treatment and prognosis of, 880–881
Plasmacytoma, 879–880, 879f
Pleomorphic adenomas, 130, 132f, 167
Ploidy
  flow cytometry of, 353–354
  in intraductal carcinoma, 294–295
Poland's syndrome, 23
Polyarteritis, 46, 46f
Polyurethane-covered implant, 52, 52f
Postmastectomy angiosarcoma, 850–856,
    851f–855f. *See also* Angiosarcoma,
    postmastectomy
  of chest wall, 829
Postradiation angiosarcoma, 829
Precancerous breast disease, 229–244
  genetic predisposition in, 229–231
  proliferative (fibrocystic) breast changes in,
      231–244
    age and, 235
    atypical hyperplasia, 236–237, 236t
      angiogenesis factor in, 243
      *bcl-2* gene in, 241
      *BRCA1* gene in, 241
      cell polarity in, 242
      classification problems in, 239
      cyclin D1 in, 241
      cytokeratins in, 243–244
      definition of, 237
      epidermal growth factor and receptor in,
          241–242
      estrogen receptor nuclear immunoreactivity
          in, 242
      flow cytometry in, 240
      fodrin in, 242–243
      frequency of, 237
      genetic and biochemical markers in,
          239–244 (*See also* specific markers)
      growth factors in, 241
      HER-2/*neu* oncogene in, 240
      insulin-like growth factors in, 242
      integrins in, 243
      interpretive differences in, 237–238
      nuclear cytology in, 239–240
      oncogenes in, 240
      p53 expression in, nuclear, 240–241
      progesterone receptor nuclear immunoreac-
          tivity in, 242
      pS2 protein in, 242
      risk of, future, 239
      stromal proteins in, 243
      telomerase in, 241
    biopsy of, 232
      breast carcinoma after, 233–234, 234t
    biopsy of, previous benign, 235
      breast carcinoma after, 236–237, 236t
      histology and, 235–236, 236t
    biopsy-proven changes in, risk in both breasts
        after, 234
    borderline lesions, 237–238
      uncertainty about, 238
    distinguishing forms of, 238–239
    etiology of, 232
    family history and, 235
    fine needle aspiration of, 232–233
    mammography of, 233
    molecular characterization of mammary
        epithelium in, 244
    risk factors for, 232, 235

Precocious puberty, 2
Pregnancy
  breast anatomy in, 11–14, 12f, 13f
  carcinoma in, 653–654
  inflammatory lesions in, 32–33, 33f
Pregnancy-like change, 15–18, 16f–18f
  calcifications, 15, 17f
Pregnancy-like hyperplasia, 15, 16f, 17f
  atypical, 15, 17f, 18f
  cystic hypersecretory hyperplasia with, 529, 532,
      532f
  laminated secretion, 15, 17f
Preinvasive carcinoma, 249
Premature thelarche, 1–2, 2f
Primary carcinoid tumor of the breast, 499. *See
    also* Mammary carcinoma with endocrine
    features
Progesterone receptors
  in breast, 11
  nuclear immunoreactivity of, in atypical
      hyperplasia, 242
Prognosis assessment, in invasive duct carcinoma,
    326–331
  bilaterality in, 327
  genetic factors in, 326–327
  incidence and mortality changes in, 331
  radiotherapy in, local, 329
  recurrence in
    early detection of, 330
    local, in conserved breast/chest wall, 329–330
    risk of, 326, 326t
  therapy on, 331
  time dependence in, 330
  tumor detection and screening methods in,
      327–328
  univariate *vs.* multivariate analysis of, 330–331
Prognostic markers, in invasive duct carcinoma,
    331–353
  microscopic histopathologic, 334–353
    angiogenesis, 345–348, 346f, 347f
    apoptosis, 339
    *bcl-2,* 340, 340f
    blood vessel invasion, 344–345, 344f
    extent of, and atypia, 351–352, 352f
    grading, 334–337, 335f, 336f, 337t (*See also*
        Grading)
    lymphatic tumor emboli, 342–343, 342f, 343f
    lymphocytic infiltrate, 341–342, 341f
    necrosis, 339, 339f
    other, 352–353
    perineural invasion, 348, 349f
    stromal characteristics, 348–351, 350f, 351f
    telomerase, 341
    vascular invasion, 345
  pathology of, gross, 331–334, 332f, 333f
    size and nodal status in, 333
    tumor configuration/shape in, 332f–335f, 334
    tumor size in, 331, 333
    tumor size in, measurement of, 333–334
Progression, 231
Prolactin-inducible protein, in apocrine carcinoma,
    493
Proliferating cell nuclear antigen (PCNA)/cyclin,
    355–356
Proliferation, immunohistochemistry of, 354–356
Proliferative (fibrocystic) breast changes, 231–244.
    *See also under* Precancerous breast disease
Proliferative phase, lobule in, 9, 9f
Prostatic carcinoma, breast metastases from, 693,
    696, 696f
pS2 protein, atypical hyperplasia with, 242
Pseudoangiomatous carcinoma, 432, 434, 436f
Pseudoangiomatous stroma, with phyllodes tumor,
    180, 181f
Pseudoangiomatous stromal hyperplasia, 757–766,
    758f–765f
  *vs.* angiosarcoma, 831, 834f
  clinical presentation of, 758
  invasive duct carcinoma in, 348, 350f

  non-Hodgkin's lymphoma in, 868, 870f
  pathology of, gross, 758–759, 758f
  pathology of, microscopic, 758f–765f, 759–763
    atypia, 763, 765f
    digital fibroma-like inclusions, 763, 764f
    giant cells and atypia, 763, 765f
    myofibroblasts, 760, 760f–762f
    myoid, 763, 764f
    spaces, 759–760, 759f, 760f
    vimentin and actin, 763, 763f
  prognosis and treatment of, 763, 766
Pseudolymphoma, 872–875, 874f
Pseudotumor, inflammatory, 42–43, 43f
pTNM staging, 253, 254
Puberty, precocious, 2
Puerperal mastitis, 32

**R**

Radial scar. *See* Radial sclerosing lesions
Radial sclerosing lesions, 87–94
  clinical presentation of, 88–89, 88f
  historical perspective on, 87–88
  intraductal carcinoma in, 284, 285f, 286f
  pathology of, gross, 89
  pathology of, microscopic, 89–93, 89f–93f
    atypical duct hyperplasia, 91, 93f
    elastosis, 89, 89f, 90f
    epithelial necrosis, 91, 92f
    epithelium trapped in stroma, 83f, 89, 91f
    with lobular carcinoma in situ, 91, 93f
    needle core biopsy, 89, 91f
    nerve entrapment, 91, 92f
    proliferative, 89, 90f
    squamous metaplasia, 91, 92f
  treatment and prognosis of, 93–94
  in tubular carcinoma, 370, 372f
Radiation, pathological effects of, 887–892
  atypia in ducts, 890f, 891
    with apocrine metaplasia, 890f, 891
  atypia in stromal fibroblasts, 889, 889f
  on ducts and lobules, 889, 889f, 890f, 891
  fat necrosis, 888f, 889
  for Hodgkin's disease, 887
  on intraductal carcinoma, 891, 891f
  on lobular carcinoma *in situ,* 891, 891f
  for mammary carcinoma, 887–888
  in normal breast, 888f–889f, 889
Radiation, sources of, 887
Radiotherapy
  for intraductal carcinoma, 311–316
    recurrences after, 313–316, 314t
  local, on prognosis, 329
Raynaud's phenomenon, in nipple, 33
Recurrence
  after breast-conserving surgery, for intraductal
      carcinoma, 313–316, 314t
  effect on prognosis
    early detection of, 330
    local, in conserved breast/chest wall, 329–330
    risk of, 326, 326t
    time to, 328–329
  of adenosquamous carcinoma, 446, 448f
  of angiomatosis, 800, 800f
  of inflammatory carcinoma, 677, 678, 678f, 681,
      681f, 682f
  of intraductal carcinoma, after radiotherapy,
      313–316, 314t
  of phyllodes tumor, 196, 196f
Renal carcinoma
  clear cell, breast metastases from, 697, 699f
  sarcomatoid, breast metastases from, 697,
      698f–699f
Residual breast, ectopic breast carcinoma in, 674,
    674f, 675f
Rhabdomyosarcoma, 823–824, 823f
  embryonal, breast metastases from, 692f, 693
  in phyllodes tumor, 183, 188f
Rosai-Dorfman disease, 875, 876f–877f
Rotter's lymph nodes, 254

# S

S-phase fraction, flow cytometry of, 353–354
Salivary gland
  acinic cell carcinoma of, breast metastases from, 690, 691f
  mucoepidermoid carcinoma of, breast metastases from, 690, 690f
Sarcoid-like granulomas in carcinoma, 41, 42f
Sarcoidosis, 40–42, 41f, 42f
Sarcoma(s), 813–856
  alveolar soft-part, 827
  angioblastic, 827, 827f
  angiosarcoma, 829–850 (See also Angiosarcoma)
    postmastectomy, 850–856, 851f–855f (See also Angiosarcoma, postmastectomy)
  chondrosarcoma, 818–819, 819f
  dermatofibrosarcoma protuberans, 825–827, 826f
  diagnosis of, 813–814
  fibrosarcoma, 821–823, 822f
  grading of, 813
  granulocytic, 881–882, 882f
  hemangiopericytoma, 823–825, 824f–826f
    clinical presentation of, 823
    metastases of, 825, 825f
    pathology of, gross, 823
    pathology of, microscopic, 823–825, 824f–826f
    prognosis and treatment of, 825, 825f
  Kaposi's, 828–829
  leiomyosarcoma, 815–816, 815f–817f
  liposarcoma, 817–818, 817f–818f
  malignant fibrous histiocytoma, 819–821, 820f, 821f
    clinical presentation of, 819
    pathology of, 820–821, 820f, 821f
    treatment and prognosis with, 821
  malignant mesenchymoma, 827
  malignant myofibroblastoma, 827–828, 828f
  myofibroblastic, 827–828, 828f
  osteogenic, 818–819, 819f
  pathology of, gross, 813, 813f
  peripheral nerve sheath, 827
  rhabdomyosarcoma, 823–824, 823f
  stromal, 814–815, 814f
  treatment of, 814
*Schistosoma japonicum* infection, 69
Schwannoma, 778–779, 779f
Scirrhous carcinoma, *vs.* adenoid cystic carcinoma, 536, 540f
Scleroderma, 46
Sclerosing adenosis, 141, 143f–145f, 145
  apocrine carcinoma in, 486, 486f
  apocrine lesions in, 486, 486f
  apocrine metaplasia in, 141, 146f, 147f
  collagenous spherulosis in, 141, 148f
  fibroadenoma with, 149, 149f, 170, 171f
  intraductal carcinoma in, 150, 150f, 151f, 282f–284, 283–284
  involving fat, 141, 144f
  lobular carcinoma *in situ* in, 149, 150f, 600, 602f–606f, 603, 606
  with marked atrophy, 141, 145f
  with microglandular adenosis, 154, 155f
  postpartum infarct in, 31, 31f, 32–33, 33f
  variants of, 145, 147f, 148f
Sclerosing duct hyperplasia, subareolar, 94–96, 94f, 95f
Sclerosing lesions, radial, 87–94. See also Radial sclerosing lesions
  intraductal carcinoma in, 284, 285f, 286f
Sclerosing lobular hyperplasia, 163, 164f
Sclerosing papillary hyperplasia of ducts, in nipple, 94–96, 94f, 95f
Sclerosing papilloma, adenosquamous carcinoma in, low-grade, 445, 446f–447f
Screening method, on prognosis, 327–328
Sebaceous adenoma of nipple, 909, 910f

Secretory carcinoma, 509–515
  age distribution of, 509, 509f
  in children and adolescents, 746f, 747
  clinical presentation of, 509–510
  metastatic, 514, 515f
  pathology of, gross, 510–511, 510f
  pathology of, microscopic, 511–514, 511f–514f
    apocrine, 511, 513f–514f
    growth patterns, 511, 511f–512f
    intraductal, 511, 511f
    solid, 511, 513f–514f
    stromal fibrosis, 511, 512f
    tumor border, 511, 512f
  prognosis and treatment of, 514–515, 515f
Secretory phase, lobule in, 10, 10f
Self-examination, breast, tumors detected by, 655
Sentinel lymph nodes
  histologic examination of, 965–966
  histopathology of, 966–971, 967f–971f
  intraoperative diagnosis of, 964–965
  mapping of, 961–964
Shape, tumor, 332f–335f, 334
Shrinkage artifact, 342, 343f
Signet-ring cells
  in intraductal carcinoma, 264, 265f
  in lobular carcinoma, 372f
  in non-Hodgkin's lymphoma, 868, 869f
  in papillary carcinoma, 395, 395f
Silicone granuloma, 49–51, 50f
Silicone lymphadenitis, 922–923, 923f
Silicone mastitis, 49–53
  clinical presentation of, 49
  etiology of, 49
  pathology of
    gross, 49, 50f
    microscopic, 49–53, 50f–52f
  treatment and prognosis of, 53
Sinus histiocytosis, 921–922, 921f
Size, tumor
  in intraductal carcinoma, 299–300
  measurement of, 333–334
  and nodal status, 333
Skin cancer. *See* Cutaneous neoplasms
Small cell carcinoma, 503–508
  in children and adolescents, 745, 746f
  pathology of, microscopic, 503–508, 503f–507f
    in dimorphic intraductal carcinoma, 503, 504f
    with focal necrosis, 503, 505f
    glandular dimorphic, 506, 506f
    hormone receptors in, 507, 507f
    with invasive tubulolobular carcinoma, 503, 505f
    metastatic, 507
    with poorly differentiated nuclear grade, 503, 504f
    with *in situ* lobular carcinoma, 503, 505f
    squamoid dimorphic, 506, 506f
    with trabecular neuroendocrine structure, 503, 505f
  treatment and prognosis with, 507–508
Small cell intraductal carcinoma, 281–283, 282f
Solid papillary carcinoma, mucinous carcinoma in, 467, 468f
Sparganosis, 70
Spherulosis, collagenous, 114–117
  clinical presentation of, 114–115
  pathology of, 114–117, 114f–116f
Spindle and squamous carcinoma, 426, 428f, 431–432, 432f, 433f
Spindle cell(s)
  in medullary carcinoma, 418f, 419
  in papillary carcinoma, 391, 392f
  in squamous carcinoma, 459, 460f
  in squamous metaplasia, 426, 428f
Spindle cell carcinoma, 431–432, 432f, 433f
  with adenocarcinoma, 431, 434f
  with chondroid differentiation, 437, 439f
  intraductal, 281, 281f
Spindle cell intraductal carcinoma, 281, 281f

Spindle cell lipoma, 786, 786f–787f
Spindle cell myoepitheliomas, 135–136, 135f
Spindle cell–keloidal carcinoma, 432, 435f
Squamous carcinoma, 425–426, 426f, 431, 431f, 432f, 455–461
  in biopsy cavity, 455, 456f
  clinical presentation of, 455, 457
  in cyst, 455, 456f–457f
  definition of, 455
  in ducts, 455, 456f
  in lobule, 455, 456f
  pathology of, gross, 457, 457f–458f
  pathology of, microscopic, 457–461, 458f–460f
    clear cell, 459, 459f
    cystic, 459, 459f
    at prosthetic breast implant site, 459, 460f
    *in situ*, 458f, 459
    spindle cell, 459, 460f
  primary, 459–460
  treatment and prognosis of, 461
Squamous metaplasia, 5–6, 5f, 425–426, 426f
  in medullary carcinoma, 418–419, 418f
  Paget's disease with, 569, 570f
  pathology of, microscopic, 431, 431f
  in phyllodes tumor, 188, 192, 192f
  spindle cell metaplasia from, 426, 428f
Stage grouping, 255–256
Staging, 253–256
  clinical, 253–254
  histopathologic grade in, 255
  histopathologic types in, 255
  historical perspective on, 254
  lymph nodes in, 254
  pathologic, 254
  rules for, 253–254
  stage grouping in, 255–256
  TNM and pTNM, 253–255
Staphylococcal abscess, 73, 73f
Stewart-Treves syndrome (postmastectomy angiosarcoma), 829, 850–856, 851f–855f
  clinical presentation of, 851, 851f
  electron microscopy of, 856
  immunohistochemistry of, 852, 854–856, 855f
  pathology of, gross, 851, 852f
  pathology of, microscopic, 852, 852f–855f
    early lesions, 852, 853f
    epithelioid, 852, 855f
    hemorrhage, 852, 853f, 854f
    lymphedema, chronic, 852, 852f
  prognosis and treatment of, 856
Stromal proteins, atypical hyperplasia with, 243
Stromal sarcoma, 813, 814–815, 814f
Stromal sclerosis, in non-Hodgkin's lymphoma, 866, 867f
Subareolar abscesses, 73–74
Subareolar sclerosing duct hyperplasia, 94–96, 94f, 95f
Superficial thrombophlebitis, 48
Supernumerary breast tissue, 25–26, 26f
Supernumerary nipples, 25–26
Sweat gland carcinoma. *See* Apocrine carcinoma
Syncytial growth, in medullary carcinoma, 413–414, 414f, 415f
Synovial metaplasia
  around breast implant, 51–53, 51f
  papillary, 51, 52f
Syringomatous adenoma of the nipple, 111–114
  clinical presentation of, 111
  historical perspective on, 111
  pathology of
    gross, 111
    microscopic, 111–113, 112f, 113f
  treatment and prognosis of, 113–114

# T

Tamoxifen, treatment effects of, 896
Telomerase, 341
  with atypical hyperplasia, 241

Teratoma, mediastinal, ectopic breast tissue carcinoma in, 674, 675f, 676
Terminal duct–lobular unit (TDLU), 264
Thelarche, premature, 1–2, 2f
Therapy, pathological effects of
  chemotherapy, 892–895 (*See also* Chemotherapy, pathological effects of)
  hormone treatment, 895–896
  radiation, 887–892 (*See also* Radiation, pathological effects of)
Thrombophlebitis, superficial, 48
Thymidine labeling index (TLI)
  for invasive duct carcinoma, 354
  menstrual cycle on, 11
Thyroid gland cancer, breast metastases from, 697, 700f
TNM staging, 253–255
  of biopsy specimens, 939–940
Transformation, 231
Transsexual breast, 26
*Trichinella,* 70
Tubercles of Morgagni, 5, 7
Tuberculous mastitis, 70–72, 71f, 72f
Tubular adenoma, 167, 167f. *See also* Fibroadenoma
Tubular adenosis, 145, 149, 149f
  lobular carcinoma *in situ* in, 603, 603f–604f
Tubular carcinoma, 365–379
  adenoid cystic carcinoma and, 546f, 547
  clinical presentation of, 365–367, 366f
  cytology of, 376–377
  defined, 365
  electron microscopy of, 376
  incidence of, 365
  mammographic findings in, 365, 366f
  metastatic, 377–379, 377f, 378f
  in nipple, 365–367, 366f
  pathology of, gross, 367
  pathology of, microscopic, 367–376
    basement membranes, 368, 370f
    calcifications, 373, 373f

columnar cell change, 373–374, 374f
    elastosis, 373, 373f
    glandular patterns, 367, 367f–368f
    immunostaining, 368, 369f–370f
    intraductal carcinoma in, 373, 373f–375f
    invasive duct, well-differentiated, 370, 372f
    with lobular carcinoma *in situ,* 374–375, 375f
    mixed, 370, 371f
    mucin forming, 367, 369f
    multifocal variant, 375–376
    needling effect, 375, 376f
    perineural invasion, 375, 375f
    radial sclerosing, 370, 372f
    "snouts" and "tufts ," 370, 371f
    tubulolobular, 370, 372f
    unicentricity, 375
  prognosis and treatment of, 377–379, 377f, 378f
Tubulolobular carcinoma, 370, 372f
  invasive, small cell carcinoma with, 503, 505f
Tumor border
  in fibromatosis, 753, 754f, 755f
  in medullary carcinoma, 413, 413f, 414f
    *vs.* nonmedullary carcinoma, 413, 414f
  in secretory carcinoma, 511, 512f
Tumor configuration, 332f–335f, 334
Tumor detection, on prognosis, 327–328
Tumor growth rate, in invasive duct carcinoma, 353–356
  clinical assessment of, 353
  immunohistochemical assessment of, 354–356
  nuclear morphometry of, 356
  S-fraction and ploidy in, flow cytometry of, 353–354
Tumor necrosis, 339, 339f
Tumor shape, 332f–335f, 334
Tumor size, 331, 333
  measurement of, 333–334
  and nodal status, 333
Turner's syndrome, 23
Typhoid mastitis, 72

**U**
Ulnar-mammary syndrome, 23
Univariate analysis, on prognosis, 330–331

**V**
Van Nuys Prognostic Index (VNPI), 288
Vascular anomalies, 800–803, 801f, 802f. *See also* Hemangiomas, venous
Vascular endothelial growth factor (VEGF), 345–347
Vascular invasion, 345
Vascular lesions, 924–95, 925f
  atypical (*See* Atypical vascular lesions)
  benign, 787, 787t
Vascular permeability factor (VPF), 345–346
Vasculitis, 43–48
  dermatomyositis, 46–47
  giant cell arteritis, 43–44, 44f
  granulomatous angiopanniculitis, 47, 47f
  lupus mastopathy, 47–48, 48f
  phlebitis, 48
  polyarteritis, 46, 46f
  scleroderma, 46
  Weber-Christian disease, 47
  Wegener's granulomatosis, 44–46, 45f
Venous drainage, 4
Venous hemangiomas, 800–803, 801f, 802f. *See also* Hemangiomas, venous
Vimentin, *vs.* cytokeratin expression, 449–450
Viral infections, 72

**W**
Weber-Christian disease, 47

**Y**
Young, carcinoma in, 654–656

**Z**
Zinc alpha 2-glycoprotein, in apocrine carcinoma, 493